Encyclopedia
of Health
Information Sources

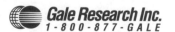

Encyclopedia of Health Information Sources

A Bibliographic Guide to Over 13,000 Citations for Publications, Organizations, and Databases on Health-Related Subjects

Includes: Abstracting, Indexing, and Current Awareness Publications; Annuals and Reviews; Associations, Professional Societies, Advocacy and Support Groups; Bibliographies; CD-ROM and Online Databases; Directories; Encyclopedias, Dictionaries, Word Books; Handbooks, Guides, Manuals, Atlases; Journals; Newsletters; Popular Works and Patient Education; Research Centers, Institutes, Clearinghouses; Standards and Statistics Sources; Textbooks and Monographs

SECOND EDITION

Edited by

Alan M. Rees
Professor Emeritus
Case Western Reserve University, Cleveland

Gale Research Inc. • *DETROIT* • *WASHINGTON, D.C.* • *LONDON*

Editor:	Alan M. Rees
Consulting Editor:	Paul Wasserman
Assistant Editor:	Constance Fawcett

Gale Research Inc. Staff

Senior Editor:	Donna Wood
Contributing Editor:	Jennifer Mossman
Project Coordinator:	Kelle S. Sisung
Associate Editors:	Jacqueline L. Longe, Rita H. Skirpan
Assistant Editors:	Erin E. Holmberg, Matt Merta, Lou Ann Shelton, Gerda Sherk, Bradford J. Wood
Data Entry Supervisor:	Benita L. Spight
Data Entry Group Leader:	Gwen Tucker
Data Entry Associates:	Gwen Johnson, Arlene Kevonian
Production Manager:	Mary Beth Trimper
Production Assistant:	Shanna Heilveil
Art Director:	Cynthia Baldwin
Keyliners:	C.J. Jonik, Yolanda Y. Latham
Supervisor of Systems and Programming:	Theresa A. Rocklin
Programmer:	Charles Beaumont

The paper used in this publication meets the minimum requirements of American National Standard for Information Sciences—Permanence Paper for Printed Library Materials, ANSI Z39.48-1984.

This book is printed on recycled paper that meets Environmental Protection Agency standards.

Library of Congress Cataloging-in-Publication Data
Encyclopedia of health information sources: a bibliographic guide to over 13,000 citations for publications, organizations, and databases on health-related subjects . . . / edited by Alan M. Rees — 2nd ed. p.   cm.
First ed. edited by Paul Wasserman and Suzanne Grefsheim.
ISBN 0-8103-6909-5: $165.00
1. Medicine–Bibliography. 2. Reference books–Medicine–Bibliography. 3. Medicine–Information services–Directories. 4. Medicine–Databases–Directories. 5. Medical care–Bibliography. 6. Reference books–Medical care–Bibliography. 7. Medical care–United States–Information services–Directories. 8. Medical care–United States–Databases–Directories.   I. Rees, Alan M.
Z6658.E54 1993
[R118]   93-22416
016.61—dc20   CIP

Printed in the United States of America

Published simultaneously in the United Kingdom
by Gale Research International Limited
(An affiliated company of Gale Research Inc.)

The trademark **ITP** is used under license.

Contents

Highlights

> 13,000 Citations
> 27 New Topics
> Extensive Revision
> CD-ROM Databases
> Telephone and Fax Numbers

Now in its second edition, the *Encyclopedia of Health Information Sources* (EHIS) offers over 13,000 citations covering a myriad of topics in the health-care field.

In response to the changing trends in research, education, and clinical practice, topics have been added, expanded, or modified to:

- reflect new and evolving medical terminology

- provide greater specificity

- represent topics of current interest and concern

27 New Topics

Biostatistics
Chronic Fatigue Syndrome
Corporate Fitness
Estrogen Replacement Therapy
Family Medicine
Fetal Development
General Medicine
Genetic Diseases
Gerontology
Health Care Fraud and Quackery
Health Education
Health Promotion
Kidney Dialysis

Lead Poisoning
Lyme Disease
Medical Consumerism
Medical and Nursing Informatics
Medical Terminology
Mood Disorders
MRI (Magnetic Resonance Imaging)
Occupational Health and Safety
Panic Disorder
Prostate Disorders
Psychoactive Drugs
Weight Control Diets

Extensive Revision of First Edition

Significant expansion of coverage has been made in such areas as:

- Education - Allied Health Education; Dental Education; Nursing Education; Patient Education

- Medical specialities - Cardiology; Emergency Medicine; Family Medicine; Neonatology

- Medical consumerism - Health Insurance; Informed Consent; Long Term Care; Malpractice; Medicare and Medicaid

- Health care administration - Health Care Financing; Health Maintenance Organizations; Hospital Mortality Rates; Quality Assurance

- Women's Health - Hysterectomy; Midwifery; Obstetrics and Gynecology; Uterine Cancer

CD-ROM Databases Added

To reflect changing technology, CD-ROM databases are now included in addition to online databases which were cited previously.

Telephone and Fax Numbers Included

Phone and fax numbers, when available, have been included to facilitate quick and easy access to information.

Introduction

The *Encyclopedia of Health Information Sources (EHIS)* has a dual purpose: to furnish comprehensive access to both print and electronic information sources in the health sciences at a specific and topical level; and to provide a menu of choices for prudent collection development. *EHIS* endeavors to answer pivotal questions posed by researchers and librarians: "Where should I look for information on chronic fatigue syndrome, artificial organs, medical ethics....?"; and, "What are the significant sources of information for the purpose of selection and acquisition?"

At present, most reference guides, bibliographies, core lists, and other collection development tools in the health sciences do not offer subject access on a topical level. Such compilations primarily identify sources for medical specialties such as clinical medicine, surgery, or pediatrics. Yet other compilations collect materials by type of format - indexes and abstracts, journals, or textbooks. Even further, separate directories must be consulted for access to popular materials, online and CD-ROM databases, government publications, research organizations, and newsletters. Consequently, it is necessary to search multiple directories and guides to identify relevant sources.

It is hoped that *EHIS* will offer unified access and serve as a preferred starting point for identifying health information sources. As the information supermarket grows in size and complexity, the need becomes more urgent for an integrated shopping guide.

What is Included?

The list of sources is by no means exhaustive. However, every effort has been made to include "classic" publications and major information sources. A source is deemed "classic" if it can be found on one of the Brandon Core Lists, the Library for Internists VII, the Core Collection of Medical Books and Journals (Medical Information Working Party U.K.); if it has received favorable book reviews; or, if it has displayed longevity as evidenced by the production of multiple editions.

Due to the rapidly moving research frontier in medicine, obsolescence of medical information is inevitable. Sources in *EHIS* are primarily those published in 1988 or later. However, some earlier materials have been included where appropriate. Alternative titles on the same topic, or multiple versions of *MEDLINE* or other databases, have been given in many instances to broaden the range of choices available to readers.

New to the second edition is the strengthened coverage of consumer literature. Several hundred popular books have been included. These are home medical guides that address questions concerning specific diseases/conditions, medical consumerism, medical ethics, drugs, etc. Newsletters that have been added are not exclusively professional, trade, or technical by nature, but also include such popular publications as the *Harvard Health Letter*.

Method of Compilation

Extensive use has been made of core lists, publishers' catalogs, book reviews, vendors' select lists, *Books in Print,* bookstore catalogs such as Dillons (London), and catalogs of professional associations such as the American Medical Association and the American Hospital Association.

Journal titles were, in many instances, identified by means of *MEDLINE* searches followed by the construction of a ranking of those journals publishing the largest number of papers on a given topic. In this manner, our listing of journals represents the publication practices of clinicians and researchers.

All in all, 6,715 unique sources were located, resulting in a total of over 13,000 distributed citations.

15 Kinds of Sources

Material under each subject heading is grouped according to the type of source or form in which information is provided. Simply look under the topic of interest to find the key information sources arranged as follows:

Abstracting, Indexing, and Current
    Awareness Publications
Annuals and Reviews
Associations, Professional Societies,
    Advocacy and Support Groups
Bibliographies
CD-ROM Databases
Directories

Encyclopedias, Dictionaries, Word Books
Handbooks, Guides, Manuals, Atlases
Journals
Newsletters
Online Databases
Popular Works and Patient Education
Research Centers, Institutes, Clearinghouses
Standards and Statistics Sources
Textbooks and Monographs

Acknowledgments

My thanks to Kelle Sisung and Jennifer Mossman of Gale Research for assistance, patience and encouragement in the accumulation, processing, and editing of vast quantities of data; to Connie Fawcett, Assistant Editor, for intelligent and creative data entry and computer support; and to medical literature maestro Alfred N. Brandon for making available to me back issues of his excellent publication, *A Majors Report*. His Core Lists were also most valuable in identifying key sources.

Available in Electronic Formats

EHIS is available for licensing on magnetic tape or diskette in a fielded format. Either the complete database or a custom selection of entries may be ordered. The database is available for internal data processing and nonpublishing purposes only. For more information, call 800-877-GALE.

Suggestions are Welcome

In spite of the considerable care that has been taken to keep errors and inconsistencies to a minimum, invariably some may have occurred. Corrections or suggestions for the improvement of future editions will be greatly appreciated. Please send to:

Editor
Encyclopedia of Health Information Sources
Gale Research Inc.
835 Penobscot Building
Detroit, MI 48226-4094

User's Guide

Entries are arranged alphabetically by ① subject, and further subdivided by ② type of source, and ③ publication title or organization name. For example:

---

① ABORTION

② ABSTRACTING, INDEXING, AND CURRENT AWARENESS PUBLICATIONS

③ *Excerpta Medica. Section 10: Obstetrics and Gynecology.* Elsevier Science Publishing Co., Inc. P.O. Box 882, Madison Square Station, New York, NY 10159-2101. Phone: (212) 989-5800. Fax: (212) 633-3990. 20/year.

Index Medicus. U.S. National Library of Medicine, 8600 Rockville Pike, Bethesda, MD 20814. Phone: (800) 638-8480. Monthly.

ASSOCIATIONS, PROFESSIONAL SOCIETIES, ADVOCACY AND SUPPORT GROUPS

National Abortion Foundation. 900 Pennsylvania Ave. S.E., Washington, DC 20003. Phone: (202) 546-9060.

Planned Parenthood Foundation of America, Inc., 810 Seventh Ave., New York, NY 10011. Phone: (212) 541-7800.

BIBLIOGRAPHIES

Abortion Bibliography. Whitston Publishing Co., P.O. Box 958, Troy, NY 12181. Phone: (518) 283-4363.

Bibliography of Bioethics. Kennedy Institute of Ethics, National Center for Bioethics Literature, Georgetown University, Washington, DC 20057. Phone: (202) 687-6771. Annual.

As the example illustrates, typical entries include the title of a publication or database, the name and address of the publisher, telephone number, fax number, frequency of issuance or year of publication.

In addition to printed and electronic data, *EHIS* also directs users to live sources of up-to-date information, providing organization names, addresses, and telephone numbers.

Locate Topic Through Outline of Contents

Rapid identification of the principal sources of health information for a particular subject can be quickly found in the Outline of Contents. Subject headings are alphabetized and an extensive linkage of cross-references provides access to preferred headings. Subject headings used reflect accepted medical terminology and include diseases and disorders, syndromes, medical specialties, tests and procedures, and a wide variety of headings relating to allied health, nursing, medical consumerism, medical ethics, mental health, and socioeconomics.

Outline of Contents

Encyclopedia
of Health
Information Sources

A

ABDOMINAL DISORDERS

See: GASTROINTESTINAL DISORDERS

ABORTION

ABSTRACTING, INDEXING, AND CURRENT AWARENESS PUBLICATIONS

Current Literature in Family Planning. Planned Parenthood Federation of America, 810 7th Ave., New York, NY 10019. Phone: (212) 603-4637.

Excerpta Medica. Section 10: Obstetrics and Gynecology. Elsevier Science Publishing Co., Inc., P.O. Box 882, Madison Square Station, New York, NY 10159-2101. Phone: (212) 989-5800. Fax: (212) 633-3990. 20/year.

Index Medicus. U.S. National Library of Medicine, 8600 Rockville Pike, Bethesda, MD 20894. Phone: (800) 638-8480. Monthly.

ASSOCIATIONS, PROFESSIONAL SOCIETIES, ADVOCACY AND SUPPORT GROUPS

National Abortion Federation. 900 Pennsylvania Ave. S.E., Washington, DC 20003. Phone: (202) 546-9060.

Planned Parenthood Foundation of America, Inc.. 810 Seventh Ave., New York, NY 10019. Phone: (212) 541-7800.

BIBLIOGRAPHIES

Abortion Bibliography. Whitston Publishing Co., P.O. Box 958, Troy, NY 12181. Phone: (518) 283-4363.

Bibliography of Bioethics. Kennedy Institute of Ethics, National Center for Bioethics Literature, Georgetown University, Washington, DC 20057. Phone: (202) 687-6771. Annual.

DIRECTORIES

National Abortion Federation-Membership Directory. National Abortion Federation, 1436 U St. N.W., Ste. 103, Washington, DC 20009. Phone: (202) 667-5881. Fax: (202) 667-5890. American.

HANDBOOKS, GUIDES, MANUALS, ATLASES

Handbook of Contraception and Abortion. Burkman. Little, Brown and Co., 34 Beacon St., Boston, MA 02108. Phone: (617) 227-0730. Fax: (617) 227-0790. 1989.

JOURNALS

Family Planning Perspectives. Alan Guttmacher Institute, 111 Fifth Ave., New York, NY 10003. Phone: (212) 254-5636.

ONLINE DATABASES

Bioethicsline. Georgetown University, Kennedy Institute of Ethics, Center for Bioethics, Washington, DC 20057. Phone: (202) 687-3885.

EMBASE. Elsevier Science Publishing Co., Inc., P.O. Box 882, Madison Square Station, New York, NY 10159-2101. Phone: (212) 989-5800. Fax: (212) 633-3990.

Human Sexuality. Clinical Communications, Inc., 132 Hutchin Hill, Shady, NY 12409. Phone: (914) 679-2217. Weekly to biweekly.

MEDLINE. National Library of Medicine, 8600 Rockville Pike, Bethesda, MD 20894. Phone: (800) 638-8480.

SciSearch. Institute for Scientific Information, 3501 Market St., Philadelphia, PA 19104. Phone: (215) 386-0100. Fax: (215) 386-6362.

RESEARCH CENTERS, INSTITUTES, CLEARINGHOUSES

Alan Guttmacher Institute. 111 5th Ave., New York, NY 10003. Phone: (212) 254-5656. Fax: (212) 254-9891.

Center for Bioethics. Clinical Research Institute of Montreal, 110 Pine Ave. W., Montreal, PQ, Canada H2W 1R7. Phone: (514) 987-5615. Fax: (514) 987-5695.

Human Life Center. University of Steubenville, Steubenville, OH 43952. Phone: (614) 282-9953.

TEXTBOOKS AND MONOGRAPHS

Psychiatric Aspects of Abortion. Nada L. Stotland (ed.). American Psychiatric Press, Inc., 1400 K St. NW, Washington, DC 20005. Phone: (202) 682-6268. Fax: (202) 789-2648. 1991.

ABUSE

See: CHILD ABUSE; SPOUSE ABUSE

ACCREDITATION, ALLIED HEALTH SCHOOLS

See: ALLIED HEALTH EDUCATION

ACCREDITATION, DENTAL SCHOOLS

See: DENTAL EDUCATION

ACCREDITATION, HOSPITALS

See: HOSPITALS

ACCREDITATION, MEDICAL SCHOOLS

See: MEDICAL EDUCATION

ACNE

See: DERMATOLOGIC DISEASES

ACQUIRED IMMUNODEFICIENCY SYNDROME

See: AIDS

ACUPUNCTURE

See also: ALTERNATIVE MEDICINE

ABSTRACTING, INDEXING, AND CURRENT AWARENESS PUBLICATIONS

Complementary Medicine Index. Medical Information Service, British Library, Boston Spa, Wetherby, W. Yorkshire LS23 7BQ, England. Phone: 0937-546039. Fax: 0937-546236. Monthly.

Index Medicus. U.S. National Library of Medicine, 8600 Rockville Pike, Bethesda, MD 20894. Phone: (800) 638-8480. Monthly.

Science Citation Index. Institute for Scientific Information, 3501 Market St., Philadelphia, PA 19104. Phone: (800) 523-1850. Fax: (215) 386-6362. Bimonthly.

ASSOCIATIONS, PROFESSIONAL SOCIETIES, ADVOCACY AND SUPPORT GROUPS

Acupuncture International Association (AIA). 2330 S. Brentwood Blvd., St. Louis, MO 63144. Phone: (314) 961-2300.

American Acupuncture Association (AAA). 4262 Kissena Blvd., Flushing, NY 11355. Phone: (718) 886-4431.

American Association for Acupuncture and Oriental Medicine (AAAOM). 1424 16th St. N.W., Ste. 501, Washington, DC 20036. Phone: (202) 265-2287.

G-Jo Institute. 4950 SW 70th Ave., Davie, FL 33314. Phone: (305) 791-1562.

International Association of Clinical Laser Acupuncturists (IACLA). 10704 Tesshire Dr., St. Louis, MO 63123. Phone: (314) 843-8520.

National Commission for the Certification of Acupuncturists (NCCA). 1424 16th St. NW, Suite 501, Washington, DC 20036. Phone: (202) 232-1404.

Traditional Acupuncture Foundation. American City Bldg., Suite 100, Columbia, MD 21044. Phone: (301) 997-4888.

CD-ROM DATABASES

SCISEARCH. Institute for Scientific Information, 3501 Market St., Philadelphia, PA 19104. Phone: (215) 386-0100. Fax: (215) 386-6362.

DIRECTORIES

Acupuncture Directory. American Business Directories, Inc., 5711 S. 86th Circle, Omaha, NE 68127. Phone: (402) 593-4600. Fax: (402) 331-1505.

HANDBOOKS, GUIDES, MANUALS, ATLASES

Cross Sectional Atlas of Commonly Used Acupuncture Points of the Arm and Leg. Alex Holland. Alex Holland, 210 Polk St. No. 3, Port Townsend, WA 98368. Phone: (206) 385-4383. 1989.

An Introduction to Basic Acupuncture: A Practical Guide for GPs and other Medical Personnel. P.F. Pearson. Kluwer Academic Publishers, P.O. Box 358, Accord Station, Hingham, MA 02018-0358. Phone: (617) 871-6600. Fax: (617) 871-6528. 1988.

JOURNALS

Acupuncture and Electro-Therapeutics Research. Pergamon Press, 660 White Plains Rd., Tarrytown, NY 10591-5153. Phone: (914) 592-7700. Fax: (914) 592-3625. Quarterly.

Alternative Medicine. V.S.P. International Science Publishers, P.O. Box 346, 3700 AH, Zeist, Netherlands. Phone: 03404-51902. Fax: 03404-58620. Quarterly.

American Journal of Acupuncture. American Journal of Acupuncture, 1840 41st Ave., Suite 102, P.O. Box 610, Capitola, CA 95010. Phone: (408) 475-1700. Quarterly.

Anaesthesia. Academic Press, Inc., 1250 Sixth Ave., San Diego, CA 92101-4311. Phone: (619) 699-6345. Fax: (619) 699-6715. Monthly.

British Journal of Acupuncture. British Acupuncture Association, Central Office, 34 Alderney St., London SW1V 4EU, England.

East West: The Journal of Natural Health and Living. East West Journal, Inc., 17 Station St., P.O. Box 1200, Brookline, MA 02146. Monthly.

Journal of Traditional Acupuncture. Traditional Acupuncture Institute, American City Bldg., Ste. 100, Columbia, MD 21044.

NEWSLETTERS

Acupuncture News. The Center for Chinese Medicine, 5266 E. Pomona Blvd., Los Angeles, CA 90022. Phone: (213) 721-0774. 6/year.

The Meridian. Acupuncture Research Institute, 313 W. Andrix St., Monterey Park, CA 91754. Phone: (213) 722-7353. 3/year.

ONLINE DATABASES

EMBASE. Elsevier Science Publishing Co., Inc., P.O. Box 882, Madison Square Station, New York, NY 10159-2101. Phone: (212) 989-5800. Fax: (212) 633-3990.

MEDLINE. National Library of Medicine, 8600 Rockville Pike, Bethesda, MD 20894. Phone: (800) 638-8480.

SciSearch. Institute for Scientific Information, 3501 Market St., Philadelphia, PA 19104. Phone: (215) 386-0100. Fax: (215) 386-6362.

RESEARCH CENTERS, INSTITUTES, CLEARINGHOUSES

Acupuncture Research Institute (ARI). 313 W. Andrix St., Monterey Park, CA 91754-6408. Phone: (213) 722-7353.

Pain Center. University of Alabama at Birmingham. UAB Medical Center, 1813 6th Ave., Birmingham, AL 35233. Phone: (205) 934-6174.

Research Institute of Acupuncture and Chinese Medicine. 66 Skyline Dr., Middlebury, CT 06762. Phone: (203) 758-9900. Fax: (203) 758-9900.

STANDARDS AND STATISTICS SOURCES

Acupuncture for Everyone. Ruth Lever. Viking Penguin, 375 Hudson St., New York, NY 10014-3657. Phone: (800) 331-4624. 1987.

TEXTBOOKS AND MONOGRAPHS

Acupuncture in Gynecology & Obstetrics. Royston Low. HarperCollins Pubs., Inc., 10 E. 53rd St., New York, NY 10022. Phone: (212) 207-7000. 1990.

Acupuncture and Moxibustion. David Tai. J.B. Lippincott Co., 227 E. Washington Square, Philadelphia, PA 19106-3780. Phone: (215) 238-4200. Fax: (215) 238-4227. 1988.

Basics of Acupuncture. G. Stux, B. Pomeranz. Springer-Verlag New York Inc., 175 Fifth Ave., New York, NY 10010. Phone: (212) 460-1500. Fax: (212) 473-6272. 1988.

The Fundamentals of Ear Acupuncture. Helmut Kropej. Medicina Biologica, 2937 NE Flanders St., Portland, OR 97232. Phone: (503) 230-7079. 1987.

Intermediate Acupuncture, Volume 2. Johannes Bischko, Alexander C. Meng. Medicina Biologica, 2937 NE Flanders St., Portland, OR 97232. Phone: (503) 230-7079. 1986.

An Introduction to Acupuncture, Volume 1. Johannes Bischko. Medicina Biologica, 2937 NE Flanders St., Portland, OR 97232. Phone: (503) 230-7079. Second revised edition 1985.

Scientific Bases of Acupuncture. B. Pomeranz, G. Stux (eds.). Springer-Verlag New York Inc., 175 Fifth Ave., New York, NY 10010. Phone: (212) 460-1500. Fax: (212) 473-6272. 1989.

Sticking to the Point: A Rational Method for the Step by Step Formulation of Administration of an Acupuncture Treatment. Bob Flaws. Blue Poppy Enterprises Press, 1775 Linden Ave., Boulder, CO 80302. Phone: (303) 442-0796. 1990.

The Workbook: An Introduction to the Meridians and Points of Acupuncture. Alex Holland, James Blair. Alex Holland, 210 Polk St. No. 3, Port Townsend, WA 98368. Phone: (206) 385-4383. 1988.

ADDICTIONS

See: ALCOHOLISM; DRUG ABUSE;
GAMBLING; SMOKING

ADDITIVES, FOOD

See: FOOD ADDITIVES

ADMINISTRATION

See: HEALTH CARE ADMINISTRATION;
HOSPITALS; NURSING HOMES

ADOLESCENT MEDICINE

See: PEDIATRICS

AFFECTIVE DISORDERS

See: DEPRESSION; MOOD DISORDERS;
PSYCHIATRIC DISORDERS

AGENT ORANGE

See: ENVIRONMENTAL POLLUTANTS;
PESTICIDES AND HERBICIDES

AGING

See also: GERONTOLOGY

ABSTRACTING, INDEXING, AND CURRENT AWARENESS PUBLICATIONS

Cumulative Subject Index to Current Literature on Aging, 1980-1988. National Council on the Aging, Inc., 600 Maryland Ave. S.W., W. Wing 100, Washington, DC 20024. Phone: (202) 479-1200. 1989.

Excerpta Medica. Section 25: Hematology. Elsevier Science Publishers, P.O. Box 882, Madison Square Station, New York, NY 10159-2101. Phone: (212) 633-3950. Fax: (212) 633-3990. 24/year.

Gerontological Abstracts. University Information Services, Inc., University of Michigan, 5212 School of Dentistry, Ann Arbor, MI 48109-1078. Phone: (313) 764-1555. Bimonthly.

Index Medicus. U.S. National Library of Medicine, 8600 Rockville Pike, Bethesda, MD 20894. Phone: (800) 638-8480. Monthly.

Index to Periodical Literature on Aging. Lorraine Publications, 2162 Chene, Detroit, MI 48207. Phone: (313) 834-4570. Biennial.

New Literature on Old Age. Center for Policy on Ageing, 25/31 Ironmonger Row, London EC1V 3QP, England. 6/year.

Psychological Abstracts. American Psychological Association, 1200 17th St. NW, Washington, DC 20036. Phone: (202) 955-7600. Monthly.

Research Alert: Aging/Geriatrics. Institute for Scientific Information, 3501 Market St., Philadelphia, PA 19104. Phone: (800) 523-1850. Fax: (215) 386-6362. Weekly.

Science Citation Index. Institute for Scientific Information, 3501 Market St., Philadelphia, PA 19104. Phone: (800) 523-1850. Fax: (215) 386-6362. Bimonthly.

ANNUALS AND REVIEWS

Annual Review of Gerontology and Geriatrics. Springer Publishing Co., Inc., 536 Broadway, 11th Floor, New York, NY 10012. Phone: (212) 431-4370.

Contemporary Geriatric Medicine. Plenum Publishing Co., 233 Spring St., New York, NY 10013-1578. Phone: (212) 620-8000. Fax: (212) 463-0742. Irregular.

In Development New Medicines for Older Americans. Pharmaceutical Manufacturers Association, 1100 15th St. N.W., Washington, DC 20005. Phone: (202) 835-3400. Annual.

In Development New Medicines for Older Americans. 1991 Annual Survey. 329 Medicines in Testing for 45 Diseases of Aging. Pharmaceutical Manufacturers Association, 1100 15th St. N.W., Washington, DC 20005. Phone: (202) 835-3400. 1991.

In Development New Medicines for Older Americans. 1991 Annual Survey. More Medicines in Testing for Cancer Than for Any Other Disease of Aging. Pharmaceutical Manufacturers Association, 1100 15th St. N.W., Washington, DC 20005. Phone: (202) 835-3400. 1991.

Year Book of Geriatrics and Gerontology. Mosby-Year Book, 11830 Westline Industrial Drive, St. Louis, MO 63146. Phone: (800) 325-4177. Fax: (314) 432-1380. Annual.

ASSOCIATIONS, PROFESSIONAL SOCIETIES, ADVOCACY AND SUPPORT GROUPS

American Aging Association (AGE). 600 S. 42nd St., Omaha, NE 68198-4635. Phone: (402) 559-4416. Fax: (402) 559-5844.

American Association of Retired Persons. 1909 K St. N.W., Washington, DC 20049. Phone: (202) 872-4700.

American Senior Citizens Association. P.O. Box 41, Fayetteville, NC 28302. Phone: (919) 323-3641.

Gerontological Society of America (GSA). 1275 K St. N.W., Ste. 350, Washington, DC 20005. Phone: (202) 842-1275.

Gray Panthers. 1424 16th St. N.W., Suite 602, Washington, DC 20036.

National Alliance of Senior Citizens. 2525 Wilson Blvd., Arlington, VA 22201. Phone: (703) 528-4380.

National Center on Rural Aging. c/o National Council on Aging, 600 Maryland Ave. S.W., Washington, DC 20024. Phone: (202) 479-1200.

National Council on Aging. 600 Maryland Ave. S.W., W. Wing 100, Washington, DC 20024. Phone: (202) 479-1200.

BIBLIOGRAPHIES

Fundamentals of Geriatrics for Health Care Professionals: An Annotated Bibliography. Joddi L. Teitelman, Iris A. Parham (eds.). Greenwood Publishing Group, Inc., 88 Post Rd. W., P.O. Box 5007, Westport, CT 06881. Phone: (203) 226-3571. 1990.

Nutri-Topics: Nutrition and the Elderly. Food and Nutrition Center, National Agricultural Library, 10301 Baltimore Blvd., Beltsville, MD 20705.

CD-ROM DATABASES

SCISEARCH. Institute for Scientific Information, 3501 Market St., Philadelphia, PA 19104. Phone: (215) 386-0100. Fax: (215) 386-6362.

ENCYCLOPEDIAS, DICTIONARIES, WORD BOOKS

The Encyclopedia of Aging and the Elderly. F. Hampton Roy, Charles Russell. Facts on File, Inc., 460 Park Ave. S., New York, NY 10016-7382. Phone: (212) 683-2244. Fax: (212) 683-3633. 1992.

HANDBOOKS, GUIDES, MANUALS, ATLASES

Merck Manual of Geriatrics. Merck & Co., Inc., P.O. Box 2000, Rahway, NJ 07065. Phone: (201) 855-4558. Irregular.

JOURNALS

Age and Aging. Oxford University Press, 200 Madison Ave., New York, NY 10016. Phone: (212) 679-7300. Bimonthly.

Aging & Neuroscience. Philadelphia College of Pharmacy and Science, Office of Professional Programs, 600 43rd St., Philadelphia, PA 19104.

Experimental Aging Research. Beech Hill Publishing Co., P.O. Box 40, Mt. Desert, ME 04660. Phone: (207) 667-5048. Fax: (207) 244-0128. Quarterly.

Mechanisms of Ageing and Development. Elsevier Science Publishing Co., Inc., P.O. Box 882, Madison Square Station, New York, NY 10159-2101. Phone: (212) 989-5800. Fax: (212) 633-3990. 18/year.

Perspective on Aging. National Council on the Aging, Inc., 600 Maryland Ave. S.W., W. Wing 100, Washington, DC 20024. Phone: (202) 479-1200. Bimonthly.

ONLINE DATABASES

EMBASE. Elsevier Science Publishing Co., Inc., P.O. Box 882, Madison Square Station, New York, NY 10159-2101. Phone: (212) 989-5800. Fax: (212) 633-3990.

MEDLINE. National Library of Medicine, 8600 Rockville Pike, Bethesda, MD 20894. Phone: (800) 638-8480.

SciSearch. Institute for Scientific Information, 3501 Market St., Philadelphia, PA 19104. Phone: (215) 386-0100. Fax: (215) 386-6362.

POPULAR WORKS AND PATIENT EDUCATION

A Consumer's Guide to Aging. David H. Solomon, Elyse Salend, Anna Nolen Rahman, and others. Johns Hopkins University Press, 701 W. 40th St., Suite 275, Baltimore, MD 21211-2190. Phone: (800) 537-5487. 1992.

RESEARCH CENTERS, INSTITUTES, CLEARINGHOUSES

Center for Geriatrics, Gerontology, and Long-Term Care. Columbia University. 100 Haven Ave., Tower 3-29F, New York, NY 10032. Phone: (212) 781-0600.

Center on Health and Aging. Atlanta University. 223 James P. Brawley Dr. S.W., Atlanta, GA 30313. Phone: (404) 653-8610.

Center for Study of Aging and Human Development. Duke University Medical Ctr., Box 3003, Durham, NC 27710. Phone: (919) 684-2248. Fax: (919) 684-8569.

Ethel Percy Andrus Gerontology Center. University of Southern California. University Park, MC 0191, Los Angeles, CA 90089-0191. Phone: (213) 740-6060. Fax: (213) 740-8241.

Gerontology Center. University of Illinois at Chicago. 2121 W. Taylor St., M/C 922, Chicago, IL 60612. Phone: (312) 996-6310.

Institute on Aging. Temple University. University Services Bldg., 1601 N. Broad St., Philadelphia, PA 19122. Phone: (215) 787-6970.

Institute on Aging. University of Pennsylvania. 3615 Chestnut St., Philadelphia, PA 19104-6006. Phone: (215) 898-3163. Fax: (215) 898-0580.

Institute of Gerontology. University of Michigan. 300 N. Ingalis, Ann Arbor, MI 48109-2007. Phone: (313) 764-3493. Fax: (313) 936-2116.

Institute for Health and Aging. University of California, San Francisco. School of Nursing, San Francisco, CA 94143-0612. Phone: (415) 476-3236. Fax: (415) 476-1253.

McGill Centre for Studies in Aging. 1650 Cedar Ave., Montreal, PQ, Canada H3Q 1A4. Phone: (514) 934-8096. Fax: (514) 937-9875.

National Institute on Aging Information Center. NIH Bldg. 31, Rm. 5C-35, 9000 Rockville Pike, Bethesda, MD 20892. Phone: (301) 496-1752. Fax: (301) 589-3014.

National Resource Center on Health Promotion and Aging. 1909 K St. N.W., 5th Flr., Washington, DC 20049. Phone: (800) 729-6686.

Sam and Rose Stein Institute for Research on Aging. University of California, San Diego. 0664, 5094 BSB, La Jolla, CA 92093. Phone: (619) 534-6299.

Sanders-Brown Center on Aging. University of Kentucky. 101 Sanders-Brown Bldg., Lexington, KY 40536. Phone: (606) 233-6040. Fax: (606) 258-2866.

University Center on Aging and Health. Case Western Reserve University. 2009 Adelbert Rd., Cleveland, OH 44106. Phone: (216) 368-2692. Fax: (216) 368-6389.

TEXTBOOKS AND MONOGRAPHS

Aging, Health, and Behavior. Marcia G. Ory, Ronald P. Abeles, Paula Darby Lipman (eds.). Sage Publications, Inc., 2455 Teller Road, P.O. Box 5084, Newbury Park, CA 91320. Phone: (805) 499-0721. Fax: (805) 499-0871. 1991.

Aging: Health Care Challenge. Lewis. F.A. Davis Co., 1915 Arch St., Philadelphia, PA 19103. Phone: (800) 523-4049. Fax: (215) 568-5065. Second edition 1990.

The Clinical Neurology of Old Age. R. Tallis. John Wiley & Sons, Inc., 605 Third Ave., New York, NY 10158-0012. Phone: (212) 850-6000. Fax: (212) 850-6088. 1989.

Dementia and Aging: Ethics, Values and Policy Choices. Robert H. Binstock, Stephen G. Post, Peter J. Whitehouse. Johns Hopkins University Press, 701 W. 40th St., Suite 275, Baltimore, MD 21211-2190. Phone: (800) 537-5487. Fax: (410) 516-6998. 1992.

Geriatric Medicine. Katz. Churchill Livingstone Inc., 650 Ave. of the Americas, New York, NY 10011. Phone: (212) 819-5400. Fax: (212) 302-6598. 1991.

Geriatrics for the Internist. Rothschild. Mosby-Year Book, 11830 Westline Industrial Drive, St. Louis, MO 63146. Phone: (800) 325-4177. Fax: (314) 432-1380. 1990.

Oxford Textbook of Geriatric Medicine. Evans. Oxford University Press, 200 Madison Ave., New York, NY 10016. Phone: (212) 679-7300. 1992.

Principles and Practice of Geriatric Medicine. Pathy. John Wiley & Sons, Inc., 605 Third Ave., New York, NY 10158-0012. Phone: (212) 850-6000. Fax: (212) 850-6088. Second edition 1992.

Textbook of Geriatric Medicine and Gerontology. Chernoff. Churchill Livingstone Inc., 650 Ave. of the Americas, New York, NY 10011. Phone: (212) 819-5400. Fax: (212) 302-6598. Fourth edition 1992.

AIDS

See also: HUMAN IMMUNODEFICIENCY VIRUS; IMMUNOLOGIC DISORDERS; SEXUALLY TRANSMITTED DISEASES

ABSTRACTING, INDEXING, AND CURRENT AWARENESS PUBLICATIONS

ATIN: AIDS Targeted Information. Williams & Wilkins, 428 E. Preston St., Baltimore, MD 21202. Phone: (800) 638-0672. Fax: (800) 447-8438. Monthly.

CA Selects: AIDS & Related Immunodeficiencies. Chemical Abstracts Service, 2540 Olentangy River Road, P.O. Box 3012, Columbus, OH 43210-0012. Phone: (800) 848-6538. Biweekly.

Current Contents/Clinical Medicine. Institute for Scientific Information, 3501 Market St., Philadelphia, PA 19104. Phone: (800) 523-1850. Fax: (215) 386-6362. Weekly.

Current Contents/Life Sciences. Institute for Scientific Information, 3501 Market St., Philadelphia, PA 19104. Phone: (215) 386-0100. Fax: (215) 386-6362.

Index Medicus. U.S. National Library of Medicine, 8600 Rockville Pike, Bethesda, MD 20894. Phone: (800) 638-8480. Monthly.

MEDOC: Index to U.S. Government Publications in the Medical and Health Sciences. Spencer S. Eccles Health Sciences Library, University of Utah, Bldg. 589, Salt Lake City, UT 84112. Phone: (801) 581-5268. Quarterly.

Research Alert: AIDS. Institute for Scientific Information, 3501 Market St., Philadelphia, PA 19104. Phone: (800) 523-1850. Fax: (215) 386-6362. Weekly.

Science Citation Index. Institute for Scientific Information, 3501 Market St., Philadelphia, PA 19104. Phone: (800) 523-1850. Fax: (215) 386-6362. Bimonthly.

Virology & AIDS Abstracts. Cambridge Scientific Abstracts, 7200 Wisconsin Ave., Bethesda, MD 20814-4823. Phone: (800) 843-7751. Fax: (301) 961-6720. Monthly.

ANNUALS AND REVIEWS

Current Topics in AIDS. John Wiley & Sons, Inc., 605 Third Ave., New York, NY 10158-0012. Phone: (212) 850-6000. Fax: (212) 850-6088. Irregular.

ASSOCIATIONS, PROFESSIONAL SOCIETIES, ADVOCACY AND SUPPORT GROUPS

American Foundation for AIDS Research. 5900 Wilshire Blvd., 2nd Fl., E. Satellite, Los Angeles, CA 90036. Phone: (213) 857-5900.

Gay Men's Health Crisis. 129 W. 20th St., New York, NY 10011. Phone: (212) 807-6664. Fax: (212) 337-3656.

National Association of People with AIDS. 2025 I St. N.W., Washington, DC 20006. Phone: (202) 429-2856.

People with AIDS Health Group. 150 W. 20th St., New York, NY 10010.

San Francisco AIDS Foundation (SFAF). P.O. Box 6182, San Francisco, CA 94101. Phone: (415) 864-5855. Fax: (415) 864-5855.

BIBLIOGRAPHIES

Acquired Immune Deficiency Syndrome. National Technical Information Service, 5285 Port Royal Rd., Springfield, VA 22161. Phone: (703) 487-4650. Fax: (703) 321-8547. Jan. 1970-Dec. 1987. PB88-855184/CBY.

Acquired Immune Deficiency Syndrome (AIDS). National Technical Information Service, 5285 Port Royal Rd., Springfield, VA 22161. Phone: (703) 487-4650. Fax: (703) 321-8547. Aug. 1983-July 1989 PB90/853862/CBY.

Acquired Immune Deficiency Syndrome: Opportunistic Infections. National Technical Information Service, 5285 Port Royal Rd., Springfield, VA 22161. Phone: (703) 487-4650. Fax: (703) 321-8547. Apr. 1987-Apr. 1988. PB88-862834/CBY.

Acquired Immune Deficiency Syndrome: Therapies and Treatments. National Technical Information Service, 5285

Port Royal Rd., Springfield, VA 22161. Phone: (703) 487-4650. Fax: (703) 321-8547. Jun. 1984-Jan. 1989. PB89-856132/CBY.

AIDS: Abstracts of the Psychological and Behavioral Literature, 1983-1990. American Psychological Association, 1200 17th St. NW, Washington, DC 20036. Phone: (202) 955-7600. Third edition 1992.

AIDS Bibliography. U.S. National Library of Medicine, Reference Section, 8600 Rockville Pike, Bethesda, MD 20894. Phone: (800) 638-8480. Monthly.

AIDS Information Sourcebook. H. Robert Malinovsky, Gerald J. Perry (eds.). Oryx Press, 4041 N. Central, Suite 700, Phoenix, AZ 85012. Phone: (800) 279-ORYX. Fax: (800) 279-4663. 3rd edition, 1991.

AIDS and Women: A Sourcebook. Sarah Watstein, Robert Laurich (eds.). Oryx Press, 4041 N. Central, Suite 700, Phoenix, AZ 85012. Phone: (800) 279-ORYX. Fax: (800) 279-4663. 1991.

How to Find Information about AIDS. Jeffrey T. Huber (ed.). Haworth Press, Inc., 10 Alice St., Binghamton, NY 13904-1580. Phone: (800) 342-9678. 1992.

Nutrition and AIDS. Food and Nutrition Center, National Agricultural Library, 10301 Baltimore Blvd., Beltsville, MD 20705. May 1991.

CD-ROM DATABASES

AIDS Compact Library. MEP, 124 Mt. Auburn St., Cambridge, MA 02138. Phone: (800) 342-1338. Fax: (617) 868-7738. Semiannual.

AIDS: Information and Education Worldwide. CD Resources, Inc., 118 W. 74th St., Suite 2A, New York, NY 10023. Phone: (212) 580-2263. Fax: (212) 877-1276. Quarterly.

AIDSLine. SilverPlatter Information, Inc., River Ridge Office Park, 100 River Ridge Rd., Norwood, MA 02062. Phone: (617) 769-2599. Fax: (617) 769-8763. Quarterly.

Excerpta Medica CD: Immunology & AIDS. SilverPlatter Information, Inc., River Ridge Office Park, 100 River Ridge Rd., Norwood, MA 02062. Phone: (617) 769-2599. Fax: (617) 769-8763. Quarterly.

Internal Medicine '92. Macmillan New Media, 124 Mt. Auburn St., Cambridge, MA 02138. Phone: (800) 342-1338. 1992.

Morbidity Mortality Weekly Report. MEP, 124 Mt. Auburn St., Cambridge, MA 02138. Phone: (800) 342-1338. Fax: (617) 868-7738. Annual.

The Physician's AIDSLINE. MEP, 124 Mt. Auburn St., Cambridge, MA 02138. Phone: (800) 342-1338. Fax: (617) 868-7738. Annual.

SCISEARCH. Institute for Scientific Information, 3501 Market St., Philadelphia, PA 19104. Phone: (215) 386-0100. Fax: (215) 386-6362.

DIRECTORIES

AIDS/HIV Treatment Directory. American Foundation for AIDS Research, 5900 Wilshire Blvd., 2nd Fl., Los Angeles, CA 90036. Phone: (213) 857-5900. Quarterly.

AIDS Information Resources Directory. American Foundation for AIDS Research, 5900 Wilshire Blvd., 2nd Flr., E. Satellite, Los Angeles, CA 90036-5032. Phone: (213) 857-5900. Quarterly.

Local AIDS Services: The National Directory. U.S. Conference of Mayors, 1620 I St. N.W., Washington, DC 20006. Phone: (202) 293-7330. Fax: (202) 293-2352. Annual.

ENCYCLOPEDIAS, DICTIONARIES, WORD BOOKS

Immunologic and AIDS Word Book. Helen E. Littrell. Springhouse Publishing Co., 1111 Bethlehem Pike, Spring House, PA 19477. Phone: (800) 331-3170. Fax: (215) 646-8716. 1992.

HANDBOOKS, GUIDES, MANUALS, ATLASES

AIDS: A Pocket Book of Diagnosis and Management. Adrian Mindel (ed.). Williams & Wilkins, 428 East Preston St., Baltimore, MD 21202. Phone: (800) 638-0672. Fax: (800) 447-8438. 1989.

The AIDS Benefits Handbook. T. McCormack. Yale University Press, 302 Temple St., New Haven, CT 06520. Phone: (203) 432-0940. 1990.

The Handbook of Immunopharmacology. Academic Press, Inc., 1250 Sixth Ave., San Diego, CA 92101-4311. Phone: (619) 699-6345. Fax: (619) 699-6715. Irregular.

JOURNALS

AIDS Education & Prevention: An Interdisciplinary Journal. Guilford Publications, Inc., 72 Spring St., New York, NY 10012. Phone: (800) 365-7006. Fax: (212) 966-6708. Quarterly.

AIDS Patient Care. Mary Ann Liebert, Inc., 1651 Third Ave., New York, NY 10128. Phone: (212) 289-2300. Fax: (212) 289-4697. Bimonthly.

AIDS Research and Human Retroviruses. Mary Ann Liebert, Inc., 1651 Third Ave., New York, NY 10128. Phone: (212) 289-2300. Fax: (212) 289-4697. Monthly.

International Journal of STD and AIDS. Royal Society of Medicine Services Ltd., 1 Wimpole St., London W1M 8AE, England. Phone: 071-408 2119. Fax: 071-355 3198. Bimonthly.

Journal of Acquired Immune Deficiency Syndromes. Raven Press, 1185 Avenue of the Americas, New York, NY 10036. Phone: (212) 930-9500. Fax: (212) 869-3495. Monthly.

Morbidity and Mortality Weekly Report. Massachusetts Medical Society, 1440 Main St., Waltham, MA 02154-1649. Phone: (617) 893-3800. Fax: (617) 893-0413. Weekly.

NEWSLETTERS

AIDS Alert. American Health Consultants, Department C1290, P.O. Box 740060, Atlanta, GA 30374. Phone: (800) 559-1032. Monthly.

AIDS Clinical Care. Massachusetts Medical Society, 1440 Main St., Waltham, MA 02154-1649. Phone: (617) 893-3800. Fax: (617) 893-0413. Monthly.

AIDS Clinical Digest. American Health Consultants, Department C1290, P.O. Box 740060, Atlanta, GA 30374. Phone: (800) 559-1032. Fax: (404) 352-1971. Semimonthly.

The AIDS Letter. Royal Society of Medicine Services Ltd., 1 Wimpole St., London W1M 8AE, England. Phone: 071-408 2119. Fax: 071-355 3198. Bimonthly.

AIDS Medical Report. American Health Consultants, Department C1290, P.O. Box 740060, Atlanta, GA 30374. Phone: (800) 559-1032. Monthly.

AIDS Treatment News. P.O. Box 411256, San Francisco, CA 94141. Phone: (800) TRE-AT12. Semimonthly.

Being Alive. 4222 Santa Monica Blvd., Ste. 105, Los Angeles, CA 90029. Phone: (213) 667-3262. Monthly.

BETA: The Bulletin of Experimental Treatments for AIDS. San Francisco AIDS Foundation, P.O. Box 2189, Berkeley, CA 94702-0189. Phone: (800) 327-9893. Fax: (415) 549-4342. Quarterly.

Common Sense about AIDS. American Health Consultants, P.O. Box 71266, Chicago, IL 60691-9987. Phone: (800) 688-2421.

Notes from the Underground. PWA Health Group, 31 W. 26th St., New York, NY 10010. Phone: (212) 532-0280. 6/year.

PI Perspective. 347 Delores St., Ste. 301, San Francisco, CA 94110. Phone: (415) 558-8669. Quarterly.

ONLINE DATABASES

AIDS Database. Bureau of Hygiene and Tropical Diseases, Keppel St., London WC1E 7HT, England. Phone: 071-636 8636. Fax: 071-580 6756. Monthly.

AIDS Knowledge Base. BRS Information Technologies, 8000 Westpark Dr., Mc Lean, VA 22102. Phone: (800) 289-4277. Fax: (703) 893-4632.

AIDSDRUGS. AIDS Clinical Trials Information Service, P.O. Box 6421, Rockville, MD 20850. Phone: (800) 874-2572. Monthly.

AIDSLINE. Division. U.S. National Library of Medicine, Specialized Information Services Division, 8600 Rockville Pike, Bethesda, MD 20894. Phone: (301) 496-6531. Weekly.

AIDSTRIALS. U.S. National AIDS Information Clearinghouse, P.O. Box 6003, Rockville, MD 20850-6003. Phone: (800) 458-5231. Biweekly.

Combined Health Information Database (CHID). U.S. National Institutes of Health, P.O. Box NDIC, Bethesda, MD 20892. Phone: (301) 496-2162. Fax: (301) 770-5164. Quarterly.

EMBASE. Elsevier Science Publishing Co., Inc., P.O. Box 882, Madison Square Station, New York, NY 10159-2101. Phone: (212) 989-5800. Fax: (212) 633-3990.

MEDLINE. National Library of Medicine, 8600 Rockville Pike, Bethesda, MD 20894. Phone: (800) 638-8480.

SciSearch. Institute for Scientific Information, 3501 Market St., Philadelphia, PA 19104. Phone: (215) 386-0100. Fax: (215) 386-6362.

POPULAR WORKS AND PATIENT EDUCATION

39 Development AIDS Medicines: Drugs and Vaccines. Pharmaceutical Manufacturers Association, 1100 15th St. N.W., Washington, DC 20005. Phone: (202) 835-3400. Annual.

AIDS: The Ultimate Challenge. Elisabeth Kubler-Ross, Mal Warshaw. Macmillan Publishing Co., 866 Third Ave., New York, NY 10011. Phone: (800) 257-5755. 1988.

Among Friends: Hospice Care for the Person with AIDS. Robert W. Buckingham. Prometheus Books, 700 E. Amherst St., Buffalo, NY 14215. Phone: (800) 421-0351. 1992.

And the Band Played On. Randy Shilts. Viking Penguin, 375 Hudson St., New York, NY 10014-3657. Phone: (800) 331-4624. 1988.

The Caregiver's Journey: When You Love Someone with AIDS. Mel Pohl, Deniston Kay, Doug Toft. HarperCollins Pubs., Inc., 10 E. 53rd St., New York, NY 10022. Phone: (212) 207-7000. 1991.

The Essential AIDS Fact Book. Paul Harding Douglas, Laura Pinsky. Pocket Books, Inc., 1230 Ave. of the Americas, New York, NY 10020. Phone: (800) 223-2348. Fax: (800) 284-0735. Revised edition 1992.

The Essential HIV Treatment Fact Book. Laura Pinsky, Paul Harding Douglas, Craig Metroka. Pocket Books, Inc., 1230 Ave. of the Americas, New York, NY 10020. Phone: (800) 223-2348. Fax: (800) 284-0735. 1992.

The Guide to Living with HIV Infection: Developed at the Johns Hopkins AIDS Clinic. John G. Bartlett, Ann K. Finkbeiner. Johns Hopkins University Press, 701 W. 40th St., Suite 275, Baltimore, MD 21211-2190. Phone: (800) 537-5487. Fax: (410) 516-6998. 1991.

The HIV Test: What You Need to Know to Make an Informed Decision. Marc Vargo. Pocket Books, Inc., 1230 Ave. of the Americas, New York, NY 10020. Phone: (800) 223-2348. Fax: (800) 284-0735. 1992.

Virus Hunting: AIDS, Cancer and the Human Retrovirus. Robert Gallo. HarperCollins Pubs., Inc., 10 E. 53rd St., New York, NY 10022-5299. Phone: (212) 207-7000. 1991.

RESEARCH CENTERS, INSTITUTES, CLEARINGHOUSES

AIDS Clinical Research Center. University of California, San Francisco. VAMC 141, 4150 Clement St., San Francisco, CA 94121. Phone: (415) 221-4810.

AIDS Clinical Trials Unit. UCLA AIDS Clinical Research Center. 10933 Le Conte Ave., Room BH-412 CHS, Los Angeles, CA 90024-1793. Phone: (213) 206-6414. Fax: (213) 206-3311.

Human Immunodeficiency Virus Center for Clinical and Behavioral Studies. New York State Psychiatric Institute, 722 W. 168th St., New York, NY 10032. Phone: (212) 960-2432. Fax: (212) 740-1774.

National AIDS Information Clearinghouse. P.O. Box 6003, Rockville, MD 20850. Phone: (800) 458-5231. Fax: (301) 738-6616. National AIDS Hotline: 800-342-AIDS.

National Cooperative Drug Discovery Group for the Treatment of AIDS. Dana Farber Cancer Institute. 44 Binney St., Boston, MA 02115. Phone: (617) 732-3068. Fax: (617) 732-3113.

National Cooperative Drug Discovery Group for the Treatment of AIDS. Duke University. Medical Center, Dept. of Surgery, P.O. BOx 2926, Durham, NC 27710. Phone: (919) 684-3103. Fax: (919) 684-4288.

National Cooperative Drug Discovery Group for the Treatment of AIDS. Emory University. Dept. of Pediatrics, 2040 Ridgewood Dr. NE, Atlanta, GA 30322. Phone: (404) 728-7711. Fax: (404) 729-7726.

National Cooperative Drug Discovery Group for the Treatment of AIDS. George Washington University. Dept. of Pharmacology, 2300 Eye St. NW, Washington, DC 20037-2313. Phone: (202) 994-2706. Fax: (202) 994-2870.

TEXTBOOKS AND MONOGRAPHS

Advances in Chemotherapy of AIDS. Robert Diasio, Jean-Pierre Sommadossi. McGraw-Hill, Inc., Health Professions Division, 1221 Avenue of the Americas, 28th Floor, New York, NY 10020. Phone: (212) 512-4228. 1990.

AIDS. Aggleton. Taylor & Francis Inc., 1900 Frost Rd., Suite 101, Bristol, PA 19007-1598. Phone: (800) 821-8312. Fax: (215) 785-5515. 1991.

AIDS: A Basic Guide in Prevention, Treatment and Understanding. M. Ross Seligson, Karen E. Peterson (eds.). Taylor & Francis Inc., 1900 Frost Rd., Suite 101, Bristol, PA 19007-1598. Phone: (800) 821-8312. Fax: (215) 785-5515. 1991.

AIDS and Alcohol/Drug Abuse: Psychosocial Research. Dennis G. Fisher (ed.). Haworth Press, 10 Alice Street, Binghamton, NY 13904-1580. Phone: (800) 342-9678. Fax: (607) 722-1424. 1991.

AIDS, Drugs, and Sexual Risk. McKegany. Taylor & Francis Inc., 1900 Frost Rd., Suite 101, Bristol, PA 19007-1598. Phone: (800) 821-8312. Fax: (215) 785-5515. 1992.

AIDS: Etiology, Diagnosis, Treatment and Prevention. Vincent T. DeVita Jr., Samuel Hellman, Steven Rosenberg. J.B. Lippincott Co., 227 E. Washington Square, Philadelphia, PA 19106-3780. Phone: (215) 238-4200. Fax: (215) 238-4227. Second edition 1988.

AIDS and HIV Diseases. Luc Montagnier. Mosby-Year Book, 11830 Westline Industrial Drive, St. Louis, MO 63146. Phone: (800) 325-4177. Fax: (314) 432-1380. 1990.

AIDS and the Hospice Community. Madalon O'Rawe, Amenta Claire Tehan (eds.). Haworth Press, 10 Alice Street, Binghamton, NY 13904-1580. Phone: (800) 342-9678. Fax: (607) 722-1424. 1991.

The AIDS Knowledge Base. P.T. Cohen, Merle A. Sande, Paul A. Volberding (eds.). Massachusetts Medical Society, 1440 Main St., Waltham, MA 02154-1649. Phone: (617) 893-3800. Fax: (617) 893-0413. 1992.

AIDS and Other Manifestations of HIV Infection. G. Wormser (ed.). Noyes Publications, Mill Rd. at Grand Ave., Park Ridge, NJ 07656. Phone: (201) 391-8484. 1987.

Cocaine, AIDS and Intravenous Drug Use. Samuel R. Friedman, Douglas S. Lipton (eds.). Haworth Press, 10 Alice Street, Binghamton, NY 13904-1580. Phone: (800) 3HA-WORTH. Fax: (607) 722-1424. 1991.

Living and Dying with AIDS. Ahmed. Plenum Publishing Co., 233 Spring St., New York, NY 10013-1578. Phone: (212) 620-8000. Fax: (212) 463-0742. 1992.

The Medical Management of AIDS. Merle A. Sande, Paul A. Volberding. W.B. Saunders Co., The Curtis Center,

Independence Square W., Philadelphia, PA 19106-3399. Phone: (215) 238-7800. Second edition 1991.

AIR POLLUTION

See: ENVIRONMENTAL POLLUTANTS

ALCOHOLISM

See also: DRUG ABUSE

ABSTRACTING, INDEXING, AND CURRENT AWARENESS PUBLICATIONS

Current Contents/Clinical Medicine. Institute for Scientific Information, 3501 Market St., Philadelphia, PA 19104. Phone: (800) 523-1850. Fax: (215) 386-6362. Weekly.

Excerpta Medica. Section 40: Drug Dependence, Alcohol Abuse and Alcoholism. Elsevier Science Publishing Co., Inc., P.O. Box 882, Madison Square Station, New York, NY 10159-2101. Phone: (212) 989-5800. Fax: (212) 633-3990. 6/year.

General Science Index. H.W. Wilson Co., 950 University Ave., Bronx, NY 10452. Phone: (800) 367-6770.

Index Medicus. U.S. National Library of Medicine, 8600 Rockville Pike, Bethesda, MD 20894. Phone: (800) 638-8480. Monthly.

MEDOC: Index to U.S. Government Publications in the Medical and Health Sciences. Spencer S. Eccles Health Sciences Library, University of Utah, Bldg. 589, Salt Lake City, UT 84112. Phone: (801) 581-5268. Quarterly.

Prevention Pipeline: An Alcohol and Drug Awareness Service. National Clearinghouse for Alcohol and Drug Information, Dept. PP, P.O. Box 2345, Rockville, MD 20852.

Psychological Abstracts. American Psychological Association, 1200 17th St. NW, Washington, DC 20036. Phone: (202) 955-7600. Monthly.

Research Alert: Alcoholism. Institute for Scientific Information, 3501 Market St., Philadelphia, PA 19104. Phone: (800) 523-1850. Fax: (215) 386-6362. Weekly.

Science Citation Index. Institute for Scientific Information, 3501 Market St., Philadelphia, PA 19104. Phone: (800) 523-1850. Fax: (215) 386-6362. Bimonthly.

ANNUALS AND REVIEWS

Advances in Alcohol and Substance Abuse. Haworth Press, 10 Alice St., Binghamton, NY 13904-1580. Phone: (803) 429-6784. Fax: (607) 722-1424.

Alcohol. Norman S. Miller (ed.). Plenum Publishing Co., 233 Spring St., New York, NY 10013-1578. Phone: (212) 620-8000. Fax: (212) 463-0742. Volume 2 1991.

Recent Developments in Alcoholism. Plenum Publishing Co., 233 Spring St., New York, NY 10013-1578. Phone: (212) 620-8000. Fax: (212) 463-0742. Annual.

Research Advances in Alcohol and Drug Problems. Plenum Publishing Co., 233 Spring St., New York, NY 10013-1578. Phone: (212) 620-8000. Fax: (212) 463-0742. Irregular.

ASSOCIATIONS, PROFESSIONAL SOCIETIES, ADVOCACY AND SUPPORT GROUPS

Al-Anon Family Group Headquarters. 1372 Broadway, New York, NY 10018-0862. Phone: (212) 245-3151.

Alcoholics Anonymous (AA). General Service Office Board, P.O. Box 459, Grand Central Station, New York, NY 10163. Phone: (212) 686-1100.

American Council on Alcoholism. 8501 LaSalle Rd., Suite 301, Towson, MD 21204.

Co-Dependents Anonymous. P.O. Box 5508, Glendale, AZ 85312-5508.

Narcotics Association for Children of Alcoholics (NACoA). 31582 Coast Highway, Ste. B, South Laguna, CA 92677-3044. Phone: (714) 499-3889.

National Association of Alcoholism and Drug Abuse Counselors (NAADAC). 3717 Columbia Pike, Ste. 300, Arlington, VA 22204. Phone: (800) 548-0497. Fax: (703) 920-4672.

National Council on Alcoholism and Drug Dependence, Inc.. 12 W. 21st St., New York, NY 10010. Phone: (212) 206-6770.

National Council on Alcoholism, Inc.. 12 W. 21st St., New York, NY 10010. Phone: (800) NCA-CALL.

Women for Sobriety. P.O. Box 618, Quakertown, PA 18951. Phone: (215) 536-8026.

BIBLIOGRAPHIES

Addiction Research Foundation Bibliographic Series. Addiction Research Foundation of Ontario, 33 Russell St., Toronto, ON, Canada M5S 2S1. Phone: (416) 595-6123. Irregular.

Bibliography and Research Guide on Alcohol and other Drugs for Social Work Educators. National Clearinghouse for Alcohol and Drug Information, Dept. PP, P.O. Box 2345, Rockville, MD 20852.

Nutri-Topics: Nutrition and Alcohol. Food and Nutrition Center, National Agricultural Library, 10301 Baltimore Blvd., Beltsville, MD 20705.

Substance Abuse Index and Abstracts: A Guide to Alcohol and Tobacco Research. Gregory Austin, William Mishkin. Comvex Scientific Co., 270 Lafayette St, Suite 705, New York, NY 10012. Phone: (212) 334-1922. 5 volumes.

CD-ROM DATABASES

PsycLit. SilverPlatter Information, Inc., River Ridge Office Park, 100 River Ridge Rd., Norwood, MA 02062. Phone: (617) 769-2599. Fax: (617) 769-8763. Quarterly.

SCISEARCH. Institute for Scientific Information, 3501 Market St., Philadelphia, PA 19104. Phone: (215) 386-0100. Fax: (215) 386-6362.

DIRECTORIES

The 100 Best Treatment Centers. Avon Books, 1350 Avenue of the Americas, 2nd Floor, New York, NY 10019. Phone: (800) 238-0658.

Alcohol, Drug Abuse, Mental Health Research Grant Awards. Alcohol, Drug Abuse, and Mental Health Administration,

5600 Fishers Lane, Rockville, MD 20857. Phone: (301) 443-1596.

Drug, Alcohol, and Other Addictions: A Directory of Treatment Centers and Prevention Programs Nationwide. Oryx Press, 4041 N. Central, Suite 700, Phoenix, AZ 85012. Phone: (800) 279-ORYX. Fax: (800) 279-4663.

ENCYCLOPEDIAS, DICTIONARIES, WORD BOOKS

Encyclopedia of Alcoholism. Robert O'Brien, Morris Evans, Glen Chafetz (eds.). Facts on File, Inc., 460 Park Ave. S., New York, NY 10016-7382. Phone: (212) 683-2244. Fax: (212) 683-3633. 1991.

HANDBOOKS, GUIDES, MANUALS, ATLASES

Concise Guide to Treatment of Alcoholism and Addictions. Richard J. Frances, John E. Franklin. American Psychiatric Press, Inc., 1400 K St. NW, Washington, DC 20005. Phone: (202) 682-6268. Fax: (202) 789-2648. 1989.

Drug and Alcohol Abuse: A Clinical Guide to Diagnosis and Treatment. Marc A. Schuckit. Plenum Publishing Co., 233 Spring St., New York, NY 10013-1578. Phone: (212) 620-8000. Fax: (212) 463-0742. Third edition 1989.

A Handbook on Drug and Alcohol Abuse. Gail Winger, Frederick G. Hofman, James H. Woods. Oxford University Press, 200 Madison Ave., New York, NY 10016. Phone: (212) 679-7300. Third edition 1992.

Handbook of Hospital Based Substance Abuse Treatment. William D. Lerner, Marjorie A. Barr. McGraw-Hill, Inc., Health Professions Division, 1221 Avenue of the Americas, 28th Floor, New York, NY 10020. Phone: (212) 512-4228. 1990.

JOURNALS

Alcholism and Addiction. IPG, 4949 Commerce Parkway, Cleveland, OH 44128. Phone: (800) 342-6237.

Alcohol Health and Research World. National Institute on Alcohol Abuse and Alcoholism, P.O. Box 2345, Rockville, MD 20852. Phone: (800) 729-6686.

Alcoholism: Clinical and Experimental Research. Williams & Wilkins, 428 E. Preston St., Baltimore, MD 21202. Phone: (800) 638-0672. Fax: (800) 447-8438. Bimonthly.

Alcoholism Treatment Quarterly. Haworth Press, 10 Alice Street, Binghamton, NY 13904-1580. Phone: (800) 342-9678. Fax: (607) 722-1424. Quarterly.

American Journal on Addictions. American Psychiatric Press, Inc., 1400 K St. NW, Washington, DC 20005. Phone: (202) 682-6268. Fax: (202) 789-2648. Quarterly.

American Journal of Drug and Alcohol Abuse. Marcel Dekker, Inc., 270 Madison Ave., New York, NY 10016. Phone: (800) 228-1160.

Drug and Alcohol Dependence. Elsevier Science Publishing Co., Inc., P.O. Box 882, Madison Square Station, New York, NY 10159-2101. Phone: (212) 989-5800. Fax: (212) 633-3990. 6/year.

Journal of Studies on Alcohol. Rutgers Center of Alcohol Studies, Box 909, Piscataway, NJ 08855. Phone: (201) 932-2190.

Journal of Substance Abuse Treatment. Pergamon Press, 660 White Plains Rd., Tarrytown, NY 10591-5153. Phone: (914) 592-7700. Fax: (914) 592-3625. 6/year.

NEWSLETTERS

Addictions Alert. American Health Consultants, Department C1290, P.O. Box 740060, Atlanta, GA 30374. Phone: (800) 559-1032. Monthly.

Alcohol Issues Insight. Bee Marketer's Insights, Inc., 51 Virginia Ave., West Nyack, NY 10994. Phone: (914) 358-7751.

The Alcoholism Report. Manisses Communications Group, 1511 K St. N.W., Suite 938, Washington, DC 20005. Phone: (202) 737-7342.

ONLINE DATABASES

Druginfo and Alcohol Use and Abuse. University of Minnesota, College of Pharmacy, Drug Information Services, 3-160 Health Sciences Center, Unit F, 308 Harvard St. Se, Minneapolis, MN 55455. Phone: (612) 624-6492. Quarterly.

EMBASE. Elsevier Science Publishing Co., Inc., P.O. Box 882, Madison Square Station, New York, NY 10159-2101. Phone: (212) 989-5800. Fax: (212) 633-3990.

ETOH (Alcohol and Alcohol Programs Science Database). National Institute on Alcohol Abuse and Alcoholism, 1400 Eye St. N.W., Ste. 600, Washington, DC 20005. Phone: (202) 842-7600.

MEDLINE. National Library of Medicine, 8600 Rockville Pike, Bethesda, MD 20894. Phone: (800) 638-8480.

PsycInfo. SilverPlatter Information, Inc., River Ridge Office Park, 100 River Ridge Rd., Norwood, MA 02062. Phone: (617) 769-2599. Fax: (617) 769-8763. Quarterly.

SciSearch. Institute for Scientific Information, 3501 Market St., Philadelphia, PA 19104. Phone: (215) 386-0100. Fax: (215) 386-6362.

POPULAR WORKS AND PATIENT EDUCATION

The 800-Cocaine Book of Drug and Alcohol Recovery. James Cocores. Random House, Inc., 201 E. 50th St., New York, NY 10022. Phone: (800) 726-0600. 1990.

Facts About Drinking. Gail G. Milgram. Consumer Reports Books, 9180 LeSaint Dr., Fairfield, OH 45014. Phone: (513) 860-1178. 1989.

Good News about Drugs and Alcohol: Curing, Treating and Preventing Substance Abuse. Mark S. Gold. Random House, Inc., 201 E. 50th St., New York, NY 10022. Phone: (800) 726-0600. 1991.

I'll Quit Tomorrow: A Practical Guide to Alcoholism Treatment. Vernon E. Johnson. HarperCollins Pubs., Inc., 10 E. 53rd St., New York, NY 10022-5299. Phone: (212) 207-7000. 1990.

True Selves: Twelve-Step Recovery from Codependency. Roseann Lloyd, Merle A. Fossum. HarperCollins Publishers, 10 E. 53rd St., New York, NY 10022-5299. Phone: (800) 242-7737. 1991.

The Twelve Steps of Alcoholics Anonymous. Karen Elliot. HarperCollins Pubs., Inc., 10 E. 53rd St., New York, NY

10022-5299. Phone: (212) 207-7000. Fax: (800) 242-7737. 1987.

RESEARCH CENTERS, INSTITUTES, CLEARINGHOUSES

Alcohol and Drug Abuse Institute. University of Washington. 3937 15th Ave. NE, NL-15, Seattle, WA 98195. Phone: (206) 543-0937. Fax: (206) 543-5473.

Alcohol Research Center. University of Connecticut. Farmington Ave., Farmington, CT 06032. Phone: (203) 679-3423. Fax: (203) 679-1296.

Alcohol Research Center. University of Michigan. 400 E. Eisenhower Pkwy., Suite 4, Ann Arbor, MI 48104. Phone: (313) 763-7952. Fax: (313) 998-7994.

Alcohol Research Group. Institute of Epidemiology and Behavioral Medicine. Medical Research Institute of San Francisco. 200 Hearst Ave., Berkeley, CA 94709. Phone: (415) 642-5208.

Alcoholism and Drug Addiction Research Foundation. 33 Russell St., Toronto, ON, Canada M5S 2S1. Phone: (416) 595-6000. Fax: (416) 979-8133.

Center for Alcohol and Addiction Studies. University of Alaska, Anchorage. 3211 Providence Dr., Anchorage, AK 99508. Phone: (907) 786-1802. Fax: (907) 786-1247.

Center of Alcohol Studies. Rutgers University. Busch Campus, Smithers Hall, Piscataway, NJ 08855-0969. Phone: (908) 932-2190. Fax: (908) 932-5944.

Hazelden Foundation. Box 176, Center City, MN 55012-0176. Phone: (800) 328-9000.

Institute of Alcoholism and Drug Dependency. Andrews University. School of Graduate Studies, Marsh Hall 100-A, Berrien Springs, MI 49104. Phone: (616) 471-3558. Fax: (616) 473-4425.

National Clearinghouse for Alcohol and Drug Information (NCADI). P.O. Box 2345, Rockville, MD 20852. Phone: (301) 468-2600.

Research Institute on Alcoholism. 1021 Main St., Buffalo, NY 14203. Phone: (716) 887-2566.

Target Research Center. P.O. Box 20626, 11724 Plaza Cir., Kansas City, MO 64195. Phone: (816) 464-5400.

STANDARDS AND STATISTICS SOURCES

The Economic Costs of Alcohol and Drug Abuse and Mental Illness: 1985. National Clearinghouse for Alcohol and Drug Information, Dept. PP, P.O. Box 2345, Rockville, MD 20852. 1990, BKD54.

Exposure to Alcoholism in the Family: United States, 1988. National Center for Health Statistics, 6525 Belcrest Rd., Rm. 1064, Hyattsville, MD 20782. Phone: (301) 436-8500. PHS 91-1250 1991.

National Household Survey on Drug Abuse: Highlights, 1988. National Clearinghouse for Alcohol and Drug Information, Dept. PP, P.O. Box 2345, Rockville, MD 20852. 1990, BKD52.

National Household Survey on Drug Abuse: Population Estimates, 1990. National Clearinghouse for Alcohol and Drug Information, Dept. PP, P.O. Box 2345, Rockville, MD 20852. 1991, BKD57.

Third Triennial Report to Congress: Drug Abuse and Alcohol Research. National Clearinghouse for Alcohol and Drug Information, Dept. PP, P.O. Box 2345, Rockville, MD 20852. 1990, BKD47.

TEXTBOOKS AND MONOGRAPHS

Addictive Disorders. Michael F. Fleming, Kristen Lawton Barry (eds.). Mosby-Year Book, 11830 Westline Industrial Drive, St. Louis, MO 63146. Phone: (800) 325-4177. Fax: (314) 432-1380. 1992.

AIDS and Alcohol/Drug Abuse: Psychosocial Research. Dennis G. Fisher (ed.). Haworth Press, 10 Alice Street, Binghamton, NY 13904-1580. Phone: (800) 342-9678. Fax: (607) 722-1424. 1991.

Alcohol, Immunomodulation, and AIDS. Daniel Seminara, Ronald Ross Watson, Albert Pawlowski (eds.). John Wiley & Sons, Inc., 605 Third Ave., New York, NY 10158-0012. Phone: (212) 850-6000. Fax: (212) 850-6088. 1990.

Alcoholism: A Practical Treatment Guide. Stanley Gitlow, Herbert Peyser. W.B. Saunders Co., The Curtis Center, Independence Sqare W., Philadelphia, PA 19106-3399. Phone: (215) 238-7800. 2nd ed., 1988.

Medical Diagnosis and Treatment of Alcoholism. Jack Mendelson, Nancy Mello. McGraw Hill, 11 W. 19th St., New York, NY 10011. Phone: (212) 337-5001. Fax: (212) 337-4092. 1992.

Substance Abuse: A Comprehensive Textbook. Joyce H. Lowinson, and others. Williams & Wilkins, 428 East Preston St., Baltimore, MD 21202. Phone: (800) 638-0672. Fax: (800) 447-8438. 2nd ed., 1992.

ALLERGIES

See also: FOOD ALLERGIES; IMMUNOLOGY

ABSTRACTING, INDEXING, AND CURRENT AWARENESS PUBLICATIONS

Biological Abstracts. BIOSIS, 2100 Arch St., Philadelphia, PA 19103-1399. Phone: (800) 523-4800. Fax: (215) 587-2016.

BIOSIS/CAS Selects: Allergy & Antiallergy. BIOSIS, 2100 Arch St., Philadelphia, PA 19103-1399. Phone: (215) 587-4800. Fax: (215) 587-2016. Biweekly.

CA Selects: Allergy & Antiallergic Agents. Chemical Abstracts Service, 2540 Olentangy River Road, P.O. Box 3012, Columbus, OH 43210-0012. Phone: (800) 848-6538. Biweekly.

Current Contents/Clinical Medicine. Institute for Scientific Information, 3501 Market St., Philadelphia, PA 19104. Phone: (800) 523-1850. Fax: (215) 386-6362. Weekly.

Excerpta Medica. Section 26: Immunology, Serology and Transplantation. Elsevier Science Publishing Co., Inc., P.O. Box 882, Madison Square Station, New York, NY 10159-2101. Phone: (212) 989-5800. Fax: (212) 633-3990. 32/year.

Index Medicus. U.S. National Library of Medicine, 8600 Rockville Pike, Bethesda, MD 20894. Phone: (800) 638-8480. Monthly.

Research Alert: Allergies, Asthma, Clinical Immunology. Institute for Scientific Information, 3501 Market St., Philadelphia, PA 19104. Phone: (800) 523-1850. Fax: (215) 386-6362. Weekly.

Research Alert: Antihistamine Agents. Institute for Scientific Information, 3501 Market St., Philadelphia, PA 19104. Phone: (800) 523-1850. Fax: (215) 386-6362. Weekly.

Science Citation Index. Institute for Scientific Information, 3501 Market St., Philadelphia, PA 19104. Phone: (800) 523-1850. Fax: (215) 386-6362. Bimonthly.

ANNUALS AND REVIEWS

Contemporary Topics in Immunobiology. Plenum Publishing Co., 233 Spring St., New York, NY 10013-1578. Phone: (212) 620-8000. Fax: (212) 463-0742. Irregular.

Immunology and Allergy Clinics. W.B. Saunders Co., The Curtis Center, Independence Square W., Philadelphia, PA 19106-3399. Phone: (215) 238-7800. Quarterly.

ASSOCIATIONS, PROFESSIONAL SOCIETIES, ADVOCACY AND SUPPORT GROUPS

American Academy of Allergy and Immunology. 611 E. Wells St., Milwaukee, WI 53202. Phone: (414) 272-6071. Fax: (414) 276-3349.

American Allergy Association. P.O. Box 7273, Menlo Park, CA 94026. Phone: (415) 322-1663.

American Board of Allergy and Immunology (ABAI). University City Science Ctr., 3624 Market St., Philadelphia, PA 19104. Phone: (215) 349-9466.

American College of Allergy and Immunology (AACIA). 800 E. Northwest Hwy., Ste. 1080, Palatine, IL 60067. Phone: (312) 255-0380.

Asthma and Allergy Foundation of America (AAFA). 1717 Massachusetts Ave., Ste. 305, Washington, DC 20036. Phone: (800) 7AS-THMA. Fax: (202) 462-2412.

CD-ROM DATABASES

Biological Abstracts on Compact Disc. BIOSIS, 2100 Arch St., Philadelphia, PA 19103-1399. Phone: (800) 523-4800. Fax: (215) 587-2016. Quarterly.

Excerpta Medica CD: Immunology & AIDS. SilverPlatter Information, Inc., River Ridge Office Park, 100 River Ridge Rd., Norwood, MA 02062. Phone: (617) 769-2599. Fax: (617) 769-8763. Quarterly.

SCISEARCH. Institute for Scientific Information, 3501 Market St., Philadelphia, PA 19104. Phone: (215) 386-0100. Fax: (215) 386-6362.

DIRECTORIES

American Academy of Allergy & Immunology-Membership Directory. American Academy of Allergy & Immunology, 611 E. Wells St., Milwaukee, WI 53202. Phone: (414) 272-6071. Fax: (414) 276-3349. Biennial.

Directory of Certified Allergists/Immunologists. American Board of Medical Specialties, 1 Rotary Center, Suite 805, Evanston, IL 60201. Phone: (708) 491-9091. Biennial.

HANDBOOKS, GUIDES, MANUALS, ATLASES

Atlas of Allergies. Philip Fireman, Raymond G. Slavin. J.B. Lippincott Co., 227 East Washington Square, Philadelphia, PA 19106-3780. Phone: (215) 238-4200. Fax: (215) 238-4227. 1991.

Color Atlas of Allergic Skin Disorders. Rino Cerio, William F. Jackson. Mosby-Year Book, 11830 Westline Industrial Drive, St. Louis, MO 63146. Phone: (800) 325-4177. Fax: (314) 432-1380. 1992.

A Color Atlas of Allergy. W.F. Jackson. Mosby-Year Book, 11830 Westline Industrial Drive, St. Louis, MO 63146. Phone: (800) 325-4177. Fax: (314) 432-1380. 1988.

Manual of Allergy and Immunology: Diagnosis and Therapy. Gleen J. Lawlor Jr., Thomas J. Fischer. Little, Brown and Co., 34 Beacon St., Boston, MA 02108. Phone: (617) 227-0730. Second edition 1988.

JOURNALS

The American Journal of Asthma & Allergy for Pediatricians. SLACK Inc., 6900 Grove Rd., Thorofare, NJ 08086-9447. Phone: (800) 257-8290. Fax: (609) 853-5991. Quarterly.

Annals of Allergy. American College of Allergy and Immunology, 800 E. Northwest Hwy., Suite 1080, Palatine, IL 60067. Phone: (708) 359-7367.

Clinical and Experimental Allergy. Blackwell Scientific Publications, Inc., 3 Cambridge Center, Cambridge, MA 02142. Phone: (800) 759-6102.

Clinical and Experimental Immunology. Blackwell Scientific Publications Ltd., Osney Mead, Oxon. OX2 OEL, England. Phone: 0865-240201. Fax: 0865-721205. Monthly.

Clinical Reviews in Allergy. Humana Press, Inc., P.O. Box 2148, Clifton, NJ 07015. Phone: (207) 773-4389.

Immunology. Blackwell Scientific Publications, Inc., 3 Cambridge Ctr., Cambridge, MA 02142. Phone: (800) 759-6102. Monthly.

Journal of Allergy and Clinical Immunology. Mosby-Year Book, 11830 Westline Industrial Drive, St. Louis, MO 63146. Phone: (800) 325-4177. Fax: (314) 432-1380. Monthly.

NEWSLETTERS

American Academy of Allergy and Immunology-News and Notes. American Academy of Allergy and Immunology, 611 E. Wells St., Milwaukee, WI 53202. Phone: (414) 272-6071. Quarterly.

ONLINE DATABASES

BIOSIS Previews. BIOSIS, 2100 Arch St., Philadelphia, PA 19103-1399. Phone: (800) 523-4800. Fax: (215) 587-2016.

EMBASE. Elsevier Science Publishing Co., Inc., P.O. Box 882, Madison Square Station, New York, NY 10159-2101. Phone: (212) 989-5800. Fax: (212) 633-3990.

Journal of Allergy and Clinical Immunology. Mosby-Year Book, 11830 Westline Industrial Drive, St. Louis, MO 63146. Phone: (800) 325-4177. Fax: (314) 432-1380.

MEDLINE. National Library of Medicine, 8600 Rockville Pike, Bethesda, MD 20894. Phone: (800) 638-8480.

SciSearch. Institute for Scientific Information, 3501 Market St., Philadelphia, PA 19104. Phone: (215) 386-0100. Fax: (215) 386-6362.

POPULAR WORKS AND PATIENT EDUCATION

Allergies. Edward Edelson. Chelsea House Pubs., 95 Madison Ave., New York, NY 10016. Phone: (212) 683-4400. 1989.

Allergies: Complete Guide to Diagnosis, Treatment, and Daily Management. Stuart Young, Bruce Dobozin, Margaret Miner. Consumer Reports Books, 9180 LeSaint Dr., Fairfield, OH 45014. Phone: (513) 860-1178. 1992.

Allergies: Random House Handbook. P. Dranov. Random House, Inc., 201 E. 50th St., New York, NY 10022. Phone: (800) 726-0600. 1990.

Complete Guide to Food Allergy and Intolerance. Brostoff. Random House, Inc., 201 E. 50th St., New York, NY 10022. Phone: (800) 726-0600. 1992.

Conquering Your Child's Allergies. M. Eric Gershwin, Edwin L. Klingelhofer. Addison-Wesley Nursing, 390 Bridge Parkway, Redwood City, CA 94065. Phone: (800) 950-5544. 1990.

Parents' Guide to Allergies & Asthma. Steinman. Bantam Doubleday Dell, Inc., 666 Fifth Ave., New York, NY 10103. Phone: (800) 223-6834. 1992.

Sneezing Your Head Off? How to Live with Your Allergic Nose. Peter B. Boggs. Simon & Schuster, Inc., 1230 Ave. of the Americas, New York, NY 10020. Phone: (212) 698-7000. 1992.

RESEARCH CENTERS, INSTITUTES, CLEARINGHOUSES

Allergy Disease Research Laboratory. Mayo Clinic and Foundation. 200 First St. SW, Rochester, MN 55905. Phone: (507) 284-2789. Fax: (507) 284-1637.

Allergy & Immunology Center. University of Colorado. Division of Immunology, 4200 E. 9th Ave., CB 164, Denver, CO 80262. Phone: (303) 270-7601.

Asthma and Allergic Center. Johns Hopkins University. 5501 Hopkins Bayview Circle, Baltimore, MD 21224. Phone: (410) 550-2300. Fax: (410) 550-2101.

Asthma & Allergic Disease Center. Brigham and Women's Hospital. 75 Francis St., Boston, MA 02115. Phone: (617) 732-1995. Fax: (617) 732-0979.

Asthma and Allergic Diseases Center. State University of New York Health Science Center at Stony Brook. Stony Brook, NY 11794. Phone: (516) 444-2272. Fax: (516) 444-2493.

Asthma and Allergic Diseases Center. University of Texas Southwestern Medical Center at Dallas.. 5323 Harry Hines Blvd., Dallas, TX 75235. Phone: (214) 688-2969. Fax: (214) 688-8275.

Asthma & Allergic Diseases Center. University of Wisconsin-Madison. 600 Highland Ave., Madison, WI 53792. Phone: (608) 263-6201.

Autoimmune Disease Center. Scripps Clinic and Research Foundation. 10666 N. Torrey Pines Rd., La Jolla, CA 92037. Phone: (619) 554-8686. Fax: (619) 554-6805.

Center for Allergy and Immunological Disorders. Baylor College of Medicine. 1 Baylor Plaza, Houston, TX 77030. Phone: (713) 791-4219.

Max Samter Institute of Allergy and Clinical Immunology. Grant Hospital of Chicago, 550 W. Webster, Chicago, IL 60614. Phone: (312) 883-3655.

National Institute of Allergy and Infectious Diseases. NIH Bldg. 31, Rm. 7A-32, 9000 Rockville Pike, Bethesda, MD 20892. Phone: (301) 496-5717.

National Jewish Center for Immunology and Respiratory Medicine. 1400 Jackson St., Denver, CO 80206. Phone: (303) 388-4461.

STANDARDS AND STATISTICS SOURCES

National Institue of Allergy and Infectious Diseases Profile. National Institute of Allergy and Infectious Diseases, Building 31, Room 7A32, 9000 Rockville Pike, Bethesda, MD 20892. Phone: (301) 496-5717. Annual.

TEXTBOOKS AND MONOGRAPHS

Allergic Diseases from Infancy to Adulthood. Charles Bierman, David Pearlman (eds.). W.B. Saunders Co., The Curtis Center, Independence Sqare W., Philadelphia, PA 19106-3399. Phone: (215) 238-7800. 2nd edition, 1988.

Allergies: Principles and Practice. Elliott Middleton Jr. (ed.). Mosby-Year Book, 11830 Westline Industrial Drive, St. Louis, MO 63146. Phone: (800) 325-4177. Fax: (314) 432-1380. 1988.

Current Therapy in Allergy, Immunology and Rheumatology. Lawrence M. Lichtenstein, Anthony Fauci. Mosby-Year Book, 11830 Westline Industrial Drive, St. Louis, MO 63146. Phone: (800) 325-4177. Fax: (314) 432-1380. Fourth edition 1991.

Fundamentals of Immunolgy and Allergy. Richard F. Lockey. W.B. Saunders Co., The Curtis Center, Independence Square W., Philadelphia, PA 19106-3399. Phone: (215) 238-7800. 1987.

Managing Asthma. Miles Weinberger. Williams & Wilkins, 428 East Preston St., Baltimore, MD 21202. Phone: (800) 638-0672. Fax: (800) 447-8438. 1990.

ALLIED HEALTH EDUCATION

See also: DENTAL ASSISTING; EMERGENCY MEDICINE; OCCUPATIONAL THERAPY; PHYSICAL THERAPY; PHYSICIANS' ASSISTANTS; RESPIRATORY THERAPY

ABSTRACTING, INDEXING, AND CURRENT AWARENESS PUBLICATIONS

Cumulative Index to Nursing and Allied Health Literature. Glendale Adventist Medical Center, P.O. Box 871, Glendale, CA 91209. Phone: (818) 409-8005. Bimonthly.

International Nursing Index. American Journal of Nursing Co., 555 W. 57th St., New York, NY 10019. Phone: (212) 582-8820. Quarterly.

Science Citation Index. Institute for Scientific Information, 3501 Market St., Philadelphia, PA 19104. Phone: (800) 523-1850. Fax: (215) 386-6362. Bimonthly.

ASSOCIATIONS, PROFESSIONAL SOCIETIES, ADVOCACY AND SUPPORT GROUPS

American Association of Medical Assistants (AAMA). 20 N. Wacker Dr., Ste. 1575, Chicago, IL 60606. Phone: (312) 899-1500.

American Society of Allied Health Professions. 1101 Connecticut Ave. N.W., Washington, DC 20036. Phone: (202) 857-1150.

American Society for Health Care Education and Training. 840 N. Lake Shore Dr., Chicago, IL 60611. Phone: (312) 280-6113.

Committee on Allied Health Education and Accreditation. 515 N. Dearborn St., Chicago, IL 60610. Phone: (312) 464-4660.

BIBLIOGRAPHIES

Core Collection in Nursing and the Allied Health Sciences: Books, Journal, Media. Oryx Press, 4041 N. Central, Suite 700, Phoenix, AZ 85012. Phone: (800) 279-ORYX. Fax: (800) 279-4663. 1990.

CD-ROM DATABASES

CD Plus/CINAHL. CD Plus, 333 7th Ave., 6th Floor, New York, NY 10001. Phone: (212) 563-3006. Monthly.

Nursing and Allied Health (CINAHL-CD) on Compact Cambridge. Cambridge Scientific Abstracts, 7200 Wisconsin Ave., Bethesda, MD 20814-4823. Phone: (800) 843-7751. Fax: (301) 961-6720. Monthly.

Nursing and Allied Health (CINAHL) on CD-ROM. CINAHL, 1509 Wilson Terrace, P.O. Box 871, Glendale, CA 91209-0871. Phone: (818) 409-8005.

Nursing and Allied Health (CINAHL-CD) on SilverPlatter. SilverPlatter Information, Inc., River Ridge Office Park, 100 River Ridge Rd., Norwood, MA 02062. Phone: (617) 769-2599. Fax: (617) 769-8763. Bimonthly.

SCISEARCH. Institute for Scientific Information, 3501 Market St., Philadelphia, PA 19104. Phone: (215) 386-0100. Fax: (215) 386-6362.

DIRECTORIES

Allied Health Education Directory. American Medical Association, 515 North State St., Chicago, IL 60610. Phone: (312) 464-0183. Fax: (312) 464-5834. Annual.

ENCYCLOPEDIAS, DICTIONARIES, WORD BOOKS

Mosby's Medical, Nursing, and Allied Health Dictionary. Kenneth N. Anderson, Lois Anderson, Walter D. Glanze (eds.). Mosby-Year Book, 11830 Westline Industrial Dr., St. Louis, MO 63146. Phone: (800) 325-4177. Fax: (314) 432-1380. Third edition 1990.

JOURNALS

Journal of Allied Health. Office of Publications Services, University of Illinois at Chicago, Box 4348, Chicago, IL 60680. Phone: (312) 996-6697. Quarterly.

Journal of the American Academy of Physician Assistants. Mosby-Year Book, 11830 Westline Industrial Drive, St. Louis,

MO 63146. Phone: (800) 325-4177. Fax: (314) 432-1380. 10/year.

NEWSLETTERS

Allied Health Education Newsletter. American Medical Association, 515 North State St., Chicago, IL 60610. Phone: (312) 464-0183. Fax: (312) 464-5834. Bimonthly.

ONLINE DATABASES

Combined Health Information Database (CHID). U.S. National Institutes of Health, P.O. Box NDIC, Bethesda, MD 20892. Phone: (301) 496-2162. Fax: (301) 770-5164. Quarterly.

Nursing and Allied Health (CINAHL). CINAHL, 1509 Wilson Terrace, P.O. Box 871, Glendale, CA 91209-0871. Phone: (818) 409-8005.

TEXTBOOKS AND MONOGRAPHS

Allied Health Education: Concepts, Organization, and Administration. Norman E. Farber, Edmund J. McTernan, Robert O. Hawkins. Charles C. Thomas, Publisher, 2600 S. First St., Springfield, IL 62794-9265. Phone: (800) 258-8900. 1989.

Twenty-Eight Allied Health Careers. American Medical Association, 515 North State St., Chicago, IL 60610. Phone: (312) 464-0183. Fax: (312) 464-5834. 1991.

ALS

See: AMYOTROPHIC LATERAL SCLEROSIS

ALTERNATIVE MEDICINE

See also: ACUPUNCTURE; BIOFEEDBACK; CHIROPRACTIC; HERBAL MEDICINE; HOLISTIC MEDICINE; HOMEOPATHY

ABSTRACTING, INDEXING, AND CURRENT AWARENESS PUBLICATIONS

Complementary Medicine Index. Medical Information Service, British Library, Boston Spa, Wetherby, W. Yorkshire LS23 7BQ, England. Phone: 0937-546039. Fax: 0937-546236. Monthly.

Consumer Health and Nutrition Index. Alan Rees. Oryx Press, 4041 N. Central, Suite 700, Phoenix, AZ 85012. Phone: (800) 279-6799. Fax: (800) 279-4663. Quarterly.

Index to Chiropractic Literature. Chiropractic Library Consortium, Western States Chiropractic College, 2900 N.E. 132nd Ave., Portland, OR 97230. Phone: (503) 256-3180. Annual.

Index Medicus. U.S. National Library of Medicine, 8600 Rockville Pike, Bethesda, MD 20894. Phone: (800) 638-8480. Monthly.

Science Citation Index. Institute for Scientific Information, 3501 Market St., Philadelphia, PA 19104. Phone: (800) 523-1850. Fax: (215) 386-6362. Bimonthly.

ASSOCIATIONS, PROFESSIONAL SOCIETIES, ADVOCACY AND SUPPORT GROUPS

Alternative Medical Association (AMA). 7909 S.E. Stark St., Portland, OR 97215. Phone: (503) 254-7555.

American Association of Naturopathic Physicians. P.O. Box 20386, Seattle, WA 98102. Phone: (206) 323-7610.

The American Botanical Council. P.O. Box 201660, Austin, TX 78720.

American Institute of Homeopathy. 1500 Massachusetts Ave., Suite 41, Washington, DC 20005. Phone: (202) 223-6182.

National Council Against Health Fraud. P.O. Box 1276, Loma Linda, CA 92354. Phone: (714) 824-4690.

BIBLIOGRAPHIES

Core Collection in Chiropractic for Health Sciences Libraries. Medical Library Association, 6 N. Michigan Ave., No. 300, Chicago, IL 60602. Phone: (312) 419-9094. Fax: (312) 419-8950. 1991.

The Guide to the American Medical Association Historical Health Fraud and Alternative Medicine Collection. American Medical Association, 515 North State St., Chicago, IL 60610. Phone: (312) 464-0183. Fax: (312) 464-5834. 1992.

Reader's Guide to Alternative Health Methods. American Medical Association, 515 N. State St., Chicago, IL 60610. Phone: (800) 621-8335. 1992.

CD-ROM DATABASES

SCISEARCH. Institute for Scientific Information, 3501 Market St., Philadelphia, PA 19104. Phone: (215) 386-0100. Fax: (215) 386-6362.

DIRECTORIES

Third Opinion: An International Directory to Alternative Therapy Centers. Avery Publishing Group, Inc., 120 Old Broadway, Garden City Park, NY 11040. Phone: (800) 548-5757. 2nd edition.

ENCYCLOPEDIAS, DICTIONARIES, WORD BOOKS

The Illustrated Dictionary of Natural Health. Nevill Drury, Susan Drury (eds.). Borgo Press, P.O. Box 2845, San Bernardino, CA 92406-2845. Phone: (909) 884-5813. Fax: (909) 888-4942. 1989.

HANDBOOKS, GUIDES, MANUALS, ATLASES

Handbook of Complementary Medicine. S. Fulder. Oxford University Press, 200 Madison Ave., New York, NY 10016. Phone: (212) 679-7300. 2nd edition 1988.

JOURNALS

Alternative Medicine. V.S.P. International Science Publishers, P.O. Box 346, 3700 AH, Zeist, Netherlands. Phone: 03404-51902. Fax: 03404-58620. Quarterly.

American Chiropractor. American Chiropractor Magazine, Inc., 3401 Lake Ave., Fort Wayne, IN 46805. Monthly.

American Journal of Acupuncture. American Journal of Acupuncture, 1840 41st Ave., Suite 102, P.O. Box 610, Capitola, CA 95010. Phone: (408) 475-1700. Quarterly.

American Journal of Chinese Medicine. American Journal of Chinese Medicine, P.O. Box 555, Garden City, NY 11530.

American Journal of Chiropractic Medicine. Mountain Spring Press, 24W 760 Geneva Rd., Carol Stream, IL 60188.

East West: The Journal of Natural Health and Living. East West Journal, Inc., 17 Station St., P.O. Box 1200, Brookline, MA 02146. Monthly.

Homeopathy. British Homeopathic Association, 27a Devonshire St., London W1N 1RJ, England. Bimonthly.

NEWSLETTERS

Acupuncture News. The Center for Chinese Medicine, 5266 E. Pomona Blvd., Los Angeles, CA 90022. Phone: (213) 721-0774. 6/year.

Alternatives. Mountain Home Publishing, P.O.Box 829, Ingram, TX 78025. Phone: (800) 527-3044. Monthly.

Edward Bach Healing Society-Newsletter. Edward Bach Healing Society, 644 Merrick Rd., Lynbrook, NY 11563-2332. Phone: (516) 825-1677. 4/year.

Holistic Medicine. American Holistic Medical Association, 4101 Lake Boone Trail, Ste. 201, Raleigh, NC 27607. Phone: (919) 787-5146. Fax: (919) 787-4916. Bimonthly.

Homeopathy Today. National Center for Homeopathy, 1500 Massachusetts Ave. N.W., No. 41, Washington, DC 20005. Phone: (202) 223-6182. Monthly.

ONLINE DATABASES

EMBASE. Elsevier Science Publishing Co., Inc., P.O. Box 882, Madison Square Station, New York, NY 10159-2101. Phone: (212) 989-5800. Fax: (212) 633-3990.

MEDLINE. National Library of Medicine, 8600 Rockville Pike, Bethesda, MD 20894. Phone: (800) 638-8480.

SciSearch. Institute for Scientific Information, 3501 Market St., Philadelphia, PA 19104. Phone: (215) 386-0100. Fax: (215) 386-6362.

POPULAR WORKS AND PATIENT EDUCATION

Alternatives in Healing. Simon Mills, Steven Finando. Penguin USA, 375 Hudson St., New York, NY 10014-3657. Phone: (800) 331-4624.

A Consumer's Guide to Alternative Medicine. Kurt Butler, Lynn Raynes. Prometheus Books, 700E. Amherst St., Buffalo, NY 14215. Phone: (800) 421-0351. 1992.

Doctor's Book of Home Remedies. Prevention Magazine Staff. Rodale Press, Inc., 33 E. Minor St., Emmaus, PA 18098. Phone: (800) 527-8200. Fax: (215) 967-6263. 1990.

The Encyclopedia of Alternative Health Care. Kristin G. Olsen. Simon & Schuster, Inc., 1230 Ave. of the Americas, New York, NY 10020. Phone: (212) 698-7000. 1990.

Healing Herbs. Michael Castleman. St. Martin's Press, 175 Fifth Ave., New York, NY 10010. Phone: (212) 674-5151. 1991.

The Natural Healing and Nutrition Annual. Mark Bricklin, Sharon Stocker (eds.). Rodale Press, Inc., 33 E. Minor St., Emmaus, PA 18098. Phone: (800) 527-8200. Fax: (215) 967-6263. Annual.

Natural Health, Natural Medicine: A Comprehensive Manual for Wellness & Self Care. Weil. Houghton Mifflin Co., 1 Beacon St., Boston, MA 02108. Phone: (800) 225-3362. 1991.

The Nutrition Desk Reference. Robert H. Garrison. Keats Publishing, Inc., P.O. Box 876, New Canaan, CT 06840. Phone: (203) 966-8721. Revised edition 1990.

Options: The Alternative Cancer Therapy Book. Richard Walters. Avery Publishing Group, Inc., 120 Old Broadway, Garden City Park, NY 11040. Phone: (800) 548-5757. 1992.

What Your Doctor Won't Tell You. Jane Heimlich. HarperCollins Publishers., Inc., 10 E. 53rd St., New York, NY 10022-5299. Phone: (212) 207-7000. Fax: (800) 242-7737. 1990.

RESEARCH CENTERS, INSTITUTES, CLEARINGHOUSES

Office for the Study of Alternative Medical Practices. National Institutes of Health, Building 31, Room B1C-35, 9000 Rockville Pike, Bethesda, MD 20892. Phone: (301) 496-4143.

ALZHEIMER'S DISEASE

See also: DEMENTIA

ABSTRACTING, INDEXING, AND CURRENT AWARENESS PUBLICATIONS

Alzheimer's Disease: Abstracts of the Psychological and Behavioral Literature. American Psychological Association, 1200 17th St. NW, Washington, DC 20036. Phone: (202) 955-7600. 1992.

BIOSIS/CAS Selects: Alzheimer's Disease & Senile Dementias. BIOSIS, 2100 Arch St., Philadelphia, PA 19103-1399. Phone: (215) 587-4800. Fax: (215) 587-2016. Biweekly.

CA Selects: Alzheimer's Disease & Related Memory Dysfunctions. Chemical Abstracts Service, 2540 Olentangy River Road, P.O. Box 3012, Columbus, OH 43210-0012. Phone: (800) 848-6538. Biweekly.

Current Contents/Clinical Medicine. Institute for Scientific Information, 3501 Market St., Philadelphia, PA 19104. Phone: (800) 523-1850. Fax: (215) 386-6362. Weekly.

Excerpta Medica. Section 25: Hematology. Elsevier Science Publishers, P.O. Box 882, Madison Square Station, New York, NY 10159-2101. Phone: (212) 633-3950. Fax: (212) 633-3990. 24/year.

Index Medicus. U.S. National Library of Medicine, 8600 Rockville Pike, Bethesda, MD 20894. Phone: (800) 638-8480. Monthly.

Research Alert: Alzheimer's Disease. Institute for Scientific Information, 3501 Market St., Philadelphia, PA 19104. Phone: (800) 523-1850. Fax: (215) 386-6362. Weekly.

Science Citation Index. Institute for Scientific Information, 3501 Market St., Philadelphia, PA 19104. Phone: (800) 523-1850. Fax: (215) 386-6362. Bimonthly.

ANNUALS AND REVIEWS

Alzheimer's Disease. Richard J. Wurtman, Suzanne Growdon, John H. Corkin, et. al.. Raven Press, 1185 Avenue of the Americas, New York, NY 10036. Phone: (212) 930-9500. Fax: (212) 869-3495. Advances in Neurology. Volume 51. 1990.

Research and Perspectives in Alzheimer's Disease. Springer-Verlag New York Inc., 175 Fifth Ave., New York, NY 10010. Phone: (212) 460-1500. Fax: (212) 473-6272. Irregular.

ASSOCIATIONS, PROFESSIONAL SOCIETIES, ADVOCACY AND SUPPORT GROUPS

Alzheimer's Association. 70 E. Lake St., Ste. 600, Chicago, IL 60601. Phone: (312) 853-3060. Fax: (312) 853-3660.

Alzheimer's Disease International. 70 E. Lake St., Ste. 600, Chicago, IL 60601. Phone: (312) 853-3060.

Alzheimer's Disease and Related Disorders Association. 70 E. Lake St., Ste. 600, Chicago, IL 60601-5997. Phone: (800) 621-0379. 800-572-6037 in IL.

BIBLIOGRAPHIES

Alzheimer's Disease: Diagnostic Tests and Drug Therapy Developments. National Technical Information Service, 5285 Port Royal Rd., Springfield, VA 22161. Phone: (703) 487-4650. Fax: (703) 321-8547. Jan. 1985-Mar. 1989 PB89-858625/CBY.

Caring and Sharing: A Catalog of Training Materials from Alzheimer's Disease Centers. Alzheimer's Disease Education and Referral Center, P.O. Box 8250, Silver Spring, MD 20907. Phone: (301) 495-3311. 1992.

CD-ROM DATABASES

Excerpta Medica CD: Neurosciences. SilverPlatter Information, Inc., River Ridge Office Park, 100 River Ridge Rd., Norwood, MA 02062. Phone: (617) 769-2599. Fax: (617) 769-8763. Quarterly.

Morbidity Mortality Weekly Report. MEP, 124 Mt. Auburn St., Cambridge, MA 02138. Phone: (800) 342-1338. Fax: (617) 868-7738. Annual.

SCISEARCH. Institute for Scientific Information, 3501 Market St., Philadelphia, PA 19104. Phone: (215) 386-0100. Fax: (215) 386-6362.

JOURNALS

Alzheimer's Disease and Associated Disorders - An International Journal. Raven Press, 1185 Avenue of the Americas, New York, NY 10036. Phone: (212) 930-9500. Fax: (212) 869-3495. Quarterly.

Dementia. S. Karger Publishers, Inc., 26 West Avon Rd., P.O. Box 529, Farmington, CT 06085. Phone: (203) 675-7834. Fax: (203) 675-7302. Bimonthly.

Morbidity and Mortality Weekly Report. Massachusetts Medical Society, 1440 Main St., Waltham, MA 02154-1649. Phone: (617) 893-3800. Fax: (617) 893-0413. Weekly.

NEWSLETTERS

Alzheimer's Association Newsletter. Alzheimer's Association, 70 W. Lake St., Ste. 600, Chicago, IL 60601-5997. Phone: (800) 621-0379. Quarterly.

The Caregiver. Duke Aging Center Alzheimer's Program, P.O. Box 3600, Duke Medical Center, Durham, NC 27710. Phone: (800) 672-4213. Quarterly.

ONLINE DATABASES

Combined Health Information Database (CHID). U.S. National Institutes of Health, P.O. Box NDIC, Bethesda, MD 20892. Phone: (301) 496-2162. Fax: (301) 770-5164. Quarterly.

EMBASE. Elsevier Science Publishing Co., Inc., P.O. Box 882, Madison Square Station, New York, NY 10159-2101. Phone: (212) 989-5800. Fax: (212) 633-3990.

MEDLINE. National Library of Medicine, 8600 Rockville Pike, Bethesda, MD 20894. Phone: (800) 638-8480.

SciSearch. Institute for Scientific Information, 3501 Market St., Philadelphia, PA 19104. Phone: (215) 386-0100. Fax: (215) 386-6362.

POPULAR WORKS AND PATIENT EDUCATION

The 36 Hour Day: A Family Guide to Caring for Persons with Alzheimer's Disease, Related Dementing Illnesses, and Memory Loss in Later Life. Nancy L. Mace, Peter V. Rabins. Johns Hopkins University Press, 701 W. 40th St., Suite 275, Baltimore, MD 21211-2190. Phone: (800) 537-5487. Second edition 1991.

Alzheimer's: A Caregiver's Guide and Sourcebook. Howard Gruetzner. John Wiley & Sons, Inc., 605 Third Ave., New York, NY 10158-0012. Phone: (212) 850-6000. Fax: (212) 850-6088. 1988.

Caring for the Alzheimer Patient: A Practical Guide. Raye L. Dippel, J. Thomas Hutton (eds.). Prometheus Books, 700 E. Amherst St., Buffalo, NY 14215. Phone: (800) 421-0351. 1991.

Confused Minds, Burdened Families: Finding Help for People with ALzheimer's and Other Dementias. U.S. Congress Office of Technology Assessment. U.S. Government Printing Office, Superintendent of Documents, P.O. Box 371954, Pittsburgh, PA 15250-7954. Phone: (202) 783-3238. Fax: (202) 512-2250. 1990.

A Consumer's Guide to Aging. David H. Solomon, Elyse Salend, Anna Nolen Rahman, and others. Johns Hopkins University Press, 701 W. 40th St., Suite 275, Baltimore, MD 21211-2190. Phone: (800) 537-5487. 1992.

Life with Charlie: Coping with an Alzheimer's Spouse or a Dementia Patient and Keeping Your Sanity. Carol Heckman-Owen. Borgo Press, P.O. Box 2845, San Bernardino, CA 92406-2845. Phone: (909) 884-5813. Fax: (909) 888-4942. 1992.

Taking Care of Caregivers: For Families and Others Who Care for People with Alzheimer's Disease and Other Forms of Dementia. D. Jeanne Roberts. Bull Publishing Co., 110 Gilbert Ave., Menlo Park, CA 94025. Phone: (800) 676-2855. 1991.

When I Grow Too Old to Dream: Coping with Alzheimer's Disease. Gerry Naughtin, Terry Laidler. Borgo Press, P.O. Box 2845, San Bernardino, CA 92406-2845. Phone: (909) 884-5813. Fax: (909) 888-4942. 1991.

When Your Loved One Has Alzheimer's: A Caregiver's Guide Based on Methods Developed by the Brookdale Center for Aging. David L. Carroll. HarperCollins Pubs., Inc., 10 E. 53rd St.,

New York, NY 10022-5299. Phone: (212) 207-7000. Fax: (800) 242-7737. 1990.

RESEARCH CENTERS, INSTITUTES, CLEARINGHOUSES

Alzheimer's Disease Center. University of Texas Southwestern Medical Center at Dallas. Dept. of Psychiatry, 5323 Harry Hines Blvd., Dallas, TX 75235-9070. Phone: (214) 688-3353. Fax: (214) 688-2405.

Alzheimer's Disease Education and Referral Center. P.O. Box 8250, Silver Spring, MD 20907. Phone: (800) 438-4380. Fax: (301) 587-4352.

Alzheimer's Disease Research Center. Mount Sinai School of Medicine of City University of New York. 1 Gustave Levy Pl., Box 1230, New York, NY 10029. Phone: (212) 241-6623. Fax: (212) 369-2344.

Alzheimer's Disease Research Center. University of California, San Diego. UCSD Medical Center, 225 Dickinson St., 8204, San Diego, CA 92103. Phone: (619) 543-5306. Fax: (619) 543-2489.

Benjamin B. Green-Field National Alzheimer's Library and Resource Center. 919 N. Michigan Ave., Ste. 1000, Chicago, IL 60611-1676. Phone: (312) 335-9602.

Center for Senility Studies, Alzheimer's Disease Treatment Research. 161 N. Dithridge St., Pittsburgh, PA 15213. Phone: (412) 683-7111.

Ethel Percy Andrus Gerontology Center. University of Southern California. University Park, MC 0191, Los Angeles, CA 90089-0191. Phone: (213) 740-6060. Fax: (213) 740-8241.

Massachusetts Alzheimer's Disease Research Center. Massachusetts General Hospital, ACC, Ste. 850, Parkman St., Boston, MA 02114. Phone: (617) 726-1728.

McGill Centre for Studies in Aging. 1650 Cedar Ave., Montreal, PQ, Canada H3Q 1A4. Phone: (514) 934-8096. Fax: (514) 937-9875.

Sanders-Brown Center on Aging. University of Kentucky. 101 Sanders-Brown Bldg., Lexington, KY 40536. Phone: (606) 233-6040. Fax: (606) 258-2866.

TEXTBOOKS AND MONOGRAPHS

Alzheimer's Disease. Carly Hellen. Butterworth-Heinemann, 80 Montvale Ave., Stoneham, MA 02180. Phone: (617) 438-8464. Fax: (617) 279-4851. 1992.

Alzheimer's Disease: Basic Mechanics, Diagnosis and Therapeutic Strategies - 1990. K. Iqbal, D.R.C. McLachlan, B. Winnblad, H.M Wisniewski. John Wiley & Sons, Inc., 605 Third Ave., New York, NY 10158-0012. Phone: (212) 850-6000. Fax: (212) 850-6088. 1991.

Alzheimer's Disease: Long Term Care. J. Edward Jackson, Robert Katzman, Phyllis Lessin (eds.). San Diego State University Press, 5189 College Ave., San Diego, CA 92182. Phone: (619) 594-6220. 1991.

Alzheimer's and Parkinson's Diseases: Recent Advances in Research and Clinical Management. H.J. Altman, B.N. Altman (eds.). Plenum Publishing Co., 233 Spring St., New York, NY 10013-1578. Phone: (212) 620-800. Fax: (212) 463-0742. 1990.

Dementia and Aging: Ethics, Values and Policy Choices. Robert H. Binstock, Stephen G. Post, Peter J. Whitehouse. Johns Hopkins University Press, 701 W. 40th St., Suite 275, Baltimore, MD 21211-2190. Phone: (800) 537-5487. Fax: (410) 516-6998. 1992.

AMBLYOPIA

See: VISION DISORDERS

AMBULATORY CARE

ABSTRACTING, INDEXING, AND CURRENT AWARENESS PUBLICATIONS

Cumulative Index to Nursing and Allied Health Literature. Glendale Adventist Medical Center, P.O. Box 871, Glendale, CA 91209. Phone: (818) 409-8005. Bimonthly.

Hospital Literature Index. American Hospital Association, 840 N. Lake Shore Dr., Chicago, IL 60611. Phone: (800) 242-2626. Fax: (312) 280-6015. Quarterly.

Index Medicus. U.S. National Library of Medicine, 8600 Rockville Pike, Bethesda, MD 20894. Phone: (800) 638-8480. Monthly.

International Nursing Index. American Journal of Nursing Co., 555 W. 57th St., New York, NY 10019. Phone: (212) 582-8820. Quarterly.

Science Citation Index. Institute for Scientific Information, 3501 Market St., Philadelphia, PA 19104. Phone: (800) 523-1850. Fax: (215) 386-6362. Bimonthly.

ASSOCIATIONS, PROFESSIONAL SOCIETIES, ADVOCACY AND SUPPORT GROUPS

Accreditation Association for Ambulatory Health Care (AAAHC). 9933 Lawler Ave., Skokie, IL 60077-3702. Phone: (708) 676-9610. Fax: (708) 676-9628.

Division of Ambulatory Care and Health Promotion (DACHP). American Hospital Association, 840 N. Lake Shore Dr., Chicago, IL 60611. Phone: (312) 280-6461. Fax: (312) 280-5979.

National Association for Ambulatory Care (NAFAC). 21 Michigan St., Grand Rapids, MI 49503. Phone: (616) 949-2138.

CD-ROM DATABASES

Nursing and Allied Health (CINAHL) on CD-ROM. CINAHL, 1509 Wilson Terrace, P.O. Box 871, Glendale, CA 91209-0871. Phone: (818) 409-8005.

SCISEARCH. Institute for Scientific Information, 3501 Market St., Philadelphia, PA 19104. Phone: (215) 386-0100. Fax: (215) 386-6362.

HANDBOOKS, GUIDES, MANUALS, ATLASES

Ambulatory Medicine: Primary Care of Families. Schwiebert. Appleton & Lange, 25 Van Zant St., East Norwalk, CT 06855. Phone: (800) 423-1359. Fax: (203) 854-9486. 1992.

Manual of Clinical Problems in Adult Ambulatory Care: With Annotated Key References. Laurie Dornbrand, Axalla J. Hoole, C. Glenn Pickard, Jr.. Little, Brown and Company, 34 Beacon St., Boston, MA 02108. Phone: (617) 227-0730. Second edition 1992.

NEWSLETTERS

Same-Day Surgery. American Health Consultants, Department C1290, P.O. Box 740060, Atlanta, GA 30374. Phone: (800) 559-1032. Fax: (404) 352-1971. Monthly.

ONLINE DATABASES

EMBASE. Elsevier Science Publishing Co., Inc., P.O. Box 882, Madison Square Station, New York, NY 10159-2101. Phone: (212) 989-5800. Fax: (212) 633-3990.

MEDLINE. National Library of Medicine, 8600 Rockville Pike, Bethesda, MD 20894. Phone: (800) 638-8480.

Nursing and Allied Health (CINAHL). CINAHL, 1509 Wilson Terrace, P.O. Box 871, Glendale, CA 91209-0871. Phone: (818) 409-8005.

SciSearch. Institute for Scientific Information, 3501 Market St., Philadelphia, PA 19104. Phone: (215) 386-0100. Fax: (215) 386-6362.

RESEARCH CENTERS, INSTITUTES, CLEARINGHOUSES

National Clearinghouse for Primary Care Information (NCPCI). 8201 Greensboro Dr., Ste. 600, Mc Lean, VA 22102. Phone: (703) 821-8955.

STANDARDS AND STATISTICS SOURCES

The National Ambulatory Medical Care Complement Survey: United States, 1980. National Center for Health Statistics. U.S. Government Printing Office, Superintendent of Documents, P.O. Box 371954, Pittsburgh, PA 15250-7954. Phone: (202) 783-3238. Fax: (202) 512-2250.

National Ambulatory Medical Care Survey: 1989 Summary. National Center for Health Statistics, 6525 Belcrest Rd., Rm. 1064, Hyattsville, MD 20782. Phone: (301) 436-8500. PHS 91-1250. 1991.

National Ambulatory Medical Care Survey: 1990 Summary. National Center for Health Statistics. U.S. Government Printing Office, Superintendent of Documents, P.O. Box 371954, Pittsburgh, PA 15250-7954. Phone: (202) 783-3238. Fax: (202) 512-2250.

The National Ambulatory Medical Care Survey, United States, 1975-81 and 1985 Trends. National Center for Health Statistics. U.S. Government Printing Office, Superintendent of Documents, P.O. Box 371954, Pittsburgh, PA 15250-7954. Phone: (202) 783-3238. Fax: (202) 512-2250.

Patterns of Ambulatory Care in General and Family Practice: The National Ambulatory Medical Care Survey, United States. National Center for Health Statistics. U.S. Government Printing Office, Superintendent of Documents, P.O. Box 371954, Pittsburgh, PA 15250-7954. Phone: (202) 783-3238. Fax: (202) 512-2250.

Patterns of Ambulatory Care in Internal Medicine: National Ambulatory Medical Care Survey, United States, January 1980-

81. National Center for Health Statistics. U.S. Government Printing Office, Superintendent of Documents, P.O. Box 371954, Pittsburgh, PA 15250-7954. Phone: (202) 783-3238. Fax: (202) 512-2250.

Patterns of Ambulatory Care in Obstetrics and Gynecology: The National Ambulatory Medical Care Survey, United States, January 1980. National Center for Health Statistics. U.S. Government Printing Office, Superintendent of Documents, P.O. Box 371954, Pittsburgh, PA 15250-7954. Phone: (202) 783-3238. Fax: (202) 512-2250.

Patterns of Ambulatory Care in Office Visits to General Surgeons: The National Ambulatory Medical Care Survey, United States. National Center for Health Statistics. U.S. Government Printing Office, Superintendent of Documents, P.O. Box 371954, Pittsburgh, PA 15250-7954. Phone: (202) 783-3238. Fax: (202) 512-2250.

Patterns of Ambulatory Care in Pediatrics: The National Ambulatory Medical Care Survey, United States, January 1980-December 1981. National Center for Health Statistics. U.S. Government Printing Office, Superintendent of Documents, P.O. Box 371954, Pittsburgh, PA 15250-7954. Phone: (202) 783-3238. Fax: (202) 512-2250.

TEXTBOOKS AND MONOGRAPHS

Ambulatory Pediatric Care. Dershewitz. J.B. Lippincott Co., 227 E. Washington Square, Philadelphia, PA 19106-3780. Phone: (215) 238-4200. Fax: (215) 238-4227. Second edition 1992.

Anesthesia for Ambulatory Surgery. Bernard Wetchler. J.B. Lippincott Co., 227 E. Washington Square, Philadelphia, PA 19106-3780. Phone: (215) 238-4200. Fax: (215) 238-4227. 2nd edition, 1991.

Current Surgical Diagnosis and Treatment. L.W. Way. Appleton & Lange, 25 Van Zant St., East Norwalk, CT 06855. Phone: (800) 423-1359. Fax: (203) 854-9486. Ninth edition 1990.

Excellence in Ambulatory Care: A Practical Guide to Developing Effective Quality Assurance Programs. Dale S. Benson Jr., Peyton G. Townes. Jossey-Bass, Inc., 350 Sansome St., San Francisco, CA 94104. Phone: (415) 433-1740. 1990.

Practical Strategies in Outpatient Medicine. Brendon Reilly. W.B. Saunders Co., The Curtis Center, Independence Sqare W., Philadelphia, PA 19106-3399. Phone: (215) 238-7800. 2nd edition, 1991.

AMBULATORY SURGERY

See: AMBULATORY CARE

AMENORRHEA

See: MENSTRUATION

AMNIOCENTESIS

See: PRENATAL TESTING

AMPHETAMINES

See: DRUGS

AMYOTROPHIC LATERAL SCLEROSIS

See also: NEUROMUSCULAR DISORDERS

ABSTRACTING, INDEXING, AND CURRENT AWARENESS PUBLICATIONS

Current Contents/Clinical Medicine. Institute for Scientific Information, 3501 Market St., Philadelphia, PA 19104. Phone: (800) 523-1850. Fax: (215) 386-6362. Weekly.

Excerpta Medica. Section 8: Neurology and Neurosurgery. Elsevier Science Publishers, P.O. Box 882, Madison Square Station, New York, NY 10159-2101. Phone: (212) 633-3950. Fax: (212) 633-3990. 32/year.

Science Citation Index. Institute for Scientific Information, 3501 Market St., Philadelphia, PA 19104. Phone: (800) 523-1850. Fax: (215) 386-6362. Bimonthly.

ANNUALS AND REVIEWS

Amyotrophic Lateral Sclerosis (and other Motor Neuron Diseases). Lewis P. Rowland. Raven Press, 1185 Avenue of the Americas, New York, NY 10036. Phone: (212) 930-9500. Fax: (212) 869-3495. Advances in Neurology. volume 56. 1991.

ASSOCIATIONS, PROFESSIONAL SOCIETIES, ADVOCACY AND SUPPORT GROUPS

ALS and Neuromuscular Research Foundation (ALSNRF). Pacific Presbyterian Medical Ctr., 2351 Clay St., No. 416, San Francisco, CA 94115. Phone: (415) 923-3604.

Amyotrophic Lateral Sclerosis Association (ALSA). 21021 Ventura Blvd., Ste. 321, Woodland Hills, CA 91364. Phone: (818) 340-7500. Fax: (818) 340-2060.

CD-ROM DATABASES

SCISEARCH. Institute for Scientific Information, 3501 Market St., Philadelphia, PA 19104. Phone: (215) 386-0100. Fax: (215) 386-6362.

NEWSLETTERS

Link. Amyotrophic Lateral Sclerosis Association, 21021 Ventura Blvd., Ste. 321, Woodland Hills, CA 91364. Phone: (818) 340-7500. Fax: (818) 340-2060.

ONLINE DATABASES

EMBASE. Elsevier Science Publishing Co., Inc., P.O. Box 882, Madison Square Station, New York, NY 10159-2101. Phone: (212) 989-5800. Fax: (212) 633-3990.

MEDLINE. National Library of Medicine, 8600 Rockville Pike, Bethesda, MD 20894. Phone: (800) 638-8480.

SciSearch. Institute for Scientific Information, 3501 Market St., Philadelphia, PA 19104. Phone: (215) 386-0100. Fax: (215) 386-6362.

POPULAR WORKS AND PATIENT EDUCATION

Love Never Ends. Jenny Richards. Lion Publishing Co., 1705 Hubbard Ave., Batavia, IL 60510. Phone: (708) 879-0707. 1991.

RESEARCH CENTERS, INSTITUTES, CLEARINGHOUSES

Jerry Lewis Neuromuscular Disease Center. New York University, 400 E. 34th St., New York, NY 10016. Phone: (212) 340-6350.

Jerry Lewis Neuromuscular Disease Research Center. Baylor College of Medicine, One Baylor Plaza, Houston, TX 77030. Phone: (713) 799-5971.

Jerry Lewis Neuromuscular Research Center. Washington University, 600 South Euclid Ave., Box 8111, St. Louis, MO 63110. Phone: (314) 362-6981.

TEXTBOOKS AND MONOGRAPHS

Amyotrophic Lateral Sclerosis: Progress in Clinical Neurologic Trials. F. Clifford Rose. Demos Publications, 156 Fifth Ave., Suite 1018, New York, NY 10010. Phone: (212) 255-8768. 1991.

Amyotrophic Lateral Sclerosis: Recent Advances in Research and Treatment. T. Tsubaki, Y. Yose (eds.). Elsevier Science Publishing Co., Inc., P.O. Box 882, Madison Square Station, New York, NY 10159-2101. Phone: (212) 989-5800. Fax: (212) 633-3990. 1988.

ANALGESICS

See: ANESTHESIOLOGY; DRUGS

ANATOMY

ABSTRACTING, INDEXING, AND CURRENT AWARENESS PUBLICATIONS

Biological Abstracts. BIOSIS, 2100 Arch St., Philadelphia, PA 19103-1399. Phone: (800) 523-4800. Fax: (215) 587-2016.

Current Contents/Life Sciences. Institute for Scientific Information, 3501 Market St., Philadelphia, PA 19104. Phone: (215) 386-0100. Fax: (215) 386-6362.

Excerpta Medica. Section 1: Anatomy, Anthropology, Embryology & Histology. Elsevier Science Publishing Co., Inc., P.O. Box 882, Madison Square Station, New York, NY 10159-2101. Phone: (212) 989-5800. Fax: (212) 633-3990. 16/year.

Excerpta Medica. Section 5: General Pathology and Pathological Anatomy. Elsevier Science Publishers, P.O. Box 882, Madison Square Station, New York, NY 10159-2101. Phone: (212) 633-3950. Fax: (212) 633-3990. 24/year.

Index Medicus. U.S. National Library of Medicine, 8600 Rockville Pike, Bethesda, MD 20894. Phone: (800) 638-8480. Monthly.

ANNUALS AND REVIEWS

Advances in Anatomy, Embryology and Cell Biology. Springer-Verlag New York Inc., 175 Fifth Ave., New York, NY 10010. Phone: (212) 460-1500. Fax: (212) 473-6272. Irregular.

Critical Reviews in Anatomy and Cell Biology. CRC Press, Inc., 2000 Corporate Blvd. N.W., Boca Raton, FL 33431. Phone: (407) 994-0555. Fax: (407) 997-0949. 4/year.

ASSOCIATIONS, PROFESSIONAL SOCIETIES, ADVOCACY AND SUPPORT GROUPS

American Association of Anatomists (AAA). Box 906, MCV Station, Richmond, VA 23298. Phone: (804) 786-9477.

International Anatomical Nomenclature Committee (IANC). 55 Hall Drive, Sydenham, London SE26 6XL, England.

International Federation of Associations of Anatomists (IFAA). Department of Anatomy, CS 10008, Medical College of Ohio, Toledo, OH 43699. Phone: (419) 381-4111.

CD-ROM DATABASES

Biological Abstracts on Compact Disc. BIOSIS, 2100 Arch St., Philadelphia, PA 19103-1399. Phone: (800) 523-4800. Fax: (215) 587-2016. Quarterly.

DIRECTORIES

Directory of Departments of Anatomy of the United States and Canada. American Association of Anatomists, 1430 Tulane Ave., New Orleans, LA 70112. Phone: (504) 584-2727.

Directory of the International Federation of Associations of Anatomists. International Federation of Associations of Anatomists, Department of Anatomy, Medical College of Ohio, POB 10008, Toledo, OH 43699. Phone: (419) 381-4111.

ENCYCLOPEDIAS, DICTIONARIES, WORD BOOKS

An Anatomical Wordbook. S.J. Lewis. Butterworth-Heinemann, 80 Montvale Ave., Stoneham, MA 02180. Phone: (617) 438-8464. Fax: (617) 279-4851. 1990.

Anatomy and Physiology Words. Stedman. Williams & Wilkins, 428 East Preston St., Baltimore, MD 21202. Phone: (800) 638-0672. Fax: (800) 447-8438. 1992.

Basic Terms of Anatomy & Physiology. Bruce P. Squires. W.B. Saunders Co., The Curtis Centerrive, Independence Square West, Philadelphia, PA 19106-3399. Phone: (215) 238-7800. Second Edition 1987.

Elsevier's Encyclopedia Dictionary of Medicine, Part B: Anatomy. A.F. Dorian. Elsevier Science Publishing Co., Inc., P.O. Box 882, Madison Square Station, New York, NY 10159-2101. Phone: (212) 989-5800. Fax: (212) 633-3990. 1988.

Glossary of Anatomy and Physiology. Diane Shaw. Springhouse Publishing Co., 1111 Bethlehem Pike, Spring House, PA 19477. Phone: (800) 331-3170. Fax: (215) 646-8716. 1992.

HANDBOOKS, GUIDES, MANUALS, ATLASES

Atlas of Human Anatomy in Cross Section. Ronald A. Bergman, Adel K. Afifi, Jean Y. Jew, and others. Williams & Wilkins, 428 East Preston St., Baltimore, MD 21202. Phone: (800) 638-0672. Fax: (800) 447-8438. 1991.

Color Atlas of the Brain and Spinal Cord. Marjorie A. England, Jennifer Wakely. Mosby-Year Book, 11830 Westline Industrial Drive, St. Louis, MO 63146. Phone: (800) 325-4177. Fax: (314) 432-1380. 1991.

Color Atlas of Human Anatomy. R.M.H. McMinn, R.T. Hutchings. Mosby-Year Book, 11830 Westline Industrial Drive, St. Louis, MO 63146. Phone: (800) 325-4177. Fax: (314) 432-1380. Second Edition 1988.

Color Atlas of Human Dissection. Colin Chumbley, Ralph T. Hutchings. Mosby-Year Book, 11830 Westline Industrial Drive, St. Louis, MO 63146. Phone: (800) 325-4177. Fax: (314) 432-1380. Second edition 1992.

Color Atlas and Textbook of Human Anatomy. Volume 1. Kahle. Thieme Medical Publishers, Inc., 381 Park Ave. S., New York, NY 10016. Phone: (212) 683-5088. Fax: (212) 779-9020. Fourth edition 1992.

Color Atlas and Textbook of Human Anatomy. Volume 2. Kahle. Thieme Medical Publishers, Inc., 381 Park Ave. S., New York, NY 10016. Phone: (212) 683-5088. Fax: (212) 779-9020. Third edition 1986.

Color Atlas and Textbook of Human Anatomy. Volume 3. Kahle. Thieme Medical Publishers, Inc., 381 Park Ave. S., New York, NY 10016. Phone: (212) 683-5088. Fax: (212) 779-9020. Third edition 1986.

Grant's Atlas of Anatomy. Anne Agur. Williams & Wilkins, 428 East Preston St., Baltimore, MD 21202. Phone: (800) 638-0672. Fax: (800) 447-8438. Ninth Edition 1991.

Gray's Anatomy. Peter L. Williams, Roger Warwick, Mary Dyson, and others. Churchill Livingstone, 650 Avenue of the Americas, New York, NY 10011. Phone: (212) 819-5400. Fax: (212) 302-6598. Thirty-seventh Edition 1989.

Human Anatomy: Text and Colour Atlas. John Arthur Gosling, P.F. Harris, I.V. Whitmore, and others. J.B. Lippincott Co., 227 East Washington Square, Philadelphia, PA 19106-3780. Phone: (215) 238-4200. Fax: (215) 238-4227. Second Edition 1991.

Neuroanatomy. Snell. Little, Brown and Co., 34 Beacon St., Boston, MA 02108. Phone: (617) 227-0730. Fax: (617) 227-0790. 1992.

JOURNALS

Acta Anatomica. S. Karger Publishers, Inc., 26 W. Avon Rd., P.O. Box 529, Farmington, CT 06085. Phone: (203) 675-7834. Fax: (203) 675-7302.

American Journal of Anatomy. Wiley-Liss, 605 Third Ave., New York, NY 10158-0012. Phone: (212) 850-6000. Fax: (212) 850-6088. Monthly.

Anatomical Record. Wiley-Liss, 605 Third Avenue, New York, NY 10158-0012. Phone: (212) 850-6000. Fax: (212) 850-6088. Monthly.

Anatomy and Embryology. Sprinter-Verlag New York Inc., 175 Fifth Ave., New York, NY 10010. Phone: (212) 460-1500. Fax: (212) 473-6272. Monthly.

Clinical Anatomy. John Wiley & Sons, Inc., 605 Third Ave., New York, NY 10158-0012. Phone: (212) 850-6000. Fax: (212) 850-6088. Bimonthly.

Journal of Anatomy. Cambridge University Press, 40 W. 20th St., New York, NY 10011. Phone: (800) 431-1580. Bimonthly.

NEWSLETTERS

Anatomical News. American Association of Anatomists, Box 101, MCV Station, Richmond, VA 23298. Phone: (804) 786-9477. Quarterly.

ONLINE DATABASES

BIOSIS Previews. BIOSIS, 2100 Arch St., Philadelphia, PA 19103-1399. Phone: (800) 523-4800. Fax: (215) 587-2016.

EMBASE. Elsevier Science Publishing Co., Inc., P.O. Box 882, Madison Square Station, New York, NY 10159-2101. Phone: (212) 989-5800. Fax: (212) 633-3990.

Gray's Anatomy. Peter L. Williams, Roger Warwick, Mary Dyson, and others. Churchill Livingstone, 650 Avenue of the Americas, New York, NY 10011. Phone: (212) 819-5400. Fax: (212) 302-6598.

MEDLINE. National Library of Medicine, 8600 Rockville Pike, Bethesda, MD 20894. Phone: (800) 638-8480.

SciSearch. Institute for Scientific Information, 3501 Market St., Philadelphia, PA 19104. Phone: (215) 386-0100. Fax: (215) 386-6362.

RESEARCH CENTERS, INSTITUTES, CLEARINGHOUSES

Center for Advanced Pathology. Pulmonary and Medistinal Pathology Department. Armed Forces Institute of Pathology. Washington, DC 20306.

Clinical Research Center. University of Minnesota. Box 504, Mayo Memorial Building, Minneapolis, MN 55455. Phone: (612) 626-0905.

Daniel Baugh Institute. Thomas Jefferson University. Jefferson Hall, 1020 Locust St., Philadelphia, PA 19107. Phone: (215) 928-7820.

Wistar Institute of Anatomy and Biology. 36th and Spruce Streets, Philadelphia, PA 19104. Phone: (215) 898-3700. Fax: (215) 573-2097.

TEXTBOOKS AND MONOGRAPHS

Anatomy as a Basis for Clinical Medicine. E.C.B. Hall-Craggs. Williams & Wilkins, 428 East Preston St., Baltimore, MD 21202. Phone: (800) 638-0672. Fax: (800) 447-8438. Second Edition 1990.

Anatomy and Physiology. Rod R. Seeley, Trent D. Stephens, Philip Tate. Mosby-Year Book, 11830 Westline Industrial Drive, St. Louis, MO 63146. Phone: (800) 325-4177. Fax: (314) 432-1380. Second Edition 1991.

Clinical Anatomy. Harold H. Lindner. Appleton & Lange, 25 Van Zant Street, East Norwalk, CT 06855. Phone: (800) 423-1359. Fax: (203) 854-9486. 1988.

Clinically Oriented Anatomy. Keith L. Moore. Williams & Wilkins, 428 East Preston St., Baltimore, MD 21202. Phone: (800) 638-0672. Fax: (800) 447-8438. Third edition 1991.

Correlative Neuroanatomy. DeGroot. Appleton & Lange, 25 Van Zant St., East Norwalk, CT 06855. Phone: (800) 423-1359. Fax: (203) 854-9486. 21st edition 1991.

Dental Anatomy. Woelfel. Williams & Wilkins, 428 E. Preston St., Baltimore, MD 21202. Phone: (800) 638-0672. Fax: (800) 447-8438. Fourth edition 1992.

Essentials of Human Anatomy & Physiology. Elaine Nicpon Marieb. Addison-Wesley Publishing Co., Rte. 128, Reading, MA 01867. Phone: (800) 447-2226. Third edition 1991.

Grant's Method of Anatomy: A Clinical Problem-Solving Approach. John V. Basmajian, Charles Slonecker. Williams & Wilkins, 428 East Preston Street, Baltimore, MD 21202. Phone: (800) 638-0672. Fax: (800) 447-8438. Eleventh Edition 1989.

Gray's Anatomy of the Human Body. Carmine D. Clemente (ed.). Lea & Febiger, 428 East Preston St., Baltimore, MD 21202. Phone: (800) 638-0672. Fax: (800) 447-8438. 1985 Thirtieth Edition.

Kraus' Dental Anatomy and Occlusion. Jordan. Mosby-Year Book, 11830 Westline Industrial Drive, St. Louis, MO 63146. Phone: (800) 325-4177. Fax: (314) 432-1380. 1991.

Laboratory Exercises in Anatomy & Physiology: Brief Edition. Gerard J. Tortora, Nicholas P. Anagnostakos. Macmillan Publishing Co., Inc., 866 Third Ave., New York, NY 10022. Phone: (800) 257-5755. Third Edition 1990.

Sectional Anatomy by MRI/CT. Georges Y. El-Khoury, and others. Churchill Livingstone, 650 Avenue of the Americas, New York, NY 10011. Phone: (212) 819-5400. Fax: (212) 302-6598. 1990.

ANEMIAS

See: HEMATOLOGY

ANESTHESIA

See: ANESTHESIOLOGY

ANESTHESIOLOGY

ABSTRACTING, INDEXING, AND CURRENT AWARENESS PUBLICATIONS

Current Contents/Clinical Medicine. Institute for Scientific Information, 3501 Market St., Philadelphia, PA 19104. Phone: (800) 523-1850. Fax: (215) 386-6362. Weekly.

Current Contents/Life Sciences. Institute for Scientific Information, 3501 Market St., Philadelphia, PA 19104. Phone: (215) 386-0100. Fax: (215) 386-6362.

Excerpta Medica. Section 24: Anesthesiology. Elsevier Science Publishers, P.O. Box 882, Madison Square Station, New York, NY 10159-2101. Phone: (212) 633-3950. Fax: (212) 633-3990. 10/year.

Index Medicus. U.S. National Library of Medicine, 8600 Rockville Pike, Bethesda, MD 20894. Phone: (800) 638-8480. Monthly.

Science Citation Index. Institute for Scientific Information, 3501 Market St., Philadelphia, PA 19104. Phone: (800) 523-1850. Fax: (215) 386-6362. Bimonthly.

ANNUALS AND REVIEWS

Advances in Anesthesia. Mosby-Year Book, 11830 Westline Industrial Drive, St. Louis, MO 63146. Phone: (800) 325-4177. Fax: (314) 432-1380. Annual.

Anesthesiology Clinics. W.B. Saunders Co., The Curtis Center, Independence Square W., Philadelphia, PA 19106-3399. Phone: (215) 238-7800. Quarterly.

Current Anaesthesia and Critical Care. Churchill Livingstone Inc., 650 Avenue of the Americas, New York, NY 10011. Phone: (212) 819-5400. Fax: (212) 302-6598. Quarterly.

Current Opinion in Anaestheiology. Current Science Group, 20 N. Third St., Philadelphia, PA 19106-2199. Phone: (800) 552-5866. Fax: (215) 574-2270. Bimonthly.

Survey of Anesthesiology. Williams & Wilkins, 428 E. Preston St., Baltimore, MD 21202. Phone: (800) 638-0672. Fax: (800) 447-8438. Bimonthly.

Year Book of Anesthesia and Pain Management. Mosby-Year Book, 11830 Westline Industrial Drive, St. Louis, MO 63146. Phone: (800) 325-4177. Fax: (314) 432-1380. Annual.

ASSOCIATIONS, PROFESSIONAL SOCIETIES, ADVOCACY AND SUPPORT GROUPS

American Board of Anesthesiology (ABA). 100 Constitution Plaza, Hartford, CT 06103. Phone: (203) 522-9857.

American Society of Anesthesiologists (ASA). 515 Busse Hwy., Park Ridge, IL 60068-3189. Phone: (708) 825-5586. Fax: (708) 825-1692.

Canadian Anaesthetists' Society. 187 Gerrard St., Toronto, ON, Canada M5A 2E5. Phone: (416) 923-1449. Fax: (416) 944-1228.

International Anesthesia Research Society. 3645 Warrensville Center Rd., Cleveland, OH 44122. Phone: (216) 295-1124.

CD-ROM DATABASES

Excerpta Medica CD: Anesthesiology. SilverPlatter Information, Inc., River Ridge Office Park, 100 River Ridge Rd., Norwood, MA 02062. Phone: (617) 769-2599. Fax: (617) 769-8763. Quarterly.

SCISEARCH. Institute for Scientific Information, 3501 Market St., Philadelphia, PA 19104. Phone: (215) 386-0100. Fax: (215) 386-6362.

DIRECTORIES

Directory of Certified Anesthesiologists. American Board of Medical Specialties, 1 Rotary Center, Suite 805, Evanston, IL 60201. Phone: (708) 491-9091. Biennial.

Directory of Medical Specialists. Marquis Who's Who, 3002 Glenview Rd., Wilmette, IL 60091. Phone: (800) 621-9669. Fax: (708) 441-2264. Biennial.

Directory of Physicians in the United States. American Medical Association, 515 North State St., Chicago, IL 60610. Phone: (312) 464-0183. Fax: (312) 464-5834. Biennial.

HANDBOOKS, GUIDES, MANUALS, ATLASES

Anesthesia Drugs Handbook. Sota Omoigui. Mosby-Year Book, 11830 Westline Industrial Drive, St. Louis, MO 63146. Phone: (800) 325-4177. Fax: (314) 432-1380. 1992.

Handbook of Clinical Anesthesia. Paul G. Barash, Bruce F. Cullen, Robert K. Stoelting. J.B. Lippincott Co., 227 East Washington Square, Philadelphia, PA 19106-3780. Phone: (215) 238-4200. Fax: (215) 238-4227. 1991.

Manual of Anesthesia. Snow. Little, Brown and Co., 34 Beacon St., Boston, MA 02108. Phone: (617) 227-0730. Fax: (617) 227-0790. Third edition 1992.

Manual of Anesthesia and the Medically Compromised Patient. Eugene Cheng, Jonathan Kay. J.B. Lippincott Co., 227 East Washington Square, Philadelphia, PA 19106-3780. Phone: (215) 238-4200. Fax: (215) 238-4227. 1990.

Manual of Complications During Anesthesia. Nikolaus Gravenstein. J.B. Lippincott Co., 227 East Washington Square, Philadelphia, PA 19106-3780. Phone: (215) 238-4200. Fax: (215) 238-4227. 1991.

The Obstetric Anesthesia Handbook. Sanjay Datta. Mosby-Year Book, 11830 Westline Industrial Drive, St. Louis, MO 63146. Phone: (800) 325-4177. Fax: (314) 432-1380. 1991.

The Pediatric Anesthesia Handbook. Charlotte Bell, Cindy Hughes, Tae Hee Oh. Mosby-Year Book, 11830 Westline Industrial Drive, St. Louis, MO 63146. Phone: (800) 325-4177. Fax: (314) 432-1380. 1991.

The Practice of Cardiac Anesthesia. Hensley. Little, Brown and Co., 34 Beacon St., Boston, MA 02108. Phone: (617) 227-0730. Fax: (617) 227-0790. 1990.

JOURNALS

Anaesthesia. Academic Press, Inc., 1250 Sixth Ave., San Diego, CA 92101-4311. Phone: (619) 699-6345. Fax: (619) 699-6715. Monthly.

Anesthesia and Analgesia. Elsevier Science Publishing Co., Inc., P.O. Box 882, Madison Square Station, New York, NY 10159-2101. Phone: (212) 989-5800. Fax: (212) 633-3990. Monthly.

Anesthesia Progress. Elsevier Science Publishing Co., Inc., P.O. Box 882, Madison Square Station, New York, NY 10159-2101. Phone: (212) 989-5800. Fax: (212) 633-3990. Bimonthly.

Anesthesiology. Journal of the American Society of Anesthesiologists, Inc.. J.B. Lippincott Co., 227 East Washington Square, Philadelphia, PA 19106-3780. Phone: (215) 238-4200. Fax: (215) 238-4227. Monthly.

British Journal of Anaesthesia. BMJ Publishing Group, BMA House, Tavistock Square, London WC1H 9JR, England. Phone: 071-383 6244/6638. Fax: 071-383 6662. Monthly.

Canadian Journal of Anaesthesia/Journal Canadien d'Anesthesie. Canadian Anaesthetists' Society, 187 Gerrard St. E., Toronto, ON, Canada M5A 2E5. Phone: (416) 923-1449. Fax: (416) 944-1228. 10/year.

International Anesthesiology Clinics. Little, Brown and Co., 34 Beacon St., Boston, MA 02108. Phone: (617) 227-0730. Fax: (617) 227-0790.

Journal of Clinical Anesthesia. Butterworth-Heinemann, 80 Montvale Ave., Stoneham, MA 02180. Phone: (617) 438-8464. Fax: (617) 279-4851. Bimonthly.

Problems in Anesthesia. J.B. Lippincott Co., 227 East Washington Square, Philadelphia, PA 19106-3780. Phone: (215) 238-4200. Fax: (215) 238-4227. Quarterly.

Regional Anesthesia. Journal of the American and European Societies of Regional Anesthesia. J.B. Lippincott Co., 227 East Washington Square, Philadelphia, PA 19106-3780. Phone: (215) 238-4200. Fax: (215) 238-4227. Bimonthly.

NEWSLETTERS

Anesthesiology Alert. American Health Consultants, Department C1290, P.O. Box 740060, Atlanta, GA 30374. Phone: (800) 559-1032. Monthly.

ONLINE DATABASES

EMBASE. Elsevier Science Publishing Co., Inc., P.O. Box 882, Madison Square Station, New York, NY 10159-2101. Phone: (212) 989-5800. Fax: (212) 633-3990.

International Pharmaceutical Abstracts. American Society of Hospital Pharmacists, 4630 Montgomery Ave., Bethesda, MD 20814. Phone: (301) 657-3000. Fax: (301) 657-1641. Monthly.

MEDLINE. National Library of Medicine, 8600 Rockville Pike, Bethesda, MD 20894. Phone: (800) 638-8480.

SciSearch. Institute for Scientific Information, 3501 Market St., Philadelphia, PA 19104. Phone: (215) 386-0100. Fax: (215) 386-6362.

RESEARCH CENTERS, INSTITUTES, CLEARINGHOUSES

American Society for the Advancement of Anesthesia in Dentistry. 6 E. Union Ave., Bound Brook, NJ 08805. Phone: (908) 469-9050.

Malignant Hypothermia Research Center. Hahnemann University, Broad & Vine St., Philadelphia, PA 19102. Phone: (215) 448-7960.

TEXTBOOKS AND MONOGRAPHS

Anesthesia. Ronald D. Miller (ed.). Churchill Livingstone Inc., 650 Avenue of the Americas, New York, NY 10011. Phone: (212) 819-5400. Fax: (212) 302-6598. Third edition. Two volumes. 1990.

Anesthesia for Ambulatory Surgery. Bernard Wetchler. J.B. Lippincott Co., 227 E. Washington Square, Philadelphia, PA 19106-3780. Phone: (215) 238-4200. Fax: (215) 238-4227. 2nd edition, 1991.

Anesthesia and Co-Existing Disease. Robert Stoelting. Churchill Livingstone Inc., 650 Ave. of the Americas, New York, NY 10011. Phone: (212) 819-5400. Fax: (212) 302-6598. 2nd edition, 1988.

The Anesthetic Plan: From Physiologic Principles to Clinical Strategies. Stanley Muravchick. Mosby-Year Book, 11830 Westline Industrial Drive, St. Louis, MO 63146. Phone: (800) 325-4177. Fax: (314) 432-1380. 1990.

Clinical Anesthesia. Paul G. Barash, Bruce F. Cullen, Robert K. Stoelting. J.B. Lippincott Co., 227 East Washington Square,

Philadelphia, PA 19106-3780. Phone: (215) 238-4200. Fax: (215) 238-4227. 1989.

Clinical Anesthesiology. Morgan. Appleton & Lange, 25 Van Zant St., East Norwalk, CT 06855. Phone: (800) 423-1359. Fax: (203) 854-9486. 1992.

Clinical Procedures in Anesthesia and Intensive Care. Jonathan L. Benumof. J.B. Lippincott Co., 227 East Washington Square, Philadelphia, PA 19106-3780. Phone: (215) 238-4200. Fax: (215) 238-4227. 1992.

Decision Making in Anesthesiology. Lois L. Bready. Mosby-Year Book, 11830 Westline Industrial Drive, St. Louis, MO 63146. Phone: (800) 325-4177. Fax: (314) 432-1380. Second edition 1992.

Introduction to Anesthesia: The Principles of Safe Practice. Robert Dripps. W.B. Saunders Co., The Curtis Center, Independence Sqare W., Philadelphia, PA 19106-3399. Phone: (215) 238-7800. 7th edition, 1988.

Principles and Practice of Anesthesiology. Mark C. Rogers, John H. Tinker, Benjamin G. Covino, et. al.. Mosby-Year Book, 11830 Westline Industrial Drive, St. Louis, MO 63146. Phone: (800) 325-4177. Fax: (314) 432-1380. 1992.

Problems in Anesthesiology: Approach to Diagnosis. Roberta E. Galford. Little, Brown and Company, 34 Beacon St., Boston, MA 02108. Phone: (617) 227-0730. 1992.

Risk and Outcome in Anesthesia. David Brown (ed.). J.B. Lippincott Co., 227 E. Washington Square, Philadelphia, PA 19106-3780. Phone: (215) 238-4200. Fax: (215) 238-4227. 1992.

Smith's Anesthesia for Infants and Children. Etsuro K. Motoyama, Peter J. Davis. Mosby-Year Book, 11830 Westline Industrial Drive, St. Louis, MO 63146. Phone: (800) 325-4177. Fax: (314) 432-1380. Fifth edition 1990.

Trauma: Anesthesia and Intensive Care. levon M. Capan, Sanford Miller, Herman Turndorf (eds.). J.B. Lippincott Co., 227 East Washington Square, Philadelphia, PA 19106-3780. Phone: (215) 238-4200. Fax: (215) 238-4227. 1991.

ANEURYSM

See: HEART DISEASES; VASCULAR DISEASES

ANGINA PECTORIS

See: HEART DISEASES

ANGIOGRAPHY

See: DIAGNOSIS; HEART DISEASES

ANGIOPLASTY

See: CARDIOVASCULAR SURGERY

ANIMAL DISEASES

See: VETERINARY MEDICINE

ANIMALS, LABORATORY

See also: VETERINARY MEDICINE

ABSTRACTING, INDEXING, AND CURRENT AWARENESS PUBLICATIONS

Animal Breeding Abstracts. C.A.B. International, Wallingford, Oxon. OX10 8DE, England. Phone: 0491-32111. Fax: 0491-33508.

Biological Abstracts. BIOSIS, 2100 Arch St., Philadelphia, PA 19103-1399. Phone: (800) 523-4800. Fax: (215) 587-2016.

Current Contents/Life Sciences. Institute for Scientific Information, 3501 Market St., Philadelphia, PA 19104. Phone: (215) 386-0100. Fax: (215) 386-6362.

Index Medicus. U.S. National Library of Medicine, 8600 Rockville Pike, Bethesda, MD 20894. Phone: (800) 638-8480. Monthly.

ASSOCIATIONS, PROFESSIONAL SOCIETIES, ADVOCACY AND SUPPORT GROUPS

American Association for the Accreditation of Laboratory Animal Care. 9650 Rockville Pike, Bethesda, MD 20814. Phone: (301) 571-1850.

American Association for Laboratory Animal Science. 70 Timber Creek, Suite 5, Cordova, TN 38018. Phone: (901) 754-8620.

American College of Laboratory Animal Medicine. Milton S. Hershey Medical Center, P.O. Box 850, Pennsylvania State University, Hershey, PA 17033.

American Society of Laboratory Animal Practitioners. 182 Grinter Hall, University of Florida, Gainesville, FL 32611.

Canadian Council on Animal Care. 151 Slater St., Suite 1000, Ottawa, ON, Canada K1P 5H3. Phone: (613) 238-4031. Fax: (613) 563-7739.

CD-ROM DATABASES

Biological Abstracts on Compact Disc. BIOSIS, 2100 Arch St., Philadelphia, PA 19103-1399. Phone: (800) 523-4800. Fax: (215) 587-2016. Quarterly.

HANDBOOKS, GUIDES, MANUALS, ATLASES

International Index of Laboratory Animals. M.F.W. Festing. Royal Society of Medicine, 1 Wimpole St., London W1M 8AE, England. Phone: 071-408 2119. Fax: 071-355 3198. Fifth edition 1987.

Parasites of Laboratory Animals. Dawn G. Owen. Royal Society of Medicine, 1 Wimpole St., London W1M 8AE, England. Phone: 071-408 2119. Fax: 071-355 3198. 1991.

JOURNALS

American Journal of Veterinary Research. American Veterinary Medical Association, 930 N. Meacham Rd., Schaumburg, IL 60196. Phone: (708) 605-8070.

Laboratory Animal Science. American Association for Laboratory Animal Science, 70 Timber Creek, Suite 5, Cordova, TN 38018. Phone: (901) 754-8620.

Laboratory Animals. Royal Society of Medicine, 1 Wimpole St., London W1M 8AE, England. Phone: 071-408 2119. Fax: 071-355 3198. Quarterly.

ONLINE DATABASES

BIOSIS Previews. BIOSIS, 2100 Arch St., Philadelphia, PA 19103-1399. Phone: (800) 523-4800. Fax: (215) 587-2016.

EMBASE. Elsevier Science Publishing Co., Inc., P.O. Box 882, Madison Square Station, New York, NY 10159-2101. Phone: (212) 989-5800. Fax: (212) 633-3990.

MEDLINE. National Library of Medicine, 8600 Rockville Pike, Bethesda, MD 20894. Phone: (800) 638-8480.

SciSearch. Institute for Scientific Information, 3501 Market St., Philadelphia, PA 19104. Phone: (215) 386-0100. Fax: (215) 386-6362.

RESEARCH CENTERS, INSTITUTES, CLEARINGHOUSES

Institute of Laboratory Animal Resources. National Research Council, 2101 Constitution Ave. N.W., Washington, DC 20418. Phone: (202) 334-2590.

Laboratory Animal Research Center. Box 2, 1230 York Ave., Rockefeller University, New York, NY 10021. Phone: (212) 590-8535.

TEXTBOOKS AND MONOGRAPHS

Animal Experimentation: The Moral Issues. Robert Baird, Stuart Rosenbaum (eds.). Prometheus Books, 700E. Amherst St., Buffalo, NY 14215. Phone: (800) 421-0351. 1990.

Guide for the Care and Use of Laboratory Animals. National Center for Research Resources, Westwood Building, National Institutes of Health, Bethesda, MD 20892. NIH Pub. No. 86-23, 1986.

ANOREXIA NERVOSA

See: EATING DISORDERS

ANTI-ARRHYTHMIA DRUGS

See: HEART DISEASES

ANTI-BACTERIAL DRUGS

See: ANTIBIOTICS

ANTI-INFLAMMATORY DRUGS

See: DRUGS

ANTIBIOTICS

See also: DRUGS; INFECTIOUS DISEASES

ABSTRACTING, INDEXING, AND CURRENT AWARENESS PUBLICATIONS

CA Selects: Antibacterial Agents. Chemical Abstracts Service, 2540 Olentangy River Road, P.O. Box 3012, Columbus, OH 43210-0012. Phone: (800) 848-6538. Biweekly.

CA Selects: Beta-Lactam Antibiotics. Chemical Abstracts Service, 2540 Olentangy River Road, P.O. Box 3012, Columbus, OH 43210-0012. Phone: (800) 848-6538. Biweekly.

CA Selects: New Antibiotics. Chemical Abstracts Service, 2540 Olentangy River Road, P.O. Box 3012, Columbus, OH 43210-0012. Phone: (800) 848-6538. Biweekly.

Chemical Abstracts. Chemical Abstracts Service, 2540 Olentangy River Rd., P.O. Box 3012, Columbus, OH 43210-0012. Phone: (800) 848-6538.

Current Contents/Clinical Medicine. Institute for Scientific Information, 3501 Market St., Philadelphia, PA 19104. Phone: (800) 523-1850. Fax: (215) 386-6362. Weekly.

Current Contents/Life Sciences. Institute for Scientific Information, 3501 Market St., Philadelphia, PA 19104. Phone: (215) 386-0100. Fax: (215) 386-6362.

Index Medicus. U.S. National Library of Medicine, 8600 Rockville Pike, Bethesda, MD 20894. Phone: (800) 638-8480. Monthly.

Microbiology Abstracts. Section B: Bacteriology. Cambridge Scientific Abstracts, 7200 Wisconsin Ave., Bethesda, MD 20814-4823. Phone: (800) 843-7751. Fax: (301) 961-6720. Monthly.

Research Alert: Antibiotics (B-Lactams-Cephalosporins, Penicillin). Institute for Scientific Information, 3501 Market St., Philadelphia, PA 19104. Phone: (800) 523-1850. Fax: (215) 386-6362. Weekly.

Research Alert: Antibiotics (Other than B-Lactams). Institute for Scientific Information, 3501 Market St., Philadelphia, PA 19104. Phone: (800) 523-1850. Fax: (215) 386-6362. Weekly.

ASSOCIATIONS, PROFESSIONAL SOCIETIES, ADVOCACY AND SUPPORT GROUPS

Alliance for the Prudent Use of Antibiotics. P.O. Box 1272, Boston, MA 02117. Phone: (617) 956-6765.

ENCYCLOPEDIAS, DICTIONARIES, WORD BOOKS

Merck Index: An Encyclopedia of Chemicals and Drugs. Merck & Co., Inc., P.O. Box 2000, Rahway, NJ 07065. Phone: (201) 855-4558. Irregular.

HANDBOOKS, GUIDES, MANUALS, ATLASES

1991-1992 Pocketbook of Infectious Disease Therapy. John Bartlett. Williams & Wilkins, 428 East Preston St., Baltimore, MD 21202. Phone: (800) 638-0672. Fax: (800) 447-8438. 1991.

Handbook of Antibiotics. Richard E. Reese, R. Gordon Douglas Jr., Robert F. Betts. Little, Brown and Company, 34 Beacon St., Boston, MA 02108. Phone: (617) 227-0730. 1988.

Manual of Antiobiotics and Infectious Disease. Conte. Williams & Wilkins, 428 East Preston St., Baltimore, MD 21202. Phone: (800) 638-0672. Fax: (800) 447-8438. Seventh edition 1992.

ONLINE DATABASES

CA File (Chemical Abstracts File). Chemical Abstracts Service, 2540 Olentangy River Rd., P.O. Box 3012, Columbus, OH 43210-0012. Phone: (800) 848-6538.

EMBASE. Elsevier Science Publishing Co., Inc., P.O. Box 882, Madison Square Station, New York, NY 10159-2101. Phone: (212) 989-5800. Fax: (212) 633-3990.

International Pharmaceutical Abstracts. American Society of Hospital Pharmacists, 4630 Montgomery Ave., Bethesda, MD 20814. Phone: (301) 657-3000. Fax: (301) 657-1641. Monthly.

MEDLINE. National Library of Medicine, 8600 Rockville Pike, Bethesda, MD 20894. Phone: (800) 638-8480.

SciSearch. Institute for Scientific Information, 3501 Market St., Philadelphia, PA 19104. Phone: (215) 386-0100. Fax: (215) 386-6362.

RESEARCH CENTERS, INSTITUTES, CLEARINGHOUSES

Office of Consumer Affairs. Food and Drug Administration. 5600 Fishers Ln., HFE-50, Rockville, MD 20857. Phone: (301) 443-3170.

TEXTBOOKS AND MONOGRAPHS

Antibiotics in Laboratory Medicine. Lorian. Williams & Wilkins, 428 East Preston St., Baltimore, MD 21202. Phone: (800) 638-0672. Fax: (800) 447-8438. Third edition 1991.

Clinical Pharmacy and Therapeutics. Eric Herfindel, and others. Williams & Wilkins, 428 East Preston St., Baltimore, MD 21202. Phone: (800) 638-0672. Fax: (800) 447-8438. 1989.

ANTICOAGULANTS

See: HEART DISEASES

ANTICONVULSANTS

See: DRUGS; EPILEPSY

ANTIDEPRESSANTS

See: DEPRESSION; PSYCHOACTIVE DRUGS

ANTIDOTES

See: POISONING

ANTIFUNGAL AGENTS

See: DRUGS

ANTIHISTAMINES

See: ALLERGIES; DRUGS

ANTIHYPERTENSIVE DRUGS

See: DRUGS; HEART DISEASES

ANTIMICROBIALS

See: ANTIBIOTICS; DRUGS

ANTINEOPLASTIC DRUGS

See: CANCER; CHEMOTHERAPY; DRUGS

ANTIVIRAL AGENTS

See: DRUGS; INFECTIOUS DISEASES

ANXIETY

ABSTRACTING, INDEXING, AND CURRENT AWARENESS PUBLICATIONS

Current Contents/Clinical Medicine. Institute for Scientific Information, 3501 Market St., Philadelphia, PA 19104. Phone: (800) 523-1850. Fax: (215) 386-6362. Weekly.

Index Medicus. U.S. National Library of Medicine, 8600 Rockville Pike, Bethesda, MD 20894. Phone: (800) 638-8480. Monthly.

Psychological Abstracts. American Psychological Association, 1200 17th St. NW, Washington, DC 20036. Phone: (202) 955-7600. Monthly.

PSYSCAN: Clinical Psychology. American Psychological Association, 1200 17th St. NW, Washington, DC 20036. Phone: (202) 955-7600. Quarterly.

Science Citation Index. Institute for Scientific Information, 3501 Market St., Philadelphia, PA 19104. Phone: (800) 523-1850. Fax: (215) 386-6362. Bimonthly.

ASSOCIATIONS, PROFESSIONAL SOCIETIES, ADVOCACY AND SUPPORT GROUPS

American Psychiatric Association (APA). 1400 K St. N.W., Washington, DC 20005. Phone: (202) 682-6000. Fax: (202) 682-6114.

Anxiety Disorders Association of America. 6000 Executive Blvd., Ste. 200, Rockville, MD 20852.

CD-ROM DATABASES

PsycLit. SilverPlatter Information, Inc., River Ridge Office Park, 100 River Ridge Rd., Norwood, MA 02062. Phone: (617) 769-2599. Fax: (617) 769-8763. Quarterly.

SCISEARCH. Institute for Scientific Information, 3501 Market St., Philadelphia, PA 19104. Phone: (215) 386-0100. Fax: (215) 386-6362.

ENCYCLOPEDIAS, DICTIONARIES, WORD BOOKS

Encyclopedia of Phobias, Fears, and Anxieties. Ronald M. Doctor, Ada P. Kahn. Facts on File, Inc., 460 Park Ave. S., New York, NY 10016-7382. Phone: (212) 683-2244. Fax: (212) 683-3633. 1989.

HANDBOOKS, GUIDES, MANUALS, ATLASES

Diagnosis and Treatment of Anxiety Disorders: A Physician's Handbook. Thomas J. McGlynn, Harry L. Metcalf (eds.). American Psychiatric Press, Inc., 1400 K St. NW, Washington, DC 20005. Phone: (202) 682-6268. Fax: (202) 789-2648. 1989.

Handbook of Anxiety. G.B. Cassano, R.R. Crowe, J.A. Gray, and others (eds.). Elsevier Science Publishing Co., Inc., P.O. Box 882, Madison Square Station, New York, NY 10159-2101. Phone: (212) 989-5800. Fax: (212) 633-3990. Irregular.

JOURNALS

American Journal of Psychiatry. American Psychiatric Press, Inc., 1400 K St. NW, Washington, DC 20005. Phone: (202) 682-6268. Fax: (202) 789-2648. Monthly.

Archives of General Psychiatry. American Medical Association, 515 North State St., Chicago, IL 60610. Phone: (312) 464-0183. Fax: (312) 464-5834. Monthly.

Psychiatric Annals. SLACK Inc., 6900 Grove Rd., Thorofare, NJ 08086-9447. Phone: (800) 257-8290. Fax: (609) 853-5991.

ONLINE DATABASES

EMBASE. Elsevier Science Publishing Co., Inc., P.O. Box 882, Madison Square Station, New York, NY 10159-2101. Phone: (212) 989-5800. Fax: (212) 633-3990.

MEDLINE. National Library of Medicine, 8600 Rockville Pike, Bethesda, MD 20894. Phone: (800) 638-8480.

PsycInfo. SilverPlatter Information, Inc., River Ridge Office Park, 100 River Ridge Rd., Norwood, MA 02062. Phone: (617) 769-2599. Fax: (617) 769-8763. Quarterly.

SciSearch. Institute for Scientific Information, 3501 Market St., Philadelphia, PA 19104. Phone: (215) 386-0100. Fax: (215) 386-6362.

POPULAR WORKS AND PATIENT EDUCATION

Anxiety Disorders and Phobias. Aaron T. Beck, Gary Emery, Ruth L. Greenberg. HarperCollins Publishers, Inc., 10 E. 53rd St., New York, NY 10022-5299. Phone: (800) 242-7737. 1990.

Good News about Panic, Anxiety and Phobias. Mark S. Gold. Bantam Books, Inc., 666 Fifth Ave., New York, NY 10103. Phone: (800) 223-6834. 1990.

Living with Stress and Anxiety. Bob Whitmore. St. Martin's Press, 175 Fifth Ave., New York, NY 10010. Phone: (212) 674-5151. 1992.

Panic Disorder in the Medical Setting. Wayne J. Katon. American Psychiatric Press, Inc., 1400 K St. N.W., Washington, DC 20005. Phone: (202) 682-6268. Fax: (202) 789-2648. 1990.

Panic Disorder: The Great Pretender. H.M. Zal. Plenum Publishing Co., 233 Spring St., New York, NY 10013-1578. Phone: (212) 620-8000. Fax: (212) 463-0742. 1990.

RESEARCH CENTERS, INSTITUTES, CLEARINGHOUSES

Affective and Anxiety Disorders Research Branch. National Institutes of Health, 5600 Fishers Lane, Room 10C24, Rockville, MD 20857.

TEXTBOOKS AND MONOGRAPHS

Anxiety and Its Disorders. D.H. Barlow. Guilford Publications, Inc., 72 Spring St., New York, NY 10012. Phone: (800) 365-7006. Fax: (212) 966-6708. 1988.

The Clinical Management of Anxiety Disorders. William Coryell, George Winokur (eds.). Oxford University Press, 200 Madison Ave., New York, NY 10016. Phone: (212) 679-7300. 1991.

Comorbitity of Mood and Anxiety Disorders. Jack D. Maser, C. Robert Cloninger (eds.). American Psychiatric Press, Inc., 1400 K St. NW, Washington, DC 20005. Phone: (202) 682-6268. Fax: (202) 789-2648. 1990.

Psychiatric Disorders in America. L.N. Robins, D.A. Regier. Macmillan Publishing Co., 866 Third Ave., New York, NY 10011. Phone: (800) 257-5755. 1991.

Psychopharmacology of Anxiolytics and Antidepressants. Sandra E. File (ed.). Pergamon Press, 660 White Plains Rd., Tarrytown, NY 10591-5153. Phone: (914) 592-7700. Fax: (914) 592-3625. 1992.

APNEA

See: SLEEP DISORDERS

APPENDECTOMY

See: GASTROINTESTINAL SURGERY

ARRHYTHMIA

See also: HEART DISEASES

ABSTRACTING, INDEXING, AND CURRENT AWARENESS PUBLICATIONS

BIOSIS/CAS Selects: Antiarrhythmic Drugs. BIOSIS, 2100 Arch St., Philadelphia, PA 19103-1399. Phone: (215) 587-4800. Fax: (215) 587-2016. Biweekly.

CA Selects: Antiarrhythmics. Chemical Abstracts Service, 2540 Olentangy River Road, P.O. Box 3012, Columbus, OH 43210-0012. Phone: (800) 848-6538. Biweekly.

Core Journals in Cardiology. Elsevier Science Publishing Co., Inc., P.O. Box 882, Madison Square Station, New York, NY 10159-2101. Phone: (212) 989-5800. Fax: (212) 633-3990. 11/year.

Current Contents/Clinical Medicine. Institute for Scientific Information, 3501 Market St., Philadelphia, PA 19104. Phone: (800) 523-1850. Fax: (215) 386-6362. Weekly.

Excerpta Medica. Section 18: Cardiovascular Disease and Cardiovascular Surgery. Elsevier Science Publishing Co., Inc., P.O. Box 882, Madison Square Station, New York, NY 10159-2101. Phone: (212) 989-5800. Fax: (212) 633-3990. 24/year.

Index Medicus. U.S. National Library of Medicine, 8600 Rockville Pike, Bethesda, MD 20894. Phone: (800) 638-8480. Monthly.

Research Alert: Antiarrhythmial Drugs. Institute for Scientific Information, 3501 Market St., Philadelphia, PA 19104. Phone: (800) 523-1850. Fax: (215) 386-6362. Weekly.

Science Citation Index. Institute for Scientific Information, 3501 Market St., Philadelphia, PA 19104. Phone: (800) 523-1850. Fax: (215) 386-6362. Bimonthly.

ANNUALS AND REVIEWS

Current Problems in Cardiology. Mosby-Year Book, 11830 Westline Industrial Drive, St. Louis, MO 63146. Phone: (800) 325-4177. Fax: (314) 432-1380. Monthly.

In Development New Medicines for Older Americans. 1991 Annual Survey. 93 Cardiovascular, Cerebrovascular Medicines in Testing for Top Causes of Death. Pharmaceutical Manufacturers Association, 1100 15th St. N.W., Washington, DC 20005. Phone: (202) 835-3400. 1991.

Year Book of Cardiology. Mosby-Year Book, 11830 Westline Industrial Drive, St. Louis, MO 63146. Phone: (800) 325-4177. Fax: (314) 432-1380. Annual.

ASSOCIATIONS, PROFESSIONAL SOCIETIES, ADVOCACY AND SUPPORT GROUPS

American College of Cardiology (ACC). 9111 Old Georgetown Rd., Bethesda, MD 20814. Phone: (800) 253-4636. Fax: (301) 897-9745.

American Heart Association (AHA). 7320 Greenville Ave., Dallas, TX 75231. Phone: (214) 373-6300.

CD-ROM DATABASES

Advanced Problems in Cardiac Arrhythmias. Hoffer. Williams & Wilkins, 428 East Preston St., Baltimore, MD 21202. Phone: (800) 638-0672. Fax: (800) 447-8438. 1990.

Cardiology MEDLINE. MEP, 124 Mt. Auburn St., Cambridge, MA 02138. Phone: (800) 342-1338. Fax: (617) 868-7738. Quarterly.

Excerpta Medica CD: Cardiology. SilverPlatter Information, Inc., River Ridge Office Park, 100 River Ridge Rd., Norwood, MA 02062. Phone: (617) 769-2599. Fax: (617) 769-8763. Quarterly.

SCISEARCH. Institute for Scientific Information, 3501 Market St., Philadelphia, PA 19104. Phone: (215) 386-0100. Fax: (215) 386-6362.

ENCYCLOPEDIAS, DICTIONARIES, WORD BOOKS

Cardiology Words. Stedman. Williams & Wilkins, 428 East Preston St., Baltimore, MD 21202. Phone: (800) 638-0672. Fax: (800) 447-8438. 1992.

HANDBOOKS, GUIDES, MANUALS, ATLASES

Handbook of Cardiac Drugs. Ralph Purdy, Robert Boucek. Little, Brown and Co., 34 Beacon St., Boston, MA 02108. Phone: (617) 227-0730. Fax: (617) 227-0790. 1988.

Manual of Cardiac Arrhythmias. Vlay. Little, Brown and Co., 34 Beacon St., Boston, MA 02108. Phone: (617) 227-0730. Fax: (617) 227-0790. 1988.

Random House Personal Medical Handbook: For People with Heart Disease. Paula Dranov. Random House, Inc., 201 E. 50th St., New York, NY 10022. Phone: (800) 726-0600. 1990.

JOURNALS

American Journal of Cardiology. Reed Publishing USA, 249 W. 17th St., New York, NY 10011. Phone: (212) 645-0067. Fax: (212) 242-6987. 22/year.

Cardiology. S. Karger Publishers, Inc., 26 W. Avon Rd., P.O. Box 529, Farmington, CT 06085. Phone: (203) 675-7834. Fax: (203) 675-7302. Bimonthly.

Coronary Artery Disease. Current Science Group, 20 N. Third St., Philadelphia, PA 19106-2199. Phone: (215) 574-2266. Fax: (215) 574-2270. Monthly.

Journal of the American College of Cardiology. Elsevier Science Publishing Co., Inc., P.O. Box 882, Madison Square Station, New York, NY 10159-2101. Phone: (212) 989-5800. Fax: (212) 633-3990. Monthly.

NEWSLETTERS

Clinical Cardiology Alert. American Health Consultants, Department C1290, P.O. Box 740060, Atlanta, GA 30374. Phone: (800) 559-1032. Fax: (404) 352-1971. Monthly.

ONLINE DATABASES

EMBASE. Elsevier Science Publishing Co., Inc., P.O. Box 882, Madison Square Station, New York, NY 10159-2101. Phone: (212) 989-5800. Fax: (212) 633-3990.

MEDLINE. National Library of Medicine, 8600 Rockville Pike, Bethesda, MD 20894. Phone: (800) 638-8480.

SciSearch. Institute for Scientific Information, 3501 Market St., Philadelphia, PA 19104. Phone: (215) 386-0100. Fax: (215) 386-6362.

POPULAR WORKS AND PATIENT EDUCATION

The Heart Attack Handbook. Joseph S. Alpert. Consumer Reports Books, 9180 LeSaint Dr., Fairfield, OH 45014. Phone: (513) 860-1178. 1993.

Yale University School of Medicine Heart Book. Barry L. Zaret, Lawrence S. Cohen, Marvin Moser, and others. William Morrow & Company, Inc., 1350 Ave. of the Americas, New York, NY 10019. Phone: (800) 237-0657. 1992.

RESEARCH CENTERS, INSTITUTES, CLEARINGHOUSES

Cleveland Clinic Foundation Research Institute. 9500 Euclid Ave., Cleveland, OH 44195-5210. Phone: (216) 444-3900. Fax: (216) 444-3279.

DeBakey Heart Center. Baylor College of Medicine. Texas Medical Center, 1 Baylor Plaza, Houston, TX 77030. Phone: (701) 797-9353. Fax: (713) 793-1192.

Framingham Heart Study. 5 Thurber St., Framingham, MA 01701. Phone: (508) 872-4386.

TEXTBOOKS AND MONOGRAPHS

Atrial Arrhythmias: Current Concepts and Management. Paul Touboul, Albert Waldo. Mosby-Year Book, 11830 Westline Industrial Drive, St. Louis, MO 63146. Phone: (800) 325-4177. Fax: (314) 432-1380. 1991.

Atrial Fibrillation. Falk. Raven Press, 1185 Ave. of the Americas, New York, NY 10036. Phone: (212) 930-9500. Fax: (212) 869-3495. 1992.

Cardiac Arrhythmias. David H. Bennett. Butterworth-Heinemann, 80 Montvale Ave., Stoneham, MA 02180. Phone: (617) 438-8464. Fax: (617) 279-4851. Third edition 1989.

Cardiac Arrhythmias and Electrophysiology. Eric N. Prystowsky, George J. Klein. McGraw-Hill, Inc., Health Professions Division, 1221 Avenue of the Americas, 28th Floor, New York, NY 10020. Phone: (212) 512-4228. 1992.

Cardiac Electrophysiology and Arrhythmias. Fisch. Elsevier Science Publishing Co., Inc., P.O. Box 882, Madison Square Station, New York, NY 10159-2101. Phone: (212) 989-5800. Fax: (212) 633-3990. 1991.

Electrical Therapy for Cardiac Arrhythmias: Pacing, Antitachycardia Devices, Catheter Ablation. Sanjeev Saksena, Nora Goldschlager. W.B. Saunders Co., The Curtis Center, Independence Square W., Philadelphia, PA 19106-3399. Phone: (215) 238-7800. 1990.

Heart Disease: A Textbook of Cardiovascular Medicine. Eugene Braunwald (ed.) W.B. Saunders Co., The Curtis Center, Independence Square W., Philadelphia, PA 19106-3399. Phone: (215) 238-7800. Third edition. Two volumes. 1988.

Pediatric Arrhythmias: Electrophysiology and Pacing. Paul C. Gillette, Arthur Garson Jr.. W.B. Saunders Co., The Curtis Center, Independence Square W., Philadelphia, PA 19106-3399. Phone: (215) 238-7800. 1990.

Perioperative Cardiac Arrhythmias. John Atlee. Mosby-Year Book, 11830 Westline Industrial Drive, St. Louis, MO 63146. Phone: (800) 325-4177. Fax: (314) 432-1380. 1989.

Principles of Cardiac Arrhythmias. Edward K. Chung. Williams & Wilkins, 428 E. Preston St., Baltimore, MD 21202. Phone: (800) 638-0672. Fax: (800) 447-8438. Fourth edition 1989.

ARTHRITIS

See also: BONE AND JOINT DISEASES; LYME DISEASE

ABSTRACTING, INDEXING, AND CURRENT AWARENESS PUBLICATIONS

CA Selects: Anti-Inflammatory Agents & Arthritis. Chemical Abstracts Service, 2540 Olentangy River Road, P.O. Box 3012, Columbus, OH 43210-0012. Phone: (800) 848-6538. Biweekly.

Current Contents/Clinical Medicine. Institute for Scientific Information, 3501 Market St., Philadelphia, PA 19104. Phone: (800) 523-1850. Fax: (215) 386-6362. Weekly.

Excerpta Medica. Section 31. Arthritis and Rheumatism. Elsevier Science Publishing Co., Inc., P.O. Box 882, Madison Square Station, New York, NY 10159-2101. Phone: (212) 989-5800. Fax: (212) 633-3990. 8/year.

Index Medicus. U.S. National Library of Medicine, 8600 Rockville Pike, Bethesda, MD 20894. Phone: (800) 638-8480. Monthly.

Research Alert: Arthritis. Institute for Scientific Information, 3501 Market St., Philadelphia, PA 19104. Phone: (800) 523-1850. Fax: (215) 386-6362. Weekly.

Science Citation Index. Institute for Scientific Information, 3501 Market St., Philadelphia, PA 19104. Phone: (800) 523-1850. Fax: (215) 386-6362. Bimonthly.

ANNUALS AND REVIEWS

Current Opinion in Rheumatology. Current Science Ltd., 20 N. Third St., Philadelphia, PA 19106-2199. Phone: (800) 552-5866. Fax: (215) 574-2270. Bimonthly.

In Development New Medicines for Arthritis. Pharmaceutical Manufacturers Association, 1100 15th St. N.W., Washington, DC 20005. Phone: (202) 835-3400. Annual.

ASSOCIATIONS, PROFESSIONAL SOCIETIES, ADVOCACY AND SUPPORT GROUPS

American College of Rheumatology (ACR). 17 Executive Park Dr. N.E., Ste. 480, Atlanta, GA 30329. Phone: (404) 633-3777. Fax: (404) 633-1870.

American Juvenile Arthritis Organization (AJAO). 1314 Spring St. N.W., Atlanta, GA 30309. Phone: (404) 872-7100. Fax: (404) 872-0457.

Arthritis Foundation (AF). 1314 Spring St. N.W., Atlanta, GA 30309. Phone: (404) 872-2100. Fax: (404) 872-0457.

Arthritis Health Professions Association. 1314 Spring St. N.W., Atlanta, GA 30309. Phone: (404) 872-7100.

International League Against Rheumatism. c/o Charles M. Plotz, SUNY Downstate Medical Center, 450 Clarkson Ave., Brooklyn, NY 11203.

Sjogren's Syndrome Foundation (SSF). 382 Main St., Port Washington, NY 11050. Phone: (516) 767-2866.

BIBLIOGRAPHIES

Antiarthritic Agents. National Technical Information Service, 5285 Port Royal Rd., Springfield, VA 22161. Phone: (703) 487-4650. Fax: (703) 321-8547. Jan. 1985-Feb. 1989 PB89-857296/CBY.

Educational Materials Exhibit Catalog.. Arthritis Health Professions Association, 1314 Spring St. N.W., Atlanta, GA 30309. Phone: (404) 872-7100. 26th National Scientific Meeting Nov. 17-21, 1991.

Rheumatoid Arthritis: Diagnosis and Clinical Treatment. National Technical Information Service, 5285 Port Royal Rd., Springfield, VA 22161. Phone: (703) 487-4650. Fax: (703) 321-8547. Jan. 1978-Feb. 1988 PB88-858915/CBY.

CD-ROM DATABASES

SCISEARCH. Institute for Scientific Information, 3501 Market St., Philadelphia, PA 19104. Phone: (215) 386-0100. Fax: (215) 386-6362.

JOURNALS

Arthritis Care and Research. Elsevier Science Publishing Co., Inc., P.O. Box 882, Madison Square Station, New York, NY 10159-2101. Phone: (212) 989-5800. Fax: (212) 633-3990. 4/year.

Arthritis and Rheumatism. American College of Rheumatology, 17 Executive Park Dr. N.E., Ste. 480, Atlanta, GA 30329. Phone: (404) 633-3777. Fax: (404) 663-1870. Monthly.

British Journal of Rheumatology. Balliere Tindall, 24-28 Oval Rd., London NW1 7DX, England. Bimonthly.

Seminars in Arthritis and Rheumatism. W.B. Saunders Co., The Curtis Center, Independence Sqare W., Philadelphia, PA 19106-3399. Phone: (215) 238-7800.

NEWSLETTERS

Arthritis Today. UAB Multipurpose Arthritis Center. University of Alabama at Birmingham, 108 Basic Health Sciences Bldg., Birmingham, AL 35294. Phone: (205) 934-0542. Quarterly.

Bulletin on the Rheumatic Diseases. Arthritis Foundation, 1314 Sprin St., N.W., Atlanta, GA 30309. Phone: (404) 872-7100. Fax: (404) 872-0457. Bimonthly.

ONLINE DATABASES

Combined Health Information Database (CHID). U.S. National Institutes of Health, P.O. Box NDIC, Bethesda, MD 20892. Phone: (301) 496-2162. Fax: (301) 770-5164. Quarterly.

EMBASE. Elsevier Science Publishing Co., Inc., P.O. Box 882, Madison Square Station, New York, NY 10159-2101. Phone: (212) 989-5800. Fax: (212) 633-3990.

MEDIS. Mead Data Central, P.O. Box 1830, Dayton, OH 45401. Phone: (800) 227-4908.

MEDLINE. National Library of Medicine, 8600 Rockville Pike, Bethesda, MD 20894. Phone: (800) 638-8480.

SciSearch. Institute for Scientific Information, 3501 Market St., Philadelphia, PA 19104. Phone: (215) 386-0100. Fax: (215) 386-6362.

POPULAR WORKS AND PATIENT EDUCATION

Arthritis: A Comprehensive Guide to Understanding Your Arthritis. James M. Fries. Addison-Wesley Nursing, 390 Bridge Parkway, Redwood City, CA 94065. Phone: (800) 950-5544. Third edition 1990.

The Arthritis Helpbook: The Tested Self-Management Program for Coping with Your Arthritis. Kate Lorig, James F. Fries. Addison-Wesley Nursing, 390 Bridge Parkway, Redwood City, CA 94065. Phone: (800) 950-5544. Third edition 1990.

Arthritis: What Works. Dava Sobel, Arthur C. Klein. St. Martin's Press, 175 Fifth Ave., New York, NY 10010. Phone: (212) 674-5151. 1989.

Comprehensive Guide to Arthritis. James F. Fries. Addison-Wesley Publishing Co., Rte. 128, Reading, MA 01867. Phone: (800) 447-2226. Third edition 1990.

The Duke University Medical Center Book of Arthritis. Susan F. Trien, David Pisetsky. Fawcett Book Group, 201 E. 50th St., New York, NY 10022. Phone: (800) 733-3000. 1992.

If It Runs in Your Family: Arthritis. Eades. Bantam Books, Inc., 666 Fifth Ave., New York, NY 10103. Phone: (800) 223-6834. 1992.

Keys to Understanding Arthritis. Elizabeth Vierck. Barron's Educational Series, Inc., P.O. Box 8040, 250 Wireless Blvd., Hauppauge, NY 11788. Phone: (516) 434-3311. Fax: (516) 434-3723. 1991.

Rheumatoid Arthritis: Its Cause and Treatment. Thomas Brown, and others. M. Evans and Co., Inc., 216 E. 49th St., New York, NY 10017. Phone: (212) 688-2810. 1992.

Take Care of Yourself: The Consumer's Guide to Medical Care. Donald Vikery, James Fries. Addison-Wesley Nursing, 390 Bridge Parkway, Redwood City, CA 94065. Phone: (800) 950-5544. Fourth edition 1989.

Taking Control of Arthritis. Fred G. Kantrowitz. HarperCollins Pubs., Inc., 10 E. 53rd St., New York, NY 10022-5299. Phone: (212) 207-7000. Fax: (800) 242-7737. 1991.

RESEARCH CENTERS, INSTITUTES, CLEARINGHOUSES

Arthritis Center. Boston University. Conte Bldg., 5th Fl., 71 E. Newton St., Boston, MA 02118. Phone: (617) 534-5154. Fax: (617) 634-3573.

Arthritis Center. University of Missouri-Columbia. MA427 Health Sciences Center, 1 Hospital Dr., Columbia, MO 65212. Phone: (314) 882-8738. Fax: (314) 884-3996.

Arthritis Clinical and Research Center. Medical University of South Carolina. 171 Ashley Ave., Charleston, SC 29425. Phone: (803) 792-2000. Fax: (803) 792-7121.

Arthritis Research Institute of America. 300 S. Duncan Ave., Ste. 240, Clearwater, FL 34615. Phone: (813) 461-4054. Fax: (813) 447-6312.

Multipurpose Arthritis Center. University of Connecticut. School of Medicine, Division of Rheumatic Diseases, Farmington, CT 06030. Phone: (203) 679-2160. Fax: (203) 679-1287.

Multipurpose Arthritis Center. University of Michigan. 3918 Taubman Center, Ann Arbor, MI 48109-0358. Phone: (313) 936-9539. Fax: (313) 763-1253.

Multipurpose Arthritis and Musculoskeletal Diseases Center. University of Alabama at Birmingham. Tinsley Harrison Tower 429 A, UAB Station, Birmingham, AL 35294. Phone: (205) 934-5306. Fax: (205) 934-1564.

National Arthritis and Musculoskeletal and Skin Diseases Information Clearinghouse (NAMSIC). 9000 Rockville Pike, P.O. Box AMS, Bethesda, MD 20892. Phone: (301) 495-4484. Fax: (301) 587-4352.

Northeast Ohio Multipurpose Arthritis Center. Case Western Reserve University. University Hospitals of Cleveland, 2074 Abington Rd., Cleveland, OH 44106. Phone: (216) 844-3168. Fax: (216) 844-5172.

Scripps Research Institute. 10666 N. Torrey Pines Rd., La Jolla, CA 92037. Phone: (619) 554-8265. Fax: (619) 554-9899.

TEXTBOOKS AND MONOGRAPHS

Arthritis and Allied Conditions. D.J. McCarty. Williams & Wilkins, 428 East Preston St., Baltimore, MD 21202. Phone: (800) 638-0672. Fax: (800) 447-8438.

Arthritis and Allied Conditions: A Textbook of Rheumatology. Daniel McCarty (ed.). Williams & Wilkins, 428 East Preston St., Baltimore, MD 21202. Phone: (800) 638-0672. Fax: (800) 447-8438. 11th ed., 1989.

Arthritis and Rheumatology in Practice. Dieppe. J.B. Lippincott Co., 227 E. Washington Square, Philadelphia, PA 19106-3780. Phone: (215) 238-4200. Fax: (215) 238-4227. 1991.

Osteoarthritis. Roland Macowitz, and others. W.B. Saunders Co., The Curtis Center, Independence Sqare W., Philadelphia, PA 19106-3399. Phone: (215) 238-7800. 2nd edition.

Rehabilitation of Early Rheumatoid Patients. Matthew H. Liang, Martha K. Logigian. Little, Brown and Company, 34 Beacon St., Boston, MA 02108. Phone: (617) 227-0730. 1992.

Rheumatoid Arthritis. Fischbach. Churchill Livingstone Inc., 650 Ave. of the Americas, New York, NY 10011. Phone: (212) 819-5400. Fax: (212) 302-6598. 1991.

Rheumatoid Arthritis: An Illustrated Guide to Pathology, Diagnosis, and Management. Ralph H. Schumacher, Eric P. Gall. J.B. Lippincott Co., 227 E. Washington Square, Philadelphia, PA 19106-3780. Phone: (215) 238-4200. Fax: (215) 238-4227. 1988.

Surgical Treatment of Rheumatoid Arthritis. Thomas Sculco (ed.). Mosby-Year Book, 11830 Westline Industrial Drive, St. Louis, MO 63146. Phone: (800) 325-4177. Fax: (314) 432-1380. 1992.

ARTHROSCOPY

See also: KNEE SURGERY

ABSTRACTING, INDEXING, AND CURRENT AWARENESS PUBLICATIONS

Index Medicus. U.S. National Library of Medicine, 8600 Rockville Pike, Bethesda, MD 20894. Phone: (800) 638-8480. Monthly.

Science Citation Index. Institute for Scientific Information, 3501 Market St., Philadelphia, PA 19104. Phone: (800) 523-1850. Fax: (215) 386-6362. Bimonthly.

ASSOCIATIONS, PROFESSIONAL SOCIETIES, ADVOCACY AND SUPPORT GROUPS

Arthroscopy Association of North America (AANA). 2250 E. Devon Ave., Ste. 101, Des Plaines, IL 60018. Phone: (708) 299-9444. Fax: (708) 299-4913.

International Arthroscopy Association. 70 W. Hubbard, Suite 202, Chicago, IL 60610. Phone: (312) 644-2623.

CD-ROM DATABASES

SCISEARCH. Institute for Scientific Information, 3501 Market St., Philadelphia, PA 19104. Phone: (215) 386-0100. Fax: (215) 386-6362.

HANDBOOKS, GUIDES, MANUALS, ATLASES

Manual of Ankle and Foot Arthroscopy. Richard O. Lundeen. Churchill Livingstone Inc., 650 Avenue of the Americas, New York, NY 10011. Phone: (212) 819-5400. Fax: (212) 302-6598. 1991.

JOURNALS

Arthroscopy. Raven Press, 1185 Avenue of the Americas, New York, NY 10036. Phone: (212) 930-9500. Fax: (212) 869-3495. Quarterly.

ONLINE DATABASES

EMBASE. Elsevier Science Publishing Co., Inc., P.O. Box 882, Madison Square Station, New York, NY 10159-2101. Phone: (212) 989-5800. Fax: (212) 633-3990.

MEDLINE. National Library of Medicine, 8600 Rockville Pike, Bethesda, MD 20894. Phone: (800) 638-8480.

SciSearch. Institute for Scientific Information, 3501 Market St., Philadelphia, PA 19104. Phone: (215) 386-0100. Fax: (215) 386-6362.

TEXTBOOKS AND MONOGRAPHS

Arthroscopic Surgery. Terry Whipple. J.B. Lippincott Co., 227 E. Washington Square, Philadelphia, PA 19106-3780. Phone: (215) 238-4200. Fax: (215) 238-4227. 1992.

Arthroscopy of the Knee. R. Aigner, J. Gillquist. Thieme Medical Publishers, Inc., 381 Park Ave. S., New York, NY 10016. Phone: (212) 683-5088. Fax: (212) 779-9020. 1991.

Arthroscopy Surgery. Orrin Sherman, Jeffrey Minkoff. Williams & Wilkins, 428 East Preston St., Baltimore, MD 21202. Phone: (800) 638-0672. Fax: (800) 447-8438. 1990.

Articular Cartilage and Knee Joint Function: Basic Science and Arthroscopy. J. Whit Ewing. Raven Press, 1185 Avenue of the Americas, New York, NY 10036. Phone: (212) 930-9500. Fax: (212) 869-3495. 1990.

Diagnostic and Surgical Arthroscopy of the Shoulder. Lanny Johnson. Mosby-Year Book, 11830 Westline Industrial Drive, St. Louis, MO 63146. Phone: (800) 325-4177. Fax: (314) 432-1380. 1992.

Operative Arthroscopy. John B. McGinty (ed.). Raven Press, 1185 Ave. of the Americas, New York, NY 10036. Phone: (212) 930-9500. Fax: (212) 869-3495. 1991.

ARTIFICIAL INSEMINATION

See: IN VITRO FERTILIZATION;
INFERTILITY

ARTIFICIAL LIMBS

See: PROSTHESES

ARTIFICIAL ORGANS

See also: TRANSPLANTATION

ABSTRACTING, INDEXING, AND CURRENT AWARENESS PUBLICATIONS

Bioengineering and Biotechnology Abstracts. Engineering Information Inc., 345 E. 47th St., New York, NY 10017-2387. Phone: (800) 221-1044. Fax: (212) 832-1857.

Current Contents/Clinical Medicine. Institute for Scientific Information, 3501 Market St., Philadelphia, PA 19104. Phone: (800) 523-1850. Fax: (215) 386-6362. Weekly.

Excerpta Medica. Section 27: Biophysics, Bioengineering and Medical Instrumentation. Elsevier Science Publishing Co., Inc., P.O. Box 882, Madison Square Station, New York, NY 10159-2101. Phone: (212) 989-5800. Fax: (212) 633-3990. 10/year.

Index Medicus. U.S. National Library of Medicine, 8600 Rockville Pike, Bethesda, MD 20894. Phone: (800) 638-8480. Monthly.

Science Citation Index. Institute for Scientific Information, 3501 Market St., Philadelphia, PA 19104. Phone: (800) 523-1850. Fax: (215) 386-6362. Bimonthly.

ASSOCIATIONS, PROFESSIONAL SOCIETIES, ADVOCACY AND SUPPORT GROUPS

American Society for Artificial Internal Organs (ASAIO). P.O. Box C, Boca Raton, FL 33429. Phone: (407) 391-8589.

International Society for Artificial Organs (ISAO). 8937 Euclid Ave., Cleveland, OH 44106. Phone: (216) 421-0757. Fax: (216) 421-1652.

BIBLIOGRAPHIES

The Artificial (Mechanical) Hearts. National Technical Information Service, 5285 Port Royal Rd., Springfield, VA 22161. Phone: (703) 487-4650. Fax: (703) 321-8547. Jan. 1970-Apr. 1989 PB89-860555/CBY.

Biomedical Engineering: Artificial Hearts and Heart Valves. National Technical Information Service, 5285 Port Royal Rd., Springfield, VA 22161. Phone: (703) 487-4650. Fax: (703) 321-8547. Jan. 1975-Nov. 1989 PB90-852971/CBY.

CD-ROM DATABASES

SCISEARCH. Institute for Scientific Information, 3501 Market St., Philadelphia, PA 19104. Phone: (215) 386-0100. Fax: (215) 386-6362.

JOURNALS

Artificial Organs. Raven Press, 1185 Avenue of the Americas, New York, NY 10036. Phone: (212) 930-9500. Fax: (212) 869-3495. Bimonthly.

Biomaterials, Artifical Cells, and Artificial Organs. Marcel Dekker, Inc., 270 Madison Ave., New York, NY 10016. Phone: (800) 228-1160.

International Journal of Artificial Organs. Wichtig Editore, Via Friuli, 72-74, 20135 Milan, Italy. Phone: 02-5452306.

Journal of Biomedical Engineering. Butterworth-Heinemann, 80 Montvale Ave., Stoneham, MA 02180. Phone: (617) 438-8464. Fax: (617) 279-4851. Bimonthly.

Transplantation Proceedings. Appleton & Lange, 25 Van Zant St., East Norwalk, CT 06855. Phone: (800) 423-1359. Fax: (203) 854-9486. Bimonthly.

NEWSLETTERS

Biomedical Technology Information Service. Quest Publishing Co., 1351 Titan Way, Brea, CA 92621. Phone: (714) 738-6400. Semimonthly.

ONLINE DATABASES

EMBASE. Elsevier Science Publishing Co., Inc., P.O. Box 882, Madison Square Station, New York, NY 10159-2101. Phone: (212) 989-5800. Fax: (212) 633-3990.

MEDLINE. National Library of Medicine, 8600 Rockville Pike, Bethesda, MD 20894. Phone: (800) 638-8480.

SciSearch. Institute for Scientific Information, 3501 Market St., Philadelphia, PA 19104. Phone: (215) 386-0100. Fax: (215) 386-6362.

POPULAR WORKS AND PATIENT EDUCATION

A Patient's Guide to Dialysis and Transplantation. Roger Gabriel. Kluwer Academic Publishers, P.O. Box 358, Accord Station, Hingham, MA 02018-0358. Phone: (617) 871-6600. Fax: (617) 871-6528. 1990.

RESEARCH CENTERS, INSTITUTES, CLEARINGHOUSES

Artificial Cells and Organs Research Centre. McGill University. 3655 Drummond St., Montreal, PQ, Canada H3G 1V6. Phone: (514) 398-3512. Fax: (514) 398-4983.

Artificial Heart Research Project. Pennsylvania State University. Milton S. Hershey Medical Ctr., 500 University Dr., Hershey, PA 17033. Phone: (717) 531-8328. Fax: (717) 531-5011.

Cleveland Clinic Foundation Research Institute. 9500 Euclid Ave., Cleveland, OH 44195-5210. Phone: (216) 444-3900. Fax: (216) 444-3279.

ASTHMA

See also: RESPIRATORY TRACT INFECTIONS

ABSTRACTING, INDEXING, AND CURRENT AWARENESS PUBLICATIONS

BIOSIS/CAS Selects: Allergy & Antiallergy. BIOSIS, 2100 Arch St., Philadelphia, PA 19103-1399. Phone: (215) 587-4800. Fax: (215) 587-2016. Biweekly.

Current Contents/Clinical Medicine. Institute for Scientific Information, 3501 Market St., Philadelphia, PA 19104. Phone: (800) 523-1850. Fax: (215) 386-6362. Weekly.

Excerpta Medica. Section 15: Chest Diseases, Thoracic Surgery and Tuberculosis. Elsevier Science Publishing Co., Inc., P.O.

Box 882, Madison Square Station, New York, NY 10159-2101. Phone: (212) 989-5800. Fax: (212) 633-3990. 20/year.

Index Medicus. U.S. National Library of Medicine, 8600 Rockville Pike, Bethesda, MD 20894. Phone: (800) 638-8480. Monthly.

Research Alert: Allergies, Asthma, Clinical Immunology. Institute for Scientific Information, 3501 Market St., Philadelphia, PA 19104. Phone: (800) 523-1850. Fax: (215) 386-6362. Weekly.

Research Alert: Asthma, Emphysema & Bronchitis; Pulmonary Diseases, Chronic (COPD). Institute for Scientific Information, 3501 Market St., Philadelphia, PA 19104. Phone: (800) 523-1850. Fax: (215) 386-6362. Weekly.

ANNUALS AND REVIEWS

Progress in Respiration Research. S. Karger Publishers, Inc., 26 West Avon Rd., P.O. Box 529, Farmington, CT 06085. Phone: (203) 675-7834. Fax: (203) 675-7302. Irregular.

ASSOCIATIONS, PROFESSIONAL SOCIETIES, ADVOCACY AND SUPPORT GROUPS

Association for the Care of Asthma. c/o Herbert Mansmann M.D., Jefferson Medical College, 1025 Walnut St., Philadelphia, PA 19107. Phone: (215) 928-8912.

Asthma and Allergy Foundation of America (AAFA). 1717 Massachusetts Ave., Ste. 305, Washington, DC 20036. Phone: (800) 7AS-THMA. Fax: (202) 462-2112.

Mothers of Asthmatics. 10875 Main St., Suite 210, Fairfax, VA 22030. Phone: (703) 385-4403.

National Foundation for Asthma (NFA). P.O. Box 30069, Tucson, AZ 85751. Phone: (602) 323-6046.

BIBLIOGRAPHIES

Asthma: Treatment and Therapy. National Technical Information Service, 5285 Port Royal Rd., Springfield, VA 22161. Phone: (703) 487-4650. Fax: (703) 321-8547. Jan. 1978-May 1989 PB89-863708/CBY.

Drugs for Bronchodilation and the Control of Bronchial Asthma. National Technical Information Service, 5285 Port Royal Rd., Springfield, VA 22161. Phone: (703) 487-4650. Fax: (703) 321-8547. Mar. 1985-Nov. 1989 PB90-854654/CBY.

DIRECTORIES

Asthma Resources Directory. Allergy Publications Inc., P.O. Box 640, Menlo Park, CA 94026. Phone: (415) 322-1663. 1990.

JOURNALS

The American Journal of Asthma & Allergy for Pediatricians. SLACK Inc., 6900 Grove Rd., Thorofare, NJ 08086-9447. Phone: (800) 257-8290. Fax: (609) 853-5991. Quarterly.

American Review of Respiratory Diseases. American Lung Association, 1740 Broadway, New York, NY 10019. Phone: (212) 315-8700. Fax: (212) 265-5642.

NEWSLETTERS

Asthma Update: A Newsletter for People with Asthma. Asthma Update, 123 Monticello Ave., Annapolis, MD 21401.

ONLINE DATABASES

Combined Health Information Database (CHID). U.S. National Institutes of Health, P.O. Box NDIC, Bethesda, MD 20892. Phone: (301) 496-2162. Fax: (301) 770-5164. Quarterly.

EMBASE. Elsevier Science Publishing Co., Inc., P.O. Box 882, Madison Square Station, New York, NY 10159-2101. Phone: (212) 989-5800. Fax: (212) 633-3990.

Journal of Allergy and Clinical Immunology. Mosby-Year Book, 11830 Westline Industrial Drive, St. Louis, MO 63146. Phone: (800) 325-4177. Fax: (314) 432-1380.

MEDLINE. National Library of Medicine, 8600 Rockville Pike, Bethesda, MD 20894. Phone: (800) 638-8480.

SciSearch. Institute for Scientific Information, 3501 Market St., Philadelphia, PA 19104. Phone: (215) 386-0100. Fax: (215) 386-6362.

POPULAR WORKS AND PATIENT EDUCATION

Asthma and Exercise. Hogshead. Holt, Rinehart & Winston, 115 W. 18th St., New York, NY 10011. Phone: (800) 488-5233. 1991.

The Asthma Self-Care Book. Geri Harrington. HarperCollins Pubs., Inc., 10 E. 53rd St., New York, NY 10022-5299. Phone: (212) 207-7000. Fax: (800) 242-7737. 1992.

The Asthma Self-Help Book: How to Live a Normal Life in Spite of Your Condition. Paul J. Hannaway. Prima Publishing, P.O. Box 1260, Rocklin, CA 95677-1260. Phone: (916) 786-0426. 1992.

Childhood Asthma: A Doctor's Complete Treatment Plan. Mike Whiteside. HarperCollins Pubs., Inc., 10 E. 53rd St., New York, NY 10022-5299. Phone: (212) 207-7000. Fax: (800) 242-7737. 1991.

Living Well with Chronic Asthma, Bronchitis, and Emphysema: A Complete Guide to Coping with Chronic Lung Disease. Myra B. Shayevitz, Berton R. Shayevitz. Consumer Reports Books, 9180 LeSaint Dr., Fairfield, OH 45014. Phone: (513) 860-1178. 1991.

Parents' Guide to Allergies & Asthma. Steinman. Bantam Doubleday Dell, Inc., 666 Fifth Ave., New York, NY 10103. Phone: (800) 223-6834. 1992.

RESEARCH CENTERS, INSTITUTES, CLEARINGHOUSES

Allergy Disease Research Laboratory. Mayo Clinic and Foundation, 200 First St. S.W., Rochester, MN 55905. Phone: (507) 284-8333.

Allergy Disease Research Laboratory. Mayo Clinic and Foundation. 200 First St. SW, Rochester, MN 55905. Phone: (507) 284-2789. Fax: (507) 284-1637.

Allergy & Immunology Center. University of Colorado. Division of Immunology, 4200 E. 9th Ave., CB 164, Denver, CO 80262. Phone: (303) 270-7601.

Asthma and Allergic Center. Johns Hopkins University. 5501 Hopkins Bayview Circle, Baltimore, MD 21224. Phone: (410) 550-2300. Fax: (410) 550-2101.

Asthma and Allergic Diseases Center. State University of New York Health Science Center at Stony Brook. Stony Brook, NY 11794. Phone: (516) 444-2272. Fax: (516) 444-2493.

Asthma & Allergic Diseases Center. University of Wisconsin-Madison. 600 Highland Ave., Madison, WI 53792. Phone: (608) 263-6201.

Autoimmune Disease Center. Scripps Clinic and Research Foundation. 10666 N. Torrey Pines Rd., La Jolla, CA 92037. Phone: (619) 554-8686. Fax: (619) 554-6805.

National Jewish Center for Immunology and Respiratory Medicine. 1400 Jackson St., Denver, CO 80206. Phone: (303) 388-4461.

TEXTBOOKS AND MONOGRAPHS

Allergic Diseases from Infancy to Adulthood. Charles Bierman, David Pearlman (eds.). W.B. Saunders Co., The Curtis Center, Independence Sqare W., Philadelphia, PA 19106-3399. Phone: (215) 238-7800. 2nd edition, 1988.

Allergies: Principles and Practice. Elliott Middleton Jr. (ed.). Mosby-Year Book, 11830 Westline Industrial Drive, St. Louis, MO 63146. Phone: (800) 325-4177. Fax: (314) 432-1380. 1988.

Asthma: Basic Mechanisms and Clinical Management. P.J. Barnes, I.W. Rodger, N.C. Thomson (eds.). Academic Press, Inc., 1250 Sixth Ave., San Diego, CA 92101-4311. Phone: (619) 699-6345. Fax: (619) 699-6715. Second edition 1992.

Managing Asthma. Miles Weinberger. Williams & Wilkins, 428 East Preston St., Baltimore, MD 21202. Phone: (800) 638-0672. Fax: (800) 447-8438. 1990.

Occupational Asthma. Emil J. Bardana Jr., Anthony Montanaro, Mark O'Hollaren. Mosby-Year Book, 11830 Westline Industrial Drive, St. Louis, MO 63146. Phone: (800) 325-4177. Fax: (314) 432-1380. 1991.

ASTIGMATISM

See: VISION DISORDERS

ATHEROSCLEROSIS

See also: HEART DISEASES

ABSTRACTING, INDEXING, AND CURRENT AWARENESS PUBLICATIONS

CA Selects: Atherosclerosis & Heart Disease. Chemical Abstracts Service, 2540 Olentangy River Road, P.O. Box 3012, Columbus, OH 43210-0012. Phone: (800) 848-6538. Biweekly.

Core Journals in Cardiology. Elsevier Science Publishing Co., Inc., P.O. Box 882, Madison Square Station, New York, NY 10159-2101. Phone: (212) 989-5800. Fax: (212) 633-3990. 11/year.

Current Contents/Clinical Medicine. Institute for Scientific Information, 3501 Market St., Philadelphia, PA 19104. Phone: (800) 523-1850. Fax: (215) 386-6362. Weekly.

Current Contents/Life Sciences. Institute for Scientific Information, 3501 Market St., Philadelphia, PA 19104. Phone: (215) 386-0100. Fax: (215) 386-6362.

Excerpta Medica. Section 18: Cardiovascular Disease and Cardiovascular Surgery. Elsevier Science Publishing Co., Inc., P.O. Box 882, Madison Square Station, New York, NY 10159-2101. Phone: (212) 989-5800. Fax: (212) 633-3990. 24/year.

Index Medicus. U.S. National Library of Medicine, 8600 Rockville Pike, Bethesda, MD 20894. Phone: (800) 638-8480. Monthly.

Research Alert: Atherosclerosis. Institute for Scientific Information, 3501 Market St., Philadelphia, PA 19104. Phone: (800) 523-1850. Fax: (215) 386-6362. Weekly.

Research Alert: Cardiovascular Diseases-Coronary Disease & Myocardial Infarction. Institute for Scientific Information, 3501 Market St., Philadelphia, PA 19104. Phone: (800) 523-1850. Fax: (215) 386-6362. Weekly.

Science Citation Index. Institute for Scientific Information, 3501 Market St., Philadelphia, PA 19104. Phone: (800) 523-1850. Fax: (215) 386-6362. Bimonthly.

ANNUALS AND REVIEWS

Acute Myocardial Infarction. Bernard Gersh, Shahbudin H. Rahimtoola (eds.). Elsevier Science Publishing Co., Inc., P.O. Box 882, Madison Square Station, New York, NY 10159-2101. Phone: (212) 989-5800. Fax: (212) 633-3990. 1991.

Atherosclerosis Reviews. Raven Press, 1185 Avenue of the Americas, New York, NY 10036. Phone: (212) 930-9500. Fax: (212) 869-3495. Irregular.

Current Opinion in Cardiology. Current Science Group, 20 N. Third St., Philadelphia, PA 19106-2199. Phone: (800) 552-5866. Fax: (215) 574-2270. Bimonthly.

Prevention and Noninvasive Therapy of Atherosclerosis. Alexander Leaf, Peter C. Weber. Raven Press, 1185 Avenue of the Americas, New York, NY 10036. Phone: (212) 930-9500. Fax: (212) 869-3495. Atherosclerosis Reviews. Volume 21. 1990.

Year Book of Cardiology. Mosby-Year Book, 11830 Westline Industrial Drive, St. Louis, MO 63146. Phone: (800) 325-4177. Fax: (314) 432-1380. Annual.

ASSOCIATIONS, PROFESSIONAL SOCIETIES, ADVOCACY AND SUPPORT GROUPS

American College of Cardiology (ACC). 9111 Old Georgetown Rd., Bethesda, MD 20814. Phone: (800) 253-4636. Fax: (301) 897-9745.

American Heart Association (AHA). 7320 Greenville Ave., Dallas, TX 75231. Phone: (214) 373-6300.

Clinical Research Institute of Montreal. 110 Pine Ave. W., Montreal, PQ, Canada H2W 1R7. Phone: (514) 987-5500. Fax: (514) 987-5679.

International Atherosclerosis Society (IAS). 6550 Fannin, No. 1423, Houston, TX 77030. Phone: (713) 790-4226. Fax: (713) 793-1080.

BIBLIOGRAPHIES

Nutri-Topics: Nutrition and Cardiovascular Disease. Food and Nutrition Center, National Agricultural Library, 10301 Baltimore Blvd., Beltsville, MD 20705.

CD-ROM DATABASES

Bibliomed Cardiology Disc. Healthcare Information Services, Inc., 2235 American River Dr., Suite 307, Sacramento, CA 95825. Phone: (800) 468-1128. Fax: (916) 648-8078. Quarterly.

Cardiology MEDLINE. MEP, 124 Mt. Auburn St., Cambridge, MA 02138. Phone: (800) 342-1338. Fax: (617) 868-7738. Quarterly.

Excerpta Medica CD: Cardiology. SilverPlatter Information, Inc., River Ridge Office Park, 100 River Ridge Rd., Norwood, MA 02062. Phone: (617) 769-2599. Fax: (617) 769-8763. Quarterly.

Hyperlipidemia. Hoffer. Williams & Wilkins, 428 East Preston St., Baltimore, MD 21202. Phone: (800) 638-0672. Fax: (800) 447-8438. 1992.

SCISEARCH. Institute for Scientific Information, 3501 Market St., Philadelphia, PA 19104. Phone: (215) 386-0100. Fax: (215) 386-6362.

ENCYCLOPEDIAS, DICTIONARIES, WORD BOOKS

Cardiology Words. Stedman. Williams & Wilkins, 428 East Preston St., Baltimore, MD 21202. Phone: (800) 638-0672. Fax: (800) 447-8438. 1992.

JOURNALS

American Journal of Cardiology. Reed Publishing USA, 249 W. 17th St., New York, NY 10011. Phone: (212) 645-0067. Fax: (212) 242-6987. 22/year.

Arteriosclerosis and Thrombosis: A Journal of Vascular Biology. American Heart Association, 7320 Greenville Ave., Dallas, TX 75231. Phone: (214) 706-1310. Fax: (214) 691-6342. Bimonthly.

Atherosclerosis. Elsevier Science Publishing Co., Inc., P.O. Box 882, Madison Square Station, New York, NY 10159-2101. Phone: (212) 989-5800. Fax: (212) 633-3990. 18/year.

British Heart Journal. BMJ Publishing Group, BMA House, Tavistock Square, London WC1H 9JR, England. Phone: 071383 6244/6638. Fax: 071383 6662. Monthly.

Coronary Artery Disease. Current Science Group, 20 N. Third St., Philadelphia, PA 19106-2199. Phone: (215) 574-2266. Fax: (215) 574-2270. Monthly.

NEWSLETTERS

Cardiac Alert. Phillips Publishing, Inc., 7811 Montrose Rd., Potomac, MD 20854. Phone: (800) 722-9000. Fax: (301) 897-9745. Monthly.

ONLINE DATABASES

EMBASE. Elsevier Science Publishing Co., Inc., P.O. Box 882, Madison Square Station, New York, NY 10159-2101. Phone: (212) 989-5800. Fax: (212) 633-3990.

MEDLINE. National Library of Medicine, 8600 Rockville Pike, Bethesda, MD 20894. Phone: (800) 638-8480.

SciSearch. Institute for Scientific Information, 3501 Market St., Philadelphia, PA 19104. Phone: (215) 386-0100. Fax: (215) 386-6362.

POPULAR WORKS AND PATIENT EDUCATION

The 8-Week Cholesterol Cure: How to Lower Your Blood Cholesterol by Up to 40 Percent Without Drugs or Deprivation.

Robert E. Kowalski. HarperCollins Publishers., Inc., 10 E. 53rd St., New York, NY 10022-5299. Phone: (212) 207-7000. Fax: (800) 242-7737. Revised edition 1990.

Coronary Heart Disease: The Facts. Desmond Julian, Claire Marley. Oxford University Press, 200 Madison Ave., New York, NY 10016. Phone: (212) 679-7300. Fax: (212) 725-2972. Second edition 1991.

Dr. Dean Ornish's Program for Reversing Heart Disease Without Drugs or Surgery. Dean Ornish. Ballantine Books, Inc., 201 E. 50th St., New York, NY 10022. Phone: (800) 726-0600. 1992.

The Heart Attack Handbook. Joseph S. Alpert. Consumer Reports Books, 9180 LeSaint Dr., Fairfield, OH 45014. Phone: (513) 860-1178. 1993.

Living with Angina: A Practical Guide to Dealing with Coronary Disease and Your Doctor. James A. Pantano. HarperCollins Pubs., Inc., 10 E. 53rd St., New York, NY 10022-5299. Phone: (212) 207-7000. Fax: (800) 242-7737. 1991.

Yale University School of Medicine Heart Book. Barry L. Zaret, Lawrence S. Cohen, Marvin Moser, and others. William Morrow & Company, Inc., 1350 Ave. of the Americas, New York, NY 10019. Phone: (800) 237-0657. 1992.

RESEARCH CENTERS, INSTITUTES, CLEARINGHOUSES

Arteriosclerosis Research Center. Wake Forest University. Dept. of Comparative Medicine, 300 S. Hawthorne Rd., Winston-Salem, NC 27103. Phone: (919) 764-3600. Fax: (919) 764-5818.

Center for Progressive Atherosclerosis Management. University of California, Berkeley. 3030 Telegraph Rd., Berkeley, CA 94705. Phone: (415) 540-1554.

Cleveland Clinic Foundation Research Institute. 9500 Euclid Ave., Cleveland, OH 44195-5210. Phone: (216) 444-3900. Fax: (216) 444-3279.

DeBakey Heart Center. Baylor College of Medicine. Texas Medical Center, 1 Baylor Plaza, Houston, TX 77030. Phone: (701) 797-9353. Fax: (713) 793-1192.

Framingham Heart Study. 5 Thurber St., Framingham, MA 01701. Phone: (508) 872-4386.

Hypertension/Atherosclerosis Unit. University of Virginia. Medical Center, Box 146, Charlottesville, VA 22908. Phone: (804) 924-2765. Fax: (804) 924-2581.

Institute of Arteriosclerosis Research. Westwood Horizon Retirement Hotel, 947 Tiverton Ave., Los Angeles, CA 90024. Phone: (213) 824-7552.

Lipoprotein and Atherosclerosis Research Program. Oklahoma Medical Research Foundation. 825 NE 13th St., Oklahoma City, OK 73104. Phone: (405) 271-7703. Fax: (405) 271-3980.

National Heart, Lung, and Blood Institute. 4733 Bethesda Ave., Ste. 530, Bethesda, MD 20814. Phone: (301) 951-3260.

Specialized Center of Research in Arteriosclerosis. University of California, San Diego. Dept. of Medicine, M-0613-D, La Jolla, CA 92093. Phone: (619) 534-0569. Fax: (619) 546-9828.

Specialized Center of Research in Atherosclerosis. University of Chicago. Dept. of Pathology, 5841 S. Maryland Ave., Box

414, Chicago, IL 60637. Phone: (312) 702-1268. Fax: (312) 702-3778.

TEXTBOOKS AND MONOGRAPHS

Atherosclerosis. Peter C. Weber. Raven Press, 1185 Ave. of the Americas, New York, NY 10036. Phone: (212) 930-9500. Fax: (212) 869-3495. 1991.

Disorders of Lipid Metabolism. Guido V. Marinetti. Plenum Publishing Co., 233 Spring St., New York, NY 10013-1578. Phone: (212) 620-8000. Fax: (212) 463-0742. 1990.

The Heart: Physiology and Metabolism. Lionel H. Opie. Raven Press, 1185 Avenue of the Americas, New York, NY 10036. Phone: (212) 930-9500. Fax: (212) 869-3495. Second edition 1991.

Heparin and the Prevention of Atherosclerosis: Basic Reserch and Clinical Application. Hyman Engelberg. John Wiley & Sons, Inc., 605 Third Ave., New York, NY 10158-0012. Phone: (212) 850-6000. Fax: (212) 850-6088. 1990.

Hyperlipidaemia. P.N. Durrington. Butterworth-Heinemann, 80 Montvale Ave., Stoneham, MA 02180. Phone: (617) 438-8464. Fax: (617) 279-4851. 1989.

Tobacco Smoking and Atherosclerosis: Pathogenesis and Cellular Mechanisms. John N. Diana (ed.). Plenum Publishing Co., 233 Spring St., New York, NY 10013-1578. Phone: (212) 620-8000. Fax: (212) 463-0742. 1990.

Working Group Report on Management of Patients with Hypertension and High Blood Cholesterol. National Heart, Lung, and Blood Institute, 4733 Bethesda Ave., Ste. 530, Bethesda, MD 20814. Phone: (301) 951-3260. NIH Pub. No. 90-2361 1990.

ATHLETE'S FOOT

See: FUNGAL DISEASES

ATHLETIC INJURIES

See: SPORTS MEDICINE

ATTENTION DEFICIT DISORDER

See also: HYPERACTIVITY

ABSTRACTING, INDEXING, AND CURRENT AWARENESS PUBLICATIONS

Index Medicus. U.S. National Library of Medicine, 8600 Rockville Pike, Bethesda, MD 20894. Phone: (800) 638-8480. Monthly.

Psychological Abstracts. American Psychological Association, 1200 17th St. NW, Washington, DC 20036. Phone: (202) 955-7600. Monthly.

Science Citation Index. Institute for Scientific Information, 3501 Market St., Philadelphia, PA 19104. Phone: (800) 523-1850. Fax: (215) 386-6362. Bimonthly.

ASSOCIATIONS, PROFESSIONAL SOCIETIES, ADVOCACY AND SUPPORT GROUPS

Attention-Deficit Disorder Association (ADDA). 8091 S. Ireland Way, Aurora, CO 80016. Phone: (303) 690-7548.

CHADD (Children with Attention Deficit Disorders). 1859 North Pine Island Rd., Suite 185, Plantation, FL 33322. Phone: (305) 587-3700.

National Center for Learning Disabilities. 99 Park Ave., New York, NY 10016. Phone: (212) 687-7211.

CD-ROM DATABASES

PsycLit. SilverPlatter Information, Inc., River Ridge Office Park, 100 River Ridge Rd., Norwood, MA 02062. Phone: (617) 769-2599. Fax: (617) 769-8763. Quarterly.

SCISEARCH. Institute for Scientific Information, 3501 Market St., Philadelphia, PA 19104. Phone: (215) 386-0100. Fax: (215) 386-6362.

HANDBOOKS, GUIDES, MANUALS, ATLASES

Attention-Deficit Hyperactivity Disorder: A Clinical Guide to Diagnosis and Treatment. Larry B. Silver. American Psychiatric Press, Inc., 1400 K St. NW, Washington, DC 20005. Phone: (202) 682-6268. Fax: (202) 789-2648. 1991.

JOURNALS

American Academy of Child and Adolescent Psychiatry Journal. Williams & Wilkins, 428 East Preston St., Baltimore, MD 21202. Phone: (800) 638-0672. Fax: (800) 447-8438.

Clinical Pediatrics. J.B. Lippincott Co., 227 E. Washington Square, Philadelphia, PA 19106-3780. Phone: (215) 238-4200. Fax: (215) 238-4227.

Journal of Pediatrics. Mosby-Year Book, 11830 Westline Industrial Drive, St. Louis, MO 63146. Phone: (800) 325-4177. Fax: (314) 432-1380. Monthly.

ONLINE DATABASES

EMBASE. Elsevier Science Publishing Co., Inc., P.O. Box 882, Madison Square Station, New York, NY 10159-2101. Phone: (212) 989-5800. Fax: (212) 633-3990.

MEDLINE. National Library of Medicine, 8600 Rockville Pike, Bethesda, MD 20894. Phone: (800) 638-8480.

SciSearch. Institute for Scientific Information, 3501 Market St., Philadelphia, PA 19104. Phone: (215) 386-0100. Fax: (215) 386-6362.

POPULAR WORKS AND PATIENT EDUCATION

The ADD Hyperactivity Workbook for Parents, Teachers, and Kids. H.C. Parker. Impact Publications, 1859 North Pine Island Rd., Suite 185, Plantation, FL 33322. Phone: (305) 587-3700.

Dr. Larry Silver's Advice to Parents on Attention-Deficit Hyperactivity Disorder. Larry B. Silver. American Psychiatric Press, Inc., 1400 K St. NW, Washington, DC 20005. Phone: (202) 682-6268. Fax: (202) 789-2648. 1992.

Help for the Hyperactive Child.. William G. Crook. Professional Books/Future Health, Inc., P.O. Box 3246, Jackson, TN 38301. Phone: (901) 423-5400. 1991.

Helping Your Hyperactive Child: From Effective Treatments and Developing Discipline and Self-Esteem to Helping Your Family Adjust. John F. Taylor. Prima Publishing, P.O. Box 1260, Rocklin, CA 95677-1260. Phone: (916) 786-0426. 1990.

Parent's Guide to Attention Deficit Disorders. Lisa J. Bain. Doubleday & Co., Inc., 666 Fifth Ave., New York, NY 10103. Phone: (800) 223-6834. 1991.

Your Hyperactive Child: A Parent's Guide to Coping with Attention Deficit Disorder. B.D. Ingersoll. Bantam Doubleday Dell, 666 Fifth Ave., New York, NY 10103. Phone: (800) 223-6834. 1988.

RESEARCH CENTERS, INSTITUTES, CLEARINGHOUSES

Carrier Foundation Division of Research. P.O. Box 147, Belle Mead, NJ 08502. Phone: (908) 281-1000.

Child Study Centre. University of Ottawa. School of Psychology, 120 University Priv., Ottawa, ON, Canada K1N 6N5. Phone: (613) 564-2249. Fax: (613) 564-7898.

AUDIOLOGY

See also: COMMUNICATION DISORDERS; HEARING DISORDERS

ABSTRACTING, INDEXING, AND CURRENT AWARENESS PUBLICATIONS

Science Citation Index. Institute for Scientific Information, 3501 Market St., Philadelphia, PA 19104. Phone: (800) 523-1850. Fax: (215) 386-6362. Bimonthly.

ASSOCIATIONS, PROFESSIONAL SOCIETIES, ADVOCACY AND SUPPORT GROUPS

American Hearing Research Foundation. 55 E. Washington St., Suite 2022, Chicago, IL 60602. Phone: (312) 726-9670.

American Speech-Language-Hearing Association (ASHA). 10801 Rockville Pike, Rockville, MD 20852. Phone: (301) 897-5700. Fax: (301) 571-0457.

National Hearing Aid Society (NHAS). 20361 Middlebelt Rd., Livonia, MI 48152. Phone: (313) 478-2610. Fax: (313) 478-4520.

CD-ROM DATABASES

SCISEARCH. Institute for Scientific Information, 3501 Market St., Philadelphia, PA 19104. Phone: (215) 386-0100. Fax: (215) 386-6362.

ENCYCLOPEDIAS, DICTIONARIES, WORD BOOKS

Encyclopedia of Deafness and Hearing Disorders. Carol Turkington, Allen Sussman. Facts on File, Inc., 460 Park Ave. S., New York, NY 10016-7382. Phone: (212) 683-2244. Fax: (212) 683-3633. 1992.

JOURNALS

British Journal of Audiology. Academic Press, Inc., 1250 Sixth Ave., San Diego, CA 92101-4311. Phone: (619) 699-6345. Fax: (619) 699-6715.

European Journal of Disorders of Communication. Whurr Publishers, P.O. Box 1897, Lawrence, KS 66044-8897. Phone: (913) 843-1221. Fax: (913) 843-1274. 4/year.

Hearing Journal. Laux Company, 63 Great Rd., Maynard, MA 01754. Phone: (617) 897-5552.

NEWSLETTERS

American Hearing Research Foundation Newsletter. American Hearing Research Foundation, 55 E. Washington St., Ste. 2022, Chicago, IL 60602. Quarterly.

POPULAR WORKS AND PATIENT EDUCATION

Living with Tinnitus. David W. Rees, Simon D. Smith. St. Martin's Press, 175 Fifth Ave., New York, NY 10010. Phone: (212) 674-5151. 1992.

RESEARCH CENTERS, INSTITUTES, CLEARINGHOUSES

Eaton-Peabody Laboratory of Auditory Physiology. Massachusetts Eye and Ear Infirmary, 243 Charles St., Boston, MA 02114. Phone: (617) 573-3745. Fax: (617) 720-4408.

Gallaudet Research Institute. Gallaudet University. 800 Florida Ave. NE, Washington, DC 20002. Phone: (202) 651-5400.

Hearing Research Laboratory. State University of New York at Buffalo. 215 parker Hall, Buffalo, NY 14214. Phone: (716) 831-2001. Fax: (716) 636-2893.

House Ear Institute. 2100 W. 3rd St., 5th Fl., Los Angeles, CA 90057. Phone: (213) 483-4431. Fax: (213) 413-6739.

Kresge Hearing Research Institute. University of Michigan. 1301 E. Ann St., Room 5032, Ann Arbor, MI 48109-0506. Phone: (313) 764-8111. Fax: (313) 764-0014.

Self-Help for Hard of Hearing People. 7800 Wisconsin Ave., Bethesda, MD 20814. Phone: (301) 657-2248.

TEXTBOOKS AND MONOGRAPHS

Hearing: An Introduction to Psychological and Physical. Marcel Dekker, Inc., 270 Madison Ave., New York, NY 10016. Phone: (800) 228-1160.

Successful Interactive Skills for Speech-Language Pathologists and Audiologists. Dorothy Molyneaux, Vera W. Lane. Aspen Publishers, Inc., 200 Orchard Ridge Dr., Gaithersburg, MD 20878. Phone: (800) 638-8437. 1990.

AUTISM

ABSTRACTING, INDEXING, AND CURRENT AWARENESS PUBLICATIONS

Core Journals in Clinical Neurology. Elsevier Science Publishing Co., Inc., P.O. Box 882, Madison Square Station, New York, NY 10159-2101. Phone: (212) 989-5800. Fax: (212) 633-3990. 11/year.

Current Contents/Clinical Medicine. Institute for Scientific Information, 3501 Market St., Philadelphia, PA 19104. Phone: (800) 523-1850. Fax: (215) 386-6362. Weekly.

Excerpta Medica. Section 32: Psychiatry. Elsevier Science Publishing Co., Inc., P.O. Box 882, Madison Square Station, New York, NY 10159-2101. Phone: (212) 989-5800. Fax: (212) 633-3990. 20/year.

Index Medicus. U.S. National Library of Medicine, 8600 Rockville Pike, Bethesda, MD 20894. Phone: (800) 638-8480. Monthly.

Psychological Abstracts. American Psychological Association, 1200 17th St. NW, Washington, DC 20036. Phone: (202) 955-7600. Monthly.

Research Alert: Autism. Institute for Scientific Information, 3501 Market St., Philadelphia, PA 19104. Phone: (800) 523-1850. Fax: (215) 386-6362. Weekly.

Science Citation Index. Institute for Scientific Information, 3501 Market St., Philadelphia, PA 19104. Phone: (800) 523-1850. Fax: (215) 386-6362. Bimonthly.

ANNUALS AND REVIEWS

Adolescent Psychiatry. American Society for Adolescent Psychiatry, 5530 Wisconsin Ave. N.W., Ste. 1149, Washington, DC 20015. Phone: (301) 652-0646. Annual.

Contemporary Psychiatry. Plenum Publishing Co., 233 Spring St., New York, NY 10013-1578. Phone: (212) 620-8000. Fax: (212) 463-0742. Quarterly.

Year Book of Psychiatry. Mosby-Year Book, 11830 Westline Industrial Drive, St. Louis, MO 63146. Phone: (800) 325-4177. Fax: (314) 432-1380. Annual.

ASSOCIATIONS, PROFESSIONAL SOCIETIES, ADVOCACY AND SUPPORT GROUPS

Autism Services Center (ASC). Douglass Educ. Bldg., 10th Ave. and Bruce St., Huntington, WV 25701. Phone: (304) 525-8014. Fax: (304) 525-8026.

Autism Society of America (ASA). 8601 Georgia Ave., Ste. 503, Silver Spring, MD 20910. Phone: (301) 565-0433.

CD-ROM DATABASES

Excerpta Medica CD: Psychiatry. SilverPlatter Information, Inc., River Ridge Office Park, 100 River Ridge Rd., Norwood, MA 02062. Phone: (617) 769-2599. Fax: (617) 769-8763. Quarterly.

PsycLit. SilverPlatter Information, Inc., River Ridge Office Park, 100 River Ridge Rd., Norwood, MA 02062. Phone: (617) 769-2599. Fax: (617) 769-8763. Quarterly.

SCISEARCH. Institute for Scientific Information, 3501 Market St., Philadelphia, PA 19104. Phone: (215) 386-0100. Fax: (215) 386-6362.

DIRECTORIES

Autism Society of Canada-Directory of Services and Resources. Autism Society Canada, 1550 Enterprise Rd., Ste. 300, Mississauga, ON, Canada L4W 4P4. Phone: (416) 795-0088. 1984.

HANDBOOKS, GUIDES, MANUALS, ATLASES

Handbook of Autism: A Guide for Parents and Professionals. Maureen Aarons, Tessa Gittens. Routledge, Chapman & Hall, Inc., 29 W. 35th St., New York, NY 10001-2291. Phone: (212) 244-3336. 1992.

JOURNALS

American Journal of Psychiatry. American Psychiatric Press, Inc., 1400 K St. NW, Washington, DC 20005. Phone: (202) 682-6268. Fax: (202) 789-2648. Monthly.

Archives of General Psychiatry. American Medical Association, 515 North State St., Chicago, IL 60610. Phone: (312) 464-0183. Fax: (312) 464-5834. Monthly.

British Journal of Psychiatry. Royal Society of Medicine Services Ltd., 1 Wimpole St., London W1M 8AE, England. Phone: 071-408 2119. Fax: 071-355 3198. Monthly.

Lancet. Williams & Wilkins, 428 East Preston St., Baltimore, MD 21202. Phone: (800) 638-0672. Fax: (800) 447-8438. Weekly.

Pediatrics. American Academy of Pediatrics, 141 Northwest Point Rd., Elk Grove Village, IL 60009-0927. Phone: (708) 228-5005. Fax: (708) 228-5097. Monthly.

Psychological Medicine. Cambridge University Press, 40 W. 20th St., New York, NY 10011. Phone: (800) 431-1580. Quarterly.

NEWSLETTERS

Autism Society of America-Advocate. Autism Society of America, 1234 Massachusetts Ave. N.W., Ste. 1017, Washington, DC 20005. Phone: (202) 783-0125. Fax: (202) 783-7435. Quarterly.

ONLINE DATABASES

EMBASE. Elsevier Science Publishing Co., Inc., P.O. Box 882, Madison Square Station, New York, NY 10159-2101. Phone: (212) 989-5800. Fax: (212) 633-3990.

MEDLINE. National Library of Medicine, 8600 Rockville Pike, Bethesda, MD 20894. Phone: (800) 638-8480.

PsycInfo. SilverPlatter Information, Inc., River Ridge Office Park, 100 River Ridge Rd., Norwood, MA 02062. Phone: (617) 769-2599. Fax: (617) 769-8763. Quarterly.

SciSearch. Institute for Scientific Information, 3501 Market St., Philadelphia, PA 19104. Phone: (215) 386-0100. Fax: (215) 386-6362.

POPULAR WORKS AND PATIENT EDUCATION

Children with Autism: A Parents' Guide. Michael Powers (ed.). Woodbine House, 5615 Fishers Ln., Rockville, MD 20852. Phone: (800) 843-7323. 1989.

RESEARCH CENTERS, INSTITUTES, CLEARINGHOUSES

Autism Research Institute. 4182 Adams Ave., San Diego, CA 92116. Phone: (619) 281-7165. Fax: (619) 563-6840.

National Autism Hotline (NAH). Prihard Bldg., 605 9th St., P.O. Box 507, Huntington, WV 25710-0507. Phone: (304) 525-8014. Fax: (304) 525-8026.

TEXTBOOKS AND MONOGRAPHS

Adapted Physical Education for Students with Autism. Kimberly Davis. Charles C. Thomas, Publisher, 2600 S. First St., Springfield, IL 62794-9265. Phone: (800) 250-8980. 1990.

Autism and Asperger Syndrome. Uta Frith. Cambridge University Press, 40 W. 20th St., New York, NY 10011. Phone: (800) 431-1580. 1991.

Autism: Nature, Diagnosis, and Treatment. Geraldine Dawson (ed.). Guilford Publications, Inc., 72 Spring St., New York, NY 10012. Phone: (800) 365-7006. Fax: (212) 966-6708. 1989.

Autistic Behaviors: Experimental Analysis and Treatment Applications. O. Ivar Lovaas. Irvington Publishers, 522 E. 82nd St., New York, NY 10028. Phone: (212) 472-4494. 1990.

Child and Adolescent Psychiatry: A Comprehensive Textbook. Melvin Lewis. Williams & Wilkins, 428 East Preston St., Baltimore, MD 21202. Phone: (800) 638-0672. Fax: (800) 447-8438. 1991.

Chronic Schizophrenia and Adult Autism: Issues in Diagnosis, Assessment and Psychological Treatment. Johnny L. Matson (ed.). Springer Publishing Co., Inc., 536 Broadway, 11th Floor, New York, NY 10012. Phone: (212) 431-4370. 1989.

Psychiatric Disorders in Children and Adolescents. Barry D. Garfinkel and others. W.B. Saunders Co., The Curtis Center, Independence Square W., Philadelphia, PA 19106-3399. Phone: (215) 238-7800. 1990.

Rett Syndrome and Autism. Haas. Mosby-Year Book, 11830 Westline Industrial Drive, St. Louis, MO 63146. Phone: (800) 325-4177. Fax: (314) 432-1380. 1988.

AUTOIMMUNE DISEASES

See also: IMMUNOLOGY

ABSTRACTING, INDEXING, AND CURRENT AWARENESS PUBLICATIONS

Current Contents/Clinical Medicine. Institute for Scientific Information, 3501 Market St., Philadelphia, PA 19104. Phone: (800) 523-1850. Fax: (215) 386-6362. Weekly.

Current Contents/Life Sciences. Institute for Scientific Information, 3501 Market St., Philadelphia, PA 19104. Phone: (215) 386-0100. Fax: (215) 386-6362.

Excerpta Medica. Section 26: Immunology, Serology and Transplantation. Elsevier Science Publishing Co., Inc., P.O. Box 882, Madison Square Station, New York, NY 10159-2101. Phone: (212) 989-5800. Fax: (212) 633-3990. 32/year.

Index Medicus. U.S. National Library of Medicine, 8600 Rockville Pike, Bethesda, MD 20894. Phone: (800) 638-8480. Monthly.

Research Alert: Immunopathology-Autoimmune Disease. Institute for Scientific Information, 3501 Market St., Philadelphia, PA 19104. Phone: (800) 523-1850. Fax: (215) 386-6362. Weekly.

Science Citation Index. Institute for Scientific Information, 3501 Market St., Philadelphia, PA 19104. Phone: (800) 523-1850. Fax: (215) 386-6362. Bimonthly.

ANNUALS AND REVIEWS

Advances in Immunology. Academic Press, Inc., 1250 Sixth Ave., San Diego, CA 92101-4311. Phone: (619) 699-6345. Fax: (619) 699-6715. Irregular.

Annual Review of Immunology. Annual Reviews Inc., 4139 El Camino Way, P.O. Box 10139, Palo Alto, CA 94303-0897. Phone: (415) 493-4400. Fax: (415) 855-9815. Annual.

Autoimmune Endocrine Disease. Anthony P. Weetman. Cambridge University Press, 40 W. 20th St., New York, NY 10011. Phone: (800) 431-1580. Cambridge Reviews in Clinical Immunology volume 1 1992.

Contemporary Topics in Immunobiology. Plenum Publishing Co., 233 Spring St., New York, NY 10013-1578. Phone: (212) 620-8000. Fax: (212) 463-0742. Irregular.

Critical Reviews in Immunology. CRC Press, Inc., 2000 Corporate Blvd. N.W., Boca Raton, FL 33431. Phone: (407) 994-0555. Fax: (407) 997-0949. Quarterly.

Current Opinion in Immunology. Current Science Group, 20 N. Third St., Philadelphia, PA 19106-2199. Phone: (800) 552-5866. Fax: (215) 574-2270. Bimonthly.

Developments in Immunology. Elsevier Science Publishing Co., Inc., P.O. Box 882, Madison Square Station, New York, NY 10159-2101. Phone: (212) 989-5800. Fax: (212) 633-3990. Irregular.

Immunological Reviews. Munksgaard International Publishers Ltd., P.O. Box 2148, DK-1016, Copenhagen K, Denmark. Phone: 33-127030. Fax: 33-129387. Bimonthly.

Immunology and Allergy Clinics. W.B. Saunders Co., The Curtis Center, Independence Square W., Philadelphia, PA 19106-3399. Phone: (215) 238-7800. Quarterly.

The Year in Immunology. S. Karger Publishers, Inc., 26 West Avon Rd., P.O. Box 529, Farmington, CT 06085. Phone: (203) 675-7834. Fax: (203) 675-7302. Annual.

CD-ROM DATABASES

Excerpta Medica CD: Immunology & AIDS. SilverPlatter Information, Inc., River Ridge Office Park, 100 River Ridge Rd., Norwood, MA 02062. Phone: (617) 769-2599. Fax: (617) 769-8763. Quarterly.

SCISEARCH. Institute for Scientific Information, 3501 Market St., Philadelphia, PA 19104. Phone: (215) 386-0100. Fax: (215) 386-6362.

DIRECTORIES

American Academy of Allergy & Immunology-Membership Directory. American Academy of Allergy & Immunology, 611 E. Wells St., Milwaukee, WI 53202. Phone: (414) 272-6071. Fax: (414) 276-3349. Biennial.

Directory of Certified Allergists/Immunologists. American Board of Medical Specialties, 1 Rotary Center, Suite 805, Evanston, IL 60201. Phone: (708) 491-9091. Biennial.

ENCYCLOPEDIAS, DICTIONARIES, WORD BOOKS

Dictionary of Immunology. F. Rosen and others (eds.). Macmillan Publishing Co., 866 Third Ave., New York, NY 10011. Phone: (800) 257-5755. 1988.

HANDBOOKS, GUIDES, MANUALS, ATLASES

The Handbook of Immunopharmacology. Academic Press, Inc., 1250 Sixth Ave., San Diego, CA 92101-4311. Phone: (619) 699-6345. Fax: (619) 699-6715. Irregular.

JOURNALS

Cellular Immunology. Academic Press, Inc., 1250 Sixth Ave., San Diego, CA 92101-4311. Phone: (619) 699-6345. Fax: (619) 699-6715. 14/year.

Clinical and Experimental Immunology. Blackwell Scientific Publications Ltd., Osney Mead, Oxon. OX2 OEL, England. Phone: 0865-240201. Fax: 0865-721205. Monthly.

Immunologic Research. S. Karger Publishers, Inc., 26 West Avon Rd., P.O. Box 529, Farmington, CT 06085. Phone: (203) 675-7834. Fax: (203) 675-7302. Quarterly.

Immunological Investigations. Marcel Dekker, Inc., 270 Madison Ave., New York, NY 10016. Phone: (800) 228-1160. 8/year.

Immunology. Blackwell Scientific Publications, Inc., 3 Cambridge Ctr., Cambridge, MA 02142. Phone: (800) 759-6102. Monthly.

Journal of Immunological Methods. Elsevier Science Publishing Co., Inc., P.O. Box 882, Madison Square Station, New York, NY 10159-2101. Phone: (212) 989-5800. Fax: (212) 633-3990. 20/year.

Journal of Immunology. Williams & Wilkins, 428 E. Preston St., Baltimore, MD 21202. Phone: (800) 638-0672. Fax: (800) 447-8438. Semimonthly.

Mediators of Inflammation. Rapid Communications of Oxford Ltd., The Old Malthouse, Paradise St., Oxford OX1 1LD, England. Phone: 44-865-790447. Fax: 44-865-244012. 6/year.

ONLINE DATABASES

CSA Life Sciences Collection. Cambridge Scientific Abstracts, 7200 Wisconsin Ave., Bethesda, MD 20814-4823. Phone: (800) 843-7751. Fax: (301) 961-6720.

EMBASE. Elsevier Science Publishing Co., Inc., P.O. Box 882, Madison Square Station, New York, NY 10159-2101. Phone: (212) 989-5800. Fax: (212) 633-3990.

MEDLINE. National Library of Medicine, 8600 Rockville Pike, Bethesda, MD 20894. Phone: (800) 638-8480.

SciSearch. Institute for Scientific Information, 3501 Market St., Philadelphia, PA 19104. Phone: (215) 386-0100. Fax: (215) 386-6362.

RESEARCH CENTERS, INSTITUTES, CLEARINGHOUSES

Arthritis Center. University of Missouri-Columbia. MA427 Health Sciences Center, 1 Hospital Dr., Columbia, MO 65212. Phone: (314) 882-8738. Fax: (314) 884-3996.

Autoimmune Disease Center. Scripps Clinic and Research Foundation. 10666 N. Torrey Pines Rd., La Jolla, CA 92037. Phone: (619) 554-8686. Fax: (619) 554-6805.

Center for Multidisciplinary Research in Immunology and DIseases at UCLA. UCLA School of Medicine, 12-262 Factor Bldg., Los Angeles, CA 90024. Phone: (213) 825-1510. Fax: (213) 206-3865.

Lupus Study Center. Hahnemann University. 221 N. Broad St., Philadelphia, PA 19107. Phone: (215) 448-7300.

Mary Imogene Bassett Medical Research Institute. 1 Atwell Rd., Cooperstown, NY 13326. Phone: (607) 547-3045. Fax: (607) 547-3061.

Scripps Research Institute. 10666 N. Torrey Pines Rd., La Jolla, CA 92037. Phone: (619) 554-8265. Fax: (619) 554-9899.

TEXTBOOKS AND MONOGRAPHS

Basic and Clinical Immunology. Daniel P. Stites, Abba T. Terr. Appleton & Lange, 25 Van Zant St., East Norwalk, CT 06855. Phone: (800) 423-1359. Fax: (203) 854-9486. Seventh edition 1990.

Basic Human Immunology. Stites, Terr (eds.). Appleton & Lange, 25 Van Zant St., East Norwalk, CT 06855. Phone: (800) 423-1359. Fax: (203) 854-9486. 1991.

Fundamental Immunology. William E. Paul. Raven Press, 1185 Avenue of the Americas, New York, NY 10036. Phone: (212) 930-9500. Fax: (212) 869-3495. Second edition 1989.

The Mosaic of Autoimmunity: The Factors Associated with Autoimmune Disease. Y. Shoenfeld, D. Isenberg. Elsevier Science Publishing Co., Inc., P.O. Box 882, Madison Square Station, New York, NY 10159-2101. Phone: (212) 989-5800. Fax: (212) 633-3990. Research Monographs in Immunology. 1989.

B

BACKACHE

ABSTRACTING, INDEXING, AND CURRENT AWARENESS PUBLICATIONS

Current Contents/Clinical Medicine. Institute for Scientific Information, 3501 Market St., Philadelphia, PA 19104. Phone: (800) 523-1850. Fax: (215) 386-6362. Weekly.

Index Medicus. U.S. National Library of Medicine, 8600 Rockville Pike, Bethesda, MD 20894. Phone: (800) 638-8480. Monthly.

Science Citation Index. Institute for Scientific Information, 3501 Market St., Philadelphia, PA 19104. Phone: (800) 523-1850. Fax: (215) 386-6362. Bimonthly.

CD-ROM DATABASES

SCISEARCH. Institute for Scientific Information, 3501 Market St., Philadelphia, PA 19104. Phone: (215) 386-0100. Fax: (215) 386-6362.

JOURNALS

East West: The Journal of Natural Health and Living. East West Journal, Inc., 17 Station St., P.O. Box 1200, Brookline, MA 02146. Monthly.

NEWSLETTERS

Back Pain Monitor. American Health Consultants, Department C1290, P.O. Box 740060, Atlanta, GA 30374. Phone: (800) 559-1032. Fax: (404) 352-1971. Monthly.

ONLINE DATABASES

EMBASE. Elsevier Science Publishing Co., Inc., P.O. Box 882, Madison Square Station, New York, NY 10159-2101. Phone: (212) 989-5800. Fax: (212) 633-3990.

MEDLINE. National Library of Medicine, 8600 Rockville Pike, Bethesda, MD 20894. Phone: (800) 638-8480.

SciSearch. Institute for Scientific Information, 3501 Market St., Philadelphia, PA 19104. Phone: (215) 386-0100. Fax: (215) 386-6362.

POPULAR WORKS AND PATIENT EDUCATION

Back in Shape: A Back Owner's Manual. Stephen Hochschuler. Houghton Mifflin Co., 1 Beacon St., Boston, MA 02108. Phone: (800) 225-3362. 1991.

The Backpower Program. David Imrie, Lu Barbuto. John Wiley & Sons, Inc., 605 Third Ave., New York, NY 10158-0012. Phone: (212) 850-6000. Fax: (212) 850-6088. 1990.

Care of the Low Back: A Patient Guide. Garth S. Russell, Thomas R. Highland. F.A. Davis Co., 1915 Arch St., Philadelphia, PA 19103. Phone: (800) 523-4049. Fax: (215) 568-5065. 1990.

No More Back Pain: A Proven Program to Free Yourself from Back Pain for Life. Alfred O. Bonati, Shirley Linde. Pharos Books, 200 Park Ave., New York, NY 10166. Phone: (212) 692-3830. 1991.

Your Aching Back: A Doctor's Guide to Relief. Augustus White. Simon & Schuster, Inc., 1230 Ave. of the Americas, New York, NY 10020. Phone: (212) 698-7000. Revised edition 1990.

RESEARCH CENTERS, INSTITUTES, CLEARINGHOUSES

Texas Back Institute Research Foundation. 3801 W. 15th St., Ste. 300, Plano, TX 75075-7788. Phone: (214) 867-2225. Fax: (214) 612-6387.

TEXTBOOKS AND MONOGRAPHS

Backache. McNab. Williams & Wilkins, 428 East Preston St., Baltimore, MD 21202. Phone: (800) 638-0672. Fax: (800) 447-8438. Second edition 1990.

Diagnosis and Treatment of Low Back Pain. Kahnovitz. Raven Press, 1185 Ave. of the Americas, New York, NY 10036. Phone: (212) 930-9500. Fax: (212) 869-3495. 1991.

Low Back Pain: An Historical and Contemporary Overview of the Occupational, Medical and Psychosocial Issues of Chronic Back Pain. Peter Mandell, Marvin H. Lipton, Joseph Burnstein, and others. SLACK Inc., 6900 Grove Rd., Thorofare, NJ 08086-9447. Phone: (800) 257-8290. Fax: (609) 853-5991. 1989.

Mechanical Low Back Pain: Perspectives in Functional Anatomy. James A. Porterfield, Carl DeRosa. W.B. Saunders Co., The Curtis Center, Independence Square W., Philadelphia, PA 19106-3399. Phone: (215) 238-7800. 1991.

Occupational Low Back Pain. Pope. Mosby-Year Book, 11830 Westline Industrial Drive, St. Louis, MO 63146. Phone: (800) 325-4177. Fax: (314) 432-1380. 1991.

BACTERIAL INFECTIONS

See: INFECTIOUS DISEASES

BACTERIOLOGY

ABSTRACTING, INDEXING, AND CURRENT AWARENESS PUBLICATIONS

Biological Abstracts. BIOSIS, 2100 Arch St., Philadelphia, PA 19103-1399. Phone: (800) 523-4800. Fax: (215) 587-2016.

BIOSIS/CAS Selects: Bacterial & Viral Genetics. BIOSIS, 2100 Arch St., Philadelphia, PA 19103-1399. Phone: (215) 587-4800. Fax: (215) 587-2016. Biweekly.

Current Contents/Life Sciences. Institute for Scientific Information, 3501 Market St., Philadelphia, PA 19104. Phone: (215) 386-0100. Fax: (215) 386-6362.

General Science Index. H.W. Wilson Co., 950 University Ave., Bronx, NY 10452. Phone: (800) 367-6770.

Index Medicus. U.S. National Library of Medicine, 8600 Rockville Pike, Bethesda, MD 20894. Phone: (800) 638-8480. Monthly.

Microbiology Abstracts. Section B: Bacteriology. Cambridge Scientific Abstracts, 7200 Wisconsin Ave., Bethesda, MD 20814-4823. Phone: (800) 843-7751. Fax: (301) 961-6720. Monthly.

CD-ROM DATABASES

Biological Abstracts on Compact Disc. BIOSIS, 2100 Arch St., Philadelphia, PA 19103-1399. Phone: (800) 523-4800. Fax: (215) 587-2016. Quarterly.

ENCYCLOPEDIAS, DICTIONARIES, WORD BOOKS

Bergey's Bacteria Words. Stedman. Williams & Wilkins, 428 East Preston St., Baltimore, MD 21202. Phone: (800) 638-0672. Fax: (800) 447-8438. 1992.

HANDBOOKS, GUIDES, MANUALS, ATLASES

Bergey's Manual of Determinative Bacteriology. Holt. Williams & Wilkins, 428 East Preston St., Baltimore, MD 21202. Phone: (800) 638-0672. Fax: (800) 447-8438. Ninth edition 1992.

Bergey's Manual of Systematic Bacteriology. John G. Holt (ed.). Williams & Wilkins, 428 E. Preston St., Baltimore, MD 21202. Phone: (800) 638-0672. Fax: (800) 447-8438. Four volumes 1989.

JOURNALS

International Journal of Systematic Bacteriology. American Society for Microbiology, 1325 Massachusetts Ave. N.W., Washington, DC 20005. Phone: (202) 737-3600.

Journal of Applied Bacteriology. Blackwell Scientific Publications, Inc., 3 Cambridge Center, Cambridge, MA 02142. Phone: (800) 759-6102.

Journal of Bacteriology. American Society for Microbiology, 1325 Massachusetts Ave. N.W., Washington, DC 20005. Phone: (202) 737-3600.

ONLINE DATABASES

BIOSIS Previews. BIOSIS, 2100 Arch St., Philadelphia, PA 19103-1399. Phone: (800) 523-4800. Fax: (215) 587-2016.

CSA Life Sciences Collection. Cambridge Scientific Abstracts, 7200 Wisconsin Ave., Bethesda, MD 20814-4823. Phone: (800) 843-7751. Fax: (301) 961-6720.

EMBASE. Elsevier Science Publishing Co., Inc., P.O. Box 882, Madison Square Station, New York, NY 10159-2101. Phone: (212) 989-5800. Fax: (212) 633-3990.

MEDLINE. National Library of Medicine, 8600 Rockville Pike, Bethesda, MD 20894. Phone: (800) 638-8480.

SciSearch. Institute for Scientific Information, 3501 Market St., Philadelphia, PA 19104. Phone: (215) 386-0100. Fax: (215) 386-6362.

RESEARCH CENTERS, INSTITUTES, CLEARINGHOUSES

Laboratory of Bacteriology and Immunology. 1230 York Ave., Rockefeller University, New York, NY 10021. Phone: (212) 570-8000.

TEXTBOOKS AND MONOGRAPHS

Medical Bacteriology. J.D. Sleigh, M.C. Timbury. Churchill Livingstone Inc., 650 Ave. of the Americas, New York, NY 10011. Phone: (212) 819-5400. Fax: (212) 302-6598. Third edition 1990.

BARBITURATES

See: DRUGS

BASAL CELL CARCINOMA

See: SKIN CANCER

BEHAVIORAL MEDICINE

ABSTRACTING, INDEXING, AND CURRENT AWARENESS PUBLICATIONS

Behavioral Medicine Abstracts. Society of Behavioral Medicine, P.O. Box 8530, University Station, Knoxville, TN 37996. Phone: (615) 974-5164. Quarterly.

Current Contents/Clinical Medicine. Institute for Scientific Information, 3501 Market St., Philadelphia, PA 19104. Phone: (800) 523-1850. Fax: (215) 386-6362. Weekly.

Index Medicus. U.S. National Library of Medicine, 8600 Rockville Pike, Bethesda, MD 20894. Phone: (800) 638-8480. Monthly.

Science Citation Index. Institute for Scientific Information, 3501 Market St., Philadelphia, PA 19104. Phone: (800) 523-1850. Fax: (215) 386-6362. Bimonthly.

ANNUALS AND REVIEWS

Developmental-Behavioral Disorders: Selected Topics. Marvin I. Gottlieb, John E. Williams (eds.). Plenum Publishing Co., 233 Spring St., New York, NY 10013-1578. Phone: (212) 620-8000. Fax: (212) 463-0742. Critical Issues in Developmental and Behavioral Pediatrics. Volume 3. 1991.

ASSOCIATIONS, PROFESSIONAL SOCIETIES, ADVOCACY AND SUPPORT GROUPS

Academy of Behavioral Medicine Research. 4301 Jones Bridge Rd., Bethesda, MD 20814. Phone: (301) 295-3270.

American Academy of Behavioral Medicine. 6750 Hillcrest Plaza, Suite 304, Dallas, TX 75230. Phone: (214) 458-8333.

Association for Advancement of Behavior Therapy (AABT). 15 W. 36th St., New York, NY 10018. Phone: (212) 279-7970. Fax: (212) 239-8038.

Society of Behavioral Medicine. P.O. Box 8530, University Station, Knoxville, TN 37996. Phone: (615) 974-5164.

CD-ROM DATABASES

PsycLit. SilverPlatter Information, Inc., River Ridge Office Park, 100 River Ridge Rd., Norwood, MA 02062. Phone: (617) 769-2599. Fax: (617) 769-8763. Quarterly.

SCISEARCH. Institute for Scientific Information, 3501 Market St., Philadelphia, PA 19104. Phone: (215) 386-0100. Fax: (215) 386-6362.

DIRECTORIES

Academy of Behavioral Medicine Research Membership Directory. Academy of Behavioral Medicine Research, 4301 Jones Bridge Rd., Bethesda, MD 20889-4799. Phone: (301) 295-3270. Fax: (301) 295-3270. Annual.

HANDBOOKS, GUIDES, MANUALS, ATLASES

Handbook of Clinical Behavior Therapy. Samuel M. Turner and others (eds.). John Wiley & Sons, Inc., 605 Third Ave., New York, NY 10158-0012. Phone: (212) 850-6000. Fax: (212) 850-6088. Second edition 1992.

JOURNALS

Annals of Behavioral Medicine. Society of Behavioral Medicine, 103 S. Adams St., Rockville, MD 20850. Phone: (301) 251-2790. Fax: (301) 279-6749. Quarterly.

Behavior Therapy. Association for the Advancement of Behavior Therapy, 15 W. 30th St., New York, NY 10018. Phone: (212) 279-7970.

Behavioral Medicine. Heldref Publications, 4000 Albermarle St. N.W., Washington, DC 20016. Phone: (202) 362-6445. Quarterly.

Behavioral Psychotherapy. Academic Press, Inc., 1250 Sixth Ave., San Diego, CA 92101-4311. Phone: (619) 699-6345. Fax: (619) 699-6715.

Behavioural Pharmacology. Rapid Communications of Oxford Ltd., The Old Malthouse, Paradise St., Oxford OX1 1LD, England. Phone: 44-865-790447. Fax: 44-865-244012. 6/year.

ONLINE DATABASES

EMBASE. Elsevier Science Publishing Co., Inc., P.O. Box 882, Madison Square Station, New York, NY 10159-2101. Phone: (212) 989-5800. Fax: (212) 633-3990.

MEDLINE. National Library of Medicine, 8600 Rockville Pike, Bethesda, MD 20894. Phone: (800) 638-8480.

SciSearch. Institute for Scientific Information, 3501 Market St., Philadelphia, PA 19104. Phone: (215) 386-0100. Fax: (215) 386-6362.

RESEARCH CENTERS, INSTITUTES, CLEARINGHOUSES

Center for Advanced Study in Behavioral Sciences. 202 Juniper Sera Blvd., Stanford, CA 94305. Phone: (415) 321-2052.

TEXTBOOKS AND MONOGRAPHS

Behavioral Pediatrics. Graydanaus. Springer-Verlag New York Inc., 175 Fifth Ave., New York, NY 10010. Phone: (212) 460-1500. Fax: (212) 473-6272. 1992.

Behavioral Science. Fadem. Williams & Wilkins, 428 East Preston St., Baltimore, MD 21202. Phone: (800) 638-0672. Fax: (800) 447-8438. 1991.

BENZODIAZEPINES

See: PSYCHOACTIVE DRUGS

BILIARY DISORDERS

See also: LIVER DISEASES

ABSTRACTING, INDEXING, AND CURRENT AWARENESS PUBLICATIONS

Core Journals in Gastroenterology. Elsevier Science Publishing Co., Inc., P.O. Box 882, Madison Square Station, New York, NY 10159-2101. Phone: (212) 989-5800. Fax: (212) 633-3990. 11/year.

Current Contents/Clinical Medicine. Institute for Scientific Information, 3501 Market St., Philadelphia, PA 19104. Phone: (800) 523-1850. Fax: (215) 386-6362. Weekly.

Excerpta Medica. Section 48: Gastroenterology. Elsevier Science Publishing Co., Inc., P.O. Box 882, Madison Square Station, New York, NY 10159-2101. Phone: (212) 989-5800. Fax: (212) 633-3990. 20/year.

Index Medicus. U.S. National Library of Medicine, 8600 Rockville Pike, Bethesda, MD 20894. Phone: (800) 638-8480. Monthly.

Science Citation Index. Institute for Scientific Information, 3501 Market St., Philadelphia, PA 19104. Phone: (800) 523-1850. Fax: (215) 386-6362. Bimonthly.

ANNUALS AND REVIEWS

Annual of Gastrointestinal Endoscopy. Current Science Group, 20 N. Third St., Philadelphia, PA 19106-2199. Phone: (800) 552-5866. Fax: (215) 574-2270. Annual.

Current Gastroenterology. Mosby-Year Book, 11830 Westline Industrial Drive, St. Louis, MO 63146. Phone: (800) 325-4177. Fax: (314) 432-1380. Annual.

Current Opinion in Gastroenterology. Current Science Group, 20 N. Third St., Philadelphia, PA 19106-2199. Phone: (800) 552-5866. Fax: (215) 574-2270. Bimonthly.

Frontiers of Gastrointestinal Research. S. Karger Publishers, Inc., 26 West Avon Rd., P.O. Box 529, Farmington, CT 06085. Phone: (203) 675-7834. Fax: (203) 675-7302. Irregular.

Gastroenterology Annual. Elsevier Science Publishing Co., Inc., P.O. Box 882, Madison Square Station, New York, NY 10159-2101. Phone: (212) 989-5800. Fax: (212) 633-3990. Annual.

Gastroenterology Clinics. W.B. Saunders Co., The Curtis Center, Independence Square W., Philadelphia, PA 19106-3399. Phone: (215) 238-7800. Quarterly.

ASSOCIATIONS, PROFESSIONAL SOCIETIES, ADVOCACY AND SUPPORT GROUPS

American Association for the Study of Liver Diseases (AASLD). 6900 Grove Rd., Thorofare, NJ 08086. Phone: (800) 257-8290. Fax: (609) 853-5991.

American Liver Foundation (ALF). 1425 Pompton Ave., Cedar Grove, NJ 07009. Phone: (201) 256-2550. Fax: (201) 661-4027.

Children's Liver Foundation (CLF). 14245 Ventura Blvd., Ste. 201, Sherman Oaks, CA 91423. Phone: (800) 526-1593.

International Biliary Association. c/o Larry C. Carey M.D., Dept. of Surgery, University Hospital, 410 W. Tenth Ave., Columbus, OH 43210.

International Hepato-Biliary-Pancreatic Association (IHBPA). c/o A.R. Moossa, University of California, San Diego, Dept. of Surgery, 225 W. Dickenson St., San Diego, CA 92103. Phone: (619) 543-5860.

CD-ROM DATABASES

Excerpta Medica CD: Gastroenterology. SilverPlatter Information, Inc., River Ridge Office Park, 100 River Ridge Rd., Norwood, MA 02062. Phone: (617) 769-2599. Fax: (617) 769-8763. Quarterly.

Gastroenterology and Hepatology MEDLINE. MEP, 124 Mt. Auburn St., Cambridge, MA 02138. Phone: (800) 342-1338. Fax: (617) 868-7738. Quarterly.

SCISEARCH. Institute for Scientific Information, 3501 Market St., Philadelphia, PA 19104. Phone: (215) 386-0100. Fax: (215) 386-6362.

HANDBOOKS, GUIDES, MANUALS, ATLASES

A Color Atlas of Liver Disease. S. Sherlock, J.A. Summerfield. Mosby-Year Book, 11830 Westline Industrial Drive, St. Louis, MO 63146. Phone: (800) 325-4177. Fax: (314) 432-1380. Second edition 1991.

Handbook of Drug Therapy in Liver and Kidney Disease. Schrier. Little, Brown and Co., 34 Beacon St., Boston, MA 02108. Phone: (617) 227-0730. Fax: (617) 227-0790. 1991.

JOURNALS

American Journal of Gastroenterology. Williams & Wilkins, 428 E. Preston St., Baltimore, MD 21202. Phone: (800) 638-0672. Fax: (800) 447-8438. Monthly.

Hepatology. Mosby-Year Book, 11830 Westline Industrial Drive, St. Louis, MO 63146. Phone: (800) 325-4177. Fax: (314) 432-1380. Monthly.

The New England Journal of Medicine. Massachusetts Medical Society, 1440 Main St., Waltham, MA 02154-1649. Phone: (617) 893-3800. Fax: (617) 893-0413. Weekly.

ONLINE DATABASES

EMBASE. Elsevier Science Publishing Co., Inc., P.O. Box 882, Madison Square Station, New York, NY 10159-2101. Phone: (212) 989-5800. Fax: (212) 633-3990.

MEDLINE. National Library of Medicine, 8600 Rockville Pike, Bethesda, MD 20894. Phone: (800) 638-8480.

SciSearch. Institute for Scientific Information, 3501 Market St., Philadelphia, PA 19104. Phone: (215) 386-0100. Fax: (215) 386-6362.

RESEARCH CENTERS, INSTITUTES, CLEARINGHOUSES

Liver Research Unit. 7601 East Imperial Highway, University of Southern California, Downey, CA 90242. Phone: (213) 940-8961.

Liver Study Unit. Billings Hospital, 950 E. 59th St., University of Chicago, Chicago, IL 60637. Phone: (312) 702-9790.

National Digestive Diseases Information Clearinghouse (NDDIC). P.O. Box NDDIC, Bethesda, MD 20892. Phone: (301) 468-6344.

TEXTBOOKS AND MONOGRAPHS

Complications of Chronic Liver Disease. Rector. Mosby-Year Book, 11830 Westline Industrial Drive, St. Louis, MO 63146. Phone: (800) 325-4177. Fax: (314) 432-1380. 1992.

Diseases of the Liver. Leon Schiff, Eugenee R. Schiff. J.B. Lippincott Co., 227 E. Washington Square, Philadelphia, PA 19106-3780. Phone: (215) 238-4200. Fax: (215) 238-4227. Sixth edition 1987.

Diseases of the Liver and Biliary System. Sherlock. Blackwell Scientific Publications, Inc., 3 Cambridge Ctr., Cambridge, MA 02142. Phone: (800) 759-6102. Ninth edition 1992.

Hepatology: A Textbook of Liver Disease. David Zakim, Thomas D. Boyer. W.B. Saunders Co., The Curtis Center, Independence Square W., Philadelphia, PA 19106-3399. Phone: (215) 238-7800. Second edition 1990.

Lithotripsy and Related Techniques for Gallstone Treatment. Paumgartner. Mosby-Year Book, 11830 Westline Industrial Drive, St. Louis, MO 63146. Phone: (800) 325-4177. Fax: (314) 432-1380. 1991.

Liver and Biliary Diseases. Neil Kaplowitz. Williams & Wilkins, 428 East Preston St., Baltimore, MD 21202. Phone: (800) 638-0672. Fax: (800) 447-8438. 1992.

The Liver and Biliary System. Gitnick. Mosby-Year Book, 11830 Westline Industrial Drive, St. Louis, MO 63146. Phone: (800) 325-4177. Fax: (314) 432-1380. 1991.

Liver Diseases. Leavy. Mosby-Year Book, 11830 Westline Industrial Drive, St. Louis, MO 63146. Phone: (800) 325-4177. Fax: (314) 432-1380. 1991.

Liver Function. Derek Cramp, Ewart Carson (eds.). Routledge, Chapman & Hall, Inc., 29 W. 35th St., New York, NY 10001-2291. Phone: (212) 244-3336. 1990.

Progress in Liver Diseases. Hans Popper, Fenton Schaffner (eds.). W.B. Saunders Co., The Curtis Center, Independence Square W., Philadelphia, PA 19106-3399. Phone: (215) 238-7800. Irregular.

Shock Wave Lithotripsy 2: Urinary and Biliary Lithotripsy. James E. Lingeman, Daniel M. Newman (eds.). Plenum Publishing Co., 233 Spring St., New York, NY 10013-1578. Phone: (212) 620-8000. Fax: (212) 463-0742. 1989.

Textbook of Liver and Biliary Surgery. William C. Meyers, R. Scott Jones. J.B. Lippincott Co., 227 E. Washington Square, Philadelphia, PA 19106-3780. Phone: (215) 238-4200. Fax: (215) 238-4227. 1990.

Wright's Liver and Biliary Disease. G.H. Millward-Sadler, M. Arthur. W.B. Saunders Co., The Curtis Center, Independence Square W., Philadelphia, PA 19106-3399. Phone: (215) 238-7800. Third edition 1991.

BIOCHEMISTRY

ABSTRACTING, INDEXING, AND CURRENT AWARENESS PUBLICATIONS

Biochemistry Abstracts. Part 1: Biological Membranes. Cambridge Scientific Abstracts, 7200 Wisconsin Ave., Bethesda, MD 20814-4823. Phone: (800) 843-7751. Fax: (301) 961-6720. Monthly.

Biochemistry Abstracts. Part 2: Nucleic Acids. Cambridge Scientific Abstracts, 7200 Wisconsin Ave., Bethesda, MD 20814-4823. Phone: (800) 843-7751. Fax: (301) 961-6720. Monthly.

Biochemistry Abstracts. Part 3: Amino-Acids, Peptides & Proteins. Cambridge Scientific Abstracts, 7200 Wisconsin Ave., Bethesda, MD 20814-4823. Phone: (800) 843-7751. Fax: (301) 961-6720. Monthly.

Biological Abstracts. BIOSIS, 2100 Arch St., Philadelphia, PA 19103-1399. Phone: (800) 523-4800. Fax: (215) 587-2016.

Biological and Agricultural Index. H W Wilson Co., 950 University Ave., Bronx, NY 10452. Phone: (800) 367-6770.

CA Selects: Antitumor Agents. Chemical Abstracts Service, 2540 Olentangy River Road, P.O. Box 3012, Columbus, OH 43210-0012. Phone: (800) 848-6538. Biweekly.

Chemical Abstracts. Chemical Abstracts Service, 2540 Olentangy River Rd., P.O. Box 3012, Columbus, OH 43210-0012. Phone: (800) 848-6538.

Chemical Abstracts: Biochemistry Sections. Chemical Abstracts Service, 2540 Olentangy River Road, P.O. Box 3012, Columbus, OH 43210-0012. Phone: (800) 848-6538. Biweekly.

Current Contents/Life Sciences. Institute for Scientific Information, 3501 Market St., Philadelphia, PA 19104. Phone: (215) 386-0100. Fax: (215) 386-6362.

Excerpta Medica. Section 29: Clinical and Experimental Biochemistry. Elsevier Science Publishing Co., Inc., P.O. Box 882, Madison Square Station, New York, NY 10159-2101. Phone: (212) 989-5800. Fax: (212) 633-3990. 40/year.

General Science Index. H.W. Wilson Co., 950 University Ave., Bronx, NY 10452. Phone: (800) 367-6770.

ANNUALS AND REVIEWS

Annual Review of Biochemistry. Annual Reviews Inc., 4139 El Camino Way, P.O. Box 10139, Palo Alto, CA 94303-0897. Phone: (415) 493-4400. Fax: (415) 855-9815. Annual.

Critical Reviews in Biochemistry and Molecular Biology. CRC Press, Inc., 2000 Corporate Blvd. N.W., Boca Raton, FL 33431. Phone: (407) 994-0555. Fax: (407) 997-0949. Bimonthly.

ASSOCIATIONS, PROFESSIONAL SOCIETIES, ADVOCACY AND SUPPORT GROUPS

American Society for Biochemistry and Molecular Biology. 9650 Rockville Pike, Bethesda, MD 20814. Phone: (301) 530-7145.

Association of Vitamin Chemists. c/o Deborah Becker, 801 Wankegan Rd., Glenview, IL 60025. Phone: (708) 998-7457.

CD-ROM DATABASES

Animated Pathways in Biochemistry. Marks. Williams & Wilkins, 428 East Preston St., Baltimore, MD 21202. Phone: (800) 638-0672. Fax: (800) 447-8438. Two parts, 1988.

Biological Abstracts on Compact Disc. BIOSIS, 2100 Arch St., Philadelphia, PA 19103-1399. Phone: (800) 523-4800. Fax: (215) 587-2016. Quarterly.

Cambridge Biochemistry Abstracts Series, Parts 1, 2, 3. Cambridge Scientific Abstracts, 7200 Wisconsin Ave., Bethesda, MD 20814-4823. Phone: (800) 843-7751. Fax: (301) 961-6720.

JOURNALS

Annals of Clinical Biochemistry. Royal Society of Medicine Services Ltd., 1 Wimpole St., London W1M 8AE, England. Phone: 071-408 2119. Fax: 071-355 3198. 6/year.

Biochemical Journal. Portland Press, Box 32, Commerce Way, Colchester, Essex C02 8HP, England. Phone: 44206-46351. Fax: 44206-549331. Semimonthly.

Biochemistry. American Chemical Society, 1155 16th St. N.W., Washington, DC 20036. Phone: (202) 872-4600. Fax: (202) 872-6005.

Biochimica et Biophysica Acta. Elsevier Science Publishing Co., Inc., P.O. Box 882, Madison Square Station, New York, NY 10159-2101. Phone: (212) 989-5800. Fax: (212) 633-3990.

Clinical Biochemistry. Pergamon Press, 660 White Plains Rd., Tarrytown, NY 10591-5153. Phone: (914) 592-7700. Fax: (914) 592-3625. 6/year.

Journal of Biological Chemistry. American Society for Biochemistry and Molecular Biology, Inc., 9650 Rockville Pike, Bethesda, MD 20814. Phone: (301) 530-7150. Fax: (301) 571-1824.

Molecular and Cellular Biochemistry: International Journal for Chemical Biology in Health and Disease. Kluwer Academic Publishers, P.O. Box 358, Accord Station, Hingham, MA 02018-0358. Phone: (617) 871-6600. Fax: (617) 871-6528. 20/year.

ONLINE DATABASES

BIOSIS Previews. BIOSIS, 2100 Arch St., Philadelphia, PA 19103-1399. Phone: (800) 523-4800. Fax: (215) 587-2016.

CA File (Chemical Abstracts File). Chemical Abstracts Service, 2540 Olentangy River Rd., P.O. Box 3012, Columbus, OH 43210-0012. Phone: (800) 848-6538.

CSA Life Sciences Collection. Cambridge Scientific Abstracts, 7200 Wisconsin Ave., Bethesda, MD 20814-4823. Phone: (800) 843-7751. Fax: (301) 961-6720.

RESEARCH CENTERS, INSTITUTES, CLEARINGHOUSES

Biochemical Epidemiology and Lipid Research Core Laboratory. Stadium Gate 27, 611 Beacon St. S.E., Minneapolis, MN 55455. Phone: (612) 624-2183.

Boston Biomedical Research Institute. 20 Staniford St., Boston, MA 02114. Phone: (617) 742-2010.

Center for Biomedical Research. University of Kansas. Smissman Research Laboratories, 2099 Constant Ave., Lawrence, KS 66046. Phone: (913) 864-5140.

General Clinical Research Center at Harbor-UCLA Medical Center. 1000 W. Carson St., Torrance, CA 90509. Phone: (213) 533-2503. Fax: (213) 320-6515.

Southwest Biomedical Research Institute. 6401 E. Thomas Rd., Scottsdale, AZ 85251. Phone: (602) 945-4363. Fax: (602) 947-8220.

TEXTBOOKS AND MONOGRAPHS

Biochemistry. Friedman. Little, Brown and Co., 34 Beacon St., Boston, MA 02108. Phone: (617) 227-0730. Fax: (617) 227-0790. Fourth edition 1992.

Biochemistry: A Review with Questions and Explanations. Paul Jay Friedman. Little, Brown and Company, 34 Beacon St., Boston, MA 02108. Phone: (617) 227-0730. Fourth edition 1992.

Biochemistry Illustrated. P.N. Campbell, A.D. Smith. Churchill Livingstone Inc., 650 Ave. of the Americas, New York, NY 10011. Phone: (212) 819-5400. Fax: (212) 302-6598. Second edition 1988.

Clinical Chemistry. Marshall. Raven Press, 1185 Ave. of the Americas, New York, NY 10036. Phone: (212) 930-9500. Fax: (212) 869-3495. 1991.

Harper's Biochemistry. Robert K. Murray, Peter A. Mayes, and others. Appleton & Lange, 25 Van Zant St., East Norwalk, CT 06855. Phone: (800) 423-1359. Fax: (203) 854-9486. 22nd edition 1990.

BIOETHICS

See: MEDICAL ETHICS

BIOFEEDBACK

See also: ALTERNATIVE MEDICINE

ABSTRACTING, INDEXING, AND CURRENT AWARENESS PUBLICATIONS

Complementary Medicine Index. Medical Information Service, British Library, Boston Spa, Wetherby, W. Yorkshire LS23 7BQ, England. Phone: 0937-546039. Fax: 0937-546236. Monthly.

Index Medicus. U.S. National Library of Medicine, 8600 Rockville Pike, Bethesda, MD 20894. Phone: (800) 638-8480. Monthly.

Psychological Abstracts. American Psychological Association, 1200 17th St. NW, Washington, DC 20036. Phone: (202) 955-7600. Monthly.

Science Citation Index. Institute for Scientific Information, 3501 Market St., Philadelphia, PA 19104. Phone: (800) 523-1850. Fax: (215) 386-6362. Bimonthly.

ASSOCIATIONS, PROFESSIONAL SOCIETIES, ADVOCACY AND SUPPORT GROUPS

American Association of Biofeedback Clinicians. 2424 Dempster St., Des Plaines, IL 60016. Phone: (312) 827-0440.

American Board of Clinical Biofeedback. 2424 Dempster St., Des Plaines, IL 60016. Phone: (312) 827-0440.

Biofeedback Society of America. c/o Francine Butler, 10200 W. 44th Ave., # 304, Wheat Ridge, CO 80033. Phone: (303) 422-8436.

BIBLIOGRAPHIES

Biofeedback Training and Instrumentation. National Technical Information Service, 5285 Port Royal Rd., Springfield, VA 22161. Phone: (703) 487-4650. Fax: (703) 321-8547. Jan. 1975-Jun. 1989 PB89-865497/CBY.

CD-ROM DATABASES

SCISEARCH. Institute for Scientific Information, 3501 Market St., Philadelphia, PA 19104. Phone: (215) 386-0100. Fax: (215) 386-6362.

DIRECTORIES

Bio Feedback Therapists Directory. American Business Directories, Inc., 5711 S. 86th Circle, Omaha, NE 68127. Phone: (402) 593-4600. Fax: (402) 331-1505. Annual.

JOURNALS

Alternative Medicine. V.S.P. International Science Publishers, P.O. Box 346, 3700 AH, Zeist, Netherlands. Phone: 03404-51902. Fax: 03404-58620. Quarterly.

Biofeedback and Self Regulation. Plenum Publishing Co., 233 Spring St., New York, NY 10013-1578. Phone: (212) 620-8000. Fax: (212) 463-0742. Quarterly.

East West: The Journal of Natural Health and Living. East West Journal, Inc., 17 Station St., P.O. Box 1200, Brookline, MA 02146. Monthly.

NEWSLETTERS

Biofeedback Clinician. American Association of Biofeedback Clinicians, 2424 Dempster, Des Plaines, IL 60016. Phone: (312) 827-0440. Quarterly.

ONLINE DATABASES

EMBASE. Elsevier Science Publishing Co., Inc., P.O. Box 882, Madison Square Station, New York, NY 10159-2101. Phone: (212) 989-5800. Fax: (212) 633-3990.

MEDLINE. National Library of Medicine, 8600 Rockville Pike, Bethesda, MD 20894. Phone: (800) 638-8480.

SciSearch. Institute for Scientific Information, 3501 Market St., Philadelphia, PA 19104. Phone: (215) 386-0100. Fax: (215) 386-6362.

RESEARCH CENTERS, INSTITUTES, CLEARINGHOUSES

Pain Center. University of Alabama at Birmingham. UAB Medical Center, 1813 6th Ave., Birmingham, AL 35233. Phone: (205) 934-6174.

TEXTBOOKS AND MONOGRAPHS

Biofeedback: Principles and Practice for Clinicians. Williams & Wilkins, 428 East Preston St., Baltimore, MD 21202. Phone: (800) 638-0672. Fax: (800) 447-8438. 1989.

BIOMECHANICS

See also: BIOMEDICAL ENGINEERING

ABSTRACTING, INDEXING, AND CURRENT AWARENESS PUBLICATIONS

Bioengineering and Biotechnology Abstracts. Engineering Information Inc., 345 E. 47th St., New York, NY 10017-2387. Phone: (800) 221-1044. Fax: (212) 832-1857.

Excerpta Medica. Section 27: Biophysics, Bioengineering and Medical Instrumentation. Elsevier Science Publishing Co., Inc., P.O. Box 882, Madison Square Station, New York, NY 10159-2101. Phone: (212) 989-5800. Fax: (212) 633-3990. 10/year.

General Science Index. H.W. Wilson Co., 950 University Ave., Bronx, NY 10452. Phone: (800) 367-6770.

Index Medicus. U.S. National Library of Medicine, 8600 Rockville Pike, Bethesda, MD 20894. Phone: (800) 638-8480. Monthly.

ASSOCIATIONS, PROFESSIONAL SOCIETIES, ADVOCACY AND SUPPORT GROUPS

Association for the Advancement of Medical Instrumentation (AAMI). 3330 Washington Blvd., Ste. 400, Arlington, VA 22201-4598. Phone: (800) 332-2264. Fax: (703) 276-0793.

CD-ROM DATABASES

Biotechnology Citation Index. Institute for Scientific Information, 3501 Market St., Philadelphia, PA 19104. Phone: (215) 386-0100. Fax: (215) 386-6362. Bimonthly.

JOURNALS

Clinical Biomechanics. Clinical Biomechanics Co., Box 35185, Los Angeles, CA 90035.

Journal of Biomechanics. Pergamon Press, 660 White Plains Rd., Tarrytown, NY 10591-5153. Phone: (914) 592-7700. Fax: (914) 592-3625. Monthly.

ONLINE DATABASES

EMBASE. Elsevier Science Publishing Co., Inc., P.O. Box 882, Madison Square Station, New York, NY 10159-2101. Phone: (212) 989-5800. Fax: (212) 633-3990.

MEDLINE. National Library of Medicine, 8600 Rockville Pike, Bethesda, MD 20894. Phone: (800) 638-8480.

SciSearch. Institute for Scientific Information, 3501 Market St., Philadelphia, PA 19104. Phone: (215) 386-0100. Fax: (215) 386-6362.

RESEARCH CENTERS, INSTITUTES, CLEARINGHOUSES

Bioengineering Research Institute. Rice University. P.O. Box 1892, Houston, TX 77251. Phone: (713) 527-4954. Fax: (713) 285-5154.

Biomedical Engineering Center. 2015 Neil Ave., Ohio State University, Columbus, OH 43210. Phone: (614) 422-6014.

Joint Program in Biomedical Engineering. University of Texas Southwestern Medical Center at Dallas. 5323 Harry Hines Blvd., Rm. G8.248, Dallas, TX 75235-9031. Phone: (214) 688-2052. Fax: (214) 688-2979.

BIOMEDICAL ENGINEERING

See also: BIOMECHANICS; PROSTHESES

ABSTRACTING, INDEXING, AND CURRENT AWARENESS PUBLICATIONS

Bioengineering and Biotechnology Abstracts. Engineering Information Inc., 345 E. 47th St., New York, NY 10017-2387. Phone: (800) 221-1044. Fax: (212) 832-1857.

Engineering Index. Engineering Information Inc., 345 E. 47th St., New York, NY 10017.

Excerpta Medica. Section 27: Biophysics, Bioengineering and Medical Instrumentation. Elsevier Science Publishing Co., Inc., P.O. Box 882, Madison Square Station, New York, NY 10159-2101. Phone: (212) 989-5800. Fax: (212) 633-3990. 10/year.

General Science Index. H.W. Wilson Co., 950 University Ave., Bronx, NY 10452. Phone: (800) 367-6770.

Index Medicus. U.S. National Library of Medicine, 8600 Rockville Pike, Bethesda, MD 20894. Phone: (800) 638-8480. Monthly.

Research Alert: Biomaterials. Institute for Scientific Information, 3501 Market St., Philadelphia, PA 19104. Phone: (800) 523-1850. Fax: (215) 386-6362. Weekly.

ANNUALS AND REVIEWS

Critical Reviews in Biomedical Engineering. CRC Press, Inc., 2000 Corporate Blvd. N.W., Boca Raton, FL 33431. Phone: (407) 994-0555. Fax: (407) 997-0949. Bimonthly.

ASSOCIATIONS, PROFESSIONAL SOCIETIES, ADVOCACY AND SUPPORT GROUPS

Association for the Advancement of Medical Instrumentation (AAMI). 3330 Washington Blvd., Ste. 400, Arlington, VA 22201-4598. Phone: (800) 332-2264. Fax: (703) 276-0793.

Biomedical Engineering Society (BMES). P.O. Box 2399, Culver City, CA 90231. Phone: (213) 206-6443.

Canadian Medical and Biological Engineering Society. Room 305, Bldg. M-50, National Research Council, Ottawa, ON,

Canada K1A 0R8. Phone: (613) 993-1686. Fax: (613) 952-7998.

Society for Biomaterials. c/o L. Rachel Sellers, SBD Box 49, University of Alabama, Birmingham, AL 35294. Phone: (205) 934-1525.

BIBLIOGRAPHIES

Biomedical Engineering: Artificial Hearts and Heart Valves. National Technical Information Service, 5285 Port Royal Rd., Springfield, VA 22161. Phone: (703) 487-4650. Fax: (703) 321-8547. Jan. 1975-Nov. 1989 PB90-852971/CBY.

CD-ROM DATABASES

Biotechnology Citation Index. Institute for Scientific Information, 3501 Market St., Philadelphia, PA 19104. Phone: (215) 386-0100. Fax: (215) 386-6362. Bimonthly.

HANDBOOKS, GUIDES, MANUALS, ATLASES

Handbook of Biomedical Engineering. Jacob Kline. Academic Press, Inc., 1250 Sixth Ave., San Diego, CA 92101-4311. Phone: (619) 699-6345. Fax: (619) 699-6715. 1988.

JOURNALS

Bio-Medical Materials and Engineering: An International Journal. Pergamon Press, Inc., 395 Saw Mill River Rd., Elmsford, NY 10523. Phone: (914) 592-7700. Fax: (914) 592-3625. 4/year.

Journal of Biomedical Engineering. Butterworth-Heinemann, 80 Montvale Ave., Stoneham, MA 02180. Phone: (617) 438-8464. Fax: (617) 279-4851. Bimonthly.

Journal of Medical Engineering & Technology. Taylor & Francis Inc., 1900 Frost Rd., Suite 101, Bristol, PA 19007-1598. Phone: (800) 821-8312. Fax: (215) 785-5515. Bimonthly.

NEWSLETTERS

Biomedical Technology Information Service. Quest Publishing Co., 1351 Titan Way, Brea, CA 92621. Phone: (714) 738-6400. Semimonthly.

ONLINE DATABASES

COMPENDEX. Engineering Information Inc., 345 E. 47th St., New York, NY 10017.

CSA Life Sciences Collection. Cambridge Scientific Abstracts, 7200 Wisconsin Ave., Bethesda, MD 20814-4823. Phone: (800) 843-7751. Fax: (301) 961-6720.

EMBASE. Elsevier Science Publishing Co., Inc., P.O. Box 882, Madison Square Station, New York, NY 10159-2101. Phone: (212) 989-5800. Fax: (212) 633-3990.

MEDLINE. National Library of Medicine, 8600 Rockville Pike, Bethesda, MD 20894. Phone: (800) 638-8480.

SciSearch. Institute for Scientific Information, 3501 Market St., Philadelphia, PA 19104. Phone: (215) 386-0100. Fax: (215) 386-6362.

RESEARCH CENTERS, INSTITUTES, CLEARINGHOUSES

Bioengineering Center. Georgia Institute of Technology. Atlanta, GA 30332-0100. Phone: (404) 894-7063. Fax: (404) 894-2291.

Bioengineering Research Institute. Rice University. P.O. Box 1892, Houston, TX 77251. Phone: (713) 527-4954. Fax: (713) 285-5154.

Biomedical Engineering Laboratories. Arizona State University.. College of Engineering, COB B-338, Tempe, AZ 85287. Phone: (602) 965-3676. Fax: (602) 965-8296.

Biomedical Engineering and Science Institute. Drexel University. 32nd and Chestnut Sts., Philadelphia, PA 19104. Phone: (215) 895-2215. Fax: (215) 895-4983.

Department of Biomedical Engineering. Rensselaer Polytechnic Institute. Jonsson Engineering Center, Troy, NY 12180-6959. Phone: (518) 276-6959. Fax: (518) 276-3035.

Engineering Research Center for Emerging Cardiovascular Technologies. Duke University. Dept. of Biomedical Engineering, 301 School of Engineering, Durham, NC 27706. Phone: (919) 684-8783. Fax: (919) 684-8886.

Institute for Biomedical Engineering. University of Utah. Dumke Bldg., Salt Lake City, UT 84112. Phone: (801) 581-6991. Fax: (801) 581-4044.

Joint Program in Biomedical Engineering. University of Texas Southwestern Medical Center at Dallas. 5323 Harry Hines Blvd., Rm. G8.248, Dallas, TX 75235-9031. Phone: (214) 688-2052. Fax: (214) 688-2979.

William A. Hillenbrand Biomedical Engineering Center. Purdue University. A.A. Potter Engineering Center, Room 204, West Lafayette, IN 47907. Phone: (317) 494-2995. Fax: (317) 494-0811.

BIOSTATISTICS

ABSTRACTING, INDEXING, AND CURRENT AWARENESS PUBLICATIONS

General Science Index. H.W. Wilson Co., 950 University Ave., Bronx, NY 10452. Phone: (800) 367-6770.

ANNUALS AND REVIEWS

Annual Review of Public Health. Annual Reviews Inc., 4139 El Camino Way, P.O. Box 10139, Palo Alto, CA 94303-0897. Phone: (415) 493-4400. Fax: (415) 855-9815. Annual.

Statistical Methods in Medical Research. Cambridge University Press, 40 W. 20th St., New York, NY 10011. Phone: (800) 431-1580. 3/year.

ASSOCIATIONS, PROFESSIONAL SOCIETIES, ADVOCACY AND SUPPORT GROUPS

Society for Epidemiologic Research. 624 N. Broadway, Suite 225, Baltimore, MD 21205. Phone: (919) 966-2110.

NEWSLETTERS

Morbidity and Mortality Weekly Report. Centers for Disease Control, 1600 Clifton Rd. N.E., Atlanta, GA 30333. Phone: (404) 488-4698.

RESEARCH CENTERS, INSTITUTES, CLEARINGHOUSES

Biostatistics Computing Laboratory. University of Michigan. School of Public Health II, Room 4317A, Ann Arbor, MI 48109. Phone: (313) 936-1017.

Department of Biostatistics and Epidemiology. University of Tennessee. Health Sciences Center, Memphis, TN 38163. Phone: (901) 528-5118.

Division of Biostatistics and Epidemiology. Dana Farber Cancer Institute. 44 Binney St., Boston, MA 02115. Phone: (617) 732-3012. Fax: (617) 737-8614.

Division of Epidemiology and Biostatistics. University of Cincinnati. ML 183, Cincinnati, OH 45267-0183. Phone: (513) 558-5631. Fax: (513) 558-1756.

Medical Biostatistics/Biometry Facility. University of Vermont. 27 Hills Science Bldg., Burlington, VT 05405. Phone: (802) 656-2526. Fax: (802) 656-0632.

TEXTBOOKS AND MONOGRAPHS

Basic and Clinical Biostatistics. Dawson-Saunders. Appleton & Lange, 25 Van Zant St., East Norwalk, CT 06855. Phone: (800) 423-1359. Fax: (203) 854-9486. 1991.

Essentials of Biostatistics. Norman. Mosby-Year Book, 11830 Westline Industrial Drive, St. Louis, MO 63146. Phone: (800) 325-4177. Fax: (314) 432-1380. 1992.

Interpretation and Use of Medical Statistics. G.J. Bourke and others. Blackwell Scientific Publications, Inc., 3 Cambridge Ctr., Cambridge, MA 02142. Phone: (800) 759-6102. Fourth edition 1991.

Medical Statistics: A Common Sense Approach. M.J. Campbell, D. Machin. John Wiley & Sons, Inc., 605 Third Ave., New York, NY 10158-0012. Phone: (212) 850-6000. Fax: (212) 850-6088. 1990.

Medical Uses of Statistics. John C. Bailar III, Frederick Mosteller (eds.). American Medical Association, 515 North State St., Chicago, IL 60610. Phone: (312) 464-0183. Fax: (312) 464-5834. 1992.

Primer of Biostatistics. Stanton A. Glantz. McGraw-Hill Inc., 11 West 19th St., New York, NY 10011. Phone: (212) 337-5001. Fax: (212) 337-4092. Third edition 1992.

Review of Biostatistics. Paul E. Leaverton. Little, Brown and Company, 34 Beacon St., Boston, MA 02108. Phone: (617) 227-0730. Fourth edition 1991.

Understanding Biostatistics. Hassard. Mosby-Year Book, 11830 Westline Industrial Drive, St. Louis, MO 63146. Phone: (800) 325-4177. Fax: (314) 432-1380. 1991.

BIOTECHNOLOGY

ABSTRACTING, INDEXING, AND CURRENT AWARENESS PUBLICATIONS

Abstract Newsletter: Biomedical Technology and Human Factors Engineering. National Technical Information Service, 5285 Port Royal Rd., Springfield, VA 22161. Phone: (703) 487-4650. Fax: (703) 321-8547. Weekly.

Bioengineering and Biotechnology Abstracts. Engineering Information Inc., 345 E. 47th St., New York, NY 10017-2387. Phone: (800) 221-1044. Fax: (212) 832-1857.

Biological Abstracts. BIOSIS, 2100 Arch St., Philadelphia, PA 19103-1399. Phone: (800) 523-4800. Fax: (215) 587-2016.

Biotechnology Research Abstracts. Cambridge Scientific Abstracts, 7200 Wisconsin Ave., Bethesda, MD 20814-4823. Phone: (800) 843-7751. Fax: (301) 961-6720. Bimonthly.

CAS BioTech Updates: Cell & Tissue Culture. Chemical Abstracts Service, 2540 Olentangy River Road, P.O. Box 3012, Columbus, OH 43210-0012. Phone: (800) 848-6538. Biweekly.

CAS BioTech Updates: DNA Formation & Repair. Chemical Abstracts Service, 2540 Olentangy River Road, P.O. Box 3012, Columbus, OH 43210-0012. Phone: (800) 848-6538. Biweekly.

CAS BioTech Updates: DNA & RNA Probes. Chemical Abstracts Service, 2540 Olentangy River Road, P.O. Box 3012, Columbus, OH 43210-0012. Phone: (800) 848-6538. Biweekly.

CAS BioTech Updates: Environmental Biotechnology. Chemical Abstracts Service, 2540 Olentangy River Road, P.O. Box 3012, Columbus, OH 43210-0012. Phone: (800) 848-6538. Biweekly.

CAS BioTech Updates: Enzymes in Biotechnology. Chemical Abstracts Service, 2540 Olentangy River Road, P.O. Box 3012, Columbus, OH 43210-0012. Phone: (800) 848-6538. Biweekly.

CAS BioTech Updates: Genetic Engineering. Chemical Abstracts Service, 2540 Olentangy River Road, P.O. Box 3012, Columbus, OH 43210-0012. Phone: (800) 848-6538. Biweekly.

CAS BioTech Updates: Pharmaceutical Applications. Chemical Abstracts Service, 2540 Olentangy River Road, P.O. Box 3012, Columbus, OH 43210-0012. Phone: (800) 848-6538. Biweekly.

CAS BioTech Updates: Slow-Release Pharmaceuticals. Chemical Abstracts Service, 2540 Olentangy River Road, P.O. Box 3012, Columbus, OH 43210-0012. Phone: (800) 848-6538. Biweekly.

Chemical Abstracts. Chemical Abstracts Service, 2540 Olentangy River Rd., P.O. Box 3012, Columbus, OH 43210-0012. Phone: (800) 848-6538.

Current Biotechnology Abstracts. Royal Society of Chemistry, Burlington House, Piccadilly, London W1V 0BN, England. Monthly.

Current Contents/Life Sciences. Institute for Scientific Information, 3501 Market St., Philadelphia, PA 19104. Phone: (215) 386-0100. Fax: (215) 386-6362.

Index Medicus. U.S. National Library of Medicine, 8600 Rockville Pike, Bethesda, MD 20894. Phone: (800) 638-8480. Monthly.

Research Alert: Genetic Engineering. Institute for Scientific Information, 3501 Market St., Philadelphia, PA 19104. Phone: (800) 523-1850. Fax: (215) 386-6362. Weekly.

ANNUALS AND REVIEWS

Critical Reviews in Biotechnology. CRC Press, Inc., 2000 Corporate Blvd. N.W., Boca Raton, FL 33431. Phone: (407) 994-0555. Fax: (407) 997-0949. Bimonthly.

Genetic Engineering. Academic Press, Inc., 1250 Sixth Ave., San Diego, CA 92101-4311. Phone: (619) 699-6345. Fax: (619) 699-6715. Irregular.

In Development Biotechnology Medicines. Pharmaceutical Manufacturers Association, 1100 15th St. N.W., Washington, DC 20005. Phone: (202) 835-3400. Annual.

ASSOCIATIONS, PROFESSIONAL SOCIETIES, ADVOCACY AND SUPPORT GROUPS

Association of Biotechnology Companies. 1666 Connecticut Ave. N.W., Suite 330, Washington, DC 20009. Phone: (202) 234-3330.

Industrial Biotechnology Association. 1625 K St. N.W., Suite 1100, Washington, DC 20006. Phone: (202) 857-0244.

BIBLIOGRAPHIES

Biotechnology in Human Health and Nutrition. National Agricultural Library, Beltsville, MD 20705. Jan. 1979-Mar. 1991.

Genetic Engineering: Monoclonal Antibodies. National Technical Information Service, 5285 Port Royal Rd., Springfield, VA 22161. Phone: (703) 487-4650. Fax: (703) 321-8547. Jan. 1978-Jan. 1989 PB88-855515/CBY.

Resource for Biomedical Sensor Technology. Case Western Reserve University. Bingham Bldg., Cleveland, OH 44106. Phone: (216) 368-2334. Fax: (216) 368-3016.

CD-ROM DATABASES

Biological Abstracts on Compact Disc. BIOSIS, 2100 Arch St., Philadelphia, PA 19103-1399. Phone: (800) 523-4800. Fax: (215) 587-2016. Quarterly.

Biotechnology Citation Index. Institute for Scientific Information, 3501 Market St., Philadelphia, PA 19104. Phone: (215) 386-0100. Fax: (215) 386-6362. Bimonthly.

ENCYCLOPEDIAS, DICTIONARIES, WORD BOOKS

Dictionary of Biotechnology: English-German. W. Babel, M. Hagemann, W. Hoehne. Elsevier Science Publishing Co., Inc., P.O. Box 882, Madison Square Station, New York, NY 10159-2101. Phone: (212) 989-5800. Fax: (212) 633-3990. 1988.

JOURNALS

Applied Microbiology and Biotechnology. Springer-Verlag New York Inc., 175 Fifth Ave., New York, NY 10010. Phone: (212) 460-1500. Fax: (212) 473-6272.

Biotechnology Advances. Pergamon Press, 660 White Plains Rd., Tarrytown, NY 10591-5153. Phone: (914) 592-7700. Fax: (914) 592-3625.

Biotechnology and Bioengineering. John Wiley & Sons, Inc., 605 Third Ave., New York, NY 10158-0012. Phone: (212) 850-6000. Fax: (212) 850-6088.

Biotechnology Therapeutics. Marcel Dekker, Inc., 270 Madison Ave., New York, NY 10016. Phone: (800) 228-1160.

Clinical Biotechnology. Mary Ann Liebert, Inc., 1651 Third Ave., New York, NY 10128. Phone: (212) 289-2300. Fax: (212) 289-4697. Quarterly.

Journal of Biotechnology. Elsevier Science Publishing Co., Inc., P.O. Box 882, Madison Square Station, New York, NY 10159-2101. Phone: (212) 989-5800. Fax: (212) 633-3990. 15/year.

Trends in Biotechnology. Elsevier Science Publishing Co., Inc., P.O. Box 882, Madison Square Station, New York, NY 10159-2101. Phone: (212) 989-5800. Fax: (212) 633-3990. 12+1/year.

World Journal of Microbiology and Biotechnology. Rapid Communications of Oxford Ltd., The Old Malthouse, Paradise St., Oxford OX1 1LD, England. Phone: 44-865-790447. Fax: 44-865-244012. 6/year.

NEWSLETTERS

Genetic Engineering News. Mary Ann Liebert, Inc., 1651 Third Ave., New York, NY 10128. Phone: (212) 289-2300. Fax: (212) 289-4697. 10/year.

ONLINE DATABASES

Biotechnology Abstracts. Derwent Publications Ltd., Rochdale House, 128 Theobalds Rd., London WC1X BRP, England. Phone: 071-242 5823. Fax: 071-405 3630. Monthly.

CA File (Chemical Abstracts File). Chemical Abstracts Service, 2540 Olentangy River Rd., P.O. Box 3012, Columbus, OH 43210-0012. Phone: (800) 848-6538.

CSA Life Sciences Collection. Cambridge Scientific Abstracts, 7200 Wisconsin Ave., Bethesda, MD 20814-4823. Phone: (800) 843-7751. Fax: (301) 961-6720.

Current Biotechnology Abstracts (CBA). Royal Society of Chemistry, Information Service, Thomas Graham House, Science Park, Milton Rd., Cambridge CB4 4WF, England. Phone: 0223 420066. Fax: 0223 423623. Monthly.

Directory of Biotechnology Information Resources. American Type Culture Collection, Bioinformatics Department, 12301 Parklawn Dr., Rockville, MD 20852-1776. Phone: (301) 881-2600. Monthly.

EMBASE. Elsevier Science Publishing Co., Inc., P.O. Box 882, Madison Square Station, New York, NY 10159-2101. Phone: (212) 989-5800. Fax: (212) 633-3990.

MEDLINE. National Library of Medicine, 8600 Rockville Pike, Bethesda, MD 20894. Phone: (800) 638-8480.

SciSearch. Institute for Scientific Information, 3501 Market St., Philadelphia, PA 19104. Phone: (215) 386-0100. Fax: (215) 386-6362.

RESEARCH CENTERS, INSTITUTES, CLEARINGHOUSES

Biomedical Engineering and Science Institute. Drexel University. 32nd and Chestnut Sts., Philadelphia, PA 19104. Phone: (215) 895-2215. Fax: (215) 895-4983.

Biotechnology Institute. University of Maryland. Microbiology Bldg., Room 1123, College Park, MD 20742. Phone: (301) 405-5189. Fax: (301) 454-8123.

Center for Advanced Biotechnology and Medicine. 679 Hoes Lane, Piscataway, NJ 08854-5638. Phone: (201) 463-5311. Fax: (201) 463-5318.

Center for Biotechnology. Baylor College of Medicine. 4000 Research Forest Dr., The Woodlands, TX 77381. Phone: (713) 363-8400. Fax: (713) 363-8475.

Center for Biotechnology. State University of New York at Stony Brook. 130 Life Sciences Bldg., Stony Brook, NY 11794-5208. Phone: (516) 632-8521. Fax: (516) 632-8577.

Institute for Molecular Biology and Biotechnology. McMaster University. Life Sciences Bldg., Room 425, 1280 Main St. W., Hamilton, ON, Canada L8S 4K1. Phone: (416) 525-9140. Fax: (416) 521-2955.

Interdisciplinary Center for Biotechnology Research. University of Florida. 1301 Filfield Hall, Gainesville, FL 32611. Phone: (904) 392-8408.

La Jolla Cancer Research Foundation. 10910 N. Torrey Pines Rd., La Jolla, CA 92037. Phone: (619) 455-6480. Fax: (619) 455-0181.

Laboratory of Genetics. University of Wisconsin-Madison. 445 Henry Mall, Madison, WI 53705. Phone: (608) 262-3112. Fax: (608) 262-2976.

TEXTBOOKS AND MONOGRAPHS

Biotechnology and Human Genetic Predisposition to Disease. Charles E. Cantor (ed.). John Wiley & Sons, Inc., 605 Third Ave., New York, NY 10158-0012. Phone: (212) 850-6000. Fax: (212) 850-6088.

Comprehensive Biotechnology: Principles, Applications & Regulations of Biotechnology in Industry, Agriculture & Medicine. M. Moo-Young (ed.). Pergamon Press, Inc., 395 Saw Mill River Rd., Elmsford, NY 10523. Phone: (914) 592-7700. Fax: (914) 592-3625. Four volumes 1985.

BIPOLAR DISORDER

See: MOOD DISORDERS

BIRTH

See: CHILDBIRTH

BIRTH CONTROL

See: CONTRACEPTION

BIRTH DEFECTS

See also: DOWN'S SYNDROME; FETAL DEVELOPMENT; GENETICS; MENTAL RETARDATION; SPINA BIFIDA

ABSTRACTING, INDEXING, AND CURRENT AWARENESS PUBLICATIONS

BIOSIS/CAS Selects: Mammalian Birth Defects. BIOSIS, 2100 Arch St., Philadelphia, PA 19103-1399. Phone: (215) 587-4800. Fax: (215) 587-2016. Biweekly.

Current Contents/Clinical Medicine. Institute for Scientific Information, 3501 Market St., Philadelphia, PA 19104. Phone: (800) 523-1850. Fax: (215) 386-6362. Weekly.

Excerpta Medica. Section 21: Developmental Biology and Teratology. Elsevier Science Publishing Co., Inc., P.O. Box 882, Madison Square Station, New York, NY 10159-2101. Phone: (212) 989-5800. Fax: (212) 633-3990. 16/year.

Excerpta Medica. Section 22: Human Genetics. Elsevier Science Publishers, P.O. Box 882, Madison Square Station, New York, NY 10159-2101. Phone: (212) 633-3950. Fax: (212) 633-3990. 24/year.

Genetics Abstracts. Cambridge Scientific Abstracts, 7200 Wisconsin Ave., Bethesda, MD 20814-4823. Phone: (800) 843-7751. Fax: (301) 961-6720. Monthly.

Index Medicus. U.S. National Library of Medicine, 8600 Rockville Pike, Bethesda, MD 20894. Phone: (800) 638-8480. Monthly.

Research Alert: Birth Defects-Congenital. Institute for Scientific Information, 3501 Market St., Philadelphia, PA 19104. Phone: (800) 523-1850. Fax: (215) 386-6362. Weekly.

Research Alert: Genetics-Human. Institute for Scientific Information, 3501 Market St., Philadelphia, PA 19104. Phone: (800) 523-1850. Fax: (215) 386-6362. Weekly.

Research Alert: Teratology & Teratogenicity. Institute for Scientific Information, 3501 Market St., Philadelphia, PA 19104. Phone: (800) 523-1850. Fax: (215) 386-6362. Weekly.

Science Citation Index. Institute for Scientific Information, 3501 Market St., Philadelphia, PA 19104. Phone: (800) 523-1850. Fax: (215) 386-6362. Bimonthly.

ANNUALS AND REVIEWS

Annual Review of Genetics. Annual Reviews Inc., 4139 El Camino Way, P.O. Box 10139, Palo Alto, CA 94303-0897. Phone: (415) 493-4400. Fax: (415) 855-9815. Annual.

Issues and Reviews in Teratology. Plenum Publishing Co., 233 Spring St., New York, NY 10013-1578. Phone: (212) 620-8000. Fax: (212) 463-0742. Irregular.

ASSOCIATIONS, PROFESSIONAL SOCIETIES, ADVOCACY AND SUPPORT GROUPS

American Academy of Pediatrics (AAP). 141 Northwest Point Blvd., P.O. Box 927, Elk Grove Village, IL 60009-0927. Phone: (708) 228-5005. Fax: (708) 228-5097.

American Cleft Palate Association. 331 Salk Hall, University of Pittsburgh, Pittsburgh, PA 15261. Phone: (800) 242-5338.

Association of Birth Defect Children (ABDC). Orlando Executive Park, 5400 Diplomat Circle, Ste. 270, Orlando, FL 32810. Phone: (407) 629-1466.

March of Dimes Birth Defects Foundation (MDBDF). 1275 Mamaroneck Ave., White Plains, NY 10605. Phone: (914) 428-7100. Fax: (914) 428-8203.

National Marfan Foundation (NMF). 382 Main St., Port Washington, NY 11050. Phone: (516) 883-8712.

Parents of Children with Down's Syndrome. P.O. Box 35268, Houston, TX 77035.

Spina Bifida Association of America (SBAA). 1700 Rockville Pike, Ste. 250, Rockville, MD 20852. Phone: (800) 621-3141. Fax: (301) 881-3392.

CD-ROM DATABASES

SCISEARCH. Institute for Scientific Information, 3501 Market St., Philadelphia, PA 19104. Phone: (215) 386-0100. Fax: (215) 386-6362.

ENCYCLOPEDIAS, DICTIONARIES, WORD BOOKS

Birth Defects Encyclopedia. Mary Louise Buyse (ed.). Mosby-Year Book, 11830 Westline Industrial Drive, St. Louis, MO 63146. Phone: (800) 325-4177. Fax: (314) 432-1380. 1990.

Encyclopedia of Genetic Disorders and Birth Defects. Mark D. Ludman, James Wynbrandt. Facts on File, Inc., 460 Park Ave. S., New York, NY 10016-7382. Phone: (212) 683-2244. Fax: (212) 683-3633. 1991.

Glossary of Genetics. Rieger. Springer-Verlag New York Inc., 175 Fifth Ave., New York, NY 10010. Phone: (212) 460-1500. Fax: (212) 473-6272. Fifth edition 1991.

HANDBOOKS, GUIDES, MANUALS, ATLASES

Chromosome Anomalies and Prenatal Development: An Atlas. Dorothy Warburton, Julianne Byrne, Nina Canki. Oxford University Press, 200 Madison Ave., New York, NY 10016. Phone: (212) 679-7300. 1991.

JOURNALS

American Journal of Human Genetics. University of Chicago Press, P.O. Box 37005, Chicago, IL 60637. Phone: (312) 753-3347. Fax: (312) 753-0811. Monthly.

Developmental Genetics. John Wiley & Sons, Inc., 605 Third Ave., New York, NY 10158-0012. Phone: (212) 850-6000. Fax: (212) 850-6088. Bimonthly.

Journal of Genetic Counseling. Human Sciences Press, 233 Spring St., New York, NY 10013-1578. Phone: (800) 221-9369. Fax: (212) 807-1047. Quarterly.

Journal of Medical Genetics. BMJ Publishing Group, BMA House, Tavistock Square, London WC1H 9JR, England. Phone: 071-383 6244/6638. Fax: 071-383 6662. Monthly.

Teratology. John Wiley & Sons, Inc., 605 Third Ave., New York, NY 10158-0012. Phone: (212) 850-6000. Fax: (212) 850-6088.

Teratology: The International Journal of Abnormal Development. John Wiley & Sons, Inc., 605 Third Ave., New York, NY 10158-0012. Phone: (212) 850-6000. Fax: (212) 850-6088. Monthly.

NEWSLETTERS

American Association on Mental Retardation-News and Notes. American Association on Mental Retardation, 1719 Kalorama Rd., N.W., Washington, DC 20009. Phone: (202) 387-1968. Bimonthly.

Down Syndrome News. National Down Syndrome Congress, 1800 Dempster St., Park Ridge, IL 60068-1146. Phone: (800) 232-6372. 10/year.

ONLINE DATABASES

Birth Defects Encyclopedia Online (BDEO). Center for Birth Defects Information Services, Inc., Dover Medical Bldg., Box 1776, Dover, MA 02030. Phone: (617) 785-2525. Quarterly.

EMBASE. Elsevier Science Publishing Co., Inc., P.O. Box 882, Madison Square Station, New York, NY 10159-2101. Phone: (212) 989-5800. Fax: (212) 633-3990.

MEDLINE. National Library of Medicine, 8600 Rockville Pike, Bethesda, MD 20894. Phone: (800) 638-8480.

SciSearch. Institute for Scientific Information, 3501 Market St., Philadelphia, PA 19104. Phone: (215) 386-0100. Fax: (215) 386-6362.

RESEARCH CENTERS, INSTITUTES, CLEARINGHOUSES

American Cleft Palate Educational Foundation. 331 Salk Hall, University of Pittsburgh, Pittsburgh, PA 15261. Phone: (800) 242-5338.

Birth Defects Center. Baylor College of Medicine, 6021 Fannin St., Houston, TX 77030. Phone: (713) 791-3261.

Birth Defects and Genetic Disorders Unit. T311 General Hospital, University of Iowa, Iowa City, IA 52242. Phone: (319) 353-6687.

California Teratogen Registry. University of California Medical Center, 225 W. Dickinson St., San Diego, CA 92103. Phone: (619) 294-6084.

Connecticut Pregnancy Exposure Information Service and Risk Line. University of Connecticut Health Center, Farmington, CT 06032. Phone: (203) 674-1465.

C.S. Mott Center for Human Growth and Development. 275 E. Hancock St., Detroit, MI 48201. Phone: (313) 577-1068. Fax: (313) 577-8554.

Teratology Information Network. University of Medicine and Dentistry of New Jersey, 401 Hadden Ave., Camden, NJ 08103. Phone: (609) 757-7869.

TEXTBOOKS AND MONOGRAPHS

Catalog of Prenatally Diagnosed Conditions. David D. Weaver. Johns Hopkins University Press, 701 W. 40th St., Suite 275, Baltimore, MD 21211-2190. Phone: (800) 537-5487. Fax: (410) 516-6998. Second edition 1992.

Catalog of Teratogenic Agents. Thomas H. Shepard. Johns Hopkins University Press, 701 W. 40th St., Suite 275, Baltimore, MD 21211-2190. Phone: (800) 537-5487. Fax: (410) 516-6998. Seventh edition 1992.

Diagnostic Dysmorphology. Jon M. Aase. Plenum Publishing Co., 233 Spring St., New York, NY 10013-1578. Phone: (212) 620-8000. Fax: (212) 463-0742. 1990.

Gait Analysis in Cerebral Palsy. James R. Gage. Cambridge University Press, 40 W. 20th St., New York, NY 10011. Phone: (800) 431-1580. 1992.

Introduction to Risk Calculation in Genetic Counseling. Young. Oxford University Press, 200 Madison Ave., New York, NY 10016. Phone: (212) 679-7300. 1991.

Prenatal Diagnosis of Congenital Abnormalities. Romero. Appleton & Lange, 25 Van Zant St., East Norwalk, CT 06855. Phone: (800) 423-1359. Fax: (203) 854-9486. 1988.

Principles and Practice of Medical Genetics. ALan E.H. Emery, David J. Rimoin (eds.). Churchill Livingstone Inc., 650 Avenue of the Americas, New York, NY 10011. Phone: (212)

819-5400. Fax: (212) 302-6598. Second edition. Two volumes. 1990.

Surgical Techniques in Cleft Lip and Cleft Palate. Bardach. Mosby-Year Book, 11830 Westline Industrial Drive, St. Louis, MO 63146. Phone: (800) 325-4177. Fax: (314) 432-1380. Second edition 1991.

What is a Cleft Lip and Palate?: A Multidisciplinary Update. O. Kriens (ed.). Thieme Medical Publishers, Inc., 381 Park Ave. S., New York, NY 10016. Phone: (212) 683-5088. Fax: (212) 779-9020. 1989.

BIRTH RATE

See: VITAL STATISTICS

BLADDER CANCER

ABSTRACTING, INDEXING, AND CURRENT AWARENESS PUBLICATIONS

Excerpta Medica. Section 16: Cancer. Elsevier Science Publishing Co., Inc., P.O. Box 882, Madison Square Station, New York, NY 10159-2101. Phone: (212) 989-5800. Fax: (212) 633-3990. 32/year.

Index Medicus. U.S. National Library of Medicine, 8600 Rockville Pike, Bethesda, MD 20894. Phone: (800) 638-8480. Monthly.

Science Citation Index. Institute for Scientific Information, 3501 Market St., Philadelphia, PA 19104. Phone: (800) 523-1850. Fax: (215) 386-6362. Bimonthly.

Statistical Reference Index. Congressional Information Service, 4520 East-West Hwy., Bethesda, MD 20814. Phone: (800) 639-8380. 1980-Present Monthly.

ASSOCIATIONS, PROFESSIONAL SOCIETIES, ADVOCACY AND SUPPORT GROUPS

American Cancer Society (ACS). 1599 Clifton Rd. N.E., Atlanta, GA 30329. Phone: (404) 320-3333.

CD-ROM DATABASES

Cancerlit. Aries Systems Corporation, One Dundee Park, Andover, MA 01810. Phone: (508) 475-7200. Fax: (508) 474-8860. Quarterly.

OncoDisc. J.B. Lippincott Co., 227 East Washington Square, Philadelphia, PA 19106-3780. Phone: (215) 238-4200. Fax: (215) 238-4227. Bimonthly.

SCISEARCH. Institute for Scientific Information, 3501 Market St., Philadelphia, PA 19104. Phone: (215) 386-0100. Fax: (215) 386-6362.

JOURNALS

CA - A Cancer Journal for Clinicians. J.B. Lippincott Co., 227 E. Washington Square, Philadelphia, PA 19106-3780. Phone: (215) 238-4200. Fax: (215) 238-4227. Bimonthly.

Cancer Research. Williams & Wilkins, 428 East Preston St., Baltimore, MD 21202. Phone: (800) 638-0672. Fax: (800) 447-8438. Semimonthly.

Journal of Clinical Oncology. W.B. Saunders Co., The Curtis Center, Independence Square W., Philadelphia, PA 19106-3399. Phone: (215) 238-7800. Monthly.

Journal of Urology. Williams & Wilkins, 428 E. Preston St., Baltimore, MD 21202. Phone: (800) 638-0672. Fax: (800) 447-8438. Monthly.

ONLINE DATABASES

Cancer Weekly. CDC AIDS Weekly/NCI Cancer Weekly, 206 Rogers St. NE, Suite 104, P.O. Box 5528, Atlanta, GA 30317. Phone: (404) 377-8895. Weekly.

EMBASE. Elsevier Science Publishing Co., Inc., P.O. Box 882, Madison Square Station, New York, NY 10159-2101. Phone: (212) 989-5800. Fax: (212) 633-3990.

MEDLINE. National Library of Medicine, 8600 Rockville Pike, Bethesda, MD 20894. Phone: (800) 638-8480.

Physician Data Query (PDQ) Cancer Information File. U.S. National Cancer Institute, International Cancer Information Center, Building 82, Room 102, Bethesda, MD 20892. Phone: (301) 496-7403. Fax: (301) 480-8105. Monthly.

Physician Data Query (PDQ) Directory File. U.S. National Cancer Institute, International Cancer Information Center, Building 82, Room 102, Bethesda, MD 20892. Phone: (301) 496-7403. Fax: (301) 480-8105. Monthly.

Physician Data Query (PDQ) Protocol File. U.S. National Cancer Institute, International Cancer Information Center, Building 82, Room 102, Bethesda, MD 20892. Phone: (301) 496-7403. Fax: (301) 480-8105. Monthly.

SciSearch. Institute for Scientific Information, 3501 Market St., Philadelphia, PA 19104. Phone: (215) 386-0100. Fax: (215) 386-6362.

POPULAR WORKS AND PATIENT EDUCATION

Everyone's Guide to Cancer Therapy: How Cancer is Diagnosed, Treated, and Managed on a Day to Day Basis. Malin Dollinger, Ernest H. Rosenbaum, Greg Cable. Andrews & McMeel, 4900 Main St., Kansas City, MO 64112. Phone: (800) 826-4216. 1991.

RESEARCH CENTERS, INSTITUTES, CLEARINGHOUSES

Cancer Information Service (CIS). Office of Cancer Communications, National Cancer Institute, Bldg. 31, Rm. 10A24, 9000 Rockville Pike, Bethesda, MD 20892. Phone: (800) 4CA-NCER.

Memorial Sloan-Kettering Cancer Center. 1275 York Ave., New York, NY 10021. Phone: (212) 355-0060.

Vincent T. Lombardi Cancer Research Center. Georgetown University. 3800 Reservoir Rd. NW, Podium Level, Washington, DC 20007. Phone: (202) 687-2110. Fax: (202) 687-6402.

TEXTBOOKS AND MONOGRAPHS

Cancer Medicine. James F. Holland, Emil Frei, Robert C. Bast Jr., and others. Williams & Wilkins, 428 East Preston St., Baltimore, MD 21202. Phone: (800) 638-0672. Fax: (800) 447-8438. Third edition 1992.

Cancer Treatment. Charles M. Haskell. W.B. Saunders Co., The Curtis Center, Independence Square W., Philadelphia, PA 19106-3399. Phone: (215) 238-7800. Third edition 1990.

Neo-Adjuvant Chemotherapy in Invasive Bladder Cancer. Ted A.W. Splinter. John Wiley & Sons, Inc., 605 Third Ave., New York, NY 10158-0012. Phone: (212) 850-6000. Fax: (212) 850-6088. 1990.

BLADDER DISEASES

See: UROLOGIC DISORDERS

BLINDNESS

See also: VISION DISORDERS

ABSTRACTING, INDEXING, AND CURRENT AWARENESS PUBLICATIONS

Excerpta Medica. Section 12: Ophthalmology. Elsevier Science Publishing Co., Inc., P.O. Box 882, Madison Square Station, New York, NY 10159-2101. Phone: (212) 989-5800. Fax: (212) 633-3990. 16/year.

Index Medicus. U.S. National Library of Medicine, 8600 Rockville Pike, Bethesda, MD 20894. Phone: (800) 638-8480. Monthly.

Science Citation Index. Institute for Scientific Information, 3501 Market St., Philadelphia, PA 19104. Phone: (800) 523-1850. Fax: (215) 386-6362. Bimonthly.

ASSOCIATIONS, PROFESSIONAL SOCIETIES, ADVOCACY AND SUPPORT GROUPS

American Council of the Blind (ACB). 1155 15th St. N.W., Ste. 720, Washington, DC 20005. Phone: (800) 424-8666. Fax: (202) 467-5085.

American Foundation for the Blind (AFB). 15 W. 16th St., New York, NY 10011. Phone: (212) 620-2000. Fax: (212) 727-7418.

Associated Services for the Blind (ASB). 919 Walnut St., Philadelphia, PA 19107. Phone: (215) 627-0600. Fax: (215) 922-0692.

Association for Education and Rehabilitation of the Blind and Visually Impaired (AER). 206 N. Washington St., Ste. 320, Alexandria, VA 22314. Phone: (703) 548-1884.

Braille Institute (BI). 741 N. Vermont Ave., Los Angeles, CA 90029. Phone: (213) 663-1111.

Canadian National Institute for the Blind. 1931 Bayview Ave., Toronto, ON, Canada M4G 4C8. Phone: (416) 480-7580.

Guide Dog Foundation for the Blind (GDFB). 371 E. Jericho Tpke., Smithtown, NY 11787. Phone: (800) 548-4337. Fax: (516) 361-5192.

Guiding Eyes for the Blind (GEB). 611 Granite Springs Rd., Yorktown Heights, NY 10598. Phone: (914) 245-4024. Fax: (914) 245-1609.

Helen Keller International (HKI). 15 W. 16th St., New York, NY 10011. Phone: (212) 807-5800. Fax: (212) 463-9341.

Helen Keller National Center for Deaf-Blind Youths and Adults (HKNC). 111 Middle Neck Rd., Sands Point, NY 11050. Phone: (516) 944-8900. Fax: (516) 944-7302.

Jewish Braille Institute of America (JBI). 110 E. 30th St., New York, NY 10016. Phone: (212) 889-2525.

National Braille Association (NBA). 1290 University Ave., Rochester, NY 14607. Phone: (716) 473-0900.

National Society to Prevent Blindness. 500 E. Remington Rd., Schaumburg, IL 60173. Phone: (800) 331-2020.

BIBLIOGRAPHIES

Library Resources for the Blind and Physically Handicapped. National Library Service for the Blind and Physically Handicapped, Library of Congress, 1291 Taylor St. N.W., Washington, DC 20542. Phone: (800) 424-8567. Fax: (202) 707-0712. Annual.

CD-ROM DATABASES

SCISEARCH. Institute for Scientific Information, 3501 Market St., Philadelphia, PA 19104. Phone: (215) 386-0100. Fax: (215) 386-6362.

ENCYCLOPEDIAS, DICTIONARIES, WORD BOOKS

Encyclopedia of Blindness and Vision Impairment. Jill Sardegna, T. Otis Paul. Facts on File, Inc., 460 Park Ave. S., New York, NY 10016-7382. Phone: (212) 683-2244. Fax: (212) 683-3633. 1992.

JOURNALS

Journal of Rehabilitation Administration. AER, 206 N. Washington St., Alexandria, VA 22314.

Journal of Vision Rehabilitation. AER, 206 N. Washington St., Alexandria, VA 22314.

Journal of Visual Impairment and Blindness. AER, 206 N. Washington St., Alexandria, VA 22314.

National Braille Association Bulletin. National Braille Association, 1290 University Ave., Rochester, NY 14607. Phone: (716) 473-0900.

NEWSLETTERS

Fighting Blindness News. RP Foundation Fighting Blindness, 1401 Mt. Royal Ave., Baltimore, MD 21217. Phone: (301) 225-9400. 3/year.

Research to Prevent Blindness-Progress Report. Research to Prevent Blindness, 598 Madison Ave., New York, NY 10022. Phone: (212) 752-4333. Annual.

ONLINE DATABASES

EMBASE. Elsevier Science Publishing Co., Inc., P.O. Box 882, Madison Square Station, New York, NY 10159-2101. Phone: (212) 989-5800. Fax: (212) 633-3990.

MEDLINE. National Library of Medicine, 8600 Rockville Pike, Bethesda, MD 20894. Phone: (800) 638-8480.

SciSearch. Institute for Scientific Information, 3501 Market St., Philadelphia, PA 19104. Phone: (215) 386-0100. Fax: (215) 386-6362.

RESEARCH CENTERS, INSTITUTES, CLEARINGHOUSES

Jules Stein Eye Institute. University of California, Los Angeles, CA 90024. Phone: (213) 825-5051.

National Library Service for the Blind and Physically Handicapped (NLS). Library of Congress, 1291 Taylor St. N.W., Washington, DC 20542. Phone: (800) 424-8567.

BLOOD BANKS

See also: TRANSFUSIONS

ABSTRACTING, INDEXING, AND CURRENT AWARENESS PUBLICATIONS

Excerpta Medica. Section 25: Hematology. Elsevier Science Publishers, P.O. Box 882, Madison Square Station, New York, NY 10159-2101. Phone: (212) 633-3950. Fax: (212) 633-3990. 24/year.

Hospital Literature Index. American Hospital Association, 840 N. Lake Shore Dr., Chicago, IL 60611. Phone: (800) 242-2626. Fax: (312) 280-6015. Quarterly.

Index Medicus. U.S. National Library of Medicine, 8600 Rockville Pike, Bethesda, MD 20894. Phone: (800) 638-8480. Monthly.

Science Citation Index. Institute for Scientific Information, 3501 Market St., Philadelphia, PA 19104. Phone: (800) 523-1850. Fax: (215) 386-6362. Bimonthly.

ASSOCIATIONS, PROFESSIONAL SOCIETIES, ADVOCACY AND SUPPORT GROUPS

American Association of Blood Banks (AABB). 1117 N. 19th St., Ste. 600, Arlington, VA 22209. Phone: (703) 528-8200. Fax: (703) 527-8036.

American Blood Commission. 700 N. Fairfax St., Suite 505, Alexandria, VA 22314. Phone: (703) 548-6262.

American Blood Resources Association. P.O. Box 3346, Annapolis, MD 21403. Phone: (301) 263-8296.

Council of Community Blood Centers. 725 15th St. N.W., No. 700, Washington, DC 20005. Phone: (202) 393-5725.

CD-ROM DATABASES

SCISEARCH. Institute for Scientific Information, 3501 Market St., Philadelphia, PA 19104. Phone: (215) 386-0100. Fax: (215) 386-6362.

DIRECTORIES

American Association of Blood Banks Membership Directory. American Association of Blood Banks, 1117 N. 19th St., Suite 600, Arlington, VA 22209. Phone: (703) 528-8200.

JOURNALS

Transfusion. J.B. Lippincott Co., 227 E. Washington Square, Philadelphia, PA 19106-3780. Phone: (215) 238-4200. Fax: (215) 238-4227.

Transfusion Medicine Reviews. W.B. Saunders Co., The Curtis Center, Independence Sqare W., Philadelphia, PA 19106-3399. Phone: (215) 238-7800.

Transfusion Science. Pergamon Press, 660 White Plains Rd., Tarrytown, NY 10591-5153. Phone: (914) 592-7700. Fax: (914) 592-3625.

ONLINE DATABASES

Combined Health Information Database (CHID). U.S. National Institutes of Health, P.O. Box NDIC, Bethesda, MD 20892. Phone: (301) 496-2162. Fax: (301) 770-5164. Quarterly.

EMBASE. Elsevier Science Publishing Co., Inc., P.O. Box 882, Madison Square Station, New York, NY 10159-2101. Phone: (212) 989-5800. Fax: (212) 633-3990.

MEDLINE. National Library of Medicine, 8600 Rockville Pike, Bethesda, MD 20894. Phone: (800) 638-8480.

SciSearch. Institute for Scientific Information, 3501 Market St., Philadelphia, PA 19104. Phone: (215) 386-0100. Fax: (215) 386-6362.

RESEARCH CENTERS, INSTITUTES, CLEARINGHOUSES

Cardeza Foundation for Hematologic Research. Thomas Jefferson University. 1015 Walnut St., Philadelphia, PA 19107. Phone: (215) 955-7786.

Foundation for Blood Research. P.O. Box 190, Scarborough, ME 04074. Phone: (207) 883-4131. Fax: (207) 883-1527.

Hematology Research Laboratory. University of Southern California. 2025 Zonal Ave., Los Angeles, CA 90033. Phone: (213) 224-6412. Fax: (213) 224-6687.

TEXTBOOKS AND MONOGRAPHS

Clinical Practice of Transfusion Medicine. Petz. Churchill Livingstone Inc., 650 Ave. of the Americas, New York, NY 10011. Phone: (212) 819-5400. Fax: (212) 302-6598. 1989.

Modern Blood Banking and Transfusion Practice. Denise Harmening. F.A. Davis Co., 1915 Arch St., Philadelphia, PA 19103. Phone: (800) 523-4049. Fax: (215) 568-5065. Second edition 1989.

Principles of Transfusion Medicine. Rossi. Williams & Wilkins, 428 East Preston St., Baltimore, MD 21202. Phone: (800) 638-0672. Fax: (800) 447-8438. 1991.

BLOOD DISEASES

See: HEMATOLOGIC DISORDERS;
HEMATOLOGY

BLOOD GROUPS

See: HEMATOLOGY

BLOOD TESTS

See: LABORATORY MEDICINE;
TRANSFUSIONS

BONE CANCER

See also: CANCER

ABSTRACTING, INDEXING, AND CURRENT AWARENESS PUBLICATIONS

Current Contents/Clinical Medicine. Institute for Scientific Information, 3501 Market St., Philadelphia, PA 19104. Phone: (800) 523-1850. Fax: (215) 386-6362. Weekly.

Excerpta Medica. Section 16: Cancer. Elsevier Science Publishing Co., Inc., P.O. Box 882, Madison Square Station, New York, NY 10159-2101. Phone: (212) 989-5800. Fax: (212) 633-3990. 32/year.

Index Medicus. U.S. National Library of Medicine, 8600 Rockville Pike, Bethesda, MD 20894. Phone: (800) 638-8480. Monthly.

Science Citation Index. Institute for Scientific Information, 3501 Market St., Philadelphia, PA 19104. Phone: (800) 523-1850. Fax: (215) 386-6362. Bimonthly.

Statistical Reference Index. Congressional Information Service, 4520 East-West Hwy., Bethesda, MD 20814. Phone: (800) 639-8380. 1980-Present Monthly.

ANNUALS AND REVIEWS

In Development New Medicines for Older Americans. 1991 Annual Survey. More Medicines in Testing for Cancer Than for Any Other Disease of Aging. Pharmaceutical Manufacturers Association, 1100 15th St. N.W., Washington, DC 20005. Phone: (202) 835-3400. 1991.

ASSOCIATIONS, PROFESSIONAL SOCIETIES, ADVOCACY AND SUPPORT GROUPS

American Cancer Society (ACS). 1599 Clifton Rd. N.E., Atlanta, GA 30329. Phone: (404) 320-3333.

Candlelighters Childhood Cancer Foundation. 1312 18th St. N.W., Suite 200, Washington, DC 20036. Phone: (800) 366-2223.

CD-ROM DATABASES

Cancer on Disc. CMC ReSearch, Inc., 7150 S.W. Hampton, Suite C-120, Portland, OR 97223. Phone: (800) 262-7668. Fax: (503) 639-1796. Annual.

OncoDisc. J.B. Lippincott Co., 227 East Washington Square, Philadelphia, PA 19106-3780. Phone: (215) 238-4200. Fax: (215) 238-4227. Bimonthly.

Physician's Data Query (PDQ). Cambridge Scientific Abstracts, 7200 Wisconsin Ave., Bethesda, MD 20814-4823. Phone: (800) 843-7751. Fax: (301) 961-6720. Quarterly.

SCISEARCH. Institute for Scientific Information, 3501 Market St., Philadelphia, PA 19104. Phone: (215) 386-0100. Fax: (215) 386-6362.

ENCYCLOPEDIAS, DICTIONARIES, WORD BOOKS

Oncology Words. Stedman. Williams & Wilkins, 428 East Preston St., Baltimore, MD 21202. Phone: (800) 638-0672. Fax: (800) 447-8438. 1992.

JOURNALS

CA - A Cancer Journal for Clinicians. J.B. Lippincott Co., 227 E. Washington Square, Philadelphia, PA 19106-3780. Phone: (215) 238-4200. Fax: (215) 238-4227. Bimonthly.

Cancer Causes and Control. Rapid Communications of Oxford Ltd., The Old Malthouse, Paradise St., Oxford OX1 1LD, England. Phone: 44-865-790447. Fax: 44-865-244012. 6/year.

Journal of Clinical Oncology. W.B. Saunders Co., The Curtis Center, Independence Square W., Philadelphia, PA 19106-3399. Phone: (215) 238-7800. Monthly.

Journal of the National Cancer Institute. Superintendent of Documents, P.O. Box 371954, Pittsburgh, PA 15250-7954. Fax: (202) 512-2233. Semimonthly.

ONLINE DATABASES

Cancer Weekly. CDC AIDS Weekly/NCI Cancer Weekly, 206 Rogers St. NE, Suite 104, P.O. Box 5528, Atlanta, GA 30317. Phone: (404) 377-8895. Weekly.

CANCERLIT. U.S. National Cancer Institute, International Cancer Information Center, Building 82, Room 102, Bethesda, MD 20892. Phone: (301) 496-7403. Fax: (301) 480-8105. Monthly.

Clinical Protocols. U.S. National Cancer Institute, International Cancer Information Center, Building 82, Room 102, Bethesda, MD 20892. Phone: (301) 496-7403. Fax: (301) 480-8105.

EMBASE. Elsevier Science Publishing Co., Inc., P.O. Box 882, Madison Square Station, New York, NY 10159-2101. Phone: (212) 989-5800. Fax: (212) 633-3990.

MEDLINE. National Library of Medicine, 8600 Rockville Pike, Bethesda, MD 20894. Phone: (800) 638-8480.

Physician Data Query (PDQ) Cancer Information File. U.S. National Cancer Institute, International Cancer Information Center, Building 82, Room 102, Bethesda, MD 20892. Phone: (301) 496-7403. Fax: (301) 480-8105. Monthly.

Physician Data Query (PDQ) Directory File. U.S. National Cancer Institute, International Cancer Information Center, Building 82, Room 102, Bethesda, MD 20892. Phone: (301) 496-7403. Fax: (301) 480-8105. Monthly.

Physician Data Query (PDQ) Protocol File. U.S. National Cancer Institute, International Cancer Information Center, Building 82, Room 102, Bethesda, MD 20892. Phone: (301) 496-7403. Fax: (301) 480-8105. Monthly.

SciSearch. Institute for Scientific Information, 3501 Market St., Philadelphia, PA 19104. Phone: (215) 386-0100. Fax: (215) 386-6362.

POPULAR WORKS AND PATIENT EDUCATION

Cancervive: The Challenge of Life After Cancer. Susan Nessim, Judith Ellis. Houghton Mifflin Co., 1 Beacon St., Boston, MA 02108. Phone: (800) 225-3362. 1991.

Everyone's Guide to Cancer Therapy: How Cancer is Diagnosed, Treated, and Managed on a Day to Day Basis. Malin Dollinger, Ernest H. Rosenbaum, Greg Cable. Andrews & McMeel, 4900 Main St., Kansas City, MO 64112. Phone: (800) 826-4216. 1991.

RESEARCH CENTERS, INSTITUTES, CLEARINGHOUSES

Cancer Information Service (CIS). Office of Cancer Communications, National Cancer Institute, Bldg. 31, Rm. 10A24, 9000 Rockville Pike, Bethesda, MD 20892. Phone: (800) 4CA-NCER.

TEXTBOOKS AND MONOGRAPHS

Bone Tumors. Mirra. Williams & Wilkins, 428 East Preston St., Baltimore, MD 21202. Phone: (800) 638-0672. Fax: (800) 447-8438. Two volumes 1989.

Cancer: Principles and Practice of Oncology. Vincent T. DeVita. J.B. Lippincott Co., 227 E. Washington Square, Philadelphia, PA 19106-3780. Phone: (215) 238-4200. Fax: (215) 238-4227. 1989 3rd edtion.

Cancer Treatment. Charles M. Haskell. W.B. Saunders Co., The Curtis Center, Independence Square W., Philadelphia, PA 19106-3399. Phone: (215) 238-7800. Third edition 1990.

BONE AND JOINT DISEASES

See also: ARTHRITIS; OSTEOPOROSIS

ABSTRACTING, INDEXING, AND CURRENT AWARENESS PUBLICATIONS

Current Contents/Clinical Medicine. Institute for Scientific Information, 3501 Market St., Philadelphia, PA 19104. Phone: (800) 523-1850. Fax: (215) 386-6362. Weekly.

Excerpta Medica. Section 31. Arthritis and Rheumatism. Elsevier Science Publishing Co., Inc., P.O. Box 882, Madison Square Station, New York, NY 10159-2101. Phone: (212) 989-5800. Fax: (212) 633-3990. 8/year.

Index Medicus. U.S. National Library of Medicine, 8600 Rockville Pike, Bethesda, MD 20894. Phone: (800) 638-8480. Monthly.

Science Citation Index. Institute for Scientific Information, 3501 Market St., Philadelphia, PA 19104. Phone: (800) 523-1850. Fax: (215) 386-6362. Bimonthly.

ANNUALS AND REVIEWS

In Development New Medicines for Arthritis. Pharmaceutical Manufacturers Association, 1100 15th St. N.W., Washington, DC 20005. Phone: (202) 835-3400. Annual.

ASSOCIATIONS, PROFESSIONAL SOCIETIES, ADVOCACY AND SUPPORT GROUPS

American College of Rheumatology (ACR). 17 Executive Park Dr. N.E., Ste. 480, Atlanta, GA 30329. Phone: (404) 633-3777. Fax: (404) 633-1870.

American Juvenile Arthritis Organization (AJAO). 1314 Spring St. N.W., Atlanta, GA 30309. Phone: (404) 872-7100. Fax: (404) 872-0457.

American Society for Bone and Mineral Research. P.O. Box 739, Kelseyville, CA 95451. Phone: (707) 279-1344.

National Osteoporosis Foundation. 1625 Eye St. N.W., Ste. 1011, Washington, DC 20006. Phone: (202) 223-2226.

Osteogenetics Imperfection Foundation. P.O. Box 14807, Clearwater, FL 34629. Phone: (813) 855-7077.

Scleroderma Association (SA). P.O. Box 910, Lynnfield, MA 01940. Phone: (508) 525-6600.

United Scleroderma Foundation (USF). P.O. Box 350, Watsonville, CA 95077. Phone: (800) 722-HOPE.

CD-ROM DATABASES

SCISEARCH. Institute for Scientific Information, 3501 Market St., Philadelphia, PA 19104. Phone: (215) 386-0100. Fax: (215) 386-6362.

HANDBOOKS, GUIDES, MANUALS, ATLASES

Handbook of Drug Therapy in Rheumatic Disease: Pharmacology and Clinical Aspects. Joe G. Hardin Jr., Gesina L. Longenecker. Little, Brown and Company, 34 Beacon St., Boston, MA 02108. Phone: (617) 227-0730. 1992.

Manual of Rheumatology and Outpatient Orthopedic Disorders: Diagnosis and Therapy. Stephen Paget, John F. Beary, Charles L. Christian, et. al.. Little, Brown and Company, 34 Beacon St., Boston, MA 02108. Phone: (617) 227-0730. Third edition 1992.

JOURNALS

Annals of the Rheumatic Diseases. BMJ Publishing Group, BMA House, Tavistock Square, London WC1H 9JR, England. Phone: 071-383 6244/6638. Fax: 071-383 6662. Monthly.

Arthritis Care and Research. Elsevier Science Publishing Co., Inc., P.O. Box 882, Madison Square Station, New York, NY 10159-2101. Phone: (212) 989-5800. Fax: (212) 633-3990. 4/year.

Journal of Back and Musculoskelatal Rehabilitation. Butterworth-Heinemann, 80 Montvale Ave., Stoneham, MA 02180. Phone: (617) 438-8464. Fax: (617) 279-4851. Quarterly.

Journal of Musculoskeletal Pain. Haworth Press, 10 Alice Street, Binghamton, NY 13904-1580. Phone: (800) 3HA-WORTH. Fax: (607) 722-1424. Quarterly.

Journal of Rheumatology. Journal of Rheumatology Publishing Co., 920 Yonge St., Ste. 115, Toronto, ON, Canada M4W 3C7. Phone: (416) 967-5155. Fax: (416) 967-7556. Monthly.

NEWSLETTERS

Bulletin on the Rheumatic Diseases. Arthritis Foundation, 1314 Sprin St., N.W., Atlanta, GA 30309. Phone: (404) 872-7100. Fax: (404) 872-0457. Bimonthly.

United Scleroderma Foundation-Newsletter. United Scleroderma Foundation, Inc., P.O. Box 350, Watsonville, CA 95077. Phone: (408) 728-2202. Quarterly.

ONLINE DATABASES

Combined Health Information Database (CHID). U.S. National Institutes of Health, P.O. Box NDIC, Bethesda, MD 20892. Phone: (301) 496-2162. Fax: (301) 770-5164. Quarterly.

EMBASE. Elsevier Science Publishing Co., Inc., P.O. Box 882, Madison Square Station, New York, NY 10159-2101. Phone: (212) 989-5800. Fax: (212) 633-3990.

MEDLINE. National Library of Medicine, 8600 Rockville Pike, Bethesda, MD 20894. Phone: (800) 638-8480.

SciSearch. Institute for Scientific Information, 3501 Market St., Philadelphia, PA 19104. Phone: (215) 386-0100. Fax: (215) 386-6362.

RESEARCH CENTERS, INSTITUTES, CLEARINGHOUSES

Multipurpose Arthritis and Musculoskeletal Diseases Center. University of Alabama at Birmingham. Tinsley Harrison Tower 429 A, UAB Station, Birmingham, AL 35294. Phone: (205) 934-5306. Fax: (205) 934-1564.

National Arthritis and Musculoskeletal and Skin Diseases Information Clearinghouse (NAMSIC). 9000 Rockville Pike, P.O. Box AMS, Bethesda, MD 20892. Phone: (301) 495-4484. Fax: (301) 587-4352.

TEXTBOOKS AND MONOGRAPHS

Diagnosis of Bone and Joint Disorders. Donald Resnick, Ken Niwayama. W.B. Saunders Co., The Curtis Center, Independence Sqare W., Philadelphia, PA 19106-3399. Phone: (215) 238-7800. 1988.

McKusick's Heritable Disorders of Connective Tissue. Peter Brighton, Victor McKusick. Mosby-Year Book, 11830 Westline Industrial Drive, St. Louis, MO 63146. Phone: (800) 325-4177. Fax: (314) 432-1380. 1992.

Metabolic Bone Disease and Clinically Related Disorders. Louis V. Avioli, Stephen M. Krane. W.B. Saunders Co., The Curtis Center, Independence Square W., Philadelphia, PA 19106-3399. Phone: (215) 238-7800. Second edition 1990.

Osteoarthritis. Roland Macowitz, and others. W.B. Saunders Co., The Curtis Center, Independence Sqare W., Philadelphia, PA 19106-3399. Phone: (215) 238-7800. 2nd edition.

Radiology of Bone Diseases. G.B. Granfield. J.B. Lippincott Co., 227 E. Washington Square, Philadelphia, PA 19106-3780. Phone: (215) 238-4200. Fax: (215) 238-4227. 5th edition, 1990.

BONE AND JOINT SURGERY

See: ORTHOPEDICS

BONE MARROW TRANSPLANTATION

See: TRANSPLANTATION

BOTULISM

See: FOOD POISONING

BOWEL CANCER

See: COLORECTAL CANCER

BRADYCARDIA

See: ARRHYTHMIA

BRAIN

See: BRAIN DISEASES

BRAIN CANCER

See also: CANCER

ABSTRACTING, INDEXING, AND CURRENT AWARENESS PUBLICATIONS

Current Contents/Clinical Medicine. Institute for Scientific Information, 3501 Market St., Philadelphia, PA 19104. Phone: (800) 523-1850. Fax: (215) 386-6362. Weekly.

Excerpta Medica. Section 16: Cancer. Elsevier Science Publishing Co., Inc., P.O. Box 882, Madison Square Station, New York, NY 10159-2101. Phone: (212) 989-5800. Fax: (212) 633-3990. 32/year.

Index Medicus. U.S. National Library of Medicine, 8600 Rockville Pike, Bethesda, MD 20894. Phone: (800) 638-8480. Monthly.

Science Citation Index. Institute for Scientific Information, 3501 Market St., Philadelphia, PA 19104. Phone: (800) 523-1850. Fax: (215) 386-6362. Bimonthly.

Statistical Reference Index. Congressional Information Service, 4520 East-West Hwy., Bethesda, MD 20814. Phone: (800) 639-8380. 1980-Present Monthly.

ANNUALS AND REVIEWS

In Development New Medicines for Older Americans. 1991 Annual Survey. More Medicines in Testing for Cancer Than for Any Other Disease of Aging. Pharmaceutical Manufacturers Association, 1100 15th St. N.W., Washington, DC 20005. Phone: (202) 835-3400. 1991.

ASSOCIATIONS, PROFESSIONAL SOCIETIES, ADVOCACY AND SUPPORT GROUPS

American Cancer Society (ACS). 1599 Clifton Rd. N.E., Atlanta, GA 30329. Phone: (404) 320-3333.

Association for Brain Tumor Research (AFBTR). 3725 N. Talman Ave., Chicago, IL 60618. Phone: (312) 286-5571. Fax: (312) 549-5561.

BIBLIOGRAPHIES

Oncology Overview: Diagnosis and Therapy of Astrocytic and Oligodendroglial Tumors. S. Clifford Schold, Jr. (ed.). U.S. Government Printing Office, Superintendent of Documents, P.O. Box 371954, Pittsburgh, PA 15250-7954. Phone: (202) 783-3238. Fax: (202) 512-2250. 1990.

CD-ROM DATABASES

Cancerlit. Aries Systems Corporation, One Dundee Park, Andover, MA 01810. Phone: (508) 475-7200. Fax: (508) 474-8860. Quarterly.

OncoDisc. J.B. Lippincott Co., 227 East Washington Square, Philadelphia, PA 19106-3780. Phone: (215) 238-4200. Fax: (215) 238-4227. Bimonthly.

Physician's Data Query (PDQ). Cambridge Scientific Abstracts, 7200 Wisconsin Ave., Bethesda, MD 20814-4823. Phone: (800) 843-7751. Fax: (301) 961-6720. Quarterly.

SCISEARCH. Institute for Scientific Information, 3501 Market St., Philadelphia, PA 19104. Phone: (215) 386-0100. Fax: (215) 386-6362.

ENCYCLOPEDIAS, DICTIONARIES, WORD BOOKS

Oncology Words. Stedman. Williams & Wilkins, 428 East Preston St., Baltimore, MD 21202. Phone: (800) 638-0672. Fax: (800) 447-8438. 1992.

JOURNALS

CA - A Cancer Journal for Clinicians. J.B. Lippincott Co., 227 E. Washington Square, Philadelphia, PA 19106-3780. Phone: (215) 238-4200. Fax: (215) 238-4227. Bimonthly.

Cancer Causes and Control. Rapid Communications of Oxford Ltd., The Old Malthouse, Paradise St., Oxford OX1 1LD, England. Phone: 44-865-790447. Fax: 44-865-244012. 6/year.

Journal of the National Cancer Institute. Superintendent of Documents, P.O. Box 371954, Pittsburgh, PA 15250-7954. Fax: (202) 512-2233. Semimonthly.

Journal of Surgical Oncology. John Wiley & Sons, Inc., 605 Third Ave., New York, NY 10158-0012. Phone: (212) 850-6000. Fax: (212) 850-6088. Monthly.

ONLINE DATABASES

Cancer Weekly. CDC AIDS Weekly/NCI Cancer Weekly, 206 Rogers St. NE, Suite 104, P.O. Box 5528, Atlanta, GA 30317. Phone: (404) 377-8895. Weekly.

CANCERLIT. U.S. National Cancer Institute, International Cancer Information Center, Building 82, Room 102, Bethesda, MD 20892. Phone: (301) 496-7403. Fax: (301) 480-8105. Monthly.

Clinical Protocols. U.S. National Cancer Institute, International Cancer Information Center, Building 82, Room 102, Bethesda, MD 20892. Phone: (301) 496-7403. Fax: (301) 480-8105.

EMBASE. Elsevier Science Publishing Co., Inc., P.O. Box 882, Madison Square Station, New York, NY 10159-2101. Phone: (212) 989-5800. Fax: (212) 633-3990.

MEDLINE. National Library of Medicine, 8600 Rockville Pike, Bethesda, MD 20894. Phone: (800) 638-8480.

Physician Data Query (PDQ) Cancer Information File. U.S. National Cancer Institute, International Cancer Information Center, Building 82, Room 102, Bethesda, MD 20892. Phone: (301) 496-7403. Fax: (301) 480-8105. Monthly.

Physician Data Query (PDQ) Directory File. U.S. National Cancer Institute, International Cancer Information Center, Building 82, Room 102, Bethesda, MD 20892. Phone: (301) 496-7403. Fax: (301) 480-8105. Monthly.

Physician Data Query (PDQ) Protocol File. U.S. National Cancer Institute, International Cancer Information Center,

Building 82, Room 102, Bethesda, MD 20892. Phone: (301) 496-7403. Fax: (301) 480-8105. Monthly.

SciSearch. Institute for Scientific Information, 3501 Market St., Philadelphia, PA 19104. Phone: (215) 386-0100. Fax: (215) 386-6362.

POPULAR WORKS AND PATIENT EDUCATION

Cancervive: The Challenge of Life After Cancer. Susan Nessim, Judith Ellis. Houghton Mifflin Co., 1 Beacon St., Boston, MA 02108. Phone: (800) 225-3362. 1991.

Everyone's Guide to Cancer Therapy: How Cancer is Diagnosed, Treated, and Managed on a Day to Day Basis. Malin Dollinger, Ernest H. Rosenbaum, Greg Cable. Andrews & McMeel, 4900 Main St., Kansas City, MO 64112. Phone: (800) 826-4216. 1991.

RESEARCH CENTERS, INSTITUTES, CLEARINGHOUSES

Brain Tumor Information Service. University of Chicago, 5841 S. Maryland Ave., Chicago, IL 60637. Phone: (312) 684-1400.

Cancer Information Service (CIS). Office of Cancer Communications, National Cancer Institute, Bldg. 31, Rm. 10A24, 9000 Rockville Pike, Bethesda, MD 20892. Phone: (800) 4CA-NCER.

Preuss Laboratory for Brain Tumor Research. Duke University. Duke Medical Ctr., Research Dr., P.O. Box 3156, Durham, NC 27710. Phone: (919) 684-4187.

TEXTBOOKS AND MONOGRAPHS

Cancer Medicine. James F. Holland, Emil Frei, Robert C. Bast Jr., and others. Williams & Wilkins, 428 East Preston St., Baltimore, MD 21202. Phone: (800) 638-0672. Fax: (800) 447-8438. Third edition 1992.

Cancer: Principles and Practice of Oncology. Vincent T. DeVita. J.B. Lippincott Co., 227 E. Washington Square, Philadelphia, PA 19106-3780. Phone: (215) 238-4200. Fax: (215) 238-4227. 1989 3rd edtion.

Cancer Treatment. Charles M. Haskell. W.B. Saunders Co., The Curtis Center, Independence Square W., Philadelphia, PA 19106-3399. Phone: (215) 238-7800. Third edition 1990.

BRAIN DEATH

See: MEDICAL ETHICS

BRAIN DISEASES

See also: NEUROLOGIC DISORDERS

ABSTRACTING, INDEXING, AND CURRENT AWARENESS PUBLICATIONS

Current Contents/Clinical Medicine. Institute for Scientific Information, 3501 Market St., Philadelphia, PA 19104. Phone: (800) 523-1850. Fax: (215) 386-6362. Weekly.

Current Contents/Life Sciences. Institute for Scientific Information, 3501 Market St., Philadelphia, PA 19104. Phone: (215) 386-0100. Fax: (215) 386-6362.

Index Medicus. U.S. National Library of Medicine, 8600 Rockville Pike, Bethesda, MD 20894. Phone: (800) 638-8480. Monthly.

Science Citation Index. Institute for Scientific Information, 3501 Market St., Philadelphia, PA 19104. Phone: (800) 523-1850. Fax: (215) 386-6362. Bimonthly.

ANNUALS AND REVIEWS

Progress in Brain Research. Elsevier Science Publishing Co., Inc., P.O. Box 882, Madison Square Station, New York, NY 10159-2101. Phone: (212) 989-5800. Fax: (212) 633-3990. Irregular.

ASSOCIATIONS, PROFESSIONAL SOCIETIES, ADVOCACY AND SUPPORT GROUPS

Association for Brain Tumor Research. 2910 W. Montrose Ave., Chicago, IL 60618. Phone: (312) 286-5571.

Brain Research Center. Children's Hospital National Medical Center, 111 Michigan Ave. N.W., Washington, DC 20010. Phone: (202) 745-3413.

Brain Research Foundation (BRF). 208 S. LaSalle St., Ste. 1426, Chicago, IL 60604. Phone: (312) 782-4311. Fax: (312) 782-6437.

Family Survival Project for Brain Damaged Adults. 44 Page St., Ste. 600, San Francisco, CA 94102. Phone: (415) 626-6556.

CD-ROM DATABASES

Neuroscience Citation Index. Institute for Scientific Information, 3501 Market St., Philadelphia, PA 19104. Phone: (800) 523-1857. Fax: (215) 386-6362. Bimonthly.

SCISEARCH. Institute for Scientific Information, 3501 Market St., Philadelphia, PA 19104. Phone: (215) 386-0100. Fax: (215) 386-6362.

HANDBOOKS, GUIDES, MANUALS, ATLASES

Color Atlas of the Brain and Spinal Cord. Marjorie A. England, Jennifer Wakely. Mosby-Year Book, 11830 Westline Industrial Drive, St. Louis, MO 63146. Phone: (800) 325-4177. Fax: (314) 432-1380. 1991.

MRI Atlas of the Brain. William G. Bradley, Graeme Bydder. Raven Press, 1185 Avenue of the Americas, New York, NY 10036. Phone: (212) 930-9500. Fax: (212) 869-3495. 1990.

Practical MRI Atlas of Neonatal Brain Development. A. James Barkovich, Charles L. Truwit. Raven Press, 1185 Avenue of the Americas, New York, NY 10036. Phone: (212) 930-9500. Fax: (212) 869-3495. 1990.

JOURNALS

Brain. Oxford University Press, 200 Madison Ave., New York, NY 10016. Phone: (212) 679-7300.

Brain Injury. Taylor & Francis Inc., 1900 Frost Rd., Suite 101, Bristol, PA 19007-1598. Phone: (800) 821-8312. Fax: (215) 785-5515. Bimonthly.

Brain Research. Elsevier Science Publishing Co., Inc., P.O. Box 882, Madison Square Station, New York, NY 10159-2101. Phone: (212) 989-5800. Fax: (212) 633-3990. 101/year.

Brain Research Reviews. Elsevier Science Publishing Co., Inc., P.O. Box 882, Madison Square Station, New York, NY 10159-2101. Phone: (212) 989-5800. Fax: (212) 633-3990.

Developmental Brain Research. Elsevier Science Publishing Co., Inc., P.O. Box 882, Madison Square Station, New York, NY 10159-2101. Phone: (212) 989-5800. Fax: (212) 633-3990.

Experimental Brain Research. Springer-Verlag New York Inc., 175 Fifth Ave., New York, NY 10010. Phone: (212) 460-1500. Fax: (212) 473-6272.

Metabolic Brain Disease. Plenum Publishing Co., 233 Spring St., New York, NY 10013-1578. Phone: (212) 620-8000. Fax: (212) 463-0742. Quarterly.

NEWSLETTERS

Brain/Mind Bulletin. Interface Press, P.O. Box 42211, Los Angeles, CA 90042. Phone: (213) 223-2500. Monthly.

ONLINE DATABASES

EMBASE. Elsevier Science Publishing Co., Inc., P.O. Box 882, Madison Square Station, New York, NY 10159-2101. Phone: (212) 989-5800. Fax: (212) 633-3990.

MEDLINE. National Library of Medicine, 8600 Rockville Pike, Bethesda, MD 20894. Phone: (800) 638-8480.

SciSearch. Institute for Scientific Information, 3501 Market St., Philadelphia, PA 19104. Phone: (215) 386-0100. Fax: (215) 386-6362.

RESEARCH CENTERS, INSTITUTES, CLEARINGHOUSES

Brain Development Research Center. University of North Carolina at Chapel Hill. CB 7250, Chapel Hill, NC 27599-7250. Phone: (919) 966-2405. Fax: (919) 966-1844.

Brain Information Service (BIS). University of California Brain Information Service, Ctr. for Health Sciences, Rm. 43-367, Los Angeles, CA 90024. Phone: (213) 825-3417.

Brain Research Foundation. 208 S. LaSalle St., Chicago, IL 60604. Phone: (312) 782-4311.

Center for Neuroscience. University of Tennessee. 875 Monroe Ave., Memphis, TN 38163. Phone: (901) 528-5956. Fax: (901) 528-7193.

TEXTBOOKS AND MONOGRAPHS

Aging Brain and Dementia: New Trends in Diagnosis and Therapy. L. Battistin, Franz Gerstenbrand (eds.). John Wiley & Sons, Inc., 605 Third Ave., New York, NY 10158-0012. Phone: (212) 850-6000. Fax: (212) 850-6088. 1989.

Chronic Encephalitis and Seizures. Frederick Andermann, Theodore Rasmussen (eds.). Butterworth-Heinemann, 80 Montvale Ave., Stoneham, MA 02180. Phone: (617) 438-8464. Fax: (617) 279-4851. 1991.

Clincal Brain Imaging. Mazziotta. F.A. Davis Co., 1915 Arch St., Philadelphia, PA 19103. Phone: (800) 523-4049. Fax: (215) 568-5065. 1992.

Magnetic Resonance Imaging of the Brain and Spine. Scott W. Atlas. Raven Press, 1185 Avenue of the Americas, New York, NY 10036. Phone: (212) 930-9500. Fax: (212) 869-3495. 1991.

BREAST CANCER

See also: CANCER; MAMMOGRAPHY

ABSTRACTING, INDEXING, AND CURRENT AWARENESS PUBLICATIONS

Current Contents/Clinical Medicine. Institute for Scientific Information, 3501 Market St., Philadelphia, PA 19104. Phone: (800) 523-1850. Fax: (215) 386-6362. Weekly.

Excerpta Medica. Section 16: Cancer. Elsevier Science Publishing Co., Inc., P.O. Box 882, Madison Square Station, New York, NY 10159-2101. Phone: (212) 989-5800. Fax: (212) 633-3990. 32/year.

ICRDB Cancergram: Breast Cancer--Diagnosis, Treatment, Preclinical Biology. U.S. Government Printing Office, Superintendent of Documents, P.O. Box 371954, Pittsburgh, PA 15250-7954. Phone: (202) 783-3238. Fax: (202) 512-2250. Monthly.

Index Medicus. U.S. National Library of Medicine, 8600 Rockville Pike, Bethesda, MD 20894. Phone: (800) 638-8480. Monthly.

Research Alert: Breast Cancer. Institute for Scientific Information, 3501 Market St., Philadelphia, PA 19104. Phone: (800) 523-1850. Fax: (215) 386-6362. Weekly.

Science Citation Index. Institute for Scientific Information, 3501 Market St., Philadelphia, PA 19104. Phone: (800) 523-1850. Fax: (215) 386-6362. Bimonthly.

ANNUALS AND REVIEWS

Breast Diseases: A Year Book Quarterly. Mosby-Year Book, 11830 Westline Industrial Drive, St. Louis, MO 63146. Phone: (800) 325-4177. Fax: (314) 432-1380. Quarterly.

In Development New Medicines for Older Americans. 1991 Annual Survey. More Medicines in Testing for Cancer Than for Any Other Disease of Aging. Pharmaceutical Manufacturers Association, 1100 15th St. N.W., Washington, DC 20005. Phone: (202) 835-3400. 1991.

ASSOCIATIONS, PROFESSIONAL SOCIETIES, ADVOCACY AND SUPPORT GROUPS

American Cancer Society (ACS). 1599 Clifton Rd. N.E., Atlanta, GA 30329. Phone: (404) 320-3333.

National Alliance of Breast Cancer Organizations (NABCO). 1180 Ave. of the Americas, 2nd Flr., New York, NY 10036. Phone: (212) 719-0154. Fax: (212) 719-0263.

BIBLIOGRAPHIES

Oncology Overview: The Management of Early Breast Cancer Non-Infiltrative Stage I and II Disease. Sandra M. Swain (ed.). U.S. Government Printing Office, Superintendent of Documents, P.O. Box 371954, Pittsburgh, PA 15250-7954. Phone: (202) 783-3238. Fax: (202) 512-2250. 1990.

CD-ROM DATABASES

Morbidity Mortality Weekly Report. MEP, 124 Mt. Auburn St., Cambridge, MA 02138. Phone: (800) 342-1338. Fax: (617) 868-7738. Annual.

OncoDisc. J.B. Lippincott Co., 227 East Washington Square, Philadelphia, PA 19106-3780. Phone: (215) 238-4200. Fax: (215) 238-4227. Bimonthly.

Physician's Data Query (PDQ). Cambridge Scientific Abstracts, 7200 Wisconsin Ave., Bethesda, MD 20814-4823. Phone: (800) 843-7751. Fax: (301) 961-6720. Quarterly.

SCISEARCH. Institute for Scientific Information, 3501 Market St., Philadelphia, PA 19104. Phone: (215) 386-0100. Fax: (215) 386-6362.

ENCYCLOPEDIAS, DICTIONARIES, WORD BOOKS

Oncology Words. Stedman. Williams & Wilkins, 428 East Preston St., Baltimore, MD 21202. Phone: (800) 638-0672. Fax: (800) 447-8438. 1992.

HANDBOOKS, GUIDES, MANUALS, ATLASES

AIDS: A Pocket Book of Diagnosis and Management. Adrian Mindel (ed.). Williams & Wilkins, 428 East Preston St., Baltimore, MD 21202. Phone: (800) 638-0672. Fax: (800) 447-8438. 1989.

Atlas of Breast Disease. Volker Barth, Klaus Prechtel. Mosby-Year Book, 11830 Westline Industrial Drive, St. Louis, MO 63146. Phone: (800) 325-4177. Fax: (314) 432-1380. Second edition 1991.

A Color Atlas of Breast Disease. R. Mansel, N. Bundred. Mosby-Year Book, 11830 Westline Industrial Drive, St. Louis, MO 63146. Phone: (800) 325-4177. Fax: (314) 432-1380. 1992.

JOURNALS

Antiviral Research. Elsevier Science Publishing Co., Inc., P.O. Box 882, Madison Square Station, New York, NY 10159-2101. Phone: (212) 989-5800. Fax: (212) 633-3990. 12/year.

Breast Cancer Research and Treatment. Kluwer Academic Publishers, P.O. Box 358, Accord Station, Hingham, MA 02018-0358. Phone: (617) 871-6600. Fax: (617) 871-6528. 12/year.

Breast Disease. Elsevier Science Publishing Co., Inc., P.O. Box 882, Madison Square Station, New York, NY 10159-2101. Phone: (212) 989-5800. Fax: (212) 633-3990. 4/year.

CA - A Cancer Journal for Clinicians. J.B. Lippincott Co., 227 E. Washington Square, Philadelphia, PA 19106-3780. Phone: (215) 238-4200. Fax: (215) 238-4227. Bimonthly.

Cancer Causes and Control. Rapid Communications of Oxford Ltd., The Old Malthouse, Paradise St., Oxford OX1 1LD, England. Phone: 44-865-790447. Fax: 44-865-244012. 6/year.

Journal of the National Cancer Institute. Superintendent of Documents, P.O. Box 371954, Pittsburgh, PA 15250-7954. Fax: (202) 512-2233. Semimonthly.

Journal of Surgical Oncology. John Wiley & Sons, Inc., 605 Third Ave., New York, NY 10158-0012. Phone: (212) 850-6000. Fax: (212) 850-6088. Monthly.

Journal of Women's Health. Mary Ann Liebert, Inc., 1651 Third Ave., New York, NY 10128. Phone: (212) 289-2300. Fax: (212) 289-4697. Quarterly.

Morbidity and Mortality Weekly Report. Massachusetts Medical Society, 1440 Main St., Waltham, MA 02154-1649. Phone: (617) 893-3800. Fax: (617) 893-0413. Weekly.

ONLINE DATABASES

Cancer Weekly. CDC AIDS Weekly/NCI Cancer Weekly, 206 Rogers St. NE, Suite 104, P.O. Box 5528, Atlanta, GA 30317. Phone: (404) 377-8895. Weekly.

Clinical Protocols. U.S. National Cancer Institute, International Cancer Information Center, Building 82, Room 102, Bethesda, MD 20892. Phone: (301) 496-7403. Fax: (301) 480-8105.

EMBASE. Elsevier Science Publishing Co., Inc., P.O. Box 882, Madison Square Station, New York, NY 10159-2101. Phone: (212) 989-5800. Fax: (212) 633-3990.

MEDLINE. National Library of Medicine, 8600 Rockville Pike, Bethesda, MD 20894. Phone: (800) 638-8480.

SciSearch. Institute for Scientific Information, 3501 Market St., Philadelphia, PA 19104. Phone: (215) 386-0100. Fax: (215) 386-6362.

POPULAR WORKS AND PATIENT EDUCATION

Dr. Susan Love's Breast Book. Susan M. Love. Addison-Wesley Nursing, 390 Bridge Parkway, Redwood City, CA 94065. Phone: (800) 950-5544. 1990.

Every Woman's Medical Handbook. Marie Stoppard. Ballantine Books, Inc., 201 E. 50th St., New York, NY 10022. Phone: (800) 733-3000. 1991.

Everyone's Guide to Cancer Therapy: How Cancer is Diagnosed, Treated, and Managed on a Day to Day Basis. Malin Dollinger, Ernest H. Rosenbaum, Greg Cable. Andrews & McMeel, 4900 Main St., Kansas City, MO 64112. Phone: (800) 826-4216. 1991.

If It Runs in Your Family: Breast Cancer, Reducing Your Risk. Mary D. Eades. Bantam Books, Inc., 666 Fifth Ave., New York, NY 10103. Phone: (800) 223-6834. 1991.

Invisible Scars: A Guide to Coping with the Emotional Impact of Breast Cancer. Mimi Greenberg. Walker Publishing Co., Inc., 720 Fifth Ave., New York, NY 10019. Phone: (212) 265-3632. 1988.

Living with Breast Cancer and Mastectomy. Nicholas Tarrier. St. Martin's Press, 175 Fifth Ave., New York, NY 10010. Phone: (212) 674-5151. 1992.

Women Talk about Breast Surgery: From Diagnosis to Recovery. Amy Gross, Dee Ito. HarperCollins Pubs., Inc., 10 E. 53rd St., New York, NY 10022-5299. Phone: (212) 207-7000. Fax: (800) 242-7737. 1991.

Women's Cancers: How to Prevent Them, How to Treat Them, How to Beat Them. Donna Dawson, Marlene Mersch (eds.). Hunter House, Inc., 2200 Central, Ste. 202, Alameda, CA 94501-4451. Phone: (510) 865-5282. 1992.

RESEARCH CENTERS, INSTITUTES, CLEARINGHOUSES

Breast Cancer Research Lab. Hahnemann University. Dept. of Microbiology and Immunology, Broad and Vine Sts., 405, Philadelphia, PA 19102-1192. Phone: (215) 448-8705.

Cancer Information Service (CIS). Office of Cancer Communications, National Cancer Institute, Bldg. 31, Rm. 10A24, 9000 Rockville Pike, Bethesda, MD 20892. Phone: (800) 4CA-NCER.

Comprehensive Breast Center. Vincent P. Lombardi Cancer Research Center, Georgetown University, Washington, DC 20007. Phone: (202) 687-2117.

Memorial Sloan-Kettering Cancer Center. 1275 York Ave., New York, NY 10021. Phone: (212) 355-0060.

National Surgical Adjuvant Breast and Bowel Project. University of Pittsburgh, Scaife Hall, Room 914, Pittsburgh, PA 15261. Phone: (412) 648-9720. Fax: (412) 648-1912.

Vincent T. Lombardi Cancer Research Center. Georgetown University. 3800 Reservoir Rd. NW, Podium Level, Washington, DC 20007. Phone: (202) 687-2110. Fax: (202) 687-6402.

STANDARDS AND STATISTICS SOURCES

Early Stage Breast Cancer. Consensus Statement. NIH Consensus Development Conference. June 18-21, 1990. National Institutes of Health, Office of Medical Applications of Research, Federal Bldg., Rm. 618, Bethesda, MD 20892. 1990.

TEXTBOOKS AND MONOGRAPHS

Breast Cancer. B.J. Kennedy (ed.). John Wiley & Sons, Inc., 605 Third Ave., New York, NY 10158-0012. Phone: (212) 850-6000. Fax: (212) 850-6088. 1989.

Breast Cancer: Conservative and Reconstructive Surgery. H. Bohmert, H.P. Leis, I.T. Jackson (eds.). Thieme Medical Publishers, Inc., 381 Park Ave. S., New York, NY 10016. Phone: (212) 683-5088. Fax: (212) 779-9020. 1989.

Breast Cancer Treatment. Fowble. Mosby-Year Book, 11830 Westline Industrial Drive, St. Louis, MO 63146. Phone: (800) 325-4177. Fax: (314) 432-1380. 1991.

The Breast: Comprehensive Management of Benign and Malignant Diseases. Kirby I. Bland, Edward M. Copeland III. W.B. Saunders Co., The Curtis Center, Independence Square W., Philadelphia, PA 19106-3399. Phone: (215) 238-7800. 1991.

Breast Diseases. Jay R. Harris, Samuel Hellman, I. Craig Henderson, et. al.. J.B. Lippincott Co., 227 E. Washington Square, Philadelphia, PA 19106-3780. Phone: (215) 238-4200. Fax: (215) 238-4227. Second edition 1991.

Cancer Medicine. James F. Holland, Emil Frei, Robert C. Bast Jr., and others. Williams & Wilkins, 428 East Preston St., Baltimore, MD 21202. Phone: (800) 638-0672. Fax: (800) 447-8438. Third edition 1992.

Cancer: Principles and Practice of Oncology. Vincent T. DeVita. J.B. Lippincott Co., 227 E. Washington Square, Philadelphia, PA 19106-3780. Phone: (215) 238-4200. Fax: (215) 238-4227. 1989 3rd edtion.

Cancer Treatment. Charles M. Haskell. W.B. Saunders Co., The Curtis Center, Independence Square W., Philadelphia, PA 19106-3399. Phone: (215) 238-7800. Third edition 1990.

Chemotherapy of Gynecological and Breast Cancer. M. Kaufmann, and others. S. Karger Publishers, Inc., 26 W. Avon

Rd., P.O. Box 529, Farmington, CT 06085. Phone: (203) 675-7834. Fax: (203) 675-7302. 1990.

The Female Breast and Its Disorders: Essentials of Diagnosis and Management. George W. Mitchell Jr., Lawrence Bassett. Williams & Wilkins, 428 East Preston St., Baltimore, MD 21202. Phone: (800) 638-0672. Fax: (800) 447-8438. 1990.

Interpretation of Breast Biopsies. Darryl Carter. Raven Press, 1185 Avenue of the Americas, New York, NY 10036. Phone: (212) 930-9500. Fax: (212) 869-3495. Second edition 1990.

Medical Management of Breast Cancer. Powles. J.B. Lippincott Co., 227 E. Washington Square, Philadelphia, PA 19106-3780. Phone: (215) 238-4200. Fax: (215) 238-4227. 1991.

Plastic and Reconstructive Surgery of the Breast. Noone. Mosby-Year Book, 11830 Westline Industrial Drive, St. Louis, MO 63146. Phone: (800) 325-4177. Fax: (314) 432-1380. 1991.

Textbook of Breast Disease. John H. Isaacs. Mosby-Year Book, 11830 Westline Industrial Drive, St. Louis, MO 63146. Phone: (800) 325-4177. Fax: (314) 432-1380. 1992.

BREAST DISEASES

See also: BREAST CANCER; GYNECOLOGIC DISORDERS

ABSTRACTING, INDEXING, AND CURRENT AWARENESS PUBLICATIONS

Current Contents/Clinical Medicine. Institute for Scientific Information, 3501 Market St., Philadelphia, PA 19104. Phone: (800) 523-1850. Fax: (215) 386-6362. Weekly.

Excerpta Medica. Section 10: Obstetrics and Gynecology. Elsevier Science Publishing Co., Inc., P.O. Box 882, Madison Square Station, New York, NY 10159-2101. Phone: (212) 989-5800. Fax: (212) 633-3990. 20/year.

Index Medicus. U.S. National Library of Medicine, 8600 Rockville Pike, Bethesda, MD 20894. Phone: (800) 638-8480. Monthly.

Science Citation Index. Institute for Scientific Information, 3501 Market St., Philadelphia, PA 19104. Phone: (800) 523-1850. Fax: (215) 386-6362. Bimonthly.

ANNUALS AND REVIEWS

Breast Diseases: A Year Book Quarterly. Mosby-Year Book, 11830 Westline Industrial Drive, St. Louis, MO 63146. Phone: (800) 325-4177. Fax: (314) 432-1380. Quarterly.

Year Book of Obstetrics and Gynecology. Mosby-Year Book, 11830 Westline Industrial Drive, St. Louis, MO 63146. Phone: (800) 325-4177. Fax: (314) 432-1380. Annual.

ASSOCIATIONS, PROFESSIONAL SOCIETIES, ADVOCACY AND SUPPORT GROUPS

American College of Obstetricians and Gynecologists (ACOG). 409 12th St. S.W., Washington, DC 20024-2188. Phone: (202) 638-5577.

Contact Lens Association of Ophthalmologists (CLAO). 523 Decatur St., Ste. 1, New Orleans, LA 70130-1027. Phone: (504) 581-4000. Fax: (504) 581-5884.

CD-ROM DATABASES

Excerpta Medica CD: Obstetrics & Gynecology. SilverPlatter Information, Inc., River Ridge Office Park, 100 River Ridge Rd., Norwood, MA 02062. Phone: (617) 769-2599. Fax: (617) 769-8763. Quarterly.

SCISEARCH. Institute for Scientific Information, 3501 Market St., Philadelphia, PA 19104. Phone: (215) 386-0100. Fax: (215) 386-6362.

HANDBOOKS, GUIDES, MANUALS, ATLASES

Atlas of Breast Disease. Volker Barth, Klaus Prechtel. Mosby-Year Book, 11830 Westline Industrial Drive, St. Louis, MO 63146. Phone: (800) 325-4177. Fax: (314) 432-1380. Second edition 1991.

A Color Atlas of Breast Disease. R. Mansel, N. Bundred. Mosby-Year Book, 11830 Westline Industrial Drive, St. Louis, MO 63146. Phone: (800) 325-4177. Fax: (314) 432-1380. 1992.

JOURNALS

American Journal of Obstetrics and Gynecology. Mosby-Year Book, 11830 Westline Industrial Drive, St. Louis, MO 63146. Phone: (800) 325-4177. Fax: (314) 432-1380. Monthly.

Antiviral Research. Elsevier Science Publishing Co., Inc., P.O. Box 882, Madison Square Station, New York, NY 10159-2101. Phone: (212) 989-5800. Fax: (212) 633-3990. 12/year.

Breast Disease. Elsevier Science Publishing Co., Inc., P.O. Box 882, Madison Square Station, New York, NY 10159-2101. Phone: (212) 989-5800. Fax: (212) 633-3990. 4/year.

Clinical Practice of Gynecology. Elsevier Science Publishing Co., Inc., P.O. Box 882, Madison Square Station, New York, NY 10159-2101. Phone: (212) 989-5800. Fax: (212) 633-3990.

Obstetrics and Gynecology. Elsevier Science Publishing Co., Inc., P.O. Box 882, Madison Square Station, New York, NY 10159-2101. Phone: (212) 989-5800. Fax: (212) 633-3990. 15/year.

NEWSLETTERS

National Women's Health Network-Network News. National Women's Health Network, 1325 G St. N.W., Washington, DC 20005. Phone: (202) 347-1140. Bimonthly.

ONLINE DATABASES

EMBASE. Elsevier Science Publishing Co., Inc., P.O. Box 882, Madison Square Station, New York, NY 10159-2101. Phone: (212) 989-5800. Fax: (212) 633-3990.

MEDLINE. National Library of Medicine, 8600 Rockville Pike, Bethesda, MD 20894. Phone: (800) 638-8480.

SciSearch. Institute for Scientific Information, 3501 Market St., Philadelphia, PA 19104. Phone: (215) 386-0100. Fax: (215) 386-6362.

POPULAR WORKS AND PATIENT EDUCATION

Dr. Susan Love's Breast Book. Susan M. Love. Addison-Wesley Nursing, 390 Bridge Parkway, Redwood City, CA 94065. Phone: (800) 950-5544. 1990.

The New Our Bodies, Ourselves: The Updated and Expanded Edition. The Boston Women's Health Book Collective. Simon & Schuster, 1230 Ave. of the Americas, New York, NY 10020. Phone: (800) 223-2348. Fax: (800) 284-0735. 1992.

Women Talk about Breast Surgery: From Diagnosis to Recovery. Amy Gross, Dee Ito. HarperCollins Pubs., Inc., 10 E. 53rd St., New York, NY 10022-5299. Phone: (212) 207-7000. Fax: (800) 242-7737. 1991.

TEXTBOOKS AND MONOGRAPHS

The Breast: Comprehensive Management of Benign and Malignant Diseases. Kirby I. Bland, Edward M. Copeland III. W.B. Saunders Co., The Curtis Center, Independence Square W., Philadelphia, PA 19106-3399. Phone: (215) 238-7800. 1991.

Breast Diseases. Jay R. Harris, Samuel Hellman, I. Craig Henderson, et. al.. J.B. Lippincott Co., 227 E. Washington Square, Philadelphia, PA 19106-3780. Phone: (215) 238-4200. Fax: (215) 238-4227. Second edition 1991.

Diagnosis and Detection of Breast Disease. Deborah E. Powell, Carol B. Stelling. Mosby-Year Book, 11830 Westline Industrial Drive, St. Louis, MO 63146. Phone: (800) 325-4177. Fax: (314) 432-1380. 1992.

The Female Breast and Its Disorders: Essentials of Diagnosis and Management. George W. Mitchell Jr., Lawrence Bassett. Williams & Wilkins, 428 East Preston St., Baltimore, MD 21202. Phone: (800) 638-0672. Fax: (800) 447-8438. 1990.

Novak's Textbook of Gynecolgy. Howard W. Wentz III, Anne Colston, Burnett, Lonnie Jones. Williams & Wilkins, 428 East Preston St., Baltimore, MD 21202. Phone: (800) 638-0672. Fax: (800) 447-8438. Eleventh edition 1988.

Textbook of Breast Disease. John H. Isaacs. Mosby-Year Book, 11830 Westline Industrial Drive, St. Louis, MO 63146. Phone: (800) 325-4177. Fax: (314) 432-1380. 1992.

BREAST FEEDING

ABSTRACTING, INDEXING, AND CURRENT AWARENESS PUBLICATIONS

Breastfeeding Abstracts. La Leche League International, Inc., 9616 Minneapolis, Franklin Park, IL 60131-8209. Phone: (312) 455-7730. Quarterly.

Index Medicus. U.S. National Library of Medicine, 8600 Rockville Pike, Bethesda, MD 20894. Phone: (800) 638-8480. Monthly.

ASSOCIATIONS, PROFESSIONAL SOCIETIES, ADVOCACY AND SUPPORT GROUPS

Boston Association for Childbirth Education. Nursing Mothers' Council, 184 Savin Hill Dr., Dorchester, MA 02125. Phone: (617) 244-5102.

Breastfeeding Support Consultants. 164 Schoolhouse Rd., Pottstown, PA 19464. Phone: (215) 326-9343.

International Lactation Consultant Association. P.O. Box 403, University of Virginia Station, Charlottesville, VA 22903.

La Leche League International. 9616 Minneapolis Ave., Franklin Park, IL 60131. Phone: (800) 525-3242.

Lactation Associates. 254 Conant Rd., Weston, MA 02193. Phone: (617) 893-3553.

BIBLIOGRAPHIES

Lactation Consultant's Topical Review and Bibliography of the Literature on Breastfeeding. Mary-Margaret Coates (ed.). La Leche League International, 9616 Minneapolis Ave., Franklin Park, IL 60131. Phone: (800) LA-LECHE. 1990.

JOURNALS

American Journal of Obstetrics and Gynecology. Mosby-Year Book, 11830 Westline Industrial Drive, St. Louis, MO 63146. Phone: (800) 325-4177. Fax: (314) 432-1380. Monthly.

Journal of Pediatric Gastroenterology and Nutrition. Raven Press, 1185 Ave. of the Americas, New York, NY 10036. Phone: (212) 930-9500. Fax: (212) 869-3495.

Pediatrics. American Academy of Pediatrics, 141 Northwest Point Rd., Elk Grove Village, IL 60009-0927. Phone: (708) 228-5005. Fax: (708) 228-5097. Monthly.

ONLINE DATABASES

EMBASE. Elsevier Science Publishing Co., Inc., P.O. Box 882, Madison Square Station, New York, NY 10159-2101. Phone: (212) 989-5800. Fax: (212) 633-3990.

MEDLINE. National Library of Medicine, 8600 Rockville Pike, Bethesda, MD 20894. Phone: (800) 638-8480.

SciSearch. Institute for Scientific Information, 3501 Market St., Philadelphia, PA 19104. Phone: (215) 386-0100. Fax: (215) 386-6362.

POPULAR WORKS AND PATIENT EDUCATION

Breastfeeding Today: A Mother's Companion. Candace Woessner, Judith Lauwers, Barbara Bernard, and others. Avery Publishing Group, Inc., 120 Old Broadway, Garden City Park, NY 11040. Phone: (800) 548-5757. Second edition 1991.

Cancervive: The Challenge of Life After Cancer. Susan Nessim, Judith Ellis. Houghton Mifflin Co., 1 Beacon St., Boston, MA 02108. Phone: (800) 225-3362. 1991.

The Nursing Mother's Companion. Harvard Common Press, 535 Albany St., Boston, MA 02118. Phone: (617) 423-5803.

Will It Hurt the Baby?: The Safe Use of Medications During Pregnancy and Breastfeeding. Richard S. Abrams. Addison-Wesley Nursing, 390 Bridge Parkway, Redwood City, CA 94065. Phone: (800) 950-5544. 1990.

The Womanly Art of Breastfeeding: Thirty-Fifth Anniversary Edition. La Leche League International Staff. Viking Penguin, 375 Hudson St., New York, NY 10014-3657. Phone: (800) 331-4624. Fifth revised edition 1991.

The Working Woman's Guide to Breastfeeding. Nancy Dana, Anne Price. Meadowbrook Press, 18318 Minnetonka Blvd., Deephaven, MN 55391. Phone: (800) 338-2232. 1987.

TEXTBOOKS AND MONOGRAPHS

Breastfeeding: A Guide for the Medical Profession. Ruth A. Lawrence. Mosby-Year Book, 11830 Westline Industrial

Drive, St. Louis, MO 63146. Phone: (800) 325-4177. Fax: (314) 432-1380. Third edition 1989.

Drug Induced Diseases in Lactation. Bennett Pov. Elsevier Science Publishing Co., Inc., P.O. Box 882, Madison Square Station, New York, NY 10159-2101. Phone: (212) 989-5800. Fax: (212) 633-3990. 1990.

Nutrition in Pregnancy and Lactation. Bonnie Worthington-Roberts, Sue Williams. Mosby-Year Book, 11830 Westline Industrial Drive, St. Louis, MO 63146. Phone: (800) 325-4177. Fax: (314) 432-1380. 1989.

BRONCHITIS

See: LUNG DISEASES; RESPIRATORY TRACT INFECTIONS

BULIMIA

See: EATING DISORDERS

BURKITT'S LYMPHOMA

See: HEMATOLOGIC DISORDERS

BURNOUT

See: STRESS

BURNS

ABSTRACTING, INDEXING, AND CURRENT AWARENESS PUBLICATIONS

Current Contents/Clinical Medicine. Institute for Scientific Information, 3501 Market St., Philadelphia, PA 19104. Phone: (800) 523-1850. Fax: (215) 386-6362. Weekly.

Index Medicus. U.S. National Library of Medicine, 8600 Rockville Pike, Bethesda, MD 20894. Phone: (800) 638-8480. Monthly.

National Bibliography on Burns. National Institute for Burn Medicine, 909 E. Ann St., Ann Arbor, MI 48104. Phone: (313) 769-9000. Annual.

Science Citation Index. Institute for Scientific Information, 3501 Market St., Philadelphia, PA 19104. Phone: (800) 523-1850. Fax: (215) 386-6362. Bimonthly.

ASSOCIATIONS, PROFESSIONAL SOCIETIES, ADVOCACY AND SUPPORT GROUPS

American Burn Association (ABA). Baltimore Regional Burn Ctr., Francis Scott Key Hospital, 4940 Eastern Ave., Baltimore, MD 21224. Phone: (301) 550-0886. Fax: (301) 550-1165.

International Society for Burn Injuries. 2005 Franklin St., Ste. 600, Denver, CO 80205. Phone: (303) 839-1694.

National Institute for Burn Medicine. 909 E. Ann St., Ann Arbor, MI 48104. Phone: (313) 769-9000.

Phoenix Society National Organization for Burn Victims. 11 Rust Hill Rd., Levittown, PA 19056. Phone: (215) 946-4788.

CD-ROM DATABASES

SCISEARCH. Institute for Scientific Information, 3501 Market St., Philadelphia, PA 19104. Phone: (215) 386-0100. Fax: (215) 386-6362.

DIRECTORIES

American Burn Association-Membership Directory. American Burn Association, Baltimore Regional Burn Center, 4940 Eastern Ave., Baltimore, MD 21224. Phone: (800) 548-BURN. Fax: (513) 751-5955. Irregular.

Burn Care Services in North America. American Burn Association, Baltimore Regional Burn Ctr., Francis Scott Key Hospital, 4940 Eastern Ave., Baltimore, MD 21224. Phone: (301) 550-0886. Fax: (301) 550-1165. Annual.

JOURNALS

Burns: Including Thermal Injury: The Journal of the International Society for Burn Injuries. Butterworth-Heinemann, 80 Montvale Ave., Stoneham, MA 02180. Phone: (617) 438-8464. Fax: (617) 279-4851. Bimonthly.

Journal of Burn Care and Rehabilitation. Mosby-Year Book, 11830 Westline Industrial Drive, St. Louis, MO 63146. Phone: (800) 325-4177. Fax: (314) 432-1380. Bimonthly.

ONLINE DATABASES

EMBASE. Elsevier Science Publishing Co., Inc., P.O. Box 882, Madison Square Station, New York, NY 10159-2101. Phone: (212) 989-5800. Fax: (212) 633-3990.

MEDLINE. National Library of Medicine, 8600 Rockville Pike, Bethesda, MD 20894. Phone: (800) 638-8480.

SciSearch. Institute for Scientific Information, 3501 Market St., Philadelphia, PA 19104. Phone: (215) 386-0100. Fax: (215) 386-6362.

RESEARCH CENTERS, INSTITUTES, CLEARINGHOUSES

Burn Trauma Center. Massachusetts General Hospital, Boston, MA 02114. Phone: (617) 726-2809.

National Burn Victim Foundation. 708 Main St., Orange, NJ 07050. Phone: (201) 731-3112.

Shriners Burn Institute. University of Cincinnati, Cincinnati, OH 45219.

University of Michigan Burn Center. 1500 E. Medical Center Dr., Ann Arbor, MI 48109. Phone: (313) 936-9666.

TEXTBOOKS AND MONOGRAPHS

Acute Management of the Burned Patient. J.A.J. Martyn. W.B. Saunders Co., The Curtis Center, Independence Square W., Philadelphia, PA 19106-3399. Phone: (215) 238-7800. 1990.

Burn Reconstruction. Bruce M. Achauer, and others. Thieme Medical Publishers, Inc., 381 Park Ave. S., New York, NY 10016. Phone: (212) 683-5088. Fax: (212) 779-9020. 1991.

Burn Trauma. R.H. Demling, C. LaLonde. Thieme Medical Publishers, Inc., 381 Park Ave. S., New York, NY 10016. Phone: (212) 683-5088. Fax: (212) 779-9020. 1989.

Critical Care of the Burn Patient: A Case Study Approach. Evelyn McLaughlin. Aspen Publishers, Inc., 200 Orchard Ridge Dr., Gaithersburg, MD 20878. Phone: (800) 638-8437. 1989.

Respiratory Injury: Smoke Inhalation and Burns. Edward F. Haponik, Andrew Munster. McGraw-Hill, Inc., 1221 Avenue of the Americas, 28th Floor, New York, NY 10020. Phone: (212) 512-4228. 1990.

BURSITIS

See: BONE AND JOINT DISEASES

BYPASS SURGERY

See: CARDIOVASCULAR SURGERY

C

CAESAREAN SECTION

See: CHILDBIRTH

CANCER

See also: BONE CANCER; BRAIN CANCER;
BREAST CANCER; COLORECTAL CANCER;
CERVICAL CANCER; HEAD AND NECK
CANCER; LEUKEMIA; LUNG CANCER;
ONCOLOGY; ORAL CANCER; OVARIAN
CANCER; PANCREATIC CANCER; SKIN
CANCER; UTERINE CANCER

ABSTRACTING, INDEXING, AND CURRENT AWARENESS PUBLICATIONS

BIOSIS/CAS Selects: Cancer Immunology. BIOSIS, 2100
Arch St., Philadelphia, PA 19103-1399. Phone: (215) 587-
4800. Fax: (215) 587-2016. Biweekly.

BIOSIS/CAS Selects: Cancer & Nutrition. BIOSIS, 2100 Arch
St., Philadelphia, PA 19103-1399. Phone: (215) 587-4800. Fax:
(215) 587-2016. Biweekly.

CA Selects: Nutritional Aspects of Cancer. Chemical Abstracts
Service, 2540 Olentangy River Road, P.O. Box 3012,
Columbus, OH 43210-0012. Phone: (800) 848-6538. Biweekly.

Cancergram. National Cancer Institute, Division of Cancer
Cause and Prevention, Bethesda, MD 20892. Phone: (301) 496-
4000. Monthly.

Current Contents/Clinical Medicine. Institute for Scientific
Information, 3501 Market St., Philadelphia, PA 19104. Phone:
(800) 523-1850. Fax: (215) 386-6362. Weekly.

Current Contents/Life Sciences. Institute for Scientific
Information, 3501 Market St., Philadelphia, PA 19104. Phone:
(215) 386-0100. Fax: (215) 386-6362.

*ICRDB Cancergram: Antitumor and Antiviral Agents--
Experimental Therapeutics, Toxicology, Pharmacology.* U.S.
Government Printing Office, Superintendent of Documents,
P.O. Box 371954, Pittsburgh, PA 15250-7954. Phone: (202)
783-3238. Fax: (202) 512-2250. Monthly.

*ICRDB Cancergram: Antitumor and Antiviral Agents--
Mechanism of Action.* U.S. Government Printing Office,
Superintendent of Documents, P.O. Box 371954, Pittsburgh,
PA 15250-7954. Phone: (202) 783-3238. Fax: (202) 512-2250.
Monthly.

*ICRDB Cancergram: Cancer Detection and Management--
Biological Markers.* U.S. Government Printing Office,

Superintendent of Documents, P.O. Box 371954, Pittsburgh,
PA 15250-7954. Phone: (202) 783-3238. Fax: (202) 512-2250.
Monthly.

ICRDB Cancergrams. U.S. National Cancer Institute,
International Cancer Information Center, Building 82, Room
102, Bethesda, MD 20892. Phone: (301) 496-7403. Fax: (301)
480-8105. Monthly.

Index Medicus. U.S. National Library of Medicine, 8600
Rockville Pike, Bethesda, MD 20894. Phone: (800) 638-8480.
Monthly.

Oncogenes & Growth Factors Abstracts. Cambridge Scientific
Abstracts, 7200 Wisconsin Ave., Bethesda, MD 20814-4823.
Phone: (800) 843-7751. Fax: (301) 961-6720. Quarterly.

Research Alert: Cancer Epidemiology. Institute for Scientific
Information, 3501 Market St., Philadelphia, PA 19104. Phone:
(800) 523-1850. Fax: (215) 386-6362. Weekly.

Research Alert: Cancer Immunology & Immunotherapy.
Institute for Scientific Information, 3501 Market St.,
Philadelphia, PA 19104. Phone: (800) 523-1850. Fax: (215)
386-6362. Weekly.

Science Citation Index. Institute for Scientific Information,
3501 Market St., Philadelphia, PA 19104. Phone: (800) 523-
1850. Fax: (215) 386-6362. Bimonthly.

ANNUALS AND REVIEWS

Advances in Cancer Research. Academic Press, Inc., 1250 Sixth
Ave., San Diego, CA 92101-4311. Phone: (619) 699-6345. Fax:
(619) 699-6715. Irregular.

*In Development New Medicines for Older Americans. 1991
Annual Survey. More Medicines in Testing for Cancer Than for
Any Other Disease of Aging.* Pharmaceutical Manufacturers
Association, 1100 15th St. N.W., Washington, DC 20005.
Phone: (202) 835-3400. 1991.

ASSOCIATIONS, PROFESSIONAL SOCIETIES, ADVOCACY AND SUPPORT GROUPS

American Cancer Society (ACS). 1599 Clifton Rd. N.E.,
Atlanta, GA 30329. Phone: (404) 320-3333.

Candlelighters Childhood Cancer Foundation. 1312 18th St.
N.W., Suite 200, Washington, DC 20036. Phone: (800) 366-
2223.

Make Today Count. 101 1/2 S. Union St., Alexandria, VA
22314. Phone: (703) 548-9674.

National Foundation for Cancer Research (NFCR). 7315 Wisconsin Ave., Ste. 332W, Bethesda, MD 20814. Phone: (800) 321-2875. Fax: (301) 654-5824.

BIBLIOGRAPHIES

Nutri-Topics: Diet and Cancer. Food and Nutrition Center, National Agricultural Library, 10301 Baltimore Blvd., Beltsville, MD 20705.

CD-ROM DATABASES

Cancer-CD. SilverPlatter Information, Inc., River Ridge Office Park, 100 River Ridge Rd., Norwood, MA 02062. Phone: (617) 769-2599. Fax: (617) 769-8763. Quarterly.

Cancer on Disc. CMC ReSearch, Inc., 7150 S.W. Hampton, Suite C-120, Portland, OR 97223. Phone: (800) 262-7668. Fax: (503) 639-1796. Annual.

Cancerlit. Aries Systems Corporation, One Dundee Park, Andover, MA 01810. Phone: (508) 475-7200. Fax: (508) 474-8860. Quarterly.

Cancerlit CD-ROM. Cambridge Scientific Abstracts, 7200 Wisconsin Ave., Bethesda, MD 20814-4823. Phone: (800) 843-7751. Fax: (301) 961-6720. Quarterly.

CD Plus/CancerLit. CD Plus, 333 7th Ave., 6th Floor, New York, NY 10001. Phone: (212) 563-3006. Monthly.

Morbidity Mortality Weekly Report. MEP, 124 Mt. Auburn St., Cambridge, MA 02138. Phone: (800) 342-1338. Fax: (617) 868-7738. Annual.

OncoDisc. J.B. Lippincott Co., 227 East Washington Square, Philadelphia, PA 19106-3780. Phone: (215) 238-4200. Fax: (215) 238-4227. Bimonthly.

Physician's Data Query (PDQ). Cambridge Scientific Abstracts, 7200 Wisconsin Ave., Bethesda, MD 20814-4823. Phone: (800) 843-7751. Fax: (301) 961-6720. Quarterly.

SCISEARCH. Institute for Scientific Information, 3501 Market St., Philadelphia, PA 19104. Phone: (215) 386-0100. Fax: (215) 386-6362.

Year Books on Disc. CMC ReSearch, Inc., 7150 S.W. Hampton, Suite C-120, Portland, OR 97223. Phone: (800) 262-7668. Fax: (503) 639-1796. Annual includes Year Books of Cardiology, Dermatology, Diagnostic Radiology, Drug Therapy, Emergency Medicine, Family Practice, Medicine, Neurology and Neurosurgery, Obstetrics and Gynecology, Oncology, Pediatrics, and Psychiatry and Applied Mental Health.

DIRECTORIES

Directory of Medical Specialists. Marquis Who's Who, 3002 Glenview Rd., Wilmette, IL 60091. Phone: (800) 621-9669. Fax: (708) 441-2264. Biennial.

Directory of Physicians in the United States. American Medical Association, 515 North State St., Chicago, IL 60610. Phone: (312) 464-0183. Fax: (312) 464-5834. Biennial.

ENCYCLOPEDIAS, DICTIONARIES, WORD BOOKS

The Cancer Dictionary. Roberta Altman, Michael J. Sarg. Facts on File, Inc., 460 Park Ave. S., New York, NY 10016-7382. Phone: (212) 683-2244. Fax: (212) 683-3633. 1992.

Oncologic Word Book. Barbara De Lorenzo. Springhouse Publishing Co., 1111 Bethlehem Pike, Spring House, PA 19477. Phone: (800) 331-3170. Fax: (215) 646-8716. 1992.

Oncology Words. Stedman. Williams & Wilkins, 428 East Preston St., Baltimore, MD 21202. Phone: (800) 638-0672. Fax: (800) 447-8438. 1992.

HANDBOOKS, GUIDES, MANUALS, ATLASES

Atlas of Cancer. Arthur T. Skarin. J.B. Lippincott Co., 227 East Washington Square, Philadelphia, PA 19106-3780. Phone: (215) 238-4200. Fax: (215) 238-4227. 1990.

Cancer: A Color Atlas. J.S. Tobias, C.J.H. Williams. J.B. Lippincott Co., 227 East Washington Square, Philadelphia, PA 19106-3780. Phone: (215) 238-4200. Fax: (215) 238-4227. 1991.

Manual of Clinical Oncology. D.K. Hossfeld, C.D. Sherman, R.R. Love, F.X. Bosch (eds.). Springer-Verlag New York Inc., 175 Fifth Ave., New York, NY 10010. Phone: (212) 460-1500. Fax: (212) 473-6272. Fifth edition 1990.

Manual of Quantitative Pathology in Cancer Diagnosis and Prognosis. J.P. Baak. Springer-Verlag New York, Inc., 175 Fifth Ave., New York, NY 10010. Phone: (212) 460-1500. Fax: (212) 473-6272. Second edition 1991.

Manual for Staging of Cancer. Oliver H. Beahrs. J.B. Lippincott Co., 227 E. Washington Square, Philadelphia, PA 19106-3780. Phone: (215) 238-4200. Fax: (215) 238-4227. Third edition 1988.

JOURNALS

CA - A Cancer Journal for Clinicians. J.B. Lippincott Co., 227 E. Washington Square, Philadelphia, PA 19106-3780. Phone: (215) 238-4200. Fax: (215) 238-4227. Bimonthly.

Cancer Causes and Control. Rapid Communications of Oxford Ltd., The Old Malthouse, Paradise St., Oxford OX1 1LD, England. Phone: 44-865-790447. Fax: 44-865-244012. 6/year.

Cancer Epidemiology, Biomarkers & Prevention. Williams & Wilkins, 428 East Preston St., Baltimore, MD 21202. Phone: (800) 638-0672. Fax: (800) 447-8438. 7/year.

Cancer Letters. Elsevier Science Publishing Co., Inc., P.O. Box 882, Madison Square Station, New York, NY 10159-2101. Phone: (212) 989-5800. Fax: (212) 633-3990. 27/year.

Cancer Research. Williams & Wilkins, 428 East Preston St., Baltimore, MD 21202. Phone: (800) 638-0672. Fax: (800) 447-8438. Semimonthly.

Cancer Therapy Update. Kluwer Academic Publishers, P.O. Box 358, Accord Station, Hingham, MA 02018-0358. Phone: (617) 871-6600. Fax: (617) 871-6528. 6/year.

Contemporary Oncology. Medical Economics, Five Paragon Dr., Montvale, NJ 07645-1742. Phone: (800) 222-3045. Fax: (201) 573-4956. 10/year.

European Journal of Cancer. Pergamon Press, 660 White Plains Rd., Tarrytown, NY 10591-5153. Phone: (914) 592-7700. Fax: (914) 592-3625. 14/year.

International Journal of Cancer. John Wiley & Sons, Inc., 605 Third Ave., New York, NY 10158-0012. Phone: (212) 850-6000. Fax: (212) 850-6088. 18/year.

Journal of Clinical Oncology. W.B. Saunders Co., The Curtis Center, Independence Square W., Philadelphia, PA 19106-3399. Phone: (215) 238-7800. Monthly.

Journal of the National Cancer Institute. Superintendent of Documents, P.O. Box 371954, Pittsburgh, PA 15250-7954. Fax: (202) 512-2233. Semimonthly.

Journal of Surgical Oncology. John Wiley & Sons, Inc., 605 Third Ave., New York, NY 10158-0012. Phone: (212) 850-6000. Fax: (212) 850-6088. Monthly.

Morbidity and Mortality Weekly Report. Massachusetts Medical Society, 1440 Main St., Waltham, MA 02154-1649. Phone: (617) 893-3800. Fax: (617) 893-0413. Weekly.

National Cancer Institute. Journal. U.S. National Cancer Institute, 9030 Old Georgetown Rd., Bldg. 82, Room 103, Bethesda, MD 20892. Phone: (301) 496-7186. Monthly.

NEWSLETTERS

AICR Newsletter. American Institute for Cancer Research (AICR), 1759 R St. N.W., Washington, DC 20009-2552. Phone: (202) 328-7744. Fax: (800) 843-8114. Quarterly.

Clinical Oncology Alert. American Health Consultants, Department C1290, P.O. Box 740060, Atlanta, GA 30374. Phone: (800) 559-1032. Fax: (404) 352-1971. Monthly.

European Cancer News. Kluwer Academic Publishers, P.O. Box 358, Accord Station, Hingham, MA 02018-0358. Phone: (617) 871-6600. Fax: (617) 871-6528. 6/year.

NCI Cancer Weekly. Charles W. Henderson, P.O. Box 5528, Atlanta, GA 30307-0527. Phone: (404) 377-8895. Weekly.

ONLINE DATABASES

Cancer Weekly. CDC AIDS Weekly/NCI Cancer Weekly, 206 Rogers St. NE, Suite 104, P.O. Box 5528, Atlanta, GA 30317. Phone: (404) 377-8895. Weekly.

CANCERLIT. U.S. National Cancer Institute, International Cancer Information Center, Building 82, Room 102, Bethesda, MD 20892. Phone: (301) 496-7403. Fax: (301) 480-8105. Monthly.

Cancerquest Online. CDC AIDS Weekly/NCI Cancer Weekly, 206 Rogers St. NE, Suite 104, P.O. Box 5528, Atlanta, GA 30317. Phone: (404) 377-8895. Weekly.

Clinical Protocols. U.S. National Cancer Institute, International Cancer Information Center, Building 82, Room 102, Bethesda, MD 20892. Phone: (301) 496-7403. Fax: (301) 480-8105.

EMBASE. Elsevier Science Publishing Co., Inc., P.O. Box 882, Madison Square Station, New York, NY 10159-2101. Phone: (212) 989-5800. Fax: (212) 633-3990.

MEDLINE. National Library of Medicine, 8600 Rockville Pike, Bethesda, MD 20894. Phone: (800) 638-8480.

Physician Data Query (PDQ) Cancer Information File. U.S. National Cancer Institute, International Cancer Information Center, Building 82, Room 102, Bethesda, MD 20892. Phone: (301) 496-7403. Fax: (301) 480-8105. Monthly.

Physician Data Query (PDQ) Directory File. U.S. National Cancer Institute, International Cancer Information Center,

Building 82, Room 102, Bethesda, MD 20892. Phone: (301) 496-7403. Fax: (301) 480-8105. Monthly.

Physician Data Query (PDQ) Protocol File. U.S. National Cancer Institute, International Cancer Information Center, Building 82, Room 102, Bethesda, MD 20892. Phone: (301) 496-7403. Fax: (301) 480-8105. Monthly.

SciSearch. Institute for Scientific Information, 3501 Market St., Philadelphia, PA 19104. Phone: (215) 386-0100. Fax: (215) 386-6362.

POPULAR WORKS AND PATIENT EDUCATION

Cancervive: The Challenge of Life After Cancer. Susan Nessim, Judith Ellis. Houghton Mifflin Co., 1 Beacon St., Boston, MA 02108. Phone: (800) 225-3362. 1991.

Everyone's Guide to Cancer Therapy: How Cancer is Diagnosed, Treated, and Managed on a Day to Day Basis. Malin Dollinger, Ernest H. Rosenbaum, Greg Cable. Andrews & McMeel, 4900 Main St., Kansas City, MO 64112. Phone: (800) 826-4216. 1991.

Options: The Alternative Cancer Therapy Book. Richard Walters. Avery Publishing Group, Inc., 120 Old Broadway, Garden City Park, NY 11040. Phone: (800) 548-5757. 1992.

Understanding Cancer. Mark Renneker. Bull Publishing Co., 110 Gilbert Ave., Menlo Park, CA 94025. Phone: (800) 676-2855. Third edition 1988.

Your Defense Against Cancer: The Complete Guide to Cancer Prevention. Henry Dreher. HarperCollins Pubs., Inc., 10 E. 53rd St., New York, NY 10022-5299. Phone: (212) 207-7000. Fax: (800) 242-7737. 1990.

RESEARCH CENTERS, INSTITUTES, CLEARINGHOUSES

Arizona Cancer Center. 1501 N. Campbell St., Tucson, AZ 85724. Phone: (602) 626-6044. Fax: (602) 626-2284.

Cancer Center. University of Iowa. 20 Medical Laboratories, Iowa City, IA 52242. Phone: (319) 335-7905.

Cancer Information Service (CIS). Office of Cancer Communications, National Cancer Institute, Bldg. 31, Rm. 10A24, 9000 Rockville Pike, Bethesda, MD 20892. Phone: (800) 4CA-NCER.

Cancer Research Center. Boston University. 80 E. Concord St., Boston, MA 02118. Phone: (617) 638-4173. Fax: (617) 638-4176.

Cancer Research Institute. New England Deaconess Hospital, 185 Pilgrim, Boston, MA 02215. Phone: (617) 732-8016.

Center for Cancer Research. Massachusetts Institute of Technology. 77 Massachusetts Ave., Cambridge, MA 02139-4307. Phone: (617) 253-8511. Fax: (617) 253-8728.

Comprehensive Cancer Center. Columbia University. 701 W. 168th St., New York, NY 10032. Phone: (212) 305-6921. Fax: (212) 305-6889.

Comprehensive Cancer Center. Ohio State University. 300 W. 10th Ave., Columbus, OH 43210. Phone: (614) 293-3304. Fax: (614) 293-3132.

Comprehensive Cancer Center. University of Alabama at Birmingham. University Station, Birmingham, AL 35294. Phone: (205) 934-5077. Fax: (205) 934-1608.

Comprehensive Cancer Center. University of Southern California. 1441 Eastlake Ave., P.O. Box 33800, Los Angeles, CA 90033-0800. Phone: (213) 224-6416.

Comprehensive Cancer Center. University of Wisconsin. 600 Highland Ave., Madison, WI 53792. Phone: (608) 263-8600. Fax: (608) 263-8613.

Coriell Institute for Medical Research (Camden). 401 Haddon Ave., Camden, NJ 08103. Phone: (609) 966-7377. Fax: (609) 964-0254.

Dana Farber Cancer Institute. 44 Binney St., Boston, MA 02115. Phone: (617) 732-3000.

Duke University Comprehensive Cancer Center. P.O. Box 3843, Durham, NC 27710.

Fox Chase Cancer Center. 7701 Burholme Ave., Philadelphia, PA 19111. Phone: (215) 728-6900. Fax: (215) 728-2571.

Fred Hutchinson Cancer Research Center. 1124 Columbia St., Seattle, WA 98104. Phone: (206) 467-5000. Fax: (206) 467-5268.

Hubert H. Humphrey Cancer Research Center. Boston University. 80 E. Concord St., Boston, MA 02118. Phone: (617) 638-4173.

La Jolla Cancer Research Foundation. 10910 N. Torrey Pines Rd., La Jolla, CA 92037. Phone: (619) 455-6480. Fax: (619) 455-0181.

Mallinckrodt Institute of Radiology. Washington University. 510 S. Kingshighway Blvd., St. Louis, MO 63110. Phone: (314) 362-2866.

Mayo Comprehensive Cancer Center. 200 First St. SW, Rochester, MN 55905. Phone: (507) 284-4718.

Memorial Sloan-Kettering Cancer Center. 1275 York Ave., New York, NY 10021. Phone: (212) 355-0060.

National Cancer Institute of Canada. 10 Alcorn Ave., Ste. 200, Toronto, ON, Canada M4V 3B1.

Oncology Center. Johns Hopkins University. 600 N. Wolfe St., Baltimore, MD 21205. Phone: (301) 955-8800. Fax: (301) 955-1904.

Ontario Cancer Institute. Princess Margaret Hospital. 500 Sherbourne St., Toronto, ON, Canada M4X 1K9. Phone: (416) 924-0671. Fax: (416) 926-6529.

Pittsburgh Cancer Institute. 200 Meyran Ave., Pittsburgh, PA 15213. Phone: (412) 647-2072. Fax: (412) 621-9354.

Radiation Therapy Oncology Center. University of Kentucky Medical Center, Rose St., Lexington, KY 40536. Phone: (606) 233-6486. Fax: (606) 257-3393.

Roswell Park Cancer Institute. 666 Elm St., Buffalo, NY 14263. Phone: (716) 845-2300. Fax: (716) 845-3545.

UNC Lineberger Comprehensive Cancer Center. University of North Carolina at Chapel Hill. Lineberger, CB 7295, Chapel Hill, NC 27599-7295. Phone: (919) 966-3036. Fax: (919) 966-3015.

Vincent T. Lombardi Cancer Research Center. Georgetown University. 3800 Reservoir Rd. NW, Podium Level, Washington, DC 20007. Phone: (202) 687-2110. Fax: (202) 687-6402.

STANDARDS AND STATISTICS SOURCES

Atlas of U.S. Cancer Mortality Among Nonwhites: 1950-1980. L.W. Pickle, T.J. Manson, and others. U.S. Government Printing Office, Superintendent of Documents, P.O. Box 371954, Pittsburgh, PA 15250-7954. Phone: (202) 783-3238. Fax: (202) 512-2250. NIH90-1582, 1990.

Cancer Facts and Figures. American Cancer Society, 1599 Clifton Rd., N.E., Atlanta, GA 30329-4251. Phone: (404) 320-3333. Annual.

Cancer Statistics. American Cancer Society, 1599 Clifton Rd., N.E., Atlanta, GA 30329-4251. Phone: (800) 227-2345. Annual.

Cancer Statistics Review. U.S. National Cancer Institute, International Cancer Information Center, Building 82, Room 102, Bethesda, MD 20892. Phone: (301) 496-7403. Fax: (301) 480-8105. Annual.

Fact Book: National Cancer Institute. U.S. National Cancer Institute, International Cancer Information Center, Building 82, Room 102, Bethesda, MD 20892. Phone: (301) 496-7403. Fax: (301) 480-8105. Annual.

National Cancer Institute Annual Report. U.S. Government Printing Office, Superintendent of Documents, P.O. Box 371954, Pittsburgh, PA 15250-7954. Phone: (202) 783-3238. Fax: (202) 512-2250. 1989.

TEXTBOOKS AND MONOGRAPHS

Cancer Medicine. James F. Holland, Emil Frei, Robert C. Bast Jr., and others. Williams & Wilkins, 428 East Preston St., Baltimore, MD 21202. Phone: (800) 638-0672. Fax: (800) 447-8438. Third edition 1992.

Cancer and Nutrition. Alfin-Slater. Plenum Publishing Co., 233 Spring St., New York, NY 10013-1578. Phone: (212) 620-8000. Fax: (212) 463-0742. 1991.

Cancer in Organ Transplant Recipients. Schmahl. Springer-Verlag New York Inc., 175 Fifth Ave., New York, NY 10010. Phone: (212) 460-1500. Fax: (212) 473-6272. 1991.

Cancer: Principles and Practice of Oncology. Vincent T. DeVita. J.B. Lippincott Co., 227 E. Washington Square, Philadelphia, PA 19106-3780. Phone: (215) 238-4200. Fax: (215) 238-4227. 1989 3rd edtion.

Cancer Treatment. Charles M. Haskell. W.B. Saunders Co., The Curtis Center, Independence Square W., Philadelphia, PA 19106-3399. Phone: (215) 238-7800. Third edition 1990.

Communicating with Cancer Patients and Their Families. Andrew Bliztwer and others (eds.). Charles Press Publishers, P.O. Box 15715, Philadelphia, PA 19123. Phone: (215) 735-3665. 1990.

Genital Papillomaviruses and Related Neoplasms. Christopher P. Crum, Gerard J. Nuovo. Raven Press, 1185 Avenue of the Americas, New York, NY 10036. Phone: (212) 930-9500. Fax: (212) 869-3495. 1991.

CANCER CENTERS

RESEARCH CENTERS, INSTITUTES, CLEARINGHOUSES

Arizona Cancer Center. 1501 N. Campbell St., Tucson, AZ 85724. Phone: (602) 626-6044. Fax: (602) 626-2284.

Cancer Research Center. Georgetown University / Howard University, 3041 Georgia Ave., N.W., Washington, DC 20007.

Columbia University Cancer Center. College of Physicians and Surgeons, 640 W. 168th St., New York, NY 10032.

Comprehensive Cancer Center. Columbia University. 701 W. 168th St., New York, NY 10032. Phone: (212) 305-6921. Fax: (212) 305-6889.

Comprehensive Cancer Center. Ohio State University. 300 W. 10th Ave., Columbus, OH 43210. Phone: (614) 293-3304. Fax: (614) 293-3132.

Comprehensive Cancer Center. University of Alabama at Birmingham. University Station, Birmingham, AL 35294. Phone: (205) 934-5077. Fax: (205) 934-1608.

Comprehensive Cancer Center. University of Southern California. 1441 Eastlake Ave., P.O. Box 33800, Los Angeles, CA 90033-0800. Phone: (213) 224-6416.

Comprehensive Cancer Center. University of Wisconsin. 600 Highland Ave., Madison, WI 53792. Phone: (608) 263-8600. Fax: (608) 263-8613.

Duke University Comprehensive Cancer Center. P.O. Box 3843, Durham, NC 27710.

Illinois Cancer Council. 36 S. Wabash Ave., Chicago, IL 60637.

Jonsson Comprehensive Cancer Center. 10-247 Factor Bldg., 10833 Le Conte Ave., University of California-Los Angeles, Los Angeles, CA 90024-1781.

Kenneth Norris Jr. Comprehensive Cancer Center. University of Southern California, 1441 Eastlake Ave., Los Angeles, CA 90033-0804.

Mayo Comprehensive Cancer Center. 200 First St. SW, Rochester, MN 55905. Phone: (507) 284-4718.

M.D. Anderson Cancer Center. 1515 Holcombe Blvd., Houston, TX 77030.

Meyer L. Prentis Comprehensive Cancer Center of Metropolitan Detroit. 110 E. Warren Ave., Detroit, MI 48201.

Ontario Cancer Institute. Princess Margaret Hospital. 500 Sherbourne St., Toronto, ON, Canada M4X 1K9. Phone: (416) 924-0671. Fax: (416) 926-6529.

Pittsburgh Cancer Institute. 200 Meyran Ave., Pittsburgh, PA 15213. Phone: (412) 647-2072. Fax: (412) 621-9354.

Sylvester Comprehensive Cancer Center. University of Miami Medical School, 1475 Northwest 12th Ave., Miami, FL 33136.

UNC Lineberger Comprehensive Cancer Center. University of North Carolina at Chapel Hill. Lineberger, CB 7295, Chapel Hill, NC 27599-7295. Phone: (919) 966-3036. Fax: (919) 966-3015.

University of Chicago Cancer Research Center. 5841 S. Maryland Ave., Chicago, IL 60637.

University of Pennsylvania Cancer Center. 3400 Spruce St., Philadelphia, PA 19104.

Vincent T. Lombardi Cancer Research Center. Georgetown University. 3800 Reservoir Rd. NW, Podium Level, Washington, DC 20007. Phone: (202) 687-2110. Fax: (202) 687-6402.

Yale University Comprehensive Cancer Center. Yale University, 333 Cedar St., New Haven, CT 06510.

CANNABIS

See: MARIJUANA

CARCINOGENS

See also: ENVIRONMENTAL POLLUTANTS

ABSTRACTING, INDEXING, AND CURRENT AWARENESS PUBLICATIONS

CA Selects: Carcinogens, Mutagens, & Teratogens. Chemical Abstracts Service, 2540 Olentangy River Road, P.O. Box 3012, Columbus, OH 43210-0012. Phone: (800) 848-6538. Biweekly.

Chemical Abstracts. Chemical Abstracts Service, 2540 Olentangy River Rd., P.O. Box 3012, Columbus, OH 43210-0012. Phone: (800) 848-6538.

Current Contents/Life Sciences. Institute for Scientific Information, 3501 Market St., Philadelphia, PA 19104. Phone: (215) 386-0100. Fax: (215) 386-6362.

Excerpta Medica. Section 16: Cancer. Elsevier Science Publishing Co., Inc., P.O. Box 882, Madison Square Station, New York, NY 10159-2101. Phone: (212) 989-5800. Fax: (212) 633-3990. 32/year.

Index Medicus. U.S. National Library of Medicine, 8600 Rockville Pike, Bethesda, MD 20894. Phone: (800) 638-8480. Monthly.

Science Citation Index. Institute for Scientific Information, 3501 Market St., Philadelphia, PA 19104. Phone: (800) 523-1850. Fax: (215) 386-6362. Bimonthly.

ANNUALS AND REVIEWS

Cancer and Metastasis Reviews. Kluwer Academic Publishers, P.O. Box 358, Accord Station, Hingham, MA 02018-0358. Phone: (617) 871-6600. Fax: (617) 871-6528. 4/year.

CD-ROM DATABASES

SCISEARCH. Institute for Scientific Information, 3501 Market St., Philadelphia, PA 19104. Phone: (215) 386-0100. Fax: (215) 386-6362.

JOURNALS

Carcinogenesis. IRL Press Ltd., Box Q, Mc Lean, VA 22101. Monthly.

Xenobiotica. Taylor & Francis Inc., 1900 Frost Rd., Suite 101, Bristol, PA 19007-1598. Phone: (800) 821-8312. Fax: (215) 785-5515.

ONLINE DATABASES

CA File (Chemical Abstracts File). Chemical Abstracts Service, 2540 Olentangy River Rd., P.O. Box 3012, Columbus, OH 43210-0012. Phone: (800) 848-6538.

EMBASE. Elsevier Science Publishing Co., Inc., P.O. Box 882, Madison Square Station, New York, NY 10159-2101. Phone: (212) 989-5800. Fax: (212) 633-3990.

MEDLINE. National Library of Medicine, 8600 Rockville Pike, Bethesda, MD 20894. Phone: (800) 638-8480.

SciSearch. Institute for Scientific Information, 3501 Market St., Philadelphia, PA 19104. Phone: (215) 386-0100. Fax: (215) 386-6362.

TOXLINE. U.S. National Library of Medicine, Toxicology Information Program, 8600 Rockville Pike, Bethesda, MD 20894. Phone: (800) 638-8480. Monthly.

TEXTBOOKS AND MONOGRAPHS

Cellular and Molecular Targets for Cancer Chemoprevention. Vernon Steele, and others. CRC Press, Inc., 2000 Corporate Blvd., N.W., Boca Raton, FL 33431. Phone: (407) 994-0555. Fax: (407) 997-0949. 1992.

Mechanisms of Environmental Carcinogenesis. J.C. Barrett. CRC Press, Inc., 2000 Corporate Blvd., N.W., Boca Raton, FL 33431. Phone: (407) 994-0555. Fax: (407) 997-0949. 1987.

CARCINOMA

See: CANCER

CARDIOLOGY

See also: CARDIOVASCULAR SURGERY;
HEART DISEASES

ABSTRACTING, INDEXING, AND CURRENT AWARENESS PUBLICATIONS

Core Journals in Cardiology. Elsevier Science Publishing Co., Inc., P.O. Box 882, Madison Square Station, New York, NY 10159-2101. Phone: (212) 989-5800. Fax: (212) 633-3990. 11/year.

Current Contents/Clinical Medicine. Institute for Scientific Information, 3501 Market St., Philadelphia, PA 19104. Phone: (800) 523-1850. Fax: (215) 386-6362. Weekly.

Excerpta Medica. Section 15: Chest Diseases, Thoracic Surgery and Tuberculosis. Elsevier Science Publishing Co., Inc., P.O. Box 882, Madison Square Station, New York, NY 10159-2101. Phone: (212) 989-5800. Fax: (212) 633-3990. 20/year.

Excerpta Medica. Section 18: Cardiovascular Disease and Cardiovascular Surgery. Elsevier Science Publishing Co., Inc., P.O. Box 882, Madison Square Station, New York, NY 10159-2101. Phone: (212) 989-5800. Fax: (212) 633-3990. 24/year.

Index Medicus. U.S. National Library of Medicine, 8600 Rockville Pike, Bethesda, MD 20894. Phone: (800) 638-8480. Monthly.

Research Alert: Cardiovascular Diseases-Interventional Cardiology. Institute for Scientific Information, 3501 Market St., Philadelphia, PA 19104. Phone: (800) 523-1850. Fax: (215) 386-6362. Weekly.

Science Citation Index. Institute for Scientific Information, 3501 Market St., Philadelphia, PA 19104. Phone: (800) 523-1850. Fax: (215) 386-6362. Bimonthly.

ANNUALS AND REVIEWS

Cardiology. Butterworth-Heinemann, 80 Montvale Ave., Stoneham, MA 02180. Phone: (617) 438-8464. Fax: (617) 279-4851. Annual.

Cardiology Clinics. W.B. Saunders Co., The Curtis Center, Independence Square W., Philadelphia, PA 19106-3399. Phone: (215) 238-7800. Quarterly.

Cardiovascular Clinics. F.A. Davis Co., 1915 Arch St., Philadelphia, PA 19103. Phone: (800) 523-4049. 3/year.

Current Opinion in Cardiology. Current Science Group, 20 N. Third St., Philadelphia, PA 19106-2199. Phone: (800) 552-5866. Fax: (215) 574-2270. Bimonthly.

Current Problems in Cardiology. Mosby-Year Book, 11830 Westline Industrial Drive, St. Louis, MO 63146. Phone: (800) 325-4177. Fax: (314) 432-1380. Monthly.

Progress in Cardiology. Lea & Febiger, 428 East Preston St., Baltimore, MD 21202. Phone: (800) 638-0672. Fax: (800) 447-8438. Semiannual.

Year Book of Cardiology. Mosby-Year Book, 11830 Westline Industrial Drive, St. Louis, MO 63146. Phone: (800) 325-4177. Fax: (314) 432-1380. Annual.

ASSOCIATIONS, PROFESSIONAL SOCIETIES, ADVOCACY AND SUPPORT GROUPS

American College of Cardiology (ACC). 9111 Old Georgetown Rd., Bethesda, MD 20814. Phone: (800) 253-4636. Fax: (301) 897-9745.

American College of Chest Physicians (ACCP). 330 Dundee Rd., Northbrook, IL 60062. Phone: (708) 498-1400.

American Heart Association (AHA). 7320 Greenville Ave., Dallas, TX 75231. Phone: (214) 373-6300.

American Medical Association (AMA). 515 N. State St., Chicago, IL 60610. Phone: (312) 464-5000. Fax: (312) 645-4184.

Association of Black Cardiologists (ABC). 2300 Garrison Blvd., Suite 150, Baltimore, MD 21216. Phone: (301) 945-2525.

Society for Vascular Surgery (SVS). 13 Elm St., P.O. Box 1565, Manchester, MA 01944. Phone: (508) 526-8330. Fax: (508) 526-4018.

BIBLIOGRAPHIES

Cardiac Pacemakers. National Technical Information Service, 5285 Port Royal Rd., Springfield, VA 22161. Phone: (703) 487-

4650. Fax: (703) 321-8547. Jan. 1976 - Oct. 1987. NTIS order no.: PB88-850797/CBY.

CD-ROM DATABASES

Bibliomed Cardiology Disc. Healthcare Information Services, Inc., 2235 American River Dr., Suite 307, Sacramento, CA 95825. Phone: (800) 468-1128. Fax: (916) 648-8078. Quarterly.

Cardiology MEDLINE. MEP, 124 Mt. Auburn St., Cambridge, MA 02138. Phone: (800) 342-1338. Fax: (617) 868-7738. Quarterly.

CardLine. Aries Systems Corporation, One Dundee Park, Andover, MA 01810. Phone: (508) 475-7200. Fax: (508) 474-8860. Monthly or quarterly.

Excerpta Medica CD: Cardiology. SilverPlatter Information, Inc., River Ridge Office Park, 100 River Ridge Rd., Norwood, MA 02062. Phone: (617) 769-2599. Fax: (617) 769-8763. Quarterly.

Heartlab. Bergeron. Williams & Wilkins, 428 East Preston St., Baltimore, MD 21202. Phone: (800) 638-0672. Fax: (800) 447-8438. 1991.

SCISEARCH. Institute for Scientific Information, 3501 Market St., Philadelphia, PA 19104. Phone: (215) 386-0100. Fax: (215) 386-6362.

Year Books on Disc. CMC ReSearch, Inc., 7150 S.W. Hampton, Suite C-120, Portland, OR 97223. Phone: (800) 262-7668. Fax: (503) 639-1796. Annual includes Year Books of Cardiology, Dermatology, Diagnostic Radiology, Drug Therapy, Emergency Medicine, Family Practice, Medicine, Neurology and Neurosurgery, Obstetrics and Gynecology, Oncology, Pediatrics, and Psychiatry and Applied Mental Health.

DIRECTORIES

Directory of Medical Specialists. Marquis Who's Who, 3002 Glenview Rd., Wilmette, IL 60091. Phone: (800) 621-9669. Fax: (708) 441-2264. Biennial.

Directory of Physicians in the United States. American Medical Association, 515 North State St., Chicago, IL 60610. Phone: (312) 464-0183. Fax: (312) 464-5834. Biennial.

ENCYCLOPEDIAS, DICTIONARIES, WORD BOOKS

Cardiology Words. Stedman. Williams & Wilkins, 428 East Preston St., Baltimore, MD 21202. Phone: (800) 638-0672. Fax: (800) 447-8438. 1992.

Clinician's Illustrated Dictionary of Cardiology. R.H. Anderson, P.J. Oldershaw, R. Dawson, E. Rowland. Science Press Ltd., 20 N. Third St., Philadelphia, PA 19106-2199. Phone: (800) 552-5866. Fax: (215) 574-2270. Second edition 1991.

HANDBOOKS, GUIDES, MANUALS, ATLASES

Manual of Cardiovascular Diagnosis and Therapy. Joseph S. Alpert, James M. Rippe. Little, Brown and Co., 34 Beacon St., Boston, MA 02108. Phone: (617) 227-0730. Third edition 1988.

Manual of Clinical Problems in Cardiology. L. David Hillis, Peter J. Wells, Michael D. Winniford (eds.). Little, Brown and

Co., 34 Beacon St., Boston, MA 02108. Phone: (617) 227-0730. Fourth edition 1992.

Manual of Coronary Care. Joseph S. Alpert, Gary S. Francis. Little, Brown and Co., 34 Beacon St., Boston, MA 02108. Phone: (617) 227-0730. Fourth edition 1987.

Pediatric Cardiology Handbook. Park. Mosby-Year Book, 11830 Westline Industrial Drive, St. Louis, MO 63146. Phone: (800) 325-4177. Fax: (314) 432-1380. 1991.

JOURNALS

Acta Cardiologica. Belgium Society for Cardiology, Avenue Circulaire, 138A, 1180 Brussels, Belgium. Phone: 375-58-92. Bimonthly.

American Heart Journal. Mosby-Year Book, 11830 Westline Industrial Drive, St. Louis, MO 63146. Phone: (800) 325-4177. Fax: (314) 432-1380. Monthly.

American Journal of Cardiology. Reed Publising USA, 249 W. 17th St., New York, NY 10011. Phone: (212) 645-0067. Fax: (212) 242-6987. 22/year.

British Heart Journal. BMJ Publishing Group, BMA House, Tavistock Square, London WC1H 9JR, England. Phone: 071383 6244/6638. Fax: 071383 6662. Monthly.

Cardiology. S. Karger Publishers, Inc., 26 W. Avon Rd., P.O. Box 529, Farmington, CT 06085. Phone: (203) 675-7834. Fax: (203) 675-7302. Bimonthly.

Cardiology in the Elderly. Current Science Group, 20 North Third St., Philadelphia, PA 19106-2199. Phone: (215) 574-2266. Fax: (215) 574-2270. Bimonthly.

Circulation. American Heart Association, 7320 Greenville Ave., Dallas, TX 75231-4599. Phone: (214) 706-1310. Fax: (214) 691-2704. Monthly.

Coronary Artery Disease. Current Science Group, 20 N. Third St., Philadelphia, PA 19106-2199. Phone: (215) 574-2266. Fax: (215) 574-2270. Monthly.

European Heart Journal. Academic Press, Inc., 1250 Sixth Ave., San Diego, CA 92101-4311. Phone: (619) 699-6345. Fax: (619) 699-6715. Monthly.

International Journal of Cardiology. Elsevier Science Publishing Co., Inc., P.O. Box 882, Madison Square Station, New York, NY 10159-2101. Phone: (212) 989-5800. Fax: (212) 633-3990. 12/year.

Journal of the American College of Cardiology. Elsevier Science Publishing Co., Inc., P.O. Box 882, Madison Square Station, New York, NY 10159-2101. Phone: (212) 989-5800. Fax: (212) 633-3990. Monthly.

Trends in Cardiovascular Medicine. Elsevier Science Publishing Co., Inc., P.O. Box 882, Madison Square Station, New York, NY 10159-2101. Phone: (212) 989-5800. Fax: (212) 633-3990. 6/year.

NEWSLETTERS

Cardiology. American College of Cardiology, 9111 Old Georgetown Rd., Bethesda, MD 20814. Phone: (800) 253-4636. Fax: (301) 897-9745. Monthly.

Clinical Cardiology Alert. American Health Consultants, Department C1290, P.O. Box 740060, Atlanta, GA 30374. Phone: (800) 559-1032. Fax: (404) 352-1971. Monthly.

Harvard Heart Letter. Harvard Medical School Publications Group, 164 Longwood Ave., Boston, MA 02115. Monthly.

ONLINE DATABASES

EMBASE. Elsevier Science Publishing Co., Inc., P.O. Box 882, Madison Square Station, New York, NY 10159-2101. Phone: (212) 989-5800. Fax: (212) 633-3990.

MEDIS. Mead Data Central, P.O. Box 1830, Dayton, OH 45401. Phone: (800) 227-4908.

MEDLINE. National Library of Medicine, 8600 Rockville Pike, Bethesda, MD 20894. Phone: (800) 638-8480.

SciSearch. Institute for Scientific Information, 3501 Market St., Philadelphia, PA 19104. Phone: (215) 386-0100. Fax: (215) 386-6362.

POPULAR WORKS AND PATIENT EDUCATION

Yale University School of Medicine Heart Book. Barry L. Zaret, Lawrence S. Cohen, Marvin Moser, and others. William Morrow & Company, Inc., 1350 Ave. of the Americas, New York, NY 10019. Phone: (800) 237-0657. 1992.

RESEARCH CENTERS, INSTITUTES, CLEARINGHOUSES

Cardiovascular Research and Training Center. University of Alabama at Birmingham. THT Room 311, Birmingham, AL 35294. Phone: (205) 934-3624. Fax: (205) 934-5596.

Cleveland Clinic Foundation Research Institute. 9500 Euclid Ave., Cleveland, OH 44195-5210. Phone: (216) 444-3900. Fax: (216) 444-3279.

DeBakey Heart Center. Baylor College of Medicine. Texas Medical Center, 1 Baylor Plaza, Houston, TX 77030. Phone: (701) 797-9353. Fax: (713) 793-1192.

Framingham Heart Study. 5 Thurber St., Framingham, MA 01701. Phone: (508) 872-4386.

Hope Heart Institute. 528 18th Ave., Seattle, WA 98122. Phone: (206) 320-2001. Fax: (206) 328-0355.

Texas Heart Institute. P.O. Box 20345, Houston, TX 77225-0345. Phone: (713) 791-3709. Fax: (713) 791-3089.

TEXTBOOKS AND MONOGRAPHS

Cardiac Catheterization, Angiography, and Intervention. Willam Grossman, Donald S. Baim (eds.). Lea & Febiger, 428 E. Preston St., Baltimore, MD 21202. Phone: (800) 638-0672. Fax: (800) 447-8438. Fourth edition 1991.

Cardiology. William W. Parmley, Kanu Chatterjee (eds.). J.B. Lippincott Co., 227 E. Washington Square, Philadelphia, PA 19106-3780. Phone: (215) 238-4200. Fax: (215) 238-4227. Two volumes 1991.

Cardiology: Fundamentals and Practice. Emilio Giuliani, Valentin Fuster, Bernard J. Gersh, et. al.. Mosby-Year Book, 11830 Westline Industrial Drive, St. Louis, MO 63146. Phone: (800) 325-4177. Fax: (314) 432-1380. Second edition 1991.

Clinical Cardiology. Maurice Sokolow, and others. Appleton & Lange, 25 Van Zant Street, East Norwalk, CT 06855. Phone: (800) 423-1359. Fax: (203) 854-9486. Fifth edition 1990.

Coronary and Peripheral Angiography and Angioplasty. Leachman Leachman. J.B. Lippincott Co., 227 East Washington Square, Philadelphia, PA 19106-3780. Phone: (215) 238-4200. Fax: (215) 238-4227. 1989.

Echocardiography in Pediatric Heart Disease. A. Rebecca Snider, Gerald A. Serwer. Mosby-Year Book, 11830 Westline Industrial Drive, St. Louis, MO 63146. Phone: (800) 325-4177. Fax: (314) 432-1380. 1990.

Essentials of Clinical Cardiology. Emmanuel Goldberger. J.B. Lippincott Co., 227 E. Washington Square, Philadelphia, PA 19106-3780. Phone: (215) 238-4200. Fax: (215) 238-4227. 1990.

The Heart. J. Willis Hurst, Robert C. Schlant, et. al.. McGraw-Hill, Inc., Health Professions Division, 1221 Avenue of the Americas, 28th Floor, New York, NY 10020. Phone: (212) 512-4228. Seventh edition 1990.

Heart Disease: A Textbook of Cardiovascular Medicine. Eugene Braunwald (ed.). W.B. Saunders Co., The Curtis Center, Independence Square W., Philadelphia, PA 19106-3399. Phone: (215) 238-7800. Third edition. Two volumes. 1988.

Interventional Cardiology. Daniel L. Kulick, Shahbudin Rahimtoola. Mosby-Year Book, 11830 Westline Industrial Drive, St. Louis, MO 63146. Phone: (800) 325-4177. Fax: (314) 432-1380. 1991.

Introduction to Clinical Cardiology. C. Richard Conti. Raven Press, 1185 Avenue of the Americas, New York, NY 10036. Phone: (212) 930-9500. Fax: (212) 869-3495. 1991.

Myocardial Infarction: Electrocardiographic Differential Diagnosis. Ary L. Goldberger. Mosby-Year Book, 11830 Westline Industrial Drive, St. Louis, MO 63146. Phone: (800) 325-4177. Fax: (314) 432-1380. Fourth edition 1991.

The Practice of Cardiology: The Medical and Surgical Cardiac Units at the Massachusetts General Hospital. Kim A. Eagle, and others (eds.). Little, Brown and Company, 34 Beacon St., Boston, MA 02108. Phone: (617) 227-0730. Second edition. Two volumes. 1989.

The Science and Practice of Pediatric Cardiology. Arthur Garson Jr., J. Timothy Bricker, Dan G. McNamara. Williams & Wilkins, 428 East Preston St., Baltimore, MD 21202. Phone: (800) 638-0672. Fax: (800) 447-8438. Three volumes 1990.

Textbook of Interventional Cardiology. Eric J. Topol (ed.). W.B. Saunders Co., The Curtis Center, Independence Square W., Philadelphia, PA 19106-3399. Phone: (215) 238-7800. 1990.

Treatment of Cardiac Emergencies. Emanuel Goldberger. Mosby-Year Book, 11830 Westline Industrial Drive, St. Louis, MO 63146. Phone: (800) 325-4177. Fax: (314) 432-1380. Fifth edition 1990.

CARDIOPULMONARY RESUSCITATION

See also: EMERGENCY MEDICINE

ABSTRACTING, INDEXING, AND CURRENT AWARENESS PUBLICATIONS

Cumulative Index to Nursing and Allied Health Literature. Glendale Adventist Medical Center, P.O. Box 871, Glendale, CA 91209. Phone: (818) 409-8005. Bimonthly.

Index Medicus. U.S. National Library of Medicine, 8600 Rockville Pike, Bethesda, MD 20894. Phone: (800) 638-8480. Monthly.

Science Citation Index. Institute for Scientific Information, 3501 Market St., Philadelphia, PA 19104. Phone: (800) 523-1850. Fax: (215) 386-6362. Bimonthly.

ASSOCIATIONS, PROFESSIONAL SOCIETIES, ADVOCACY AND SUPPORT GROUPS

American Heart Association (AHA). 7320 Greenville Ave., Dallas, TX 75231. Phone: (214) 373-6300.

National Registry of Emergency Medical Technicians (NREMT). P.O. Box 29233, Columbus, OH 43229. Phone: (614) 888-4484.

CD-ROM DATABASES

CPR Training by Computer. Hoffer. Williams & Wilkins, 428 East Preston St., Baltimore, MD 21202. Phone: (800) 638-0672. Fax: (800) 447-8438. Second edition 1992.

Emergency Medicine MEDLINE. MEP, 124 Mt. Auburn St., Cambridge, MA 02138. Phone: (800) 342-1338. Fax: (617) 868-7738. Quarterly.

Nursing and Allied Health (CINAHL) on CD-ROM. CINAHL, 1509 Wilson Terrace, P.O. Box 871, Glendale, CA 91209-0871. Phone: (818) 409-8005.

SCISEARCH. Institute for Scientific Information, 3501 Market St., Philadelphia, PA 19104. Phone: (215) 386-0100. Fax: (215) 386-6362.

Year Books on Disc. CMC ReSearch, Inc., 7150 S.W. Hampton, Suite C-120, Portland, OR 97223. Phone: (800) 262-7668. Fax: (503) 639-1796. Annual includes Year Books of Cardiology, Dermatology, Diagnostic Radiology, Drug Therapy, Emergency Medicine, Family Practice, Medicine, Neurology and Neurosurgery, Obstetrics and Gynecology, Oncology, Pediatrics, and Psychiatry and Applied Mental Health.

HANDBOOKS, GUIDES, MANUALS, ATLASES

Handbook of Emergency Care Procedures. Harvey Grant, Dwight Lodge. Prentice Hall, 113 Sylvan Ave., Rt. 9W, Prentice Hall Bldg., Englewood Cliffs, NJ 07632. Phone: (201) 767-5937. 1988.

JOURNALS

Archives of Emergency Medicine. Blackwell Scientific Publications, Inc., 3 Cambridge Ctr., Cambridge, MA 02142. Phone: (800) 759-6102. Quarterly.

Resuscitation. Elsevier Science Publishing Co., Inc., P.O. Box 882, Madison Square Station, New York, NY 10159-2101. Phone: (212) 989-5800. Fax: (212) 633-3990. 6/year.

ONLINE DATABASES

EMBASE. Elsevier Science Publishing Co., Inc., P.O. Box 882, Madison Square Station, New York, NY 10159-2101. Phone: (212) 989-5800. Fax: (212) 633-3990.

MEDLINE. National Library of Medicine, 8600 Rockville Pike, Bethesda, MD 20894. Phone: (800) 638-8480.

Nursing and Allied Health (CINAHL). CINAHL, 1509 Wilson Terrace, P.O. Box 871, Glendale, CA 91209-0871. Phone: (818) 409-8005.

SciSearch. Institute for Scientific Information, 3501 Market St., Philadelphia, PA 19104. Phone: (215) 386-0100. Fax: (215) 386-6362.

POPULAR WORKS AND PATIENT EDUCATION

The American Red Cross First Aid and Safety Handbook. Kathleen A. Handal. Little, Brown and Co., 34 Beacon St., Boston, MA 02108. Phone: (617) 227-0730. 1992.

RESEARCH CENTERS, INSTITUTES, CLEARINGHOUSES

Resuscitation Research Center. 3434 Fifth Ave., 2nd Floor, University of Pittsburgh, Pittsburgh, PA 15260. Phone: (412) 624-6735.

TEXTBOOKS AND MONOGRAPHS

Cardiopulmonary Resuscitation. P.J.F. Baskett (ed.). Elsevier Science Publishing Co., Inc., P.O. Box 882, Madison Square Station, New York, NY 10159-2101. Phone: (212) 989-5800. Fax: (212) 633-3990. 1989.

Cardiopulmonary Resuscitation: Scientific Basis, Current Standards and Future Trends. William Kaye, Nicholas Bircher. Churchill Livingstone Inc., 650 Ave. of the Americas, New York, NY 10011. Phone: (212) 819-5400. Fax: (212) 302-6598. 1989.

Paramedic Emergency Care. Bryan E. Bledsoe, Robert S. Porter, Bruce R. Shade. Prentice Hall, 113 Sylvan Ave., Rt. 9W, Prentice Hall Bldg., Englewood Cliffs, NJ 07632. Phone: (201) 767-5937. 1991.

CARDIOVASCULAR DISEASES

See: HEART DISEASES

CARDIOVASCULAR SURGERY

See also: CARDIOLOGY; HEART DISEASES; SURGERY; THORACIC SURGERY

ABSTRACTING, INDEXING, AND CURRENT AWARENESS PUBLICATIONS

Core Journals in Cardiology. Elsevier Science Publishing Co., Inc., P.O. Box 882, Madison Square Station, New York, NY 10159-2101. Phone: (212) 989-5800. Fax: (212) 633-3990. 11/year.

Current Contents/Clinical Medicine. Institute for Scientific Information, 3501 Market St., Philadelphia, PA 19104. Phone: (800) 523-1850. Fax: (215) 386-6362. Weekly.

Excerpta Medica. Section 18: Cardiovascular Disease and Cardiovascular Surgery. Elsevier Science Publishing Co., Inc., P.O. Box 882, Madison Square Station, New York, NY 10159-2101. Phone: (212) 989-5800. Fax: (212) 633-3990. 24/year.

Index Medicus. U.S. National Library of Medicine, 8600 Rockville Pike, Bethesda, MD 20894. Phone: (800) 638-8480. Monthly.

Research Alert: Surgery-Heart-Thoracic. Institute for Scientific Information, 3501 Market St., Philadelphia, PA 19104. Phone: (800) 523-1850. Fax: (215) 386-6362. Weekly.

Science Citation Index. Institute for Scientific Information, 3501 Market St., Philadelphia, PA 19104. Phone: (800) 523-1850. Fax: (215) 386-6362. Bimonthly.

ANNUALS AND REVIEWS

Advances in Cardiac Surgery. Mosby-Year Book, 11830 Westline Inustrial Drive, St. Louis, MO 63146. Phone: (800) 325-4177. Fax: (314) 432-1380. Annual.

Annual of Cardiac Surgery. Current Science Group, 20 N. Third St,, Philadelphia, PA 19106-2199. Phone: (800) 552-5866. Fax: (215) 574-2266. Annual.

Cardiology. Butterworth-Heinemann, 80 Montvale Ave., Stoneham, MA 02180. Phone: (617) 438-8464. Fax: (617) 279-4851. Annual.

Cardiology Clinics. W.B. Saunders Co., The Curtis Center, Independence Square W., Philadelphia, PA 19106-3399. Phone: (215) 238-7800. Quarterly.

Cardiovascular Clinics. F.A. Davis Co., 1915 Arch St., Philadelphia, PA 19103. Phone: (800) 523-4049. 3/year.

Chest Surgery Clinics of North America. W.B. Saunders Co., The Curtis Center, Independence Square W., Philadelphia, PA 19106-3399. Phone: (215) 238-7800. Quarterly.

Current Problems in Cardiology. Mosby-Year Book, 11830 Westline Industrial Drive, St. Louis, MO 63146. Phone: (800) 325-4177. Fax: (314) 432-1380. Monthly.

Progress in Cardiology. Lea & Febiger, 428 East Preston St., Baltimore, MD 21202. Phone: (800) 638-0672. Fax: (800) 447-8438. Semiannual.

Year Book of Cardiology. Mosby-Year Book, 11830 Westline Industrial Drive, St. Louis, MO 63146. Phone: (800) 325-4177. Fax: (314) 432-1380. Annual.

Year Book of Vascular Surgery. Mosby-Year Book, 11830 Westline Industrial Drive, St. Louis, MO 63146. Phone: (800) 325-4177. Fax: (314) 432-1380. Annual.

ASSOCIATIONS, PROFESSIONAL SOCIETIES, ADVOCACY AND SUPPORT GROUPS

American Heart Association (AHA). 7320 Greenville Ave., Dallas, TX 75231. Phone: (214) 373-6300.

Association of Physician's Assistants in Cardiovascular Surgery (APACVS). 2000 Tate Springs Rd., P.O. Box 2242, Lynchburg, VA 24501-2242. Phone: (407) 839-1752.

International Society for Cardiovascular Surgery (ICVS). 13 Elm St., P.O. Box 1565, Manchester, MA 01944. Phone: (508) 526-8330. Fax: (508) 526-4018.

Mended Hearts. c/o American Heart Association, 7320 Greenville Ave., Dallas, TX 75231. Phone: (214) 706-1442.

Michael E. DeBakey International Surgical Society (MEDISS). 1 Baylor Plaza, Dept. of Surgery, Houston, TX 77030. Phone: (713) 798-4557.

Society for Vascular Surgery (SVS). 13 Elm St., P.O. Box 1565, Manchester, MA 01944. Phone: (508) 526-8330. Fax: (508) 526-4018.

CD-ROM DATABASES

Bibliomed Cardiology Disc. Healthcare Information Services, Inc., 2235 American River Dr., Suite 307, Sacramento, CA 95825. Phone: (800) 468-1128. Fax: (916) 648-8078. Quarterly.

Cardiology MEDLINE. MEP, 124 Mt. Auburn St., Cambridge, MA 02138. Phone: (800) 342-1338. Fax: (617) 868-7738. Quarterly.

CardLine. Aries Systems Corporation, One Dundee Park, Andover, MA 01810. Phone: (508) 475-7200. Fax: (508) 474-8860. Monthly or quarterly.

Excerpta Medica CD: Cardiology. SilverPlatter Information, Inc., River Ridge Office Park, 100 River Ridge Rd., Norwood, MA 02062. Phone: (617) 769-2599. Fax: (617) 769-8763. Quarterly.

SCISEARCH. Institute for Scientific Information, 3501 Market St., Philadelphia, PA 19104. Phone: (215) 386-0100. Fax: (215) 386-6362.

Year Books on Disc. CMC ReSearch, Inc., 7150 S.W. Hampton, Suite C-120, Portland, OR 97223. Phone: (800) 262-7668. Fax: (503) 639-1796. Annual includes Year Books of Cardiology, Dermatology, Diagnostic Radiology, Drug Therapy, Emergency Medicine, Family Practice, Medicine, Neurology and Neurosurgery, Obstetrics and Gynecology, Oncology, Pediatrics, and Psychiatry and Applied Mental Health.

DIRECTORIES

Directory of Certified Thoracic Surgeons. American Board of Medical Specialties, 1 Rotary Center, Suite 805, Evanston, IL 60201. Phone: (708) 491-9091. Biennial.

ENCYCLOPEDIAS, DICTIONARIES, WORD BOOKS

Cardiology Words. Stedman. Williams & Wilkins, 428 East Preston St., Baltimore, MD 21202. Phone: (800) 638-0672. Fax: (800) 447-8438. 1992.

HANDBOOKS, GUIDES, MANUALS, ATLASES

Atlas of Adult Cardiac Surgery. William A. Gay. Churchill Livingstone Inc., 650 Avenue of the Americas, New York, NY 10011. Phone: (212) 819-5400. Fax: (212) 302-6598. 1990.

Cardiothoracic Handbook: A Pocket Companion. A. Hedly Brown, Fernando Guzman. Butterworth-Heinemann, 80 Montvale Ave., Stoneham, MA 02180. Phone: (617) 438-8464. Fax: (617) 279-4851. 1989.

The Johns Hopkins Manual of Cardiac Surgical Care. William A. Baumgartner, Sharon Gallagher-Owens, et. al.. Mosby-Year Book, 11830 Westline Industrial Drive, St. Louis, MO 63146. Phone: (800) 325-4177. Fax: (314) 432-1380. 1992.

Manual of Cardiovascular Diagnosis and Therapy. Joseph S. Alpert, James M. Rippe. Little, Brown and Co., 34 Beacon St., Boston, MA 02108. Phone: (617) 227-0730. Third edition 1988.

Manual of Clinical Problems in Cardiology. L. David Hillis, Peter J. Wells, Michael D. Winniford (eds.). Little, Brown and Co., 34 Beacon St., Boston, MA 02108. Phone: (617) 227-0730. Fourth edition 1992.

Manual of Coronary Care. Joseph S. Alpert, Gary S. Francis. Little, Brown and Co., 34 Beacon St., Boston, MA 02108. Phone: (617) 227-0730. Fourth edition 1987.

Manual of Postoperative Management in Adult Cardiac Surgery. Carlos Moreno-Cabral. Williams & Wilkins, 428 E. Preston St., Baltimore, MD 21202. Phone: (800) 638-0672. Fax: (800) 447-8438. 1988.

The Practice of Cardiac Anesthesia. Hensley. Little, Brown and Co., 34 Beacon St., Boston, MA 02108. Phone: (617) 227-0730. Fax: (617) 227-0790. 1990.

Vascular Surgical Techniques: An Atlas. R.M. Greenhalgh. W.B. Saunders Co., The Curtis Center, Independence Square W., Philadelphia, PA 19106-3399. Phone: (215) 238-7800. 1989.

Wylie's Atlas of Vascular Surgery: 6 Volume Set. Stoney. J.B. Lippincott Co., 227 E. Washington Square, Philadelphia, PA 19106-3780. Phone: (215) 238-4200. Fax: (215) 238-4227. 1993.

JOURNALS

American Heart Journal. Mosby-Year Book, 11830 Westline Industrial Drive, St. Louis, MO 63146. Phone: (800) 325-4177. Fax: (314) 432-1380. Monthly.

American Journal of Cardiology. Reed Publishing USA, 249 W. 17th St., New York, NY 10011. Phone: (212) 645-0067. Fax: (212) 242-6987. 22/year.

Annals of Thoracic Surgery. Elsevier Science Publishing Co., Inc., P.O. Box 882, Madison Square Station, New York, NY 10159-2101. Phone: (212) 989-5800. Fax: (212) 633-3990. Monthly.

Cardiology. S. Karger Publishers, Inc., 26 W. Avon Rd., P.O. Box 529, Farmington, CT 06085. Phone: (203) 675-7834. Fax: (203) 675-7302. Bimonthly.

Circulation. American Heart Association, 7320 Greenville Ave., Dallas, TX 75231-4599. Phone: (214) 706-1310. Fax: (214) 691-2704. Monthly.

Coronary Artery Disease. Current Science Group, 20 N. Third St., Philadelphia, PA 19106-2199. Phone: (215) 574-2266. Fax: (215) 574-2270. Monthly.

Journal of the American College of Cardiology. Elsevier Science Publishing Co., Inc., P.O. Box 882, Madison Square Station, New York, NY 10159-2101. Phone: (212) 989-5800. Fax: (212) 633-3990. Monthly.

The Journal of Heart and Lung Transplantation. Mosby-Year Book, 11830 Westline Industrial Drive, St. Louis, MO 63146. Phone: (800) 325-4177. Fax: (314) 432-1380. Bimonthly.

Journal of Thoracic and Cardiovascular Surgery. Mosby-Year Book, 11830 Westline Industrial Drive, St. Louis, MO 63146. Phone: (800) 325-4177. Fax: (314) 432-1380. Monthly.

Journal of Vascular Nursing. Mosby-Year Book, 11830 Westline Industrial Drive, St. Louis, MO 63146. Phone: (800) 325-4177. Fax: (314) 432-1380. Quarterly.

The Journal of Vascular Surgery. Mosby-Year Book, 11830 Westline Industrial Drive, St. Louis, MO 63146. Phone: (800) 325-4177. Fax: (314) 432-1380. Monthly.

NEWSLETTERS

Cardiac Alert. Phillips Publishing, Inc., 7811 Montrose Rd., Potomac, MD 20854. Phone: (800) 722-9000. Fax: (301) 897-9745. Monthly.

Cardiology. American College of Cardiology, 9111 Old Georgetown Rd., Bethesda, MD 20814. Phone: (800) 253-4636. Fax: (301) 897-9745. Monthly.

ONLINE DATABASES

EMBASE. Elsevier Science Publishing Co., Inc., P.O. Box 882, Madison Square Station, New York, NY 10159-2101. Phone: (212) 989-5800. Fax: (212) 633-3990.

MEDLINE. National Library of Medicine, 8600 Rockville Pike, Bethesda, MD 20894. Phone: (800) 638-8480.

SciSearch. Institute for Scientific Information, 3501 Market St., Philadelphia, PA 19104. Phone: (215) 386-0100. Fax: (215) 386-6362.

POPULAR WORKS AND PATIENT EDUCATION

Confronting Mitral Valve Prolapse. Frederickson. Warner Books, Inc., 666 Fifth Ave., 9th Fl., New York, NY 10103. Phone: (212) 484-2900. 1992.

Coronary Bypass Surgery: Who Needs It?. Siegfried Kra. W.W. Norton & Co., Inc., 500 Fifth Ave., New York, NY 10110. Phone: (800) 223-2584. 1987.

Eight Steps to a Healthy Heart: The Complete Guide to Recovering from Heart Attack, Bypass Surgery, and Heart Disease. Robert E. Kowalski. Warner Books, Inc., 666 Fifth Ave., 9th Flr., New York, NY 10103. Phone: (212) 484-2900. 1992.

The Healing Way: Adult Recovery from Childhood Sexual Abuse. Kristin A. Kunzman. HarperCollins Publishers, 10 E. 53rd St., New York, NY 10022-5299. Phone: (800) 242-7737. 1990.

The Heart Attack Handbook. Joseph S. Alpert. Consumer Reports Books, 9180 LeSaint Dr., Fairfield, OH 45014. Phone: (513) 860-1178. 1993.

The Heart Surgery Trap: Why Most Invasive Procedures Are Unnecessary and How to Avoid Them. Julian Whitaker. Simon & Schuster, Inc., 1230 Ave. of the Americas, New York, NY 10020. Phone: (212) 698-7000. 1992.

Mr. King, You're Having a Heart Attack: How a Heart Attack & Bypass Surgery Changed My Life. Larry King, B.D. Colen.

Dell Publishing Co., Inc., 666 Fifth Ave., New York, NY 10103. Phone: (800) 255-4133. 1990.

A Patient's Guide to Heart Surgery: Understanding the Practical and Emotional Aspects of Heart Surgery. Carol Cohan, June B. Pimm, James R. Jude. HarperCollins Pubs., Inc., 10 E. 53rd St., New York, NY 10022-5299. Phone: (212) 207-7000. Fax: (800) 242-7737. 1991.

Well-Informed Patient's Guide to Coronary Bypass Surgery. Jeffrey Gold. Bantam Doubleday Dell, 666 Fifth Ave., New York, NY 10103. Phone: (800) 223-6834. 1991.

Yale University School of Medicine Heart Book. Barry L. Zaret, Lawrence S. Cohen, Marvin Moser, and others. William Morrow & Company, Inc., 1350 Ave. of the Americas, New York, NY 10019. Phone: (800) 237-0657. 1992.

RESEARCH CENTERS, INSTITUTES, CLEARINGHOUSES

Artificial Heart Research Laboratory. University of Utah. 803 North 300 West, N.W. Wing, Salt Lake City, UT 84103. Phone: (801) 581-6991.

Cardiovascular Research Institute. University of California, San Francisco. San Francisco, CA 94143-0130. Phone: (415) 476-2226. Fax: (415) 476-2283.

Cardiovascular Surgical Research Laboratory. University of Texas. Room 15, University of Texas Medical Branch, Galveston, TX 77550. Phone: (409) 761-1203.

Cleveland Clinic Foundation Research Institute. 9500 Euclid Ave., Cleveland, OH 44195-5210. Phone: (216) 444-3900. Fax: (216) 444-3279.

DeBakey Heart Center. Baylor College of Medicine. Texas Medical Center, 1 Baylor Plaza, Houston, TX 77030. Phone: (701) 797-9353. Fax: (713) 793-1192.

Heart and Vascular Institute. Henry Ford Hospital, 2799 W. Grand Blvd., Detroit, MI 48202. Phone: (313) 876-2695. Fax: (313) 876-2687.

Hope Heart Institute. 528 18th Ave., Seattle, WA 98122. Phone: (206) 320-2001. Fax: (206) 328-0355.

Iowa Cardiovascular Center. University of Iowa. College of Medicine, 616 MRC, Iowa City, IA 52242. Phone: (319) 335-8588. Fax: (319) 335-6969.

Likoff Cardiovascular Institute. Hahnemann University. Broad and Vine Streets, Philadelphia, PA 19102. Phone: (215) 448-8790.

National Heart, Lung, and Blood Institute. 4733 Bethesda Ave., Ste. 530, Bethesda, MD 20814. Phone: (301) 951-3260.

Nora Eccles Harrison Cardiovascular Research and Training Institute. University of Utah. Nora Eccles Harrison Bldg., Salt Lake City, UT 84112. Phone: (801) 581-8183.

Texas Heart Institute. P.O. Box 20345, Houston, TX 77225-0345. Phone: (713) 791-3709. Fax: (713) 791-3089.

Whitaker Cardiovascular Institute. Boston University. 80 E. Concord St., Boston, MA 02118. Phone: (917) 638-4018. Fax: (617) 638-5258.

STANDARDS AND STATISTICS SOURCES

National Heart, Lung, and Blood Institute Fact Book. National Heart, Lung, and Blood Institute, NIH Bldg. 31, 9000 Rockville Pike, Bethesda, MD 20892. Phone: (301) 496-5166. Annual.

TEXTBOOKS AND MONOGRAPHS

Adult Cardiac Surgery. Bojar. Blackwell Scientific Publications, Inc., 3 Cambridge Ctr., Cambridge, MA 02142. Phone: (800) 759-6102. 1992.

Angioplasty. G. David Jang. McGraw-Hill Inc., 11 West 19th St., New York, NY 10011. Phone: (212) 337-5001. Fax: (212) 337-4092. Third edition 1993.

Cardiac Catheterization, Angiography, and Intervention. Willam Grossman, Donald S. Baim (eds.). Lea & Febiger, 428 E. Preston St., Baltimore, MD 21202. Phone: (800) 638-0672. Fax: (800) 447-8438. Fourth edition 1991.

Cardiac Surgery. Dwight C. McGoon (ed.). F.A. Davis Co., 1915 Arch St., Philadelphia, PA 19103. Phone: (800) 523-4049. Second edition 1987.

Cardiac Surgery: A Looseleaf Workbook & Update Service. Donald Doty. Mosby-Year Book, 11830 Westline Industrial Drive, St. Louis, MO 63146. Phone: (800) 325-4177. Fax: (314) 432-1380. 1991.

Cardiomyopathies and Heart-Lung Transplantation. Amar S. Kapoor, Hillel Laks, John S. Schroeder, et. al.. McGraw-Hill, Inc., Health Professions Division, 1221 Avenue of the Americas, 28th Floor, New York, NY 10020. Phone: (212) 512-4228. 1991.

Care of the Patient with Previous Coronary Bypass Surgery. David Waters, Martial G. Bourassa. F.A. Davis Co., 1915 Arch St., Philadelphia, PA 19103. Phone: (800) 523-4049. 1991.

Case Presentations in Vascular Surgery. D. Bouchier-Hayes, P. Broe, D. Mehigan. Butterworth-Heinemann, 80 Montvale Ave., Stoneham, MA 02180. Phone: (617) 438-8464. Fax: (617) 279-4851. 1991.

Complications in Cardiothoracic Surgery. John A. Waldhausen, Mark B. Orringer. Mosby-Year Book, 11830 Westline Industrial Drive, St. Louis, MO 63146. Phone: (800) 325-4177. Fax: (314) 432-1380. 1991.

Coronary Angioplasty. Clark. John Wiley & Sons, Inc., 605 Third Ave., New York, NY 10158-0012. Phone: (212) 850-6000. Fax: (212) 850-6088. Second edition 1991.

Coronary Artery Bypass Surgery. Lawrie Morris. Mosby-Year Book, 11830 Westline Industrial Drive, St. Louis, MO 63146. Phone: (800) 325-4177. Fax: (314) 432-1380. 1991.

Current Surgical Diagnosis and Treatment. L.W. Way. Appleton & Lange, 25 Van Zant St., East Norwalk, CT 06855. Phone: (800) 423-1359. Fax: (203) 854-9486. Ninth edition 1990.

Current Therapy in Vascular Surgery. Calvin B. Ernst, James C. Stanley. Mosby-Year Book, 11830 Westline Industrial Drive, St. Louis, MO 63146. Phone: (800) 325-4177. Fax: (314) 432-1380. Second edition 1991.

Glenn's Thoracic and Cardiovascular Surgery. Arthur Baue, Alexander S. Geha, Graeme L. Hammond, and others.

Appleton & Lange, 25 Van Zant St., East Norwalk, CT 06855. Phone: (800) 423-1359. Fax: (203) 854-9486. Fifth edition 1991.

Impact of Cardiac Surgery on the Quality of Life: Neurological & Psychological Aspects. A.E. Wilner, G. Rodewald (eds.). Plenum Publishing Co., 233 Spring St., New York, NY 10013-1578. Phone: (212) 620-8000. Fax: (212) 463-0742. 1990.

Laser Angioplasty. Timothy A. Sanborn (ed.). John Wiley & Sons, Inc., 605 Third Ave., New York, NY 10158-0012. Phone: (212) 850-6000. Fax: (212) 850-6088. 1989.

Prospects of Heart Surgery. A. Radley. Springer-Verlag New York Inc., 175 Fifth Ave., New York, NY 10010. Phone: (212) 460-1500. Fax: (212) 473-6272. 1988.

Quality of Life After Open Heart Surgery. Paul J. Walter (ed.). Kluwer Academic Publishers, P.O. Box 358, Accord Station, Hingham, MA 02018-0358. Phone: (617) 871-6600. Fax: (617) 871-6528. 1992.

Reoperations in Cardiac Surgery. J. Stark, A.D. Pacifico (eds.). Springer-Verlag New York Inc., 175 Fifth Ave., New York, NY 10010. Phone: (212) 460-1500. Fax: (212) 473-6272. 1989.

Replacement Cardiac Valves. Endre Bodnar, Robert Frater. McGraw-Hill, Inc., Health Professions Division, 1221 Avenue of the Americas, 28th Floor, New York, NY 10020. Phone: (212) 512-4228. 1992.

Surgery of the Third Ventricle. Michael Apuzzo. Williams & Wilkins, 438 E. Preston St., Baltimore, MD 21202. Phone: (800) 638-0672. Fax: (800) 447-8438. 1987.

Surgical Treatment of Congenital Heart Disease. Grady L. Hallman, Denton A. Cooley, Howard P. Gutgesell. Lea & Febiger, 428 E. Preston St., Baltimore, MD 21202. Phone: (800) 638-0672. Fax: (800) 447-8438. Third edition 1987.

Vascular Surgery in Infancy and Childhood. J. Leonel Villavicenzio. Williams & Wilkins, 428 East Preston St., Baltimore, MD 21202. Phone: (800) 638-0672. Fax: (800) 447-8438. 1992.

Vascular Surgery: Principles and Practice. Frank J. Veith, Robert W. Hobson II, Russell A. Williams. McGraw-Hill Inc., 11 West 19th St., New York, NY 10011. Phone: (212) 337-5001. Fax: (212) 337-4092. Second edition 1992.

CARIES

See: DENTISTRY

CARPAL TUNNEL SYNDROME

See: NEUROLOGIC DISORDERS

CATARACTS

See also: EYE DISEASES; EYE SURGERY; VISION DISORDERS

ABSTRACTING, INDEXING, AND CURRENT AWARENESS PUBLICATIONS

Core Journals in Ophthalmology. Elsevier Science Publishing Co., Inc., P.O. Box 882, Madison Square Station, New York,

NY 10159-2101. Phone: (212) 989-5800. Fax: (212) 633-3990. 11/year.

Current Contents/Clinical Medicine. Institute for Scientific Information, 3501 Market St., Philadelphia, PA 19104. Phone: (800) 523-1850. Fax: (215) 386-6362. Weekly.

Excerpta Medica. Section 12: Ophthalmology. Elsevier Science Publishing Co., Inc., P.O. Box 882, Madison Square Station, New York, NY 10159-2101. Phone: (212) 989-5800. Fax: (212) 633-3990. 16/year.

Index Medicus. U.S. National Library of Medicine, 8600 Rockville Pike, Bethesda, MD 20894. Phone: (800) 638-8480. Monthly.

Key Ophthalmology: Current Literature in Perspective. Mosby-Year Book, 11830 Westline Industrial Drive, St. Louis, MO 63146. Phone: (800) 325-4177. Fax: (314) 432-1380. Quarterly.

Ophthalmic Literature. Institute of Ophthalmology, Judd St., London WC1H 9QS, England. 7/year.

Science Citation Index. Institute for Scientific Information, 3501 Market St., Philadelphia, PA 19104. Phone: (800) 523-1850. Fax: (215) 386-6362. Bimonthly.

ANNUALS AND REVIEWS

Year Book of Ophthalmology. Mosby-Year Book, 11830 Westline Industrial Drive, St. Louis, MO 63146. Phone: (800) 325-4177. Fax: (314) 432-1380. Annual.

ASSOCIATIONS, PROFESSIONAL SOCIETIES, ADVOCACY AND SUPPORT GROUPS

American Academy of Ophthalmology (AAO). 655 Beach St., San Francisco, CA 94109. Phone: (415) 561-8500. Fax: (415) 561-8533.

American Society of Cataract and Refractive Surgery (ASCRS). 3702 Pender Dr., Ste. 250, Fairfax, VA 22030. Phone: (703) 591-2220. Fax: (703) 591-0614.

American Society of Contemporary Ophthalmology (ASCO). 233 E. Erie St., St. 710, Chicago, IL 60611. Phone: (312) 951-1400.

CD-ROM DATABASES

SCISEARCH. Institute for Scientific Information, 3501 Market St., Philadelphia, PA 19104. Phone: (215) 386-0100. Fax: (215) 386-6362.

DIRECTORIES

American Society of Bariatric Physicians-Directory. American Society of Bariatric Physicians, 5600 S. Quebec, Ste. 160-D, Englewood, CO 80111. Phone: (303) 779-4833. Fax: (303) 779-4834. Annual.

HANDBOOKS, GUIDES, MANUALS, ATLASES

Phacoemulsification Surgery. Terence M. Devine, William Banko, Edward Wakin. McGraw-Hill, Inc., Health Professions Division, 1221 Avenue of the Americas, 28th Floor, New York, NY 10020. Phone: (212) 512-4228. 1990.

Sutureless Cataract Surgery. James P. Gills, Donald R. Sanders (eds.). SLACK Inc., 6900 Grove Rd., Thorofare, NJ 08086-9447. Phone: (800) 257-8290. Fax: (609) 853-5991. 1991.

JOURNALS

Journal of Cataract and Refractive Surgery. Waverly Press, 428 E. Preston St., Baltimore, MD 21202. Phone: (800) 638-0672. Fax: (800) 447-8438. Bimonthly.

ONLINE DATABASES

Combined Health Information Database (CHID). U.S. National Institutes of Health, P.O. Box NDIC, Bethesda, MD 20892. Phone: (301) 496-2162. Fax: (301) 770-5164. Quarterly.

EMBASE. Elsevier Science Publishing Co., Inc., P.O. Box 882, Madison Square Station, New York, NY 10159-2101. Phone: (212) 989-5800. Fax: (212) 633-3990.

MEDLINE. National Library of Medicine, 8600 Rockville Pike, Bethesda, MD 20894. Phone: (800) 638-8480.

SciSearch. Institute for Scientific Information, 3501 Market St., Philadelphia, PA 19104. Phone: (215) 386-0100. Fax: (215) 386-6362.

POPULAR WORKS AND PATIENT EDUCATION

Cataract Surgery: Before and After. Robert I. Johnson. SLACK Inc., 6900 Grove Rd., Thorofare, NJ 08086-9447. Phone: (800) 257-8290. Fax: (609) 853-5991. Two volumes 1989.

The Well-Informed Patient's Guide to Cataract and Other Eye Surgery. Mark Speaker, Karyn Feiden. Bantam Doubleday Dell, 666 Fifth Ave., New York, NY 10103. Phone: (800) 223-6834. 1991.

RESEARCH CENTERS, INSTITUTES, CLEARINGHOUSES

Hermann Eye Center. University of Texas Health Science Center at Houston. Dept. of Ophthalmology, 6411 Fannin St., Houston, TX 77030. Phone: (713) 797-1777.

Wilmer Ophthalmological Institute. Johns Hopkins University. 601 N. Broadway, Baltimore, MD 21205. Phone: (301) 955-6846. Fax: (301) 955-0675.

TEXTBOOKS AND MONOGRAPHS

Age-Related Cataract. Richard W. Young. Oxford University Press, 200 Madison Ave., New York, NY 10016. Phone: (212) 679-7300. 1991.

Cataract Surgery and Its Complications. Jaffe. Mosby-Year Book, 11830 Westline Industrial Drive, St. Louis, MO 63146. Phone: (800) 325-4177. Fax: (314) 432-1380. Fifth edition 1990.

Ophthalmic Surgery: Principles and Concepts. George Spaeth (ed.). W.B. Saunders Co., The Curtis Center, Independence Sqare W., Philadelphia, PA 19106-3399. Phone: (215) 238-7800. 1990.

Ophthalmology: Principles and Concepts. Frank Newell. Mosby-Year Book, 11830 Westline Industrial Drive, St. Louis, MO 63146. Phone: (800) 325-4177. Fax: (314) 432-1380. 7th edition, 1992.

The Physician's Guide to Cataracts, Glaucoma and Other Eye Problems. John Eden. Consumer Reports Books, 9180 LeSaint Dr., Fairfield, OH 45014. Phone: (513) 860-1178. 1992.

Will's Treatment of Eye Disease. Friedberg. J.B. Lippincott Co., 227 E. Washington Square, Philadelphia, PA 19106-3780. Phone: (215) 238-4200. Fax: (215) 238-4227. 1990.

CELIAC DISEASE

See: GASTROINTESTINAL DISORDERS

CEREBRAL PALSY

ABSTRACTING, INDEXING, AND CURRENT AWARENESS PUBLICATIONS

General Science Index. H.W. Wilson Co., 950 University Ave., Bronx, NY 10452. Phone: (800) 367-6770.

ASSOCIATIONS, PROFESSIONAL SOCIETIES, ADVOCACY AND SUPPORT GROUPS

American Academy of Cerebral Palsy and Developmental Medicine. 1910 Byrd Ave., Suite 118, Richmond, VA 23230.

National Easter Seal Society. 70 E. Lake St., Chicago, IL 60601. Phone: (312) 726-6200.

United Cerebral Palsy Association (UCPA). 7 Penn Plaza, Ste. 804, New York, NY 100010. Phone: (212) 268-6655. Fax: (212) 268-5960.

NEWSLETTERS

Word from Washington. United Cerebral Palsy Associations, Inc (UCP), 1522 K St. N.W., Ste. 112, Washington, DC 20005. Phone: (202) 842-1266. Monthly.

POPULAR WORKS AND PATIENT EDUCATION

Children with Cerebral Palsy: A Parents' Guide. Elaine Geralis (ed.). Woodbine House, 5615 Fishers Ln., Rockville, MD 20852. Phone: (800) 843-7323. Fax: (301) 468-5784. 1991.

Handling the Young Cerebral Palsied Child at Home. Nancy Finnie. Penguin USA, 375 Hudson St., New York, NY 10014-3657. Phone: (800) 331-4624. 1989.

TEXTBOOKS AND MONOGRAPHS

Developmental Disabilities: Delivery of Medical Care for Children and Adults. I.L Rubin, A.C. Crocker. Williams & Wilkins, 428 East Preston St., Baltimore, MD 21202. Phone: (800) 638-0672. Fax: (800) 447-8438. 1989.

Easy Diagnosis and Therapy in Cerebral Palsy: A Primer on Infant Development Problems. A.L Scherzer, T. Tschanuter. Marcel Dekker, Inc., 270 Madison Ave., New York, NY 10016. Phone: (800) 228-1160. 2nd edition, 1990.

Gait Analysis in Cerebral Palsy. James R. Gage. Cambridge University Press, 40 W. 20th St., New York, NY 10011. Phone: (800) 431-1580. 1992.

CEREBROVASCULAR DISEASES

See also: NEUROLOGIC DISORDERS

ABSTRACTING, INDEXING, AND CURRENT AWARENESS PUBLICATIONS

Current Contents/Clinical Medicine. Institute for Scientific Information, 3501 Market St., Philadelphia, PA 19104. Phone: (800) 523-1850. Fax: (215) 386-6362. Weekly.

Excerpta Medica. Section 8: Neurology and Neurosurgery. Elsevier Science Publishers, P.O. Box 882, Madison Square Station, New York, NY 10159-2101. Phone: (212) 633-3950. Fax: (212) 633-3990. 32/year.

Index Medicus. U.S. National Library of Medicine, 8600 Rockville Pike, Bethesda, MD 20894. Phone: (800) 638-8480. Monthly.

Research Alert: Cerebrovascular Diseases-Strokes & TIA. Institute for Scientific Information, 3501 Market St., Philadelphia, PA 19104. Phone: (800) 523-1850. Fax: (215) 386-6362. Weekly.

Science Citation Index. Institute for Scientific Information, 3501 Market St., Philadelphia, PA 19104. Phone: (800) 523-1850. Fax: (215) 386-6362. Bimonthly.

ASSOCIATIONS, PROFESSIONAL SOCIETIES, ADVOCACY AND SUPPORT GROUPS

National Stroke Association (NSA). 300 E. Hampden Ave., Ste. 240, Englewood, CO 80110. Phone: (303) 762-9922.

Stroke Club International. 805 12th St., Galveston, TX 77550. Phone: (409) 762-1022.

CD-ROM DATABASES

SCISEARCH. Institute for Scientific Information, 3501 Market St., Philadelphia, PA 19104. Phone: (215) 386-0100. Fax: (215) 386-6362.

HANDBOOKS, GUIDES, MANUALS, ATLASES

The Adult Stroke Patient: A Manual for Evaluation and Treatment of Perceptual and Cognitive Dysfunction. Barbara Zoltan, Ellen Siev, Brenda Freishtat. SLACK Inc., 6900 Grove Rd., Thorofare, NJ 08086-9447. Phone: (800) 257-8290. Fax: (609) 853-5991. Revised second edition. 1991.

JOURNALS

Circulation Research. American Heart Association, 7320 Greenville Ave., Dallas, TX 75231. Phone: (214) 706-1310. Fax: (214) 691-6342. Monthly.

Haemostasis. S. Karger Publishers, Inc., 26 W. Avon Rd., P.O. Box 529, Farmington, CT 06085. Phone: (203) 675-7834. Fax: (203) 675-7302.

Stroke: A Journal of Cerebral Circulation. American Heart Association, 7320 Greenville Ave., Dallas, TX 75231. Phone: (214) 706-1310. Fax: (214) 691-6342. Monthly.

Thrombosis and Hemostasis. F.K. Schattauer Verlagsgesellschaft mbH, Lenzhalde 3, Postfach 104545, D-7000 Stuttgart 1, Germany. Phone: 0711-22987-0. Bimonthly.

Thrombosis Research. Pergamon Press, 660 White Plains Rd., Tarrytown, NY 10591-5153. Phone: (914) 592-7700. Fax: (914) 592-3625.

NEWSLETTERS

Stroke Clubs, International-Bulletin. Stroke Clubs, International, 805 12th St., Galveston, TX 77550. Phone: (713) 762-1022. Irregular.

ONLINE DATABASES

EMBASE. Elsevier Science Publishing Co., Inc., P.O. Box 882, Madison Square Station, New York, NY 10159-2101. Phone: (212) 989-5800. Fax: (212) 633-3990.

MEDLINE. National Library of Medicine, 8600 Rockville Pike, Bethesda, MD 20894. Phone: (800) 638-8480.

SciSearch. Institute for Scientific Information, 3501 Market St., Philadelphia, PA 19104. Phone: (215) 386-0100. Fax: (215) 386-6362.

POPULAR WORKS AND PATIENT EDUCATION

After a Stroke: A Support Book for Patients, Caregivers, Families and Friends. Geoffrey A. Donnan, Carol Burton. North Atlantic Books, 2800 Woolsey St., Berkeley, CA 94705. Phone: (510) 652-5309. Second edition 1992.

Living with Stroke. Paul King. St. Martin's Press, 175 Fifth Ave., New York, NY 10010. Phone: (212) 674-5151. 1992.

Stroke: A Guide for Patients and Their Families. John E. Sarno, Martha Sarno. Sterling Publishing Co., Inc., 387 Park Ave. S., New York, NY 10016-8810. Phone: (800) 367-9692.

Stroke: A Self-Help Manual for Stroke Sufferers and Their Relatives. R.M. Youngson. Borgo Press, P.O. Box 2845, San Bernardino, CA 92406-2845. Phone: (909) 884-5813. Fax: (909) 888-4942. 1990.

Stroke Fact Book: Everything You Want and Need to Know about Stroke--From Prevention to Rehabilitation. Conn Foley, H.F. Pizer. Courage Ct., 3915 Golden Valley Rd., Golden Valley, MN 55422. Phone: (612) 520-0261.

Strokes: What Families Should Know. Shimberg. Ballantine Books, Inc., 201 E. 50th St., New York, NY 10022. Phone: (800) 733-3000. 1990.

RESEARCH CENTERS, INSTITUTES, CLEARINGHOUSES

Center for the Study of Cerebrovascular Disease and Stroke. 22 S. Green St., University of Maryland, Baltimore, MD 21201. Phone: (301) 328-5080.

Cerebral Vascular Disease Research Center. P.O. Box 016960, Dept. of Neurology, University of Miami, Miami, FL 33101. Phone: (302) 547-6449.

Cerebrovascular Research Center. 3600 Hamilton Walk, University of Pennsylvania, Philadelphia, PA 19104. Phone: (215) 662-2632.

Hypertension/Atherosclerosis Unit. University of Virginia. Medical Center, Box 146, Charlottesville, VA 22908. Phone: (804) 924-2765. Fax: (804) 924-2581.

TEXTBOOKS AND MONOGRAPHS

The Aftermath of Stroke: The Experience of Patients and Their Families. Robert Anderson. Cambridge University Press, 40 W. 20th St., New York, NY 10011. Phone: (800) 431-1580. 1992.

Cerebral Vascular Disease. J.S. Meyer (ed.). Elsevier Science Publishing Co., Inc., P.O. Box 882, Madison Square Station, New York, NY 10159-2101. Phone: (212) 989-5800. Fax: (212) 633-3990. Volume 7, 1989.

Cerebrovascular Disorders. James F. Toole. Raven Press, 1185 Avenue of the Americas, New York, NY 10036. Phone: (212) 930-9500. Fax: (212) 869-3495. Fourth edition 1990.

Progress in Cerebrovascular Disease: Current Concepts in Stroke and Vascular Dementia. J.S. Chopra, K. Jagannathan, Lechner and others (eds.). Elsevier Science Publishing Co., Inc., P.O. Box 882, Madison Square Station, New York, NY 10159-2101. Phone: (212) 989-5800. Fax: (212) 633-3990. 1990.

Vascular Surgery. Robert Rutherford. W.B. Saunders Co., The Curtis Center, Independence Sqare W., Philadelphia, PA 19106-3399. Phone: (215) 238-7800. 3rd edition, 1989.

CERVICAL CANCER

See also: CANCER

ABSTRACTING, INDEXING, AND CURRENT AWARENESS PUBLICATIONS

Current Contents/Clinical Medicine. Institute for Scientific Information, 3501 Market St., Philadelphia, PA 19104. Phone: (800) 523-1850. Fax: (215) 386-6362. Weekly.

Excerpta Medica. Section 16: Cancer. Elsevier Science Publishing Co., Inc., P.O. Box 882, Madison Square Station, New York, NY 10159-2101. Phone: (212) 989-5800. Fax: (212) 633-3990. 32/year.

ICRDB Cancergram: Gynecologic Tumors--Diagnosis, Treatment. U.S. Government Printing Office, Superintendent of Documents, P.O. Box 371954, Pittsburgh, PA 15250-7954. Phone: (202) 783-3238. Fax: (202) 512-2250. Monthly.

Index Medicus. U.S. National Library of Medicine, 8600 Rockville Pike, Bethesda, MD 20894. Phone: (800) 638-8480. Monthly.

ANNUALS AND REVIEWS

In Development New Medicines for Older Americans. 1991 Annual Survey. More Medicines in Testing for Cancer Than for Any Other Disease of Aging. Pharmaceutical Manufacturers Association, 1100 15th St. N.W., Washington, DC 20005. Phone: (202) 835-3400. 1991.

ASSOCIATIONS, PROFESSIONAL SOCIETIES, ADVOCACY AND SUPPORT GROUPS

American Cancer Society (ACS). 1599 Clifton Rd. N.E., Atlanta, GA 30329. Phone: (404) 320-3333.

American College of Obstetricians and Gynecologists (ACOG). 409 12th St. S.W., Washington, DC 20024-2188. Phone: (202) 638-5577.

National Women's Health Network (NWHN). 1325 G St. N.W., Washington, DC 20005. Phone: (202) 347-1140. Fax: (202) 347-1168.

BIBLIOGRAPHIES

Cervical Cancer: Risk Assessment and Preventive Care. National Technical Information Service, 5285 Port Royal Rd., Springfield, VA 22161. Phone: (703) 487-4650. Fax: (703) 321-8547. Jan. 1978-Nov. 1988 PB89-851679/CBY.

CD-ROM DATABASES

Cancerlit. Aries Systems Corporation, One Dundee Park, Andover, MA 01810. Phone: (508) 475-7200. Fax: (508) 474-8860. Quarterly.

OncoDisc. J.B. Lippincott Co., 227 East Washington Square, Philadelphia, PA 19106-3780. Phone: (215) 238-4200. Fax: (215) 238-4227. Bimonthly.

Physician's Data Query (PDQ). Cambridge Scientific Abstracts, 7200 Wisconsin Ave., Bethesda, MD 20814-4823. Phone: (800) 843-7751. Fax: (301) 961-6720. Quarterly.

ENCYCLOPEDIAS, DICTIONARIES, WORD BOOKS

Oncology Words. Stedman. Williams & Wilkins, 428 East Preston St., Baltimore, MD 21202. Phone: (800) 638-0672. Fax: (800) 447-8438. 1992.

JOURNALS

American Journal of Obstetrics and Gynecology. Mosby-Year Book, 11830 Westline Industrial Drive, St. Louis, MO 63146. Phone: (800) 325-4177. Fax: (314) 432-1380. Monthly.

CA - A Cancer Journal for Clinicians. J.B. Lippincott Co., 227 E. Washington Square, Philadelphia, PA 19106-3780. Phone: (215) 238-4200. Fax: (215) 238-4227. Bimonthly.

Cancer Causes and Control. Rapid Communications of Oxford Ltd., The Old Malthouse, Paradise St., Oxford OX1 1LD, England. Phone: 44-865-790447. Fax: 44-865-244012. 6/year.

Gynecologic Oncology. Academic Press, Inc., 1250 Sixth Ave., San Diego, CA 92101-4311. Phone: (619) 699-6345. Fax: (619) 699-6715. Monthly.

Journal of the National Cancer Institute. Superintendent of Documents, P.O. Box 371954, Pittsburgh, PA 15250-7954. Fax: (202) 512-2233. Semimonthly.

Journal of Surgical Oncology. John Wiley & Sons, Inc., 605 Third Ave., New York, NY 10158-0012. Phone: (212) 850-6000. Fax: (212) 850-6088. Monthly.

Obstetrics and Gynecology. Elsevier Science Publishing Co., Inc., P.O. Box 882, Madison Square Station, New York, NY 10159-2101. Phone: (212) 989-5800. Fax: (212) 633-3990. 15/year.

ONLINE DATABASES

Cancer Weekly. CDC AIDS Weekly/NCI Cancer Weekly, 206 Rogers St. NE, Suite 104, P.O. Box 5528, Atlanta, GA 30317. Phone: (404) 377-8895. Weekly.

CANCERLIT. U.S. National Cancer Institute, International Cancer Information Center, Building 82, Room 102, Bethesda,

MD 20892. Phone: (301) 496-7403. Fax: (301) 480-8105. Monthly.

Clinical Protocols. U.S. National Cancer Institute, International Cancer Information Center, Building 82, Room 102, Bethesda, MD 20892. Phone: (301) 496-7403. Fax: (301) 480-8105.

EMBASE. Elsevier Science Publishing Co., Inc., P.O. Box 882, Madison Square Station, New York, NY 10159-2101. Phone: (212) 989-5800. Fax: (212) 633-3990.

MEDLINE. National Library of Medicine, 8600 Rockville Pike, Bethesda, MD 20894. Phone: (800) 638-8480.

Physician Data Query (PDQ) Cancer Information File. U.S. National Cancer Institute, International Cancer Information Center, Building 82, Room 102, Bethesda, MD 20892. Phone: (301) 496-7403. Fax: (301) 480-8105. Monthly.

Physician Data Query (PDQ) Directory File. U.S. National Cancer Institute, International Cancer Information Center, Building 82, Room 102, Bethesda, MD 20892. Phone: (301) 496-7403. Fax: (301) 480-8105. Monthly.

Physician Data Query (PDQ) Protocol File. U.S. National Cancer Institute, International Cancer Information Center, Building 82, Room 102, Bethesda, MD 20892. Phone: (301) 496-7403. Fax: (301) 480-8105. Monthly.

SciSearch. Institute for Scientific Information, 3501 Market St., Philadelphia, PA 19104. Phone: (215) 386-0100. Fax: (215) 386-6362.

POPULAR WORKS AND PATIENT EDUCATION

Cancervive: The Challenge of Life After Cancer. Susan Nessim, Judith Ellis. Houghton Mifflin Co., 1 Beacon St., Boston, MA 02108. Phone: (800) 225-3362. 1991.

Everyone's Guide to Cancer Therapy: How Cancer is Diagnosed, Treated, and Managed on a Day to Day Basis. Malin Dollinger, Ernest H. Rosenbaum, Greg Cable. Andrews & McMeel, 4900 Main St., Kansas City, MO 64112. Phone: (800) 826-4216. 1991.

RESEARCH CENTERS, INSTITUTES, CLEARINGHOUSES

Cancer Information Service (CIS). Office of Cancer Communications, National Cancer Institute, Bldg. 31, Rm. 10A24, 9000 Rockville Pike, Bethesda, MD 20892. Phone: (800) 4CA-NCER.

Mayo Comprehensive Cancer Center. 200 First St. SW, Rochester, MN 55905. Phone: (507) 284-4718.

Memorial Sloan-Kettering Cancer Center. 1275 York Ave., New York, NY 10021. Phone: (212) 355-0060.

Oncology Center. Johns Hopkins University. 600 N. Wolfe St., Baltimore, MD 21205. Phone: (301) 955-8800. Fax: (301) 955-1904.

TEXTBOOKS AND MONOGRAPHS

Cancer Medicine. James F. Holland, Emil Frei, Robert C. Bast Jr., and others. Williams & Wilkins, 428 East Preston St., Baltimore, MD 21202. Phone: (800) 638-0672. Fax: (800) 447-8438. Third edition 1992.

Cancer: Principles and Practice of Oncology. Vincent T. DeVita. J.B. Lippincott Co., 227 E. Washington Square, Philadelphia, PA 19106-3780. Phone: (215) 238-4200. Fax: (215) 238-4227. 1989 3rd edtion.

Cancer Treatment. Charles M. Haskell. W.B. Saunders Co., The Curtis Center, Independence Square W., Philadelphia, PA 19106-3399. Phone: (215) 238-7800. Third edition 1990.

Clinical Gynecologic Oncology. Philip DiSaia, William Grosman. Mosby-Year Book, 11830 Westline Industrial Drive, St. Louis, MO 63146. Phone: (800) 325-4177. Fax: (314) 432-1380. 3rd edition, 1989.

Genital Papillomaviruses and Related Neoplasms. Christopher P. Crum, Gerard J. Nuovo. Raven Press, 1185 Avenue of the Americas, New York, NY 10036. Phone: (212) 930-9500. Fax: (212) 869-3495. 1991.

Gynecologic Oncology. Robert C. Knapp, Ross Berkowitz. McGraw-Hill Inc., 11 West 19th St., New York, NY 10011. Phone: (212) 337-5001. Fax: (212) 337-4092. Second edition 1992.

CESAREAN SECTION

See: CHILDBIRTH

CHEMOTHERAPY

ABSTRACTING, INDEXING, AND CURRENT AWARENESS PUBLICATIONS

Biological Abstracts. BIOSIS, 2100 Arch St., Philadelphia, PA 19103-1399. Phone: (800) 523-4800. Fax: (215) 587-2016.

CA Selects: Antitumor Agents. Chemical Abstracts Service, 2540 Olentangy River Road, P.O. Box 3012, Columbus, OH 43210-0012. Phone: (800) 848-6538. Biweekly.

Cumulative Index to Nursing and Allied Health Literature. Glendale Adventist Medical Center, P.O. Box 871, Glendale, CA 91209. Phone: (818) 409-8005. Bimonthly.

Current Contents/Clinical Medicine. Institute for Scientific Information, 3501 Market St., Philadelphia, PA 19104. Phone: (800) 523-1850. Fax: (215) 386-6362. Weekly.

Current Contents/Life Sciences. Institute for Scientific Information, 3501 Market St., Philadelphia, PA 19104. Phone: (215) 386-0100. Fax: (215) 386-6362.

Excerpta Medica. Section 16: Cancer. Elsevier Science Publishing Co., Inc., P.O. Box 882, Madison Square Station, New York, NY 10159-2101. Phone: (212) 989-5800. Fax: (212) 633-3990. 32/year.

Index Medicus. U.S. National Library of Medicine, 8600 Rockville Pike, Bethesda, MD 20894. Phone: (800) 638-8480. Monthly.

Research Alert: Cancer Chemotherapy. Institute for Scientific Information, 3501 Market St., Philadelphia, PA 19104. Phone: (800) 523-1850. Fax: (215) 386-6362. Weekly.

Science Citation Index. Institute for Scientific Information, 3501 Market St., Philadelphia, PA 19104. Phone: (800) 523-1850. Fax: (215) 386-6362. Bimonthly.

ANNUALS AND REVIEWS

In Development New Medicines for Older Americans. 1991 Annual Survey. More Medicines in Testing for Cancer Than for Any Other Disease of Aging. Pharmaceutical Manufacturers Association, 1100 15th St. N.W., Washington, DC 20005. Phone: (202) 835-3400. 1991.

ASSOCIATIONS, PROFESSIONAL SOCIETIES, ADVOCACY AND SUPPORT GROUPS

Chemotherapy Foundation (CF). 183 Madison Ave., Rm. 403, New York, NY 10016. Phone: (212) 213-9292. Fax: (212) 689-5164.

CD-ROM DATABASES

Biological Abstracts on Compact Disc. BIOSIS, 2100 Arch St., Philadelphia, PA 19103-1399. Phone: (800) 523-4800. Fax: (215) 587-2016. Quarterly.

Cancerlit. Aries Systems Corporation, One Dundee Park, Andover, MA 01810. Phone: (508) 475-7200. Fax: (508) 474-8860. Quarterly.

Nursing and Allied Health (CINAHL) on CD-ROM. CINAHL, 1509 Wilson Terrace, P.O. Box 871, Glendale, CA 91209-0871. Phone: (818) 409-8005.

SCISEARCH. Institute for Scientific Information, 3501 Market St., Philadelphia, PA 19104. Phone: (215) 386-0100. Fax: (215) 386-6362.

HANDBOOKS, GUIDES, MANUALS, ATLASES

Cancer Chemotherapy Handbook. Fischer. Mosby-Year Book, 11830 Westline Industrial Drive, St. Louis, MO 63146. Phone: (800) 325-4177. Fax: (314) 432-1380. Third edition 1989.

JOURNALS

American Journal of Clinical Oncology. Raven Press, 1185 Ave. of the Americas, New York, NY 10036. Phone: (212) 930-9500. Fax: (212) 869-3495. Bimonthly.

Anti-Cancer Drugs. Rapid Communications of Oxford Ltd., The Old Malthouse, Paradise St., Oxford OX1 1LD, England. Phone: 44-865-790447. Fax: 44-865-244012. 6/year.

Journal of Clinical Oncology. W.B. Saunders Co., The Curtis Center, Independence Square W., Philadelphia, PA 19106-3399. Phone: (215) 238-7800. Monthly.

Journal of Surgical Oncology. John Wiley & Sons, Inc., 605 Third Ave., New York, NY 10158-0012. Phone: (212) 850-6000. Fax: (212) 850-6088. Monthly.

ONLINE DATABASES

BIOSIS Previews. BIOSIS, 2100 Arch St., Philadelphia, PA 19103-1399. Phone: (800) 523-4800. Fax: (215) 587-2016.

CANCERLIT. U.S. National Cancer Institute, International Cancer Information Center, Building 82, Room 102, Bethesda, MD 20892. Phone: (301) 496-7403. Fax: (301) 480-8105. Monthly.

EMBASE. Elsevier Science Publishing Co., Inc., P.O. Box 882, Madison Square Station, New York, NY 10159-2101. Phone: (212) 989-5800. Fax: (212) 633-3990.

MEDLINE. National Library of Medicine, 8600 Rockville Pike, Bethesda, MD 20894. Phone: (800) 638-8480.

Nursing and Allied Health (CINAHL). CINAHL, 1509 Wilson Terrace, P.O. Box 871, Glendale, CA 91209-0871. Phone: (818) 409-8005.

Physician Data Query (PDQ) Cancer Information File. U.S. National Cancer Institute, International Cancer Information Center, Building 82, Room 102, Bethesda, MD 20892. Phone: (301) 496-7403. Fax: (301) 480-8105. Monthly.

Physician Data Query (PDQ) Directory File. U.S. National Cancer Institute, International Cancer Information Center, Building 82, Room 102, Bethesda, MD 20892. Phone: (301) 496-7403. Fax: (301) 480-8105. Monthly.

Physician Data Query (PDQ) Protocol File. U.S. National Cancer Institute, International Cancer Information Center, Building 82, Room 102, Bethesda, MD 20892. Phone: (301) 496-7403. Fax: (301) 480-8105. Monthly.

SciSearch. Institute for Scientific Information, 3501 Market St., Philadelphia, PA 19104. Phone: (215) 386-0100. Fax: (215) 386-6362.

POPULAR WORKS AND PATIENT EDUCATION

Everyone's Guide to Cancer Therapy: How Cancer is Diagnosed, Treated, and Managed on a Day to Day Basis. Malin Dollinger, Ernest H. Rosenbaum, Greg Cable. Andrews & McMeel, 4900 Main St., Kansas City, MO 64112. Phone: (800) 826-4216. 1991.

The Facts about Chemotherapy. Paul Reich. Consumer Reports Books, 101 Truman Ave., Yonkers, NY 10703. Phone: (914) 378-2000. 1991.

Managing the Side Effects of Chemotherapy and Radiation Therapy. Marilyn J. Dodd. Prentice Hall, 113 Sylvan Ave., Rt. 9W, Prentice Hall Bldg., Englewood Cliffs, NJ 07632. Phone: (201) 767-5937. 1991.

Nutrition for the Chemotherapy Patient. Janet Ramstack. Bull Publishing Co., 110 Gilbert Ave., Menlo Park, CA 94025. Phone: (800) 676-2855. 1990.

RESEARCH CENTERS, INSTITUTES, CLEARINGHOUSES

Cancer Research Center. Boston University. 80 E. Concord St., Boston, MA 02118. Phone: (617) 638-4173. Fax: (617) 638-4176.

Center for Basic Cancer Research. Kansas State University. Division of Biology, Ackert Hall, Manhattan, KS 66506. Phone: (913) 532-6705.

Charity Hospital Oncology Treatment Unit. Tulane University. Charity Hospital of New Orleans, 1532 Tulane Ave., New Orleans, LA 70112. Phone: (504) 568-8131.

Comprehensive Cancer Center. Ohio State University. 300 W. 10th Ave., Columbus, OH 43210. Phone: (614) 293-3304. Fax: (614) 293-3132.

Dana Farber Cancer Institute. 44 Binney St., Boston, MA 02115. Phone: (617) 732-3000.

Fox Chase Cancer Center. 7701 Burholme Ave., Philadelphia, PA 19111. Phone: (215) 728-6900. Fax: (215) 728-2571.

Grace Cancer Drug Center. Roswell Park Cancer Institute. Elm & Carlton Sts., Buffalo, NY 14263. Phone: (716) 845-5860. Fax: (716) 845-8857.

Hubert H. Humphrey Cancer Research Center. Boston University. 80 E. Concord St., Boston, MA 02118. Phone: (617) 638-4173.

Laboratory of Experimental Chemotherapy for Parasitology. Rockefeller University, 1230 York Ave., New York, NY 10021. Phone: (212) 570-8232.

LCF Foundation, Inc.. 41 Mall Rd., Burlington, MA 01805. Phone: (617) 273-5100. Fax: (617) 273-8999.

Mayo Comprehensive Cancer Center. 200 First St. SW, Rochester, MN 55905. Phone: (507) 284-4718.

Oncology Center. Johns Hopkins University. 600 N. Wolfe St., Baltimore, MD 21205. Phone: (301) 955-8800. Fax: (301) 955-1904.

Research Office. John L. McClellan Memorial Veterans' Hospital. 4300 W. Seventh St., Little Rock, AR 72205. Phone: (501) 661-1202. Fax: (501) 671-2510.

Roswell Park Cancer Institute. 666 Elm St., Buffalo, NY 14263. Phone: (716) 845-2300. Fax: (716) 845-3545.

University of Maryland Cancer Center. University of Maryland at Baltimore. 22 S. Greene St., Baltimore, MD 21201. Phone: (301) 328-5506. Fax: (301) 328-6896.

TEXTBOOKS AND MONOGRAPHS

Advances in Chemotherapy of AIDS. Robert Diasio, Jean-Pierre Sommadossi. McGraw-Hill, Inc., Health Professions Division, 1221 Avenue of the Americas, 28th Floor, New York, NY 10020. Phone: (212) 512-4228. 1990.

Cancer Chemotherapy: Principles and Practice. Bruce Chabner, Jerry Collins. J.B. Lippincott Co., 227 E. Washington Square, Philadelphia, PA 19106-3780. Phone: (215) 238-4200. Fax: (215) 238-4227. 1990.

Chemotherapy of Gynecologic Cancer. Gunter Deppe (ed.). John Wiley & Sons, Inc., 605 Third Ave., New York, NY 10158-0012. Phone: (212) 850-6000. Fax: (212) 850-6088. Second edition 1989.

Chemotherapy of Gynecological and Breast Cancer. M. Kaufmann, and others. S. Karger Publishers, Inc., 26 W. Avon Rd., P.O. Box 529, Farmington, CT 06085. Phone: (203) 675-7834. Fax: (203) 675-7302. 1990.

Chemotherapy Source Book. Perry. Williams & Wilkins, 428 East Preston St., Baltimore, MD 21202. Phone: (800) 638-0672. Fax: (800) 447-8438. 1992.

CHEST DISEASES

See: LUNG DISEASES

CHICKENPOX

See: INFECTIOUS DISEASES

CHILD ABUSE

See also: SPOUSE ABUSE

ABSTRACTING, INDEXING, AND CURRENT AWARENESS PUBLICATIONS

Child Abuse: Abstracts of the Psychological and Behavioral Literature, Volume 2, 1986-1990. American Psychological Association, 1200 17th St. NW, Washington, DC 20036. Phone: (202) 955-7600. 1992.

ASSOCIATIONS, PROFESSIONAL SOCIETIES, ADVOCACY AND SUPPORT GROUPS

Child Welfare League of America. 440 First St. N.W., Suite 310, Washington, DC 20001-2085. Phone: (202) 638-2952.

International Society for Prevention of Child Abuse and Neglect. 1205 Oneida St., Denver, CO 80220. Phone: (303) 321-3963.

Molesters Anonymous. 1209 N.E. St., San Bernardino, CA 92405. Phone: (714) 355-1100.

National Committee for Prevention of Child Abuse. 332 S. Michigan Ave., Ste. 1600, Chicago, IL 60604. Phone: (312) 663-3520.

National Exchange Club Foundation for the Prevention of Child Abuse. 3050 Central Ave., Toledo, OH 43606. Phone: (419) 525-3232.

BIBLIOGRAPHIES

Child Abuse and Neglect. National Technical Information Service, 5285 Port Royal Rd., Springfield, VA 22161. Phone: (703) 487-4650. Fax: (703) 321-8547. Jan. 1971-Apr. 1989 PB89-861207/CBY.

DIRECTORIES

Sexual Assault and Child Sexual Abuse: A Directory of Victim/ Survivor Services and Prevention Programs. Linda Webster (ed.). Oryx Press, 4041 N. Central, Suite 700, Phoenix, AZ 85012. Phone: (800) 279-ORYX. Fax: (800) 279-4663. 1989.

ENCYCLOPEDIAS, DICTIONARIES, WORD BOOKS

Encyclopedia of Child Abuse. Robin E. Clark, Judith Clark. Facts on File, Inc., 460 Park Ave. S., New York, NY 10016-7382. Phone: (212) 683-2244. Fax: (212) 683-3633. 1989.

HANDBOOKS, GUIDES, MANUALS, ATLASES

Color Atlas of Child Sexual Abuse. Chadwick. Mosby-Year Book, 11830 Westline Industrial Drive, St. Louis, MO 63146. Phone: (800) 325-4177. Fax: (314) 432-1380. 1989.

ONLINE DATABASES

Child Abuse and Neglect. Clearinghouse on Child Abuse and Neglect Information, P.O. Box 1182, Washington, DC 20013. Phone: (703) 821-2086.

POPULAR WORKS AND PATIENT EDUCATION

Allies in Healing: When the Person You Love Was Sexually Abused as a Child, a Support Book for Partners. Laura Davis.

HarperCollins Pubs., Inc., 10 E. 53rd St., New York, NY 10022-5299. Phone: (212) 207-7000. 1991.

Child Abuse: A Practical Guide for Those Who Help Others. E. Clay Jorgenson. Continuum Publishing Co., 370 Lexington Ave., New York, NY 10017. Phone: (212) 532-3650. 1990.

The Courage to Heal: A Guide for Women Survivors of Child Sexual Abuse. Ellen Bass, Laura Davis. HarperCollins Pubs., Inc., 10 E. 53rd St., New York, NY 10022-5299. Phone: (212) 207-7000. Revised edition 1992.

The Healing Way: Adult Recovery from Childhood Sexual Abuse. Kristin A. Kunzman. HarperCollins Publishers, 10 E. 53rd St., New York, NY 10022-5299. Phone: (800) 242-7737. 1990.

Strong at the Broken Places: Overcoming the Trauma of Childhood Abuse. Linda T. Sanford. Random House, Inc., 201 E. 50th St., New York, NY 10022. Phone: (800) 726-0600. 1990.

Trauma and Recovery: The Aftermath of Violence--from Domestic Abuse to Political Terror. Judith Lewis Herman. Basic Books, 10 E. 53rd St., New York, NY 10022. Phone: (800) 242-7737. 1993.

RESEARCH CENTERS, INSTITUTES, CLEARINGHOUSES

Clearinghouse on Child Abuse and Neglect Information. P.O. Box 1182, Washington, DC 20013. Phone: (703) 821-2086.

National Clearinghouse on Child Abuse and Neglect and Family Violence Information. P.O. Box 1182, Washington, DC 20013. Phone: (800) FYI-3366. Fax: (703) 385-3206.

TEXTBOOKS AND MONOGRAPHS

Child Abuse. Ludwig. Churchill Livingstone Inc., 650 Ave. of the Americas, New York, NY 10011. Phone: (212) 819-5400. Fax: (212) 302-6598. Second edition 1992.

Child Advocacy for the Clinician: An Approach to Child Abuse and Neglect. Lawrence S. Wilson. Williams & Wilkins, 428 East Preston St., Baltimore, MD 21202. Phone: (800) 638-0672. Fax: (800) 447-8438. 1989.

Child Sexual Abuse: The Initial Effects. Beverly Gomes-Schwartz, Jonathan M. Horowitz, et. al.. Sage Publications, Inc., 2455 Teller Road, P.O. Box 5084, Newbury Park, CA 91320. Phone: (805) 499-0721. Fax: (805) 499-0871. 1990.

CHILDBIRTH

See also: MIDWIFERY; OBSTETRICS AND GYNECOLOGY; PREGNANCY

ABSTRACTING, INDEXING, AND CURRENT AWARENESS PUBLICATIONS

Cumulative Index to Nursing and Allied Health Literature. Glendale Adventist Medical Center, P.O. Box 871, Glendale, CA 91209. Phone: (818) 409-8005. Bimonthly.

Current Contents/Clinical Medicine. Institute for Scientific Information, 3501 Market St., Philadelphia, PA 19104. Phone: (800) 523-1850. Fax: (215) 386-6362. Weekly.

Excerpta Medica. Section 10: Obstetrics and Gynecology. Elsevier Science Publishing Co., Inc., P.O. Box 882, Madison

Square Station, New York, NY 10159-2101. Phone: (212) 989-5800. Fax: (212) 633-3990. 20/year.

Index Medicus. U.S. National Library of Medicine, 8600 Rockville Pike, Bethesda, MD 20894. Phone: (800) 638-8480. Monthly.

Nursing and Midwifery Index. CLN Publications, c/o Bournemouth University, Dorset House Library, Talbot Campus, Fern Barrow, Poole, Dorset BH12 5BB, England. Monthly.

Science Citation Index. Institute for Scientific Information, 3501 Market St., Philadelphia, PA 19104. Phone: (800) 523-1850. Fax: (215) 386-6362. Bimonthly.

ANNUALS AND REVIEWS

Obstetrics and Gynecology Clinics. W.B. Saunders Co., The Curtis Center, Independence Square W., Philadelphia, PA 19106-3399. Phone: (215) 238-7800. Quarterly.

ASSOCIATIONS, PROFESSIONAL SOCIETIES, ADVOCACY AND SUPPORT GROUPS

American College of Nurse-Midwives (ACNM). 1522 K St. N.W., Ste. 1000, Washington, DC 20005. Phone: (202) 289-0171. Fax: (202) 289-4395.

American College of Obstetricians and Gynecologists (ACOG). 409 12th St. S.W., Washington, DC 20024-2188. Phone: (202) 638-5577.

American Society for Prophylaxis in Obstetrics (ASPO/LAMAZE). 1840 Wilson Blvd., Ste. 204, Arlington, VA 22201. Phone: (800) 368-4404. Fax: (703) 524-8743.

American Society of Psychoprophylaxis in Obstetrics. 1840 Wilson Blvd., Ste. 204, Arlington, VA 22201. Phone: (703) 524-7802.

C/SEC Inc.. Cesarean/Support Education and Concern, 22 Forest Rd., Framingham, MA 01701. Phone: (508) 877-8266.

Cesarean Support, Education and Concern (C/SEC). 22 Forest Rd., Framingham, MA 01701. Phone: (508) 877-8266.

Childbirth Education Foundation (CEF). P.O. Box 5, Richboro, PA 18954. Phone: (215) 357-2792.

Consortium for Nurse-Midwifery, Inc. (CNMI). 1911 W. 233rd St., Torrance, CA 90501. Phone: (213) 539-9801.

International Cesarean Awareness Network (ICAN). P.O. Box 152, Syracuse, NY 13210. Phone: (315) 424-1942.

International Childbirth Education Association (ICEA). P.O. Box 20048, Minneapolis, MN 55420-0048. Phone: (612) 854-8660.

Midwives Alliance of North America (MANA). 30 S. Main, Concord, NH 03301. Phone: (603) 225-9586.

National Association of Childbearing Centers. 3123 Gottschalk Rd., Perkiomenville, PA 18074. Phone: (215) 234-8068.

National Association of Parents and Professionals for Safe Alternatives in Childbirth. Route 1, Box 646, Marble Hill, MO 63764. Phone: (314) 238-2010.

Vaginal Birth after Cesarean. 10 Great Plain Terrace, Needham, MA 02192. Phone: (617) 449-2490.

CD-ROM DATABASES

Excerpta Medica CD: Obstetrics & Gynecology. SilverPlatter Information, Inc., River Ridge Office Park, 100 River Ridge Rd., Norwood, MA 02062. Phone: (617) 769-2599. Fax: (617) 769-8763. Quarterly.

Maternal Fetal Medicine: Labor Management. Valerion A. Catanzarite. Williams & Wilkins, 428 East Preston St., Baltimore, MD 21202. Phone: (800) 638-0672. Fax: (800) 447-8438. 1990.

Nursing and Allied Health (CINAHL) on CD-ROM. CINAHL, 1509 Wilson Terrace, P.O. Box 871, Glendale, CA 91209-0871. Phone: (818) 409-8005.

OBGLine. Aries Systems Corporation, One Dundee Park, Andover, MA 01810. Phone: (508) 475-7200. Fax: (508) 474-8860. Monthly or quarterly.

SCISEARCH. Institute for Scientific Information, 3501 Market St., Philadelphia, PA 19104. Phone: (215) 386-0100. Fax: (215) 386-6362.

ENCYCLOPEDIAS, DICTIONARIES, WORD BOOKS

Bailliere's Midwive's Dictionary. Margaret Adams. W.B. Saunders Co., The Curtis Center, Independence Square W., Philadelphia, PA 19106-3399. Phone: (215) 238-7800. Seventh edition 1991.

Obstetric and Gynecologic Word Book. Helen E. Littrell. Springhouse Publishing Co., 1111 Bethlehem Pike, Spring House, PA 19477. Phone: (800) 331-3170. Fax: (215) 646-8716. 1992.

Obstetric and Gynecological Words. Stedman. Williams & Wilkins, 428 East Preston St., Baltimore, MD 21202. Phone: (800) 638-0672. Fax: (800) 447-8438. 1992.

HANDBOOKS, GUIDES, MANUALS, ATLASES

Color Atlas of Childbirth and Obstetric Techniques. F.A. Al-Azzawi. Mosby-Year Book, 11830 Westline Industrial Drive, St. Louis, MO 63146. Phone: (800) 325-4177. Fax: (314) 432-1380. 1991.

Nurse's Clinical Guide to Maternity Care. Aileen MacLaren. Springhouse Publishing Co., 1111 Bethlehem Pike, Spring House, PA 19477. Phone: (800) 331-3170. Fax: (215) 646-8716. 1992.

Pregnancy, Childbirth and the Newborn: The Complete Guide. Penny Simkin, and others. Meadowbrook Press, 18318 Minnetonka Blvd., Deephaven, MN 55391. Phone: (800) 338-2232. 1991.

Zuspan and Quilligan's Manual of Obstetrics and Gynecology. Jay D. Iams, Frederick P. Zuspan, Edward J. Quilligan. Mosby-Year Book, 11830 Westline Industrial Drive, St. Louis, MO 63146. Phone: (800) 325-4177. Fax: (314) 432-1380. Second edition 1990.

JOURNALS

American Journal of Obstetrics and Gynecology. Mosby-Year Book, 11830 Westline Industrial Drive, St. Louis, MO 63146. Phone: (800) 325-4177. Fax: (314) 432-1380. Monthly.

Birth. Blackwell Scientific Publications, Inc., 3 Cambridge Center, Cambridge, MA 02142. Phone: (800) 759-6102.

The Birth Gazette. The Birth Gazette, 42 The Farm, Summertown, TN 38483. Phone: (615) 904-2519.

Journal of Nurse-Midwifery. Elsevier Science Publishing Co., Inc., P.O. Box 882, Madison Square Station, New York, NY 10159-2101. Phone: (212) 989-5800. Fax: (212) 633-3990. 6/year.

Midwifery Today. Midwifery Today, Box 2072, Eugene, OR 97402.

NEWSLETTERS

ACOG Newsletter. American College of Obstetricians and Gynecologists, 409 12th St. S.W., Washington, DC 20024-2188. Phone: (202) 638-5577. Monthly.

National Women's Health Network-Network News. National Women's Health Network, 1325 G St. N.W., Washington, DC 20005. Phone: (202) 347-1140. Bimonthly.

OB/GYN Clinical Alert. American Health Consultants, Department C1290, P.O. Box 740060, Atlanta, GA 30374. Phone: (800) 559-1032. Fax: (404) 352-1971. Monthly.

ONLINE DATABASES

EMBASE. Elsevier Science Publishing Co., Inc., P.O. Box 882, Madison Square Station, New York, NY 10159-2101. Phone: (212) 989-5800. Fax: (212) 633-3990.

MEDLINE. National Library of Medicine, 8600 Rockville Pike, Bethesda, MD 20894. Phone: (800) 638-8480.

Nursing and Allied Health (CINAHL). CINAHL, 1509 Wilson Terrace, P.O. Box 871, Glendale, CA 91209-0871. Phone: (818) 409-8005.

SciSearch. Institute for Scientific Information, 3501 Market St., Philadelphia, PA 19104. Phone: (215) 386-0100. Fax: (215) 386-6362.

POPULAR WORKS AND PATIENT EDUCATION

Alternative Birth: The Complete Guide. Carl Jones. Jeremy P. Tarcher, Inc., 5858 Wilshire Blvd., Suite 200, Los Angeles, CA 90036. Phone: (213) 935-9980. 1991.

Birth after Cesarean: The Medical Facts. Bruce L. Flamm. Simon & Schuster, 1230 Ave. of the Americas, New York, NY 10020. Phone: (800) 223-2348. Fax: (800) 284-0735. 1990.

The Birth Partner. Penny Simkin. Harvard Common Press, 535 Albany St., Boston, MA 02118. Phone: (617) 423-5803. 1989.

Birth-Tech: Tests and Technology in Pregnancy and Birth. Anne Charlish, Linda Hughey Holt. Facts on File, Inc., 460 Park Ave. S., New York, NY 10016-7382. Phone: (212) 683-2244. Fax: (212) 683-3633. 1990.

The Cesarean Myth: Choosing the Best Way to Have Your Baby. Mortimer Rosen, Lillian Thomas. Viking Penguin, 375 Hudson St., New York, NY 10014-3657. Phone: (800) 331-4624. 1989.

A Child Is Born: The Completely New Edition. Lennart Nilsson. Bantam Doubleday Dell, 666 Fifth Ave., New York, NY 10103. Phone: (800) 223-6834. 1990.

The Complete Mothercare Manual. Rosalind Y. Ting, Herbert Brant, Kenneth S. Holt. Simon & Schuster, 1230 Ave. of the Americas, New York, NY 10020. Phone: (800) 223-2348. Fax: (800) 284-0735. Revised edition, 1992.

A Good Birth, A Safe Birth. Diana Korte, Roberta Scaer. Harvard Common Press, 535 Albany St., Boston, MA 02118. Phone: (617) 423-5803. 3rd edition, 1992.

Having a Cesarean Baby: The Complete Guide for a Happy and Safe Cesarean Childbirth Experience. Richard Hausknecht, Joan R. Heilman. Viking Penguin, 375 Hudson St., New York, NY 10014-3657. Phone: (800) 331-4624. Second revised edition 1991.

Homebirth. Sheila Kitzinger. Dorling Kindersley, Inc., 232 Madison Ave., Ste. 1206, New York, NY 10016. Phone: (212) 684-0404. 1991.

Husband-Coached Birth. Robert A. Bradley. HarperCollins Pubs., Inc., 10 E. 53rd St., New York, NY 10022-5299. Phone: (212) 207-7000. Fax: (800) 242-7737. Third edition 1981.

The Illustrated Book of Pregnancy and Childbirth. Margaret Martin. Facts on File, Inc., 460 Park Ave. S., New York, NY 10016-7382. Phone: (212) 683-2244. Fax: (212) 683-3633. 1991.

Methods of Childbirth: A Classic Work for Today's Woman. Constance A. Bean. William Morrow & Company, Inc., 1350 Ave. of the Americas, New York, NY 10019. Phone: (800) 237-0657. Revised edition 1990.

A New Life: Pregnancy, Birth and Your Child's First Year - A Comprehensive Guide. John T. Queenan, Carrie N. Queenan (eds.). Little, Brown and Co., 34 Beacon St., Boston, MA 02108. Phone: (617) 227-0730. Second edition 1992.

Open Season: A Survival Guide for Natural Childbirth in the 1990s. Nancy W. Cohen. Greenwood Publishing Group, Inc., 88 Post Rd. W., P.O. Box 5007, Westport, CT 06881. Phone: (203) 226-3571. 1991.

Understanding Pregnancy and Childbirth. Sheldon H. Cherry. Macmillan Publishing Co., 866 Third Ave., New York, NY 10011. Phone: (800) 257-5755. 1992.

TEXTBOOKS AND MONOGRAPHS

Forcep Deliveries. Dennen. F.A. Davis Co., 1915 Arch St., Philadelphia, PA 19103. Phone: (800) 523-4049. Fax: (215) 568-5065. Third editio 1989.

Instrument Assisted Vaginal Delivery. Leonard E. Laufe, Michael Berkus. McGraw-Hill, Inc., Health Professions Division, 1221 Avenue of the Americas, 28th Floor, New York, NY 10020. Phone: (212) 512-4228. 1992.

Practical Guide to High-Risk Pregnancy and Delivery. Fernando Arias. Mosby-Year Book, 11830 Westline Industrial Drive, St. Louis, MO 63146. Phone: (800) 325-4177. Fax: (314) 432-1380. Second edition 1992.

Surgical Obstetrics. Warren Plauche, John Memson, Mary Jo O'Sullivan. W.B. Saunders Co., The Curtis Center, Independence Sqare W., Philadelphia, PA 19106-3399. Phone: (215) 238-7800. 1992.

CHIROPRACTIC

See also: ALTERNATIVE MEDICINE

ABSTRACTING, INDEXING, AND CURRENT AWARENESS PUBLICATIONS

Complementary Medicine Index. Medical Information Service, British Library, Boston Spa, Wetherby, W. Yorkshire LS23 7BQ, England. Phone: 0937-546039. Fax: 0937-546236. Monthly.

Current Contents/Clinical Medicine. Institute for Scientific Information, 3501 Market St., Philadelphia, PA 19104. Phone: (800) 523-1850. Fax: (215) 386-6362. Weekly.

Index to Chiropractic Literature. Chiropractic Library Consortium, Western States Chiropractic College, 2900 N.E. 132nd Ave., Portland, OR 97230. Phone: (503) 256-3180. Annual.

Index Medicus. U.S. National Library of Medicine, 8600 Rockville Pike, Bethesda, MD 20894. Phone: (800) 638-8480. Monthly.

Science Citation Index. Institute for Scientific Information, 3501 Market St., Philadelphia, PA 19104. Phone: (800) 523-1850. Fax: (215) 386-6362. Bimonthly.

ASSOCIATIONS, PROFESSIONAL SOCIETIES, ADVOCACY AND SUPPORT GROUPS

American Black Chiropractors Association. 1918 E. Grand Blvd., St. Louis, MO 63107. Phone: (314) 531-0615.

American Chiropractic Association. 1701 Clarendon Blvd., Arlington, VA 22209. Phone: (202) 276-8800. Fax: (703) 243-2593.

American College of Chiropractic Orthopedists. 910 Grand Ave., Suite 112, San Diego, CA 92109.

Canadian Chiropractic Association. 1396 Eglinton Ave. W., Toronto, ON, Canada M6C 2E4. Phone: (416) 781-5656. Fax: (416) 781-7344.

Council on Chiropractic Education. 4401 Westown Parkway, Suite 120, West Des Moines, IA 50265. Phone: (515) 226-9001.

Foundation for Chiropractic Education and Research (FCER). 1701 Clarendon Blvd., Arlington, VA 22209. Phone: (703) 276-7445.

International Chiropractors Association (ICA). 1110 N. Glebe Rd., Ste. 1000, Arlington, VA 22201. Phone: (703) 528-5000.

CD-ROM DATABASES

SCISEARCH. Institute for Scientific Information, 3501 Market St., Philadelphia, PA 19104. Phone: (215) 386-0100. Fax: (215) 386-6362.

DIRECTORIES

American Chiropractic Association-Membership Directory. American Chiropractic Association, 1701 Clarendon Blvd., Arlington, VA 22209. Phone: (703) 276-8800. Fax: (703) 243-2593.

JOURNALS

Alternative Medicine. V.S.P. International Science Publishers, P.O. Box 346, 3700 AH, Zeist, Netherlands. Phone: 03404-51902. Fax: 03404-58620. Quarterly.

American Chiropractor. American Chiropractor Magazine, Inc., 3401 Lake Ave., Fort Wayne, IN 46805. Monthly.

American Journal of Chiropractic Medicine. Mountain Spring Press, 24W 760 Geneva Rd., Carol Stream, IL 60188.

Chiropractic. American Chiropractor Magazine, Inc., 3401 Lake Ave., Fort Wayne, IN 46805. Quarterly.

Chiropractic Sports Medicine. Williams & Wilkins, 428 E. Preston St., Baltimore, MD 21202. Phone: (800) 638-0672. Fax: (800) 447-8438. Quarterly.

Chiropractic Technique. Williams & Wilkins, 428 E. Preston St., Baltimore, MD 21202. Phone: (800) 638-0672. Fax: (800) 447-8438. Quarterly.

East West: The Journal of Natural Health and Living. East West Journal, Inc., 17 Station St., P.O. Box 1200, Brookline, MA 02146. Monthly.

European Journal of Chiropractic. Blackwell Scientific Publications, Inc., 3 Cambridge Ctr., Cambridge, MA 02142. Phone: (800) 759-6102. Quarterly.

JMPT: The Journal of Manipulative and Physiological Therapeutics. Williams & Wilkins, 428 E. Preston St., Baltimore, MD 21202. Phone: (800) 638-0672. Fax: (800) 447-8438. 9/year.

ONLINE DATABASES

EMBASE. Elsevier Science Publishing Co., Inc., P.O. Box 882, Madison Square Station, New York, NY 10159-2101. Phone: (212) 989-5800. Fax: (212) 633-3990.

MEDLINE. National Library of Medicine, 8600 Rockville Pike, Bethesda, MD 20894. Phone: (800) 638-8480.

SciSearch. Institute for Scientific Information, 3501 Market St., Philadelphia, PA 19104. Phone: (215) 386-0100. Fax: (215) 386-6362.

POPULAR WORKS AND PATIENT EDUCATION

The Backpower Program. David Imrie, Lu Barbuto. John Wiley & Sons, Inc., 605 Third Ave., New York, NY 10158-0012. Phone: (212) 850-6000. Fax: (212) 850-6088. 1990.

The Encyclopedia of Alternative Health Care. Kristin G. Olsen. Simon & Schuster, Inc., 1230 Ave. of the Americas, New York, NY 10020. Phone: (212) 698-7000. 1990.

Everybody's Guide to Chiropractic Health Care. Nathaniel Altman. Jeremy P. Tarcher, Inc., 5858 Wilshire Blvd., Suite 200, Los Angeles, CA 90036. Phone: (213) 935-9980. 1990.

RESEARCH CENTERS, INSTITUTES, CLEARINGHOUSES

Institute for Chiropractic Research. Northwestern College of Chiropractic, 2501 W. 84th St., Bloomington, MN 55431. Phone: (612) 888-4777.

TEXTBOOKS AND MONOGRAPHS

Chiropractic Management of Spine Related Disorders. Meridel Gateman. Williams & Wilkins, 428 East Preston St., Baltimore, MD 21202. Phone: (800) 638-0672. Fax: (800) 447-8438. 1990.

Chiropractic Treatment of Spinal Deformities. Donald Aspegren. Williams & Wilkins, 428 East Preston St., Baltimore, MD 21202. Phone: (800) 638-0672. Fax: (800) 447-8438. 1991.

Chiropractor's Manual of Low Back and Leg Pain. J.E. Thomas. Appleton & Lange, 25 Van Zant St., East Norwalk, CT 06855. Phone: (800) 423-1359. Fax: (203) 854-9486. 1991.

Fundamentals of Chiropractic Diagnosis and Management. Dana Lawrence (ed.). Williams & Wilkins, 428 East Preston St., Baltimore, MD 21202. Phone: (800) 638-0672. Fax: (800) 447-8438. 1990.

Ganstead's Textbook of Chiropractic. Gregory Plaugher. Williams & Wilkins, 428 East Preston St., Baltimore, MD 21202. Phone: (800) 638-0672. Fax: (800) 447-8438. 1992.

Low Back Pain: Mechanisms, Diagnosis, and Treatment. Jamel M. Cox. Williams & Wilkins, 428 East Preston St., Baltimore, MD 21202. Phone: (800) 638-0672. Fax: (800) 447-8438. 1990.

Modern Developments in the Principles and Practice of Chiropractic. Scott Haldeman. Appleton & Lange, 25 Van Zant St., East Norwalk, CT 06855. Phone: (800) 423-1359. Fax: (203) 854-9486. 1991.

CHLAMYDIA INFECTIONS

See: SEXUALLY TRANSMITTED DISEASES

CHOKING

See: EMERGENCY MEDICINE

CHOLECYSTECTOMY

See: GASTROINTESTINAL DISORDERS

CHOLERA

See: INFECTIOUS DISEASES

CHOLESTEROL

ABSTRACTING, INDEXING, AND CURRENT AWARENESS PUBLICATIONS

Current Contents/Clinical Medicine. Institute for Scientific Information, 3501 Market St., Philadelphia, PA 19104. Phone: (800) 523-1850. Fax: (215) 386-6362. Weekly.

BIBLIOGRAPHIES

Cholesterol: Cardiac Risk Assessment. National Technical Information Service, 5285 Port Royal Rd., Springfield, VA 22161. Phone: (703) 487-4650. Fax: (703) 321-8547. Jan. 1970-Apr. 1988 PB88-863691/CBY.

Cholesterol in Foods and Its Effects on Animals and Humans. National Technical Information Service, 5285 Port Royal Rd., Springfield, VA 22161. Phone: (703) 487-4650. Fax: (703) 321-8547. May 1986-Sept. 1988 PB88-870167/CBY.

JOURNALS

American Journal of Cardiology. Reed Publising USA, 249 W. 17th St., New York, NY 10011. Phone: (212) 645-0067. Fax: (212) 242-6987. 22/year.

American Journal of Clinical Nutrition. Waverly Press, 428 E. Preston St., Baltimore, MD 21202. Phone: (800) 638-0672. Fax: (800) 447-8438. Monthly.

Circulation. American Heart Association, 7320 Greenville Ave., Dallas, TX 75231-4599. Phone: (214) 706-1310. Fax: (214) 691-2704. Monthly.

Journal of Lipid Research. Federation of American Societies for Experimental Biology, 9650 Rockville Pike, Bethesda, MD 20814. Phone: (301) 530-7100.

Lipids. American Oil Chemists' Society, 1608 Broadmoor Dr., Champaign, IL 61821. Phone: (217) 359-2344.

POPULAR WORKS AND PATIENT EDUCATION

The Eight Week Cholesterol Cure: How to Lower Your Cholesterol by Up to 40 Percent without Drugs or Deprivation. Robert E. Kowalski. HarperCollins Publishers, Inc., 10 E. 53rd St., New York, NY 10022-5299. Phone: (212) 207-7000. Fax: (800) 242-7737.

Heart Failure. Thomas J. Moore. Simon & Schuster, 1230 Ave. of the Americas, New York, NY 10020. Phone: (800) 223-2348. Fax: (800) 284-0735.

RESEARCH CENTERS, INSTITUTES, CLEARINGHOUSES

Arizona Heart Institute. 2632 N. 20th St., Phoenix, AZ 85006. Phone: (602) 266-2200.

Arteriosclerosis Research Center. Wake Forest University. Dept. of Comparative Medicine, 300 S. Hawthorne Rd., Winston-Salem, NC 27103. Phone: (919) 764-3600. Fax: (919) 764-5818.

Biochemical Epidemiology and Lipid Research Core Laboratory. Stadium Gate 27, 611 Beacon St. S.E., Minneapolis, MN 55455. Phone: (612) 624-2183.

Cholesterol Research Center. University of California, Berkeley. 3031 Telegraph Rd., Berkeley, CA 94705. Phone: (415) 540-1554.

Department of Biochemistry. L-11, The Cleveland Clinic Foundation, 9500 Euclid Ave., Cleveland, OH 44106. Phone: (216) 444-5744.

Lipid Laboratory. University of Kansas. Medical Center, 3800 Cambridge, Kansas City, KS 66103. Phone: (913) 588-6025.

Lipid Research Center. 4566 Scott Ave., Box 8046, Washington University School of Medicine, St. Louis, MO 63110. Phone: (314) 362-3522.

Lipid Research Clinic. University of Iowa. Dept. of Internal Medicine, Westlawn S-219, Iowa City, IA 52242. Phone: (319) 335-8201.

National Heart, Lung, and Blood Institute Education Programs Information Center. 4733 Bethesda Ave., Ste. 530, Bethesda, MD 20814. Phone: (301) 951-3260.

Northwest Lipid Research Center. Room 732, Harborview Hall, 326 Ninth Ave., Seattle, WA 98104. Phone: (206) 223-3236.

Specialized Center of Research in Arteriosclerosis. University of California, San Diego. Dept. of Medicine, M-0613-D, La Jolla, CA 92093. Phone: (619) 534-0569. Fax: (619) 546-9828.

TEXTBOOKS AND MONOGRAPHS

Disorders of Lipid Metabolism. Guido V. Marinetti. Plenum Publishing Co., 233 Spring St., New York, NY 10013-1578. Phone: (212) 620-8000. Fax: (212) 463-0742. 1990.

CHRONIC FATIGUE SYNDROME

ABSTRACTING, INDEXING, AND CURRENT AWARENESS PUBLICATIONS

Current Contents/Clinical Medicine. Institute for Scientific Information, 3501 Market St., Philadelphia, PA 19104. Phone: (800) 523-1850. Fax: (215) 386-6362. Weekly.

Index Medicus. U.S. National Library of Medicine, 8600 Rockville Pike, Bethesda, MD 20894. Phone: (800) 638-8480. Monthly.

Research Alert: Chronic Fatigue Syndrome. Institute for Scientific Information, 3501 Market St., Philadelphia, PA 19104. Phone: (800) 523-1850. Fax: (215) 386-6362. Weekly.

Science Citation Index. Institute for Scientific Information, 3501 Market St., Philadelphia, PA 19104. Phone: (800) 523-1850. Fax: (215) 386-6362. Bimonthly.

ASSOCIATIONS, PROFESSIONAL SOCIETIES, ADVOCACY AND SUPPORT GROUPS

Chronic Fatigue and Immune Dysfunction Association. P.O. Box 220398, Charlotte, NC 28222-0398. Phone: (704) 362-2343.

Chronic Fatigue Syndrome Society, International (CFSS). P.O. Box 230108, Portland, OR 97223. Phone: (503) 684-5261.

National Chronic Fatigue Syndrome Association. 3521 Broadway, Ste. 222, Kansas City, MO 64111. Phone: (816) 931-4777.

United CFS/CFIDS/CEBV Federation. 2141 W. Fairlane Ave., Milwaukee, WI 53209. Phone: (414) 351-5837.

CD-ROM DATABASES

SCISEARCH. Institute for Scientific Information, 3501 Market St., Philadelphia, PA 19104. Phone: (215) 386-0100. Fax: (215) 386-6362.

JOURNALS

Annals of Internal Medicine. American College of Physicians, Independence Mall W., Sixth St. at Race, Philadelphia, PA 19106-1572. Phone: (800) 523-1546. Fax: (215) 351-2594. Semimonthly.

Journal of the Chronic Fatigue Syndromes. Haworth Press, 10 Alice Street, Binghamton, NY 13904-1580. Phone: (800) 342-9678. Fax: (607) 722-1424. Quarterly.

Journal of Infectious Diseases. University of Chicago Press, P.O. Box 37005, Chicago, IL 60637. Phone: (312) 753-3347. Fax: (312) 753-0811. Monthly.

The New England Journal of Medicine. Massachusetts Medical Society, 1440 Main St., Waltham, MA 02154-1649. Phone: (617) 893-3800. Fax: (617) 893-0413. Weekly.

ONLINE DATABASES

EMBASE. Elsevier Science Publishing Co., Inc., P.O. Box 882, Madison Square Station, New York, NY 10159-2101. Phone: (212) 989-5800. Fax: (212) 633-3990.

MEDLINE. National Library of Medicine, 8600 Rockville Pike, Bethesda, MD 20894. Phone: (800) 638-8480.

SciSearch. Institute for Scientific Information, 3501 Market St., Philadelphia, PA 19104. Phone: (215) 386-0100. Fax: (215) 386-6362.

POPULAR WORKS AND PATIENT EDUCATION

Chronic Fatigue Syndrome: A Victim's Guide to Understanding, Treating, and Coping with the Debilitating Illness. E.C. Fisher. Warner Books, Inc., 666 Fifth Ave., 9th Floor, New York, NY 10103. Phone: (212) 484-2900. 1989.

Chronic Fatigue Syndrome: The Hidden Epidemic. Jesse Stoff, Charles R. Pellegrino. HarperCollins Pubs., Inc., 10 E. 53rd St., New York, NY 10022-5299. Phone: (212) 207-7000. Revised edition 1992.

Hope and Help for Chronic Fatigue Syndrome. Karyn Feiden. Simon & Schuster, Inc., 1230 Ave. of the Americas, New York, NY 10020. Phone: (212) 698-7000. 1992.

RESEARCH CENTERS, INSTITUTES, CLEARINGHOUSES

CFS Research Foundation. P.O. Box 6747 Cherry Creek, Denver, CO 80206.

Chronic Fatigue and Immune Disorder Center. 1200 Bin 2, Suite 170, Houston, TX 77004. Phone: (713) 529-5454.

Chronic Fatigue Syndrome Clinic of Miriam Hospital. 164 Summit Ave., Providence, RI 02906. Phone: (401) 331-8500.

Chronic Fatigue Syndrome Information Institute. 5840 Cameron Run Terrace #1413, Alexandria, VA 22303.

CIRRHOSIS

See: LIVER DISEASES

CLASSIFICATION OF DISEASES

See: DISEASE CLASSIFICATION

CLEFT LIP AND CLEFT PALATE

See: BIRTH DEFECTS

CLINICAL PHARMACOLOGY

ABSTRACTING, INDEXING, AND CURRENT AWARENESS PUBLICATIONS

BIOSIS/CAS Selects: Drug Interactions. BIOSIS, 2100 Arch St., Philadelphia, PA 19103-1399. Phone: (215) 587-4800. Fax: (215) 587-2016. Biweekly.

CA Selects: Drug Delivery Systems & Dosage Forms. Chemical Abstracts Service, 2540 Olentangy River Road, P.O. Box 3012, Columbus, OH 43210-0012. Phone: (800) 848-6538. Biweekly.

Current Contents/Life Sciences. Institute for Scientific Information, 3501 Market St., Philadelphia, PA 19104. Phone: (215) 386-0100. Fax: (215) 386-6362.

Excerpta Medica. Section 30: Clinical and Experimental Pharmacology. Elsevier Science Publishing Co., Inc., P.O. Box 882, Madison Square Station, New York, NY 10159-2101. Phone: (212) 989-5800. Fax: (212) 633-3990. 32/year.

Excerpta Medica. Section 52: Toxicology. Elsevier Science Publishing Co., Inc., P.O. Box 882, Madison Square Station, New York, NY 10159-2101. Phone: (212) 989-5800. Fax: (212) 633-3990. 20/year.

Index Medicus. U.S. National Library of Medicine, 8600 Rockville Pike, Bethesda, MD 20894. Phone: (800) 638-8480. Monthly.

International Pharmaceutical Abstracts. American Society of Hospital Pharmacists, 4630 Montgomery Ave., Bethesda, MD 20814. Phone: (301) 657-3000. Fax: (301) 657-1641. Semimonthly.

PharmIndex. Skyline Publishers, Inc., P.O. Box 1029, University Station, Portland, OR 97207. Phone: (503) 228-6568. Monthly.

Science Citation Index. Institute for Scientific Information, 3501 Market St., Philadelphia, PA 19104. Phone: (800) 523-1850. Fax: (215) 386-6362. Bimonthly.

ANNUALS AND REVIEWS

Advances in Pharmacology. Academic Press, Inc., 1250 Sixth Ave., San Diego, CA 92101-4311. Phone: (619) 699-6345. Fax: (619) 699-6715. Irregular.

Annual Review of Pharmacology and Toxicology. Annual Reviews Inc., 4139 El Camino Way, P.O. Box 10139, Palo Alto, CA 94303-0897. Phone: (415) 493-4400. Fax: (415) 855-9815. Annual.

Year Book of Drug Therapy. Mosby-Year Book, 11830 Westline Industrial Drive, St. Louis, MO 63146. Phone: (800) 325-4177. Fax: (314) 432-1380. Annual.

Year Book of Pharmacology. CRC Press, Inc., 2000 Corporate Blvd. N.W., Boca Raton, FL 33431. Phone: (407) 994-0555. Fax: (407) 997-0949. Annual.

ASSOCIATIONS, PROFESSIONAL SOCIETIES, ADVOCACY AND SUPPORT GROUPS

American College of Clinical Pharmacology. 175 Stafford Ave., Suite 1, Wayne, PA 19087. Phone: (215) 687-7711.

American Society for Clinical Pharmacology and Therapeutics. 1718 Gallagher Rd., Norristown, PA 19401. Phone: (215) 825-3838.

BIBLIOGRAPHIES

Lecture Notes on Clinical Pharmacology. John L. Reid. Blackwell Scientific Publications, Inc., 3 Cambridge Center, Cambridge, MA 02142. Phone: (800) 759-6102. 1989.

CD-ROM DATABASES

Excerpta Medica CD: Drugs & Pharmacology. SilverPlatter Information, Inc., River Ridge Office Park, 100 River Ridge Rd., Norwood, MA 02062. Phone: (617) 769-2599. Fax: (617) 769-8763. Quarterly.

International Pharmaceutical Abstracts. SilverPlatter Information, Inc., River Ridge Office Park, 100 River Ridge Rd., Norwood, MA 02062. Phone: (617) 769-2599. Fax: (617) 769-8763. Quarterly.

SCISEARCH. Institute for Scientific Information, 3501 Market St., Philadelphia, PA 19104. Phone: (215) 386-0100. Fax: (215) 386-6362.

SEDBASE (Side Effects of Drugs). SilverPlatter Information, Inc., River Ridge Office Park, 100 River Ridge Rd., Norwood, MA 02062. Phone: (617) 769-2599. Fax: (617) 769-8763. Semiannual.

ENCYCLOPEDIAS, DICTIONARIES, WORD BOOKS

Merck Index: An Encyclopedia of Chemicals and Drugs. Merck & Co., Inc., P.O. Box 2000, Rahway, NJ 07065. Phone: (201) 855-4558. Irregular.

JOURNALS

Clinical Neuropharmacology. Raven Press, 1185 Avenue of the Americas, New York, NY 10036. Phone: (212) 930-9500. Fax: (212) 869-3495. Bimonthly.

Journal of Clinical Pharmacology. J.B. Lippincott Co., 227 E. Washington Square, Philadelphia, PA 19106-3780. Phone: (215) 238-4200. Fax: (215) 238-4227.

Journal of Pharmaceutical Sciences. American Pharmaceutical Association, 2215 Constitution Ave. NW, Washington, DC 200037. Phone: (800) 237-2742. Fax: (202) 783-2351. Monthly.

Pharmaceutical Physician. British Association of Pharmaceutical Physicians, 1 Wimpole St., London W1M 8AE, England. Phone: (44) 71 491 8610. Fax: (44) 71 499 2405. Bimonthly.

ONLINE DATABASES

EMBASE. Elsevier Science Publishing Co., Inc., P.O. Box 882, Madison Square Station, New York, NY 10159-2101. Phone: (212) 989-5800. Fax: (212) 633-3990.

International Pharmaceutical Abstracts. American Society of Hospital Pharmacists, 4630 Montgomery Ave., Bethesda, MD 20814. Phone: (301) 657-3000. Fax: (301) 657-1641. Monthly.

MEDLINE. National Library of Medicine, 8600 Rockville Pike, Bethesda, MD 20894. Phone: (800) 638-8480.

Pharmline. Regional Drug Information Service, The London Hospital, Whitechapel Rd., London E1 1BB, England. Phone: 071-377 7489. Weekly.

SciSearch. Institute for Scientific Information, 3501 Market St., Philadelphia, PA 19104. Phone: (215) 386-0100. Fax: (215) 386-6362.

RESEARCH CENTERS, INSTITUTES, CLEARINGHOUSES

Center for Biomedical Research. University of Kansas. Smissman Research Laboratories, 2099 Constant Ave., Lawrence, KS 66046. Phone: (913) 864-5140.

Department of Pharmacology and Therapeutics. McGill University. 3655 Rue Drummond, Montreal, PQ, Canada H3G 1Y6. Phone: (514) 398-3621. Fax: (514) 398-6690.

STANDARDS AND STATISTICS SOURCES

Clinical Pharmacology and Therapeutics. Mosby-Year Book, 11830 Westline Industrial Drive, St. Louis, MO 63146. Phone: (800) 325-4177. Fax: (314) 432-1380.

TEXTBOOKS AND MONOGRAPHS

Basic and Clinical Pharmacology. Katzung. Appleton & Lange, 25 Van Zant St., East Norwalk, CT 06855. Phone: (800) 423-1359. Fax: (203) 854-9486. Fifth edition 1992.

Clinical Pharmacology and Nursing. Charold L. Baer, Bradley R. Williams. Springhouse Publishing Co., 1111 Bethlehem Pike, Spring House, PA 19477. Phone: (800) 331-3170. Fax: (215) 646-8716. Second edition 1992.

Essentials of Medical Pharmacology. Kalant. Mosby-Year Book, 11830 Westline Industrial Drive, St. Louis, MO 63146. Phone: (800) 325-4177. Fax: (314) 432-1380. 1991.

Goodman and Gilman's The Pharmacological Basis of Therapeutics. Alfred Goodman Gilman, Theodore W. Rall, Alan S. Nies, et. al.. McGraw-Hill, Inc., 1221 Avenue of the Americas, 28th Floor, New York, NY 10020. Phone: (212) 512-4228. Eighth edition 1990.

Melmon and Morrelli's Clinical Pharmacology: Basic Principles of Therapeutics. Kenneth L. Melmon, Howard F. Morrelli, Brian B. Hoffman. McGraw-Hill, Inc., 11 West 19th St., New York, NY 10011. Phone: (212) 337-5001. Fax: (212) 337-4092. Third edition 1992.

Therapeutic Drugs. Sir Colin Dollery (ed.). Churchill Livingstone Inc., 650 Avenue of the Americas, New York, NY 10011. Phone: (212) 819-5400. Fax: (212) 302-6598. Two volumes 1991.

CLUSTER HEADACHE

See: HEADACHE

COCAINE

See also: DRUG ABUSE

ABSTRACTING, INDEXING, AND CURRENT AWARENESS PUBLICATIONS

Excerpta Medica. Section 40: Drug Dependence, Alcohol Abuse and Alcoholism. Elsevier Science Publishing Co., Inc., P.O. Box 882, Madison Square Station, New York, NY 10159-2101. Phone: (212) 989-5800. Fax: (212) 633-3990. 6/year.

Index Medicus. U.S. National Library of Medicine, 8600 Rockville Pike, Bethesda, MD 20894. Phone: (800) 638-8480. Monthly.

Psychological Abstracts. American Psychological Association, 1200 17th St. NW, Washington, DC 20036. Phone: (202) 955-7600. Monthly.

Research Alert: Drug Addiction & Abuse. Institute for Scientific Information, 3501 Market St., Philadelphia, PA 19104. Phone: (800) 523-1850. Fax: (215) 386-6362. Weekly.

Science Citation Index. Institute for Scientific Information, 3501 Market St., Philadelphia, PA 19104. Phone: (800) 523-1850. Fax: (215) 386-6362. Bimonthly.

ASSOCIATIONS, PROFESSIONAL SOCIETIES, ADVOCACY AND SUPPORT GROUPS

American Council for Drug Education. 204 Monroe St., Suite 110, Rockville, MD 20850. Phone: (301) 294-0600.

Cocaine Anonymous. 6125 Washington Blvd., Ste. 202, Culver City, CA 90232. Phone: (213) 839-1141.

Narcotics Anonymous. World Service Office, P.O. Box 9999, Van Nuys, CA 91409. Phone: (818) 780-3951.

BIBLIOGRAPHIES

Cocaine: Properties, Effects, and Modes of Actions. National Technical Information Service, 5285 Port Royal Rd., Springfield, VA 22161. Phone: (703) 487-4650. Fax: (703) 321-8547. Jan. 1970-Nov. 1988.

Cocaine: Toxicity, Abuse, and Treatment. National Technical Information Service, 5285 Port Royal Rd., Springfield, VA 22161. Phone: (703) 487-4650. Fax: (703) 321-8547. Jan. 1978-Nov. 1988 PB89-852065/CBY.

Drug Abuse Bibliography. Whitston Publishing Co., P.O. Box 958., Troy, NY 12181. Phone: (518) 283-4363. Annual.

CD-ROM DATABASES

PsycLit. SilverPlatter Information, Inc., River Ridge Office Park, 100 River Ridge Rd., Norwood, MA 02062. Phone: (617) 769-2599. Fax: (617) 769-8763. Quarterly.

SCISEARCH. Institute for Scientific Information, 3501 Market St., Philadelphia, PA 19104. Phone: (215) 386-0100. Fax: (215) 386-6362.

DIRECTORIES

Drug, Alcohol, and Other Addictions: A Directory of Treatment Centers and Prevention Programs Nationwide. Oryx Press, 4041 N. Central, Suite 700, Phoenix, AZ 85012. Phone: (800) 279-ORYX. Fax: (800) 279-4663.

ENCYCLOPEDIAS, DICTIONARIES, WORD BOOKS

Encyclopedia of Drug Abuse. Glen Evans, Robert O'Brien, Sidney Cohen, James Fine. Facts on File, Inc., 460 Park Ave. S., New York, NY 10016-7382. Phone: (212) 683-2244. Fax: (212) 683-3633. Third edition 1992.

HANDBOOKS, GUIDES, MANUALS, ATLASES

A Handbook on Drug and Alcohol Abuse. Gail Winger, Frederick G. Hofman, James H. Woods. Oxford University Press, 200 Madison Ave., New York, NY 10016. Phone: (212) 679-7300. Third edition 1992.

JOURNALS

Journal of Substance Abuse Treatment. Pergamon Press, 660 White Plains Rd., Tarrytown, NY 10591-5153. Phone: (914) 592-7700. Fax: (914) 592-3625. 6/year.

ONLINE DATABASES

Drug and Alcohol Abuse Prevention Centers. Oryx Press, 4041 N. Central, Suite 700, Phoenix, AZ 85012. Phone: (800) 279-6799. Fax: (800) 279-4663.

EMBASE. Elsevier Science Publishing Co., Inc., P.O. Box 882, Madison Square Station, New York, NY 10159-2101. Phone: (212) 989-5800. Fax: (212) 633-3990.

MEDLINE. National Library of Medicine, 8600 Rockville Pike, Bethesda, MD 20894. Phone: (800) 638-8480.

PsycInfo. SilverPlatter Information, Inc., River Ridge Office Park, 100 River Ridge Rd., Norwood, MA 02062. Phone: (617) 769-2599. Fax: (617) 769-8763. Quarterly.

SciSearch. Institute for Scientific Information, 3501 Market St., Philadelphia, PA 19104. Phone: (215) 386-0100. Fax: (215) 386-6362.

POPULAR WORKS AND PATIENT EDUCATION

The 800-Cocaine Book of Drug and Alcohol Recovery. James Cocores. Random House, Inc., 201 E. 50th St., New York, NY 10022. Phone: (800) 726-0600. 1990.

RESEARCH CENTERS, INSTITUTES, CLEARINGHOUSES

Hazelden Foundation. Box 176, Center City, MN 55012-0176. Phone: (800) 328-9000.

National Clearinghouse for Alcohol and Drug Information (NCADI). P.O. Box 2345, Rockville, MD 20852. Phone: (301) 468-2600.

TEXTBOOKS AND MONOGRAPHS

Cocaine, AIDS and Intravenous Drug Use. Samuel R. Friedman, Douglas S. Lipton (eds.). Haworth Press, 10 Alice Street, Binghamton, NY 13904-1580. Phone: (800) 3HA-WORTH. Fax: (607) 722-1424. 1991.

Cocaine: Pharmacology, Physiology and Clinical Strategies. Joan M. Lakoski, Matthew P. Galloway, Francis J. White. CRC Press, Inc., 2000 Corporate Blvd. N.W., Boca Raton, FL 33431. Phone: (407) 994-0555. Fax: (407) 997-0949. 1992.

Cocaine Solutions: Help for Cocaine Abusers and Their Families. Jennifer Rice-Licare, Katharine Delaney-

McLoughlin. Haworth Press, Inc., 10 Alice St., Binghamton, NY 13904-1580. Phone: (800) 342-9678. 1990.

Substance Abuse: A Comprehensive Textbook. Hoyce H. Lowinson, Pedro Ruiz, Robert B. Millman (eds.). Williams & Wilkins, 428 East Preston St., Baltimore, MD 21202. Phone: (800) 638-0672. Fax: (800) 447-8438. Second edition 1992.

COLITIS

See: GASTROINTESTINAL DISORDERS

COLONOSCOPY

See: ENDOSCOPY

COLOR BLINDNESS

See: VISION DISORDERS

COLORECTAL CANCER

See also: CANCER

ABSTRACTING, INDEXING, AND CURRENT AWARENESS PUBLICATIONS

Current Contents/Clinical Medicine. Institute for Scientific Information, 3501 Market St., Philadelphia, PA 19104. Phone: (800) 523-1850. Fax: (215) 386-6362. Weekly.

Excerpta Medica. Section 16: Cancer. Elsevier Science Publishing Co., Inc., P.O. Box 882, Madison Square Station, New York, NY 10159-2101. Phone: (212) 989-5800. Fax: (212) 633-3990. 32/year.

Excerpta Medica. Section 48: Gastroenterology. Elsevier Science Publishing Co., Inc., P.O. Box 882, Madison Square Station, New York, NY 10159-2101. Phone: (212) 989-5800. Fax: (212) 633-3990. 20/year.

ICRDB Cancergram: Colorectal Cancer--Diagnosis, Treatment. U.S. Government Printing Office, Superintendent of Documents, P.O. Box 371954, Pittsburgh, PA 15250-7954. Phone: (202) 783-3238. Fax: (202) 512-2250. Monthly.

Index Medicus. U.S. National Library of Medicine, 8600 Rockville Pike, Bethesda, MD 20894. Phone: (800) 638-8480. Monthly.

Science Citation Index. Institute for Scientific Information, 3501 Market St., Philadelphia, PA 19104. Phone: (800) 523-1850. Fax: (215) 386-6362. Bimonthly.

ANNUALS AND REVIEWS

Advances in Cancer Research. Academic Press, Inc., 1250 Sixth Ave., San Diego, CA 92101-4311. Phone: (619) 699-6345. Fax: (619) 699-6715. Irregular.

Critical Reviews in Oncogenesis. CRC Press, Inc., 2000 Corporate Blvd. N.W., Boca Raton, FL 33431. Phone: (407) 994-0555. Fax: (407) 997-0949. 6/year.

Critical Reviews in Oncology/Hematology. Elsevier Science Publishing Co., Inc., P.O. Box 882, Madison Square Station, New York, NY 10159-2101. Phone: (212) 989-5800. Fax: (212) 633-3990. Quarterly.

Current Opinion in Oncology. Current Science Ltd., 20 N. Third St., Philadelphia, PA 19106-2199. Phone: (800) 552-5866. Fax: (215) 574-2270. Bimonthly.

Current Problems in Cancer. Mosby-Year Book, 11830 Westline Industrial Drive, St. Louis, MO 63146. Phone: (800) 325-4177. Fax: (314) 432-1380. Bimonthly.

Important Advances in Oncology. Vincent T. Devita, Samuel Hellman, Steven A. Rosenberg, et. al.. J.B. Lippincott Co., 227 East Washington Square, Philadelphia, PA 19106-3780. Phone: (215) 238-4200. Fax: (215) 238-4227. Annual.

In Development New Medicines for Older Americans. 1991 Annual Survey. More Medicines in Testing for Cancer Than for Any Other Disease of Aging. Pharmaceutical Manufacturers Association, 1100 15th St. N.W., Washington, DC 20005. Phone: (202) 835-3400. 1991.

Progress in Cancer Research and Therapy. Raven Press, 1185 Avenue of the Americas, New York, NY 10036. Phone: (212) 930-9500. Fax: (212) 869-3495. Irregular.

Seminars in Oncology. W.B. Saunders Co., The Curtis Center, Independence Square W., Philadelphia, PA 19106-3399. Phone: (215) 238-7800. Bimonthly.

Seminars in Surgical Oncology. John Wiley & Sons, Inc., 605 Third Ave., New York, NY 10158-0012. Phone: (212) 850-6000. Fax: (212) 850-6088. Quarterly.

Year Book of Oncology. Mosby-Year Book, 11830 Westline Industrial Drive, St. Louis, MO 63146. Phone: (800) 325-4177. Fax: (314) 432-1380. Annual.

ASSOCIATIONS, PROFESSIONAL SOCIETIES, ADVOCACY AND SUPPORT GROUPS

American Cancer Society (ACS). 1599 Clifton Rd. N.E., Atlanta, GA 30329. Phone: (404) 320-3333.

American Gastroenterological Association (AGA). 6900 Grove Rd., Thorofare, NJ 08086. Phone: (609) 848-9218. Fax: (609) 853-5991.

American Society of Colon and Rectal Surgeons (ASCRS). 615 Griswold, No. 1717, Detroit, MI 48226. Phone: (313) 961-7880.

United Ostomy Association (UOA). 36 Executive Park, Ste. 120, Irvine, CA 92714. Phone: (714) 660-8624. Fax: (714) 660-9262.

BIBLIOGRAPHIES

Oncology Overview: Management of Colorectal Neoplasms. Daniel Haller (ed.). U.S. Government Printing Office, Superintendent of Documents, P.O. Box 371954, Pittsburgh, PA 15250-7954. Phone: (202) 783-3238. Fax: (202) 512-2250. 1990.

CD-ROM DATABASES

Cancer-CD. SilverPlatter Information, Inc., River Ridge Office Park, 100 River Ridge Rd., Norwood, MA 02062. Phone: (617) 769-2599. Fax: (617) 769-8763. Quarterly.

Cancer on Disc. CMC ReSearch, Inc., 7150 S.W. Hampton, Suite C-120, Portland, OR 97223. Phone: (800) 262-7668. Fax: (503) 639-1796. Annual.

Cancerlit. Aries Systems Corporation, One Dundee Park, Andover, MA 01810. Phone: (508) 475-7200. Fax: (508) 474-8860. Quarterly.

Cancerlit CD-ROM. Cambridge Scientific Abstracts, 7200 Wisconsin Ave., Bethesda, MD 20814-4823. Phone: (800) 843-7751. Fax: (301) 961-6720. Quarterly.

OncoDisc. J.B. Lippincott Co., 227 East Washington Square, Philadelphia, PA 19106-3780. Phone: (215) 238-4200. Fax: (215) 238-4227. Bimonthly.

Physician's Data Query (PDQ). Cambridge Scientific Abstracts, 7200 Wisconsin Ave., Bethesda, MD 20814-4823. Phone: (800) 843-7751. Fax: (301) 961-6720. Quarterly.

SCISEARCH. Institute for Scientific Information, 3501 Market St., Philadelphia, PA 19104. Phone: (215) 386-0100. Fax: (215) 386-6362.

Year Books on Disc. CMC ReSearch, Inc., 7150 S.W. Hampton, Suite C-120, Portland, OR 97223. Phone: (800) 262-7668. Fax: (503) 639-1796. Annual includes Year Books of Cardiology, Dermatology, Diagnostic Radiology, Drug Therapy, Emergency Medicine, Family Practice, Medicine, Neurology and Neurosurgery, Obstetrics and Gynecology, Oncology, Pediatrics, and Psychiatry and Applied Mental Health.

ENCYCLOPEDIAS, DICTIONARIES, WORD BOOKS

Oncology Words. Stedman. Williams & Wilkins, 428 East Preston St., Baltimore, MD 21202. Phone: (800) 638-0672. Fax: (800) 447-8438. 1992.

JOURNALS

American Journal of Clinical Oncology. Raven Press, 1185 Ave. of the Americas, New York, NY 10036. Phone: (212) 930-9500. Fax: (212) 869-3495. Bimonthly.

CA - A Cancer Journal for Clinicians. J.B. Lippincott Co., 227 E. Washington Square, Philadelphia, PA 19106-3780. Phone: (215) 238-4200. Fax: (215) 238-4227. Bimonthly.

Cancer. J.B. Lippincott Co., 227 East Washington Square, Philadelphia, PA 19106-3780. Phone: (215) 238-4200. Fax: (215) 238-4227. Semimonthly.

Cancer Causes and Control. Rapid Communications of Oxford Ltd., The Old Malthouse, Paradise St., Oxford OX1 1LD, England. Phone: 44-865-790447. Fax: 44-865-244012. 6/year.

Diseases of the Colon and Rectum. Williams & Wilkins, 428 E. Preston St., Baltimore, MD 21202. Phone: (800) 638-0672. Fax: (800) 447-8438. Monthly.

Gastroenterology. W.B. Saunders Co., The Curtis Center, Independence Sqare W., Philadelphia, PA 19106-3399. Phone: (215) 238-7800.

International Journal of Cancer. John Wiley & Sons, Inc., 605 Third Ave., New York, NY 10158-0012. Phone: (212) 850-6000. Fax: (212) 850-6088. 18/year.

International Journal of Colorectal Disease. Springer-Verlag New York Inc., 175 Fifth Ave., New York, NY 10010. Phone: (212) 460-1500. Fax: (212) 473-6272. 4/year.

Journal of Clinical Gastroenterology. Raven Press, 1185 Avenue of the Americas, New York, NY 10036. Phone: (212) 930-9500. Fax: (212) 869-3495. Bimonthly.

Journal of Clinical Oncology. W.B. Saunders Co., The Curtis Center, Independence Square W., Philadelphia, PA 19106-3399. Phone: (215) 238-7800. Monthly.

Journal of the National Cancer Institute. Superintendent of Documents, P.O. Box 371954, Pittsburgh, PA 15250-7954. Fax: (202) 512-2233. Semimonthly.

National Cancer Institute. Journal. U.S. National Cancer Institute, 9030 Old Georgetown Rd., Bldg. 82, Room 103, Bethesda, MD 20892. Phone: (301) 496-7186. Monthly.

ONLINE DATABASES

Cancer Weekly. CDC AIDS Weekly/NCI Cancer Weekly, 206 Rogers St. NE, Suite 104, P.O. Box 5528, Atlanta, GA 30317. Phone: (404) 377-8895. Weekly.

Clinical Protocols. U.S. National Cancer Institute, International Cancer Information Center, Building 82, Room 102, Bethesda, MD 20892. Phone: (301) 496-7403. Fax: (301) 480-8105.

EMBASE. Elsevier Science Publishing Co., Inc., P.O. Box 882, Madison Square Station, New York, NY 10159-2101. Phone: (212) 989-5800. Fax: (212) 633-3990.

MEDLINE. National Library of Medicine, 8600 Rockville Pike, Bethesda, MD 20894. Phone: (800) 638-8480.

Physician Data Query (PDQ) Cancer Information File. U.S. National Cancer Institute, International Cancer Information Center, Building 82, Room 102, Bethesda, MD 20892. Phone: (301) 496-7403. Fax: (301) 480-8105. Monthly.

Physician Data Query (PDQ) Directory File. U.S. National Cancer Institute, International Cancer Information Center, Building 82, Room 102, Bethesda, MD 20892. Phone: (301) 496-7403. Fax: (301) 480-8105. Monthly.

Physician Data Query (PDQ) Protocol File. U.S. National Cancer Institute, International Cancer Information Center, Building 82, Room 102, Bethesda, MD 20892. Phone: (301) 496-7403. Fax: (301) 480-8105. Monthly.

SciSearch. Institute for Scientific Information, 3501 Market St., Philadelphia, PA 19104. Phone: (215) 386-0100. Fax: (215) 386-6362.

POPULAR WORKS AND PATIENT EDUCATION

Cancervive: The Challenge of Life After Cancer. Susan Nessim, Judith Ellis. Houghton Mifflin Co., 1 Beacon St., Boston, MA 02108. Phone: (800) 225-3362. 1991.

Everyone's Guide to Cancer Therapy: How Cancer is Diagnosed, Treated, and Managed on a Day to Day Basis. Malin Dollinger, Ernest H. Rosenbaum, Greg Cable. Andrews & McMeel, 4900 Main St., Kansas City, MO 64112. Phone: (800) 826-4216. 1991.

If It Runs in Your Family: Colorectal Cancer, Reducing Your Risk. Norman Sohn. Bantam Books, Inc., 666 Fifth Ave., New York, NY 10103. Phone: (800) 223-6834. 1992.

RESEARCH CENTERS, INSTITUTES, CLEARINGHOUSES

Cancer Information Service (CIS). Office of Cancer Communications, National Cancer Institute, Bldg. 31, Rm. 10A24, 9000 Rockville Pike, Bethesda, MD 20892. Phone: (800) 4CA-NCER.

National Surgical Adjuvant Breast and Bowel Project. University of Pittsburgh, Scaife Hall, Room 914, Pittsburgh, PA 15261. Phone: (412) 648-9720. Fax: (412) 648-1912.

STANDARDS AND STATISTICS SOURCES

Adjuvant Therapy for Patients with Colon and Rectum Cancer. Consensus Statement. NIH Consensus Development Conference. April 16-18, 1990. National Institutes of Health, Office of Medical Applications of Research, Federal Bldg., Rm. 618, Bethesda, MD 20892. 1990.

TEXTBOOKS AND MONOGRAPHS

Adenomatous Polyps of the Colon. R. Lev. Springer-Verlag New York Inc., 175 Fifth Ave., New York, NY 10010. Phone: (212) 460-1500. Fax: (212) 473-6272. 1989.

Cancer Medicine. James F. Holland, Emil Frei, Robert C. Bast Jr., and others. Williams & Wilkins, 428 East Preston St., Baltimore, MD 21202. Phone: (800) 638-0672. Fax: (800) 447-8438. Third edition 1992.

Cancer: Principles and Practice of Oncology. Vincent T. DeVita. J.B. Lippincott Co., 227 E. Washington Square, Philadelphia, PA 19106-3780. Phone: (215) 238-4200. Fax: (215) 238-4227. 1989 3rd edtion.

Cancer Treatment. Charles M. Haskell. W.B. Saunders Co., The Curtis Center, Independence Square W., Philadelphia, PA 19106-3399. Phone: (215) 238-7800. Third edition 1990.

Causation & Prevention of Colorectal Cancer. J. Faivre, M.J. Hill. Elsevier Science Publishers, P.O. Box 882, Madison Square Station, New York, NY 10159-2101. Phone: (212) 633-3950. Fax: (212) 633-3990. 1987.

Cell & Molecular Biology of Colon Cancer. Leonard H. Augenlicht (ed.). CRC Press, Inc., 2000 Corporate Blvd. N.W., Boca Raton, FL 33431. Phone: (407) 994-0555. Fax: (407) 997-0949. 1989.

Colon and Rectal Surgery. Marvin L. Corman. J.B. Lippincott Co., 227 East Washington Square, Philadelphia, PA 19106-3780. Phone: (215) 238-4200. Fax: (215) 238-4227. Third edition 1992.

Colorectal Cancer. H.K. Seitz, and others (eds.). Springer-Verlag New York Inc., 175 Fifth Ave., New York, NY 10010. Phone: (212) 460-1500. Fax: (212) 473-6272. 1989.

Current Therapy in Colon and Rectal Surgery. Victor W. Fazio. Mosby-Year Book, 11830 Westline Industrial Drive, St. Louis, MO 63146. Phone: (800) 325-4177. Fax: (314) 432-1380. 1990.

Flexible Sigmoidoscopy: Techniques and Utilization. Melvin Schapiro, Glen A. Lehman (eds.). Williams & Wilkins, 428 E. Preston St., Baltimore, MD 21202. Phone: (800) 638-0672. Fax: (800) 447-8438. 1990.

High Risk Pregnancy. A.A. Calder, W. Dunlop. Butterworth-Heinemann, 80 Montvale Ave., Stoneham, MA 02180. Phone: (617) 438-8464. Fax: (617) 279-4851. 1991.

Ostomy Care and the Cancer Patient. Dorothy B. Smith, Douglas E. Johnson. W.B. Saunders Co., The Curtis Center, Independence Square W., Philadelphia, PA 19106-3399. Phone: (215) 238-7800. 1986.

Pathology of the Colon, Small Intestine, and Anus. Norris. Churchill Livingstone Inc., 650 Ave. of the Americas, New York, NY 10011. Phone: (212) 819-5400. Fax: (212) 302-6598. 1991.

COLORECTAL SURGERY

See also: STOMA; SURGERY

ABSTRACTING, INDEXING, AND CURRENT AWARENESS PUBLICATIONS

Core Journals in Gastroenterology. Elsevier Science Publishing Co., Inc., P.O. Box 882, Madison Square Station, New York, NY 10159-2101. Phone: (212) 989-5800. Fax: (212) 633-3990. 11/year.

Current Contents/Clinical Medicine. Institute for Scientific Information, 3501 Market St., Philadelphia, PA 19104. Phone: (800) 523-1850. Fax: (215) 386-6362. Weekly.

Excerpta Medica. Section 16: Cancer. Elsevier Science Publishing Co., Inc., P.O. Box 882, Madison Square Station, New York, NY 10159-2101. Phone: (212) 989-5800. Fax: (212) 633-3990. 32/year.

Excerpta Medica. Section 48: Gastroenterology. Elsevier Science Publishing Co., Inc., P.O. Box 882, Madison Square Station, New York, NY 10159-2101. Phone: (212) 989-5800. Fax: (212) 633-3990. 20/year.

Index Medicus. U.S. National Library of Medicine, 8600 Rockville Pike, Bethesda, MD 20894. Phone: (800) 638-8480. Monthly.

Science Citation Index. Institute for Scientific Information, 3501 Market St., Philadelphia, PA 19104. Phone: (800) 523-1850. Fax: (215) 386-6362. Bimonthly.

ASSOCIATIONS, PROFESSIONAL SOCIETIES, ADVOCACY AND SUPPORT GROUPS

American Society of Colon and Rectal Surgeons (ASCRS). 615 Griswold, No. 1717, Detroit, MI 48226. Phone: (313) 961-7880.

International Academy of Proctology. c/o George Donnally M.D., 1203 Hadley Rd., Mooresville, IN 46158. Phone: (317) 831-9300.

United Ostomy Association (UOA). 36 Executive Park, Ste. 120, Irvine, CA 92714. Phone: (714) 660-8624. Fax: (714) 660-9262.

CD-ROM DATABASES

SCISEARCH. Institute for Scientific Information, 3501 Market St., Philadelphia, PA 19104. Phone: (215) 386-0100. Fax: (215) 386-6362.

DIRECTORIES

Directory of Certified Colon and Rectal Surgeons. American Board of Medical Specialties, 1 Rotary Center, Suite 805, Evanston, IL 60201. Phone: (708) 491-9091.

HANDBOOKS, GUIDES, MANUALS, ATLASES

Atlas of Surgical Management of Anorectal Malformations. A. Pena. Springer-Verlag New York Inc., 175 Fifth Ave., New York, NY 10010. Phone: (212) 460-1500. Fax: (212) 473-6272. 1989.

JOURNALS

American Journal of Surgery. Reed Publishing USA, 249 W. 17th St., New York, NY 10011. Phone: (212) 645-0067. Fax: (212) 242-6987. Monthly.

Archives of Surgery. American Medical Association, 515 North State St., Chicago, IL 60610. Phone: (312) 464-0183. Fax: (312) 464-5834. Monthly.

British Journal of Surgery. Butterworth-Heinemann, 80 Montvale Ave., Stoneham, MA 02180. Phone: (617) 438-8464. Fax: (617) 279-4851. Monthly Monthly.

Cancer. J.B. Lippincott Co., 227 East Washington Square, Philadelphia, PA 19106-3780. Phone: (215) 238-4200. Fax: (215) 238-4227. Semimonthly.

Diseases of the Colon and Rectum. Williams & Wilkins, 428 E. Preston St., Baltimore, MD 21202. Phone: (800) 638-0672. Fax: (800) 447-8438. Monthly.

Journal of Clinical Gastroenterology. Raven Press, 1185 Avenue of the Americas, New York, NY 10036. Phone: (212) 930-9500. Fax: (212) 869-3495. Bimonthly.

Journal of Surgical Oncology. John Wiley & Sons, Inc., 605 Third Ave., New York, NY 10158-0012. Phone: (212) 850-6000. Fax: (212) 850-6088. Monthly.

ONLINE DATABASES

EMBASE. Elsevier Science Publishing Co., Inc., P.O. Box 882, Madison Square Station, New York, NY 10159-2101. Phone: (212) 989-5800. Fax: (212) 633-3990.

MEDLINE. National Library of Medicine, 8600 Rockville Pike, Bethesda, MD 20894. Phone: (800) 638-8480.

SciSearch. Institute for Scientific Information, 3501 Market St., Philadelphia, PA 19104. Phone: (215) 386-0100. Fax: (215) 386-6362.

POPULAR WORKS AND PATIENT EDUCATION

The Ostomy Book: Living Comfortably with Colostomies, Ileostomies & Urostomies. Barbara D. Mullen, Kerry A. McGinn. Bull Publishing Co., 110 Gilbert Ave., Menlo Park, CA 94025. Phone: (800) 676-2855. 1992.

TEXTBOOKS AND MONOGRAPHS

Colorectal Surgery Illustrated. Joel Bauer. Mosby-Year Book, 11830 Westline Industrial Drive, St. Louis, MO 63146. Phone: (800) 325-4177. Fax: (314) 432-1380. 1992.

Current Surgical Diagnosis and Treatment. L.W. Way. Appleton & Lange, 25 Van Zant St., East Norwalk, CT 06855.

Phone: (800) 423-1359. Fax: (203) 854-9486. Ninth edition 1990.

Current Therapy in Colon and Rectal Surgery. Victor W. Fazio. Mosby-Year Book, 11830 Westline Industrial Drive, St. Louis, MO 63146. Phone: (800) 325-4177. Fax: (314) 432-1380. 1990.

Pathology of the Colon, Small Intestine, and Anus. Norris. Churchill Livingstone Inc., 650 Ave. of the Americas, New York, NY 10011. Phone: (212) 819-5400. Fax: (212) 302-6598. 1991.

Shackelford's Surgery of the Alimentary Tract. E. Zuidema, and others (eds.). W.B. Saunders Co., The Curtis Center, Independence Sqare W., Philadelphia, PA 19106-3399. Phone: (215) 238-7800. 1991.

COLOSTOMY

See: COLORECTAL CANCER

COMMON COLD

See: INFECTIOUS DISEASES

COMMUNICABLE DISEASES

See: INFECTIOUS DISEASES

COMMUNICATION DISORDERS

See also: AUDIOLOGY

ABSTRACTING, INDEXING, AND CURRENT AWARENESS PUBLICATIONS

Excerpta Medica. Section 11: Otorhinolaryngology. Elsevier Science Publishing Co., Inc., P.O. Box 882, Madison Square Station, New York, NY 10159-2101. Phone: (212) 989-5800. Fax: (212) 633-3990. 16/year.

Index Medicus. U.S. National Library of Medicine, 8600 Rockville Pike, Bethesda, MD 20894. Phone: (800) 638-8480. Monthly.

Psychological Abstracts. American Psychological Association, 1200 17th St. NW, Washington, DC 20036. Phone: (202) 955-7600. Monthly.

Science Citation Index. Institute for Scientific Information, 3501 Market St., Philadelphia, PA 19104. Phone: (800) 523-1850. Fax: (215) 386-6362. Bimonthly.

ASSOCIATIONS, PROFESSIONAL SOCIETIES, ADVOCACY AND SUPPORT GROUPS

American Hearing Research Foundation. 55 E. Washington St., Suite 2022, Chicago, IL 60602. Phone: (312) 726-9670.

American Speech-Language-Hearing Association (ASHA). 10801 Rockville Pike, Rockville, MD 20852. Phone: (301) 897-5700. Fax: (301) 571-0457.

Communication Disorders and Sciences. 555 Manoogian Hall, Wayne State University, Detroit, MI 48202. Phone: (313) 577-3337.

International Foundation for Stutterers (IFS). P.O. Box 462, Belle Mead, NJ 08502. Phone: (201) 359-6469.

National Center for Stuttering (NCS). 200 E. 33rd St., New York, NY 10016. Phone: (212) 532-1460.

National Hearing Association. 711 Enterprise Dr., Suite 101, Oak Brook, IL 60521.

National Stuttering Project (NSP). 4601 Irving St., San Francisco, CA 94122-1020.

Orton Dyslexia Society (ODS). 724 York Rd., Baltimore, MD 21204. Phone: (800) ABC-D123.

CD-ROM DATABASES

SCISEARCH. Institute for Scientific Information, 3501 Market St., Philadelphia, PA 19104. Phone: (215) 386-0100. Fax: (215) 386-6362.

ENCYCLOPEDIAS, DICTIONARIES, WORD BOOKS

Encyclopedia of Deafness and Hearing Disorders. Carol Turkington, Allen Sussman. Facts on File, Inc., 460 Park Ave. S., New York, NY 10016-7382. Phone: (212) 683-2244. Fax: (212) 683-3633. 1992.

JOURNALS

British Journal of Disorders of Communication. Whurr Publishers Ltd., 19b Compton Terrace, London N1 2UN, England. Phone: 01-359-5979. 3/year.

European Journal of Disorders of Communication. Whurr Publishers, P.O. Box 1897, Lawrence, KS 66044-8897. Phone: (913) 843-1221. Fax: (913) 843-1274. 4/year.

Hearing Journal. Laux Company, 63 Great Rd., Maynard, MA 01754. Phone: (617) 897-5552.

Journal of Communication Disorders. Elsevier Science Publishing Co., Inc., P.O. Box 882, Madison Square Station, New York, NY 10159-2101. Phone: (212) 989-5800. Fax: (212) 633-3990. 4/year.

NEWSLETTERS

American Hearing Research Foundation Newsletter. American Hearing Research Foundation, 55 E. Washington St., Ste. 2022, Chicago, IL 60602. Quarterly.

ONLINE DATABASES

EMBASE. Elsevier Science Publishing Co., Inc., P.O. Box 882, Madison Square Station, New York, NY 10159-2101. Phone: (212) 989-5800. Fax: (212) 633-3990.

MEDLINE. National Library of Medicine, 8600 Rockville Pike, Bethesda, MD 20894. Phone: (800) 638-8480.

SciSearch. Institute for Scientific Information, 3501 Market St., Philadelphia, PA 19104. Phone: (215) 386-0100. Fax: (215) 386-6362.

POPULAR WORKS AND PATIENT EDUCATION

Living Well with Hearing Loss: A Guide for the Hearing Impaired and Their Families. Debbie Huning. John Wiley & Sons, Inc., 605 Third Ave., New York, NY 10158-0012. Phone: (212) 850-6000. Fax: (212) 850-6088. 1992.

Stutter No More: The Fast, Simple, Proven Technique with an Astonishing Long-Term Success Rate. Martin F. Schwartz. Simon & Schuster, Inc., 1230 Ave. of the Americas, New York, NY 10020. Phone: (212) 698-7000. 1992.

Turning Around: The Upside-Down Kids, Helping Dyslexic Kids Overcome Their Disorder. Harold N. Levinson. M. Evans and Co., Inc., 216 E. 49th St., New York, NY 10017. Phone: (212) 688-2810. 1992.

RESEARCH CENTERS, INSTITUTES, CLEARINGHOUSES

Center for Research in Speech and Hearing Sciences. 33 West 42nd St., City University of New York, New York, NY 10036. Phone: (212) 790-4366.

Communication Disorders Clinic. Communication Disorders & Speech Science Dept., University of Colorado-Boulder, Boulder, CO 80309. Phone: (303) 492-5375.

David T. Siegel Institute for Communicative Disorders. Michael Reese Hospital & Medical Center, 3033 South Cottage Grove Ave., Chicago, IL 60616. Phone: (312) 791-2900.

Division of Communication Disorders. Department of Speech, Louisiana State University, Baton Rouge, LA 70803. Phone: (504) 388-2545.

National Institute on Deafness and Other Communication Disorders Information Clearinghouse. P.O. Box 37777, Washington, DC 20013. Phone: (800) 241-1044. Fax: (301) 565-5112.

Self-Help for Hard of Hearing People. 7800 Wisconsin Ave., Bethesda, MD 20814. Phone: (301) 657-2248.

TEXTBOOKS AND MONOGRAPHS

Children with Specific Speech and Language Impairment. Corinne Haynes, Sandhya Naidoo. Cambridge University Press, 40 W. 20th St., New York, NY 10011. Phone: (800) 431-1580. 1992.

Diagnosis and Evaluation in Speech Pathology. William O. Haynes, and others. Prentice Hall, 113 Sylvan Ave., Rt. 9W, Prentice Hall Bldg., Englewood Cliffs, NJ 07632. Phone: (201) 767-5937. Fourth edition 1992.

Hearing: An Introduction to Psychological and Physical. Marcel Dekker, Inc., 270 Madison Ave., New York, NY 10016. Phone: (800) 228-1160.

An Introduction to Neurogenic Communication Disorders. Robert H. Brookshire. Mosby-Year Book, 11830 Westline Industrial Drive, St. Louis, MO 63146. Phone: (800) 325-4177. Fax: (314) 432-1380. Fourth edition 1992.

Language and Speech Disorders: A Neurophysiological Approach. E.M.R. Critchley. Rapid Communications of Oxford Ltd., The Old Malthouse, Paradise St., Oxford OX1 1LD, England. Phone: 44-865-790447. Fax: 44-865-244012. 1987.

Survey of Communication Disorders. John M. Palmer, Phillip A. Yantis. Williams & Wilkins, 428 East Preston St., Baltimore, MD 21202. Phone: (800) 638-0672. Fax: (800) 447-8438. 1990.

COMPUTED TOMOGRAPHY (CT)

See: RADIOLOGY; TOMOGRAPHY

CONGENITAL DISORDERS

See: BIRTH DEFECTS

CONGESTIVE HEART FAILURE

See: HEART DISEASES

CONJUNCTIVITIS

See: EYE DISEASES

CONSTIPATION

See: GASTROINTESTINAL DISORDERS

CONSUMER HEALTH INFORMATION

See also: PATIENT EDUCATION

ABSTRACTING, INDEXING, AND CURRENT AWARENESS PUBLICATIONS

Consumer Health and Nutrition Index. Alan Rees. Oryx Press, 4041 N. Central, Suite 700, Phoenix, AZ 85012. Phone: (800) 279-6799. Fax: (800) 279-4663. Quarterly.

Cumulative Index to Nursing and Allied Health Literature. Glendale Adventist Medical Center, P.O. Box 871, Glendale, CA 91209. Phone: (818) 409-8005. Bimonthly.

Medical Abstracts Newsletter. Communi-T Publications, P.O. Box 2170, Teaneck, NJ 07666. Phone: (201) 836-5030. Monthly.

ASSOCIATIONS, PROFESSIONAL SOCIETIES, ADVOCACY AND SUPPORT GROUPS

National Women's Health Network (NWHN). 1325 G St. N.W., Washington, DC 20005. Phone: (202) 347-1140. Fax: (202) 347-1168.

People's Medical Society. 462 Walnut St., Allentown, PA 18102. Phone: (215) 770-1670.

Public Citizen Health Research Group (PCHRG). 2000 P St. N.W., Ste. 700, Washington, DC 20036. Phone: (202) 872-0320.

BIBLIOGRAPHIES

Consumer Health Information Source Book. Alan Rees, Catherine Hoffman. Oryx Press, 4041 N. Central, Suite 700, Phoenix, AZ 85012. Phone: (800) 279-6799. Fax: (800) 279-4663. Third edition 1990.

Health Information Resources in the Federal Government. OOPHP National Health Information Ctr., Office of Disease Prevention and Health Promotion, Public Health Service, 330 C St. S.W., Rm. 2132, Washington, DC 20201. Phone: (800) 336-4797. Fax: (301) 565-5112. Irregular.

Patient Education Sourcebook: Volume II. Christine Frank (ed.). Health Sciences Communications Association, 6105 Lindell Blvd., St. Louis, MO 63112. Phone: (314) 725-4722. 1990.

CD-ROM DATABASES

Family Doctor. CMC ReSearch, Inc., 7150 S.W. Hampton, Suite C-120, Portland, OR 97223. Phone: (800) 262-7668. Fax: (503) 639-1796. Irregular.

Health Reference Center. Information Access Company, 362 Lakeside Dr., Foster City, CA 94404. Phone: (800) 227-8431. Monthly.

MDX-Health Digest. SilverPlatter Information, Inc., River Ridge Office Park, 100 River Ridge Rd., Norwood, MA 02062. Phone: (617) 769-2599. Fax: (617) 769-8763.

Nursing and Allied Health (CINAHL) on CD-ROM. CINAHL, 1509 Wilson Terrace, P.O. Box 871, Glendale, CA 91209-0871. Phone: (818) 409-8005.

Personal Medical Library CD-ROM. EBSCO Publishing, P.O. Box 325, Topsfield, MA 01983. Phone: (800) 221-1826. Fax: (508) 887-3923.

DIRECTORIES

National Healthlines Directory. Louanne Marinos. Information Resources Press, 1110 N. Glebe Rd., Ste. 550, Arlington, VA 22201. Phone: (703) 558-8270. Fax: (703) 558-4979. 1992.

JOURNALS

FDA Consumer. U.S. Government Printing Office, Superintendent of Documents, P.O. Box 371954, Pittsburgh, PA 15250-7954. Phone: (202) 783-3238. Fax: (202) 512-2250. Monthly.

NEWSLETTERS

Health Facts. Center for Medical Consumers, 237 Thompson St., New York, NY 10012. Phone: (212) 674-7105. Monthly.

Health Letter. Public Citizen Health Research Group, 2000 P St. N.W., Ste. 700, Washington, DC 20036. Phone: (202) 872-0320. Monthly.

Health News. Faculty of Medicine. University of Toronto, Medical Sciences Bldg., Toronto, ON, Canada M5S 1A8. Phone: (416) 948-5411. Fax: (416) 978-4552. Bimonthly.

Health & You. Health Ink Co., One Executive Dr., Moorestown, NJ 08057. Quarterly.

Healthline. Mosby-Year Book, 11830 Westline Industrial Drive, St. Louis, MO 63146. Phone: (800) 325-4177. Fax: (314) 432-1380. Monthly.

Johns Hopkins Medical Letter: Health After 50. Medletter Associates, Inc., P.O. Box 359179, Palm Coast, FL 32137. Monthly.

Mayo Clinic Health Letter. Mayo Foundation for Medical Education and Research, 200 First St. N.W., Rochester, MN 55905. Phone: (507) 284-4587. Fax: (507) 284-5410. Monthly.

People's Medical Society-Newsletter. People's Medical Society, 462 Walnut St., Allentown, PA 18102. Phone: (215) 770-1670. Bimonthly.

University of California, Berkeley Wellness Letter. Health Letter Associates, Box 412, Prince St. Sta., New York, NY 10003-0007. Phone: (212) 505-2255. Fax: (212) 505-5462. Monthly.

The University of Texas Lifetime Health Letter. Health Science Center. University of Texas, 1100 Holcombe Blvd., P.O. Box 20036, Houston, TX 77225. Phone: (800) 274-6377. Monthly.

ONLINE DATABASES

Health Periodicals Database. Information Access Company, 362 Lakeside Dr., Foster City, CA 94404. Phone: (800) 227-8431. Weekly.

Nursing and Allied Health (CINAHL). CINAHL, 1509 Wilson Terrace, P.O. Box 871, Glendale, CA 91209-0871. Phone: (818) 409-8005.

POPULAR WORKS AND PATIENT EDUCATION

9000 Questionable Doctors. Sidney Wolfe. Public Citizen Health Resource Group, 2000 P St. N.W., Suite 700, Washington, DC 20036. Phone: (202) 872-0320. 1993.

Patient Drug Facts. Bernie R. Olin III (ed.). J.B. Lippincott Co., 227 E. Washington Square, Philadelphia, PA 19106-3780. Phone: (215) 238-4200. Fax: (215) 238-4227. Quarterly.

Personal Health Reporter. Alan Rees, Charlene Wiley. Gale Research, Inc., 835 Penobscot Bldg., Detroit, MI 48226-4094. Phone: (800) 877-GALE. Fax: (313) 961-6083. 1992.

RESEARCH CENTERS, INSTITUTES, CLEARINGHOUSES

Center for Medical Consumers and Health Care Information (CMC). 237 Thompson St., New York, NY 10012. Phone: (212) 674-7105. Fax: (212) 674-7100.

Consumer Information Center. Pueblo, CO 81009.

National Health Information Center. Office of Disease Prevention and Health Promotion, P.O. Box 1133, Washington, DC 20013-1133. Phone: (800) 336-4797.

National Second Surgical Opinion Program. Health Care Financing Administration, 200 Independence Ave. S.W., Washington, DC 20201. Phone: (800) 638-6833.

TEXTBOOKS AND MONOGRAPHS

Consumer Health Information: Managing Hospital Based Centers. Salvinija Kemaghan, Barbara Gilott. American Hospital Association, 840 N. Lake Shore Dr., Chicago, IL 60611. Phone: (312) 280-6000. Fax: (312) 280-5979. 1991.

Locating Resources for Healthy People 2000 Health Promotion Projects. Public Health Service, Office of Disease Prevention and Health Promotion, Washington, DC 20201. 1991.

Managing Consumer Health Information Services. Alan Rees. Oryx Press, 4041 N. Central, Suite 700, Phoenix, AZ 85012. Phone: (800) 279-ORYX. Fax: (800) 279-4663. 1991.

CONTACT LENSES

ABSTRACTING, INDEXING, AND CURRENT AWARENESS PUBLICATIONS

Core Journals in Ophthalmology. Elsevier Science Publishing Co., Inc., P.O. Box 882, Madison Square Station, New York, NY 10159-2101. Phone: (212) 989-5800. Fax: (212) 633-3990. 11/year.

Excerpta Medica. Section 12: Ophthalmology. Elsevier Science Publishing Co., Inc., P.O. Box 882, Madison Square Station, New York, NY 10159-2101. Phone: (212) 989-5800. Fax: (212) 633-3990. 16/year.

Index Medicus. U.S. National Library of Medicine, 8600 Rockville Pike, Bethesda, MD 20894. Phone: (800) 638-8480. Monthly.

Ophthalmic Literature. Institute of Ophthalmology, Judd St., London WC1H 9QS, England. 7/year.

Research Alert: Ophthalmology. Institute for Scientific Information, 3501 Market St., Philadelphia, PA 19104. Phone: (800) 523-1850. Fax: (215) 386-6362. Weekly.

ANNUALS AND REVIEWS

Year Book of Ophthalmology. Mosby-Year Book, 11830 Westline Industrial Drive, St. Louis, MO 63146. Phone: (800) 325-4177. Fax: (314) 432-1380. Annual.

ASSOCIATIONS, PROFESSIONAL SOCIETIES, ADVOCACY AND SUPPORT GROUPS

American Academy of Ophthalmology (AAO). 655 Beach St., San Francisco, CA 94109. Phone: (415) 561-8500. Fax: (415) 561-8533.

Contact Lens Association of Ophthalmologists (CLAO). 523 Decatur St., Ste. 1, New Orleans, LA 70130-1027. Phone: (504) 581-4000. Fax: (504) 581-5884.

National Contact Lens Examiners (NCLE). 10341 Democracy Ln., Fairfax, VA 22030. Phone: (703) 691-1060. Fax: (703) 691-3929.

BIBLIOGRAPHIES

Contact Lens Solutions. National Technical Information Service, 5285 Port Royal Rd., Springfield, VA 22161. Phone: (703) 487-4650. Fax: (703) 321-8547. Jan. 1970-Apr. 1989 PB89-860043/CBY.

Contact Lenses and the Risk of Infection. National Technical Information Service, 5285 Port Royal Rd., Springfield, VA 22161. Phone: (703) 487-4650. Fax: (703) 321-8547. Jan. 1978-May 1989 PB89-863070/CBY.

HANDBOOKS, GUIDES, MANUALS, ATLASES

Color Atlas of Contact Lenses. W. Ehrich, D. Epstein. Thieme Medical Publishers, Inc., 381 Park Ave. S., New York, NY 10016. Phone: (212) 683-5088. Fax: (212) 779-9020. 1988.

A Colour Atlas of Contact Lenses. Montague Ruben. Appleton & Lange, 25 Van Zant St., East Norwalk, CT 06855. Phone: (800) 423-1359. Fax: (203) 854-9486. 2nd edition 1988.

The Contact Lens Manual. Andrew Gasson, Judith Morris. Butterworth-Heinemann, 80 Montvale Ave., Stoneham, MA 02180. Phone: (617) 438-8464. Fax: (617) 279-4851. 1991.

Manual of Clinical Problems in Opththalmology. Gittinger. Little, Brown and Co., 34 Beacon St., Boston, MA 02108. Phone: (617) 227-0730. 1988.

JOURNALS

Archives of Ophthalmology. American Medical Association, 515 North State St., Chicago, IL 60610. Phone: (312) 464-0183. Fax: (312) 464-5834. Monthly.

International Contact Lens Clinic. Butterworth-Heinemann, 80 Montvale Ave., Stoneham, MA 02180. Phone: (617) 438-8464. Fax: (617) 279-4851. Bimonthly.

The Journal of the British Contact Lens Association. Mosby-Year Book, 11830 Westline Industrial Drive, St. Louis, MO 63146. Phone: (800) 325-4177. Fax: (314) 432-1380. Quarterly.

Survey of Ophthalmology. Survey of Ophthalmology, Inc., Suite 4, 7 Kent St., Brookline, MA 02146. Phone: (617) 566-2138. Fax: (617) 566-4019. Bimonthly.

ONLINE DATABASES

EMBASE. Elsevier Science Publishing Co., Inc., P.O. Box 882, Madison Square Station, New York, NY 10159-2101. Phone: (212) 989-5800. Fax: (212) 633-3990.

MEDLINE. National Library of Medicine, 8600 Rockville Pike, Bethesda, MD 20894. Phone: (800) 638-8480.

SciSearch. Institute for Scientific Information, 3501 Market St., Philadelphia, PA 19104. Phone: (215) 386-0100. Fax: (215) 386-6362.

TEXTBOOKS AND MONOGRAPHS

Complications of Contact Lens Wear. Alan Tomlinson. Mosby-Year Book, 11830 Westline Industrial Drive, St. Louis, MO 63146. Phone: (800) 325-4177. Fax: (314) 432-1380. 1992.

Contact Lenses. J. Stone, A.J. Phillips. Butterworth-Heinemann, 80 Montvale Ave., Stoneham, MA 02180. Phone: (617) 438-8464. Fax: (617) 279-4851. 3rd edition 1989.

Contact Lenses: A Textbook for Practitioner and Student. A.J. Phillips, J. Stone. Butterworth-Heinemann, 80 Montvale Ave., Stoneham, MA 02180. Phone: (617) 438-8464. Fax: (617) 279-4851. 1989.

Contact Lenses: Guide to Selection, Fitting, and Management of Complications. Susan Svenson. Appleton & Lange, 25 Van Zant St., East Norwalk, CT 06855. Phone: (800) 423-1359. Fax: (203) 854-9486. 1987.

Malpractice and Contact Lenses. Harvey M. Rosenwasser. Butterworth-Heinemann, 80 Montvale Ave., Stoneham, MA 02180. Phone: (617) 438-8464. Fax: (617) 279-4851. Updated edition 1991.

CONTRACEPTION

See also: FAMILY PLANNING

ABSTRACTING, INDEXING, AND CURRENT AWARENESS PUBLICATIONS

Current Contents/Clinical Medicine. Institute for Scientific Information, 3501 Market St., Philadelphia, PA 19104. Phone: (800) 523-1850. Fax: (215) 386-6362. Weekly.

Current Literature in Family Planning. Planned Parenthood Federation of America, 810 7th Ave., New York, NY 10019. Phone: (212) 603-4637.

Excerpta Medica. Section 10: Obstetrics and Gynecology. Elsevier Science Publishing Co., Inc., P.O. Box 882, Madison Square Station, New York, NY 10159-2101. Phone: (212) 989-5800. Fax: (212) 633-3990. 20/year.

Index Medicus. U.S. National Library of Medicine, 8600 Rockville Pike, Bethesda, MD 20894. Phone: (800) 638-8480. Monthly.

Latest Literature in Family Planning. Family Planning Information Service, 27-35 Mortimer St., London W1N 7RJ, England. Bimonthly.

Research Alert: Contraceptive Drugs & Devices. Institute for Scientific Information, 3501 Market St., Philadelphia, PA 19104. Phone: (800) 523-1850. Fax: (215) 386-6362. Weekly.

Science Citation Index. Institute for Scientific Information, 3501 Market St., Philadelphia, PA 19104. Phone: (800) 523-1850. Fax: (215) 386-6362. Bimonthly.

ASSOCIATIONS, PROFESSIONAL SOCIETIES, ADVOCACY AND SUPPORT GROUPS

The Couple to Couple League International, Inc.. P.O. Box 111184, Cincinnati, OH 45211.

Planned Parenthood Foundation of America, Inc.. 810 Seventh Ave., New York, NY 10019. Phone: (212) 541-7800.

BIBLIOGRAPHIES

Abortion Bibliography. Whitston Publishing Co., P.O. Box 958, Troy, NY 12181. Phone: (518) 283-4363.

Condoms: Manufacturing, Marketing, and Use. National Technical Information Service, 5285 Port Royal Rd., Springfield, VA 22161. Phone: (703) 487-4650. Fax: (703) 321-8547. Apr. 1979-Oct. 1989. PB90-850801/CBY.

Contraceptives: Devices, and Contraceptive Methods and Formulations. National Technical Information Service, 5285 Port Royal Rd., Springfield, VA 22161. Phone: (703) 487-4650. Fax: (703) 321-8547. Oct. 1970-Oct. 1989 PB90-855131/CBY.

Pregnancy Products: Contraceptives, Pregnancy and Ovulation Kits. National Technical Information Service, 5285 Port Royal Rd., Springfield, VA 22161. Phone: (703) 487-4650. Fax: (703) 321-8547. Jan. 1985-Feb. 1989 PB89-857353/CBY.

CD-ROM DATABASES

Excerpta Medica CD: Obstetrics & Gynecology. SilverPlatter Information, Inc., River Ridge Office Park, 100 River Ridge Rd., Norwood, MA 02062. Phone: (617) 769-2599. Fax: (617) 769-8763. Quarterly.

SCISEARCH. Institute for Scientific Information, 3501 Market St., Philadelphia, PA 19104. Phone: (215) 386-0100. Fax: (215) 386-6362.

HANDBOOKS, GUIDES, MANUALS, ATLASES

Handbook of Contraception and Abortion. Burkman. Little, Brown and Co., 34 Beacon St., Boston, MA 02108. Phone: (617) 227-0730. Fax: (617) 227-0790. 1989.

JOURNALS

Advances in Contraception. Kluwer Academic Publishers, P.O. Box 358, Accord Station, Hingham, MA 02018-0358. Phone: (617) 871-6600. Fax: (617) 871-6528. 4/year.

Contraception. Butterworth-Heinemann, 80 Montvale Ave., Stoneham, MA 02180. Phone: (617) 438-8464. Fax: (617) 279-4851. Monthly.

Contraceptive Technology Update. American Health Consultants, P.O. Box 71266, Chicago, IL 60691. Phone: (800) 688-2421. Fax: (404) 352-1971.

Family Planning Perspectives. Alan Guttmacher Institute, 111 Fifth Ave., New York, NY 10003. Phone: (212) 254-5636.

NEWSLETTERS

Contraceptive Technology Update. American Health Consultants, Department C1290, P.O. Box 740060, Atlanta, GA 30374. Phone: (800) 559-1032. Fax: (404) 352-1971. Monthly.

ONLINE DATABASES

EMBASE. Elsevier Science Publishing Co., Inc., P.O. Box 882, Madison Square Station, New York, NY 10159-2101. Phone: (212) 989-5800. Fax: (212) 633-3990.

Human Sexuality. Clinical Communications, Inc., 132 Hutchin Hill, Shady, NY 12409. Phone: (914) 679-2217. Weekly to biweekly.

MEDLINE. National Library of Medicine, 8600 Rockville Pike, Bethesda, MD 20894. Phone: (800) 638-8480.

POPLINE. U.S. National Library of Medicine, MEDLARS Management Section, 8600 Rockville Pike, Bethesda, MD 20894. Phone: (800) 638-8480. Monthly.

SciSearch. Institute for Scientific Information, 3501 Market St., Philadelphia, PA 19104. Phone: (215) 386-0100. Fax: (215) 386-6362.

POPULAR WORKS AND PATIENT EDUCATION

Contraception. V.L. Bullough, B. Bullough. Prometheus Books, 700E. Amherst St., Buffalo, NY 14215. Phone: (800) 421-0351. 1990.

Contraception: A Guide to Birth Control Methods. Vern L. Bullough, Bonnie Bullough. Prometheus Books, 700 E. Amherst St., Buffalo, NY 14215. Phone: (800) 421-0351. 1990.

The Contraceptive Handbook: A Guide to Safe and Effective Choices for Men and Women. Beverly Winikoff, Suzanne Wymelenberg, and others. Consumer Reports Books, 9180 LeSaint Dr., Fairfield, OH 45014. Phone: (513) 860-1178. 1992.

Contraceptive Technology, 1990-1992: With Two Special Sections: AIDS and Condoms. Robert A. Hatcher. Irvington Publishers, 522 E. 82nd St., New York, NY 10028. Phone: (212) 472-4494. 15th edition 1990.

The New Our Bodies, Ourselves: The Updated and Expanded Edition. The Boston Women's Health Book Collective. Simon & Schuster, 1230 Ave. of the Americas, New York, NY 10020. Phone: (800) 223-2348. Fax: (800) 284-0735. 1992.

RESEARCH CENTERS, INSTITUTES, CLEARINGHOUSES

Alan Guttmacher Institute. 111 5th Ave., New York, NY 10003. Phone: (212) 254-5656. Fax: (212) 254-9891.

Center for Population and Family Health. Columbia University. Level B-3, 60 Haven Ave., New York, NY 10032. Phone: (212) 305-6960. Fax: (212) 305-7024.

Contraceptive Research and Development Program (CONRAD). 1611 N. Kent St., Ste. 806, Arlington, VA 22209. Phone: (703) 524-4744. Fax: (703) 524-4770.

Family Health International. P.O. Box 13950, Research Triangle Park, NC 27709. Phone: (919) 544-7040. Fax: (919) 544-7261.

Population Information Program. 527 St. Paul Place, Johns Hopkins University, Baltimore, MD 21202. Phone: (410) 659-6300. Fax: (410) 659-6266.

STANDARDS AND STATISTICS SOURCES

Population Reports, Series A: Oral Contraception. Population Information Program, 527 St. Paul Place, Johns Hopkins University, Baltimore, MD 21202. Phone: (410) 659-6300. Fax: (410) 659-6266. Irregular.

Population Reports, Series B: Intrauterine Devices. Population Information Program, 527 St. Paul Place, Johns Hopkins University, Baltimore, MD 21202. Phone: (410) 659-6300. Fax: (410) 659-6266. Irregular.

Population Reports, Series C: Female Sterilization. Population Information Program, 527 St. Paul Place, Johns Hopkins University, Baltimore, MD 21202. Phone: (410) 659-6300. Fax: (410) 659-6266. Irregular.

Population Reports, Series D: Male Sterilization. Population Information Program, 527 St. Paul Place, Johns Hopkins University, Baltimore, MD 21202. Phone: (410) 659-6300. Fax: (410) 659-6266. Irregular.

Population Reports, Series E: Law and Policy. Population Information Program, 527 St. Paul Place, Johns Hopkins University, Baltimore, MD 21202. Phone: (410) 659-6300. Fax: (410) 659-6266. Irregular.

Population Reports, Series H: Barrier Methods. Population Information Program, 527 St. Paul Place, Johns Hopkins University, Baltimore, MD 21202. Phone: (410) 659-6300. Fax: (410) 659-6266. Irregular.

Population Reports, Series I: Rhythm, Periodic Abstinence. Population Information Program, 527 St. Paul Place, Johns Hopkins University, Baltimore, MD 21202. Phone: (410) 659-6300. Fax: (410) 659-6266. Irregular.

Population Reports, Series J: Family Planning Programs. Population Information Program, 527 St. Paul Place, Johns

Hopkins University, Baltimore, MD 21202. Phone: (410) 659-6300. Fax: (410) 659-6266. Irregular.

Population Reports, Series L: Issues in World Health. Population Information Program, 527 St. Paul Place, Johns Hopkins University, Baltimore, MD 21202. Phone: (410) 659-6300. Fax: (410) 659-6266. Irregular.

Population Reports, Series M: Special Topics. Population Information Program, 527 St. Paul Place, Johns Hopkins University, Baltimore, MD 21202. Phone: (410) 659-6300. Fax: (410) 659-6266. Irregular.

TEXTBOOKS AND MONOGRAPHS

Clinical Guide to Contraception. Speroff. Williams & Wilkins, 428 East Preston St., Baltimore, MD 21202. Phone: (800) 638-0672. Fax: (800) 447-8438. 1992.

Contraception and Mechanisms of Endometrial Bleeding. C. D'Arcangues, I.S. Fraser, J.R. Newton, V. Odlind (eds.). Cambridge University Press, 40 W. 20th St., New York, NY 10011. Phone: (800) 431-1580. 1990.

CONVULSIONS

See: NEUROLOGIC DISORDERS

CORONARY ARTERY DISEASE

See: ATHEROSCLEROSIS

CORONARY BYPASS SURGERY

See: CARDIOVASCULAR SURGERY

CORONARY DISEASES

See: HEART DISEASES

CORPORATE FITNESS

See also: HEALTH PROMOTION

ABSTRACTING, INDEXING, AND CURRENT AWARENESS PUBLICATIONS

Cumulative Index to Nursing and Allied Health Literature. Glendale Adventist Medical Center, P.O. Box 871, Glendale, CA 91209. Phone: (818) 409-8005. Bimonthly.

Health Education Index. B. Edsall & Co., Ltd., Greater London House, Hampstead Rd., London NW1, England. 2/year.

ASSOCIATIONS, PROFESSIONAL SOCIETIES, ADVOCACY AND SUPPORT GROUPS

Wellness Councils of America. 1823 Harney St., Ste. 201, Omaha, NE 68102. Phone: (402) 444-1711.

CD-ROM DATABASES

Nursing and Allied Health (CINAHL) on CD-ROM. CINAHL, 1509 Wilson Terrace, P.O. Box 871, Glendale, CA 91209-0871. Phone: (818) 409-8005.

JOURNALS

Business and Health. Medical Economics, Five Paragon Dr., Montvale, NJ 07645-1742. Phone: (800) 222-3045. Fax: (201) 573-4956. Monthly.

Health Values: The Journal of Health Behavior, Education & Promotion. PNG Publications, P.O. Box 4593, Star City, WV 26504-4593. Phone: (304) 293-4699. Fax: (304) 293-4693. Bimonthly.

NEWSLETTERS

Employee Health and Fitness. American Health Consultants, Department C1290, P.O. Box 740060, Atlanta, GA 30374. Phone: (800) 559-1032. Monthly.

Executive Good Health Report. Executive Good Health Report, P.O. Box 8800, Chapel Hill, NC 27515.

ONLINE DATABASES

Nursing and Allied Health (CINAHL). CINAHL, 1509 Wilson Terrace, P.O. Box 871, Glendale, CA 91209-0871. Phone: (818) 409-8005.

RESEARCH CENTERS, INSTITUTES, CLEARINGHOUSES

American Institute for Preventive Medicine. 244450 Evergreen Road, Southfield, MI 48075. Phone: (313) 971-6077.

Corporate Health Designs. P.O. Box 55056, Seattle, WA 98155. Phone: (206) 364-3448.

National Center for Health Promotion. 3920 Varsity Dr., Ann Arbor, MI 48108. Phone: (313) 971-6077.

National Resource Center for Worksite Health Promotion. 777 N. Capitol St. N.E., Ste. 800, Washington, DC 20002. Phone: (202) 408-9320.

Washington Business Group on Health. 777 N. Capitol St. N.E., Suite 800, Washington, DC 20002. Phone: (202) 408-9320.

TEXTBOOKS AND MONOGRAPHS

How Employers Are Saving Through Wellness and Fitness Programs. American Business Publishers, 3100 Highway 138, Wall, NJ 07719. Phone: (201) 681-1133.

COSMETIC SURGERY

See: PLASTIC AND COSMETIC SURGERY

COUNSELING

See: FAMILY THERAPY; PSYCHIATRY; PSYCHOLOGY

CPR

See: CARDIOPULMONARY RESUSCITATION

CRACK

See: COCAINE

CRIB DEATH

See: SUDDEN INFANT DEATH SYNDROME

CRITICAL CARE

ABSTRACTING, INDEXING, AND CURRENT AWARENESS PUBLICATIONS

AACN Nursing Scan in Critical Care. NURSECOM, Inc., 1211 Locust St., Philadelphia, PA 19107. Phone: (215) 545-7222. Bimonthly.

Current Contents/Clinical Medicine. Institute for Scientific Information, 3501 Market St., Philadelphia, PA 19104. Phone: (800) 523-1850. Fax: (215) 386-6362. Weekly.

Hospital Literature Index. American Hospital Association, 840 N. Lake Shore Dr., Chicago, IL 60611. Phone: (800) 242-2626. Fax: (312) 280-6015. Quarterly.

Science Citation Index. Institute for Scientific Information, 3501 Market St., Philadelphia, PA 19104. Phone: (800) 523-1850. Fax: (215) 386-6362. Bimonthly.

ANNUALS AND REVIEWS

Advances in Trauma and Critical Care Medicine. Mosby-Year Book, 11830 Westline Industrial Drive, St. Louis, MO 63146. Phone: (800) 325-4177. Fax: (314) 432-1380. Annual.

Contemporary Management in Critical Care. Churchill Livingstone Inc., 650 Avenue of the Americas, New York, NY 10011. Phone: (212) 819-5400. Fax: (212) 302-6598. Quarterly.

Critical Care Clinics. W.B. Saunders Co., The Curtis Center, Independence Square W., Philadelphia, PA 19106-3399. Phone: (215) 238-7800. Quarterly.

Critical Care Nursing Clinics of North America. W.B. Saunders Co., The Curtis Center, Independence Square W., Philadelphia, PA 19106-3399. Phone: (215) 238-7800. Quarterly.

Current Anaesthesia and Critical Care. Churchill Livingstone Inc., 650 Avenue of the Americas, New York, NY 10011. Phone: (212) 819-5400. Fax: (212) 302-6598. Quarterly.

Year Book of Critical Care Medicine. Mosby-Year Book, 11830 Westline Industrial Drive, St. Louis, MO 63146. Phone: (800) 325-4177. Fax: (314) 432-1380. Annual.

ASSOCIATIONS, PROFESSIONAL SOCIETIES, ADVOCACY AND SUPPORT GROUPS

American Association of Critical-Care Nurses (AACN). 1 Civic Plaza, Newport Beach, CA 92660. Phone: (714) 644-9310. Fax: (714) 640-4903.

Society for Critical Care Medicine (SCCM). 251 E. Imperial Hwy., Ste. 480, Fullerton, CA 92635. Phone: (714) 449-8700. Fax: (714) 870-5243.

CD-ROM DATABASES

Basic Life Support. Hoffer. Williams & Wilkins, 428 East Preston St., Baltimore, MD 21202. Phone: (800) 638-0672. Fax: (800) 447-8438. 1989.

Clinical Problems in Obstetrics: Critical Care Obstetrics. Catanzarite. Williams & Wilkins, 428 East Preston St., Baltimore, MD 21202. Phone: (800) 638-0672. Fax: (800) 447-8438. 1989.

Critical Care Medicine: Diagnosis and Management of Patients with Acute Myocardial Infarction and It's Complications. Edward P. Hoffer. Williams & Wilkins, 428 East Preston St., Baltimore, MD 21202. Phone: (800) 638-0672. Fax: (800) 447-8438. 1992.

Critical Care MEDLINE. MEP, 124 Mt. Auburn St., Cambridge, MA 02138. Phone: (800) 342-1338. Fax: (617) 868-7738. Quarterly.

Critical Care Obstetrics: Clinical Cases. Valerion A. Catanzarite. Williams & Wilkins, 428 East Preston St., Baltimore, MD 21202. Phone: (800) 638-0672. Fax: (800) 447-8438. 1989.

Critical Care Obstetrics: Obstetric Infections. Valerion A. Catanzarite. Williams & Wilkins, 428 East Preston St., Baltimore, MD 21202. Phone: (800) 638-0672. Fax: (800) 447-8438. 1989.

SCISEARCH. Institute for Scientific Information, 3501 Market St., Philadelphia, PA 19104. Phone: (215) 386-0100. Fax: (215) 386-6362.

DIRECTORIES

Critical Care Choices. Springhouse Publishing Co., 1111 Bethlehem Pike, Spring House, PA 19477. Phone: (800) 331-3170. Fax: (215) 646-8716. Annual.

HANDBOOKS, GUIDES, MANUALS, ATLASES

The Critical Care Drug Handbook. Gary P. Zaloga. Mosby-Year Book, 11830 Westline Industrial Drive, St. Louis, MO 63146. Phone: (800) 325-4177. Fax: (314) 432-1380. 1991.

Critical Care Manual: Applied Physiology and Principles of Therapy. Robert Francis Wilson. F.A. Davis Co., 1915 Arch St., Philadelphia, PA 19103. Phone: (800) 523-4049. Fax: (215) 568-5065. Second edition 1992.

Handbook of Critical Care. James L. Berk, James Sampliner. Little, Brown and Company, 34 Beacon St., Boston, MA 02108. Phone: (617) 227-0730. Third edition 1990.

Handbook of Critical Care Procedures and Therapy. Roy D. Cane, Richard Davison, Michael H. Albrink. Mosby-Year Book, 11830 Westline Industrial Drive, St. Louis, MO 63146. Phone: (800) 325-4177. Fax: (314) 432-1380. 1992.

Handbook of Pediatric Intensive Care. Mark C. Rogers (ed.). Williams & Wilkins, 428 East Preston St., Baltimore, MD 21202. Phone: (800) 638-0672. Fax: (800) 447-8438. 1989.

Postoperative Critical Care Procedures of the Massachusetts General Hospital. William Hoffman, John D. Wasnick (eds.).

Little, Brown and Company, 34 Beacon St., Boston, MA 02108. Phone: (617) 227-0730. Second edition 1992.

JOURNALS

American Journal of Critical Care. American Association of Critical Care Nurses, 101 Columbia, Aliso Viejo, CA 92656-1491. Phone: (714) 362-2000. Fax: (714) 362-2020. Bimonthly.

Care of the Critically Ill. Mosby-Year Book, 11830 Westline Industrial Drive, St. Louis, MO 63146. Phone: (800) 325-4177. Fax: (314) 432-1380. Bimonthly.

Critical Care Medicine. Williams & Wilkins, 428 E. Preston St., Baltimore, MD 21202. Phone: (800) 638-0672. Fax: (800) 447-8438. Monthly.

Heart & Lung: The Journal of Critical Care. Mosby-Year Book, 11830 Westline Industrial Drive, St. Louis, MO 63146. Phone: (800) 325-4177. Fax: (314) 432-1380. Bimonthly.

RESEARCH CENTERS, INSTITUTES, CLEARINGHOUSES

Institute of Critical Care Medicine. 1975 Zonal Ave., KAM 307B, Los Angeles, CA 90033. Phone: (213) 225-9633.

TEXTBOOKS AND MONOGRAPHS

Acute Management of the Burned Patient. J.A.J. Martyn. W.B. Saunders Co., The Curtis Center, Independence Square W., Philadelphia, PA 19106-3399. Phone: (215) 238-7800. 1990.

Chest Medicine: Essentials of Pulmonary and Critical Care Medicine. George. Williams & Wilkins, 428 East Preston St., Baltimore, MD 21202. Phone: (800) 638-0672. Fax: (800) 447-8438. Second edition 1990.

Clinical Problems in Acute Care Medicine. James J. Heffernan, Robert A. Witzburg, Alan S. Cohen. W.B. Saunders Co., The Curtis Center, Independence Square W., Philadelphia, PA 19106-3399. Phone: (215) 238-7800. 1989.

Critical Care. Joseph M. Civetta, Robert W. Taylor, Robert R. Kirby (eds.). J.B. Lippincott Co., 227 E. Washington Square, Philadelphia, PA 19106-3780. Phone: (215) 238-4200. Fax: (215) 238-4227. 1988.

Critical Care Procedures. Roy D. Crane, Michael Albrink. Mosby-Year Book, 11830 Westline Industrial Drive, St. Louis, MO 63146. Phone: (800) 325-4177. Fax: (314) 432-1380. 1992.

Critical Care Toxicology. Lewis Goldfrank, Robert Hoffman (eds.). Churchill Livingstone Inc., 650 Avenue of the Americas, New York, NY 10011. Phone: (212) 819-5400. Fax: (212) 302-6598. 1991.

Current Emergency Diagnosis and Treatment. Mary T. Ho, Charles E. Saunders. Appleton & Lange, 25 Van Zant St., East Norwalk, CT 06855. Phone: (800) 423-1359. Fax: (203) 854-9486. Fourth edition 1992.

Current Therapy in Critical Care Medicine. Joseph E. Parrillo. Mosby-Year Book, 11830 Westline Industrial Drive, St. Louis, MO 63146. Phone: (800) 325-4177. Fax: (314) 432-1380. 1991.

Intensive Care Medicine. James M. Rippe, Richard S. Irwin, Joseph S. Alpert, et. al.. Little, Brown and Company, 34 Beacon St., Boston, MA 02108. Phone: (617) 227-0730. Second edition 1991.

Pediatric Critical Care. Fuhrman. Mosby-Year Book, 11830 Westline Industrial Drive, St. Louis, MO 63146. Phone: (800) 325-4177. Fax: (314) 432-1380. 1992.

Principles of Critical Care. Jesse B. Hall, Gregory A. Schmidt, Lawrence D.H. Wood. McGraw-Hill, Inc., 1221 Avenue of the Americas, 28th Floor, New York, NY 10020. Phone: (212) 512-4228. 1992.

Pulmonary and Critical Care Medicine. Roger C. Bone (ed.). Mosby-Year Book, 11830 Westline Industrial Drive, St. Louis, MO 63146. Phone: (800) 325-4177. Fax: (314) 432-1380. 1992.

The Society of Critical Care Medicine: Textbook of Critical Care. William C. Shoemaker, Stephen Ayres, Ake Grenvik, and others. W.B. Saunders Co., The Curtis Center, Independence Square W., Philadelphia, PA 19106-3399. Phone: (215) 238-7800. Second edition 1989.

CROHN'S DISEASE

See: GASTROINTESTINAL DISORDERS

CVS (CHORIONIC VILLUS SAMPLING)

See: PRENATAL TESTING

CYSTIC FIBROSIS

ABSTRACTING, INDEXING, AND CURRENT AWARENESS PUBLICATIONS

Current Contents/Clinical Medicine. Institute for Scientific Information, 3501 Market St., Philadelphia, PA 19104. Phone: (800) 523-1850. Fax: (215) 386-6362. Weekly.

Excerpta Medica. Section 15: Chest Diseases, Thoracic Surgery and Tuberculosis. Elsevier Science Publishing Co., Inc., P.O. Box 882, Madison Square Station, New York, NY 10159-2101. Phone: (212) 989-5800. Fax: (212) 633-3990. 20/year.

Excerpta Medica. Section 22: Human Genetics. Elsevier Science Publishers, P.O. Box 882, Madison Square Station, New York, NY 10159-2101. Phone: (212) 633-3950. Fax: (212) 633-3990. 24/year.

Index Medicus. U.S. National Library of Medicine, 8600 Rockville Pike, Bethesda, MD 20894. Phone: (800) 638-8480. Monthly.

Research Alert: Cystic Fibrosis/Endocrine Disorders. Institute for Scientific Information, 3501 Market St., Philadelphia, PA 19104. Phone: (800) 523-1850. Fax: (215) 386-6362. Weekly.

Science Citation Index. Institute for Scientific Information, 3501 Market St., Philadelphia, PA 19104. Phone: (800) 523-1850. Fax: (215) 386-6362. Bimonthly.

ASSOCIATIONS, PROFESSIONAL SOCIETIES, ADVOCACY AND SUPPORT GROUPS

Cystic Fibrosis Foundation (CFF). 6931 Arlington Rd., No. 200, Bethesda, MD 20814. Phone: (800) 344-4823. Fax: (301) 951-6378.

CD-ROM DATABASES

SCISEARCH. Institute for Scientific Information, 3501 Market St., Philadelphia, PA 19104. Phone: (215) 386-0100. Fax: (215) 386-6362.

JOURNALS

American Journal of Human Genetics. University of Chicago Press, P.O. Box 37005, Chicago, IL 60637. Phone: (312) 753-3347. Fax: (312) 753-0811. Monthly.

ONLINE DATABASES

EMBASE. Elsevier Science Publishing Co., Inc., P.O. Box 882, Madison Square Station, New York, NY 10159-2101. Phone: (212) 989-5800. Fax: (212) 633-3990.

MEDLINE. National Library of Medicine, 8600 Rockville Pike, Bethesda, MD 20894. Phone: (800) 638-8480.

SciSearch. Institute for Scientific Information, 3501 Market St., Philadelphia, PA 19104. Phone: (215) 386-0100. Fax: (215) 386-6362.

POPULAR WORKS AND PATIENT EDUCATION

Cystic Fibrosis. Peter Goodfellow. Oxford University Press, 200 Madison Ave., New York, NY 10016. Phone: (212) 679-7300. 1989.

Cystic Fibrosis: A Guide for Patient and Family. David M. Orenstein. Raven Press, 1185 Ave. of the Americas, New York, NY 10036. Phone: (212) 930-9500. Fax: (212) 869-3495. 1989.

Cystic Fibrosis: The Facts. Ann Harris, Maurice Super. Oxford University Press, 200 Madison Ave., New York, NY 10016. Phone: (212) 679-7300. Fax: (212) 725-2972. Second edition 1991.

RESEARCH CENTERS, INSTITUTES, CLEARINGHOUSES

Cystic Fibrosis Care, Teaching and Research Center. Emory University. 2040 Ridgewood N.E., Atlanta, GA 30322. Phone: (404) 727-5728.

Cystic Fibrosis Center. Cedars-Sinai Medical Center, Room 4430, 8700 Beverly Blvd., Los Angeles, CA 90048. Phone: (213) 855-6390. Fax: (213) 657-1778.

Cystic Fibrosis Center. University of Colorado. 4200 E. Ninth Ave., C-220, Denver, CO 80262. Phone: (303) 270-7518.

Cystic Fibrosis and Pediatric Pulmonary Center. Case Western Reserve University. 2101 Adelbert Rd., Cleveland, OH 44106. Phone: (216) 844-3267. Fax: (216) 844-5916.

Cystic Fibrosis and Pediatric Pulmonary Clinic. Indiana University. 702 Barnhill Dr., Rm. 293, Indianapolis, IN 46202. Phone: (317) 274-7208. Fax: (317) 274-4471.

Cystic Fibrosis Research Center (Chicago). Northwestern University, 2300 Children's Plaza, Chicago, IL 60614. Phone: (312) 880-4354.

Cystic Fibrosis Research Center. Duke University. P.O. Box 2994, Durham, NC 27710. Phone: (919) 684-3364.

Cystic Fibrosis Research Center. Johns Hopkins University. 212 Wood Basic Science, 725 N. Wolfe St., Baltimore, MD 21205. Phone: (301) 955-7166.

Cystic Fibrosis Research Center and Pediatric Pulmonary Disease Center. Tulane University. 1430 Tulane Ave., New Orleans, LA 70122. Phone: (504) 588-5601. Fax: (504) 588-5490.

Cystic Fibrosis Research Center. University of Pittsburgh. 3705 Fifth Ave., Pittsburgh, PA 15213. Phone: (412) 692-5630. Fax: (412) 692-6645.

Gregory Fleming James Cystic Fibrosis Research Center. University of Alabama at Birmingham. 1918 University Blvd., UAB Station, Birmingham, AL 35294-0005. Phone: (205) 934-0982. Fax: (205) 934-7593.

Pediatric Pulmonary and Cystic Fibrosis Care, Research & Teaching Center. Albany Medical College. 22 New Scotland Ave., Albany, NY 12208. Phone: (518) 432-1392. Fax: (518) 432-1395.

CYSTITIS

See: UROLOGIC DISORDERS

D

D AND C

See: GYNECOLOGIC DISORDERS;
OBSTETRICS AND GYNECOLOGY

DEAFNESS

See also: HEARING DISORDERS

ABSTRACTING, INDEXING, AND CURRENT AWARENESS PUBLICATIONS

Index Medicus. U.S. National Library of Medicine, 8600 Rockville Pike, Bethesda, MD 20894. Phone: (800) 638-8480. Monthly.

Psychological Abstracts. American Psychological Association, 1200 17th St. NW, Washington, DC 20036. Phone: (202) 955-7600. Monthly.

Science Citation Index. Institute for Scientific Information, 3501 Market St., Philadelphia, PA 19104. Phone: (800) 523-1850. Fax: (215) 386-6362. Bimonthly.

ASSOCIATIONS, PROFESSIONAL SOCIETIES, ADVOCACY AND SUPPORT GROUPS

Alexander Graham Bell Association for the Deaf (AGBAD). 3417 Volta Pl. N.W., Washington, DC 20007. Phone: (202) 337-5220.

American Society for Deaf Children. 814 Thayer Ave., Silver Spring, MD 20910. Phone: (301) 585-5400.

Better Hearing Institute. Box 1840, Washington, DC 20013. Phone: (703) 642-0580.

Deafness Research Foundation (DRF). 9 E. 38th St., 7th Flr., New York, NY 10016. Phone: (800) 535-3323. Fax: (212) 779-2125.

Helen Keller National Center for Deaf-Blind Youths and Adults (HKNC). 111 Middle Neck Rd., Sands Point, NY 11050. Phone: (516) 944-8900. Fax: (516) 944-7302.

National Association for the Deaf. 814 Thayer Rd., Silver Spring, MD 20910. Phone: (301) 587-1788.

National Hearing Aid Society (NHAS). 20361 Middlebelt Rd., Livonia, MI 48152. Phone: (313) 478-2610. Fax: (313) 478-4520.

CD-ROM DATABASES

SCISEARCH. Institute for Scientific Information, 3501 Market St., Philadelphia, PA 19104. Phone: (215) 386-0100. Fax: (215) 386-6362.

ENCYCLOPEDIAS, DICTIONARIES, WORD BOOKS

Encyclopedia of Deafness and Hearing Disorders. Carol Turkington, Allen Sussman. Facts on File, Inc., 460 Park Ave. S., New York, NY 10016-7382. Phone: (212) 683-2244. Fax: (212) 683-3633. 1992.

JOURNALS

American Annals of the Deaf. American Annals of the Deaf, KDES PAS 6, 800 Florida Ave. N.E., Washington, DC 20002. Phone: (202) 651-5340. Quarterly.

Ear and Hearing. Williams & Wilkins, 428 E. Preston St., Baltimore, MD 21202. Phone: (800) 638-0672. Fax: (800) 447-8438. Bimonthly.

Hearing Rehabilitation Quarterly. New York League for the Hard of Hearing, 71 W. 23rd St., New York, NY 10010. Phone: (212) 741-7650.

NEWSLETTERS

American Hearing Research Foundation Newsletter. American Hearing Research Foundation, 55 E. Washington St., Ste. 2022, Chicago, IL 60602. Quarterly.

Receiver. Deafness Research Foundation, 9 E. 38th St., New York, NY 10016. Phone: (212) 684-6556. Irregular.

ONLINE DATABASES

EMBASE. Elsevier Science Publishing Co., Inc., P.O. Box 882, Madison Square Station, New York, NY 10159-2101. Phone: (212) 989-5800. Fax: (212) 633-3990.

MEDLINE. National Library of Medicine, 8600 Rockville Pike, Bethesda, MD 20894. Phone: (800) 638-8480.

SciSearch. Institute for Scientific Information, 3501 Market St., Philadelphia, PA 19104. Phone: (215) 386-0100. Fax: (215) 386-6362.

POPULAR WORKS AND PATIENT EDUCATION

Living with Tinnitus. David W. Rees, Simon D. Smith. St. Martin's Press, 175 Fifth Ave., New York, NY 10010. Phone: (212) 674-5151. 1992.

RESEARCH CENTERS, INSTITUTES, CLEARINGHOUSES

Gallaudet Research Institute. Gallaudet University. 800 Florida Ave. NE, Washington, DC 20002. Phone: (202) 651-5400.

House Ear Institute. 2100 W. 3rd St., 5th Fl., Los Angeles, CA 90057. Phone: (213) 483-4431. Fax: (213) 413-6739.

National Information Center on Deafness (NICD). Gallaudet University, 800 Florida Ave. N.E., Washington, DC 20002-3625. Phone: (202) 651-5051. Fax: (202) 651-5463.

National Institute on Deafness and Other Communication Disorders Information Clearinghouse. P.O. Box 37777, Washington, DC 20013. Phone: (800) 241-1044. Fax: (301) 565-5112.

DEATH AND DYING

See also: MEDICAL ETHICS; TERMINAL CARE

ABSTRACTING, INDEXING, AND CURRENT AWARENESS PUBLICATIONS

Cumulative Index to Nursing and Allied Health Literature. Glendale Adventist Medical Center, P.O. Box 871, Glendale, CA 91209. Phone: (818) 409-8005. Bimonthly.

Index Medicus. U.S. National Library of Medicine, 8600 Rockville Pike, Bethesda, MD 20894. Phone: (800) 638-8480. Monthly.

Palliative Care Index. Medical Information Service, British Library, Boston Spa, Wetherby, W. Yorkshire LS23 7BQ, England. Phone: 0937-546039. Fax: 0937-546236. Monthly.

Psychological Abstracts. American Psychological Association, 1200 17th St. NW, Washington, DC 20036. Phone: (202) 955-7600. Monthly.

Science Citation Index. Institute for Scientific Information, 3501 Market St., Philadelphia, PA 19104. Phone: (800) 523-1850. Fax: (215) 386-6362. Bimonthly.

ASSOCIATIONS, PROFESSIONAL SOCIETIES, ADVOCACY AND SUPPORT GROUPS

Compassionate Friends. P.O. Box 3696, Oak Brook, IL 60521. Phone: (312) 990-0010.

Concern for Dying. 250 W. 57th St., New York, NY 10107. Phone: (212) 246-6962.

Foundation of Thanatology. 630 W. 168th St., New York, NY 10032. Phone: (212) 928-2066.

Hemlock Society. P.O. Box 11830, Eugene, OR 97440. Phone: (503) 342-5748.

Society for the Right to Die. 250 W. 57th St., New York, NY 10107. Phone: (212) 246-6973.

BIBLIOGRAPHIES

Bibliography of Bioethics. Kennedy Institute of Ethics, National Center for Bioethics Literature, Georgetown University, Washington, DC 20057. Phone: (202) 687-6771. Annual.

CD-ROM DATABASES

Nursing and Allied Health (CINAHL) on CD-ROM. CINAHL, 1509 Wilson Terrace, P.O. Box 871, Glendale, CA 91209-0871. Phone: (818) 409-8005.

PsycLit. SilverPlatter Information, Inc., River Ridge Office Park, 100 River Ridge Rd., Norwood, MA 02062. Phone: (617) 769-2599. Fax: (617) 769-8763. Quarterly.

SCISEARCH. Institute for Scientific Information, 3501 Market St., Philadelphia, PA 19104. Phone: (215) 386-0100. Fax: (215) 386-6362.

ONLINE DATABASES

Bioethicsline. Georgetown University, Kennedy Institute of Ethics, Center for Bioethics, Washington, DC 20057. Phone: (202) 687-3885.

EMBASE. Elsevier Science Publishing Co., Inc., P.O. Box 882, Madison Square Station, New York, NY 10159-2101. Phone: (212) 989-5800. Fax: (212) 633-3990.

MEDLINE. National Library of Medicine, 8600 Rockville Pike, Bethesda, MD 20894. Phone: (800) 638-8480.

Nursing and Allied Health (CINAHL). CINAHL, 1509 Wilson Terrace, P.O. Box 871, Glendale, CA 91209-0871. Phone: (818) 409-8005.

PsycInfo. SilverPlatter Information, Inc., River Ridge Office Park, 100 River Ridge Rd., Norwood, MA 02062. Phone: (617) 769-2599. Fax: (617) 769-8763. Quarterly.

SciSearch. Institute for Scientific Information, 3501 Market St., Philadelphia, PA 19104. Phone: (215) 386-0100. Fax: (215) 386-6362.

POPULAR WORKS AND PATIENT EDUCATION

AIDS: The Ultimate Challenge. Elisabeth Kubler-Ross, Mal Warshaw. Macmillan Publishing Co., 866 Third Ave., New York, NY 10011. Phone: (800) 257-5755. 1988.

Comforting Those Who Grieve: A Guide for Helping Others. Doug Manning. HarperCollins Publishers, Inc., 10 E. 53rd St., New York, NY 10022-5299. Phone: (800) 242-7737. 1987.

Dying with Dignity: Understanding Euthanasia. Derek Humphry. Carol Publishing Group, 600 Madison Ave., 11th Flr., New York, NY 10022. Phone: (212) 486-2200. 1992.

Dying at Home: A Family Guide for Caregiving. Andrea Sankar. Johns Hopkins University Press, 701 W. 40th St., Suite 275, Baltimore, MD 21211-2190. Phone: (800) 537-5487. 1991.

Euthanasia: The Moral Issues. Robert M. Baird, Stuart E. Rosenbaum (eds.). Prometheus Books, 700 E. Amherst St., Buffalo, NY 14215. Phone: (800) 421-0351. 1989.

Final Exit: The Practicalities of Self-Deliverance and Assisted Suicide for the Dying. Derek Humphry. Bantam Books, Inc., 666 Fifth Ave., New York, NY 10103. Phone: (800) 223-6834. 1993.

The Grief Recovery Handbook: A Step-by-Step Program for Moving Beyond Loss. John W. James, Frank Cherry. HarperCollins Publishers, Inc., 10 E. 53rd St., New York, NY 10022-5299. Phone: (800) 242-7737. 1989.

The Grieving Child: A Parent's Guide. Fitzgerald. Simon & Schuster, Inc., 1230 Ave. of the Americas, New York, NY 10020. Phone: (800) 223-2348. Fax: (800) 284-0735. 1992.

Grieving: Surviving the Pain & Learning to Live Again. Catherine M. Sanders. John Wiley & Sons, Inc., 605 Third Ave., New York, NY 10158-0012. Phone: (212) 850-6000. Fax: (212) 850-6088. 1992.

How to Survive the Loss of a Love. Colgrove. Bantam Doubleday Dell, Inc., 666 Fifth Ave., New York, NY 10103. Phone: (800) 223-6834. 1991.

Living with Dying: A Loving Guide for Family and Close Friends. David Carroll. Paragon House Publishers, 90 Fifth Ave., New York, NY 10011. Phone: (800) 727-2466. Revised edition 1991.

Suddenly Alone. Gates. HarperCollins Pubs., Inc., 10 E. 53rd St., New York, NY 10022-5299. Phone: (212) 207-7000. Fax: (800) 242-7737. 1991.

Your Living Will: Why, When and How to Write One. Eileen P. Flynn. Carol Publishing Group, 600 Madison Ave., 11th Flr., New York, NY 10022. Phone: (212) 486-2200. 1992.

RESEARCH CENTERS, INSTITUTES, CLEARINGHOUSES

Center for Bioethics. Clinical Research Institute of Montreal, 110 Pine Ave. W., Montreal, PQ, Canada H2W 1R7. Phone: (514) 987-5615. Fax: (514) 987-5695.

Human Life Center. University of Steubenville, Steubenville, OH 43952. Phone: (614) 282-9953.

TEXTBOOKS AND MONOGRAPHS

Caring for the Dying Patient and the Family. J. Robbins. HarperCollins Pubs., Inc., 10 E. 53rd St., New York, NY 10022-5299. Phone: (212) 207-7000. Fax: (800) 242-7737. 2nd edition 1989.

Death, Dying, and Bereavement. L. Sherr. Blackwell Scientific Publications, Inc., 3 Cambridge Ctr., Cambridge, MA 02142. Phone: (800) 759-6102. 1989.

DEMENTIA

See also: ALZHEIMER'S DISEASE;
NEUROLOGIC DISORDERS

ABSTRACTING, INDEXING, AND CURRENT AWARENESS PUBLICATIONS

BIOSIS/CAS Selects: Alzheimer's Disease & Senile Dementias. BIOSIS, 2100 Arch St., Philadelphia, PA 19103-1399. Phone: (215) 587-4800. Fax: (215) 587-2016. Biweekly.

CA Selects: Alzheimer's Disease & Related Memory Dysfunctions. Chemical Abstracts Service, 2540 Olentangy River Road, P.O. Box 3012, Columbus, OH 43210-0012. Phone: (800) 848-6538. Biweekly.

Current Contents/Clinical Medicine. Institute for Scientific Information, 3501 Market St., Philadelphia, PA 19104. Phone: (800) 523-1850. Fax: (215) 386-6362. Weekly.

Current Contents/Life Sciences. Institute for Scientific Information, 3501 Market St., Philadelphia, PA 19104. Phone: (215) 386-0100. Fax: (215) 386-6362.

Index Medicus. U.S. National Library of Medicine, 8600 Rockville Pike, Bethesda, MD 20894. Phone: (800) 638-8480. Monthly.

Psychological Abstracts. American Psychological Association, 1200 17th St. NW, Washington, DC 20036. Phone: (202) 955-7600. Monthly.

Science Citation Index. Institute for Scientific Information, 3501 Market St., Philadelphia, PA 19104. Phone: (800) 523-1850. Fax: (215) 386-6362. Bimonthly.

CD-ROM DATABASES

Neuroscience Citation Index. Institute for Scientific Information, 3501 Market St., Philadelphia, PA 19104. Phone: (800) 523-1857. Fax: (215) 386-6362. Bimonthly.

SCISEARCH. Institute for Scientific Information, 3501 Market St., Philadelphia, PA 19104. Phone: (215) 386-0100. Fax: (215) 386-6362.

JOURNALS

Alzheimer's Disease and Associated Disorders - An International Journal. Raven Press, 1185 Avenue of the Americas, New York, NY 10036. Phone: (212) 930-9500. Fax: (212) 869-3495. Quarterly.

Dementia. S. Karger Publishers, Inc., 26 West Avon Rd., P.O. Box 529, Farmington, CT 06085. Phone: (203) 675-7834. Fax: (203) 675-7302. Bimonthly.

ONLINE DATABASES

EMBASE. Elsevier Science Publishing Co., Inc., P.O. Box 882, Madison Square Station, New York, NY 10159-2101. Phone: (212) 989-5800. Fax: (212) 633-3990.

MEDLINE. National Library of Medicine, 8600 Rockville Pike, Bethesda, MD 20894. Phone: (800) 638-8480.

SciSearch. Institute for Scientific Information, 3501 Market St., Philadelphia, PA 19104. Phone: (215) 386-0100. Fax: (215) 386-6362.

POPULAR WORKS AND PATIENT EDUCATION

The 36 Hour Day: A Family Guide to Caring for Persons with Alzheimer's Disease, Related Dementing Illnesses, and Memory Loss in Later Life. Nancy L. Mace, Peter V. Rabins. Johns Hopkins University Press, 701 W. 40th St., Suite 275, Baltimore, MD 21211-2190. Phone: (800) 537-5487. Second edition 1991.

Life with Charlie: Coping with an Alzheimer's Spouse or a Dementia Patient and Keeping Your Sanity. Carol Heckman-Owen. Borgo Press, P.O. Box 2845, San Bernardino, CA 92406-2845. Phone: (909) 884-5813. Fax: (909) 888-4942. 1992.

Living with Dementia. John Riordan, Bob Whitmore. St. Martin's Press, 175 Fifth Ave., New York, NY 10010. Phone: (212) 674-5151. 1992.

Taking Care of Caregivers: For Families and Others Who Care for People with Alzheimer's Disease and Other Forms of Dementia. D. Jeanne Roberts. Bull Publishing Co., 110 Gilbert Ave., Menlo Park, CA 94025. Phone: (800) 676-2855. 1991.

RESEARCH CENTERS, INSTITUTES, CLEARINGHOUSES

Center for Neurological Diseases. University of Miami. 1501 N.W. 9th Ave., P.O. Box 016960, Miami, FL 33136. Phone: (305) 547-6732.

Dementia Study Laboratory. University of Western Ontario. Dept. of Pathology, Health Sciences Center, London, ON, Canada N6A 5C1.

Winifred Masterson Burke Medical Research Institute, Inc., Dementia Research Service. Cornell University. 785 Mamaroneck Ave., White Plains, NY 10605. Phone: (914) 337-2443. Fax: (914) 946-1722.

TEXTBOOKS AND MONOGRAPHS

Aging Brain and Dementia: New Trends in Diagnosis and Therapy. L. Battistin, Franz Gerstenbrand (eds.). John Wiley & Sons, Inc., 605 Third Ave., New York, NY 10158-0012. Phone: (212) 850-6000. Fax: (212) 850-6088. 1989.

Alzheimer's Disease: Long Term Care. J. Edward Jackson, Robert Katzman, Phyllis Lessin (eds.). San Diego State University Press, 5189 College Ave., San Diego, CA 92182. Phone: (619) 594-6220. 1991.

Care-Giving in Dementia: Research and Applications. Gemma M. Jones, Bere M. Miesen (eds.). Routledge, Chapman & Hall, Inc., 29 W. 35th St., New York, NY 10001-2291. Phone: (212) 244-3336. 1991.

Dementia. Peter J. Whitehouse. F.A. Davis Co., 1915 Arch St., Philadelphia, PA 19103. Phone: (800) 523-4049. Fax: (215) 568-5065. Contemporary Neurology. Series No. 42. 1992.

Dementia and Aging: Ethics, Values and Policy Choices. Robert H. Binstock, Stephen G. Post, Peter J. Whitehouse. Johns Hopkins University Press, 701 W. 40th St., Suite 275, Baltimore, MD 21211-2190. Phone: (800) 537-5487. Fax: (410) 516-6998. 1992.

Dementia Care: Patient, Family and Community. Nancy L. Mace (ed.). Johns Hopkins University Press, 701 W. 40th St., Suite 275, Baltimore, MD 21211-2190. Phone: (800) 537-5487. Fax: (410) 516-6998. 1984.

The Dementias: Diagnosis and Treatment. Myron F. Weiner (ed.). American Psychiatric Press, Inc., 1400 K St. NW, Washington, DC 20005. Phone: (202) 682-6268. Fax: (202) 789-2648. 1991.

DENTAL ASSISTING

See also: ALLIED HEALTH EDUCATION

ABSTRACTING, INDEXING, AND CURRENT AWARENESS PUBLICATIONS

Cumulative Index to Nursing and Allied Health Literature. Glendale Adventist Medical Center, P.O. Box 871, Glendale, CA 91209. Phone: (818) 409-8005. Bimonthly.

Dental Abstracts. Mosby-Year Book, 11830 Westline Industrial Drive, St. Louis, MO 63146. Phone: (800) 325-4177. Fax: (314) 432-1380. Bimonthly.

Index to Dental Literature. American Dental Association, 211 E. Chicago Ave., Chicago, IL 60611-2678. Phone: (800) 947-4746. Fax: (312) 440-3542. Quarterly.

ASSOCIATIONS, PROFESSIONAL SOCIETIES, ADVOCACY AND SUPPORT GROUPS

American Dental Assistants Association (ADAA). 919 N. Michigan Ave., Ste. 3400, Chicago, IL 60611. Phone: (312) 664-3327. Fax: (312) 664-5288.

American Dental Hygienists' Association (ADHA). 444 N. Michigan Ave., Ste. 3400, Chicago, IL 60611. Phone: (800) 243-ADHA. Fax: (312) 440-8929.

Dental Assisting National Board (DANB). 216 E. Ontario St., Chicago, IL 60611. Phone: (312) 642-3368.

National Association of Dental Assistants. 900 S. Washington St., No. G-13, Falls Church, VA 22046. Phone: (703) 237-8616.

BIBLIOGRAPHIES

Current Titles in Dentistry. Munksgaard International Publishers Ltd., P.O. Box 2148, DK-1016, Copenhagen K, Denmark. Phone: 33-127030. Fax: 33-129387. Monthly.

CD-ROM DATABASES

Nursing and Allied Health (CINAHL) on CD-ROM. CINAHL, 1509 Wilson Terrace, P.O. Box 871, Glendale, CA 91209-0871. Phone: (818) 409-8005.

ENCYCLOPEDIAS, DICTIONARIES, WORD BOOKS

A Concise Illustrated Dental Dictionary. F.J. Harty, R. Ogston. Butterworth-Heinemann, 80 Montvale Ave., Stoneham, MA 02180. Phone: (617) 438-8464. Fax: (617) 279-4851. 1987.

Jablonski's Dictionary of Dentistry. Stanley Jablonski. Krieger Publishing Co., P.O. Box 9542, Melbourne, FL 32902-9542. Phone: (407) 724-9542. Fax: (407) 951-3671. 2993.

Mosby's Medical, Nursing, and Allied Health Dictionary. Kenneth N. Anderson, Lois Anderson, Walter D. Glanze (eds.). Mosby-Year Book, 11830 Westline Industrial Dr., St. Louis, MO 63146. Phone: (800) 325-4177. Fax: (314) 432-1380. Third edition 1990.

ONLINE DATABASES

Nursing and Allied Health (CINAHL). CINAHL, 1509 Wilson Terrace, P.O. Box 871, Glendale, CA 91209-0871. Phone: (818) 409-8005.

TEXTBOOKS AND MONOGRAPHS

Clinical Practice of the Dental Hygienist. Esther M. Wilkins. Williams & Wilkins, 428 E. Preston St., Baltimore, MD 21202. Phone: (800) 638-0672. Fax: (800) 447-8438. Sixth edition 1989.

The Dental Assistant. Roger E. Barton, Stephen R. Matteson, Richard Richardson. Williams & Wilkins, 428 E. Preston St., Baltimore, MD 21202. Phone: (800) 638-0672. Fax: (800) 447-8438. Sixth edition 1988.

Essentials of Dental Assisting. Ann Ehrlich, Hazel O. Torres. W.B. Saunders Co., The Curtis Center, Independence Square W., Philadelphia, PA 19106-3399. Phone: (215) 238-7800. 1992.

Essentials of Dental Radiography for Dental Assistants and Hygienists. Wolf R. DeLyre, Orlen N. Johnson. Appleton &

Lange, 25 Van Zant St., East Norwalk, CT 06855. Phone: (800) 423-1359. Fax: (203) 854-9486. Fourth edition 1990.

Modern Dental Assisting. Hazel O. Torres, Ann Ehrlich. W.B. Saunders Co., The Curtis Center, Independence Square W., Philadelphia, PA 19106-3399. Phone: (215) 238-7800. Fourth edition 1990.

Mosby's Comprehensive Review of Dental Hygiene. Michele Leonardi Darby, Eleanor J. Bushee (eds.). Mosby-Year Book, 11830 Westline Industrial Drive, St. Louis, MO 63146. Phone: (800) 325-4177. Fax: (314) 432-1380. Second edition 1991.

Oral Pathology for the Dental Hygienist. Olga A.C. Ibsen, Joan Andersen Phelan. W.B. Saunders Co., The Curtis Center, Independence Square W., Philadelphia, PA 19106-3399. Phone: (215) 238-7800. 1992.

Radiology for Dental Auxiliaries. Herbert H. Frommer. Mosby-Year Book, 11830 Westline Industrial Drive, St. Louis, MO 63146. Phone: (800) 325-4177. Fax: (314) 432-1380. Fifth edition 1992.

DENTAL CARE

See: DENTISTRY

DENTAL CARIES

See: DENTISTRY

DENTAL EDUCATION

ABSTRACTING, INDEXING, AND CURRENT AWARENESS PUBLICATIONS

Cumulative Index to Nursing and Allied Health Literature. Glendale Adventist Medical Center, P.O. Box 871, Glendale, CA 91209. Phone: (818) 409-8005. Bimonthly.

Dental Abstracts. Mosby-Year Book, 11830 Westline Industrial Drive, St. Louis, MO 63146. Phone: (800) 325-4177. Fax: (314) 432-1380. Bimonthly.

Index to Dental Literature. American Dental Association, 211 E. Chicago Ave., Chicago, IL 60611-2678. Phone: (800) 947-4746. Fax: (312) 440-3542. Quarterly.

Index Medicus. U.S. National Library of Medicine, 8600 Rockville Pike, Bethesda, MD 20894. Phone: (800) 638-8480. Monthly.

ASSOCIATIONS, PROFESSIONAL SOCIETIES, ADVOCACY AND SUPPORT GROUPS

American Association of Dental Schools. 1625 Massachusetts Ave. N.W., Washington, DC 20036. Phone: (202) 667-9433.

American Student Dental Association. 211 E. Chicago Ave., Suite 840, Chicago, IL 60611. Phone: (312) 440-2795.

CD-ROM DATABASES

Nursing and Allied Health (CINAHL) on CD-ROM. CINAHL, 1509 Wilson Terrace, P.O. Box 871, Glendale, CA 91209-0871. Phone: (818) 409-8005.

DIRECTORIES

American Dental Directory. American Dental Association, 211 E. Chicago Ave., Chicago, IL 60611-2678. Phone: (800) 947-4746. Fax: (312) 440-3542. Annual.

Barron's Guide to Medical and Dental Schools. Barron's Educational Series, Inc., P.O. Box 8040, 250 Wireless Blvd., Hauppauge, NY 11788. Phone: (516) 434-3311. Fax: (516) 434-3723. Biennial.

Directory of Association Offices. American Association of Dental Schools, 1625 Massachusetts Ave. N.W., Washington, DC 20036. Phone: (202) 667-9433.

Directory of Dental Educators. American Association of Dental Schools, 1625 Massachusetts Ave. N.W., Washington, DC 20036. Phone: (202) 667-9433.

JOURNALS

Journal of Dental Education. American Associatoin of Dental Schools, 1625 Massachusetts Ave. N.W., Washington, DC 20036. Phonc: (202) 667-9433. Monthly.

ONLINE DATABASES

EMBASE. Elsevier Science Publishing Co., Inc., P.O. Box 882, Madison Square Station, New York, NY 10159-2101. Phone: (212) 989-5800. Fax: (212) 633-3990.

MEDLINE. National Library of Medicine, 8600 Rockville Pike, Bethesda, MD 20894. Phonc: (800) 638-8480.

Nursing and Allied Health (CINAHL). CINAHL, 1509 Wilson Terrace, P.O. Box 871, Glendale, CA 91209-0871. Phone: (818) 409-8005.

SciSearch. Institute for Scientific Information, 3501 Market St., Philadelphia, PA 19104. Phone: (215) 386-0100. Fax: (215) 386-6362.

STANDARDS AND STATISTICS SOURCES

American Report on Dental Education. American Dental Association, 211 E. Chicago Ave., Chicago, IL 60611. Phone: (312) 440-2500. Annual.

TEXTBOOKS AND MONOGRAPHS

Dental Health Education: Theory and Practice. Christina De Biase. Williams & Wilkins, 428 E. Preston St., Baltimore, MD 21202. Phone: (800) 638-0672. Fax: (800) 447-8438. 1991.

DENTAL HYGIENE

See: DENTAL ASSISTING; DENTAL EDUCATION

DENTAL IMPLANTS

See: ORAL SURGERY

DENTAL SCHOOLS

See: DENTAL EDUCATION

DENTISTRY

See also: ENDODONTICS; MOUTH DISEASES;
ORAL SURGERY; ORTHODONTICS;
PERIODONTICS; PROSTHODONTICS

ABSTRACTING, INDEXING, AND CURRENT AWARENESS PUBLICATIONS

Current Contents/Clinical Medicine. Institute for Scientific Information, 3501 Market St., Philadelphia, PA 19104. Phone: (800) 523-1850. Fax: (215) 386-6362. Weekly.

Dental Abstracts. Mosby-Year Book, 11830 Westline Industrial Drive, St. Louis, MO 63146. Phone: (800) 325-4177. Fax: (314) 432-1380. Bimonthly.

Index to Dental Literature. American Dental Association, 211 E. Chicago Ave., Chicago, IL 60611-2678. Phone: (800) 947-4746. Fax: (312) 440-3542. Quarterly.

Index Medicus. U.S. National Library of Medicine, 8600 Rockville Pike, Bethesda, MD 20894. Phone: (800) 638-8480. Monthly.

Research Alert: Dental Medicine. Institute for Scientific Information, 3501 Market St., Philadelphia, PA 19104. Phone: (800) 523-1850. Fax: (215) 386-6362. Weekly.

ANNUALS AND REVIEWS

Dental Clinics. W.B. Saunders Co., The Curtis Center, Independence Square W., Philadelphia, PA 19106-3399. Phone: (215) 238-7800. Quarterly.

Year Book of Dentistry. Mosby-Year Book, 11830 Westline Industrial Drive, St. Louis, MO 63146. Phone: (800) 325-4177. Fax: (314) 432-1380. Annual.

ASSOCIATIONS, PROFESSIONAL SOCIETIES, ADVOCACY AND SUPPORT GROUPS

Academy of General Dentistry (AGD). 211 E. Chicago Ave., Ste. 1200, Chicago, IL 60611. Phone: (312) 440-4300.

American Academy of Pediatric Dentistry (AAPD). 211 E. Chicago Ave., Ste. 1036, Chicago, IL 60611. Phone: (312) 337-2169.

American Dental Association (ADA). 211 E. Chicago Ave., Chicago, IL 60611. Phone: (312) 440-2500.

American Society of Dentistry for Children. 211 E. Chicago Ave., Ste. 1430, Chicago, IL 60611. Phone: (312) 943-1244. Fax: (312) 943-5341.

Canadian Dental Association. 1815 Alta Vista Dr., Ottawa, ON, Canada KIG 3Y6. Phone: (613) 523-1770.

BIBLIOGRAPHIES

Current Titles in Dentistry. Munksgaard International Publishers Ltd., P.O. Box 2148, DK-1016, Copenhagen K, Denmark. Phone: 33-127030. Fax: 33-129387. Monthly.

Dentistry Journals and Serials: An Analytical Guide. Greenwood Publishing Group, Inc., 88 Post Rd. W., P.O. Box 5007, Westport, CT 06881. Phone: (203) 226-3571. 1985.

DIRECTORIES

American Dental Directory. American Dental Association, 211 E. Chicago Ave., Chicago, IL 60611-2678. Phone: (800) 947-4746. Fax: (312) 440-3542. Annual.

ENCYCLOPEDIAS, DICTIONARIES, WORD BOOKS

A Concise Illustrated Dental Dictionary. F.J. Harty, R. Ogston. Butterworth-Heinemann, 80 Montvale Ave., Stoneham, MA 02180. Phone: (617) 438-8464. Fax: (617) 279-4851. 1987.

Dental and Otolaryngology Word Book. Helen E. Littrell. Springhouse Publishing Co., 1111 Bethlehem Pike, Spring House, PA 19477. Phone: (800) 331-3170. Fax: (215) 646-8716. 1992.

Jablonski's Dictionary of Dentistry. Stanley Jablonski. Krieger Publishing Co., P.O. Box 9542, Melbourne, FL 32902-9542. Phone: (407) 724-9542. Fax: (407) 951-3671. 2993.

HANDBOOKS, GUIDES, MANUALS, ATLASES

A Color Atlas of Conservative Dentistry. J. Ralph Grundy, John Glyn Jones. Mosby-Year Book, 11830 Westline Industrial Drive, St. Louis, MO 63146. Phone: (800) 325-4177. Fax: (314) 432-1380. Second edition 1992.

JOURNALS

Anesthesia Progress. Elsevier Science Publishing Co., Inc., P.O. Box 882, Madison Square Station, New York, NY 10159-2101. Phone: (212) 989-5800. Fax: (212) 633-3990. Bimonthly.

British Dental Journal. BMJ Publishing Group, BMA House, Tavistock Square, London WC1H 9JR, England. Phone: 071-383 6244/6638. Fax: 071-383 6662. 22/year.

General Dentistry: Journal of the Academy of General Dentistry. Academy of General Dentistry, 211 E. Chicago Ave., Suite 1200, Chicago, IL 60611-2670. Phone: (312) 440-4300. Fax: (312) 440-4315. Bimonthly.

Implant Dentistry. Williams & Wilkins, 428 E. Preston St., Baltimore, MD 21202. Phone: (800) 638-0672. Fax: (800) 447-8438. Quarterly.

Journal of the American Dental Association. American Dental Association, 211 E. Chicago Ave., Chicago, IL 60611-2678. Phone: (800) 947-4746. Fax: (312) 440-3542. Monthly.

Journal of Dental Research. American Association for Dental Research, 1111 14th St. N.W., Suite 1000, Washington, DC 20005. Phone: (202) 898-1050.

Journal of Dentistry. Butterworth-Heinemann, 80 Montvale Ave., Stoneham, MA 02180. Phone: (617) 438-8464. Fax: (617) 279-4851. Bimonthly.

Oral Surgery, Oral Medicine, Oral Pathology. Mosby-Year Book, 11830 Westline Industrial Drive, St. Louis, MO 63146. Phone: (800) 325-4177. Fax: (314) 432-1380. Monthly.

NEWSLETTERS

Cosmetic Dentistry for GPs. American Health Consultants, Department C1290, P.O. Box 740060, Atlanta, GA 30374. Phone: (800) 559-1032. Monthly.

ONLINE DATABASES

EMBASE. Elsevier Science Publishing Co., Inc., P.O. Box 882, Madison Square Station, New York, NY 10159-2101. Phone: (212) 989-5800. Fax: (212) 633-3990.

MEDLINE. National Library of Medicine, 8600 Rockville Pike, Bethesda, MD 20894. Phone: (800) 638-8480.

SciSearch. Institute for Scientific Information, 3501 Market St., Philadelphia, PA 19104. Phone: (215) 386-0100. Fax: (215) 386-6362.

POPULAR WORKS AND PATIENT EDUCATION

Complete Guide to Dental Health: How to Avoid Being Overcharged and Overtreated. Jay Friedman. Consumer Reports Books, 9180 LeSaint Dr., Fairfield, OH 45014. Phone: (513) 860-1178. 1991.

The Mount Sinai Medical Center Family Guide to Dental Health. Jack Klatell, Andrew Kaplan, Gray Williams Jr.. Macmillan Publishing Co., Inc., 866 Third Ave., New York, NY 10022. Phone: (800) 257-5755. 1992.

TMJ Book. Andrew Kaplan, Gray Williams, Jr.. Pharos Books, 200 Park Ave., New York, NY 10166. Phone: (212) 692-3830. 1988.

RESEARCH CENTERS, INSTITUTES, CLEARINGHOUSES

National Institute of Dental Research. NIH Bldg. 31, Rm. 2C-35, 9000 Rockville Pike, Bethesda, MD 20892. Phone: (301) 496-4261.

TEXTBOOKS AND MONOGRAPHS

Burket's Oral Medicine. Malcolm A. Lynch, Vernon J. Brightman, Martin Greenberg. J.B. Lippincott Co., 227 East Washington Square, Philadelphia, PA 19106-3780. Phone: (215) 238-4200. Fax: (215) 238-4227. Ninth edition 1992.

Clark's Clinical Dentistry. Jefferson F. Hardon (ed.). J.B. Lippincott Co., 227 East Washington Square, Philadelphia, PA 19106-3780. Phone: (215) 238-4200. Fax: (215) 238-4227. Five volumes. 1992. Annual update.

Dental Anatomy. Woelfel. Williams & Wilkins, 428 E. Preston St., Baltimore, MD 21202. Phone: (800) 638-0672. Fax: (800) 447-8438. Fourth edition 1992.

Kraus' Dental Anatomy and Occlusion. Jordan. Mosby-Year Book, 11830 Westline Industrial Drive, St. Louis, MO 63146. Phone: (800) 325-4177. Fax: (314) 432-1380. 1991.

Principles and Practice of Operative Dentistry. Charbeneau. Williams & Wilkins, 428 East Preston St., Baltimore, MD 21202. Phone: (800) 638-0672. Fax: (800) 447-8438. 1988.

Risk Markers for Oral Diseases. Volume 1: Dental Caries. N.W. Johnson (ed.). Cambridge University Press, 40 W. 20th St., New York, NY 10011. Phone: (800) 431-1580. 1991.

Skinner's Science of Dental Materials. Ralph W. Phillips. W.B. Saunders Co., The Curtis Center, Independence Square W.,

Philadelphia, PA 19106-3399. Phone: (215) 238-7800. Ninth edition 1991.

DEPRESSION

See also: MOOD DISORDERS; PSYCHIATRIC DISORDERS

ABSTRACTING, INDEXING, AND CURRENT AWARENESS PUBLICATIONS

Current Contents/Clinical Medicine. Institute for Scientific Information, 3501 Market St., Philadelphia, PA 19104. Phone: (800) 523-1850. Fax: (215) 386-6362. Weekly.

Index Medicus. U.S. National Library of Medicine, 8600 Rockville Pike, Bethesda, MD 20894. Phone: (800) 638-8480. Monthly.

Psychological Abstracts. American Psychological Association, 1200 17th St. NW, Washington, DC 20036. Phone: (202) 955-7600. Monthly.

Research Alert: Antidepressants. Institute for Scientific Information, 3501 Market St., Philadelphia, PA 19104. Phone: (800) 523-1850. Fax: (215) 386-6362. Weekly.

Science Citation Index. Institute for Scientific Information, 3501 Market St., Philadelphia, PA 19104. Phone: (800) 523-1850. Fax: (215) 386-6362. Bimonthly.

ASSOCIATIONS, PROFESSIONAL SOCIETIES, ADVOCACY AND SUPPORT GROUPS

American Psychiatric Association (APA). 1400 K St. N.W., Washington, DC 20005. Phone: (202) 682-6000. Fax: (202) 682-6114.

Canadian Psychiatric Association. 294 Albert St., Suite 204, Ottawa, ON, Canada K1P 6E6. Phone: (613) 234-2815. Fax: (613) 234-9857.

Canadian Psychological Association. Chemin Vincent, Old Chelsea, PQ, Canada J0X 2N0. Phone: (819) 827-3927. Fax: (819) 827-4639.

Foundation for Depression and Manic Depression (FDMD). 7 E. 67th St., New York, NY 10021. Phone: (212) 772-3400.

National Alliance for the Mentally Ill (NAMI). 2101 Wilson Blvd., Ste. 302, Arlington, VA 22201. Phone: (703) 524-7600. Fax: (703) 524-9094.

National Depressive and Manic Depressive Association (NDMDA). 53 W. Jackson Blvd., Ste. 505, Chicago, IL 60604. Phone: (312) 939-2442. Fax: (312) 939-1241.

National Foundation for Depressive Illness. 245 Seventh Ave., New York, NY 10001. Phone: (212) 620-7637.

National Mental Health Association (NMHA). 1021 Prince St., Alexandria, VA 22314-2971. Phone: (703) 684-7722. Fax: (703) 684-5968.

CD-ROM DATABASES

Excerpta Medica CD: Psychiatry. SilverPlatter Information, Inc., River Ridge Office Park, 100 River Ridge Rd., Norwood, MA 02062. Phone: (617) 769-2599. Fax: (617) 769-8763. Quarterly.

PsycLit. SilverPlatter Information, Inc., River Ridge Office Park, 100 River Ridge Rd., Norwood, MA 02062. Phone: (617) 769-2599. Fax: (617) 769-8763. Quarterly.

SCISEARCH. Institute for Scientific Information, 3501 Market St., Philadelphia, PA 19104. Phone: (215) 386-0100. Fax: (215) 386-6362.

ENCYCLOPEDIAS, DICTIONARIES, WORD BOOKS

The Encyclopedia of Depression. Roberta Roesch, Stanley W. Jackson. Facts on File, Inc., 460 Park Ave. S., New York, NY 10016-7382. Phone: (212) 683-2244. Fax: (212) 683-3633. 1990.

Psychiatry Words. Stedman. Williams & Wilkins, 428 East Preston St., Baltimore, MD 21202. Phone: (800) 638-0672. Fax: (800) 447-8438. 1992.

HANDBOOKS, GUIDES, MANUALS, ATLASES

Getting Help: A Consumer's Guide to Therapy. Christine Amner. Paragon House Publishers, 90 Fifth Ave., New York, NY 10011. Phone: (800) 727-2466. 1991.

JOURNALS

Harvard Review of Psychiatry. Mosby-Year Book, 11830 Westline Industrial Drive, St. Louis, MO 63146. Phone: (800) 325-4177. Fax: (314) 432-1380. Bimonthly.

Journal of Affective Disorders. Elsevier Science Publishing Co., Inc., P.O. Box 882, Madison Square Station, New York, NY 10159-2101. Phone: (212) 989-5800. Fax: (212) 633-3990. 12/year.

NEWSLETTERS

Harvard Mental Health Letter. Harvard Medical School Publications Group, 164 Longwood Ave., Boston, MA 02115. Monthly.

ONLINE DATABASES

EMBASE. Elsevier Science Publishing Co., Inc., P.O. Box 882, Madison Square Station, New York, NY 10159-2101. Phone: (212) 989-5800. Fax: (212) 633-3990.

MEDLINE. National Library of Medicine, 8600 Rockville Pike, Bethesda, MD 20894. Phone: (800) 638-8480.

Mental Health Abstracts. IFI/Plenum Data Company, 302 Swann Ave., Alexandria, VA 22301. Phone: (800) 368-3093. Monthly.

PsycInfo. SilverPlatter Information, Inc., River Ridge Office Park, 100 River Ridge Rd., Norwood, MA 02062. Phone: (617) 769-2599. Fax: (617) 769-8763. Quarterly.

SciSearch. Institute for Scientific Information, 3501 Market St., Philadelphia, PA 19104. Phone: (215) 386-0100. Fax: (215) 386-6362.

POPULAR WORKS AND PATIENT EDUCATION

Depression. Dianne Hales. Chelsea House Pubs., 95 Madison Ave., New York, NY 10016. Phone: (212) 683-4400. 1989.

Depression after Childbirth: How to Recognize and Treat Postnatal Depression. Katharina Dalton. Oxford University

Press, 200 Madison Ave., New York, NY 10016. Phone: (212) 679-7300. 1989.

Depression and Its Treatment. John H. Greist, James W. Jefferson. American Psychiatric Press, Inc., 1400 K St. NW, Washington, DC 20005. Phone: (202) 682-6268. Fax: (202) 789-2648. Revised edition 1992.

Feeling Good: The New Mood Therapy. Burns. Avon Books, 1350 Ave. of the Americas, 2nd Flr., New York, NY 10019. Phone: (800) 238-0658. 1992.

Free Yourself from Depression. Michael D. Yapko. Rodale Press, Inc., 33 E. Minor St., Emmaus, PA 18098. Phone: (800) 527-8200. Fax: (215) 967-6263. 1992.

Overcoming Depression. Demitri Papolos, Janice Papolos. HarperCollins Pubs., Inc., 10 E. 53rd St., New York, NY 10022-5299. Phone: (212) 207-7000. Fax: (800) 242-7737. Revised edition 1992.

Seasonal Affective Disorder: Winter Depression: Who Gets It, What Causes It, How to Cure It. Angela Smyth, Chris Thompson. HarperCollins Pubs., Inc., 10 E. 53rd St., New York, NY 10022-5299. Phone: (212) 207-7000. Fax: (800) 242-7737. 1992.

Your Skin: From Acne to Zits. Jerome Z. Litt. W.W. Norton & Co., Inc., 500 Fifth Ave., New York, NY 10110. Phone: (800) 223-2584. 1989.

RESEARCH CENTERS, INSTITUTES, CLEARINGHOUSES

Depression Research Unit. University of Pennsylvania. School of Medicine, Dept. of Psychiatry, 3600 Spruce St., Philadelphia, PA 19104. Phone: (215) 662-3462. Fax: (215) 662-6443.

Hogg Foundation for Mental Health. University of Texas. Austin, TX 78713-7998. Phone: (512) 471-5041. Fax: (512) 471-9608.

Langley Porter Psychiatric Institute. University of California, San Francisco. 401 Parnassus Ave., San Francisco, CA 94143. Phone: (415) 476-7000.

Menninger Clinic Department of Research. Box 829, Topeka, KS 66601. Phone: (913) 273-7500. Fax: (913) 273-8625.

Missouri Institute of Mental Health. University of Missouri-Columbia. 5247 Fyler Ave., St. Louis, MO 63139-1494. Phone: (314) 644-8787. Fax: (314) 644-8834.

Psoriasis Research Institute (PRI). 600 Town and Country Village, Palo Alto, CA 94301. Phone: (415) 326-1848. Fax: (415) 326-1262.

Western Psychiatric Institute and Clinic. University of Pittsburgh. 3811 O'Hara St., Pittsburgh, PA 15213. Phone: (412) 624-2360. Fax: (412) 624-1881.

TEXTBOOKS AND MONOGRAPHS

Antidepressants: Thirty Years On. B. Leonard, P.S.J. Spencer (eds.). Rapid Communications of Oxford Ltd., The Old Malthouse, Paradise St., Oxford OX1 1LD, England. Phone: 44-865-790447. Fax: 44-865-244012. 1992.

Clinical Guide to Depression in Children and Adolescents. Mohammad Shafii, Sharon Lee Shafii (eds.). American

Psychiatric Press, Inc., 1400 K St. NW, Washington, DC 20005. Phone: (202) 682-6268. Fax: (202) 789-2648. 1991.

Combined Pharmacotherapy and Psychotherapy for Depression. Donna Manning, Allen J. Frances (eds.). American Psychiatric Press, Inc., 1400 K St. NW, Washington, DC 20005. Phone: (202) 682-6268. Fax: (202) 789-2648. 1990.

Depression and Mania. Anastasios Georgotas, Robert Cancro (eds.). Elsevier Science Publishing Co., Inc., P.O. Box 882, Madison Square Station, New York, NY 10159-2101. Phone: (212) 989-5800. Fax: (212) 633-3990. 1988.

Depressive Disorders: Facts, Theories, and Treatment Methods. Benjamin B. Wolman, George Striker (eds.). John Wiley & Sons, Inc., 605 Third Ave., New York, NY 10158-0012. Phone: (212) 850-6000. Fax: (212) 850-6088. 1990.

Refractory Depression. Jay D. Amsterdam. Raven Press, 1185 Avenue of the Americas, New York, NY 10036. Phone: (212) 930-9500. Fax: (212) 869-3495. Advances in Neuropsychiatry and Psychopharmacology. Volume 2. 1991.

Treatment Strategies for Refractory Depression. Steven P. Roose, Alexander H. Glassman (eds.). American Psychiatric Press, Inc., 1400 K St. NW, Washington, DC 20005. Phone: (202) 682-6268. Fax: (202) 789-2648. 1990.

DERMABRASION

See: PLASTIC AND COSMETIC SURGERY

DERMATITIS

See: DERMATOLOGIC DISEASES

DERMATOLOGIC DISEASES

ABSTRACTING, INDEXING, AND CURRENT AWARENESS PUBLICATIONS

Current Contents/Clinical Medicine. Institute for Scientific Information, 3501 Market St., Philadelphia, PA 19104. Phone: (800) 523-1850. Fax: (215) 386-6362. Weekly.

Excerpta Medica. Section 13: Dermatology and Venereology. Elsevier Science Publishing Co., Inc., P.O. Box 882, Madison Square Station, New York, NY 10159-2101. Phone: (212) 989-5800. Fax: (212) 633-3990. 16/year.

Index Medicus. U.S. National Library of Medicine, 8600 Rockville Pike, Bethesda, MD 20894. Phone: (800) 638-8480. Monthly.

Research Alert: Dermatology. Institute for Scientific Information, 3501 Market St., Philadelphia, PA 19104. Phone: (800) 523-1850. Fax: (215) 386-6362. Weekly.

ANNUALS AND REVIEWS

Current Problems in Dermatology. Mosby-Year Book, 11830 Westline Industrial Drive, St. Louis, MO 63146. Phone: (800) 325-4177. Fax: (314) 432-1380. Bimonthly.

Dermatologic Clinics. W.B. Saunders Co., The Curtis Center, Independence Square W., Philadelphia, PA 19106-3399. Phone: (215) 238-7800. Quarterly.

ASSOCIATIONS, PROFESSIONAL SOCIETIES, ADVOCACY AND SUPPORT GROUPS

National Alopecia Areata Foundation (NAAF). 714 C St., Ste. 216, San Rafael, CA 94901. Phone: (415) 456-4644. Fax: (415) 456-4274.

National Psoriasis Foundation (NPF). 6443 S.W. Beaverton Hwy., Ste. 210, Portland, OR 97221. Phone: (503) 297-1545. Fax: (503) 292-9341.

CD-ROM DATABASES

Year Books on Disc. CMC ReSearch, Inc., 7150 S.W. Hampton, Suite C-120, Portland, OR 97223. Phone: (800) 262-7668. Fax: (503) 639-1796. Annual includes Year Books of Cardiology, Dermatology, Diagnostic Radiology, Drug Therapy, Emergency Medicine, Family Practice, Medicine, Neurology and Neurosurgery, Obstetrics and Gynecology, Oncology, Pediatrics, and Psychiatry and Applied Mental Health.

ENCYCLOPEDIAS, DICTIONARIES, WORD BOOKS

Dictionary of Dermatological Terms. Carter. Williams & Wilkins, 428 East Preston St., Baltimore, MD 21202. Phone: (800) 638-0672. Fax: (800) 447-8438. Fourth edition 1992.

HANDBOOKS, GUIDES, MANUALS, ATLASES

An Atlas of Psoriasis. L. Fry. The Parthenon Publishing Group, Inc., 120 Mill Rd., Park Ridge, NJ 07656. Phone: (201) 391-6796. 1992.

Color Atlas of Allergic Skin Disorders. Rino Cerio, William F. Jackson. Mosby-Year Book, 11830 Westline Industrial Drive, St. Louis, MO 63146. Phone: (800) 325-4177. Fax: (314) 432-1380. 1992.

Color Atlas of Pediatric Dermatology. Samuel Weinberg, Neil S. Prose. McGraw-Hill, Inc., Health Professions Division, 1221 Avenue of the Americas, 28th Floor, New York, NY 10020. Phone: (212) 512-4228. Second edition 1990.

Color Atlas and Synopsis of Clinical Dermatology. Thomas B. Fitzpatrick, Richard A. Johnson, Machie Polano. McGraw-Hill, Inc., 1221 Avenue of the Americas, 28th Floor, New York, NY 10020. Phone: (212) 512-4228. Second edition 1992.

CRC Handbook of Contact Dermatitis. Howard Maibach, Daniel Hogan, Christopher Dannaker. CRC Press, Inc., 2000 Corporate Blvd. N.W., Boca Raton, FL 33431. Phone: (407) 994-0555. Fax: (407) 997-0949. 1992.

Handbook of Skin Clues of Systemic Diseases. Paul H. Jacobs, Todd S. Anhalt. Williams & Wilkins, 428 East Preston St., Baltimore, MD 21202. Phone: (800) 638-0672. Fax: (800) 447-8438. 1992.

Manual of Skin Diseases. Gordon C. Sauer. J.B. Lippincott Co., 227 East Washington Square, Philadelphia, PA 19106-3780. Phone: (215) 238-4200. Fax: (215) 238-4227. Sixth edition 1991.

Pinkus' Guide to Dermatohistopathology. Amir Mehregan, Ken Hashimoto. Appleton & Lange, 25 Van Zant St., East Norwalk, CT 06855. Phone: (800) 423-1359. Fax: (203) 854-9486. 1991.

JOURNALS

Clinics in Dermatolgy. Elsevier Science Publishing Co., Inc., P.O. Box 882, Madison Square Station, New York, NY 10159-2101. Phone: (212) 989-5800. Fax: (212) 633-3990. 4/year.

Journal of the American Academy of Dermatology. Mosby-Year Book, 11830 Westline Industrial Drive, St. Louis, MO 63146. Phone: (800) 325-4177. Fax: (314) 432-1380. Monthly.

Journal of the European Academy of Dermatology and Venereology. Elsevier Science Publishing Co., Inc., P.O. Box 882, Madison Square Station, New York, NY 10159-2101. Phone: (212) 989-5800. Fax: (212) 633-3990. 4/year.

NEWSLETTERS

National Psoriasis Foundation-Bulletin. National Psoriasis Foundation, 6553 S.W. Beaverton Hwy., Ste. 210, Portland, OR 97221. Phone: (503) 297-1545. Fax: (503) 292-9341. Bimonthly.

ONLINE DATABASES

Combined Health Information Database (CHID). U.S. National Institutes of Health, P.O. Box NDIC, Bethesda, MD 20892. Phone: (301) 496-2162. Fax: (301) 770-5164. Quarterly.

EMBASE. Elsevier Science Publishing Co., Inc., P.O. Box 882, Madison Square Station, New York, NY 10159-2101. Phone: (212) 989-5800. Fax: (212) 633-3990.

MEDLINE. National Library of Medicine, 8600 Rockville Pike, Bethesda, MD 20894. Phone: (800) 638-8480.

SciSearch. Institute for Scientific Information, 3501 Market St., Philadelphia, PA 19104. Phone: (215) 386-0100. Fax: (215) 386-6362.

POPULAR WORKS AND PATIENT EDUCATION

Healthy Skin. Consumer Reports Books, 9180 LeSaint Dr., Fairfield, OH 45014. Phone: (513) 860-1178. 1989.

Take Care of Your Skin. Elaine Brumberg. HarperCollins Publishers, Inc., 10 E. 53rd St., New York, NY 10022-5299. Phone: (800) 242-7737. 1990.

Treating Acne: A Guide for Teens and Adults. Richard A. Walzer. Consumer Reports Books, 9180 LeSaint Dr., Fairfield, OH 45014. Phone: (513) 860-1178. 1992.

RESEARCH CENTERS, INSTITUTES, CLEARINGHOUSES

Laboratory of Dermatology Research. Memorial Sloan-Kettering Cancer Center, 1275 York Ave., New York, NY 10021. Phone: (212) 794-8143.

Laboratory of Investigative Dermatology. Rockefeller University, 1230 York Ave., New York, NY 10021. Phone: (212) 870-8000.

National Arthritis and Musculoskeletal and Skin Diseases Information Clearinghouse (NAMSIC). 9000 Rockville Pike, P.O. Box AMS, Bethesda, MD 20892. Phone: (301) 495-4484. Fax: (301) 587-4352.

TEXTBOOKS AND MONOGRAPHS

Andrews' Diseases of the Skin: Clinical Dermatology. Harry L. Arnold, Richard B. Odom, William D. James. W.B. Saunders Co., The Curtis Center, Independence Square W., Philadelphia, PA 19106-3399. Phone: (215) 238-7800. Eighth edition 1990.

Clinical Dermatology. Harvey Baker. W.B. Saunders Co., The Curtis Center, Independence Square W., Philadelphia, PA 19106-3399. Phone: (215) 238-7800. Fourth edition 1989.

Clinical Dermatology: A Color Guide to Diagnosis and Therapy. Thomas P. Habif. Mosby-Year Book, 11830 Westline Industrial Drive, St. Louis, MO 63146. Phone: (800) 325-4177. Fax: (314) 432-1380. Second edition 1990.

Clinical Dermatology: An Illustrated Textbook. Rona M. Mackie. Oxford University Press, 200 Madison Ave., New York, NY 10016. Phone: (212) 679-7300. Third edition 1991.

Cosmetic Surgery of the Skin. Coleman. Mosby-Year Book, 11830 Westline Industrial Drive, St. Louis, MO 63146. Phone: (800) 325-4177. Fax: (314) 432-1380. 1991.

Current Dermatologic Therapy 2. Stuart Maddin. W.B. Saundres Co., The Curtis Center, Independence Square W., Philadelphia, PA 19106-3399. Phone: (215) 238-7800. 1991.

Dermatology. Milton Orkin, Howard I. Maibach, Mark V. Dahl (eds.). Appleton & Lange, 25 Van Zant Street, East Norwalk, CT 06855. Phone: (800) 423-1359. Fax: (203) 854-9486. 1990.

Dermatology: Diagnosis and Therapy. Edward E. Bondi, Brian V. Jegasothy, Gerald S. Lazarus (eds.). Appleton & Lange, 25 Van Zant Street, East Norwalk, CT 06855. Phone: (800) 423-1359. Fax: (203) 854-9486. 1991.

Differential Diagnosis in Dermatology. Richard Ashton, Barbara Leppard. J.B. Lippincott Co., 227 E. Washington Square, Philadelphia, PA 19106-3780. Phone: (215) 238-4200. Fax: (215) 238-4227. 1990.

Mohs Micrographic Surgery. George R. Mikhail (ed.). W.B. Saunders Co., The Curtis Center, Independence Square W., Philadelphia, PA 19106-3399. Phone: (215) 238-7800. 1991.

Practical Dermatology. Adam O. Glodstein, Beth G. Goldstein. Mosby-Year Book, 11830 Westline Industrial Drive, St. Louis, MO 63146. Phone: (800) 325-4177. Fax: (314) 432-1380. 1992.

Principles of Dermatology. Donald P. Lookingbill, James G. Marks. W.B. Saunders Company, The Curtis Center, Independence Square W., Philadelphia, PA 19106-3399. Phone: (215) 238-7800. 1986.

Principles and Practice of Dermatology. W. Mitchell Sams Jr., Peter J. Lynch (eds.). Churchill Livingstone Inc., 650 Avenue of the Americas, New York, NY 10011. Phone: (212) 819-5400. Fax: (212) 302-6598. 1990.

Systemic Drugs for Skin Disease. Stephen E. Wolverton, Jonathan K. Wilkin (eds.). W.B. Saunders Co., The Curtis Center, Independence Sqare W., Philadelphia, PA 19106-3399. Phone: (215) 238-7800. 1991.

Textbook of Dermatology. A. Rook. Mosby-Year Book, 11830 Westline Industrial Drive, St. Louis, MO 63146. Phone: (800) 325-4177. Fax: (314) 432-1380. Fourth edition 1986.

DERMATOLOGY

See also: SKIN CANCER

ABSTRACTING, INDEXING, AND CURRENT AWARENESS PUBLICATIONS

Core Journals in Dermatology. Elsevier Science Publishing Co., Inc., P.O. Box 882, Madison Square Station, New York, NY 10159-2101. Phone: (212) 989-5800. Fax: (212) 633-3990. 11/year.

Excerpta Medica. Section 13: Dermatology and Venereology. Elsevier Science Publishing Co., Inc., P.O. Box 882, Madison Square Station, New York, NY 10159-2101. Phone: (212) 989-5800. Fax: (212) 633-3990. 16/year.

Index Medicus. U.S. National Library of Medicine, 8600 Rockville Pike, Bethesda, MD 20894. Phone: (800) 638-8480. Monthly.

Research Alert: Dermatology. Institute for Scientific Information, 3501 Market St., Philadelphia, PA 19104. Phone: (800) 523-1850. Fax: (215) 386-6362. Weekly.

Science Citation Index. Institute for Scientific Information, 3501 Market St., Philadelphia, PA 19104. Phone: (800) 523-1850. Fax: (215) 386-6362. Bimonthly.

ANNUALS AND REVIEWS

Advances in Dermatology. Mosby-Year Book, 11830 Westline Inustrial Drive, St. Louis, MO 63146. Phone: (800) 325-4177. Fax: (314) 432-1380. Annual.

Current Problems in Dermatology. Mosby-Year Book, 11830 Westline Industrial Drive, St. Louis, MO 63146. Phone: (800) 325-4177. Fax: (314) 432-1380. Bimonthly.

Dermatologic Clinics. W.B. Saunders Co., The Curtis Center, Independence Square W., Philadelphia, PA 19106-3399. Phone: (215) 238-7800. Quarterly.

Recent Advances in Dermatology. Churchill Livingstone Inc., 650 Avenue of the Americas, New York, NY 10011. Phone: (212) 819-5400. Fax: (212) 302-6598. Irregular.

Year Book of Dermatologic Surgery. Mosby-Year Book, 11830 Westline Industrial Drive, St. Louis, MO 63146. Phone: (800) 325-4177. Fax: (314) 432-1380. Annual.

Year Book of Dermatology. Mosby-Year Book, 11830 Westline Industrial Drive, St. Louis, MO 63146. Phone: (800) 325-4177. Fax: (314) 432-1380. Annual.

ASSOCIATIONS, PROFESSIONAL SOCIETIES, ADVOCACY AND SUPPORT GROUPS

American Academy of Dermatology (AAD). 1567 Maple Ave., P.O. Box 3116, Evanston, IL 60201. Phone: (708) 869-3954. Fax: (708) 869-4382.

American Board of Dermatology (ABD). Henry Ford Hospital, Detroit, MI 48202. Phone: (313) 871-8739.

American Dermatological Association (ADA). Department of Dermatology, University Hospitals BT 2045-1, Iowa City, IA 52242. Phone: (319) 356-2274.

American Society for Dermatologic Surgery (ASDS). P.O. Box 3116, Evanston, IL 60204. Phone: (312) 869-3954.

Dermatology Foundation (DF). 1563 Maple Ave., Evanston, IL 60201. Phone: (312) 328-2256.

Society for Investigative Dermatology (SID). Building 100, Room 269, San Francisco General Hospital, San Francisco, CA 94110. Phone: (415) 647-3992.

Society for Pediatric Dermatology (SPD). University of Michigan Hospitals, 1910 Taubman Health Care Center, Ann Arbor, MI 48109. Phone: (313) 936-4086.

CD-ROM DATABASES

SCISEARCH. Institute for Scientific Information, 3501 Market St., Philadelphia, PA 19104. Phone: (215) 386-0100. Fax: (215) 386-6362.

Year Books on Disc. CMC ReSearch, Inc., 7150 S.W. Hampton, Suite C-120, Portland, OR 97223. Phone: (800) 262-7668. Fax: (503) 639-1796. Annual includes Year Books of Cardiology, Dermatology, Diagnostic Radiology, Drug Therapy, Emergency Medicine, Family Practice, Medicine, Neurology and Neurosurgery, Obstetrics and Gynecology, Oncology, Pediatrics, and Psychiatry and Applied Mental Health.

DIRECTORIES

Directory of Certified Dermatologists. American Board of Medical Specialties, 1 Rotary Center, Suite 805, Evanston, IL 60201. Phone: (708) 491-9091. Fax: (708) 328-3596.

Directory of Medical Specialists. Marquis Who's Who, 3002 Glenview Rd., Wilmette, IL 60091. Phone: (800) 621-9669. Fax: (708) 441-2264. Biennial.

Directory of Physicians in the United States. American Medical Association, 515 North State St., Chicago, IL 60610. Phone: (312) 464-0183. Fax: (312) 464-5834. Biennial.

ENCYCLOPEDIAS, DICTIONARIES, WORD BOOKS

Dictionary of Dermatological Terms. Carter. Williams & Wilkins, 428 East Preston St., Baltimore, MD 21202. Phone: (800) 638-0672. Fax: (800) 447-8438. Fourth edition 1992.

HANDBOOKS, GUIDES, MANUALS, ATLASES

Clinical Atlas of Dermatology. C. Ferrandiz. Mosby-Year Book, 11830 Westline Industrial Drive, St. Louis, MO 63146. Phone: (800) 325-4177. Fax: (314) 432-1380. 1987.

Color Atlas of Dermatology. G.M. Levene, D.C. Calnan. Mosby-Year Book, 11830 Westline Industrial Drive, St. Louis, MO 63146. Phone: (800) 325-4177. Fax: (314) 432-1380. 1984.

Dermatology in General Medicine. Thomas B. Fitzpatrick, Arthur Z. Eisen, Klaus Wolff, et. al.. McGraw-Hill Inc., 11 W. 19th St., New York, NY 10011. Phone: (212) 337-5001. Fax: (212) 337-4092. 2 vols. Fourth edition. 1992.

Manual of Clinical Problems in Dermatology: With Annotated Key References. Suzanne M. Olbricht, Michael E. Bigby, Kenneth A. Arndt. Little, Brown and Company, 34 Beacon St., Boston, MA 02108. Phone: (617) 227-0730. 1992.

Manual of Dermatologic Therapeutics: With Essentials of Diagnosis. Kenneth A. Arndt. Little, Brown and Company, 34 Beacon St., Boston, MA 02108. Phone: (617) 227-0730. Fourth edition 1988.

Manual of Skin Diseases. Gordon C. Sauer. J.B. Lippincott Co., 227 East Washington Square, Philadelphia, PA 19106-3780. Phone: (215) 238-4200. Fax: (215) 238-4227. Sixth edition 1991.

Pocket Guide to Dermatology. Andrew J. Scheman. Williams & Wilkins, 428 East Preston Street, Baltimore, MD 21202. Phone: (800) 638-0672. Fax: (800) 447-8438. 1990.

JOURNALS

American Academy of Dermatology Journal. Mosby-Year Book, 11830 Westline Industrial Drive, St. Louis, MO 63146. Phone: (800) 325-4177. Fax: (314) 432-1380. Monthly.

Archives of Dermatology. American Medical Association, 515 N. State St., Chicago, IL 60610. Phone: (312) 464-0183. Fax: (312) 464-5834. Monthly.

British Journal of Dermatology. Blackwell Scientific Publications Ltd., Osney Mead, Oxon. OX2 OEL, England. Phone: 0865-240201. Fax: 0865-721205. Monthly.

Clinical and Experimental Dermatology. Blackwell Scientific Publications Ltd., Osney Mead, Oxon. OX2 OEL, England. Phone: 0865-240201. Fax: 0865-721205. Bimonthly.

Clinics in Dermatolgy. Elsevier Science Publishing Co., Inc., P.O. Box 882, Madison Square Station, New York, NY 10159-2101. Phone: (212) 989-5800. Fax: (212) 633-3990. 4/year.

Cutis. Cahners Publishing Co., 249 W. 17th St., New York, NY 10011. Phone: (212) 645-0067. Fax: (212) 242-6987. Monthly.

International Journal of Dermatology. J.B. Lippincott Co., 227 East Washington Square, Philadelphia, PA 19106-3780. Phone: (215) 238-4200. Fax: (215) 238-4227. 10/year.

Journal of the American Academy of Dermatology. Mosby-Year Book, 11830 Westline Industrial Drive, St. Louis, MO 63146. Phone: (800) 325-4177. Fax: (314) 432-1380. Monthly.

Journal of Dermatologic Surgery and Oncology. Journal of Dermatologic Surgery, Inc., 245 Fifth Ave., New York, NY 10016. Phone: (212) 721-5175. Monthly.

Journal of the European Academy of Dermatology and Venereology. Elsevier Science Publishing Co., Inc., P.O. Box 882, Madison Square Station, New York, NY 10159-2101. Phone: (212) 989-5800. Fax: (212) 633-3990. 4/year.

Journal of Investigative Dermatology. Elsevier Science Publishing Co., Inc., P.O. Box 882, Madison Square Station, New York, NY 10159-2101. Phone: (212) 989-5800. Fax: (212) 633-3990. Monthly.

Seminars in Dermatology. W.B. Saunders Co., The Curtis Center, Independence Square W., Philadelphia, PA 19106-3399. Phone: (215) 238-7800. Quarterly.

ONLINE DATABASES

EMBASE. Elsevier Science Publishing Co., Inc., P.O. Box 882, Madison Square Station, New York, NY 10159-2101. Phone: (212) 989-5800. Fax: (212) 633-3990.

MEDIS. Mead Data Central, P.O. Box 1830, Dayton, OH 45401. Phone: (800) 227-4908.

MEDLINE. National Library of Medicine, 8600 Rockville Pike, Bethesda, MD 20894. Phone: (800) 638-8480.

SciSearch. Institute for Scientific Information, 3501 Market St., Philadelphia, PA 19104. Phone: (215) 386-0100. Fax: (215) 386-6362.

POPULAR WORKS AND PATIENT EDUCATION

Your Skin: From Acne to Zits. Jerome Z. Litt. W.W. Norton & Co., Inc., 500 Fifth Ave., New York, NY 10110. Phone: (800) 223-2584. 1989.

RESEARCH CENTERS, INSTITUTES, CLEARINGHOUSES

Immunodermatology Center. University of Texas. Southwestern Medical Center, 5323 Harry Hines Blvd., Dermatology Department, Dallas, TX 75235. Phone: (214) 688-2969.

Psoriasis Research Institute (PRI). 600 Town and Country Village, Palo Alto, CA 94301. Phone: (415) 326-1848. Fax: (415) 326-1262.

DIABETES

ABSTRACTING, INDEXING, AND CURRENT AWARENESS PUBLICATIONS

Current Contents/Clinical Medicine. Institute for Scientific Information, 3501 Market St., Philadelphia, PA 19104. Phone: (800) 523-1850. Fax: (215) 386-6362. Weekly.

Excerpta Medica. Section 3: Endocrinology. Elsevier Science Publishing Co., Inc., P.O. Box 882, Madison Square Station, New York, NY 10159-2101. Phone: (212) 989-5800. Fax: (212) 633-3990. 24/year.

Research Alert: Diabetes & Glucose Metabolism. Institute for Scientific Information, 3501 Market St., Philadelphia, PA 19104. Phone: (800) 523-1850. Fax: (215) 386-6362. Weekly.

Research Alert: Hypoglycemic Agents. Institute for Scientific Information, 3501 Market St., Philadelphia, PA 19104. Phone: (800) 523-1850. Fax: (215) 386-6362. Weekly.

ASSOCIATIONS, PROFESSIONAL SOCIETIES, ADVOCACY AND SUPPORT GROUPS

American Association for Diabetes Education. 560 N. Michigan Ave., Suite 1400, Chicago, IL 60611. Phone: (312) 661-1700.

American Diabetes Association (ADA). P.O. Box 25757, 1660 Duke St., Alexandria, VA 22314. Phone: (800) 232-3472. Fax: (703) 836-7439.

Juvenile Diabetes Foundation International (JDFI). 432 Park Ave. S., New York, NY 10016. Phone: (800) 223-1138. Fax: (212) 725-7259.

National Hypoglycemia Association (NHA). P.O. Box 120, Ridgewood, NJ 07451. Phone: (201) 670-1189.

BIBLIOGRAPHIES

Nutri-Topics: Nutrition and Diabetes. Food and Nutrition Center, National Agricultural Library, 10301 Baltimore Blvd., Beltsville, MD 20705.

HANDBOOKS, GUIDES, MANUALS, ATLASES

Color Atlas of Diabetes. Arnold Bloom, Peter Watkins, John Ireland. Mosby-Year Book, 11830 Westline Industrial Drive, St. Louis, MO 63146. Phone: (800) 325-4177. Fax: (314) 432-1380. Second edition 1991.

Handbook of Diabetes. Williams. Blackwell Scientific Publications, Inc., 3 Cambridge Ctr., Cambridge, MA 02142. Phone: (800) 759-6102. 1992.

Joslin Diabetes Manual. Leo P. Krall, Richard Beaser. Chronimed Publishing, 13911 Ridgedale Dr., Suite 250, Minnetonka, MN 55343. Phone: (800) 444-5951. 12th edition 1989.

Random House Personal Medical Handbook: For People with Diabetes. Paula Dranov. Random House, Inc., 201 E. 50th St., New York, NY 10022. Phone: (800) 726-0600. 1990.

JOURNALS

Diabetes Care. American Diabetes Association, P.O. Box 25757, 1600 Duke St., Alexandria, VA 22314. Phone: (800) 232-3472. Fax: (703) 836-7439.

Diabetes Forecast. American Diabetes Association, P.O. Box 25757, 1600 Duke St., Alexandria, VA 22314. Phone: (800) 232-3472. Fax: (703) 836-7439.

Diabetes Research and Clinical Practice. Elsevier Science Publishing Co., Inc., P.O. Box 882, Madison Square Station, New York, NY 10159-2101. Phone: (212) 989-5800. Fax: (212) 633-3990. 12/year.

Diabetic Medicine. John Wiley & Sons, Inc., 605 Third Ave., New York, NY 10158-0012. Phone: (212) 850-6000. Fax: (212) 850-6088. 10/year.

Journal of Diabetes and its Complications. Elsevier Science Publishing Co., Inc., P.O. Box 882, Madison Square Station, New York, NY 10159-2101. Phone: (212) 989-5800. Fax: (212) 633-3990. 4/year.

NEWSLETTERS

Diabetes. American Diabetes Association, National Service Center, 1660 Duke St., Alexandria, VA 22314. Phone: (800) 232-2172. Fax: (703) 836-7439. Quarterly.

ONLINE DATABASES

Combined Health Information Database (CHID). U.S. National Institutes of Health, P.O. Box NDIC, Bethesda, MD 20892. Phone: (301) 496-2162. Fax: (301) 770-5164. Quarterly.

EMBASE. Elsevier Science Publishing Co., Inc., P.O. Box 882, Madison Square Station, New York, NY 10159-2101. Phone: (212) 989-5800. Fax: (212) 633-3990.

MEDLINE. National Library of Medicine, 8600 Rockville Pike, Bethesda, MD 20894. Phone: (800) 638-8480.

SciSearch. Institute for Scientific Information, 3501 Market St., Philadelphia, PA 19104. Phone: (215) 386-0100. Fax: (215) 386-6362.

POPULAR WORKS AND PATIENT EDUCATION

American Diabetes Association Special Celebrations and Parties Cookbook. Betty Wedman. Prentice Hall, Prentice Hall Bldg.,

113 Sylvan Ave., Rt. 9W, Englewood Cliffs, NJ 07632. Phone: (201) 767-5937. 1989.

Diabetes A to Z. American Diabetes Association, P.O. Box 25757, 1600 Duke St., Alexandria, VA 22314. Phone: (800) 232-3472. Fax: (703) 836-7439. 1988.

Diabetes Mellitus: A Practical Handbook. Suellyn K. Milchovich, Barbara D. Long. Bull Publishing Co., 110 Gilbert Ave., Menlo Park, CA 94025. Phone: (800) 676-2855. 1990.

Diabetes and Pregnancy: What to Expect. American Diabetes Association, P.O. Box 25757, 1600 Duke St., Alexandria, VA 22314. Phone: (800) 232-3472. Fax: (703) 836-7439. 1989.

The Diabetic's Book: All Your Questions Answered. June Biermann, Barbara Toohey. Jeremy P. Tarcher, Inc., 5858 Wilshire Blvd., Suite 200, Los Angeles, CA 90036. Phone: (213) 935-9980. 1990.

Gestational Diabetes: What to Expect. American Diabetes Association, P.O. Box 25757, 1600 Duke St., Alexandria, VA 22314. Phone: (800) 232-3472. Fax: (703) 836-7439. 1989.

If Your Child Has Diabetes: An Answer Book for Parents. Putnam Publishing Group, 200 Madison Ave., New York, NY 10016. Phone: (800) 631-8571. 1990.

RESEARCH CENTERS, INSTITUTES, CLEARINGHOUSES

Banting and Best Department of Medical Research. University of Toronto. 112 College St., Toronto, ON, Canada M5G 1L6. Phone: (416) 978-2429. Fax: (416) 978-8528.

Diabetes and Endocrinology Research Center. University of Iowa. 3E19 VA Hospital, Iowa City, IA 52240. Phone: (319) 338-0581.

Diabetes-Endocrinology Research Center. University of Massachusetts. Medical School, Dept. of Biochemistry, 55 Lake Ave. N, Worcester, MA 01655. Phone: (508) 856-3047. Fax: (508) 856-6231.

Diabetes Research Center. University of Virginia Diabetes Center, Health Sciences Center, Box 423, Charlottesville, VA 22908. Phone: (804) 924-5246.

Diabetes Research Institute. University of Miami. P.O. Box 016960, Miami, FL 33101. Phone: (305) 547-6657.

Diabetes Research and Training Center. University of Michigan. University of Michigan Hospital, 1331 E. Ann St., Room 5111, Ann Arbor, MI 48109-0580. Phone: (313) 763-5256.

Diabetes Research and Training Center. Washington University. School of Medicine, 660 S. Euclid Ave., St. Louis, MO 63110. Phone: (314) 454-6046. Fax: (314) 454-6225.

Joslin Diabetes Center. 1 Joslin Pl., Boston, MA 02215. Phone: (617) 732-2400. Fax: (617) 732-2487.

Julia McFarlane Diabetes Research Center. University of Calgary. Faculty of Medicine, 3330 Hospital Dr. NW, Calgara, AB, Canada T2N 4N1. Phone: (403) 220-3011.

National Diabetes Information Clearinghouse (NDIC). P.O. Box NDIC, Bethesda, MD 20892. Phone: (301) 468-2162.

Scripps Research Institute. 10666 N. Torrey Pines Rd., La Jolla, CA 92037. Phone: (619) 554-8265. Fax: (619) 554-9899.

STANDARDS AND STATISTICS SOURCES

Diabetes Surveillance. Centers for Disease Control, 1600 Clifton Rd. N.E., Atlanta, GA 30333. Phone: (404) 488-4698. Annual.

TEXTBOOKS AND MONOGRAPHS

Clinical Diabetes Mellitus: A Problem-Oriented Approach. J.K. Davidson (ed.). Thieme Medical Publishers, Inc., 381 Park Ave. S., New York, NY 10016. Phone: (212) 683-5088. Fax: (212) 779-9020. Second revised edition 1991.

Diabetes Complicating Pregnancy: The Joslin Clinic Method. John W. Hare. John Wiley & Sons, Inc., 605 Third Ave., New York, NY 10158-0012. Phone: (212) 850-6000. Fax: (212) 850-6088. 1989.

Diabetes Mellitus: Diagnosis and Treatment. Mayer B. Davidson. Churchill Livingstone Inc., 650 Avenue of the Americas, New York, NY 10011. Phone: (212) 819-5400. Fax: (212) 302-6598. Third edition 1991.

Diabetes in Practice. H. Connor, A.J.M. Boulton. John Wiley & Sons, Inc., 605 Third Ave., New York, NY 10158-0012. Phone: (212) 850-6000. Fax: (212) 850-6088. 1989.

Management and Education of the Diabetic Patient. Robert J. Metz, James W. Benson. W.B. Saunders Co., The Curtis Center, Independence Square W., Philadelphia, PA 19106-3399. Phone: (215) 238-7800. 1988.

Nutrition Care of People with Diabetes Mellitus: A Nutrition Reference for Health Professionals. Penelope S. Easton, Charlotte S. Harker, Catherine Higgins. Haworth Press, 10 Alice Street, Binghamton, NY 13904-1580. Phone: (800) 3HA-WORTH. Fax: (607) 722-1424. 1991.

Textbook of Diabetes. Pickup. Blackwell Scientific Publications, Inc., 3 Cambridge Ctr., Cambridge, MA 02142. Phone: (800) 759-6102. Two volumes 1991.

DIAGNOSIS

See also: ENDOSCOPY; LABORATORY MEDICINE; MAMMOGRAPHY; MRI (MAGNETIC RESONANCE IMAGING); NUCLEAR MEDICINE; RADIOLOGY; ULTRASOUND

ABSTRACTING, INDEXING, AND CURRENT AWARENESS PUBLICATIONS

Current Contents/Clinical Medicine. Institute for Scientific Information, 3501 Market St., Philadelphia, PA 19104. Phone: (800) 523-1850. Fax: (215) 386-6362. Weekly.

Excerpta Medica. Section 14: Radiology. Elsevier Science Publishing Co., Inc., P.O. Box 882, Madison Square Station, New York, NY 10159-2101. Phone: (212) 989-5800. Fax: (212) 633-3990. 24/year.

Index Medicus. U.S. National Library of Medicine, 8600 Rockville Pike, Bethesda, MD 20894. Phone: (800) 638-8480. Monthly.

Science Citation Index. Institute for Scientific Information, 3501 Market St., Philadelphia, PA 19104. Phone: (800) 523-1850. Fax: (215) 386-6362. Bimonthly.

ANNUALS AND REVIEWS

Advances in Gastrointestinal Radiology. Mosby-Year Book, 11830 Westline Industrial Drive, St. Louis, MO 63146. Phone: (800) 325-4177. Fax: (314) 432-1380. Annual.

Critical Reviews in Diagnostic Imaging. CRC Press, Inc., 2000 Corporate Blvd. N.W., Boca Raton, FL 33431. Phone: (407) 994-0555. Fax: (407) 997-0949. Bimonthly.

Current Medical Diagnosis and Treatment. Appleton & Lange, 25 Van Zant St., East Norwalk, CT 06855. Phone: (800) 423-1359. Fax: (203) 854-9486. Annual.

Current Problems in Diagnostic Radiology. Mosby-Year Book, 11830 Westline Industrial Drive, St. Louis, MO 63146. Phone: (800) 325-4177. Fax: (314) 432-1380. Bimonthly.

Year Book of Diagnostic Radiology. Mosby-Year Book, 11830 Westline Industrial Drive, St. Louis, MO 63146. Phone: (800) 325-4177. Fax: (314) 432-1380. Annual.

Year Book of Ultrasound. Mosby-Year Book, 11830 Westline Industrial Drive, St. Louis, MO 63146. Phone: (800) 325-4177. Fax: (314) 432-1380. Annual.

ASSOCIATIONS, PROFESSIONAL SOCIETIES, ADVOCACY AND SUPPORT GROUPS

American Association of Gynecological Laparoscopists. 13021 E. Florence Ave., Santa Fe Springs, CA 90670. Phone: (213) 946-8774.

American Institute of Ultrasound in Medicine (AIUM). 4405 East-West Hwy., Ste. 504, Bethesda, MD 20814. Phone: (800) 638-5352. Fax: (301) 652-2408.

American Registry of Diagnostic Medical Sonographers (ARDMS). 2368 Victory Pkwy., No. 510, Cincinnati, OH 45206-2810. Phone: (513) 281-7111. Fax: (513) 721-6670.

Council on Diagnostic Imaging. P.O. Box 1655, Ashtabula, OH 44004. Phone: (216) 993-7213.

Society of Diagnostic Medical Sonographers (SDMS). 12225 Greenville Ave., Ste. 434, Dallas, TX 75243. Phone: (214) 235-7980. Fax: (214) 235-7369.

BIBLIOGRAPHIES

Computer Aided Medical Diagnosis. National Technical Information Service, 5285 Port Royal Rd., Springfield, VA 22161. Phone: (703) 487-4650. Fax: (703) 321-8547. May 1986-Jan. 1989 PB89-855100/CBY.

CD-ROM DATABASES

Excerpta Medica CD: Radiology & Nuclear Medicine. SilverPlatter Information, Inc., River Ridge Office Park, 100 River Ridge Rd., Norwood, MA 02062. Phone: (617) 769-2599. Fax: (617) 769-8763. Quarterly.

MAXX: Maximum Access to Diagnosis and Therapy. Little, Brown and Company, 34 Beacon St., Boston, MA 02108. Phone: (617) 227-0730. The Electronic Library of Medicine.

Scientific American Medicine CONSULT. Scientific American, Inc., 415 Madison Ave., New York, NY 10017. Phone: (212) 754-0550. Fax: (212) 980-3062. Quarterly.

SCISEARCH. Institute for Scientific Information, 3501 Market St., Philadelphia, PA 19104. Phone: (215) 386-0100. Fax: (215) 386-6362.

Year Books on Disc. CMC ReSearch, Inc., 7150 S.W. Hampton, Suite C-120, Portland, OR 97223. Phone: (800) 262-7668. Fax: (503) 639-1796. Annual includes Year Books of Cardiology, Dermatology, Diagnostic Radiology, Drug Therapy, Emergency Medicine, Family Practice, Medicine, Neurology and Neurosurgery, Obstetrics and Gynecology, Oncology, Pediatrics, and Psychiatry and Applied Mental Health.

DIRECTORIES

Directory of Certified Radiologists. American Board of Medical Specialties, 1 Rotary Center, Suite 805, Evanston, IL 60201. Phone: (708) 491-9091. Biennial.

ENCYCLOPEDIAS, DICTIONARIES, WORD BOOKS

A Dictionary of Clinical Tests. O. Potparie, J. Gibson. The Parthenon Publishing Group, Inc., 120 Mill Rd., Park Ridge, NJ 07656. Phone: (201) 391-6796. 1992.

HANDBOOKS, GUIDES, MANUALS, ATLASES

Atlas of Diagnostic Oncology. Skarin. Raven Press, 1185 Ave. of the Americas, New York, NY 10036. Phone: (212) 930-9500. Fax: (212) 869-3495. 1991.

Atlas of Surgical Endoscopy. Ponsky. Mosby-Year Book, 11830 Westline Industrial Drive, St. Louis, MO 63146. Phone: (800) 325-4177. Fax: (314) 432-1380. 1992.

Color Atlas of Clinical Applications of Fiberoptic Bronchoscopy. Kitamura. Mosby-Year Book, 11830 Westline Industrial Drive, St. Louis, MO 63146. Phone: (800) 325-4177. Fax: (314) 432-1380. 1991.

The Common Symptom Guide. John Wasson, B. Timothy Walsh, Richard Tompkins, and others. McGraw-Hill, Inc., Health Professions Division, 1221 Avenue of the Americas, 28th Floor, New York, NY 10020. Phone: (212) 512-4228. Third edition 1992.

Diagnostic Handbook of Clinical Decision Making. Goldenberg. Mosby-Year Book, 11830 Westline Industrial Drive, St. Louis, MO 63146. Phone: (800) 325-4177. Fax: (314) 432-1380. 1989.

Diagnostic Procedure Handbook with Key Work Index. Joseph A. Golish (ed.). Williams & Wilkins, 428 East Preston St., Baltimore, MD 21202. Phone: (800) 638-0672. Fax: (800) 447-8438. 1992.

A Guide to Physical Examination and History Taking. Barbara Bates, and others. J.B. Lippincott Co., 227 E. Washington Square, Philadelphia, PA 19106-3780. Phone: (215) 238-4200. Fax: (215) 238-4227. 1991.

Laboratory Test Handbook. David S. Jacobs, Bernard L. Kasten Jr., Wayne R. DeMott. Williams & Wilkins, 428 E. Preston St., Baltimore, MD 21202. Phone: (800) 638-0672. Fax: (800) 447-8438. Second edition 19990.

Manual of Clinical Evaluation. Aronson. Little, Brown and Co., 34 Beacon St., Boston, MA 02108. Phone: (617) 227-0730. Fax: (617) 227-0790. 1988.

Manual of Diagnostic Imaging. Straub. Little, Brown and Co., 34 Beacon St., Boston, MA 02108. Phone: (617) 227-0730. Fax: (617) 227-0790. Second edition 1989.

A Manual of Laboratory and Diagnostic Tests. Frances Fischbach. J.B. Lippincott Co., 227 East Washington Square, Philadelphia, PA 19106-3780. Phone: (215) 238-4200. Fax: (215) 238-4227. 1992.

Manual of Nursing Diagnosis. Marjory Gordon. Mosby-Year Book, 11830 Westline Industrial Drive, St. Louis, MO 63146. Phone: (800) 325-4177. Fax: (314) 432-1380. Irregular.

Manual of Pediatric Physical Diagnosis. Barness. Mosby-Year Book, 11830 Westline Industrial Drive, St. Louis, MO 63146. Phone: (800) 325-4177. Fax: (314) 432-1380. Sixth edition 1991.

Manual of Pulmonary Function Testing. Gregg Rupper. Mosby-Year Book, 11830 Westline Industrial Drive, St. Louis, MO 63146. Phone: (800) 325-4177. Fax: (314) 432-1380. 5th edition, 1991.

Merck Manual of Diagnosis and Therapy. Robert Berkow (ed.). Merck & Co., Inc., P.O. Box 2000, Rahway, NJ 07065. Phone: (201) 855-4558. 16th edition. 1992.

Mosby's Guide to Physical Examination. Henry M. Seidel, Jane W. Ball, Joyce E. Dains, et. al.. Mosby-Year Book, 11830 Westline Industrial Drive, St. Louis, MO 63146. Phone: (800) 325-4177. Fax: (314) 432-1380. Second edition 1991.

Office and Bedside Diagnosis. Cooke. Appleton & Lange, 25 Van Zant St., East Norwalk, CT 06855. Phone: (800) 423-1359. Fax: (203) 854-9486. 1992.

Practical Manual of Operative Laparoscopy and Hysteroscopy. Azziz. Springer-Verlag New York Inc., 175 Fifth Ave., New York, NY 10010. Phone: (212) 460-1500. Fax: (212) 473-6272. 1992.

Signs and Symptoms Handbook. Springhouse Publishing Co., 1111 Bethlehem Pike, Spring House, PA 19477. Phone: (800) 331-3170. Fax: (215) 646-8716. 1988.

JOURNALS

Imaging. Rapid Communications of Oxford Ltd., The Old Malthouse, Paradise St., Oxford OX1 1LD, England. Phone: 44-865-790447. Fax: 44-865-244012. 4/year.

Journal of Laparoendoscopic Surgery. Mary Ann Liebert, Inc., 1651 Third Ave., New York, NY 10128. Phone: (212) 289-2300. Fax: (212) 289-4697. Bimonthly.

Nursing Diagnosis. J.B. Lippincott Co., 227 E. Washington Square, Philadelphia, PA 19106-3780. Phone: (215) 238-4200. Fax: (215) 238-4227. Quarterly.

Prenatal Diagnosis. John Wiley & Sons, Inc., 605 Third Ave., New York, NY 10158-0012. Phone: (212) 850-6000. Fax: (212) 850-6088. Monthly.

NEWSLETTERS

Diagnostic Testing Alert. American Health Consultants, Department C1290, P.O. Box 740060, Atlanta, GA 30374. Phone: (800) 559-1032. Monthly.

ONLINE DATABASES

EMBASE. Elsevier Science Publishing Co., Inc., P.O. Box 882, Madison Square Station, New York, NY 10159-2101. Phone: (212) 989-5800. Fax: (212) 633-3990.

MEDLINE. National Library of Medicine, 8600 Rockville Pike, Bethesda, MD 20894. Phone: (800) 638-8480.

SciSearch. Institute for Scientific Information, 3501 Market St., Philadelphia, PA 19104. Phone: (215) 386-0100. Fax: (215) 386-6362.

POPULAR WORKS AND PATIENT EDUCATION

Complete Guide to Symptoms, Illness and Surgery for People over Fifty. H. Winter Griffith. Putnam Publishing Group, 200 Madison Ave., New York, NY 10016. Phone: (800) 631-8571. 1992.

Medical Choices, Medical Chances: How Patients, Families and Physicians Can Cope with Uncertainty. Harold Bursztajn, Richard I. Feinbloom, Robert M. Hamm. Routledge, Chapman & Hall, Inc., 29 W. 35th St., New York, NY 10001-2291. Phone: (212) 244-3336. 1990.

Medical Tests and Diagnostic Procedures: A Patient's Guide to Just What the Doctor Ordered. Philip Shtasel. HarperCollins Publishers., Inc., 10 E. 53rd St., New York, NY 10022-5299. Phone: (212) 207-7000. Fax: (800) 242-7737. 1990.

TEXTBOOKS AND MONOGRAPHS

Clinical Methods: The History, Physical and Laboratory Examinations. H. Kenneth Walker, W. Dallas Hall, J. Willis Hurst. Butterworth-Heinemann, 80 Montvale Ave., Stoneham, MA 02180. Phone: (617) 438-8464. Fax: (617) 279-4851. Third edition 1990.

Clinical Sonography: A Practical Guide. Roger C. Sanders. Little, Brown and Co., 34 Beacon St., Boston, MA 02108. Phone: (617) 227-0730. Fax: (617) 227-0790. Second edition 1991.

Common Diagnostic Tests: Use and Interpretation. Harold C. Sox Jr. (ed.). American Medical Association, 515 North State St., Chicago, IL 60610. Phone: (312) 464-0183. Fax: (312) 464-5834. Second edition 1990.

Common Screening Tests. David M. Eddy (ed.). American Medical Association, 515 North State St., Chicago, IL 60610. Phone: (312) 464-0183. Fax: (312) 464-5834. 1991.

The Complete Patient History. Maurice Kraytman. McGraw-Hill, Inc., Health Professions Division, 1221 Avenue of the Americas, 28th Floor, New York, NY 10020. Phone: (212) 512-4228. Second edition 1990.

Current Diagnosis 8. Rex Conn (ed.). Williams & Wilkins, 428 East Preston St., Baltimore, MD 21202. Phone: (800) 638-0672. Fax: (800) 447-8438. 1991.

Current Surgical Diagnosis and Treatment. L.W. Way. Appleton & Lange, 25 Van Zant St., East Norwalk, CT 06855. Phone: (800) 423-1359. Fax: (203) 854-9486. Ninth edition 1990.

Decision Making in Medicine. Harry L. Greene. Mosby-Year Book, 11830 Westline Industrial Drive, St. Louis, MO 63146. Phone: (800) 325-4177. Fax: (314) 432-1380. 1992.

Diagnostic Bronchoscopy: A Teaching Manual. Stradling. Churchill Livingstone Inc., 650 Ave. of the Americas, New York, NY 10011. Phone: (212) 819-5400. Fax: (212) 302-6598. Sixth edition 1991.

Diagnostic Radiology. R.G. Grainger, D. Allison. Churchill Livingstone Inc., 650 Ave. of the Americas, New York, NY 10011. Phone: (212) 819-5400. Fax: (212) 302-6598. Second edition 1991.

Diagnostic Radiology in Emergency Medicine. Rosen. Mosby-Year Book, 11830 Westline Industrial Drive, St. Louis, MO 63146. Phone: (800) 325-4177. Fax: (314) 432-1380. 1992.

Diagnostic Ultrasonics: Principles and Use of Instruments. W.N. McDicken. Churchill Livingstone Inc., 650 Avenue of the Americas, New York, NY 10011. Phone: (212) 819-5400. Fax: (212) 302-6598. 1991.

Diagnostic Ultrasound: Principles, Instruments, and Exercises. Frederick W. Kremkau. W.B. Saunders Co., The Curtis Center, Independence Square W., Philadelphia, PA 19106-3399. Phone: (215) 238-7800. Third edition 1989.

Differential Diagnosis in Conventional Radiology. F.A. Burgener, M. Kormano. Thieme Medical Publishers, Inc., 381 Park Ave. S., New York, NY 10016. Phone: (212) 683-5088. Fax: (212) 779-9020. Second edition 1991.

Difficult Diagnosis 2. Robert B. Taylor (ed.). W.B. Saunders Co., The Curtis Center, Independence Square W., Philadelphia, PA 19106-3399. Phone: (215) 238-7800. 1992.

Learning Clinical Reasoning. Kassirer. Williams & Wilkins, 428 East Preston St., Baltimore, MD 21202. Phone: (800) 638-0672. Fax: (800) 447-8438. 1991.

Operative Laparoscopy. Maurice-Antoine Bruhat, Gerard Mage, Jean-Luc Pouly. McGraw-Hill, Inc., Health Professions Division, 1221 Avenue of the Americas, 28th Floor, New York, NY 10020. Phone: (212) 512-4228. 1992.

Physical Diagnosis. Norton Grenberger, Daniel Hinthorn. Mosby-Year Book, 11830 Westline Industrial Drive, St. Louis, MO 63146. Phone: (800) 325-4177. Fax: (314) 432-1380. 1992.

Problem-Oriented Medical Diagnosis. H. Harold Friedman (ed.). Little, Brown and Company, 34 Beacon St., Boston, MA 02108. Phone: (617) 227-0730. Fifth edition 1991.

Textbook of Diagnostic Ultrasonography. Sandra L. Hagen-Ansert. Mosby-Year Book, 11830 Westline Industrial Drive, St. Louis, MO 63146. Phone: (800) 325-4177. Fax: (314) 432-1380. Third edition 1989.

Transvaginal Ultrasound. Nyberg. Mosby-Year Book, 11830 Westline Industrial Drive, St. Louis, MO 63146. Phone: (800) 325-4177. Fax: (314) 432-1380. Second edition 1992.

DIAGNOSTIC RELATED GROUPS

See also: HEALTH CARE FINANCING;
HEALTH INSURANCE

ABSTRACTING, INDEXING, AND CURRENT AWARENESS PUBLICATIONS

Cumulative Index to Nursing and Allied Health Literature. Glendale Adventist Medical Center, P.O. Box 871, Glendale, CA 91209. Phone: (818) 409-8005. Bimonthly.

Hospital Literature Index. American Hospital Association, 840 N. Lake Shore Dr., Chicago, IL 60611. Phone: (800) 242-2626. Fax: (312) 280-6015. Quarterly.

Index Medicus. U.S. National Library of Medicine, 8600 Rockville Pike, Bethesda, MD 20894. Phone: (800) 638-8480. Monthly.

MEDOC: Index to U.S. Government Publications in the Medical and Health Sciences. Spencer S. Eccles Health Sciences Library, University of Utah, Bldg. 589, Salt Lake City, UT 84112. Phone: (801) 581-5268. Quarterly.

CD-ROM DATABASES

HFCA --On CD-ROM. FD Inc., 600 New Hampshire Ave. NW, Suite 355, Washington, DC 20037. Phone: (800) 332-6623. Fax: (202) 337 0457. Monthly.

Nursing and Allied Health (CINAHL) on CD-ROM CINAHL, 1509 Wilson Terrace, P.O. Box 871, Glendale, CA 91209-0871. Phone: (818) 409-8005.

HANDBOOKS, GUIDES, MANUALS, ATLASES

Medicare DRG Handbook: Comparative Clinical & Financial Standards. Health Care Investment Analysts, Inc., 300 E. Lombard St., Baltimore, MD 21202. Phone: (410) 576-9600. Fax: (410) 783-0575. 1992.

NEWSLETTERS

DRG Monitor. Hanley & Belfus, Inc., 210 S. 13th St., Philadelphia, PA 19107. Phone: (215) 546-7293. Monthly.

ONLINE DATABASES

Diagnosis Related Groups Database. Health Care Investment Analysts, Inc., 300 E. Lombard St., Baltimore, MD 21202. Phone: (410) 576-9600. Fax: (410) 783-0575.

EMBASE. Elsevier Science Publishing Co., Inc., P.O. Box 882, Madison Square Station, New York, NY 10159-2101. Phone: (212) 989-5800. Fax: (212) 633-3990.

MEDLINE. National Library of Medicine, 8600 Rockville Pike, Bethesda, MD 20894. Phone: (800) 638-8480.

Nursing and Allied Health (CINAHL). CINAHL, 1509 Wilson Terrace, P.O. Box 871, Glendale, CA 91209-0871. Phone: (818) 409-8005.

SciSearch. Institute for Scientific Information, 3501 Market St., Philadelphia, PA 19104. Phone: (215) 386-0100. Fax: (215) 386-6362.

STANDARDS AND STATISTICS SOURCES

Length of Stay by DRG and Payment Source, 1992-93. HCIA Inc., P.O. Box 303, Ann Arbor, MI 48106-0303. 5 vols..

TEXTBOOKS AND MONOGRAPHS

DRGs: Their Design and Development. Robert B. Fetter (ed.). Health Administration Press, 1021 E. Huron St., Ann Arbor, MI 48104-9990. Phone: (313) 764-1380. Fax: (313) 763-1105. 1991.

DIALYSIS

See: KIDNEY DIALYSIS

DIAPHRAGM

See: CONTRACEPTION

DIARRHEA

See: GASTROINTESTINAL DISORDERS

DIET

See: NUTRITION

DIETETICS

See: NUTRITION; NUTRITIONAL DISORDERS

DIGESTIVE SYSTEM DISEASES

See: GASTROINTESTINAL DISORDERS

DILATION AND CURETTAGE

See: GYNECOLOGIC DISORDERS;
OBSTETRICS AND GYNECOLOGY

DIPTHERIA

See: INFECTIOUS DISEASES

DISABLED

See: HANDICAPPED

DISEASE CLASSIFICATION

ABSTRACTING, INDEXING, AND CURRENT AWARENESS PUBLICATIONS

MEDOC: Index to U.S. Government Publications in the Medical and Health Sciences. Spencer S. Eccles Health Sciences Library, University of Utah, Bldg. 589, Salt Lake City, UT 84112. Phone: (801) 581-5268. Quarterly.

BIBLIOGRAPHIES

Annotated Bibliography of DSM-III. Andrew Skodol, Robert Spitzer. American Psychiatric Association, 1400 K St. N.W., Washington, DC 20005. Phone: (202) 682-6000. Fax: (202) 682-6114. 1987.

CD-ROM DATABASES

Morbidity Mortality Weekly Report. MEP, 124 Mt. Auburn St., Cambridge, MA 02138. Phone: (800) 342-1338. Fax: (617) 868-7738. Annual.

ENCYCLOPEDIAS, DICTIONARIES, WORD BOOKS

Professional Guide to Diseases. Springhouse Publishing Co., 1111 Bethlehem Pike, Spring House, PA 19477. Phone: (800) 331-3170. Fax: (215) 646-8716. Fourth edition 1992.

HANDBOOKS, GUIDES, MANUALS, ATLASES

Current Procedural Terminology (CPT). American Medical Association, 515 N. State St., Chicago, IL 60610. Phone: (312) 464-5000. Fax: (312) 645-4184. 1993.

Diagnostic and Statistical Manual of Mental Disorders, Third Edition, Revised. American Psychiatric Association, 1400 K St. N.W., Washington, DC 20005. Phone: (202) 682-6000. Fax: (202) 682-6114. 1987.

ICD-10: The International Statistical Classification of Diseases & Related Health Problems. American Psychiatric Press, Inc., 1400 K St. N.W., Washington, DC 20005. Phone: (202) 682-6268. Fax: (202) 789-2648. Three volumes 1992.

TNM Atlas: Illustrated Guide to the TNM-PTNM Classification of Malignant Tumors. B. Spiessl (ed.). Springer-Verlag New York Inc., 175 Fifth Ave., New York, NY 10010. Phone: (212) 460-1500. Fax: (212) 473-6272. 1989.

TNM Classification of Malignant Tumors. Springer-Verlag New York Inc., 175 Fifth Ave., New York, NY 10010. Phone: (212) 460-1500. Fax: (212) 473-6272. 4th ed., rev..

JOURNALS

Morbidity and Mortality Weekly Report. Massachusetts Medical Society, 1440 Main St., Waltham, MA 02154-1649. Phone: (617) 893-3800. Fax: (617) 893-0413. Weekly.

NEWSLETTERS

CPT Assistant. American Medical Association, 515 N. State St., Chicago, IL 60610. Phone: (312) 464-5000. Fax: (312) 645-4184.

ONLINE DATABASES

Rare Disease Database. National Organization for Rare Disorders, P.O. Box 8923, New Fairfield, CT 06812. Phone: (800) 999-6673. Fax: (203) 746-6481. Weekly.

TEXTBOOKS AND MONOGRAPHS

International Classification of Diseases. Revisionist Press, P.O. Box 2009, Brooklyn, NY 11202. Phone: (212) 532-7827. Three volumes 1984.

DISLOCATIONS

See: ORTHOPEDICS

DIVERTICULITIS

See: GASTROINTESTINAL DISORDERS

DIVING MEDICINE

See: UNDERSEA MEDICINE

DOMESTIC VIOLENCE

See: CHILD ABUSE; SPOUSE ABUSE

DOWN'S SYNDROME

See also: BIRTH DEFECTS

ABSTRACTING, INDEXING, AND CURRENT AWARENESS PUBLICATIONS

Current Contents/Clinical Medicine. Institute for Scientific Information, 3501 Market St., Philadelphia, PA 19104. Phone: (800) 523-1850. Fax: (215) 386-6362. Weekly.

Excerpta Medica. Section 22: Human Genetics. Elsevier Science Publishers, P.O. Box 882, Madison Square Station, New York, NY 10159-2101. Phone: (212) 633-3950. Fax: (212) 633-3990. 24/year.

Index Medicus. U.S. National Library of Medicine, 8600 Rockville Pike, Bethesda, MD 20894. Phone: (800) 638-8480. Monthly.

Science Citation Index. Institute for Scientific Information, 3501 Market St., Philadelphia, PA 19104. Phone: (800) 523-1850. Fax: (215) 386-6362. Bimonthly.

ASSOCIATIONS, PROFESSIONAL SOCIETIES, ADVOCACY AND SUPPORT GROUPS

March of Dimes Birth Defects Foundation (MDBDF). 1275 Mamaroneck Ave., White Plains, NY 10605. Phone: (914) 428-7100. Fax: (914) 428-8203.

National Association for Down Syndrome. P.O. Box 4542, Oak Brook, IL 60521. Phone: (312) 325-9112.

National Down Syndrome Congress. 1800 Dempster St., Park Ridge, IL 60068. Phone: (312) 823-7550.

National Down Syndrome Society. 141 Fifth Ave., New York, NY 10010. Phone: (800) 221-4602.

Parents of Children with Down's Syndrome. P.O. Box 35268, Houston, TX 77035.

CD-ROM DATABASES

SCISEARCH. Institute for Scientific Information, 3501 Market St., Philadelphia, PA 19104. Phone: (215) 386-0100. Fax: (215) 386-6362.

DIRECTORIES

Babies with Down's Syndrome: A New Parents' Guide. Woodbine House, 5615 Fishers Ln., Rockville, MD 20852. Phone: (800) 843-7323. Fax: (301) 468-5784. 1986.

JOURNALS

Journal of Genetic Counseling. Human Sciences Press, 233 Spring St., New York, NY 10013-1578. Phone: (800) 221-9369. Fax: (212) 807-1047. Quarterly.

Pediatrics. American Academy of Pediatrics, 141 Northwest Point Rd., Elk Grove Village, IL 60009-0927. Phone: (708) 228-5005. Fax: (708) 228-5097. Monthly.

NEWSLETTERS

Down Syndrome News. National Down Syndrome Congress, 1800 Dempster St., Park Ridge, IL 60068-1146. Phone: (800) 232-6372. 10/year.

ONLINE DATABASES

EMBASE. Elsevier Science Publishing Co., Inc., P.O. Box 882, Madison Square Station, New York, NY 10159-2101. Phone: (212) 989-5800. Fax: (212) 633-3990.

MEDLINE. National Library of Medicine, 8600 Rockville Pike, Bethesda, MD 20894. Phone: (800) 638-8480.

SciSearch. Institute for Scientific Information, 3501 Market St., Philadelphia, PA 19104. Phone: (215) 386-0100. Fax: (215) 386-6362.

POPULAR WORKS AND PATIENT EDUCATION

Down Syndrome: The Facts. Mark Selikowitz. Oxford University Press, 200 Madison Ave., New York, NY 10016. Phone: (212) 679-7300. 1990.

TEXTBOOKS AND MONOGRAPHS

Children with Down Syndrome: A Developmental Perspective. Dante Cicchetti, Marjorie Beeghly (eds.). Cambridge University Press, 40 W. 20th St., New York, NY 10011. Phone: (800) 431-1580. 1990.

DRGS

See: DIAGNOSTIC RELATED GROUPS

DRUG ABUSE

See also: ALCOHOLISM; COCAINE; MARIJUANA

ABSTRACTING, INDEXING, AND CURRENT AWARENESS PUBLICATIONS

Excerpta Medica. Section 38: Adverse Reactions Titles. Elsevier Science Publishing Co., Inc., P.O. Box 882, Madison Square Station, New York, NY 10159-2101. Phone: (212) 989-5800. Fax: (212) 633-3990. 12/year.

Excerpta Medica. Section 40: Drug Dependence, Alcohol Abuse and Alcoholism. Elsevier Science Publishing Co., Inc., P.O. Box 882, Madison Square Station, New York, NY 10159-2101. Phone: (212) 989-5800. Fax: (212) 633-3990. 6/year.

Index Medicus. U.S. National Library of Medicine, 8600 Rockville Pike, Bethesda, MD 20894. Phone: (800) 638-8480. Monthly.

MEDOC: Index to U.S. Government Publications in the Medical and Health Sciences. Spencer S. Eccles Health Sciences Library, University of Utah, Bldg. 589, Salt Lake City, UT 84112. Phone: (801) 581-5268. Quarterly.

Prevention Pipeline: An Alcohol and Drug Awareness Service. National Clearinghouse for Alcohol and Drug Information, Dept. PP, P.O. Box 2345, Rockville, MD 20852.

Psychological Abstracts. American Psychological Association, 1200 17th St. NW, Washington, DC 20036. Phone: (202) 955-7600. Monthly.

Research Alert: Drug Addiction & Abuse. Institute for Scientific Information, 3501 Market St., Philadelphia, PA 19104. Phone: (800) 523-1850. Fax: (215) 386-6362. Weekly.

Science Citation Index. Institute for Scientific Information, 3501 Market St., Philadelphia, PA 19104. Phone: (800) 523-1850. Fax: (215) 386-6362. Bimonthly.

ANNUALS AND REVIEWS

Advances in Alcohol and Substance Abuse. Haworth Press, 10 Alice St., Binghamton, NY 13904-1580. Phone: (803) 429-6784. Fax: (607) 722-1424.

Marijuana. Mark S. Gold. Plenum Publishing Co., 233 Spring St., New York, NY 10013-1578. Phone: (212) 620-8000. Fax: (212) 463-0742. Volume 1 1989.

Research Advances in Alcohol and Drug Problems. Plenum Publishing Co., 233 Spring St., New York, NY 10013-1578. Phone: (212) 620-8000. Fax: (212) 463-0742. Irregular.

ASSOCIATIONS, PROFESSIONAL SOCIETIES, ADVOCACY AND SUPPORT GROUPS

American Council for Drug Education. 204 Monroe St., Suite 110, Rockville, MD 20850. Phone: (301) 294-0600.

Co-Dependents Anonymous. P.O. Box 5508, Glendale, AZ 85312-5508.

Cocaine Anonymous. 6125 Washington Blvd., Ste. 202, Culver City, CA 90232. Phone: (213) 839-1141.

Do It Now Foundation. P.O. Box 21126, Phoenix, AZ 85036.

Nar-Anon Family Group Headquarters. World Service Office, P.O. Box 2562, Palos Verdes Peninsula, CA 90274. Phone: (213) 547-5800.

Narcotics Anonymous. World Service Office, P.O. Box 9999, Van Nuys, CA 91409. Phone: (818) 780-3951.

National Association of Alcoholism and Drug Abuse Counselors (NAADAC). 3717 Columbia Pike, Ste. 300, Arlington, VA 22204. Phone: (800) 548-0497. Fax: (703) 920-4672.

National Council on Alcoholism and Drug Dependence, Inc.. 12 W. 21st St., New York, NY 10010. Phone: (212) 206-6770.

BIBLIOGRAPHIES

Addiction Research Foundation Bibliographic Series. Addiction Research Foundation of Ontario, 33 Russell St., Toronto, ON, Canada M5S 2S1. Phone: (416) 595-6123. Irregular.

Bibliography and Research Guide on Alcohol and other Drugs for Social Work Educators. National Clearinghouse for Alcohol and Drug Information, Dept. PP, P.O. Box 2345, Rockville, MD 20852.

Drug Abuse. National Technical Information Service, 5285 Port Royal Rd., Springfield, VA 22161. Phone: (703) 487-4650. Fax: (703) 321-8547. Jan. 1975-Sept. 1989 PB89-872600/CBY.

Drug Abuse Bibliography. Whitston Publishing Co., P.O. Box 958., Troy, NY 12181. Phone: (518) 283-4363. Annual.

Drug Abuse, Drug Abuse Prevention, and Drug Testing. National Technical Information Service, 5285 Port Royal Rd., Springfield, VA 22161. Phone: (703) 487-4650. Fax: (703) 321-8547. Jan. 1985-Feb. 1989 PB88-862444/CBY.

CD-ROM DATABASES

PsycLit. SilverPlatter Information, Inc., River Ridge Office Park, 100 River Ridge Rd., Norwood, MA 02062. Phone: (617) 769-2599. Fax: (617) 769-8763. Quarterly.

SCISEARCH. Institute for Scientific Information, 3501 Market St., Philadelphia, PA 19104. Phone: (215) 386-0100. Fax: (215) 386-6362.

DIRECTORIES

The 100 Best Treatment Centers. Avon Books, 1350 Avenue of the Americas, 2nd Floor, New York, NY 10019. Phone: (800) 238-0658.

Alcohol, Drug Abuse, Mental Health Research Grant Awards. Alcohol, Drug Abuse, and Mental Health Administration, 5600 Fishers Lane, Rockville, MD 20857. Phone: (301) 443-1596.

Drug, Alcohol, and Other Addictions: A Directory of Treatment Centers and Prevention Programs Nationwide. Oryx Press, 4041 N. Central, Suite 700, Phoenix, AZ 85012. Phone: (800) 279-ORYX. Fax: (800) 279-4663.

ENCYCLOPEDIAS, DICTIONARIES, WORD BOOKS

Encyclopedia of Drug Abuse. Glen Evans, Robert O'Brien, Sidney Cohen, James Fine. Facts on File, Inc., 460 Park Ave. S., New York, NY 10016-7382. Phone: (212) 683-2244. Fax: (212) 683-3633. Third edition 1992.

HANDBOOKS, GUIDES, MANUALS, ATLASES

Concise Guide to Treatment of Alcoholism and Addictions. Richard J. Frances, John E. Franklin. American Psychiatric Press, Inc., 1400 K St. NW, Washington, DC 20005. Phone: (202) 682-6268. Fax: (202) 789-2648. 1989.

Drug and Alcohol Abuse: A Clinical Guide to Diagnosis and Treatment. Marc A. Schuckit. Plenum Publishing Co., 233 Spring St., New York, NY 10013-1578. Phone: (212) 620-8000. Fax: (212) 463-0742. Third edition 1989.

A Handbook on Drug and Alcohol Abuse. Gail Winger, Frederick G. Hofman, James H. Woods. Oxford University Press, 200 Madison Ave., New York, NY 10016. Phone: (212) 679-7300. Third edition 1992.

Handbook of Hospital Based Substance Abuse Treatment. William D. Lerner, Marjorie A. Barr. McGraw-Hill, Inc., Health Professions Division, 1221 Avenue of the Americas, 28th Floor, New York, NY 10020. Phone: (212) 512-4228. 1990.

JOURNALS

Addictive Behaviors. Pergamon Press, 660 White Plains Rd., Tarrytown, NY 10591-5153. Phone: (914) 592-7700. Fax: (914) 592-3625.

Alcholism and Addiction. IPG, 4949 Commerce Parkway, Cleveland, OH 44128. Phone: (800) 342-6237.

American Journal on Addictions. American Psychiatric Press, Inc., 1400 K St. NW, Washington, DC 20005. Phone: (202) 682-6268. Fax: (202) 789-2648. Quarterly.

American Journal of Drug and Alcohol Abuse. Marcel Dekker, Inc., 270 Madison Ave., New York, NY 10016. Phone: (800) 228-1160.

Drug and Alcohol Dependence. Elsevier Science Publishing Co., Inc., P.O. Box 882, Madison Square Station, New York, NY 10159-2101. Phone: (212) 989-5800. Fax: (212) 633-3990. 6/year.

Drugs and Society. Haworth Press, 10 Alice Street, Binghamton, NY 13904-1580. Phone: (800) 342-9678. Fax: (607) 722-1424. Quarterly.

Journal of Addictive Diseases. Haworth Press, 10 Alice Street, Binghamton, NY 13904-1580. Phone: (800) 3HA-WORTH. Fax: (607) 722-1424. Quarterly.

Journal of Substance Abuse. Ablex Publishing Co., 355 Chestnut St., Norwood, NJ 07648. Phone: (201) 767-8450. Fax: (201) 767-6717. Quarterly.

Journal of Substance Abuse Treatment. Pergamon Press, 660 White Plains Rd., Tarrytown, NY 10591-5153. Phone: (914) 592-7700. Fax: (914) 592-3625. 6/year.

NEWSLETTERS

Addictions Alert. American Health Consultants, Department C1290, P.O. Box 740060, Atlanta, GA 30374. Phone: (800) 559-1032. Monthly.

ONLINE DATABASES

Druginfo and Alcohol Use and Abuse. University of Minnesota, College of Pharmacy, Drug Information Services, 3-160 Health

Sciences Center, Unit F, 308 Harvard St. Se, Minneapolis, MN 55455. Phone: (612) 624-6492. Quarterly.

EMBASE. Elsevier Science Publishing Co., Inc., P.O. Box 882, Madison Square Station, New York, NY 10159-2101. Phone: (212) 989-5800. Fax: (212) 633-3990.

MEDLINE. National Library of Medicine, 8600 Rockville Pike, Bethesda, MD 20894. Phone: (800) 638-8480.

PsycInfo. SilverPlatter Information, Inc., River Ridge Office Park, 100 River Ridge Rd., Norwood, MA 02062. Phone: (617) 769-2599. Fax: (617) 769-8763. Quarterly.

SciSearch. Institute for Scientific Information, 3501 Market St., Philadelphia, PA 19104. Phone: (215) 386-0100. Fax: (215) 386-6362.

POPULAR WORKS AND PATIENT EDUCATION

The 800-Cocaine Book of Drug and Alcohol Recovery. James Cocores. Random House, Inc., 201 E. 50th St., New York, NY 10022. Phone: (800) 726-0600. 1990.

The Facts about Drug Use. Barry Stimmel. Consumer Reports Books, 101 Truman Ave., Yonkers, NY 10703. Phone: (914) 378-2000. 1991.

Good News about Drugs and Alcohol: Curing, Treating and Preventing Substance Abuse. Mark S. Gold. Random House, Inc., 201 E. 50th St., New York, NY 10022. Phone: (800) 726-0600. 1991.

Staying Clean: Living Without Drugs. Hazelden Staff. HarperCollins Publishers, 10 E. 53rd St., New York, NY 10022-5299. Phone: (800) 242-7737. 1990.

RESEARCH CENTERS, INSTITUTES, CLEARINGHOUSES

Addiction Research and Treatment Corporation. 22 Chapel St., Brooklyn, NY 11201. Phone: (718) 260-2917. Fax: (718) 522-3186.

Alcohol and Drug Abuse Institute. University of Washington. 3937 15th Ave. NE, NL-15, Seattle, WA 98195. Phone: (206) 543-0937. Fax: (206) 543-5473.

Alcoholism and Drug Addiction Research Foundation. 33 Russell St., Toronto, ON, Canada M5S 2S1. Phone: (416) 595-6000. Fax: (416) 979-8133.

Center for Alcohol and Addiction Studies. University of Alaska, Anchorage. 3211 Providence Dr., Anchorage, AK 99508. Phone: (907) 786-1802. Fax: (907) 786-1247.

Center for Alcohol and Drug Education. University of Alabama. Box 870219, Tuscaloosa, AL 35487-0219. Phone: (205) 348-1943.

The Drugsource Information Clearinghouse. 3700 Forest Dr., Columbia, SC 29204. Phone: (803) 734-9559.

Hazelden Foundation. Box 176, Center City, MN 55012-0176. Phone: (800) 328-9000.

Housing and Urban Development Drug Information and Strategy Clearinghouse. P.O. Box 6424, Rockville, MD 20850. Phone: (800) 955-2232.

Institute of Alcoholism and Drug Dependency. Andrews University. School of Graduate Studies, Marsh Hall 100-A,

Berrien Springs, MI 49104. Phone: (616) 471-3558. Fax: (616) 473-4425.

Narcotic and Drug Research, Inc.. 11 Beach St., New York, NY 10013. Phone: (212) 966-8700. Fax: (212) 334-8058.

Research Institute on Alcoholism. 1021 Main St., Buffalo, NY 14203. Phone: (716) 887-2566.

Target Research Center. P.O. Box 20626, 11724 Plaza Cir., Kansas City, MO 64195. Phone: (816) 464-5400.

STANDARDS AND STATISTICS SOURCES

Anabolic Steroid Abuse. National Institute on Drug Abuse, 5600 Fishers Lane, Rockville, MD 20857. Phone: (301) 443-6480. 1990.

Drugs in the Workplace: Research and Evaluation Data. National Institute on Drug Abuse, 5600 Fishers Lane, Rockville, MD 20857. Phone: (301) 443-6480. 1989.

The Economic Costs of Alcohol and Drug Abuse and Mental Illness: 1985. National Clearinghouse for Alcohol and Drug Information, Dept. PP, P.O. Box 2345, Rockville, MD 20852. 1990, BKD54.

Epidemiology of Cocaine Use and Abuse. National Institute on Drug Abuse, 5600 Fishers Lane, Rockville, MD 20857. Phone: (301) 443-6480. 1991.

National Household Survey on Drug Abuse: Highlights 1988. National Clearinghouse for Alcohol and Drug Information, Dept. PP, P.O. Box 2345, Rockville, MD 20852. 1990, BKD52.

National Household Survey on Drug Abuse: Population Estimates, 1990. National Clearinghouse for Alcohol and Drug Information, Dept. PP, P.O. Box 2345, Rockville, MD 20852. 1991, BKD57.

Third Triennial Report to Congress: Drug Abuse and Alcohol Research. National Clearinghouse for Alcohol and Drug Information, Dept. PP, P.O. Box 2345, Rockville, MD 20852. 1990, BKD47.

TEXTBOOKS AND MONOGRAPHS

Addictive Disorders. Michael F. Fleming, Kristen Lawton Barry (eds.). Mosby-Year Book, 11830 Westline Industrial Drive, St. Louis, MO 63146. Phone: (800) 325-4177. Fax: (314) 432-1380. 1992.

AIDS and Alcohol/Drug Abuse: Psychosocial Research. Dennis G. Fisher (ed.). Haworth Press, 10 Alice Street, Binghamton, NY 13904-1580. Phone: (800) 342-9678. Fax: (607) 722-1424. 1991.

AIDS, Drugs, and Sexual Risk. McKegany. Taylor & Francis Inc., 1900 Frost Rd., Suite 101, Bristol, PA 19007-1598. Phone: (800) 821-8312. Fax: (215) 785-5515. 1992.

Cocaine, AIDS and Intravenous Drug Use. Samuel R. Friedman, Douglas S. Lipton (eds.). Haworth Press, 10 Alice Street, Binghamton, NY 13904-1580. Phone: (800) 3HA-WORTH. Fax: (607) 722-1424. 1991.

Cocaine Solutions: Help for Cocaine Abusers and Their Families. Jennifer Rice-Licare, Katharine Delaney-McLoughlin. Haworth Press, Inc., 10 Alice St., Binghamton, NY 13904-1580. Phone: (800) 342-9678. 1990.

Substance Abuse: A Comprehensive Textbook. Hoyce H. Lowinson, Pedro Ruiz, Robert B. Millman (eds.). Williams & Wilkins, 428 East Preston St., Baltimore, MD 21202. Phone: (800) 638-0672. Fax: (800) 447-8438. Second edition 1992.

DRUG COMPANIES

See: PHARMACEUTICAL INDUSTRY

DRUG HYPERSENSITIVITY

See also: DRUG INTERACTIONS; DRUG TOXICITY; PHARMACOLOGY

ABSTRACTING, INDEXING, AND CURRENT AWARENESS PUBLICATIONS

Current Contents/Life Sciences. Institute for Scientific Information, 3501 Market St., Philadelphia, PA 19104. Phone: (215) 386-0100. Fax: (215) 386-6362.

Excerpta Medica. Section 26: Immunology, Serology and Transplantation. Elsevier Science Publishing Co., Inc., P.O. Box 882, Madison Square Station, New York, NY 10159-2101. Phone: (212) 989-5800. Fax: (212) 633-3990. 32/year.

Excerpta Medica. Section 38: Adverse Reactions Titles. Elsevier Science Publishing Co., Inc., P.O. Box 882, Madison Square Station, New York, NY 10159-2101. Phone: (212) 989-5800. Fax: (212) 633-3990. 12/year.

Index Medicus. U.S. National Library of Medicine, 8600 Rockville Pike, Bethesda, MD 20894. Phone: (800) 638-8480. Monthly.

International Pharmaceutical Abstracts. American Society of Hospital Pharmacists, 4630 Montgomery Ave., Bethesda, MD 20814. Phone: (301) 657-3000. Fax: (301) 657-1641. Semimonthly.

CD-ROM DATABASES

1993 PDR Library on CD-ROM. Medical Economics, Five Paragon Dr., Montvale, NJ 07645-1742. Phone: (800) 232-7379. Fax: (201) 573-4956. 1993.

International Pharmaceutical Abstracts. SilverPlatter Information, Inc., River Ridge Office Park, 100 River Ridge Rd., Norwood, MA 02062. Phone: (617) 769-2599. Fax: (617) 769-8763. Quarterly.

PDR on CD-ROM. Medical Economics, Five Paragon Dr., Montvale, NJ 07645-1742. Phone: (800) 222-3045. Fax: (201) 573-4956. 3/year.

Year Books on Disc. CMC ReSearch, Inc., 7150 S.W. Hampton, Suite C-120, Portland, OR 97223. Phone: (800) 262-7668. Fax: (503) 639-1796. Annual includes Year Books of Cardiology, Dermatology, Diagnostic Radiology, Drug Therapy, Emergency Medicine, Family Practice, Medicine, Neurology and Neurosurgery, Obstetrics and Gynecology, Oncology, Pediatrics, and Psychiatry and Applied Mental Health.

DIRECTORIES

AFHS Drug Information. American Society of Hospital Pharmacists, 4630 Montgomery Ave., Bethesda, MD 20814.

Phone: (301) 657-3000. Fax: (301) 652-8278. Annual, updated irregularly.

HANDBOOKS, GUIDES, MANUALS, ATLASES

PDR Drug Interactions and Side Effects Index. Medical Economics, Five Paragon Dr., Montvale, NJ 07645-1742. Phone: (800) 222-3045. Fax: (201) 573-4956. Annual.

Physician's Desk Reference. Medical Economics, Five Paragon Dr., Montvale, NJ 07645-1742. Phone: (800) 222-3045. Fax: (201) 573-4956. Annual.

USP DI Volume I: Drug Information for the Health Care Professional. United States Pharmacopeial Convention, Inc., 12601 Twinbrook Parkway, Rockville, MD 20852. Phone: (800) 227-8772. Fax: (301) 816-8148. Annual Two volumes.

USP DI Volume II. Advice for the Patient: Drug Information in Lay Language. United States Pharmacopeial Convention, Inc., 12601 Twinbrook Parkway, Rockville, MD 20852. Phone: (800) 227-8772. Fax: (301) 816-8148. Annual.

JOURNALS

Medical Letter on Drugs and Therapeutics. Medical Letter Inc., 56 Hamilton St., New Rochelle, NY 10801. Phone: (914) 235-0500.

ONLINE DATABASES

ADRID: Adverse Drug Reactions and Interactions Database. Paul de Haen International, 2750 S. Shoshone St., Englewood, CO 80110. Phone: (800) 438-0296.

Drug Information Full Text. American Society of Hospital Pharmacists, 4630 Montgomery Ave., Bethesda, MD 20814. Phone: (301) 657-3000. Fax: (301) 652-8278.

EMBASE. Elsevier Science Publishing Co., Inc., P.O. Box 882, Madison Square Station, New York, NY 10159-2101. Phone: (212) 989-5800. Fax: (212) 633-3990.

International Pharmaceutical Abstracts. American Society of Hospital Pharmacists, 4630 Montgomery Ave., Bethesda, MD 20814. Phone: (301) 657-3000. Fax: (301) 657-1641. Monthly.

MEDLINE. National Library of Medicine, 8600 Rockville Pike, Bethesda, MD 20894. Phone: (800) 638-8480.

Pharmline. Regional Drug Information Service, The London Hospital, Whitechapel Rd., London E1 1BB, England. Phone: 071-377 7489. Weekly.

Physician's Desk Reference. Medical Economics, Five Paragon Dr., Montvale, NJ 07645-1742. Phone: (800) 222-3045. Fax: (201) 573-4956. Monthly.

SciSearch. Institute for Scientific Information, 3501 Market St., Philadelphia, PA 19104. Phone: (215) 386-0100. Fax: (215) 386-6362.

DRUG INTERACTIONS

See also: DRUG TOXICITY; PHARMACOLOGY

ABSTRACTING, INDEXING, AND CURRENT AWARENESS PUBLICATIONS

BIOSIS/CAS Selects: Drug Interactions. BIOSIS, 2100 Arch St., Philadelphia, PA 19103-1399. Phone: (215) 587-4800. Fax: (215) 587-2016. Biweekly.

Current Contents/Life Sciences. Institute for Scientific Information, 3501 Market St., Philadelphia, PA 19104. Phone: (215) 386-0100. Fax: (215) 386-6362.

Excerpta Medica. Section 38: Adverse Reactions Titles. Elsevier Science Publishing Co., Inc., P.O. Box 882, Madison Square Station, New York, NY 10159-2101. Phone: (212) 989-5800. Fax: (212) 633-3990. 12/year.

Index Medicus. U.S. National Library of Medicine, 8600 Rockville Pike, Bethesda, MD 20894. Phone: (800) 638-8480. Monthly.

International Pharmaceutical Abstracts. American Society of Hospital Pharmacists, 4630 Montgomery Ave., Bethesda, MD 20814. Phone: (301) 657-3000. Fax: (301) 657-1641. Semimonthly.

Science Citation Index. Institute for Scientific Information, 3501 Market St., Philadelphia, PA 19104. Phone: (800) 523-1850. Fax: (215) 386-6362. Bimonthly.

ANNUALS AND REVIEWS

Year Book of Drug Therapy. Mosby-Year Book, 11830 Westline Industrial Drive, St. Louis, MO 63146. Phone: (800) 325-4177. Fax: (314) 432-1380. Annual.

ASSOCIATIONS, PROFESSIONAL SOCIETIES, ADVOCACY AND SUPPORT GROUPS

American Pharmaceutical Association (APhA). 2215 Constitution Ave. N.W., Washington, DC 20037. Phone: (202) 628-4410. Fax: (202) 783-2351.

American Society of Hospital Pharmacists (ASHP). 4630 Montgomery Ave., Bethesda, MD 20814. Phone: (301) 657-3000. Fax: (301) 652-8278.

National Mental Health Association (NMHA). 1021 Prince St., Alexandria, VA 22314-2971. Phone: (703) 684-7722. Fax: (703) 684-5968.

CD-ROM DATABASES

1993 PDR Library on CD-ROM. Medical Economics, Five Paragon Dr., Montvale, NJ 07645-1742. Phone: (800) 232-7379. Fax: (201) 573-4956. 1993.

Drug Information Source on CD-ROM. Cambridge Scientific Abstracts, 7200 Wisconsin Ave., Bethesda, MD 20814-4823. Phone: (800) 843-7751. Fax: (301) 961-6720. Quarterly.

Hansten and Horn's Drug Interactions. Borin. Williams & Wilkins, 428 East Preston St., Baltimore, MD 21202. Phone: (800) 638-0672. Fax: (800) 447-8438. 1991.

International Pharmaceutical Abstracts. SilverPlatter Information, Inc., River Ridge Office Park, 100 River Ridge Rd., Norwood, MA 02062. Phone: (617) 769-2599. Fax: (617) 769-8763. Quarterly.

PDR on CD-ROM. Medical Economics, Five Paragon Dr., Montvale, NJ 07645-1742. Phone: (800) 222-3045. Fax: (201) 573-4956. 3/year.

SCISEARCH. Institute for Scientific Information, 3501 Market St., Philadelphia, PA 19104. Phone: (215) 386-0100. Fax: (215) 386-6362.

SEDBASE (Side Effects of Drugs). SilverPlatter Information, Inc., River Ridge Office Park, 100 River Ridge Rd., Norwood, MA 02062. Phone: (617) 769-2599. Fax: (617) 769-8763. Semiannual.

Year Books on Disc. CMC ReSearch, Inc., 7150 S.W. Hampton, Suite C-120, Portland, OR 97223. Phone: (800) 262-7668. Fax: (503) 639-1796. Annual includes Year Books of Cardiology, Dermatology, Diagnostic Radiology, Drug Therapy, Emergency Medicine, Family Practice, Medicine, Neurology and Neurosurgery, Obstetrics and Gynecology, Oncology, Pediatrics, and Psychiatry and Applied Mental Health.

DIRECTORIES

AFHS Drug Information. American Society of Hospital Pharmacists, 4630 Montgomery Ave., Bethesda, MD 20814. Phone: (301) 657-3000. Fax: (301) 652-8278. Annual, updated irregularly.

ENCYCLOPEDIAS, DICTIONARIES, WORD BOOKS

Merck Index: An Encyclopedia of Chemicals and Drugs. Merck & Co., Inc., P.O. Box 2000, Rahway, NJ 07065. Phone: (201) 855-4558. Irregular.

HANDBOOKS, GUIDES, MANUALS, ATLASES

Drug-Test Interactions Handbook. Jack G. Salway. Raven Press, 1185 Avenue of the Americas, New York, NY 10036. Phone: (212) 930-9500. Fax: (212) 869-3495. 1990.

Drug Therapy. Katzung. Appleton & Lange, 25 Van Zant St., East Norwalk, CT 06855. Phone: (800) 423-1359. Fax: (203) 854-9486. Second edition 1991.

PDR Drug Interactions and Side Effects Index. Medical Economics, Five Paragon Dr., Montvale, NJ 07645-1742. Phone: (800) 222-3045. Fax: (201) 573-4956. Annual.

USP DI Volume I: Drug Information for the Health Care Professional. United States Pharmacopeial Convention, Inc., 12601 Twinbrook Parkway, Rockville, MD 20852. Phone: (800) 227-8772. Fax: (301) 816-8148. Annual Two volumes.

USP DI Volume II. Advice for the Patient: Drug Information in Lay Language. United States Pharmacopeial Convention, Inc., 12601 Twinbrook Parkway, Rockville, MD 20852. Phone: (800) 227-8772. Fax: (301) 816-8148. Annual.

JOURNALS

Drug Metabolism and Disposition. Williams & Wilkins, 428 East Preston St., Baltimore, MD 21202. Phone: (800) 638-0672. Fax: (800) 447-8438.

Journal of Pharmacology. J.B. Lippincott Co., 227 E. Washington Square, Philadelphia, PA 19106-3780. Phone: (215) 238-4200. Fax: (215) 238-4227.

Medical Letter on Drugs and Therapeutics. Medical Letter Inc., 56 Hamilton St., New Rochelle, NY 10801. Phone: (914) 235-0500.

ONLINE DATABASES

EMBASE. Elsevier Science Publishing Co., Inc., P.O. Box 882, Madison Square Station, New York, NY 10159-2101. Phone: (212) 989-5800. Fax: (212) 633-3990.

International Pharmaceutical Abstracts. American Society of Hospital Pharmacists, 4630 Montgomery Ave., Bethesda, MD 20814. Phone: (301) 657-3000. Fax: (301) 657-1641. Monthly.

MEDLINE. National Library of Medicine, 8600 Rockville Pike, Bethesda, MD 20894. Phone: (800) 638-8480.

SciSearch. Institute for Scientific Information, 3501 Market St., Philadelphia, PA 19104. Phone: (215) 386-0100. Fax: (215) 386-6362.

DRUG REHABILITATION

See: DRUG ABUSE

DRUG TOXICITY

See also: DRUG HYPERSENSITIVITY; DRUG
INTERACTIONS; PHARMACOLOGY;
POISONING; TOXICOLOGY

ABSTRACTING, INDEXING, AND CURRENT AWARENESS PUBLICATIONS

Biological Abstracts. BIOSIS, 2100 Arch St., Philadelphia, PA 19103-1399. Phone: (800) 523-4800. Fax: (215) 587-2016.

CA Selects: Drug & Cosmetic Toxicity. Chemical Abstracts Service, 2540 Olentangy River Road, P.O. Box 3012, Columbus, OH 43210-0012. Phone: (800) 848-6538. Biweekly.

Chemical Abstracts. Chemical Abstracts Service, 2540 Olentangy River Rd., P.O. Box 3012, Columbus, OH 43210-0012. Phone: (800) 848-6538.

Current Contents/Life Sciences. Institute for Scientific Information, 3501 Market St., Philadelphia, PA 19104. Phone: (215) 386-0100. Fax: (215) 386-6362.

Excerpta Medica. Section 38: Adverse Reactions Titles. Elsevier Science Publishing Co., Inc., P.O. Box 882, Madison Square Station, New York, NY 10159-2101. Phone: (212) 989-5800. Fax: (212) 633-3990. 12/year.

Excerpta Medica. Section 52: Toxicology. Elsevier Science Publishing Co., Inc., P.O. Box 882, Madison Square Station, New York, NY 10159-2101. Phone: (212) 989-5800. Fax: (212) 633-3990. 20/year.

Index Medicus. U.S. National Library of Medicine, 8600 Rockville Pike, Bethesda, MD 20894. Phone: (800) 638-8480. Monthly.

International Pharmaceutical Abstracts. American Society of Hospital Pharmacists, 4630 Montgomery Ave., Bethesda, MD 20814. Phone: (301) 657-3000. Fax: (301) 657-1641. Semimonthly.

Science Citation Index. Institute for Scientific Information, 3501 Market St., Philadelphia, PA 19104. Phone: (800) 523-1850. Fax: (215) 386-6362. Bimonthly.

Toxicology Abstracts. Cambridge Scientific Abstracts, 7200 Wisconsin Ave., Bethesda, MD 20814-4823. Phone: (800) 843-7751. Fax: (301) 961-6720. Monthly.

CD-ROM DATABASES

1993 PDR Library on CD-ROM. Medical Economics, Five Paragon Dr., Montvale, NJ 07645-1742. Phone: (800) 232-7379. Fax: (201) 573-4956. 1993.

Biological Abstracts on Compact Disc. BIOSIS, 2100 Arch St., Philadelphia, PA 19103-1399. Phone: (800) 523-4800. Fax: (215) 587-2016. Quarterly.

PDR on CD-ROM. Medical Economics, Five Paragon Dr., Montvale, NJ 07645-1742. Phone: (800) 222-3045. Fax: (201) 573-4956. 3/year.

PolTox. Cambridge Scientific Abstracts, 7200 Wisconsin Ave., Bethesda, MD 20814-4823. Phone: (800) 843-7751. Fax: (301) 961-6720. Quarterly.

SCISEARCH. Institute for Scientific Information, 3501 Market St., Philadelphia, PA 19104. Phone: (215) 386-0100. Fax: (215) 386-6362.

TOXLINE. SilverPlatter Information, Inc., River Ridge Office Park, 100 River Ridge Rd., Norwood, MA 02062. Phone: (617) 769-2599. Fax: (617) 769-8763. Quarterly.

TOXLINE Plus. SilverPlatter Information, Inc., River Ridge Office Park, 100 River Ridge Rd., Norwood, MA 02062. Phone: (617) 769-2599. Fax: (617) 769-8763. Quarterly.

Year Books on Disc. CMC ReSearch, Inc., 7150 S.W. Hampton, Suite C-120, Portland, OR 97223. Phone: (800) 262-7668. Fax: (503) 639-1796. Annual includes Year Books of Cardiology, Dermatology, Diagnostic Radiology, Drug Therapy, Emergency Medicine, Family Practice, Medicine, Neurology and Neurosurgery, Obstetrics and Gynecology, Oncology, Pediatrics, and Psychiatry and Applied Mental Health.

DIRECTORIES

AFHS Drug Information. American Society of Hospital Pharmacists, 4630 Montgomery Ave., Bethesda, MD 20814. Phone: (301) 657-3000. Fax: (301) 652-8278. Annual, updated irregularly.

ENCYCLOPEDIAS, DICTIONARIES, WORD BOOKS

Merck Index: An Encyclopedia of Chemicals and Drugs. Merck & Co., Inc., P.O. Box 2000, Rahway, NJ 07065. Phone: (201) 855-4558. Irregular.

HANDBOOKS, GUIDES, MANUALS, ATLASES

Handbook of Medical Toxicology. Peter Viccellio (ed.). Little, Brown and Company, 34 Beacon St., Boston, MA 02108. Phone: (617) 227-0730. 1992.

Handbook of Toxicology. Viccellio. Little, Brown and Co., 34 Beacon St., Boston, MA 02108. Phone: (617) 227-0730. Fax: (617) 227-0790. 1992.

PDR Drug Interactions and Side Effects Index. Medical Economics, Five Paragon Dr., Montvale, NJ 07645-1742. Phone: (800) 222-3045. Fax: (201) 573-4956. Annual.

JOURNALS

Drug Metabolism and Disposition. Williams & Wilkins, 428 East Preston St., Baltimore, MD 21202. Phone: (800) 638-0672. Fax: (800) 447-8438.

Journal of Clinical Pharmacology. J.B. Lippincott Co., 227 E. Washington Square, Philadelphia, PA 19106-3780. Phone: (215) 238-4200. Fax: (215) 238-4227.

Medical Letter on Drugs and Therapeutics. Medical Letter Inc., 56 Hamilton St., New Rochelle, NY 10801. Phone: (914) 235-0500.

ONLINE DATABASES

BIOSIS Previews. BIOSIS, 2100 Arch St., Philadelphia, PA 19103-1399. Phone: (800) 523-4800. Fax: (215) 587-2016.

CA File (Chemical Abstracts File). Chemical Abstracts Service, 2540 Olentangy River Rd., P.O. Box 3012, Columbus, OH 43210-0012. Phone: (800) 848-6538.

CSA Life Sciences Collection. Cambridge Scientific Abstracts, 7200 Wisconsin Ave., Bethesda, MD 20814-4823. Phone: (800) 843-7751. Fax: (301) 961-6720.

EMBASE. Elsevier Science Publishing Co., Inc., P.O. Box 882, Madison Square Station, New York, NY 10159-2101. Phone: (212) 989-5800. Fax: (212) 633-3990.

MEDLINE. National Library of Medicine, 8600 Rockville Pike, Bethesda, MD 20894. Phone: (800) 638-8480.

Physician's Desk Reference. Medical Economics, Five Paragon Dr., Montvale, NJ 07645-1742. Phone: (800) 222-3045. Fax: (201) 573-4956. Monthly.

SciSearch. Institute for Scientific Information, 3501 Market St., Philadelphia, PA 19104. Phone: (215) 386-0100. Fax: (215) 386-6362.

TOXLINE. U.S. National Library of Medicine, Toxicology Information Program, 8600 Rockville Pike, Bethesda, MD 20894. Phone: (800) 638-8480. Monthly.

TEXTBOOKS AND MONOGRAPHS

Goldfrank's Toxicologic Emergencies. Lewis R. Goldfrank, Neal E. Fomenbaum, Neal A. Lewin, and others. Appleton & Lange, 25 Van Zant St., East Norwalk, CT 06855. Phone: (800) 423-1359. Fax: (203) 854-9486. Fourth edition 1990.

Medical Toxicology: Diagnosis and Treatment of Human Poisoning. Ellerhorn. Elsevier Science Publishing Co., Inc., P.O. Box 882, Madison Square Station, New York, NY 10159-2101. Phone: (212) 989-5800. Fax: (212) 633-3990. 1988.

Poisoning and Drug Overdose. Kent R. Olson. Appleton & Lange, 25 Van Zant St., East Norwalk, CT 06855. Phone: (800) 423-1359. Fax: (203) 854-9486. Biennial 1990.

Principles and Practice of Clinical Toxicology. Gossel. Raven Press, 1185 Ave. of the Americas, New York, NY 10036. Phone: (212) 930-9500. Fax: (212) 869-3495. Second edition 1990.

Toxicologic Emergencies. Goldfrank. Appleton & Lange, 25 Van Zant St., East Norwalk, CT 06855. Phone: (800) 423-1359. Fax: (203) 854-9486. Fourth edition 1990.

DRUGS

See also: ANTIBIOTICS; NON-PRESCRIPTION DRUGS; ORPHAN DRUGS; PHARMACEUTICAL INDUSTRY; PHARMACOLOGY; PHARMACY; PSYCHOACTIVE DRUGS; PSYCHOPHARMACOLOGY

ABSTRACTING, INDEXING, AND CURRENT AWARENESS PUBLICATIONS

BIOSIS/CAS Selects: Antiarrhythmic Drugs. BIOSIS, 2100 Arch St., Philadelphia, PA 19103-1399. Phone: (215) 587-4800. Fax: (215) 587-2016. Biweekly.

BIOSIS/CAS Selects: Anticonvulsants. BIOSIS, 2100 Arch St., Philadelphia, PA 19103-1399. Phone: (215) 587-4800. Fax: (215) 587-2016. Biweekly.

BIOSIS/CAS Selects: Antifungal Agents. BIOSIS, 2100 Arch St., Philadelphia, PA 19103-1399. Phone: (215) 587-4800. Fax: (215) 587-2016. Biweekly.

BIOSIS/CAS Selects: Antiulcer Agents. BIOSIS, 2100 Arch St., Philadelphia, PA 19103-1399. Phone: (215) 587-4800. Fax: (215) 587-2016. Biweekly.

BIOSIS/CAS Selects: Antiviral Agents. BIOSIS, 2100 Arch St., Philadelphia, PA 19103-1399. Phone: (215) 587-4800. Fax: (215) 587-2016. Biweekly.

CA Selects: Anti-Inflammatory Agents & Arthritis. Chemical Abstracts Service, 2540 Olentangy River Road, P.O. Box 3012, Columbus, OH 43210-0012. Phone: (800) 848-6538. Biweekly.

CA Selects: Anticonvulsants & Antiepileptics. Chemical Abstracts Service, 2540 Olentangy River Road, P.O. Box 3012, Columbus, OH 43210-0012. Phone: (800) 848-6538. Biweekly.

CA Selects: Antifungal & Antimycotic Agents. Chemical Abstracts Service, 2540 Olentangy River Road, P.O. Box 3012, Columbus, OH 43210-0012. Phone: (800) 848-6538. Biweekly.

CA Selects: Drug Delivery Systems & Dosage Forms. Chemical Abstracts Service, 2540 Olentangy River Road, P.O. Box 3012, Columbus, OH 43210-0012. Phone: (800) 848-6538. Biweekly.

CA Selects: Drug Interactions. Chemical Abstracts Service, 2540 Olentangy River Road, P.O. Box 3012, Columbus, OH 43210-0012. Phone: (800) 848-6538. Biweekly.

CA Selects: Hypertension & Antihypertensives. Chemical Abstracts Service, 2540 Olentangy River Road, P.O. Box 3012, Columbus, OH 43210-0012. Phone: (800) 848-6538. Biweekly.

CA Selects: Prostaglandins. Chemical Abstracts Service, 2540 Olentangy River Road, P.O. Box 3012, Columbus, OH 43210-0012. Phone: (800) 848-6538. Biweekly.

CA Selects: Ulcer Inhibitors. Chemical Abstracts Service, 2540 Olentangy River Road, P.O. Box 3012, Columbus, OH 43210-0012. Phone: (800) 848-6538. Biweekly.

CA Selects: Virucides & Virustats. Chemical Abstracts Service, 2540 Olentangy River Road, P.O. Box 3012, Columbus, OH 43210-0012. Phone: (800) 848-6538. Biweekly.

CAS BioTech Updates: Pharmaceutical Applications. Chemical Abstracts Service, 2540 Olentangy River Road, P.O. Box 3012, Columbus, OH 43210-0012. Phone: (800) 848-6538. Biweekly.

CAS BioTech Updates: Slow-Release Pharmaceuticals. Chemical Abstracts Service, 2540 Olentangy River Road, P.O. Box 3012, Columbus, OH 43210-0012. Phone: (800) 848-6538. Biweekly.

Chemical Abstracts. Chemical Abstracts Service, 2540 Olentangy River Rd., P.O. Box 3012, Columbus, OH 43210-0012. Phone: (800) 848-6538.

Clin-Alert. Learned Information, Inc., 143 Old Marlton Pike, Medford, NJ 08055. Phone: (609) 654-6266. 24/year.

Excerpta Medica. Section 38: Adverse Reactions Titles. Elsevier Science Publishing Co., Inc., P.O. Box 882, Madison Square Station, New York, NY 10159-2101. Phone: (212) 989-5800. Fax: (212) 633-3990. 12/year.

ICRDB Cancergram: Cancer Detection and Management-- Nuclear Medicine. U.S. Government Printing Office, Superintendent of Documents, P.O. Box 371954, Pittsburgh, PA 15250-7954. Phone: (202) 783-3238. Fax: (202) 512-2250. Monthly.

Index Medicus. U.S. National Library of Medicine, 8600 Rockville Pike, Bethesda, MD 20894. Phone: (800) 638-8480. Monthly.

International Pharmaceutical Abstracts. American Society of Hospital Pharmacists, 4630 Montgomery Ave., Bethesda, MD 20814. Phone: (301) 657-3000. Fax: (301) 657-1641. Semimonthly.

PharmIndex. Skyline Publishers, Inc., P.O. Box 1029, University Station, Portland, OR 97207. Phone: (503) 228-6568. Monthly.

Research Alert: Angina Pectoris/Antianginal Drugs. Institute for Scientific Information, 3501 Market St., Philadelphia, PA 19104. Phone: (800) 523-1850. Fax: (215) 386-6362. Weekly.

Research Alert: Antiarrhythmial Drugs. Institute for Scientific Information, 3501 Market St., Philadelphia, PA 19104. Phone: (800) 523-1850. Fax: (215) 386-6362. Weekly.

Research Alert: Anticonvulsant Agents/Epilepsy & Seizure Disorders. Institute for Scientific Information, 3501 Market St., Philadelphia, PA 19104. Phone: (800) 523-1850. Fax: (215) 386-6362. Weekly.

Research Alert: Antihistamine Agents. Institute for Scientific Information, 3501 Market St., Philadelphia, PA 19104. Phone: (800) 523-1850. Fax: (215) 386-6362. Weekly.

Research Alert: Antihypertensive Agents. Institute for Scientific Information, 3501 Market St., Philadelphia, PA 19104. Phone: (800) 523-1850. Fax: (215) 386-6362. Weekly.

Research Alert: Antiulcer Agents. Institute for Scientific Information, 3501 Market St., Philadelphia, PA 19104. Phone: (800) 523-1850. Fax: (215) 386-6362. Weekly.

Research Alert: Antiviral Agents. Institute for Scientific Information, 3501 Market St., Philadelphia, PA 19104. Phone: (800) 523-1850. Fax: (215) 386-6362. Weekly.

Research Alert: Hypoglycemic Agents. Institute for Scientific Information, 3501 Market St., Philadelphia, PA 19104. Phone: (800) 523-1850. Fax: (215) 386-6362. Weekly.

Research Alert: Prostaglandins, Leukotrienes, Thromboxanes. Institute for Scientific Information, 3501 Market St., Philadelphia, PA 19104. Phone: (800) 523-1850. Fax: (215) 386-6362. Weekly.

ANNUALS AND REVIEWS

Advanced Drug Delivery Reviews. Elsevier Science Publishing Co., Inc., P.O. Box 882, Madison Square Station, New York, NY 10159-2101. Phone: (212) 989-5800. Fax: (212) 633-3990. 6/year.

Advances in Drug Research. Academic Press, Inc., 1250 Sixth Ave., San Diego, CA 92101-4311. Phone: (619) 699-6345. Fax: (619) 699-6715. Irregular.

Drug Facts and Comparisons. J.B. Lippincott Co., 227 E. Washington Square, Philadelphia, PA 19106-3780. Phone: (215) 238-4200. Fax: (215) 238-4227. Annual.

In Development Biotechnology Medicines. Pharmaceutical Manufacturers Association, 1100 15th St. N.W., Washington, DC 20005. Phone: (202) 835-3400. Annual.

In Development New Medicines for Arthritis. Pharmaceutical Manufacturers Association, 1100 15th St. N.W., Washington, DC 20005. Phone: (202) 835-3400. Annual.

In Development New Medicines for Children. Pharmaceutical Manufacturers Association, 1100 15th St. N.W., Washington, DC 20005. Phone: (202) 835-3400. Quarterly.

In Development New Medicines for Older Americans. Pharmaceutical Manufacturers Association, 1100 15th St. N.W., Washington, DC 20005. Phone: (202) 835-3400. Annual.

In Development New Medicines for Older Americans. 1991 Annual Survey. 93 Cardiovascular, Cerebrovascular Medicines in Testing for Top Causes of Death. Pharmaceutical Manufacturers Association, 1100 15th St. N.W., Washington, DC 20005. Phone: (202) 835-3400. 1991.

In Development New Medicines for Older Americans. 1991 Annual Survey. 116 Medicines Target 19 Debilitating Diseases. Pharmaceutical Manufacturers Association, 1100 15th St. N.W., Washington, DC 20005. Phone: (202) 835-3400. 1991.

In Development New Medicines for Older Americans. 1991 Annual Survey. 329 Medicines in Testing for 45 Diseases of Aging. Pharmaceutical Manufacturers Association, 1100 15th St. N.W., Washington, DC 20005. Phone: (202) 835-3400. 1991.

In Development New Medicines for Older Americans. 1991 Annual Survey. More Medicines in Testing for Cancer Than for Any Other Disease of Aging. Pharmaceutical Manufacturers Association, 1100 15th St. N.W., Washington, DC 20005. Phone: (202) 835-3400. 1991.

In Development New Medicines for Women. Pharmaceutical Manufacturers Association, 1100 15th St. N.W., Washington, DC 20005. Phone: (202) 835-3400. Annual.

In Development Orphan Drugs. Pharmaceutical Manufacturers Association, 1100 15th St. N.W., Washington, DC 20005. Phone: (202) 835-3400. Annual.

Prostaglandins and Related Compounds: Seventh International Conference, Florence, Italy. Bengt Samuelsson, Peter W Ramwell, Rodolfo Paoletti, et. al.. Raven Press, 1185 Avenue of the Americas, New York, NY 10036. Phone: (212) 930-9500. Fax: (212) 869-3495. Advances in Prostaglandin, Thromboxane, and Leukotriene Research, Volumes 21A and 21B. Two volumes. 1991.

Year Book of Drug Therapy. Mosby-Year Book, 11830 Westline Industrial Drive, St. Louis, MO 63146. Phone: (800) 325-4177. Fax: (314) 432-1380. Annual.

ASSOCIATIONS, PROFESSIONAL SOCIETIES, ADVOCACY AND SUPPORT GROUPS

American Pharmaceutical Association (APhA). 2215 Constitution Ave. N.W., Washington, DC 20037. Phone: (202) 628-4410. Fax: (202) 783-2351.

American Society of Hospital Pharmacists (ASHP). 4630 Montgomery Ave., Bethesda, MD 20814. Phone: (301) 657-3000. Fax: (301) 652-8278.

Drug Information Association (DIA). P.O. Box 3113, Maple Glen, PA 19002. Phone: (215) 628-2288.

United States Pharmacopeial Convention (USP). 12601 Twinbrook Pkwy., Rockville, MD 20852. Phone: (800) 227-8772. Fax: (301) 816-8375.

BIBLIOGRAPHIES

New Drug Approvals in 1991. Pharmaceutical Manufacturers Association, 1100 15th St. N.W., Washington, DC 20005. Phone: (202) 835-3400. 1992.

CD-ROM DATABASES

1993 PDR Library on CD-ROM. Medical Economics, Five Paragon Dr., Montvale, NJ 07645-1742. Phone: (800) 232-7379. Fax: (201) 573-4956. 1993.

Drug Data Report on CD-ROM. Prous Science Publishers, Apdo. de Correos 540, E-08080 Barcelona, Spain. Phone: 03 4592220. Fax: 03 2581535. Quarterly.

Drug Information Source on CD-ROM. Cambridge Scientific Abstracts, 7200 Wisconsin Ave., Bethesda, MD 20814-4823. Phone: (800) 843-7751. Fax: (301) 961-6720. Quarterly.

Excerpta Medica CD: Drugs & Pharmacology. SilverPlatter Information, Inc., River Ridge Office Park, 100 River Ridge Rd., Norwood, MA 02062. Phone: (617) 769-2599. Fax: (617) 769-8763. Quarterly.

International Pharmaceutical Abstracts. SilverPlatter Information, Inc., River Ridge Office Park, 100 River Ridge Rd., Norwood, MA 02062. Phone: (617) 769-2599. Fax: (617) 769-8763. Quarterly.

PDR on CD-ROM. Medical Economics, Five Paragon Dr., Montvale, NJ 07645-1742. Phone: (800) 222-3045. Fax: (201) 573-4956. 3/year.

Physician's Desk Reference. Medical Economics, Five Paragon Dr., Montvale, NJ 07645-1742. Phone: (800) 222-3045. Fax: (201) 573-4956. 3/year.

SEDBASE (Side Effects of Drugs). SilverPlatter Information, Inc., River Ridge Office Park, 100 River Ridge Rd., Norwood, MA 02062. Phone: (617) 769-2599. Fax: (617) 769-8763. Semiannual.

Year Books on Disc. CMC ReSearch, Inc., 7150 S.W. Hampton, Suite C-120, Portland, OR 97223. Phone: (800) 262-7668. Fax: (503) 639-1796. Annual includes Year Books of Cardiology, Dermatology, Diagnostic Radiology, Drug Therapy, Emergency Medicine, Family Practice, Medicine, Neurology and Neurosurgery, Obstetrics and Gynecology, Oncology, Pediatrics, and Psychiatry and Applied Mental Health.

DIRECTORIES

AFHS Drug Information. American Society of Hospital Pharmacists, 4630 Montgomery Ave., Bethesda, MD 20814. Phone: (301) 657-3000. Fax: (301) 652-8278. Annual, updated irregularly.

American Druggist Blue Book. Hearst Corporation, 60 E. 42nd St., New York, NY 10165. Phone: (212) 297-9680. Fax: (415) 588-6867. Annual.

Drugs Available Abroad. Jerry L. Schlesser. Gale Research, Inc., 835 Penobscot Bldg., Detroit, MI 48226-4094. Phone: (800) 877-GALE. Fax: (313) 961-6083. Annual.

Edmund's Prescription Drug Prices. St. Martin's Press, 175 Fifth Ave., New York, NY 10010. Phone: (212) 674-5151. Annual.

Red Book. Medical Economics, Five Paragon Dr., Montvale, NJ 07645-1742. Phone: (800) 222-3045. Fax: (201) 573-4956. Annual.

ENCYCLOPEDIAS, DICTIONARIES, WORD BOOKS

Merck Index: An Encyclopedia of Chemicals and Drugs. Merck & Co., Inc., P.O. Box 2000, Rahway, NJ 07065. Phone: (201) 855-4558. Irregular.

Pharmaceutical Word Book. Barbara De Lorenzo. Springhouse Publishing Co., 1111 Bethlehem Pike, Spring House, PA 19477. Phone: (800) 331-3170. Fax: (215) 646-8716. Second edition 1992.

Pharmaceutical Words. Stedman. Williams & Wilkins, 428 East Preston St., Baltimore, MD 21202. Phone: (800) 638-0672. Fax: (800) 447-8438. 1992.

USAN and the USP Dictionary of Drug Names. United States Pharmacopeial Convention, Inc., 12601 Twinbrook Parkway, Rockville, MD 20852. Phone: (800) 227-8772. Fax: (301) 816-8148. Annual.

HANDBOOKS, GUIDES, MANUALS, ATLASES

American Drug Index. J.B. Lippincott Co., 227 E. Washington Square, Philadelphia, PA 19106-3780. Phone: (215) 238-4200. Fax: (215) 238-4227. Annual.

Cardiology Drug Facts. Ezra A. Amsterdam, Jonathan Abrams, Dale Berg, and others. J.B. Lippincott Co., 227 E. Washington Square, Philadelphia, PA 19106-3780. Phone: (215) 238-4200. Fax: (215) 238-4227. 1990.

Dosage Calculations Manual. Catherine M. Todd, Belle Erickson. Springhouse Publishing Co., 1111 Bethlehem Pike, Spring House, PA 19477. Phone: (800) 331-3170. Fax: (215) 646-8716. Second edition 1992.

Drug Evaluations Annual. American Medical Association, 515 North State St., Chicago, IL 60610. Phone: (312) 464-0183. Fax: (312) 464-5834. Annual.

Drug-Test Interactions Handbook. Jack G. Salway. Raven Press, 1185 Avenue of the Americas, New York, NY 10036. Phone: (212) 930-9500. Fax: (212) 869-3495. 1990.

Drug Therapy. Katzung. Appleton & Lange, 25 Van Zant St., East Norwalk, CT 06855. Phone: (800) 423-1359. Fax: (203) 854-9486. Second edition 1991.

Handbook of Cardiac Drugs. Ralph Purdy, Robert Boucek. Little, Brown and Co., 34 Beacon St., Boston, MA 02108. Phone: (617) 227-0730. Fax: (617) 227-0790. 1988.

Handbook of Ocular Drugs. Pavan-Langst. Little, Brown and Co., 34 Beacon St., Boston, MA 02108. Phone: (617) 227-0730. Fax: (617) 227-0790. 1991.

Handbook of Prescribing Medications for Geriatric Patients. Ahronheim. Little, Brown and Co., 34 Beacon St., Boston, MA 02108. Phone: (617) 227-0730. Fax: (617) 227-0790. 1992.

Introduction to Drug Therapy. Springhouse Publishing Co., 1111 Bethlehem Pike, Spring House, PA 19477. Phone: (800) 331-3170. Fax: (215) 646-8716. 1992.

Ophthalmic Drug Facts. Jimmy D. Bartlett, N. Rex Ghormley, Siret Jaanus, and others. J.B. Lippincott Co., 227 E. Washington Square, Philadelphia, PA 19106-3780. Phone: (215) 238-4200. Fax: (215) 238-4227. 1992.

PDR Drug Interactions and Side Effects Index. Medical Economics, Five Paragon Dr., Montvale, NJ 07645-1742. Phone: (800) 222-3045. Fax: (201) 573-4956. Annual.

PDR Indications Index. Medical Economics, Five Paragon Dr., Montvale, NJ 07645-1742. Phone: (800) 222-3045. Fax: (201) 573-4956. Annual.

Pediatric Drug Handbook. Benitz. Mosby-Year Book, 11830 Westline Industrial Drive, St. Louis, MO 63146. Phone: (800) 325-4177. Fax: (314) 432-1380. Second edition 1988.

Physician's 1992 Drug Handbook. Springhouse Publishing Co., 1111 Bethlehem Pike, Spring House, PA 19477. Phone: (800) 331-3170. Fax: (215) 646-8716. 1992.

Physician's Desk Reference. Medical Economics, Five Paragon Dr., Montvale, NJ 07645-1742. Phone: (800) 222-3045. Fax: (201) 573-4956. Annual.

Physician's Desk Reference for Nonprescription Drugs. Medical Economics, Five Paragon Dr., Montvale, NJ 07645-1742. Phone: (800) 222-3045. Fax: (201) 573-4956. Annual.

USP DI Volume I: Drug Information for the Health Care Professional. United States Pharmacopeial Convention, Inc., 12601 Twinbrook Parkway, Rockville, MD 20852. Phone: (800) 227-8772. Fax: (301) 816-8148. Annual Two volumes.

USP DI Volume II. Advice for the Patient: Drug Information in Lay Language. United States Pharmacopeial Convention, Inc., 12601 Twinbrook Parkway, Rockville, MD 20852. Phone: (800) 227-8772. Fax: (301) 816-8148. Annual.

JOURNALS

Clinical Pharmacy. American Society of Hospital Pharmacists, 4630 Montgomery Ave., Bethesda, MD 20814. Phone: (301) 657-3000. Fax: (301) 652-8278. Monthly.

Medical Letter on Drugs and Therapeutics. Medical Letter Inc., 56 Hamilton St., New Rochelle, NY 10801. Phone: (914) 235-0500.

Prostaglandins. Butterworth-Heinemann, 80 Montvale Ave., Stoneham, MA 02180. Phone: (617) 438-8464. Fax: (617) 279-4851. Monthly.

NEWSLETTERS

Drug Utilization Review. American Health Consultants, Department C1290, P.O. Box 740060, Atlanta, GA 30374. Phone: (800) 559-1032. Fax: (404) 352-1971. Monthly.

Facts and Comparisons Drug Newsletter. J.B. Lippincott Co., 227 E. Washington Square, Philadelphia, PA 19106-3780. Phone: (215) 238-4200. Fax: (215) 238-4227. Monthly.

FDA Drug Bulletin. Food and Drug Administration. Department of Health and Human Services, 5600 Fishers Ln., Rockville, MD 20857. Phone: (301) 443-3220. 3-4/year.

ONLINE DATABASES

CA File (Chemical Abstracts File). Chemical Abstracts Service, 2540 Olentangy River Rd., P.O. Box 3012, Columbus, OH 43210-0012. Phone: (800) 848-6538.

EMBASE. Elsevier Science Publishing Co., Inc., P.O. Box 882, Madison Square Station, New York, NY 10159-2101. Phone: (212) 989-5800. Fax: (212) 633-3990.

International Pharmaceutical Abstracts. American Society of Hospital Pharmacists, 4630 Montgomery Ave., Bethesda, MD 20814. Phone: (301) 657-3000. Fax: (301) 657-1641. Monthly.

MEDLINE. National Library of Medicine, 8600 Rockville Pike, Bethesda, MD 20894. Phone: (800) 638-8480.

Pharmline. Regional Drug Information Service, The London Hospital, Whitechapel Rd., London E1 1BB, England. Phone: 071-377 7489. Weekly.

Physician's Desk Reference. Medical Economics, Five Paragon Dr., Montvale, NJ 07645-1742. Phone: (800) 222-3045. Fax: (201) 573-4956. Monthly.

SciSearch. Institute for Scientific Information, 3501 Market St., Philadelphia, PA 19104. Phone: (215) 386-0100. Fax: (215) 386-6362.

POPULAR WORKS AND PATIENT EDUCATION

39 Development AIDS Medicines: Drugs and Vaccines. Pharmaceutical Manufacturers Association, 1100 15th St. N.W., Washington, DC 20005. Phone: (202) 835-3400. Annual.

AARP Pharmacy Service Prescription Drug Handbook. AARP. HarperCollins Pubs., Inc., 10 E. 53rd St., New York, NY 10022-5299. Phone: (212) 207-7000. Fax: (800) 242-7737. Revised edition 1992.

About Your Medicines. United States Pharmacopeial Convention, Inc., 12601 Twinbrook Parkway, Rockville, MD 20852. Phone: (800) 227-8772. Fax: (301) 816-8148. Sixth edition 1992.

Advice for the Patient. United States Pharmacopeial Convention, Inc., 12601 Twinbrook Parkway, Rockville, MD 20852. Phone: (800) 227-8772. Fax: (301) 816-8148. 1989.

The Complete Drug Reference. United States Pharmacopeia. Consumer Reports Books, 9180 LeSaint Dr., Fairfield, OH 45014. Phone: (513) 860-1178. Annual.

Complete Guide to Prescription & Non-Prescription Drugs. H. Winter Griffith. Putnam Publishing Group, 200 Madison Ave., New York, NY 10016. Phone: (800) 631-8571. Revised edition 1992.

The Essential Guide to Prescription Drugs. James W. Long. HarperCollins Pubs., Inc., 10 E. 53rd St., New York, NY 10022-5299. Phone: (212) 207-7000. Annual.

Graedons' Best Medicine: From Herbal Remedies to High-Tech Rx Breakthroughs. Joe Graedon, Teresa Graedon. Bantam Books, Inc., 666 Fifth Ave., New York, NY 10103. Phone: (800) 223-6834. 1991.

Guide to Prescription and Over-the-Counter Drugs: Brand Name Drugs, Generic Drugs, Vitamins, Minerals, Food Additives. American Medical Association Staff. Random House, Inc., 201 E. 50th St., New York, NY 10022. Phone: (800) 726-0600. 1988.

The Handbook of Heart Drugs: A Consumer's Guide to Safe and Effective Use. Martin Goldman. Holt, Rinehart & Winston, 115 W. 18th St., New York, NY 10011. Phone: (800) 488-5233. 1992.

The Pill Book: The Illustrated Guide to the Most Prescribed Drugs in the U.S.. Harold M. Silverman. Bantam Books, Inc., 666 Fifth Ave., New York, NY 10103. Phone: (800) 223-6834. Fourth edition 1990.

Prescription Drug Reference Guide. Consumer Guide Eds.. Outlet Book Co., 225 Park Ave. S., New York, NY 10003. Phone: (212) 254-1600. 1990.

Prescription Drugs & Their Side Effects. Edward L. Stern. Putnam Publishing Group, 200 Madison Ave., New York, NY 10016. Phone: (800) 631-8571. Sixth edition 1991.

Worst Pills, Best Pills. Sidney Wolf and others. 2000 P St. N.W., Ste. 700, Washington, DC 20036. Phone: (202) 872-0320. 1988.

RESEARCH CENTERS, INSTITUTES, CLEARINGHOUSES

Center for Biomedical Research. University of Kansas. Smissman Research Laboratories, 2099 Constant Ave., Lawrence, KS 66046. Phone: (913) 864-5140.

Food and Drug Administration. 5600 Fishers Lane, Rockville, MD 20857. Phone: (301) 443-2410.

Office of Consumer Affairs. Food and Drug Administration. 5600 Fishers Ln., HFE-50, Rockville, MD 20857. Phone: (301) 443-3170.

TEXTBOOKS AND MONOGRAPHS

British National Formulary. Pharmaceutical Press, Rittenhouse Book Distributors, 511 Feheley Dr., King of Prussia, PA 19406. Phone: (800) 345-6425. Fax: (800) 223-7488. No. 23 1992.

European Pharmacopeia. Pharmaceutical Press, Rittenhouse Book Distributors, 511 Feheley Dr., King of Prussia, PA 19406. Phone: (800) 345-6425. Fax: (800) 223-7488. Second edition. Part II-15. 1992.

Family Physician's Compendium of Drug Therapy. McGraw-Hill Inc., 11 West 19th St., New York, NY 10011. Phone: (212) 337-5001. Fax: (212) 337-4092. 1989.

Pharmacological Basis of Therapeutics. L. Goodman, A. Gilman. McGraw-Hill Inc., 11 West 19th St., New York, NY 10011. Phone: (212) 337-5001. Fax: (212) 337-4092. 8th edition 1990.

Prostaglandins in Clinical Practice. W. David Watikins, Myron B. Peterson, J. Raymon Fletcher. Raven Press, 1185 Avenue of the Americas, New York, NY 10036. Phone: (212) 930-9500. Fax: (212) 869-3495. 1989.

Therapeutic Drugs. Sir Colin Dollery (ed.). Churchill Livingstone Inc., 650 Avenue of the Americas, New York, NY 10011. Phone: (212) 819-5400. Fax: (212) 302-6598. Two volumes 1991.

DRUGS, NON-PRESCRIPTION

See: NON-PRESCRIPTION DRUGS

DUODENAL ULCER

See: ULCERS

DYSENTERY

See: GASTROINTESTINAL DISORDERS

DYSLEXIA

See: COMMUNICATION DISORDERS

E

EAR DISORDERS

See: OTOLARYNGOLOGY

EATING DISORDERS

ABSTRACTING, INDEXING, AND CURRENT AWARENESS PUBLICATIONS

Current Contents/Clinical Medicine. Institute for Scientific Information, 3501 Market St., Philadelphia, PA 19104. Phone: (800) 523-1850. Fax: (215) 386-6362. Weekly.

Index Medicus. U.S. National Library of Medicine, 8600 Rockville Pike, Bethesda, MD 20894. Phone: (800) 638-8480. Monthly.

Psychological Abstracts. American Psychological Association, 1200 17th St. NW, Washington, DC 20036. Phone: (202) 955-7600. Monthly.

Science Citation Index. Institute for Scientific Information, 3501 Market St., Philadelphia, PA 19104. Phone: (800) 523-1850. Fax: (215) 386-6362. Bimonthly.

ASSOCIATIONS, PROFESSIONAL SOCIETIES, ADVOCACY AND SUPPORT GROUPS

American Anorexia/Bulimia Association (AA/BA). 418 E. 76th St., New York, NY 10021. Phone: (212) 734-1114.

Anorexia Nervosa and Related Eating Disorders (ANRED). P.O. Box 5102, Eugene, OR 97405. Phone: (503) 344-1144.

Bulimia Anorexia Self-Help. 6125 Clayton Ave., Ste. 215, St. Louis, MO 63139. Phone: (800) 227-4785. 24-hour Crisis Line: 800-762-3334.

International Association of Eating Disorders Professionals (IAEDP). 34213 Coast Hwy., Ste. E, Dana Point, CA 92629. Phone: (714) 248-1150. Fax: (714) 248-8851.

National Anorexic Aid Society, Inc.. P.O. Box 29461, Columbus, OH 43229. Phone: (614) 436-1112.

National Association of Anorexia Nervosa and Associated Disorders. P.O. Box 7, Highland Park, IL 60035. Phone: (312) 831-3438.

Overeaters Anonymous. 1246 S. LaCienega Blvd., Rm. 203, Los Angeles, CA 90035. Phone: (213) 618-8835.

BIBLIOGRAPHIES

Anorexia Nervosa and Other Eating Disorders (Excluding Obesity). National Technical Information Service, 5285 Port

Royal Rd., Springfield, VA 22161. Phone: (703) 487-4650. Fax: (703) 321-8547. Jan. 1978-May 1989 PB89-863419/CBY.

Nutri-Topics: Anorexia Nervosa and Bulimia. Food and Nutrition Center, National Agricultural Library, 10301 Baltimore Blvd., Beltsville, MD 20705.

CD-ROM DATABASES

PsycLit. SilverPlatter Information, Inc., River Ridge Office Park, 100 River Ridge Rd., Norwood, MA 02062. Phone: (617) 769-2599. Fax: (617) 769-8763. Quarterly.

SCISEARCH. Institute for Scientific Information, 3501 Market St., Philadelphia, PA 19104. Phone: (215) 386-0100. Fax: (215) 386-6362.

JOURNALS

Archives of General Psychiatry. American Medical Association, 515 North State St., Chicago, IL 60610. Phone: (312) 464-0183. Fax: (312) 464-5834. Monthly.

Eating Disorders Review. P.M. Inc., 14545 Friar St. No. 209, Box 2468, Van Nuys, CA 91404. Phone: (213) 873-4394.

Journal of Psychiatric Research. Pergamon Press, 660 White Plains Rd., Tarrytown, NY 10591-5153. Phone: (914) 592-7700. Fax: (914) 592-3625.

NEWSLETTERS

American Anorexia/Bulimia Association-Newsletter. American Anorexia/Bulimia Association, Inc., 418 E. 76th St., New York, NY 10021. Phone: (201) 734-1114. 4/year.

ONLINE DATABASES

EMBASE. Elsevier Science Publishing Co., Inc., P.O. Box 882, Madison Square Station, New York, NY 10159-2101. Phone: (212) 989-5800. Fax: (212) 633-3990.

MEDLINE. National Library of Medicine, 8600 Rockville Pike, Bethesda, MD 20894. Phone: (800) 638-8480.

PsycInfo. SilverPlatter Information, Inc., River Ridge Office Park, 100 River Ridge Rd., Norwood, MA 02062. Phone: (617) 769-2599. Fax: (617) 769-8763. Quarterly.

SciSearch. Institute for Scientific Information, 3501 Market St., Philadelphia, PA 19104. Phone: (215) 386-0100. Fax: (215) 386-6362.

POPULAR WORKS AND PATIENT EDUCATION

Anorexia Nervosa: A Guide for Sufferers and Their Families. R.L. Palmer. Penguin USA, 375 Hudson St., New York, NY 10014-3657. Phone: (800) 331-4624. 1989.

Anorexia Nervosa and Recovery: Hunger for Meaning. Karen Way. Haworth Press, 10 Alice Street, Binghamton, NY 13904-1580. Phone: (800) 342-9678. Fax: (607) 722-1424. 1992.

Bulimarexia. Boskind-White. W.W. Norton & Co., Inc., 500 Fifth Ave., New York, NY 10110. Phone: (800) 223-2584. Second edition 1991.

Bulimia: A Guide to Recovery. Lindsey Hall, Leigh Cohn. Gurze Books, P.O. Box 2238, Carlsbad, CA 92008. Phone: (619) 434-7533. 1992.

Controlling Eating Disorders with Facts, Advice and Resources. Raymond Lemberg (ed.). Oryx Press, 4041 N. Central, Suite 700, Phoenix, AZ 85012. Phone: (800) 279-6799. Fax: (800) 279-4663. 1992.

Living with Anorexia and Bulimia. James Moorey. St. Martin's Press, 175 Fifth Ave., New York, NY 10010. Phone: (212) 674-5151. 1992.

Overcoming Eating Disorders: Recovery from Anorexia, Bulimia and Compulsive Overeating. Kathleen Zraly, David Swift. Continuum Publishing Co., 370 Lexington Ave., New York, NY 10017. Phone: (212) 532-3650. 1992.

Overcoming Overeating. Jane R. Hirschman, Carol H. Munter. Addison-Wesley Publishing Co., Rte. 128, Reading, MA 01867. Phone: (800) 447-2226. 1988.

A Parent's Guide to Eating Disorders and Obesity. Martha M. Jablow. Bantam Doubleday Dell, 666 Fifth Ave., New York, NY 10103. Phone: (800) 223-6834. 1992.

Surviving an Eating Disorder: Strategies for Family and Friends. Michele Siegel, Judith Brisman, Margot Weinshel. HarperCollins Pubs., Inc., 10 E. 53rd St., New York, NY 10022-5299. Phone: (212) 207-7000. Fax: (800) 242-7737. 1989.

RESEARCH CENTERS, INSTITUTES, CLEARINGHOUSES

Center for the Research and Treatment of Anorexia Nervosa. 10921 Wilshire Blvd., Ste. 702, Los Angeles, CA 90024. Phone: (213) 824-5881.

Center for the Study of Anorexia and Bulimia. 1 W. 91st St., New York, NY 10024. Phone: (212) 595-3449.

Eating Disorders Research and Treatment Program. Michael Reese Hospital and Medical Center, Lake Shore Dr. at 31st St., Chicago, IL 60616. Phone: (312) 791-3878.

TEXTBOOKS AND MONOGRAPHS

Conversations with Anorexics. Hilde Bruch, Danita Czyzewski, Melanie A. Suhr (eds.). HarperCollins Publishers, Inc., 10 E. 53rd St., New York, NY 10022-5299. Phone: (800) 242-7737. 1989.

Eating Behavior in Eating Disorders. B. Timothy Walsh. American Psychiatric Press, 1400 K St. N.W., Washington, DC 20005. Phone: (202) 682-6000. Fax: (202) 682-6114. 1988.

Eating Disorders. L. George Hsu. Guilford Publications, Inc., 72 Spring St., New York, NY 10012. Phone: (800) 365-7006. Fax: (212) 366-6708.

Eating and Growth Disorders in Infants and Children. Joseph L. Woolston. Sage Publications, Inc., 2455 Teller Road, P.O. Box 5084, Newbury Park, CA 91320. Phone: (805) 499-0721. Fax: (805) 499-0871. 1991.

Family Approaches in Treatment of Eating Disorders. D. Blake Woodside, Lorie Shekter-Wolfson (eds.). American Psychiatric Press, Inc., 1400 K St. NW, Washington, DC 20005. Phone: (202) 682-6268. Fax: (202) 789-2648. 1991.

Medical Aspects of Anorexia Nervosa. S. Bhanji, D. Mattingly. Butterworth-Heinemann, 80 Montvale Ave., Stoneham, MA 02180. Phone: (617) 438-8464. Fax: (617) 279-4851. 1988.

ECG

See: ELECTROCARDIOGRAPHY

ECHOCARDIOGRAPHY

See: CARDIOLOGY; HEART DISEASES

ECLAMPSIA

See: PREGNANCY COMPLICATIONS

ECONOMICS OF HEALTH CARE

See: HEALTH CARE FINANCING

ECTOPIC PREGNANCY

See: PREGNANCY COMPLICATIONS

ECZEMA

See: DERMATOLOGIC DISEASES

EDUCATION

See: ALLIED HEALTH EDUCATION; DENTAL EDUCATION; MEDICAL EDUCATION; NURSING EDUCATION

EEG

See: ELECTROENCEPHALOGRAPHY

EKG

See: ELECTROCARDIOGRAPHY

ELECTROCARDIOGRAPHY

ABSTRACTING, INDEXING, AND CURRENT AWARENESS PUBLICATIONS

Excerpta Medica. Section 18: Cardiovascular Disease and Cardiovascular Surgery. Elsevier Science Publishing Co., Inc., P.O. Box 882, Madison Square Station, New York, NY 10159-2101. Phone: (212) 989-5800. Fax: (212) 633-3990. 24/year.

Index Medicus. U.S. National Library of Medicine, 8600 Rockville Pike, Bethesda, MD 20894. Phone: (800) 638-8480. Monthly.

Research Alert: Cardiovascular Diseases-Interventional Cardiology. Institute for Scientific Information, 3501 Market St., Philadelphia, PA 19104. Phone: (800) 523-1850. Fax: (215) 386-6362. Weekly.

Research Alert: Electrocardiography. Institute for Scientific Information, 3501 Market St., Philadelphia, PA 19104. Phone: (800) 523-1850. Fax: (215) 386-6362. Weekly.

CD-ROM DATABASES

Cardiology MEDLINE. MEP, 124 Mt. Auburn St., Cambridge, MA 02138. Phone: (800) 342-1338. Fax: (617) 868-7738. Quarterly.

HANDBOOKS, GUIDES, MANUALS, ATLASES

ECG Ready Reference. Henry Mamott. Mosby-Year Book, 11830 Westline Industrial Drive, St. Louis, MO 63146. Phone: (800) 325-4177. Fax: (314) 432-1380. 1990.

Guide to Basic Electrocardiography. John Wagner Beasley, E. Wayne Grogan Jr.. Plenum Publishing Co., 233 Spring St., New York, NY 10013-1578. Phone: (212) 620-8000. Fax: (212) 463-0742. 1990.

Manual of Cardiovascular Diagnosis and Therapy. Joseph S. Alpert, James M. Rippe. Little, Brown and Co., 34 Beacon St., Boston, MA 02108. Phone: (617) 227-0730. Third edition 1988.

Simplified EKG Analysis: A Sequential Guide to Interpretation and Diagnosis. Charles B. Seelig. Mosby-Year Book, 11830 Westline Industrial Drive, St. Louis, MO 63146. Phone: (800) 325-4177. Fax: (314) 432-1380. 1991.

JOURNALS

American Journal of Cardiology. Reed Publishing USA, 249 W. 17th St., New York, NY 10011. Phone: (212) 645-0067. Fax: (212) 242-6987. 22/year.

Cardiology. S. Karger Publishers, Inc., 26 W. Avon Rd., P.O. Box 529, Farmington, CT 06085. Phone: (203) 675-7834. Fax: (203) 675-7302. Bimonthly.

Journal of the American College of Cardiology. Elsevier Science Publishing Co., Inc., P.O. Box 882, Madison Square Station, New York, NY 10159-2101. Phone: (212) 989-5800. Fax: (212) 633-3990. Monthly.

Journal of Electrocardiology. Churchill Livingstone Inc., 650 Avenue of the Americas, New York, NY 10011. Phone: (212) 819-5400. Fax: (212) 302-6598. Quarterly.

Trends in Cardiovascular Medicine. Elsevier Science Publishing Co., Inc., P.O. Box 882, Madison Square Station, New York, NY 10159-2101. Phone: (212) 989-5800. Fax: (212) 633-3990. 6/year.

ONLINE DATABASES

EMBASE. Elsevier Science Publishing Co., Inc., P.O. Box 882, Madison Square Station, New York, NY 10159-2101. Phone: (212) 989-5800. Fax: (212) 633-3990.

MEDLINE. National Library of Medicine, 8600 Rockville Pike, Bethesda, MD 20894. Phone: (800) 638-8480.

SciSearch. Institute for Scientific Information, 3501 Market St., Philadelphia, PA 19104. Phone: (215) 386-0100. Fax: (215) 386-6362.

TEXTBOOKS AND MONOGRAPHS

Basic Arrhythmias. Iris Gail Walraven. Prentice Hall, 113 Sylvan Ave., Rt. 9W, Prentice Hall Bldg., Englewood Cliffs, NJ 07632. Phone: (201) 767-5937. Third edition 1991.

Electrocardiogram. Klinge. Thieme Medical Publishers, Inc., 381 Park Ave. S., New York, NY 10016. Phone: (212) 683-5088. Fax: (212) 779-9020. 1988.

Electrocardiography: 100 Diagnostic Criteria. Harold Brooks. Mosby-Year Book, 11830 Westline Industrial Drive, St. Louis, MO 63146. Phone: (800) 325-4177. Fax: (314) 432-1380. 1987.

Electrocardiography: Essentials of Interpretation. Nora Goldschlager, Mervin Goldman. Appleton & Lange, 25 Van Zant St., East Norwalk, CT 06855. Phone: (800) 423-1359. Fax: (203) 854-9486. 1984.

Electrocardiology in Clinical Practice. T-Chuan Chou. W.B. Saunders Co., The Curtis Center, Independence Square W., Philadelphia, PA 19106-3399. Phone: (215) 238-7800. Third edition 1991.

An Introduction to Electrocardiography. L. Schamroth, C. Schamroth. BMJ Publishing Group, BMA House, Tavistock Square, London WC1H 9JR, England. Phone: 071383 6244. Fax: 071383 6662. Seventh edition 1990.

Myocardial Infarction: Electrocardiographic Differential Diagnosis. Ary L. Goldberger. Mosby-Year Book, 11830 Westline Industrial Drive, St. Louis, MO 63146. Phone: (800) 325-4177. Fax: (314) 432-1380. Fourth edition 1991.

Principles of Electrocardiography. Nora Goldschlager, Mervin J. Goldman. Appleton & Lange, 25 Van Zant St., East Norwalk, CT 06855. Phone: (800) 423-1359. Fax: (203) 854-9486. Thirteenth edition 1989.

Textbook of Interventional Cardiology. Eric J. Topol (ed.). W.B. Saunders Co., The Curtis Center, Independence Square W., Philadelphia, PA 19106-3399. Phone: (215) 238-7800. 1990.

ELECTROENCEPHALOGRAPHY

ABSTRACTING, INDEXING, AND CURRENT AWARENESS PUBLICATIONS

Index Medicus. U.S. National Library of Medicine, 8600 Rockville Pike, Bethesda, MD 20894. Phone: (800) 638-8480. Monthly.

ASSOCIATIONS, PROFESSIONAL SOCIETIES, ADVOCACY AND SUPPORT GROUPS

American Board of Registration of EEG Technologists (ABRET). Davis Medical Ctr., EEG Lab, 2315 Stockton Blvd., Sacramento, CA 95817.

American Electroencephalographic Soceity (AEEGS). 2579 Melinda Dr., Atlanta, GA 30345. Phone: (404) 320-1746.

American Medical Electroencephalographic Association (AMEEGA). 850 Grove Rd., Ste. 11, Elm Grove, WI 53122. Phone: (414) 797-7800.

American Society of Electroneurodiagnostic Technologists, Inc. (ASET). Sixth at Quint, Carroll, IA 51401. Phone: (712) 792-2978.

HANDBOOKS, GUIDES, MANUALS, ATLASES

EEG Handbook. Dyro. Little, Brown and Co., 34 Beacon St., Boston, MA 02108. Phone: (617) 227-0730. Fax: (617) 227-0790. 1989.

JOURNALS

American Journal of EEG Technology. American Society of Electroneurodiagnostic Technologists, Inc., Sixth at Quint, Carroll, IA 51401. Phone: (712) 792-2978. Quarterly.

Clinical Electroencephalography. American Medical Electroencephalographic Assoc., 850 Grove Rd., Ste. 11, Elm Grove, WI 53122. Phone: (414) 797-7800. Quarterly.

Electroencephalography and Clinical Neurophysiology. Elsevier Science Publishing Co., Inc., P.O. Box 882, Madison Square Station, New York, NY 10159-2101. Phone: (212) 989-5800. Fax: (212) 633-3990. 18/year.

ONLINE DATABASES

EMBASE. Elsevier Science Publishing Co., Inc., P.O. Box 882, Madison Square Station, New York, NY 10159-2101. Phone: (212) 989-5800. Fax: (212) 633-3990.

MEDLINE. National Library of Medicine, 8600 Rockville Pike, Bethesda, MD 20894. Phone: (800) 638-8480.

SciSearch. Institute for Scientific Information, 3501 Market St., Philadelphia, PA 19104. Phone: (215) 386-0100. Fax: (215) 386-6362.

TEXTBOOKS AND MONOGRAPHS

Current Practice of Clinical Electroencephalography. David Daly, Timothy Pedley. Raven Press, 1185 Ave. of the Americas, New York, NY 10036. Phone: (212) 930-9500. Fax: (212) 869-3495. Second edition 1990.

Electroencephalography. Ernst Niedermeyer, F.H. Lopes da Silva. Williams & Wilkins, 428 East Preston St., Baltimore, MD 21202. Phone: (800) 638-0672. Fax: (800) 447-8438. 1987.

Fundamentals of EEG Technology. Fay S. Tyner and others. Raven Press, 1185 Ave. of the Americas, New York, NY 10036. Phone: (212) 930-9500. Fax: (212) 869-3495. Two volumes 1983-1989.

Rapid Interpretation of EKG. Dubin. Cover Publishing Co., P.O. Box 1092, Tampa, FL 33601. Phone: (813) 237-0266. Fourth edition 1989.

Spehlmann's EEG Primer. Fisch. Elsevier Science Publishing Co., Inc., P.O. Box 882, Madison Square Station, New York, NY 10159-2101. Phone: (212) 989-5800. Fax: (212) 633-3990. Second edition 1991.

EMBOLISM

See: VASCULAR DISEASES

EMBRYO TRANSFER

See: IN VITRO FERTILIZATION; INFERTILITY

EMBRYOLOGY

See also: FETAL DEVELOPMENT

ABSTRACTING, INDEXING, AND CURRENT AWARENESS PUBLICATIONS

Current Contents/Life Sciences. Institute for Scientific Information, 3501 Market St., Philadelphia, PA 19104. Phone: (215) 386-0100. Fax: (215) 386-6362.

Excerpta Medica. Section 1: Anatomy, Anthropology, Embryology & Histology. Elsevier Science Publishing Co., Inc., P.O. Box 882, Madison Square Station, New York, NY 10159-2101. Phone: (212) 989-5800. Fax: (212) 633-3990. 16/year.

Excerpta Medica. Section 21: Developmental Biology and Teratology. Elsevier Science Publishing Co., Inc., P.O. Box 882, Madison Square Station, New York, NY 10159-2101. Phone: (212) 989-5800. Fax: (212) 633-3990. 16/year.

Excerpta Medica. Section 22: Human Genetics. Elsevier Science Publishers, P.O. Box 882, Madison Square Station, New York, NY 10159-2101. Phone: (212) 633-3950. Fax: (212) 633-3990. 24/year.

General Science Index. H.W. Wilson Co., 950 University Ave., Bronx, NY 10452. Phone: (800) 367-6770.

Index Medicus. U.S. National Library of Medicine, 8600 Rockville Pike, Bethesda, MD 20894. Phone: (800) 638-8480. Monthly.

Science Citation Index. Institute for Scientific Information, 3501 Market St., Philadelphia, PA 19104. Phone: (800) 523-1850. Fax: (215) 386-6362. Bimonthly.

CD-ROM DATABASES

SCISEARCH. Institute for Scientific Information, 3501 Market St., Philadelphia, PA 19104. Phone: (215) 386-0100. Fax: (215) 386-6362.

JOURNALS

Acta Anatomica. S. Karger Publishers, Inc., 26 W. Avon Rd., P.O. Box 529, Farmington, CT 06085. Phone: (203) 675-7834. Fax: (203) 675-7302.

Cell Differentiation and Development. Elsevier Science Publishing Co., Inc., P.O. Box 882, Madison Square Station, New York, NY 10159-2101. Phone: (212) 989-5800. Fax: (212) 633-3990.

Development. Company of Biologists Ltd., Box 32, Commerce Way, Colchester, Essex CO2 8HP, England. Phone: 0206-46351. Fax: 0206-549331. 13/year.

Developmental Biology. Academic Press, Inc., 1250 Sixth Ave., San Diego, CA 92101-4311. Phone: (619) 699-6345. Fax: (619) 699-6715.

ONLINE DATABASES

EMBASE. Elsevier Science Publishing Co., Inc., P.O. Box 882, Madison Square Station, New York, NY 10159-2101. Phone: (212) 989-5800. Fax: (212) 633-3990.

MEDLINE. National Library of Medicine, 8600 Rockville Pike, Bethesda, MD 20894. Phone: (800) 638-8480.

SciSearch. Institute for Scientific Information, 3501 Market St., Philadelphia, PA 19104. Phone: (215) 386-0100. Fax: (215) 386-6362.

RESEARCH CENTERS, INSTITUTES, CLEARINGHOUSES

Carnegie Institution of Washington. Department of Embryology, 115 W. University Parkway, Baltimore, MD 21210. Phone: (301) 467-1414.

Carnegie Laboratories of Embryology. CPRC, University of California, Davis, CA 95616. Phone: (916) 752-0210.

TEXTBOOKS AND MONOGRAPHS

A Coloring Book of Embryology. George Matsumura, Marjorie A. England. Mosby-Year Book, 11830 Westline Industrial Drive, St. Louis, MO 63146. Phone: (800) 325-4177. Fax: (314) 432-1380. 1992.

The Developing Human. K.L. Moore. W.B. Saunders Co., The Curtis Center, Independence Square W., Philadelphia, PA 19106-3399. Phone: (215) 238-7800. Fourth edition 1988.

Developmental Pathology of the Embryo and Fetus. James E. Dimmick, Dagmar K. Kalousek (eds.). J.B. Lippincott Co., 227 E. Washington Square, Philadelphia, PA 19106-3780. Phone: (215) 238-4200. Fax: (215) 238-4227. 1992.

Embryo Experimentation. Peter Singer, Helga Kuhse, Stephen Buckle, and others. Cambridge University Press, 40 W. 20th St., New York, NY 10011. Phone: (800) 431-1580. 1990.

Embryology for Surgeons. Stephen W. Gray, John E. Skonadalakis. Williams & Wilkins, 428 East Preston St., Baltimore, MD 21202. Phone: (800) 638-0672. Fax: (800) 447-8438. 1992.

Fetal Tissue Transplants in Medicine. Robert G. Edwards. Cambridge University Press, 40 W. 20th St., New York, NY 10011. Phone: (800) 431-1580. 1992.

Langman's Medical Embryology. Thomas W. Sadler. Williams & Wilkins, 428 East Preston St., Baltimore, MD 21202. Phone: (800) 638-0672. Fax: (800) 447-8438. 1990.

Medical Embryology. J. Langman, T.W. Sadler. Williams & Wilkins, 428 East Preston St., Baltimore, MD 21202. Phone: (800) 638-0672. Fax: (800) 447-8438. Sixth edition 1990.

EMERGENCY CARE

See: EMERGENCY MEDICINE

EMERGENCY MEDICAL TECHNICIANS

ABSTRACTING, INDEXING, AND CURRENT AWARENESS PUBLICATIONS

Cumulative Index to Nursing and Allied Health Literature. Glendale Adventist Medical Center, P.O. Box 871, Glendale, CA 91209. Phone: (818) 409-8005. Bimonthly.

ASSOCIATIONS, PROFESSIONAL SOCIETIES, ADVOCACY AND SUPPORT GROUPS

International Rescue and Emergency Care Association. 8107 Ensign Curve, Bloomington, MN 55438. Phone: (612) 941-2926.

National Association of Emergency Medical Technicians. 9140 Ward Pwky., Kansas City, MO 64114. Phone: (816) 444-3500. Fax: (816) 444-0330.

National Flight Paramedics Association. c/o David J. Samuels, Samaritan Air Evacuation, 1242 E. McDowell Rd., Phoenix, AZ 85006.

National Registry of Emergency Medical Technicians (NREMT). P.O. Box 29233, Columbus, OH 43229. Phone: (614) 888-4484.

CD-ROM DATABASES

CPR Training by Computer. Hoffer. Williams & Wilkins, 428 East Preston St., Baltimore, MD 21202. Phone: (800) 638-0672. Fax: (800) 447-8438. Second edition 1992.

Nursing and Allied Health (CINAHL) on CD-ROM. CINAHL, 1509 Wilson Terrace, P.O. Box 871, Glendale, CA 91209-0871. Phone: (818) 409-8005.

HANDBOOKS, GUIDES, MANUALS, ATLASES

Handbook of Emergency Care Procedures. Harvey Grant, Dwight Lodge. Prentice Hall, 113 Sylvan Ave., Rt. 9W, Prentice Hall Bldg., Englewood Cliffs, NJ 07632. Phone: (201) 767-5937. 1988.

Manual of Prehospital Emergency Medicine. Robert Miller. Mosby-Year Book, 11830 Westline Industrial Drive, St. Louis, MO 63146. Phone: (800) 325-4177. Fax: (314) 432-1380. 1992.

Paramedic Skills Manual. Charles Phillips and others. Prentice Hall, 113 Sylvan Ave., Rt. 9W, Prentice Hall Bldg., Englewood Cliffs, NJ 07632. Phone: (201) 767-5937. Second edition 1990.

ONLINE DATABASES

Nursing and Allied Health (CINAHL). CINAHL, 1509 Wilson Terrace, P.O. Box 871, Glendale, CA 91209-0871. Phone: (818) 409-8005.

TEXTBOOKS AND MONOGRAPHS

Advanced Emergency Care for Paramedic Practice. Shirley Jones, Al Weigel, Roger White, and others. J.B. Lippincott Co., 227 E. Washington Square, Philadelphia, PA 19106-3780. Phone: (215) 238-4200. Fax: (215) 238-4227. 1991.

Emergency Care. Harvey Grant, Robert Murray Jr., J. David Bergeron. Prentice Hall, 113 Sylvan Ave., Rt. 9W, Prentice Hall Bldg., Englewood Cliffs, NJ 07632. Phone: (201) 767-5937. Fifth edition 1990.

Emergency Care in the Streets. Nancy L. Caroline. Little, Brown and Company, 34 Beacon St., Boston, MA 02108. Phone: (617) 227-0730. Fourth edition 1991.

Emergency Medical Treatment: A Text for EMT-As and EMT-Intermediates. Nancy L. Caroline. Little, Brown and Company, 34 Beacon St., Boston, MA 02108. Phone: (617) 227-0730. Third edition 1991.

EMS Street Strategies: Effective Patient Interaction. Stephen M. Soreff, Robert T. Cadigan. F.A. Davis Co., 1915 Arch St., Philadelphia, PA 19103. Phone: (800) 523-4049. Fax: (215) 568-5065. 1992.

Paramedic Emergency Care. Bryan E. Bledsoe, Robert S. Porter, Bruce R. Shade. Prentice Hall, 113 Sylvan Ave., Rt. 9W, Prentice Hall Bldg., Englewood Cliffs, NJ 07632. Phone: (201) 767-5937. 1991.

EMERGENCY MEDICINE

See also: ALLIED HEALTH EDUCATION;
CARDIOPULMONARY RESUSCITATION

ABSTRACTING, INDEXING, AND CURRENT AWARENESS PUBLICATIONS

Cumulative Index to Nursing and Allied Health Literature. Glendale Adventist Medical Center, P.O. Box 871, Glendale, CA 91209. Phone: (818) 409-8005. Bimonthly.

Current Contents/Clinical Medicine. Institute for Scientific Information, 3501 Market St., Philadelphia, PA 19104. Phone: (800) 523-1850. Fax: (215) 386-6362. Weekly.

ENA's Nursing Scan in Emergency Care. NURSECOM, Inc., 1211 Locust St., Philadelphia, PA 19107. Phone: (215) 545-7222. Bimonthly.

Index Medicus. U.S. National Library of Medicine, 8600 Rockville Pike, Bethesda, MD 20894. Phone: (800) 638-8480. Monthly.

Science Citation Index. Institute for Scientific Information, 3501 Market St., Philadelphia, PA 19104. Phone: (800) 523-1850. Fax: (215) 386-6362. Bimonthly.

ANNUALS AND REVIEWS

Current Therapy of Trauma. Mosby-Year Book, 11830 Westline Industrial Drive, St. Louis, MO 63146. Phone: (800) 325-4177. Fax: (314) 432-1380. Irregular.

Emergency Medicine Clinics. W.B. Saunders Co., The Curtis Center, Independence Square W., Philadelphia, PA 19106-3399. Phone: (215) 238-7800. Quarterly.

Year Book of Emergency Medicine. Mosby-Year Book, 11830 Westline Industrial Drive, St. Louis, MO 63146. Phone: (800) 325-4177. Fax: (314) 432-1380. Annual.

ASSOCIATIONS, PROFESSIONAL SOCIETIES, ADVOCACY AND SUPPORT GROUPS

American Board of Emergency Medicine (ABEM). 200 Woodland Pass, Ste. D, East Lansing, MI 48823. Phone: (517) 332-4800. Fax: (517) 332-2234.

American College of Emergency Physicians (ACEP). P.O. Box 619911, Dallas, TX 75261-9911. Phone: (214) 550-0911.

Emergency Medicine Foundation. P.O. Box 61911, Dallas, TX 75261. Phone: (214) 550-0911.

Emergency Nurses Association (ENA). 230 E. Ohio, No. 600, Chicago, IL 60611. Phone: (312) 649-0297. Fax: (312) 649-9430.

National Emergency Medicine Association (NEMA). 306 W. Joppa Rd., Towson, MD 21204. Phone: (800) 332-6362.

CD-ROM DATABASES

Clinical Problems in Emergency Medicine: Acute Respiratory Distress. Smith. Williams & Wilkins, 428 East Preston St., Baltimore, MD 21202. Phone: (800) 638-0672. Fax: (800) 447-8438. 1989.

Clinical Problems in Emergency Medicine: Alcoholic Patient. Smith. Williams & Wilkins, 428 East Preston St., Baltimore, MD 21202. Phone: (800) 638-0672. Fax: (800) 447-8438. 1989.

Clinical Problems in Emergency Medicine: Unresponsive Patient. Smith. Williams & Wilkins, 428 East Preston St., Baltimore, MD 21202. Phone: (800) 638-0672. Fax: (800) 447-8438. 1989.

CPR Training by Computer. Hoffer. Williams & Wilkins, 428 East Preston St., Baltimore, MD 21202. Phone: (800) 638-0672. Fax: (800) 447-8438. Second edition 1992.

Emergency Medicine MEDLINE. MEP, 124 Mt. Auburn St., Cambridge, MA 02138. Phone: (800) 342-1338. Fax: (617) 868-7738. Quarterly.

Nursing and Allied Health (CINAHL) on CD-ROM. CINAHL, 1509 Wilson Terrace, P.O. Box 871, Glendale, CA 91209-0871. Phone: (818) 409-8005.

SCISEARCH. Institute for Scientific Information, 3501 Market St., Philadelphia, PA 19104. Phone: (215) 386-0100. Fax: (215) 386-6362.

Year Books on Disc. CMC ReSearch, Inc., 7150 S.W. Hampton, Suite C-120, Portland, OR 97223. Phone: (800) 262-7668. Fax: (503) 639-1796. Annual includes Year Books of Cardiology, Dermatology, Diagnostic Radiology, Drug Therapy, Emergency Medicine, Family Practice, Medicine, Neurology and Neurosurgery, Obstetrics and Gynecology, Oncology, Pediatrics, and Psychiatry and Applied Mental Health.

DIRECTORIES

Directory of Certified Emergency Physicians. American Board of Medical Specialties, 1 Rotary Center, Suite 805, Evanston, IL 60201. Phone: (708) 491-9091. Biennial.

Directory of Medical Specialists. Marquis Who's Who, 3002 Glenview Rd., Wilmette, IL 60091. Phone: (800) 621-9669. Fax: (708) 441-2264. Biennial.

Directory of Physicians in the United States. American Medical Association, 515 North State St., Chicago, IL 60610. Phone: (312) 464-0183. Fax: (312) 464-5834. Biennial.

ENCYCLOPEDIAS, DICTIONARIES, WORD BOOKS

Mosby's Emergency Dictionary: Quick Reference for Emergency Responders. James G. Yvorra (ed.). Mosby-Year Book, 11830 Westline Industrial Drive, St. Louis, MO 63146. Phone: (800) 325-4177. Fax: (314) 432-1380. 1989.

Mosby's Medical, Nursing, and Allied Health Dictionary. Kenneth N. Anderson, Lois Anderson, Walter D. Glanze (eds.). Mosby-Year Book, 11830 Westline Industrial Dr., St. Louis, MO 63146. Phone: (800) 325-4177. Fax: (314) 432-1380. Third edition 1990.

HANDBOOKS, GUIDES, MANUALS, ATLASES

The American Medical Association Handbook of First Aid and Emergency Care. Random House, Inc., 201 E. 50th St., New York, NY 10022. Phone: (800) 726-0600. Revised edition 1990.

Color Atlas of Diagnosis After Recent Injury. P.S. London. Mosby-Year Book, 11830 Westline Industrial Drive, St. Louis, MO 63146. Phone: (800) 325-4177. Fax: (314) 432-1380. 1991.

Emergency Pediatrics On Call. Ellen Crain, Jeffrey C. Gershel, E. John Gallagher. McGraw-Hill, Inc., 1221 Avenue of the Americas, 28th Floor, New York, NY 10020. Phone: (212) 512-4228. Second edition 1992.

Emergency Procedures. Michael Jostremski, and others. W.B. Saunders Co., The Curtis Center, Independence Squre W., Philadelphia, PA 19106-3399. Phone: (215) 238-7800. 1992.

EMT Manual. Michael K. Copass, Roy G. Soper, Mickey S. Eisenberg. W.B. Saunders Co., The Curtis Center, Independence Square W., Philadelphia, PA 19106-3399. Phone: (215) 238-7800. Second edition 1991.

Handbook of Neonatal Intensive Care. Merenstein. Mosby-Year Book, 11830 Westline Industrial Drive, St. Louis, MO 63146. Phone: (800) 325-4177. Fax: (314) 432-1380. Second edition 1989.

Handbook of Pediatric Emergencies. Baldwin. Little, Brown and Co., 34 Beacon St., Boston, MA 02108. Phone: (617) 227-0730. Fax: (617) 227-0790. 1989.

Immediate Eye Care: An Illustrated Manual. Nicola Ragge, David L. Easty. Mosby-Year Book, 11830 Westline Industrial Drive, St. Louis, MO 63146. Phone: (800) 325-4177. Fax: (314) 432-1380. 1991.

Manual of Acute Therapeutics. Iverson. Little, Brown and Co., 34 Beacon St., Boston, MA 02108. Phone: (617) 227-0730. Third edition 1987.

Manual of Emergency Medical Therapeutics. Gideon Bosker, Jeffrey S. Jones. Mosby-Year Book, 11830 Westline Industrial

Drive, St. Louis, MO 63146. Phone: (800) 325-4177. Fax: (314) 432-1380. 1992.

Manual of Emergency Medicine. Michael Eliastam and others (eds.). Mosby-Year Book, 11830 Westline Industrial Drive, St. Louis, MO 63146. Phone: (800) 325-4177. Fax: (314) 432-1380. Fifth edition 1989.

Manual of Emergency Medicine: Diagnosis and Treatment. Jon L. Jenkins, Joseph Loscalzo. Little, Brown and Company, 34 Beacon St., Boston, MA 02108. Phone: (617) 227-0730. Second edition 1990.

Manual of Emergency Orthopedics. William M. Green, Robert W. Derlet, Timothy Bray. Williams & Wilkins, 428 East Preston St., Baltimore, MD 21202. Phone: (800) 638-0672. Fax: (800) 447-8438. 1992.

Manual of Emergency and Outpatient Techniques. ALlen P. Klippel, Charles Anderson. Little, Brown and Co., 34 Beacon St., Boston, MA 02108. Phone: (617) 227-0730. 1979.

Manual of Psychiatric Emergencies. Steven E. Hyman (ed.). Little, Brown and Co., 34 Beacon St., Boston, MA 02108. Phone: (617) 227-0730. Fax: (617) 227-0790. Second edition 1988.

JOURNALS

Annals of Emergency Medicine. American College of Emergency Physicians, P.O. Box 619911, Dallas, TX 75261. Phone: (214) 550-0911. Monthly.

Archives of Emergency Medicine. Blackwell Scientific Publications, Inc., 3 Cambridge Ctr., Cambridge, MA 02142. Phone: (800) 759-6102. Quarterly.

Critical Care Medicine. Williams & Wilkins, 428 E. Preston St., Baltimore, MD 21202. Phone: (800) 638-0672. Fax: (800) 447-8438. Monthly.

Emergency. Hare Publications, P.O. Box 159, Carlsbad, CA 92008. Phone: (619) 438-2511. Monthly.

Emergency Care Quarterly. Aspen Publishers, Inc., 200 Orchard Ridge Dr., Gaithersburg, MD 20878. Phone: (800) 638-8437. Quarterly.

Emergency Medical Services. Creative Age Publications, 7628 Densmore Ave., Van Nuys, CA 91406. Phone: (818) 782-7328. 10/year.

Emergency Medicine. Reed Publishing USA, 249 W. 17th St., New York, NY 10011. Phone: (212) 645-0067. Fax: (212) 242-6987. 21/year.

Injury: British Journal of Accident Surgery. Butterworth-Heinemann, 80 Montvale Ave., Stoneham, MA 02180. Phone: (617) 438-8464. Fax: (617) 279-4851. 8/year.

Journal of Emergency Nursing. Mosby-Year Book, 11830 Westline Industrial Drive, St. Louis, MO 63146. Phone: (800) 325-4177. Fax: (314) 432-1380. Bimonthly.

Pediatric Emergency Care. Williams & Wilkins, 428 E. Preston St., Baltimore, MD 21202. Phone: (800) 638-0672. Fax: (800) 447-8438. Bimonthly.

Resuscitation. Elsevier Science Publishing Co., Inc., P.O. Box 882, Madison Square Station, New York, NY 10159-2101. Phone: (212) 989-5800. Fax: (212) 633-3990. 6/year.

Topics in Emergency Medicine. Aspen Publishers, Inc., 1600 Research Blvd., Rockville, MD 20850. Phone: (301) 251-5554. Quarterly.

NEWSLETTERS

Emergency Medicine Reports. American Health Consultants, Department C1290, P.O. Box 740060, Atlanta, GA 30374. Phone: (800) 559-1032. Fax: (404) 352-1971. Biweekly.

ONLINE DATABASES

EMBASE. Elsevier Science Publishing Co., Inc., P.O. Box 882, Madison Square Station, New York, NY 10159-2101. Phone: (212) 989-5800. Fax: (212) 633-3990.

Emergency Medicine Reports. American Health Consultants, Department C1290, P.O. Box 740060, Atlanta, GA 30374. Phone: (800) 559-1032. Fax: (404) 352-1971. Biweekly.

MEDLINE. National Library of Medicine, 8600 Rockville Pike, Bethesda, MD 20894. Phone: (800) 638-8480.

Nursing and Allied Health (CINAHL). CINAHL, 1509 Wilson Terrace, P.O. Box 871, Glendale, CA 91209-0871. Phone: (818) 409-8005.

SciSearch. Institute for Scientific Information, 3501 Market St., Philadelphia, PA 19104. Phone: (215) 386-0100. Fax: (215) 386-6362.

POPULAR WORKS AND PATIENT EDUCATION

The Baby & Child Emergency First-Aid Handbook. Mitchell Einzig (ed.). Simon & Schuster, 1230 Ave. of the Americas, New York, NY 10020. Phone: (800) 223-2348. Fax: (800) 284-0735. 1992.

Childhood Emergencies-What to Do: A Quick Reference Guide. Project Care for Children Staff. Bull Publishing Co., 110 Gilbert Ave., Menlo Park, CA 94025. Phone: (800) 676-2855. 1989.

Knife and Gun Club: Scenes from an Emergency Room. Eugene Richards. Atlantic Monthly Press, 19 Union Sq. W., 11th Flr., New York, NY 10003. Phone: (212) 645-4462. 1991.

RESEARCH CENTERS, INSTITUTES, CLEARINGHOUSES

Center for Emergency Medicine of Western Pennsylvania. 230 McKee Place, Suite 500, Pittsburgh, PA 15213. Phone: (412) 647-5790. Fax: (412) 578-3200.

Institute of Critical Care Medicine. 1975 Zonal Ave., KAM 307B, Los Angeles, CA 90033. Phone: (213) 225-9633.

TEXTBOOKS AND MONOGRAPHS

Asthma: Basic Mechanisms and Clinical Management. P.J. Barnes, I.W. Rodger, N.C. Thomson (eds.). Academic Press, Inc., 1250 Sixth Ave., San Diego, CA 92101-4311. Phone: (619) 699-6345. Fax: (619) 699-6715. Second edition 1992.

Cardiac Emergency Care. Edward K. Chung (ed.). Williams & Wilkins, 428 East Preston St., Baltimore, MD 21202. Phone: (800) 638-0672. Fax: (800) 447-8438. Fourth edition 1991.

The Clinical Practice of Emergency Medicine. Ann L. Harwood-Nuss, Christopher H. Linden, Robert Luten. J.B. Lippincott Co., 227 East Washington Square, Philadelphia, PA 19106-3780. Phone: (215) 238-4200. Fax: (215) 238-4227. 1991.

Clinical Procedures in Emergency Medicine. James R. Roberts, Jerris R. Hedges. W.B. Saunders Co., The Curtis Center, Independence Square W., Philadelphia, PA 19106-3399. Phone: (215) 238-7800. Second edition 1991.

Critical Care. Joseph M. Civetta, Robert W. Taylor, Robert R. Kirby (eds.). J.B. Lippincott Co., 227 E. Washington Square, Philadelphia, PA 19106-3780. Phone: (215) 238-4200. Fax: (215) 238-4227. 1988.

Current Emergency Diagnosis and Treatment. Mary T. Ho, Charles E. Saunders. Appleton & Lange, 25 Van Zant St., East Norwalk, CT 06855. Phone: (800) 423-1359. Fax: (203) 854-9486. Fourth edition 1992.

Current Practice in Emergency Medicine. Michael Callaham. Mosby-Year Book, 11830 Westline Industrial Drive, St. Louis, MO 63146. Phone: (800) 325-4177. Fax: (314) 432-1380. Second edition 1991.

Diagnostic Radiology in Emergency Medicine. Rosen. Mosby-Year Book, 11830 Westline Industrial Drive, St. Louis, MO 63146. Phone: (800) 325-4177. Fax: (314) 432-1380. 1992.

Emergency Medical Treatment: A Text for EMT-As and EMT-Intermediates. Nancy L. Caroline. Little, Brown and Company, 34 Beacon St., Boston, MA 02108. Phone: (617) 227-0730. Third edition 1991.

Emergency Medicine. Harold L. May, Richard V. Aghababian, Gary R. Fleisher (eds.). Little, Brown and Company, 34 Beacon St., Boston, MA 02108. Phone: (617) 227-0730. Second edition Two volumes 1992.

Emergency Medicine: A Comprehensive Study Guide. Judith E. Tintinalli, Ernest Ruiz, Ronald L. Krome. McGraw-Hill, Inc., 1221 Avenue of the Americas, 28th Floor, New York, NY 10020. Phone: (212) 512-4228. 1990.

Emergency Medicine: An Approach to Clinical Problem-Solving. Glenn C. Hamilton, Alexander Trott, Arthur B. Sanders, et. al.. W.B. Saunders Co., The Curtis Center, Independence Square W., Philadelphia, PA 19106-3399. Phone: (215) 238-7800. 1991.

Emergency Medicine: Concepts and Clinical Practice. Peter Rosen, Roger M. Barkin, Richard Brain, and others. Mosby-Year Book, 11830 Westline Industrial Drive, St. Louis, MO 63146. Phone: (800) 325-4177. Fax: (314) 432-1380. Third edition 1992.

Emergency Plastic Surgery. Richard J. Greco. Little, Brown and Company, 34 Beacon St., Boston, MA 02108. Phone: (617) 227-0730. 1991.

Emergency Radiology. Keats. Mosby-Year Book, 11830 Westline Industrial Drive, St. Louis, MO 63146. Phone: (800) 325-4177. Fax: (314) 432-1380. Second edition.

First Aid Responding to Emergencies. American Red Cross. Mosby-Year Book, 11830 Westline Industrial Drive, St. Louis, MO 63146. Phone: (800) 325-4177. Fax: (314) 432-1380. 1991.

Geriatric Emergency Medicine. Gideon Bosker, George Schwartz, Jeffrey S. Jones, et. al.. Mosby-Year Book, 11830 Westline Industrial Drive, St. Louis, MO 63146. Phone: (800) 325-4177. Fax: (314) 432-1380. 1990.

Infectious Disease in Emergency Medicine. Judith C. Brillman, Ronald W. Quenzer. Little, Brown and Company, 34 Beacon St., Boston, MA 02108. Phone: (617) 227-0730. 1992.

The Management of Major Trauma. Colin Robertson, Anthony D. Redmond. Oxford University Press, 200 Madison Ave., New York, NY 10016. Phone: (212) 679-7300. 1991.

Neonatal Emergencies. Donn. Futura Publishing Co., Inc., P.O. Box 330, Mount Kisco, NY 10549. Phone: (914) 666-7528. 1991.

Neurologic Emergencies: Recognition and Management. Michael Salcman. Raven Press, 1185 Avenue of the Americas, New York, NY 10036. Phone: (212) 930-9500. Fax: (212) 869-3495. Second edition 1990.

Pediatric Emergency Medicine. Barkin. Mosby-Year Book, 11830 Westline Industrial Drive, St. Louis, MO 63146. Phone: (800) 325-4177. Fax: (314) 432-1380. 1992.

Pediatric Trauma. Martin R. Eichelberger. Mosby-Year Book, 11830 Westline Industrial Drive, St. Louis, MO 63146. Phone: (800) 325-4177. Fax: (314) 432-1380. 1992.

Prehospital Emergency Pharmacolgy. Bryan E. Bledsoe and others. Prentice Hall, 113 Sylvan Ave., Rt. 9W, Prentice Hall Bldg., Englewood Cliffs, NJ 07632. Phone: (201) 767-5937. Third edition 1992.

Principles and Practice of Emergency Medicine. Goerge R. Schwartz, and others (eds.). Williams & Wilkins, 428 East Preston St., Baltimore, MD 21202. Phone: (800) 638-0672. Fax: (800) 447-8438. Third edition 1992.

Radiology of Emergency Medicine. Harris. Williams & Wilkins, 428 East Preston St., Baltimore, MD 21202. Phone: (800) 638-0672. Fax: (800) 447-8438. Third edition 1992.

Textbook of Pediatric Emergency Medicine. Gary Fleisher, Stephen Ludwig (eds.). Williams & Wilkins, 428 East Preston St., Baltimore, MD 21202. Phone: (800) 638-0672. Fax: (800) 447-8438. Second edition 1988.

Trauma: Anesthesia and Intensive Care. Ievon M. Capan, Sanford Miller, Herman Turndorf (eds.). J.B. Lippincott Co., 227 East Washington Square, Philadelphia, PA 19106-3780. Phone: (215) 238-4200. Fax: (215) 238-4227. 1991.

Wounds and Lacerations: Emergency Care and Closure. Alexander Trott. Mosby-Year Book, 11830 Westline Industrial Drive, St. Louis, MO 63146. Phone: (800) 325-4177. Fax: (314) 432-1380. Second edition 1991.

EMPHYSEMA

See: LUNG DISEASES

ENCEPHALITIS

See: BRAIN DISEASES

ENDOCARDITIS

See: HEART DISEASES

ENDOCRINE DISORDERS

See also: ENDOCRINOLOGY; THYROID
DISEASES

ABSTRACTING, INDEXING, AND CURRENT AWARENESS PUBLICATIONS

Current Contents/Clinical Medicine. Institute for Scientific Information, 3501 Market St., Philadelphia, PA 19104. Phone: (800) 523-1850. Fax: (215) 386-6362. Weekly.

Current Contents/Life Sciences. Institute for Scientific Information, 3501 Market St., Philadelphia, PA 19104. Phone: (215) 386-0100. Fax: (215) 386-6362.

Endocrinology Abstracts. Cambridge Scientific Abstracts, 7200 Wisconsin Ave., Bethesda, MD 20814-4823. Phone: (800) 843-7751. Fax: (301) 961-6720. Monthly.

Excerpta Medica. Section 3: Endocrinology. Elsevier Science Publishing Co., Inc., P.O. Box 882, Madison Square Station, New York, NY 10159-2101. Phone: (212) 989-5800. Fax: (212) 633-3990. 24/year.

Index Medicus. U.S. National Library of Medicine, 8600 Rockville Pike, Bethesda, MD 20894. Phone: (800) 638-8480. Monthly.

Research Alert: Cystic Fibrosis/Endocrine Disorders. Institute for Scientific Information, 3501 Market St., Philadelphia, PA 19104. Phone: (800) 523-1850. Fax: (215) 386-6362. Weekly.

ANNUALS AND REVIEWS

Autoimmune Endocrine Disease. Anthony P. Weetman. Cambridge University Press, 40 W. 20th St., New York, NY 10011. Phone: (800) 431-1580. Cambridge Reviews in Clinical Immunology volume 1 1992.

Endocrinology and Metabolism Clinics. W.B. Saunders Co., The Curtis Center, Independence Square W., Philadelphia, PA 19106-3399. Phone: (215) 238-7800. Quarterly.

CD-ROM DATABASES

CSA Life Sciences Collection. Cambridge Scientific Abstracts, 7200 Wisconsin Ave., Bethesda, MD 20814-4823. Phone: (800) 843-7751. Fax: (301) 961-6720.

MAXX: Maximum Access to Diagnosis and Therapy. Little, Brown and Company, 34 Beacon St., Boston, MA 02108. Phone: (617) 227-0730. The Electronic Library of Medicine.

HANDBOOKS, GUIDES, MANUALS, ATLASES

Color Atlas of Obesity. Roland Jung. Mosby-Year Book, 11830 Westline Industrial Drive, St. Louis, MO 63146. Phone: (800) 325-4177. Fax: (314) 432-1380. 1991.

Handbook of Clinical Endocrinology. Fitzgerald. Appleton & Lange, 25 Van Zant St., East Norwalk, CT 06855. Phone: (800) 423-1359. Fax: (203) 854-9486. Second edition 1992.

Handbook of Diabetes. Williams. Blackwell Scientific Publications, Inc., 3 Cambridge Ctr., Cambridge, MA 02142. Phone: (800) 759-6102. 1992.

Handbook of Drug Therapy in Reproductive Endocrinology. Rivlin. Little, Brown and Co., 34 Beacon St., Boston, MA 02108. Phone: (617) 227-0730. Fax: (617) 227-0790. 1990.

JOURNALS

Endocrine Reviews. Williams & Wilkins, 428 E. Preston St., Baltimore, MD 21202. Phone: (800) 638-0672. Fax: (800) 447-8438. Quarterly.

Trends in Endocrinology and Metabolism. Elsevier Science Publishing Co., Inc., P.O. Box 882, Madison Square Station, New York, NY 10159-2101. Phone: (212) 989-5800. Fax: (212) 633-3990. 10/year.

ONLINE DATABASES

CSA Life Sciences Collection. Cambridge Scientific Abstracts, 7200 Wisconsin Ave., Bethesda, MD 20814-4823. Phone: (800) 843-7751. Fax: (301) 961-6720.

EMBASE. Elsevier Science Publishing Co., Inc., P.O. Box 882, Madison Square Station, New York, NY 10159-2101. Phone: (212) 989-5800. Fax: (212) 633-3990.

MEDLINE. National Library of Medicine, 8600 Rockville Pike, Bethesda, MD 20894. Phone: (800) 638-8480.

SciSearch. Institute for Scientific Information, 3501 Market St., Philadelphia, PA 19104. Phone: (215) 386-0100. Fax: (215) 386-6362.

RESEARCH CENTERS, INSTITUTES, CLEARINGHOUSES

Center for Endocrinology, Metabolism and Nutrition. 10-555 Searle, 303 Chicago Ave., Chicago, IL 60611. Phone: (708) 908-8023. Fax: (312) 908-9032.

TEXTBOOKS AND MONOGRAPHS

Basic and Clinical Endocrinology. Francis S. Greenspan, Peter H. Forsham. Appleton & Lange, 25 Van Zant St., East Norwalk, CT 06855. Phone: (800) 423-1359. Fax: (203) 854-9486. Third edition 1990.

Clinical Pediatric Endocrinology. Hung. Mosby-Year Book, 11830 Westline Industrial Drive, St. Louis, MO 63146. Phone: (800) 325-4177. Fax: (314) 432-1380. 1992.

Current Therapy in Endocrinology and Metabolism. C. Wayne Bardin (ed.). Mosby-Year Book, 11830 Westline Industrial Drive, St. Louis, MO 63146. Phone: (800) 325-4177. Fax: (314) 432-1380. Fourth edition 1991.

Endocrine Toxicology. Christopher K. Atterwill, J.D. Flack (eds.). Cambridge University Press, 40 W. 20th St., New York, NY 10011. Phone: (800) 431-1580. 1992.

Endocrinology and Metabolism. Philip Felig, John D. Baxter, Lawrence A. Frohman. McGraw-Hill, Inc., Health Professions Division, 1221 Avenue of the Americas, 28th Floor, New York, NY 10020. Phone: (212) 512-4228. Third edition 1992.

Immunogenetics of Endocrine Disorders. Nadir R. Farid (ed.). John Wiley & Sons, Inc., 605 Third Ave., New York, NY 10158-0012. Phone: (212) 850-6000. Fax: (212) 850-6088. 1988.

Metabolic Bone Disease and Clinically Related Disorders. Louis V. Avioli, Stephen M. Krane. W.B. Saunders Co., The Curtis Center, Independence Square W., Philadelphia, PA 19106-3399. Phone: (215) 238-7800. Second edition 1990.

Practical Approach to Pediatric Endocrinology. Bacon. Mosby-Year Book, 11830 Westline Industrial Drive, St. Louis, MO 63146. Phone: (800) 325-4177. Fax: (314) 432-1380. Third edition 1990.

Principles and Practice of Endocrinology and Metabolism. Kenneth L. Becker, John P. Bilezikian, William J Bremner. J.B. Lippincott Co., 227 East Washington Square, Philadelphia, PA 19106-3780. Phone: (215) 238-4200. Fax: (215) 238-4227. 1990.

Textbook of Diabetes. Pickup. Blackwell Scientific Publications, Inc., 3 Cambridge Ctr., Cambridge, MA 02142. Phone: (800) 759-6102. Two volumes 1991.

Thyroid Disease in Clinical Practice. McDougall. Oxford University Press, 200 Madison Ave., New York, NY 10016. Phone: (212) 679-7300. 1992.

Werner and Ingbar's The Thyroid: A Fundamental and Clinical Text. Lewis E. Braverman, Robert D. Utiger. J.B. Lippincott Co., 227 E. Washington Square, Philadelphia, PA 19106-3780. Phone: (215) 238-4200. Fax: (215) 238-4227. Sixth edition 1992.

ENDOCRINOLOGY

See also: ENDOCRINE DISORDERS; HORMONES

ABSTRACTING, INDEXING, AND CURRENT AWARENESS PUBLICATIONS

Current Contents/Life Sciences. Institute for Scientific Information, 3501 Market St., Philadelphia, PA 19104. Phone: (215) 386-0100. Fax: (215) 386-6362.

Endocrinology Abstracts. Cambridge Scientific Abstracts, 7200 Wisconsin Ave., Bethesda, MD 20814-4823. Phone: (800) 843-7751. Fax: (301) 961-6720. Monthly.

Excerpta Medica. Section 3: Endocrinology. Elsevier Science Publishing Co., Inc., P.O. Box 882, Madison Square Station, New York, NY 10159-2101. Phone: (212) 989-5800. Fax: (212) 633-3990. 24/year.

Index Medicus. U.S. National Library of Medicine, 8600 Rockville Pike, Bethesda, MD 20894. Phone: (800) 638-8480. Monthly.

Science Citation Index. Institute for Scientific Information, 3501 Market St., Philadelphia, PA 19104. Phone: (800) 523-1850. Fax: (215) 386-6362. Bimonthly.

ANNUALS AND REVIEWS

Advances in Endocrinology and Metabolism. Mosby-Year Book, 11830 Westline Industrial Drive, St. Louis, MO 63146. Phone: (800) 325-4177. Fax: (314) 432-1380. Annual.

Advances in Human Fertility and Reproductive Endocrinology. Raven Press, 1185 Ave. of the Americas, New York, NY 10036. Phone: (212) 930-9500. Fax: (212) 869-3495.

Endocrinology and Metabolism Clinics. W.B. Saunders Co., The Curtis Center, Independence Square W., Philadelphia, PA 19106-3399. Phone: (215) 238-7800. Quarterly.

Year Book of Endocrinology. Mosby-Year Book, 11830 Westline Industrial Drive, St. Louis, MO 63146. Phone: (800) 325-4177. Fax: (314) 432-1380. Annual.

ASSOCIATIONS, PROFESSIONAL SOCIETIES, ADVOCACY AND SUPPORT GROUPS

Endocrine Society (ES). 9650 Rockville Pike, Bethesda, MD 20814. Phone: (301) 571-1802.

CD-ROM DATABASES

SCISEARCH. Institute for Scientific Information, 3501 Market St., Philadelphia, PA 19104. Phone: (215) 386-0100. Fax: (215) 386-6362.

DIRECTORIES

Directory of Medical Specialists. Marquis Who's Who, 3002 Glenview Rd., Wilmette, IL 60091. Phone: (800) 621-9669. Fax: (708) 441-2264. Biennial.

Directory of Physicians in the United States. American Medical Association, 515 North State St., Chicago, IL 60610. Phone: (312) 464-0183. Fax: (312) 464-5834. Biennial.

JOURNALS

Acta Endocrinologica. Rhodos International Publishing, Strandgade 36, DK-1401 Copenhagen, Denmark.

Clinical Endocrinology. Blackwell Scientific Publications, Inc., 3 Cambridge Ctr., Cambridge, MA 02142. Phone: (800) 759-6102. Monthly.

Diabetes. American Diabetes Association, P.O. Box 25757, 1600 Duke St., Alexandria, VA 22314. Phone: (800) 232-3472. Fax: (703) 836-7439.

Endocrine Reviews. Williams & Wilkins, 428 E. Preston St., Baltimore, MD 21202. Phone: (800) 638-0672. Fax: (800) 447-8438. Quarterly.

The Endocrinologist. Williams & Wilkins, 428 E. Preston St., Baltimore, MD 21202. Phone: (800) 638-0672. Fax: (800) 447-8438. Bimonthly.

Endocrinology. Williams & Wilkins, 428 E. Preston St., Baltimore, MD 21202. Phone: (800) 638-0672. Fax: (800) 447-8438. Monthly.

General and Comparative Endocrinology. Academic Press, Inc., 1250 Sixth Ave., San Diego, CA 92101-4311. Phone: (619) 699-6345. Fax: (619) 699-6715.

Journal of Clinical Endocrinology & Metabolism. Williams & Wilkins, 428 E. Preston St., Baltimore, MD 21202. Phone: (800) 638-0672. Fax: (900) 447-8438. Monthly.

Journal of Endocrinology. Journal of Endocrinology Ltd., 23 Richmond Hill, Bristol, Avon BS8 1EN, England. Phone: 0462-672555. Fax: 0272-237489.

Molecular Endocrinology. The Endocrine Society, 9650 Rockville Pike, Bethesda, MD 20814. Phone: (301) 571-1802. Fax: (301) 571-1869. Monthly.

ONLINE DATABASES

CSA Life Sciences Collection. Cambridge Scientific Abstracts, 7200 Wisconsin Ave., Bethesda, MD 20814-4823. Phone: (800) 843-7751. Fax: (301) 961-6720.

EMBASE. Elsevier Science Publishing Co., Inc., P.O. Box 882, Madison Square Station, New York, NY 10159-2101. Phone: (212) 989-5800. Fax: (212) 633-3990.

MEDLINE. National Library of Medicine, 8600 Rockville Pike, Bethesda, MD 20894. Phone: (800) 638-8480.

SciSearch. Institute for Scientific Information, 3501 Market St., Philadelphia, PA 19104. Phone: (215) 386-0100. Fax: (215) 386-6362.

RESEARCH CENTERS, INSTITUTES, CLEARINGHOUSES

Diabetes and Endocrinology Research Center. University of Iowa. 3E19 VA Hospital, Iowa City, IA 52240. Phone: (319) 338-0581.

Diabetes-Endocrinology Research Center. University of Massachusetts. Medical School, Dept. of Biochemistry, 55 Lake Ave. N, Worcester, MA 01655. Phone: (508) 856-3047. Fax: (508) 856-6231.

Diabetes Research Center. New York Medical College. Metropolitan Hospital, 1900 Second Ave., Room 13M3, New York, NY 10029. Phone: (212) 369-5490.

Endocrine Research Group. University of Calgary. 3330 Hospital Dr. NW, Calgary, AB, Canada T2N 4N1. Phone: (403) 220-6870. Fax: (403) 270-0737.

Endocrinology Research Laboratories. Indiana University. Emerson Hall 421, 545 Barnhill Dr., Indianapolis, IN 46202-5124. Phone: (317) 274-8554. Fax: (317) 274-4311.

Joslin Diabetes Center. 1 Joslin Pl., Boston, MA 02215. Phone: (617) 732-2400. Fax: (617) 732-2487.

McGill Centre for Research on Endocrine Mechanisms. McGill University. Royal Victoria Hospital, Endocrine Laboratory, 687 Pine Ave. W., L205, Montreal, PQ, Canada H3A 2B4. Phone: (514) 842-1231. Fax: (514) 842-2376.

TEXTBOOKS AND MONOGRAPHS

Basic and Clinical Endocrinology. Francis S. Greenspan, Peter H. Forsham. Appleton & Lange, 25 Van Zant St., East Norwalk, CT 06855. Phone: (800) 423-1359. Fax: (203) 854-9486. Third edition 1990.

Clinical Pediatric Endocrinology. Solomon A. Kaplan. W.B. Saunders Co., The Curtis Center, Independence Square W., Philadelphia, PA 19106-3399. Phone: (215) 238-7800. Second edition 1990.

Endocrinology. Leslie J. DeGroot (ed.). W.B. Saunders Co., The Curtis Center, Independence Square W., Philadelphia, PA 19106-3399. Phone: (215) 238-7800. Second edition Three volumes 1989.

Endocrinology and Metabolism. Philip Felig, John D. Baxter, Lawrence A. Frohman. McGraw-Hill, Inc., Health Professions Division, 1221 Avenue of the Americas, 28th Floor, New York, NY 10020. Phone: (212) 512-4228. Third edition 1992.

Introduction to Clinical Reproductive Endocrinology. Gillian C.L. Lachelin. Butterworth-Heinemann, 80 Montvale Ave., Stoneham, MA 02180. Phone: (617) 438-8464. Fax: (617) 279-4851. 1991.

Principles and Practice of Endocrinology and Metabolism. Kenneth L. Becker, John P. Bilezikian, William J Bremner. J.B. Lippincott Co., 227 East Washington Square, Philadelphia, PA 19106-3780. Phone: (215) 238-4200. Fax: (215) 238-4227. 1990.

Williams' Textbook of Endocrinology. Jean D. Wilson, Daniel W. Foster. W.B. Saunders Co., The Curtis Center, Independence Square W., Philadelphia, PA 19106-3399. Phone: (215) 238-7800. Eighth edition 1991.

ENDODONTICS

See also: DENTISTRY; ORAL SURGERY

ABSTRACTING, INDEXING, AND CURRENT AWARENESS PUBLICATIONS

Current Contents/Clinical Medicine. Institute for Scientific Information, 3501 Market St., Philadelphia, PA 19104. Phone: (800) 523-1850. Fax: (215) 386-6362. Weekly.

Dental Abstracts. Mosby-Year Book, 11830 Westline Industrial Drive, St. Louis, MO 63146. Phone: (800) 325-4177. Fax: (314) 432-1380. Bimonthly.

Index to Dental Literature. American Dental Association, 211 E. Chicago Ave., Chicago, IL 60611-2678. Phone: (800) 947-4746. Fax: (312) 440-3542. Quarterly.

Index Medicus. U.S. National Library of Medicine, 8600 Rockville Pike, Bethesda, MD 20894. Phone: (800) 638-8480. Monthly.

Science Citation Index. Institute for Scientific Information, 3501 Market St., Philadelphia, PA 19104. Phone: (800) 523-1850. Fax: (215) 386-6362. Bimonthly.

ANNUALS AND REVIEWS

Dental Clinics. W.B. Saunders Co., The Curtis Center, Independence Square W., Philadelphia, PA 19106-3399. Phone: (215) 238-7800. Quarterly.

Year Book of Dentistry. Mosby-Year Book, 11830 Westline Industrial Drive, St. Louis, MO 63146. Phone: (800) 325-4177. Fax: (314) 432-1380. Annual.

ASSOCIATIONS, PROFESSIONAL SOCIETIES, ADVOCACY AND SUPPORT GROUPS

American Association of Endodontists (AAE). 211 E. Chicago Ave., Ste. 1201, Chicago, IL 60611. Phone: (312) 266-7255. Fax: (312) 266-9867.

American Board of Endodontics. 211 E. Chicago Ave., Suite 1501, Chicago, IL 60611. Phone: (312) 266-7310.

American Dental Association (ADA). 211 E. Chicago Ave., Chicago, IL 60611. Phone: (312) 440-2500.

American Endodontic Society. 1440 N. Harbor Blvd., Suite 719, Fullerton, CA 92635. Phone: (714) 870-5590.

CD-ROM DATABASES

SCISEARCH. Institute for Scientific Information, 3501 Market St., Philadelphia, PA 19104. Phone: (215) 386-0100. Fax: (215) 386-6362.

DIRECTORIES

American Dental Directory. American Dental Association, 211 E. Chicago Ave., Chicago, IL 60611-2678. Phone: (800) 947-4746. Fax: (312) 440-3542. Annual.

HANDBOOKS, GUIDES, MANUALS, ATLASES

Color Atlas of Endodontics. J.J. Messing, C.J.R. Stock. Mosby-Year Book, 11830 Westline Industrial Drive, St. Louis, MO 63146. Phone: (800) 325-4177. Fax: (314) 432-1380. 1988.

Surgical Endodontics: A Colour Manual. Ian E. Barnes. Butterworth-Heinemann, 80 Montvale Ave., Stoneham, MA 02180. Phone: (617) 438-8464. Fax: (617) 279-4851. Second edition 1990.

JOURNALS

American Journal of Human Genetics. University of Chicago Press, P.O. Box 37005, Chicago, IL 60637. Phone: (312) 753-3347. Fax: (312) 753-0811. Monthly.

International Endodontic Journal. Blackwell Scientific Publications, Inc., 3 Cambridge Center, Cambridge, MA 02142. Phone: (800) 759-6102.

Journal of the American Dental Association. American Dental Association, 211 E. Chicago Ave., Chicago, IL 60611-2678. Phone: (800) 947-4746. Fax: (312) 440-3542. Monthly.

Journal of Endodontics. Williams & Wilkins, 428 E. Preston St., Baltimore, MD 21202. Phone: (800) 638-0672. Fax: (800) 447-8438. Monthly.

NEWSLETTERS

Endodontics for GPs. American Health Consultants, Department C1290, P.O. Box 740060, Atlanta, GA 30374. Phone: (800) 559-1032. Monthly.

ONLINE DATABASES

EMBASE. Elsevier Science Publishing Co., Inc., P.O. Box 882, Madison Square Station, New York, NY 10159-2101. Phone: (212) 989-5800. Fax: (212) 633-3990.

MEDLINE. National Library of Medicine, 8600 Rockville Pike, Bethesda, MD 20894. Phone: (800) 638-8480.

SciSearch. Institute for Scientific Information, 3501 Market St., Philadelphia, PA 19104. Phone: (215) 386-0100. Fax: (215) 386-6362.

POPULAR WORKS AND PATIENT EDUCATION

The Mount Sinai Medical Center Family Guide to Dental Health. Jack Klatell, Andrew Kaplan, Gray Williams Jr.. Macmillan Publishing Co., Inc., 866 Third Ave., New York, NY 10022. Phone: (800) 257-5755. 1992.

RESEARCH CENTERS, INSTITUTES, CLEARINGHOUSES

National Institute of Dental Research. NIH Bldg. 31, Rm. 2C-35, 9000 Rockville Pike, Bethesda, MD 20892. Phone: (301) 496-4261.

TEXTBOOKS AND MONOGRAPHS

Endodontic Practice. Louis I. Grossman, and others. Williams & Wilkins, 428 East Preston St., Baltimore, MD 21202. Phone: (800) 638-0672. Fax: (800) 447-8438. 1988.

Endodontic Therapy. Franklin S. Weine. Mosby-Year Book, 11830 Westline Industrial Drive, St. Louis, MO 63146. Phone: (800) 325-4177. Fax: (314) 432-1380. 1984.

Principles and Practice of Endodontics. Richard E. Walton, Mahmoud Torabinejad. W.B. Saunders Co., The Curtis Center, Independence Square W., Philadelphia, PA 19106-3399. Phone: (215) 238-7800. 1989.

Principles and Practice of Operative Dentistry. Charbeneau. Williams & Wilkins, 428 East Preston St., Baltimore, MD 21202. Phone: (800) 638-0672. Fax: (800) 447-8438. 1988.

Problem Solving in Endodontics. James L. Gutmann, Thom C. Dumsha, Paul E. Lovdahl, et. al.. Mosby-Year Book, 11830 Westline Industrial Drive, St. Louis, MO 63146. Phone: (800) 325-4177. Fax: (314) 432-1380. Second edition 1992.

Textbook of Traumatic Injuries to the Teeth. J.O. Andreasen. Mosby-Year Book, 11830 Westline Industrial Drive, St. Louis, MO 63146. Phone: (800) 325-4177. Fax: (314) 432-1380. Third edition 1992.

ENDOMETRIOSIS

See: GYNECOLOGIC DISORDERS

ENDOSCOPY

See also: DIAGNOSIS

ABSTRACTING, INDEXING, AND CURRENT AWARENESS PUBLICATIONS

Current Contents/Clinical Medicine. Institute for Scientific Information, 3501 Market St., Philadelphia, PA 19104. Phone: (800) 523-1850. Fax: (215) 386-6362. Weekly.

Index Medicus. U.S. National Library of Medicine, 8600 Rockville Pike, Bethesda, MD 20894. Phone: (800) 638-8480. Monthly.

Science Citation Index. Institute for Scientific Information, 3501 Market St., Philadelphia, PA 19104. Phone: (800) 523-1850. Fax: (215) 386-6362. Bimonthly.

ANNUALS AND REVIEWS

Annual of Gastrointestinal Endoscopy. Current Science Group, 20 N. Third St., Philadelphia, PA 19106-2199. Phone: (800) 552-5866. Fax: (215) 574-2270. Annual.

Gastrointestinal Endoscopy Clinics of North America. W.B. Saunders Co., The Curtis Center, Independence Square W., Philadelphia, PA 19106-3399. Phone: (215) 238-7800. Quarterly.

ASSOCIATIONS, PROFESSIONAL SOCIETIES, ADVOCACY AND SUPPORT GROUPS

American Society for Gastrointestinal Endoscopy (ASGE). 13 Elm St., P.O. Box 1565, Manchester, MA 01944. Phone: (508) 526-8330.

Society of American Gastrointestinal Endoscopic Surgeons (SAGES). 1271 Stoner Ave., Suite 409, Los Angeles, CA 90025. Phone: (213) 479-3249.

CD-ROM DATABASES

SCISEARCH. Institute for Scientific Information, 3501 Market St., Philadelphia, PA 19104. Phone: (215) 386-0100. Fax: (215) 386-6362.

HANDBOOKS, GUIDES, MANUALS, ATLASES

Atlas of Endourology. Kurt Amplatz. Mosby-Year Book, 11830 Westline Industrial Drive, St. Louis, MO 63146. Phone: (800) 325-4177. Fax: (314) 432-1380. 1991.

Atlas of Gastrointestinal Endoscopy. Fred E. Silverstein, Guido Tytgat. J.B. Lippincott Co., 227 E. Washington Square, Philadelphia, PA 19106-3780. Phone: (215) 238-4200. Fax: (215) 238-4227. Second edition 1991.

Atlas of Surgical Endoscopy. Ponsky. Mosby-Year Book, 11830 Westline Industrial Drive, St. Louis, MO 63146. Phone: (800) 325-4177. Fax: (314) 432-1380. 1992.

Color Atlas of Clinical Applications of Fiberoptic Bronchoscopy. Kitamura. Mosby-Year Book, 11830 Westline Industrial Drive, St. Louis, MO 63146. Phone: (800) 325-4177. Fax: (314) 432-1380. 1991.

A Color Atlas of Gastrointestinal Endoscopy. K.F.R. Schiller and others. W.B. Saunders Co., The Curtis Center, Independence Sqare W., Philadelphia, PA 19106-3399. Phone: (215) 238-7800. 1987.

Practical Manual of Operative Laparoscopy and Hysteroscopy. Azziz. Springer-Verlag New York Inc., 175 Fifth Ave., New York, NY 10010. Phone: (212) 460-1500. Fax: (212) 473-6272. 1992.

Slide Atlas of Gastrointestinal Endoscopy 1992. P.B. Cotton, G.N. Tytgat, C.B. Williams. Science Press Ltd., 20 N. Third St., Philadelphia, PA 19106-2199. Phone: (800) 552-5866. Fax: (215) 574-2270. 1992.

JOURNALS

Endoscopy. Thieme Medical Publishers, Inc., 381 Park Ave. S., New York, NY 10016. Phone: (212) 683-5088. Fax: (212) 779-9020. Bimonthly.

Gastroenterology. W.B. Saunders Co., The Curtis Center, Independence Sqare W., Philadelphia, PA 19106-3399. Phone: (215) 238-7800.

Gastrointestinal Endoscopy. Mosby-Year Book, 11830 Westline Industrial Drive, St. Louis, MO 63146. Phone: (800) 325-4177. Fax: (314) 432-1380. Bimonthly.

Journal of Laparoendoscopic Surgery. Mary Ann Liebert, Inc., 1651 Third Ave., New York, NY 10128. Phone: (212) 289-2300. Fax: (212) 289-4697. Bimonthly.

Surgical Laparoscopy and Endoscopy. Raven Press, 1185 Avenue of the Americas, New York, NY 10036. Phone: (212) 930-9500. Fax: (212) 869-3495. Quarterly.

ONLINE DATABASES

EMBASE. Elsevier Science Publishing Co., Inc., P.O. Box 882, Madison Square Station, New York, NY 10159-2101. Phone: (212) 989-5800. Fax: (212) 633-3990.

MEDLINE. National Library of Medicine, 8600 Rockville Pike, Bethesda, MD 20894. Phone: (800) 638-8480.

SciSearch. Institute for Scientific Information, 3501 Market St., Philadelphia, PA 19104. Phone: (215) 386-0100. Fax: (215) 386-6362.

TEXTBOOKS AND MONOGRAPHS

Advanced Therapeutic Endoscopy. Jamie S. Barkin, Cesar A. O'Phelan (eds.). Raven Press, 1185 Avenue of the Americas, New York, NY 10036. Phone: (212) 930-9500. Fax: (212) 869-3495. 1990.

Endoscopic Surgery. Rodney A. WHite, Stanley R. Klein. Mosby-Year Book, 11830 Westline Industrial Drive, St. Louis, MO 63146. Phone: (800) 325-4177. Fax: (314) 432-1380. 1991.

Endosonography in Obstetrics & Gynecology. G. Bernascheck, and others. Springer-Verlag New York Inc., 175 Fifth Ave., New York, NY 10010. Phone: (212) 460-1500. Fax: (212) 473-6272. 1990.

Gynecological Endoscopy. Alan G. Gordon, B. Victor Lewis. J.B. Lippincott Co., 227 E. Washington Square, Philadelphia, PA 19106-3780. Phone: (215) 238-4200. Fax: (215) 238-4227. 1988.

An Introduction to Gastrointestinal Endoscopy. J. Baillie, W. Hogan. Butterworth-Heinemann, 80 Montvale Ave., Stoneham, MA 02180. Phone: (617) 438-8464. Fax: (617) 279-4851. 1991.

Office Endoscopy. Bergein F. Overholt, Sarkis J. Chobanian. Williams & Wilkins, 428 E. Preston St., Baltimore, MD 21202. Phone: (800) 638-0672. Fax: (800) 447-8438. 1990.

Operative Laparoscopy. Maurice-Antoine Bruhat, Gerard Mage, Jean-Luc Pouly. McGraw-Hill, Inc., Health Professions Division, 1221 Avenue of the Americas, 28th Floor, New York, NY 10020. Phone: (212) 512-4228. 1992.

Practical Gastrointestinal Endoscopy. Peter B. Cotton, Christopher B. Williams. Mosby-Year Book, 11830 Westline Industrial Drive, St. Louis, MO 63146. Phone: (800) 325-4177. Fax: (314) 432-1380. Third edition 1990.

Techniques in Therapeutic Endoscopy. Jerome D. Waye, and others. W.B. Saunders Co., The Curtis Center, Independence Square W., Philadelphia, PA 19106-3399. Phone: (215) 238-7800. 1987.

Therapeutic Alimentary Endoscopy and Radiology. John R. Bennett, Richard H. Hunt (eds.). Williams & Wilkins, 428 E. Preston St., Baltimore, MD 21202. Phone: (800) 638-0672. Fax: (800) 447-8438. Second edition 1990.

ENT

See: OTOLARYNGOLOGY

ENVIRONMENTAL HEALTH

See also: ENVIRONMENTAL POLLUTANTS

ABSTRACTING, INDEXING, AND CURRENT AWARENESS PUBLICATIONS

Excerpta Medica. Section 46: Environmental Health and Pollution Control. Elsevier Science Publishing Co., Inc., P.O. Box 882, Madison Square Station, New York, NY 10159-2101. Phone: (212) 989-5800. Fax: (212) 633-3990. 10/year.

Index Medicus. U.S. National Library of Medicine, 8600 Rockville Pike, Bethesda, MD 20894. Phone: (800) 638-8480. Monthly.

Pollution Abstracts. Cambridge Scientific Abstracts, 7200 Wisconsin Ave., Bethesda, MD 20814-4823. Phone: (800) 843-7751. Fax: (301) 961-6720. Bimonthly.

Science Citation Index. Institute for Scientific Information, 3501 Market St., Philadelphia, PA 19104. Phone: (800) 523-1850. Fax: (215) 386-6362. Bimonthly.

ANNUALS AND REVIEWS

Year Book of Occupational and Environmental Medicine. Mosby-Year Book, 11830 Westline Industrial Drive, St. Louis, MO 63146. Phone: (800) 325-4177. Fax: (314) 432-1380. Annual.

ASSOCIATIONS, PROFESSIONAL SOCIETIES, ADVOCACY AND SUPPORT GROUPS

Air Pollution Control Association. P.O. Box 2801, Pittsburgh, PA 15230.

Environmental Action Foundation. 1525 New Hampshire Ave., Washington, DC 20036.

National Environmental Health Association (NEHA). 720 S. Colorado Blvd., Ste. 970, S. Tower, Denver, CO 80222. Phone: (303) 456-9090.

Society for Occupational and Environmental Health. 2021 K St. N.W., Suite 305, Washington, DC 20006.

CD-ROM DATABASES

PolTox. Cambridge Scientific Abstracts, 7200 Wisconsin Ave., Bethesda, MD 20814-4823. Phone: (800) 843-7751. Fax: (301) 961-6720. Quarterly.

SCISEARCH. Institute for Scientific Information, 3501 Market St., Philadelphia, PA 19104. Phone: (215) 386-0100. Fax: (215) 386-6362.

TOXLINE. SilverPlatter Information, Inc., River Ridge Office Park, 100 River Ridge Rd., Norwood, MA 02062. Phone: (617) 769-2599. Fax: (617) 769-8763. Quarterly.

JOURNALS

Archives of Environmental Health. Heldref Publications, 4000 Albemarle St. N.W., Washington, DC 20016. Phone: (202) 362-6445. Bimonthly.

ONLINE DATABASES

TOXLINE. U.S. National Library of Medicine, Toxicology Information Program, 8600 Rockville Pike, Bethesda, MD 20894. Phone: (800) 638-8480. Monthly.

RESEARCH CENTERS, INSTITUTES, CLEARINGHOUSES

Center for Environmental Health Sciences. Massachusetts Institute of Technology, Cambridge, MA 02139. Phone: (617) 253-6220.

Environmental Health Institute. Pharmacy Building, Purdue University, Lafayette, IN 47907. Phone: (317) 494-1436.

Kresge Center for Environmental Health. Harvard University, 655 Huntington Ave., Boston, MA 02115. Phone: (617) 732-1272.

Public Information Center. Environmental Protection Agency. PM-211B, 401 M. St. S.W., Washington, DC 20460. Phone: (202) 382-2080.

TEXTBOOKS AND MONOGRAPHS

Environmental and Occupational Medicine. William N. Rom (ed.). Little, Brown and Company, 34 Beacon St., Boston, MA 02108. Phone: (617) 227-0730. Second edition 1992.

Primer of Environmental Toxicology. Smith. Williams & Wilkins, 428 East Preston St., Baltimore, MD 21202. Phone: (800) 638-0672. Fax: (800) 447-8438. 1992.

ENVIRONMENTAL POLLUTANTS

See also: CARCINOGENS; ENVIRONMENTAL
HEALTH; PESTICIDES AND HERBICIDES

ABSTRACTING, INDEXING, AND CURRENT AWARENESS PUBLICATIONS

Abstracts in Health Effects of Environmental Pollutants. BIOSIS, 2100 Arch St., Philadelphia, PA 19103-1399. Phone: (215) 587-4800. Fax: (215) 587-2016. Monthly.

Chemical Abstracts. Chemical Abstracts Service, 2540 Olentangy River Rd., P.O. Box 3012, Columbus, OH 43210-0012. Phone: (800) 848-6538.

Current Contents/Life Sciences. Institute for Scientific Information, 3501 Market St., Philadelphia, PA 19104. Phone: (215) 386-0100. Fax: (215) 386-6362.

Environmental Pollution and Control: An Abstract Newsletter. U.S. National Technical Information Service, 5285 Port Royal Rd., Springfield, VA 22161. Phone: (703) 487-4929. Fax: (703) 321-8199. Weekly.

Index Medicus. U.S. National Library of Medicine, 8600 Rockville Pike, Bethesda, MD 20894. Phone: (800) 638-8480. Monthly.

MEDOC: Index to U.S. Government Publications in the Medical and Health Sciences. Spencer S. Eccles Health Sciences Library, University of Utah, Bldg. 589, Salt Lake City, UT 84112. Phone: (801) 581-5268. Quarterly.

Pollution Abstracts. Cambridge Scientific Abstracts, 7200 Wisconsin Ave., Bethesda, MD 20814-4823. Phone: (800) 843-7751. Fax: (301) 961-6720. Bimonthly.

Science Citation Index. Institute for Scientific Information, 3501 Market St., Philadelphia, PA 19104. Phone: (800) 523-1850. Fax: (215) 386-6362. Bimonthly.

ANNUALS AND REVIEWS

Reviews of Environmental Contamination and Toxicology. Ware. Springer-Verlag New York, Inc., 175 Fifth Ave., New York, NY 10010. Phone: (212) 460-1500. Fax: (212) 473-6272. 1991.

BIBLIOGRAPHIES

Pesticide Residues in Foods. Food and Nutrition Center, National Agricultural Library, 10301 Baltimore Blvd., Beltsville, MD 20705. August 1990.

CD-ROM DATABASES

PolTox. Cambridge Scientific Abstracts, 7200 Wisconsin Ave., Bethesda, MD 20814-4823. Phone: (800) 843-7751. Fax: (301) 961-6720. Quarterly.

SCISEARCH. Institute for Scientific Information, 3501 Market St., Philadelphia, PA 19104. Phone: (215) 386-0100. Fax: (215) 386-6362.

TOXLINE. SilverPlatter Information, Inc., River Ridge Office Park, 100 River Ridge Rd., Norwood, MA 02062. Phone: (617) 769-2599. Fax: (617) 769-8763. Quarterly.

TOXLINE Plus. SilverPlatter Information, Inc., River Ridge Office Park, 100 River Ridge Rd., Norwood, MA 02062. Phone: (617) 769-2599. Fax: (617) 769-8763. Quarterly.

ONLINE DATABASES

CA File (Chemical Abstracts File). Chemical Abstracts Service, 2540 Olentangy River Rd., P.O. Box 3012, Columbus, OH 43210-0012. Phone: (800) 848-6538.

EMBASE. Elsevier Science Publishing Co., Inc., P.O. Box 882, Madison Square Station, New York, NY 10159-2101. Phone: (212) 989-5800. Fax: (212) 633-3990.

MEDLINE. National Library of Medicine, 8600 Rockville Pike, Bethesda, MD 20894. Phone: (800) 638-8480.

Pollution Abstracts. Cambridge Scientific Abstracts, 7200 Wisconsin Ave., Bethesda, MD 20814-4823. Phone: (800) 843-7751. Fax: (301) 961-6720.

SciSearch. Institute for Scientific Information, 3501 Market St., Philadelphia, PA 19104. Phone: (215) 386-0100. Fax: (215) 386-6362.

RESEARCH CENTERS, INSTITUTES, CLEARINGHOUSES

Air Pollution Health Effects Laboratory. University of California, Irvine. Dept. of Community and Environmental Medicine, Irvine, CA 92717. Phone: (714) 856-5860. Fax: (714) 856-4763.

Center for Environmental Toxicology. Colorado State University Center for Environmental Toxicology, Fort Collins, CO 80521. Phone: (303) 491-8522.

Institute of Toxicology and Environmental Health. University of California, Davis. Davis, CA 95616. Phone: (916) 752-1340. Fax: (916) 752-5300.

TEXTBOOKS AND MONOGRAPHS

Primer of Environmental Toxicology. Smith. Williams & Wilkins, 428 East Preston St., Baltimore, MD 21202. Phone: (800) 638-0672. Fax: (800) 447-8438. 1992.

EPIDEMIOLOGY

See also: PUBLIC HEALTH

ABSTRACTING, INDEXING, AND CURRENT AWARENESS PUBLICATIONS

American Statistics Index: A Comprehensive Guide and Index to the Statistical Publications of the United States Government. Congressional Information Service, 4520 East-West Hwy., Bethesda, MD 20814. Phone: (800) 639-8380. 1973-Present Monthly.

Current Contents/Clinical Medicine. Institute for Scientific Information, 3501 Market St., Philadelphia, PA 19104. Phone: (800) 523-1850. Fax: (215) 386-6362. Weekly.

Current Contents/Life Sciences. Institute for Scientific Information, 3501 Market St., Philadelphia, PA 19104. Phone: (215) 386-0100. Fax: (215) 386-6362.

Excerpta Medica. Section 17: Public Health, Social Medicine and Epidemiology. Elsevier Science Publishing Co., Inc., P.O. Box 882, Madison Square Station, New York, NY 10159-2101. Phone: (212) 989-5800. Fax: (212) 633-3990. 24/year.

Index to Health Information. Congressional Information Service, 4520 East-West Hwy., Bethesda, MD 20814. Phone: (800) 639-8380. Quarterly.

Index Medicus. U.S. National Library of Medicine, 8600 Rockville Pike, Bethesda, MD 20894. Phone: (800) 638-8480. Monthly.

Science Citation Index. Institute for Scientific Information, 3501 Market St., Philadelphia, PA 19104. Phone: (800) 523-1850. Fax: (215) 386-6362. Bimonthly.

Statistical Reference Index. Congressional Information Service, 4520 East-West Hwy., Bethesda, MD 20814. Phone: (800) 639-8380. 1980-Present Monthly.

ANNUALS AND REVIEWS

Annual Review of Public Health. Annual Reviews Inc., 4139 El Camino Way, P.O. Box 10139, Palo Alto, CA 94303-0897. Phone: (415) 493-4400. Fax: (415) 855-9815. Annual.

ASSOCIATIONS, PROFESSIONAL SOCIETIES, ADVOCACY AND SUPPORT GROUPS

American College of Epidemiology (ACE). Michigan Cancer Foundation, 110 E. Warren, Detroit, MI 48201. Phone: (313) 833-0710. Fax: (313) 831-8714.

American Epidemiological Society. 735 Gatewood Rd. N.E., Emory University School of Medicine, Atlanta, GA 30322. Phone: (404) 727-0199.

Canadian Public Health Association. 1565 Carling Ave., Suite 400, Ottawa, ON, Canada K1Z 8R1. Phone: (613) 725-3769. Fax: (613) 725-9826.

International Epidemiological Association (IEA). University of California, Los Angeles, School of Public Health, Rm. 71-269CHS, Los Angeles, CA 90024. Phone: (213) 206-2837. Fax: (213) 206-6039.

CD-ROM DATABASES

Health for All. CD Resources, Inc., 118 W. 74th St., Suite 2A, New York, NY 10023. Phone: (212) 580-2263. Fax: (212) 877-1276. Semiannual.

Morbidity Mortality Weekly Report. MEP, 124 Mt. Auburn St., Cambridge, MA 02138. Phone: (800) 342-1338. Fax: (617) 868-7738. Annual.

SCISEARCH. Institute for Scientific Information, 3501 Market St., Philadelphia, PA 19104. Phone: (215) 386-0100. Fax: (215) 386-6362.

Statistical Masterfile. Congressional Information Service, 4520 East-West Highway, Bethesda, MD 20814-3389. Phone: (800) 638-8380. Quarterly.

ENCYCLOPEDIAS, DICTIONARIES, WORD BOOKS

A Dictionary of Epidemiology. John M. Last (ed.). Oxford University Press, 200 Madison Ave., New York, NY 10016. Phone: (212) 679-7300. Second edition 1988.

JOURNALS

American Journal of Epidemiology. Johns Hopkins University School of Hygiene and Public Health, 2007 E. Monument St., Baltimore, MD 21205. Phone: (301) 955-3441.

American Journal of Public Health. American Public Health Association, 1015 15th St. NW, Washington, DC 20005. Phone: (202) 789-5666. Monthly.

Annals of Epidemiology. Elsevier Science Publishing Co., Inc., P.O. Box 882, Madison Square Station, New York, NY 10159-2101. Phone: (212) 989-5800. Fax: (212) 633-3990. Bimonthly.

Cancer Epidemiology, Biomarkers & Prevention. Williams & Wilkins, 428 East Preston St., Baltimore, MD 21202. Phone: (800) 638-0672. Fax: (800) 447-8438. 7/year.

Epidemiological Bulletin. Pan American Health Organization, 525 23rd St., N.W., Washington, DC 20037. Phone: (202) 861-3200. Bimonthly.

Epidemiology and Infection. Cambridge University Press, 40 W. 20th St., New York, NY 10011. Phone: (800) 431-1580. Bimonthly.

Journal of Clinical Epidemiology. Pergamon Press, 660 White Plains Rd., Tarrytown, NY 10591-5153. Phone: (914) 592-7700. Fax: (914) 592-3625.

Journal of Epidemiology & Community Health. BMJ Publishing Group, BMA House, Tavistock Square, London WC1H 9JR, England. Phone: 071-383 6244/6638. Fax: 071-383 6662. 6/year.

Morbidity and Mortality Weekly Report. Massachusetts Medical Society, 1440 Main St., Waltham, MA 02154-1649. Phone: (617) 893-3800. Fax: (617) 893-0413. Weekly.

NEWSLETTERS

Morbidity and Mortality Weekly Report. Centers for Disease Control, 1600 Clifton Rd. N.E., Atlanta, GA 30333. Phone: (404) 488-4698.

ONLINE DATABASES

EMBASE. Elsevier Science Publishing Co., Inc., P.O. Box 882, Madison Square Station, New York, NY 10159-2101. Phone: (212) 989-5800. Fax: (212) 633-3990.

MEDLINE. National Library of Medicine, 8600 Rockville Pike, Bethesda, MD 20894. Phone: (800) 638-8480.

SciSearch. Institute for Scientific Information, 3501 Market St., Philadelphia, PA 19104. Phone: (215) 386-0100. Fax: (215) 386-6362.

RESEARCH CENTERS, INSTITUTES, CLEARINGHOUSES

Center for Epidemiological Research. Oak Ridge Associated Universities, 210 Badger Rd., P.O. Box 117, Oak Ridge, TN 37830-0117. Phone: (615) 576-2866.

Centers for Disease Control. 1600 Clifton Rd. N.E., Atlanta, GA 30333. Phone: (404) 488-4698.

Clinical Epidemiology Unit. University of Pennsylvania. School of Medicine, 2L NEB/S2, Philadelphia, PA 19104-6095. Phone: (215) 898-4623. Fax: (215) 573-5315.

Department of Biostatistics and Epidemiology. University of Tennessee. Health Sciences Center, Memphis, TN 38163. Phone: (901) 528-5118.

Division of Biostatistics and Epidemiology. Dana Farber Cancer Institute. 44 Binney St., Boston, MA 02115. Phone: (617) 732-3012. Fax: (617) 737-8614.

Division of Epidemiology and Biostatistics. University of Cincinnati. ML 183, Cincinnati, OH 45267-0183. Phone: (513) 558-5631. Fax: (513) 558-1756.

Medical Biostatistics/Biometry Facility. University of Vermont. 27 Hills Science Bldg., Burlington, VT 05405. Phone: (802) 656-2526. Fax: (802) 656-0632.

Tecumseh Community Health Study. University of Michigan. School of Public Health, Dept. of Epidemiology, Ann Arbor, MI 48109-2029. Phone: (313) 764-5435. Fax: (313) 764-3192.

STANDARDS AND STATISTICS SOURCES

Statistical Abstract of the United States. U.S. Government Printing Office, Superintendent of Documents, Washington, DC 20402. Phone: (202) 783-3238. Annual.

TEXTBOOKS AND MONOGRAPHS

Clinical Epidemiology. Fletcher. Williams & Wilkins, 428 East Preston St., Baltimore, MD 21202. Phone: (800) 638-0672. Fax: (800) 447-8438. Second edition 1988.

Clinical Epidemiology: A Basic Science for Clinical Medicine. David Sackett, R. Brian Haynes, Peter Tugwell, et. al.. Little, Brown and Company, 34 Beacon St., Boston, MA 02108. Phone: (617) 227-0730. Second edition 1991.

Epidemiology in Medical Practice. D.J.P. Barker, G. Rose. Churchill Livingstone Inc., 650 Ave. of the Americas, New York, NY 10011. Phone: (212) 819-5400. Fax: (212) 302-6598. Fourth edition 1990.

Practical Epidemiology. D.J.P. Barker, A.J. Hall. Churchill Livingstone Inc., 650 Ave. of the Americas, New York, NY 10011. Phone: (212) 819-5400. Fax: (212) 302-6598. Fourth edition 1991.

Short Course in Epidemiology. Norell. Raven Press, 1185 Ave. of the Americas, New York, NY 10036. Phone: (212) 930-9500. Fax: (212) 869-3495. 1992.

EPILEPSY

ABSTRACTING, INDEXING, AND CURRENT AWARENESS PUBLICATIONS

BIOSIS/CAS Selects: Anticonvulsants. BIOSIS, 2100 Arch St., Philadelphia, PA 19103-1399. Phone: (215) 587-4800. Fax: (215) 587-2016. Biweekly.

CA Selects: Anticonvulsants & Antiepileptics. Chemical Abstracts Service, 2540 Olentangy River Road, P.O. Box 3012, Columbus, OH 43210-0012. Phone: (800) 848-6538. Biweekly.

Current Contents/Clinical Medicine. Institute for Scientific Information, 3501 Market St., Philadelphia, PA 19104. Phone: (800) 523-1850. Fax: (215) 386-6362. Weekly.

Current Contents/Life Sciences. Institute for Scientific Information, 3501 Market St., Philadelphia, PA 19104. Phone: (215) 386-0100. Fax: (215) 386-6362.

Excerpta Medica. Section 50: Epilepsy Abstracts. Elsevier Science Publishing Co., Inc., P.O. Box 882, Madison Square Station, New York, NY 10159-2101. Phone: (212) 989-5800. Fax: (212) 633-3990. 6/year.

Index Medicus. U.S. National Library of Medicine, 8600 Rockville Pike, Bethesda, MD 20894. Phone: (800) 638-8480. Monthly.

National Epilepsy Library Quarterly Update. Epilepsy Foundation of America, 4351 Garden City Dr., Landover, MD 20785. Phone: (301) 459-3700. Fax: (301) 577-2684. Quarterly.

Research Alert: Anticonvulsant Agents/Epilepsy & Seizure Disorders. Institute for Scientific Information, 3501 Market St., Philadelphia, PA 19104. Phone: (800) 523-1850. Fax: (215) 386-6362. Weekly.

Science Citation Index. Institute for Scientific Information, 3501 Market St., Philadelphia, PA 19104. Phone: (800) 523-1850. Fax: (215) 386-6362. Bimonthly.

ANNUALS AND REVIEWS

Advances in the Neurobiology of Epilepsy. Demos Publications, Inc., 386 Park Ave. S., Suite 201, New York, NY 10016. Phone: (212) 683-0072. Irregular.

Recent Advances in Epilepsy. Churchill Livingstone Inc., 650 Ave. of the Americas, New York, NY 10011. Phone: (212) 819-5400. Fax: (212) 302-6598. Irregular.

ASSOCIATIONS, PROFESSIONAL SOCIETIES, ADVOCACY AND SUPPORT GROUPS

American Epilepsy Society (AES). 638 Prospect Ave., Hartford, CT 06105. Phone: (203) 232-4825. Fax: (203) 232-0819.

Epilepsy Foundation of America (EFA). 4351 Garden City Dr., Landover, MD 20785. Phone: (301) 459-3700. Fax: (301) 577-2684.

CD-ROM DATABASES

SCISEARCH. Institute for Scientific Information, 3501 Market St., Philadelphia, PA 19104. Phone: (215) 386-0100. Fax: (215) 386-6362.

HANDBOOKS, GUIDES, MANUALS, ATLASES

A Practical Guide to Epilepsy. Mogens Dam. McGraw-Hill, Inc., Health Professions Division, 1221 Avenue of the Americas, 28th Floor, New York, NY 10020. Phone: (212) 512-4228. 1992.

JOURNALS

Brain Research. Elsevier Science Publishing Co., Inc., P.O. Box 882, Madison Square Station, New York, NY 10159-2101. Phone: (212) 989-5800. Fax: (212) 633-3990. 101/year.

Epilepsia. Raven Press, 1185 Avenue of the Americas, New York, NY 10036. Phone: (212) 930-9500. Fax: (212) 869-3495. Bimonthly.

Epilepsy Research. Elsevier Science Publishing Co., Inc., P.O. Box 882, Madison Square Station, New York, NY 10159-2101. Phone: (212) 989-5800. Fax: (212) 633-3990. 9/year.

Journal of Epilepsy. Demos Publications, Inc., 156 Fifth Ave., Ste. 1018, New York, NY 10010. Phone: (212) 255-8768. Quarterly.

Neuroscience. Pergamon Press, 660 White Plains Rd., Tarrytown, NY 10591-5153. Phone: (914) 592-7700. Fax: (914) 592-3625.

ONLINE DATABASES

EMBASE. Elsevier Science Publishing Co., Inc., P.O. Box 882, Madison Square Station, New York, NY 10159-2101. Phone: (212) 989-5800. Fax: (212) 633-3990.

EPIL. Epilepsy Foundation of America, National Epilepsy Library, 4351 Garden City Dr., Landover, MD 20785. Phone: (800) EFA-4050. Fax: (301) 577-2684.

MEDLINE. National Library of Medicine, 8600 Rockville Pike, Bethesda, MD 20894. Phone: (800) 638-8480.

SciSearch. Institute for Scientific Information, 3501 Market St., Philadelphia, PA 19104. Phone: (215) 386-0100. Fax: (215) 386-6362.

POPULAR WORKS AND PATIENT EDUCATION

Children with Epilepsy: A Parents' Guide. Helen Reisner (ed.). Woodbine House, 5615 Fishers Ln., Rockville, MD 20852. Phone: (800) 843-7323. Fax: (301) 468-5784. 1988.

Does Your Child Have Epilepsy?. James E. Jan. PRO-ED, 8700 Shoal Creek Blvd., Austin, TX 78758-6897. Phone: (512) 451-3246. Second edition 1991.

Epilepsy: A New Approach. Adrienne Richard. Prentice Hall, 113 Sylvan Ave., Rt. 9W, Prentice Hall Bldg., Englewood Cliffs, NJ 07632. Phone: (201) 767-5937. 1990.

Seizures and Epilepsy in Childhood: A Guide for Parents. John M. Freeman, Eileen P. Vining, Diana J. Pillas. Johns Hopkins University Press, 701 W. 40th St., Suite 275, Baltimore, MD 21211-2190. Phone: (800) 537-5487. 1990.

What You Can Do about Epilepsy. Goldberg. Bantam Doubleday Dell, Inc., 666 Fifth Ave., New York, NY 10103. Phone: (800) 223-6834. 1991.

RESEARCH CENTERS, INSTITUTES, CLEARINGHOUSES

Epilepsy Research Center. Duke University. Box 3676, 401 Brain Research Bldg., Durham, NC 27710. Phone: (919) 286-6111.

STANDARDS AND STATISTICS SOURCES

Surgery for Epilepsy. Consensus Statement. *NIH Consensus Development Conference. March 19-20, 1990.* National Institutes of Health, Office of Medical Applications of Research, Federal Bldg., Rm. 618, Bethesda, MD 20892. 1990.

TEXTBOOKS AND MONOGRAPHS

Antiepileptic Drugs. Rene H. Levy, F.E. Dreifuss, Richard H. Mattson, and others. Raven Press, 1185 Avenue of the Americas, New York, NY 10036. Phone: (212) 930-9500. Fax: (212) 869-3495. Third edition 1989.

Chronic Epilepsy: Its Prognosis and Management. Michael R. Trimble (ed.). John Wiley & Sons, Inc., 605 Third Ave., New York, NY 10158-0012. Phone: (212) 850-6000. Fax: (212) 850-6088. 1989.

Epilepsies. Niedermeyer. Williams & Wilkins, 428 East Preston St., Baltimore, MD 21202. Phone: (800) 638-0672. Fax: (800) 447-8438. 1990.

The Epilepsies: Diagnosis and Management. Ernst Niedermeyer. Williams & Wilkins, 428 E. Preston St., Baltimore, MD 21202. Phone: (800) 638-0672. Fax: (800) 447-8438. 1990.

Epilepsy: 100 Elementary Principles. Roger J. Porter. W.B. Saunders Co., The Curtis Center, Independence Sqare W., Philadelphia, PA 19106-3399. Phone: (215) 238-7800. 1989.

Epilepsy: Current Approaches to Diagnosis and Management. Dennis B. Smith. Raven Press, 1185 Avenue of the Americas, New York, NY 10036. Phone: (212) 930-9500. Fax: (212) 869-3495. 1991.

Epilepsy, Sleep and Sleep Deprivation. Rolf Degen, Ernst Rodin (eds.). Elsevier Science Publishing Co., Inc., P.O. Box 882, Madison Square Station, New York, NY 10159-2101. Phone: (212) 989-5800. Fax: (212) 633-3990. 1991.

Epilepsy Surgery. Luders. Raven Press, 1185 Ave. of the Americas, New York, NY 10036. Phone: (212) 930-9500. Fax: (212) 869-3495. 1992.

The Medical Treatment of Epilepsy. S.R. Resor, H. Kutt (eds.). Marcel Dekker, Inc., 270 Madison Ave., New York, NY 10016. Phone: (800) 228-1160. 1992.

Neurotransmitters and Epilepsy. Coyle Fisher (ed.). John Wiley & Sons, Inc., 605 Third Ave., New York, NY 10158-0012. Phone: (212) 850-6000. Fax: (212) 850-6088. 1991.

Pediatric Epilepsy. Dodson. Demos Publications, Inc., 156 Fifth Ave., Ste. 1018, New York, NY 10010. Phone: (212) 255-8768. 1992.

Seizures and Epilepsy. Jerome Engel, Jr.. F.A. Davis Co., 1915 Arch St., Philadelphia, PA 19103. Phone: (800) 523-4049. Fax: (215) 568-5065. Contemporary Neurology. Series No. 31. 1989.

ESOPHAGEAL CANCER

See: CANCER

ESTROGEN REPLACEMENT THERAPY

ABSTRACTING, INDEXING, AND CURRENT AWARENESS PUBLICATIONS

Current Contents/Clinical Medicine. Institute for Scientific Information, 3501 Market St., Philadelphia, PA 19104. Phone: (800) 523-1850. Fax: (215) 386-6362. Weekly.

Current Contents/Life Sciences. Institute for Scientific Information, 3501 Market St., Philadelphia, PA 19104. Phone: (215) 386-0100. Fax: (215) 386-6362.

Index Medicus. U.S. National Library of Medicine, 8600 Rockville Pike, Bethesda, MD 20894. Phone: (800) 638-8480. Monthly.

Science Citation Index. Institute for Scientific Information, 3501 Market St., Philadelphia, PA 19104. Phone: (800) 523-1850. Fax: (215) 386-6362. Bimonthly.

ASSOCIATIONS, PROFESSIONAL SOCIETIES, ADVOCACY AND SUPPORT GROUPS

American College of Obstetricians and Gynecologists (ACOG). 409 12th St. S.W., Washington, DC 20024-2188. Phone: (202) 638-5577.

National Women's Health Network (NWHN). 1325 G St. N.W., Washington, DC 20005. Phone: (202) 347-1140. Fax: (202) 347-1168.

North American Menopause Society (NAMS). University Hospitals of Cleveland, 2074 Abington Rd., Cleveland, OH 44106. Phone: (216) 844-3334. Fax: (216) 844-3348.

CD-ROM DATABASES

Excerpta Medica CD: Obstetrics & Gynecology. SilverPlatter Information, Inc., River Ridge Office Park, 100 River Ridge Rd., Norwood, MA 02062. Phone: (617) 769-2599. Fax: (617) 769-8763. Quarterly.

SCISEARCH. Institute for Scientific Information, 3501 Market St., Philadelphia, PA 19104. Phone: (215) 386-0100. Fax: (215) 386-6362.

JOURNALS

Acta Obstetrica et Gynecologica Scandanavica. Scandinavian Association of Obstetricians and Gynecologists, Box 443, S-901, 09, Umeaa, Sweden. 8/year.

American Journal of Obstetrics and Gynecology. Mosby-Year Book, 11830 Westline Industrial Drive, St. Louis, MO 63146. Phone: (800) 325-4177. Fax: (314) 432-1380. Monthly.

British Journal of Obstetrics & Gynaecology. Blackwell Publishers, Three Cambridge Center, Cambridge, MA 02142. Phone: (617) 225-0430. Fax: (617) 494-1437. Monthly.

Journal of Clinical Endocrinology & Metabolism. Williams & Wilkins, 428 E. Preston St., Baltimore, MD 21202. Phone: (800) 638-0672. Fax: (900) 447-8438. Monthly.

Maturitas. Elsevier Science Publishing Co., Inc., P.O. Box 882, Madison Square Station, New York, NY 10159-2101. Phone: (212) 989-5800. Fax: (212) 633-3990. 4/year.

Obstetrics and Gynecology. Elsevier Science Publishing Co., Inc., P.O. Box 882, Madison Square Station, New York, NY 10159-2101. Phone: (212) 989-5800. Fax: (212) 633-3990. 15/year.

NEWSLETTERS

Menopause News. Menopause News, 2074 Union St., San Francisco, CA 94123. 6/year.

National Women's Health Network-Network News. National Women's Health Network, 1325 G St. N.W., Washington, DC 20005. Phone: (202) 347-1140. Bimonthly.

ONLINE DATABASES

EMBASE. Elsevier Science Publishing Co., Inc., P.O. Box 882, Madison Square Station, New York, NY 10159-2101. Phone: (212) 989-5800. Fax: (212) 633-3990.

MEDLINE. National Library of Medicine, 8600 Rockville Pike, Bethesda, MD 20894. Phone: (800) 638-8480.

SciSearch. Institute for Scientific Information, 3501 Market St., Philadelphia, PA 19104. Phone: (215) 386-0100. Fax: (215) 386-6362.

POPULAR WORKS AND PATIENT EDUCATION

Doctor Discusses Menopause and Estrogens. Edward M. Davis, Dona Meilach. Budlong Press, 5915 Northwest Hwy., Chicago, IL 60631. 1990.

Estrogen: A Complete Guide to Reversing the Effects of Menopause Using Hormone Replacement Therapy. Lila Nachtigall, Joan R. Heilman. HarperCollins Pubs., Inc., 10 E. 53rd St., New York, NY 10022-5299. Phone: (212) 207-7000. Fax: (800) 242-7737. Revised edition 1991.

Hormones, Hot Flashes & Mood Swings: Living Through the Ups & Downs of Menopause. Clark Gillespie. HarperCollins Pubs., Inc., 10 E. 53rd St., New York, NY 10022-5299. Phone: (212) 207-7000. Fax: (800) 242-7737. 1989.

Managing Your Menopause. Wulf H. Utian. Prentice Hall, 113 Sylvan Ave., Rt. 9W, Prentice Hall Bldg., Englewood Cliffs, NJ 07632. Phone: (201) 767-5937. 1991.

Menopause: A Guide for Women and the Men Who Love Them. Winnifred B. Cutler. W.W. Norton & Co., Inc., 500 Fifth Ave., New York, NY 10110. Phone: (800) 223-2584. 1991.

Menopause: All Your Questions Answered. Contemporary Books, Inc., 180 N. Michigan Ave., Chicago, IL 60601. Phone: (312) 782-9181. 1987.

Menopause: Naturally Preparing for the Second Half of Life. Sadia Greenwood. Volcano Press, Inc., P.O. Box 270, Volcano, CA 95689. Phone: (209) 296-3445. 1989.

Menopause and the Years Ahead. Mary Beard, Lindsay Curtis. Fisher Books, P.O. Box 38040, Tucson, AZ 85740-8040. Phone: (602) 292-9080. Revised edition 1991.

Natural Menopause: The Complete Guide to a Woman's Most Misunderstood Passage. Susan Perry, Katherine O'Harlan. Addison-Wesley Publishing Co., Rte. 128, Reading, MA 01867. Phone: (800) 447-2226. 1992.

RESEARCH CENTERS, INSTITUTES, CLEARINGHOUSES

Center for the Mature Woman. Medical College of Pennsylvania. 3300 Henry Ave., Philadelphia, PA 19129. Phone: (215) 842-7180.

Division of Reproductive Endocrinology. University of Tennessee. 956 Ct. Ave., Room D328, Memphis, TN 38163. Phone: (901) 528-5859.

Queen Elizabeth Hospital Research Institute. 550 University Ave., Toronto, ON, Canada M5G 2A2. Phone: (416) 672-4218.

TEXTBOOKS AND MONOGRAPHS

Menopause: Evaluation, Treatment and Health Concerns. Charles B. Hammond, Florence P. Haseltine, Isaac Schiff. John Wiley & Sons, Inc., 605 Third Ave., New York, NY 10158-0012. Phone: (212) 850-6000. Fax: (212) 850-6088. 1989.

Perimenopausal & Geriatric Gynecology. Hugh R. Barber. Macmillan Publishing Co., 866 Third Ave., New York, NY 10011. Phone: (800) 257-5755. 1988.

Transdermal Estrogen Replacement for Menopausal Women. George F. Birdwood (ed.). Hogrefe & Huber Publishers, P.O. Box 51, Lewiston, NY 14092. Phone: (716) 282-1610. 1988.

ESTROGENS

See: ESTROGEN REPLACEMENT THERAPY; HORMONES

ETHICS

See: MEDICAL ETHICS

EUTHANASIA

See: DEATH AND DYING; MEDICAL ETHICS

EXERCISE

ABSTRACTING, INDEXING, AND CURRENT AWARENESS PUBLICATIONS

Consumer Health and Nutrition Index. Alan Rees. Oryx Press, 4041 N. Central, Suite 700, Phoenix, AZ 85012. Phone: (800) 279-6799. Fax: (800) 279-4663. Quarterly.

Health, Physical Education and Recreation Microform Publications Bulletin. Microform Publications, College of Human Development and Performance, University of Oregon, 1479 Moss St., Eugene, OR 97403. Semiannual.

Kirby's Guide to Fitness and Motor Performance Tests. BenOak Publishing Co., P.O. Box 474, Cape Girardeau, MO 63702-0474. Phone: (314) 334-8789. 1991.

Physical Education Index. BenOak Publishing Co., P.O. Box 474, Cape Girardeau, MO 63702-0474. Phone: (314) 334-8789. Quarterly.

Physical Fitness/Sports Medicine. President's Council on Physical Fitness and Sports, 450 Fifth St. NW, Suite 7130, Washington, DC 20001. Phone: (202) 272-3421. Quarterly.

ANNUALS AND REVIEWS

The Perspective Series. William C. Brown Communications, Inc., 2460 Kerper Blvd., Dubuque, IA 52001. Phone: (800) 338-5578. Irregular.

ASSOCIATIONS, PROFESSIONAL SOCIETIES, ADVOCACY AND SUPPORT GROUPS

Aerobics and Fitness Association of America (AFAA). 15250 Ventura Blvd., Ste. 310, Sherman Oaks, CA 91403. Phone: (818) 905-0040. Fax: (818) 990-5468.

Institute for Aerobics Research (IAR). 12330 Preston Rd., Dallas, TX 75230. Phone: (800) 635-7050.

National Association for Sport and Physical Education. 1900 Association Dr., Reston, VA 22091. Phone: (800) 321-0789.

BIBLIOGRAPHIES

Exercise Machines: Rowing, Cycling, and Skiing Types. National Technical Information Service, 5285 Port Royal Rd., Springfield, VA 22161. Phone: (703) 487-4650. Fax: (703) 321-8547. Jan. 1970-Nov. 1988 PB89-851331/CBY.

Physical Fitness: Subject, Reference and Research Guidebook. Felix M. Terrence. ABBE Publishers Association, 4111 Gallows Rd., Annondale, VA 22003-1862. Phone: (703) 750-0255.

ONLINE DATABASES

Sport and Leisure Database. Faculty of Human Kinetics and Leisure Studies, University of Waterloo, Waterloo, ON, Canada N2L 3G1. Phone: (519) 885-1211.

POPULAR WORKS AND PATIENT EDUCATION

The 35-Plus Good Health Guide for Women: The Prime of Life Program Developed at Kaiser-Permanente for Women Over 35. Jean Perry Spodnik, David P. Cogan. HarperCollins Publishers, Inc., 10 E. 53rd St., New York, NY 10022-5299. Phone: (800) 242-7737. Revised edition 1990.

Walking Medicine: The Lifetime Guide to Preventive and Rehabilitative Exercisewalking Programs. Gary Yanker, Kathy Burton. McGraw-Hill Inc., 11 West 19th St., New York, NY 10011. Phone: (212) 337-5001. Fax: (212) 337-4092. 1990.

Your Personal Fitness Survey: A Guide to Your Current State of Health. David Gamon, Kathleen O'Brien. Borgo Press, P.O. Box 2845, San Bernardino, CA 92406-2845. Phone: (909) 884-5813. Fax: (909) 888-4942. 1991.

RESEARCH CENTERS, INSTITUTES, CLEARINGHOUSES

Exercise Physiology Laboratory. 129 Larkins Hall, 337 W. 17th Ave., Ohio State University, Columbus, OH 43210. Phone: (614) 292-6687.

Exercise Physiology Laboratory, University of Louisville. Belknap Campus, Louisville, KY 40208. Phone: (502) 588-6649.

National Institute for Fitness and Sport. 250 S. Agnes, Indianapolis, IN 46223. Phone: (317) 274-3432.

President's Council on Physical Fitness and Sports (PCPFS). 450 Fifth St. N.W., Ste. 7103, Washington, DC 20001. Phone: (202) 272-3430.

TEXTBOOKS AND MONOGRAPHS

Nutrition, Weight Control, and Exercise. Frank I. Katch, William D. McArdle. Williams & Wilkins, 428 East Preston St., Baltimore, MD 21202. Phone: (800) 638-0672. Fax: (800) 447-8438. 1988.

Stretching and Strengthening Exercises. H. Spring, U. Illi, H.R. Kunz, and others. Thieme Medical Publishers, Inc., 381 Park Ave. S., New York, NY 10016. Phone: (212) 683-5088. Fax: (212) 779-9020. 1991.

EYE CANCER

See: CANCER; EYE DISEASES

EYE DISEASES

See also: CATARACTS; GLAUCOMA;
OPHTHALMOLOGY; VISION DISORDERS

ABSTRACTING, INDEXING, AND CURRENT AWARENESS PUBLICATIONS

Core Journals in Ophthalmology. Elsevier Science Publishing Co., Inc., P.O. Box 882, Madison Square Station, New York, NY 10159-2101. Phone: (212) 989-5800. Fax: (212) 633-3990. 11/year.

Current Contents/Clinical Medicine. Institute for Scientific Information, 3501 Market St., Philadelphia, PA 19104. Phone: (800) 523-1850. Fax: (215) 386-6362. Weekly.

Excerpta Medica. Section 12: Ophthalmology. Elsevier Science Publishing Co., Inc., P.O. Box 882, Madison Square Station, New York, NY 10159-2101. Phone: (212) 989-5800. Fax: (212) 633-3990. 16/year.

Index Medicus. U.S. National Library of Medicine, 8600 Rockville Pike, Bethesda, MD 20894. Phone: (800) 638-8480. Monthly.

Key Ophthalmology: Current Literature in Perspective. Mosby-Year Book, 11830 Westline Industrial Drive, St. Louis, MO 63146. Phone: (800) 325-4177. Fax: (314) 432-1380. Quarterly.

Ophthalmic Literature. Institute of Ophthalmology, Judd St., London WC1H 9QS, England. 7/year.

Research Alert: Glaucoma, Diabetic Retinopathy & Related Diseases. Institute for Scientific Information, 3501 Market St., Philadelphia, PA 19104. Phone: (800) 523-1850. Fax: (215) 386-6362. Weekly.

Research Alert: Ophthalmology. Institute for Scientific Information, 3501 Market St., Philadelphia, PA 19104. Phone: (800) 523-1850. Fax: (215) 386-6362. Weekly.

Science Citation Index. Institute for Scientific Information, 3501 Market St., Philadelphia, PA 19104. Phone: (800) 523-1850. Fax: (215) 386-6362. Bimonthly.

ANNUALS AND REVIEWS

Current Opinion in Ophthalmology. Current Science Ltd., 20 N. Third St., Philadelphia, PA 19106-2199. Phone: (800) 552-5866. Fax: (215) 574-2270. Bimonthly.

Ophthalmology Clinics. W.B. Saunders Co., The Curtis Center, Independence Square W., Philadelphia, PA 19106-3399. Phone: (215) 238-7800. Quarterly.

Year Book of Ophthalmology. Mosby-Year Book, 11830 Westline Industrial Drive, St. Louis, MO 63146. Phone: (800) 325-4177. Fax: (314) 432-1380. Annual.

ASSOCIATIONS, PROFESSIONAL SOCIETIES, ADVOCACY AND SUPPORT GROUPS

Association for Macular Diseases (AMD). 210 E. 64th St., New York, NY 10021. Phone: (212) 605-3719.

Canadian Ophthalmological Society. 1525 Carling Ave., No. 610, Ottawa, ON, Canada K1Z 8R9. Phone: (613) 729-6779. Fax: (613) 729-7209.

Eye Bank Association of America, Inc.. 1001 Connecticut Ave. N.W., Ste. 601, Washington, DC 20036-5504. Phone: (202) 775-499.

International Eye Foundation (IEF). 7801 Norfolk Ave., Bethesda, MD 20814. Phone: (301) 986-1830.

CD-ROM DATABASES

SCISEARCH. Institute for Scientific Information, 3501 Market St., Philadelphia, PA 19104. Phone: (215) 386-0100. Fax: (215) 386-6362.

DIRECTORIES

Directory of Certified Ophthalmologists. American Board of Medical Specialties, 1 Rotary Center, Suite 805, Evanston, IL 60201. Phone: (708) 491-9091. Biennial.

ENCYCLOPEDIAS, DICTIONARIES, WORD BOOKS

Ophthalmic Terminology. Stein. Mosby-Year Book, 11830 Westline Industrial Drive, St. Louis, MO 63146. Phone: (800) 325-4177. Fax: (314) 432-1380. Third edition 1992.

Ophthalmic Word Book. Barbara De Lorenzo. Springhouse Publishing Co., 1111 Bethlehem Pike, Spring House, PA 19477. Phone: (800) 331-3170. Fax: (215) 646-8716. 1992.

Ophthalmology Words. Stedman. Williams & Wilkins, 428 East Preston St., Baltimore, MD 21202. Phone: (800) 638-0672. Fax: (800) 447-8438. 1992.

HANDBOOKS, GUIDES, MANUALS, ATLASES

Color Atlas of Corneal Dystrophies and Degenerations. Casey. Mosby-Year Book, 11830 Westline Industrial Drive, St. Louis, MO 63146. Phone: (800) 325-4177. Fax: (314) 432-1380. 1991.

Color Atlas of Eye Systemic Diseases. Kritzinger. Mosby-Year Book, 11830 Westline Industrial Drive, St. Louis, MO 63146. Phone: (800) 325-4177. Fax: (314) 432-1380. Second edition 1993.

Handbook of Ocular Drugs. Pavan-Langst. Little, Brown and Co., 34 Beacon St., Boston, MA 02108. Phone: (617) 227-0730. Fax: (617) 227-0790. 1991.

Handbook of Ophthalmology. Gardner. Appleton & Lange, 25 Van Zant St., East Norwalk, CT 06855. Phone: (800) 423-1359. Fax: (203) 854-9486. 1987.

Manual of Clinical Problems in Opththalmology. Gittinger. Little, Brown and Co., 34 Beacon St., Boston, MA 02108. Phone: (617) 227-0730. 1988.

Manual of Ocular Diagnosis and Therapy. Deborah Pavan-Langstone (ed.). Little, Brown and Company, 34 Beacon St., Boston, MA 02108. Phone: (617) 227-0730. Third edition 1991.

Ophthalmic Drug Facts. Jimmy D. Bartlett, N. Rex Ghormley, Siret Jaanus, and others. J.B. Lippincott Co., 227 E. Washington Square, Philadelphia, PA 19106-3780. Phone: (215) 238-4200. Fax: (215) 238-4227. 1992.

JOURNALS

American Journal of Ophthalmology. Ophthalmic Publishing Co., 435 N. Michigan Ave., Chicago, IL 60611. Phone: (312) 787-3853.

Annals of Ophthalmology. Altiers and Maynard Communications, 59 Oakwood Dr., Madison, CT 06443. Phone: (203) 421-3494.

Archives of Ophthalmology. American Medical Association, 515 North State St., Chicago, IL 60610. Phone: (312) 464-0183. Fax: (312) 464-5834. Monthly.

Clinical Eye and Vision Care. Butterworth-Heinemann, 80 Montvale Ave., Stoneham, MA 02180. Phone: (617) 438-8464. Fax: (617) 279-4851. Quarterly.

Eye. BMJ Publishing Group, BMA House, Tavistock Square, London WC1H 9JR, England. Phone: 071-383 6244/6638. Fax: 071-383 6662. 6/year.

Survey of Ophthalmology. Survey of Ophthalmology, Inc., Suite 4, 7 Kent St., Brookline, MA 02146. Phone: (617) 566-2138. Fax: (617) 566-4019. Bimonthly.

NEWSLETTERS

Ophthalmology Alert. American Health Consultants, Department C1290, P.O. Box 740060, Atlanta, GA 30374. Phone: (800) 559-1032. Monthly.

ONLINE DATABASES

Combined Health Information Database (CHID). U.S. National Institutes of Health, P.O. Box NDIC, Bethesda, MD 20892. Phone: (301) 496-2162. Fax: (301) 770-5164. Quarterly.

EMBASE. Elsevier Science Publishing Co., Inc., P.O. Box 882, Madison Square Station, New York, NY 10159-2101. Phone: (212) 989-5800. Fax: (212) 633-3990.

MEDLINE. National Library of Medicine, 8600 Rockville Pike, Bethesda, MD 20894. Phone: (800) 638-8480.

SciSearch. Institute for Scientific Information, 3501 Market St., Philadelphia, PA 19104. Phone: (215) 386-0100. Fax: (215) 386-6362.

POPULAR WORKS AND PATIENT EDUCATION

20/20: A Total Guide to Improving Your Vision and Preventing Eye Disease. Mitchell H. Friedlaender. Rodale Press, Inc., 33 E. Minor St., Emmaus, PA 18098. Phone: (800) 527-8200. Fax: (215) 967-6263. 1991.

RESEARCH CENTERS, INSTITUTES, CLEARINGHOUSES

Hermann Eye Center. University of Texas Health Science Center at Houston. Dept. of Ophthalmology, 6411 Fannin St., Houston, TX 77030. Phone: (713) 797-1777.

Wills Eye Hospital. 9th & Walnut St., Philadelphia, PA 19107. Phone: (215) 928-3272.

Wilmer Ophthalmological Institute. Johns Hopkins University. 601 N. Broadway, Baltimore, MD 21205. Phone: (301) 955-6846. Fax: (301) 955-0675.

W.K. Kellogg Eye Center. University of Michigan. 1000 Wall St., Ann Arbor, MI 48105-1994. Phone: (313) 763-1415. Fax: (313) 936-2340.

TEXTBOOKS AND MONOGRAPHS

Age-Related Cataract. Richard W. Young. Oxford University Press, 200 Madison Ave., New York, NY 10016. Phone: (212) 679-7300. 1991.

Applied Pharmacology of Glaucoma. Stephen M. Drance, Michael Vanbuskirk, Arthur H. Neufeld. Williams & Wilkins, 428 East Preston St., Baltimore, MD 21202. Phone: (800) 638-0672. Fax: (800) 447-8438. 1991.

Decision Making in Ophthalmology. Richard van Heuven, Johan T. Zwaan. Mosby-Year Book, 11830 Westline Industrial Drive, St. Louis, MO 63146. Phone: (800) 325-4177. Fax: (314) 432-1380. 1992.

Diseases of the External Eye, Ocular Adnexa, and Orbit. H. Bruce Ostler, Marian W. Ostler. Williams & Wilkins, 428 East Preston St., Baltimore, MD 21202. Phone: (800) 638-0672. Fax: (800) 447-8438. 1991.

The Eye in Systemic Disease. Jack J. Kanski, D. Thomas. Butterworth-Heinemann, 80 Montvale Ave., Stoneham, MA

02180. Phone: (617) 438-8464. Fax: (617) 279-4851. Second edition 1990.

Ophthalmic Surgery: Principles and Concepts. George Spaeth (ed.). W.B. Saunders Co., The Curtis Center, Independence Sqare W., Philadelphia, PA 19106-3399. Phone: (215) 238-7800. 1990.

Ophthalmology: A Diagnostic Text. William H. Coles. Williams & Wilkins, 428 East Preston St., Baltimore, MD 21202. Phone: (800) 638-0672. Fax: (800) 447-8438. 1989.

Ophthalmology: Principles and Concepts. Frank Newell. Mosby-Year Book, 11830 Westline Industrial Drive, St. Louis, MO 63146. Phone: (800) 325-4177. Fax: (314) 432-1380. 7th edition, 1992.

Parson's Diseases of the Eye. Stephen J.H. Miller. Churchill Livingstone Inc., 650 Avenue of the Americas, New York, NY 10011. Phone: (212) 819-5400. Fax: (212) 302-6598. 18th edition 1990.

The Physician's Guide to Cataracts, Glaucoma and Other Eye Problems. John Eden. Consumer Reports Books, 9180 LeSaint Dr., Fairfield, OH 45014. Phone: (513) 860-1178. 1992.

A Text and Atlas of Strabismus Surgery. Renee Richards. Williams & Wilkins, 428 East Preston St., Baltimore, MD 21202. Phone: (800) 638-0672. Fax: (800) 447-8438. 1991.

Will's Treatment of Eye Disease. Friedberg. J.B. Lippincott Co., 227 E. Washington Square, Philadelphia, PA 19106-3780. Phone: (215) 238-4200. Fax: (215) 238-4227. 1990.

EYE SURGERY

See also: CATARACTS; GLAUCOMA; LASER SURGERY; OPHTHALMOLOGY; SURGERY; VISION DISORDERS

ABSTRACTING, INDEXING, AND CURRENT AWARENESS PUBLICATIONS

Core Journals in Ophthalmology. Elsevier Science Publishing Co., Inc., P.O. Box 882, Madison Square Station, New York, NY 10159-2101. Phone: (212) 989-5800. Fax: (212) 633-3990. 11/year.

Current Contents/Clinical Medicine. Institute for Scientific Information, 3501 Market St., Philadelphia, PA 19104. Phone: (800) 523-1850. Fax: (215) 386-6362. Weekly.

Excerpta Medica. Section 12: Ophthalmology. Elsevier Science Publishing Co., Inc., P.O. Box 882, Madison Square Station, New York, NY 10159-2101. Phone: (212) 989-5800. Fax: (212) 633-3990. 16/year.

Index Medicus. U.S. National Library of Medicine, 8600 Rockville Pike, Bethesda, MD 20894. Phone: (800) 638-8480. Monthly.

Key Ophthalmology: Current Literature in Perspective. Mosby-Year Book, 11830 Westline Industrial Drive, St. Louis, MO 63146. Phone: (800) 325-4177. Fax: (314) 432-1380. Quarterly.

Science Citation Index. Institute for Scientific Information, 3501 Market St., Philadelphia, PA 19104. Phone: (800) 523-1850. Fax: (215) 386-6362. Bimonthly.

ANNUALS AND REVIEWS

Complications in Ophthalmic Surgery. Gilbert Smolin, Mitchell H. Friedlaender (eds.). Little, Brown and Company, 34 Beacon St., Boston, MA 02108. Phone: (617) 227-0730. International Ophthalmology Clinics. vol. 32, no. 4 1992.

Current Opinion in Ophthalmology. Current Science Ltd., 20 N. Third St., Philadelphia, PA 19106-2199. Phone: (800) 552-5866. Fax: (215) 574-2270. Bimonthly.

Ophthalmology Clinics. W.B. Saunders Co., The Curtis Center, Independence Square W., Philadelphia, PA 19106-3399. Phone: (215) 238-7800. Quarterly.

ASSOCIATIONS, PROFESSIONAL SOCIETIES, ADVOCACY AND SUPPORT GROUPS

American Society of Cataract and Refractive Surgery (ASCRS). 3702 Pender Dr., Ste. 250, Fairfax, VA 22030. Phone: (703) 591-2220. Fax: (703) 591-0614.

Canadian Ophthalmological Society. 1525 Carling Ave., No. 610, Ottawa, ON, Canada K1Z 8R9. Phone: (613) 729-6779. Fax: (613) 729-7209.

BIBLIOGRAPHIES

Laser Eye Surgery. National Technical Information Service, 5285 Port Royal Rd., Springfield, VA 22161. Phone: (703) 487-4650. Fax: (703) 321-8547. Jan. 1975-Apr. 1989 PB89-859763/CBY.

CD-ROM DATABASES

SCISEARCH. Institute for Scientific Information, 3501 Market St., Philadelphia, PA 19104. Phone: (215) 386-0100. Fax: (215) 386-6362.

DIRECTORIES

Directory of Certified Ophthalmologists. American Board of Medical Specialties, 1 Rotary Center, Suite 805, Evanston, IL 60201. Phone: (708) 491-9091. Biennial.

ENCYCLOPEDIAS, DICTIONARIES, WORD BOOKS

Ophthalmic Terminology. Stein. Mosby-Year Book, 11830 Westline Industrial Drive, St. Louis, MO 63146. Phone: (800) 325-4177. Fax: (314) 432-1380. Third edition 1992.

Ophthalmic Word Book. Barbara De Lorenzo. Springhouse Publishing Co., 1111 Bethlehem Pike, Spring House, PA 19477. Phone: (800) 331-3170. Fax: (215) 646-8716. 1992.

Ophthalmology Words. Stedman. Williams & Wilkins, 428 East Preston St., Baltimore, MD 21202. Phone: (800) 638-0672. Fax: (800) 447-8438. 1992.

Surgery on File: Eye, Ear, Nose and Throat Surgery. The Diagram Group. Facts on File, Inc., 460 Park Ave. S., New York, NY 10016-7382. Phone: (212) 683-2244. 1988.

HANDBOOKS, GUIDES, MANUALS, ATLASES

Atlas of Neuro-Ophthalmic Surgery. Thomas C. Spoor, James A. Garrity, John M. Ramocki (eds.). Little, Brown and Company, 34 Beacon St., Boston, MA 02108. Phone: (617) 227-0730. 1992.

Atlas of Ophthalmic Surgery. Jaffe. Raven Press, 1185 Ave. of the Americas, New York, NY 10036. Phone: (212) 930-9500. Fax: (212) 869-3495. 1990.

Color Atlas of Ophthalmic Surgery. Minckler. J.B. Lippincott Co., 227 E. Washington Square, Philadelphia, PA 19106-3780. Phone: (215) 238-4200. Fax: (215) 238-4227. 1992.

Immediate Eye Care: An Illustrated Manual. Nicola Ragge, David L. Easty. Mosby-Year Book, 11830 Westline Industrial Drive, St. Louis, MO 63146. Phone: (800) 325-4177. Fax: (314) 432-1380. 1991.

Manual of Pediatric Ophthalmology and Strabismus Surgery. Monte A. Del Monte. Churchill Livingstone Inc., 650 Ave. of the Americas, New York, NY 10011. Phone: (212) 819-5400. Fax: (212) 302-6598. 1991.

Ophthalmic Surgery: Cataracts. Richard P. Kratz, and others. J.B. Lippincott Co., 227 E. Washington Square, Philadelphia, PA 19106-3780. Phone: (215) 238-4200. Fax: (215) 238-4227. 1991.

Sutureless Cataract Surgery. James P. Gills, Donald R. Sanders (eds.). SLACK Inc., 6900 Grove Rd., Thorofare, NJ 08086-9447. Phone: (800) 257-8290. Fax: (609) 853-5991. 1991.

JOURNALS

American Journal of Ophthalmology. Ophthalmic Publishing Co., 435 N. Michigan Ave., Chicago, IL 60611. Phone: (312) 787-3853.

Eye. BMJ Publishing Group, BMA House, Tavistock Square, London WC1H 9JR, England. Phone: 071-383 6244/6638. Fax: 071-383 6662. 6/year.

Journal of Cataract and Refractive Surgery. Waverly Press, 428 E. Preston St., Baltimore, MD 21202. Phone: (800) 638-0672. Fax: (800) 447-8438. Bimonthly.

Ophthalmic Surgery. SLACK Inc., 6900 Grove Rd., Thorofare, NJ 08086-9447. Phone: (800) 257-8290. Fax: (609) 853-5991. Monthly.

Refractive and Corneal Surgery. SLACK Inc., 6900 Grove Rd., Thorofare, NJ 08086-9447. Phone: (800) 257-8290. Fax: (609) 853-5991. Bimonthly.

Survey of Ophthalmology. Survey of Ophthalmology, Inc., Suite 4, 7 Kent St., Brookline, MA 02146. Phone: (617) 566-2138. Fax: (617) 566-4019. Bimonthly.

ONLINE DATABASES

EMBASE. Elsevier Science Publishing Co., Inc., P.O. Box 882, Madison Square Station, New York, NY 10159-2101. Phone: (212) 989-5800. Fax: (212) 633-3990.

MEDLINE. National Library of Medicine, 8600 Rockville Pike, Bethesda, MD 20894. Phone: (800) 638-8480.

SciSearch. Institute for Scientific Information, 3501 Market St., Philadelphia, PA 19104. Phone: (215) 386-0100. Fax: (215) 386-6362.

POPULAR WORKS AND PATIENT EDUCATION

Cataract Surgery: Before and After. Robert I. Johnson. SLACK Inc., 6900 Grove Rd., Thorofare, NJ 08086-9447.

Phone: (800) 257-8290. Fax: (609) 853-5991. Two volumes 1989.

RESEARCH CENTERS, INSTITUTES, CLEARINGHOUSES

Hermann Eye Center. University of Texas Health Science Center at Houston. Dept. of Ophthalmology, 6411 Fannin St., Houston, TX 77030. Phone: (713) 797-1777.

Wills Eye Hospital. 9th & Walnut St., Philadelphia, PA 19107. Phone: (215) 928-3272.

TEXTBOOKS AND MONOGRAPHS

Cataract Surgery and Its Complications. Jaffe. Mosby-Year Book, 11830 Westline Industrial Drive, St. Louis, MO 63146. Phone: (800) 325-4177. Fax: (314) 432-1380. Fifth edition 1990.

Cosmetic Blepharoplasty. Stephen L. Bosniak. Raven Press, 1185 Avenue of the Americas, New York, NY 10036. Phone: (212) 930-9500. Fax: (212) 869-3495. 1991.

Current Surgical Diagnosis and Treatment. L.W. Way. Appleton & Lange, 25 Van Zant St., East Norwalk, CT 06855. Phone: (800) 423-1359. Fax: (203) 854-9486. Ninth edition 1990.

Eye Surgery. Eisner. Springer-Verlag New York Inc., 175 Fifth Ave., New York, NY 10010. Phone: (212) 460-1500. Fax: (212) 473-6272. Second edition 1990.

Glaucoma Surgery. Obstbaum. Appleton & Lange, 25 Van Zant St., East Norwalk, CT 06855. Phone: (800) 423-1359. Fax: (203) 854-9486. 1991.

Laser Surgery in Ophthalmology. Weingeist. Appleton & Lange, 25 Van Zant St., East Norwalk, CT 06855. Phone: (800) 423-1359. Fax: (203) 854-9486. 1992.

Ophthalmic Lasers. Wayne F. March (ed.). SLACK Inc., 6900 Grove Rd., Thorofare, NJ 08086-9447. Phone: (800) 257-8290. Fax: (609) 853-5991. Second edition 1990.

Ophthalmic Surgery: Principles and Concepts. George Spaeth (ed.). W.B. Saunders Co., The Curtis Center, Independence Sqare W., Philadelphia, PA 19106-3399. Phone: (215) 238-7800. 1990.

Ophthalmology: Principles and Concepts. Frank Newell. Mosby-Year Book, 11830 Westline Industrial Drive, St. Louis, MO 63146. Phone: (800) 325-4177. Fax: (314) 432-1380. 7th edition, 1992.

The Physician's Guide to Cataracts, Glaucoma and Other Eye Problems. John Eden. Consumer Reports Books, 9180 LeSaint Dr., Fairfield, OH 45014. Phone: (513) 860-1178. 1992.

Stallards' Eye Surgery. M.J. Roper Hall (ed.). Butterworth-Heinemann, 80 Montvale Ave., Stoneham, MA 02180. Phone: (617) 438-8464. Fax: (617) 279-4851. Seventh edition 1989.

Surgery of the Eyelids and Orbit: An Anatomical Approach. Bradley N. Lemke, Robert C. Della Rocca. Appleton & Lange, 25 Van Zant St., East Norwalk, CT 06855. Phone: (800) 423-1359. Fax: (203) 854-9486. 1990.

Surgical Anatomy of the Orbit. Barry M. Zide, Glenn W. Jelks. Raven Press, 1185 Avenue of the Americas, New York, NY 10036. Phone: (212) 930-9500. Fax: (212) 869-3495. 1985.

A Text and Atlas of Strabismus Surgery. Renee Richards. Williams & Wilkins, 428 East Preston St., Baltimore, MD 21202. Phone: (800) 638-0672. Fax: (800) 447-8438. 1991.

Will's Treatment of Eye Disease. Friedberg. J.B. Lippincott Co., 227 E. Washington Square, Philadelphia, PA 19106-3780. Phone: (215) 238-4200. Fax: (215) 238-4227. 1990.

F

FAINTING

See: NEUROMUSCULAR DISORDERS

FAMILY MEDICINE

ABSTRACTING, INDEXING, AND CURRENT AWARENESS PUBLICATIONS

Current Contents/Clinical Medicine. Institute for Scientific Information, 3501 Market St., Philadelphia, PA 19104. Phone: (800) 523-1850. Fax: (215) 386-6362. Weekly.

FAMLI (Family Medicine Literature Index). College of Family Physicians of Canada, 4000 Leslie St., Willowdale, ON, Canada M2K 2R9. Annual.

Index Medicus. U.S. National Library of Medicine, 8600 Rockville Pike, Bethesda, MD 20894. Phone: (800) 638-8480. Monthly.

Science Citation Index. Institute for Scientific Information, 3501 Market St., Philadelphia, PA 19104. Phone: (800) 523-1850. Fax: (215) 386-6362. Bimonthly.

ANNUALS AND REVIEWS

Year Book of Family Practice. Mosby-Year Book, 11830 Westline Industrial Drive, St. Louis, MO 63146. Phone: (800) 325-4177. Fax: (314) 432-1380. Annual.

ASSOCIATIONS, PROFESSIONAL SOCIETIES, ADVOCACY AND SUPPORT GROUPS

American Academy of Family Physicians (AAFP). 8880 Ward Pkwy., Kansas City, MO 64114. Phone: (816) 333-9700. Fax: (816) 822-0580.

American Board of Family Practice (ABFP). 2228 Young Dr., Lexington, KY 40505. Phone: (606) 269-5626.

College of Family Physicians of Canada. 2630 Skymark Ave., Mississaugua, ON, Canada L4W 5A4.

CD-ROM DATABASES

1993 PDR Library on CD-ROM. Medical Economics, Five Paragon Dr., Montvale, NJ 07645-1742. Phone: (800) 232-7379. Fax: (201) 573-4956. 1993.

American Family Physician. CMC ReSearch, Inc., 7150 S.W. Hampton, Suite C-120, Portland, OR 97223. Phone: (800) 262-7668. Fax: (503) 639-1796. Annual.

Family Practice Library. CMC ReSearch, Inc., 7150 S.W. Hampton, Suite C-120, Portland, OR 97223. Phone: (800) 262-7668. Fax: (503) 639-1796. Annual.

Family Practice MEDLINE. MEP, 124 Mt. Auburn St., Cambridge, MA 02138. Phone: (800) 342-1338. Fax: (617) 868-7738. Quarterly.

Internal Medicine '92. Macmillan New Media, 124 Mt. Auburn St., Cambridge, MA 02138. Phone: (800) 342-1338. 1992.

Oxford Textbook of Medicine. Oxford University Press, 200 Madison Ave., New York, NY 10016. Phone: (212) 679-7300. Irregular.

PDR on CD-ROM. Medical Economics, Five Paragon Dr., Montvale, NJ 07645-1742. Phone: (800) 222-3045. Fax: (201) 573-4956. 3/year.

SCISEARCH. Institute for Scientific Information, 3501 Market St., Philadelphia, PA 19104. Phone: (215) 386-0100. Fax: (215) 386-6362.

Year Books on Disc. CMC ReSearch, Inc., 7150 S.W. Hampton, Suite C-120, Portland, OR 97223. Phone: (800) 262-7668. Fax: (503) 639-1796. Annual includes Year Books of Cardiology, Dermatology, Diagnostic Radiology, Drug Therapy, Emergency Medicine, Family Practice, Medicine, Neurology and Neurosurgery, Obstetrics and Gynecology, Oncology, Pediatrics, and Psychiatry and Applied Mental Health.

DIRECTORIES

Directory of Certified Family Physicians. American Board of Medical Specialties, 1 Rotary Center, Suite 805, Evanston, IL 60201. Phone: (708) 491-9091. Biennial.

ENCYCLOPEDIAS, DICTIONARIES, WORD BOOKS

Dictionary of Modern Medicine. Segen. The Parthenon Publishing Group, Inc., 120 Mill Rd., Park Ridge, NJ 07656. Phone: (201) 391-6796. 1992.

Encyclopedia of Health. Chelsea House Publishers, 95 Madison Ave., New York, NY 10016. Phone: (800) 848-2665. Irregular.

Melloni's Illustrated Medical Dictionary. Dox. Williams & Wilkins, 428 East Preston St., Baltimore, MD 21202. Phone: (800) 638-0672. Fax: (800) 447-8438. Second edition 1985.

Mosby's Medical, Nursing, and Allied Health Dictionary. Kenneth N. Anderson, Lois Anderson, Walter D. Glanze (eds.). Mosby-Year Book, 11830 Westline Industrial Dr., St. Louis, MO 63146. Phone: (800) 325-4177. Fax: (314) 432-1380. Third edition 1990.

HANDBOOKS, GUIDES, MANUALS, ATLASES

The Family Practice Desk Reference. Charles E. Driscoll, Edward T. Bope, Charles W. Smith, Jr.. Mosby-Year Book, 11830 Westline Industrial Drive, St. Louis, MO 63146. Phone: (800) 325-4177. Fax: (314) 432-1380. Second edition 1991.

Family Practice Drug Handbook. Ellsworth. Mosby-Year Book, 11830 Westline Industrial Drive, St. Louis, MO 63146. Phone: (800) 325-4177. Fax: (314) 432-1380. 1991.

Family Practice Handbook. Littler. Mosby-Year Book, 11830 Westline Industrial Drive, St. Louis, MO 63146. Phone: (800) 325-4177. Fax: (314) 432-1380. 1990.

The Family Practice Handbook: The Iowa Manual for Residents. John E. Littler, Timothy Momany. Mosby-Year Book, 11830 Westline Industrial Drive, St. Louis, MO 63146. Phone: (800) 325-4177. Fax: (314) 432-1380. 1990.

JOURNALS

Family Medicine. Society of Teachers of Family Medicine, Box 8729, 8880 Ward Pwky., Kansas City, MO 64114. Phone: (816) 333-9700. Fax: (816) 822-0580. 8/year.

Family Practice. Oxford University Press, 200 Madison Ave., New York, NY 10016. Phone: (212) 679-7300. Quarterly.

Family Practice Research Journal. American Academy of Family Physicians, 8880 Ward Pkwy., Kansas City, MO 64114-2797. Phone: (816) 333-9700. Fax: (816) 822-0580. Quarterly.

Journal of the American Board of Family Practice. Massachusetts Medical Society, 1440 Main St., Waltham, MA 02154-1649. Phone: (617) 893-3800. Fax: (617) 893-0413. Bimonthly.

Journal of Family Practice. Appleton & Lange, 25 Van Zant St., East Norwalk, CT 06855. Phone: (800) 423-1359. Fax: (203) 854-9486. Monthly.

NEWSLETTERS

Family Practice Alert. American Health Consultants, Department C1290, P.O. Box 740060, Atlanta, GA 30374. Phone: (800) 559-1032. Monthly.

Harvard Family Health Letter. Harvard Medical School Publications Group, 164 Longwood Ave., Boston, MA 02115. Monthly.

ONLINE DATABASES

EMBASE. Elsevier Science Publishing Co., Inc., P.O. Box 882, Madison Square Station, New York, NY 10159-2101. Phone: (212) 989-5800. Fax: (212) 633-3990.

MEDIS. Mead Data Central, P.O. Box 1830, Dayton, OH 45401. Phone: (800) 227-4908.

MEDLINE. National Library of Medicine, 8600 Rockville Pike, Bethesda, MD 20894. Phone: (800) 638-8480.

SciSearch. Institute for Scientific Information, 3501 Market St., Philadelphia, PA 19104. Phone: (215) 386-0100. Fax: (215) 386-6362.

POPULAR WORKS AND PATIENT EDUCATION

New Good Housekeeping Family Health and Medical Guide. Hearst Corporation, 60 E. 42nd St., New York, NY 10165. Phone: (212) 297-9680. Fax: (415) 588-6867. Revised edition 1988.

TEXTBOOKS AND MONOGRAPHS

Difficult Medical Management. Robert B. Taylor. W.B. Saunders Co., The Curtis Center, Independence Square W., Philadelphia, PA 19106-3399. Phone: (215) 238-7800. 1991.

Essentials of Family Medicine. Philip B. Sloane, Richard M. Baker, Lisa M. Slatt (eds.). Williams & Wilkins, 428 E. Preston St., Baltimore, MD 21202. Phone: (800) 638-0672. Fax: (800) 447-8438. 1988.

Family Medicine. Taylor. Springer-Verlag New York Inc., 175 Fifth Ave., New York, NY 10010. Phone: (212) 460-1500. Fax: (212) 473-6272. Third edition 1988.

Family Medicine: Principles and Practice. Robert B. Taylor. Springer-Verlag New York Inc., 175 Fifth Ave., New York, NY 10010. Phone: (212) 460-1500. Fax: (212) 473-6272. 3rd edition, 1988.

Family Practice Review. Swanson. Mosby-Year Book, 11830 Westline Industrial Drive, St. Louis, MO 63146. Phone: (800) 325-4177. Fax: (314) 432-1380. Second edition 1991.

Oxford Textbook of Medicine. D.J. Weatherall, J.G.G. Ledingham, D.A. Warrell. Oxford University Press, 200 Madison Ave., New York, NY 10016. Phone: (212) 679-7300. Fax: (212) 725-2972. Second edition 1987.

Principles of Ambulatory Medicine. L. Randol Barker, John R. Burton, Philip D. Zieve. Williams & Wilkins, 428 East Preston St., Baltimore, MD 21202. Phone: (800) 638-0672. Fax: (800) 447-8438. 1990.

Scientific American Medicine. Scientific American, 415 Madison Ave., New York, NY 10017. Phone: (800) 545-0554. Monthly.

A Textbook of Family Medicine. Ian R. McWhinney. Oxford University Press, 200 Madison Ave., New York, NY 10016. Phone: (212) 679-7300. 1989.

Textbook of Family Practice. Robert E. Rakel. W.B. Saunders Co., The Curtis Center, Independence Square W., Philadelphia, PA 19106-3399. Phone: (215) 238-7800. Fourth edition 1990.

FAMILY PLANNING

See also: CONTRACEPTION

ABSTRACTING, INDEXING, AND CURRENT AWARENESS PUBLICATIONS

Current Literature in Family Planning. Planned Parenthood Federation of America, 810 7th Ave., New York, NY 10019. Phone: (212) 603-4637.

Index Medicus. U.S. National Library of Medicine, 8600 Rockville Pike, Bethesda, MD 20894. Phone: (800) 638-8480. Monthly.

Latest Literature in Family Planning. Family Planning Information Service, 27-35 Mortimer St., London W1N 7RJ, England. Bimonthly.

ASSOCIATIONS, PROFESSIONAL SOCIETIES, ADVOCACY AND SUPPORT GROUPS

Association for Voluntary Surgical Contraception. 122 E. 42nd St., New York, NY 10168. Phone: (212) 351-2500.

The Couple to Couple League International, Inc.. P.O. Box 111184, Cincinnati, OH 45211.

National Family Planning and Reproductive Health Association. 122 C St. N.W., Suite 380, Washington, DC 20001. Phone: (202) 628-3535.

BIBLIOGRAPHIES

Abortion Bibliography. Whitston Publishing Co., P.O. Box 958, Troy, NY 12181. Phone: (518) 283-4363.

HANDBOOKS, GUIDES, MANUALS, ATLASES

Handbook of Contraception and Abortion. Burkman. Little, Brown and Co., 34 Beacon St., Boston, MA 02108. Phone: (617) 227-0730. Fax: (617) 227-0790. 1989.

JOURNALS

British Journal of Family Planning. National Association of Family Planning Doctors, 27 Sussex Pl., Regent's Park, London NW1 4RG, England.

Contraception. Butterworth-Heinemann, 80 Montvale Ave., Stoncham, MA 02180. Phone: (617) 438-8464. Fax: (617) 279-4851. Monthly.

Family Planning Perspectives. Alan Guttmacher Institute, 111 Fifth Ave., New York, NY 10003. Phone: (212) 254-5636.

ONLINE DATABASES

EMBASE. Elsevier Science Publishing Co., Inc., P.O. Box 882, Madison Square Station, New York, NY 10159-2101. Phone: (212) 989-5800. Fax: (212) 633-3990.

MEDLINE. National Library of Medicine, 8600 Rockville Pike, Bethesda, MD 20894. Phone: (800) 638-8480.

POPLINE. U.S. National Library of Medicine, MEDLARS Management Section, 8600 Rockville Pike, Bethesda, MD 20894. Phone: (800) 638-8480. Monthly.

SciSearch. Institute for Scientific Information, 3501 Market St., Philadelphia, PA 19104. Phone: (215) 386-0100. Fax: (215) 386-6362.

POPULAR WORKS AND PATIENT EDUCATION

Contraception. V.L. Bullough, B. Bullough. Prometheus Books, 700E. Amherst St., Buffalo, NY 14215. Phone: (800) 421-0351. 1990.

Contraception: A Guide to Birth Control Methods. Vern L. Bullough, Bonnie Bullough. Prometheus Books, 700 E. Amherst St., Buffalo, NY 14215. Phone: (800) 421-0351. 1990.

The Contraceptive Handbook: A Guide to Safe and Effective Choices for Men and Women. Beverly Winikoff, Suzanne Wymelenberg, and others. Consumer Reports Books, 9180 LeSaint Dr., Fairfield, OH 45014. Phone: (513) 860-1178. 1992.

Contraceptive Technology, 1990-1992: With Two Special Sections: AIDS and Condoms. Robert A. Hatcher. Irvington Publishers, 522 E. 82nd St., New York, NY 10028. Phone: (212) 472-4494. 15th edition 1990.

RESEARCH CENTERS, INSTITUTES, CLEARINGHOUSES

Alan Guttmacher Institute. 111 5th Ave., New York, NY 10003. Phone: (212) 254-5656. Fax: (212) 254-9891.

Center for Population and Family Health. Columbia University. Level B-3, 60 Haven Ave., New York, NY 10032. Phone: (212) 305-6960. Fax: (212) 305-7024.

Family Health International. P.O. Box 13950, Research Triangle Park, NC 27709. Phone: (919) 544-7040. Fax: (919) 544-7261.

Human Life Center. University of Steubenville, Steubenville, OH 43952. Phone: (614) 282-9953.

STANDARDS AND STATISTICS SOURCES

International Family Planning Perspectives. Alan Guttmacher Institute, 111 Fifth Ave., New York, NY 10003. Phone: (212) 254-5636. Quarterly.

Population Reports, Series A: Oral Contraception. Population Information Program, 527 St. Paul Place, Johns Hopkins University, Baltimore, MD 21202. Phone: (410) 659-6300. Fax: (410) 659-6266. Irregular.

Population Reports, Series B: Intrauterine Devices. Population Information Program, 527 St. Paul Place, Johns Hopkins University, Baltimore, MD 21202. Phone: (410) 659-6300. Fax: (410) 659-6266. Irregular.

Population Reports, Series C: Female Sterilization. Population Information Program, 527 St. Paul Place, Johns Hopkins University, Baltimore, MD 21202. Phone: (410) 659-6300. Fax: (410) 659-6266. Irregular.

Population Reports, Series D: Male Sterilization. Population Information Program, 527 St. Paul Place, Johns Hopkins University, Baltimore, MD 21202. Phone: (410) 659-6300. Fax: (410) 659-6266. Irregular.

Population Reports, Series E: Law and Policy. Population Information Program, 527 St. Paul Place, Johns Hopkins University, Baltimore, MD 21202. Phone: (410) 659-6300. Fax: (410) 659-6266. Irregular.

Population Reports, Series H: Barrier Methods. Population Information Program, 527 St. Paul Place, Johns Hopkins University, Baltimore, MD 21202. Phone: (410) 659-6300. Fax: (410) 659-6266. Irregular.

Population Reports, Series I: Rhythm, Periodic Abstinence. Population Information Program, 527 St. Paul Place, Johns Hopkins University, Baltimore, MD 21202. Phone: (410) 659-6300. Fax: (410) 659-6266. Irregular.

Population Reports, Series J: Family Planning Programs. Population Information Program, 527 St. Paul Place, Johns Hopkins University, Baltimore, MD 21202. Phone: (410) 659-6300. Fax: (410) 659-6266. Irregular.

Population Reports, Series L: Issues in World Health. Population Information Program, 527 St. Paul Place, Johns Hopkins University, Baltimore, MD 21202. Phone: (410) 659-6300. Fax: (410) 659-6266. Irregular.

Population Reports, Series M: Special Topics. Population Information Program, 527 St. Paul Place, Johns Hopkins University, Baltimore, MD 21202. Phone: (410) 659-6300. Fax: (410) 659-6266. Irregular.

TEXTBOOKS AND MONOGRAPHS

Clinical Guide to Contraception. Speroff. Williams & Wilkins, 428 East Preston St., Baltimore, MD 21202. Phone: (800) 638-0672. Fax: (800) 447-8438. 1992.

FAMILY THERAPY

See also: MARITAL THERAPY; PSYCHOLOGY

ABSTRACTING, INDEXING, AND CURRENT AWARENESS PUBLICATIONS

Psychological Abstracts. American Psychological Association, 1200 17th St. NW, Washington, DC 20036. Phone: (202) 955-7600. Monthly.

ASSOCIATIONS, PROFESSIONAL SOCIETIES, ADVOCACY AND SUPPORT GROUPS

American Association for Marriage and Family Therapy (AAMFT). 1100 17th St. N.W., 10th Flr., Washington, DC 20036. Phone: (202) 452-0109.

Family Therapy Network (FTN). 7705 13th St. N.W., Washington, DC 20012. Phone: (202) 829-2452. Fax: (202) 726-7983.

National Academy of Counselors and Family Therapists. 55 Morris Ave., Springfield, NJ 07081. Phone: (201) 379-7496.

National Council on Family Relations. 3989 Central Ave. N.E., Suite 550, Minneapolis, MN 55421. Phone: (612) 781-9331.

BIBLIOGRAPHIES

Family Therapy: A Bibliography. Bernard Lubin, and others. Greenwood Publishing Group, Inc., 88 Post Rd. W., P.O. Box 5007, Westport, CT 06881. Phone: (203) 226-3571.

CD-ROM DATABASES

PsycLit. SilverPlatter Information, Inc., River Ridge Office Park, 100 River Ridge Rd., Norwood, MA 02062. Phone: (617) 769-2599. Fax: (617) 769-8763. Quarterly.

JOURNALS

American Association for Marital and Family Therapy. 1100 17th St. N.W., Washington, DC 20036. Phone: (202) 452-0109.

Family Process. Family Process, 841 Broadway, No. 504, New York, NY 10003. Phone: (212) 565-6517.

Family Systems Medicine. Family Systems Medicine, P.O. Box 6452, Syracuse, NY 13217. Phone: (212) 879-4900.

Family Therapy. Libra Publishers, Inc., 3089C Claremont Dr., Suite 383, San Diego, CA 92117. Phone: (619) 581-9449.

Journal of Sex and Marital Therapy. Brunner/Mazel Pubs., 19 Union Sq. W., New York, NY 10003. Phone: (212) 924-3344.

ONLINE DATABASES

Family Research. National Council on Family Relations, 3989 Central Ave. N.E., Suite 550, Minneapolis, MN 55421. Phone: (612) 781-9331.

PsycInfo. SilverPlatter Information, Inc., River Ridge Office Park, 100 River Ridge Rd., Norwood, MA 02062. Phone: (617) 769-2599. Fax: (617) 769-8763. Quarterly.

RESEARCH CENTERS, INSTITUTES, CLEARINGHOUSES

Ackerman Institute for Family Therapy. 149 E. 78th St., New York, NY 10021. Phone: (212) 879-4900.

TEXTBOOKS AND MONOGRAPHS

Family Therapy: An Overview. Irene Goldenberg, Herbert Goldenberg. Brooks/Cole Publishing Co., 10 Davis Dr., Belmont, CA 94002. Phone: (415) 595-2350.

FARSIGHTEDNESS

See: VISION DISORDERS

FEES

See: HEALTH CARE FINANCING

FERTILITY

See: INFERTILITY

FETAL ALCOHOL SYNDROME

ABSTRACTING, INDEXING, AND CURRENT AWARENESS PUBLICATIONS

Index Medicus. U.S. National Library of Medicine, 8600 Rockville Pike, Bethesda, MD 20894. Phone: (800) 638-8480. Monthly.

Prevention Pipeline: An Alcohol and Drug Awareness Service. National Clearinghouse for Alcohol and Drug Information, Dept. PP, P.O. Box 2345, Rockville, MD 20852.

Psychological Abstracts. American Psychological Association, 1200 17th St. NW, Washington, DC 20036. Phone: (202) 955-7600. Monthly.

Research Alert: Alcoholism. Institute for Scientific Information, 3501 Market St., Philadelphia, PA 19104. Phone: (800) 523-1850. Fax: (215) 386-6362. Weekly.

Science Citation Index. Institute for Scientific Information, 3501 Market St., Philadelphia, PA 19104. Phone: (800) 523-1850. Fax: (215) 386-6362. Bimonthly.

ANNUALS AND REVIEWS

Research Advances in Alcohol and Drug Problems. Plenum Publishing Co., 233 Spring St., New York, NY 10013-1578. Phone: (212) 620-8000. Fax: (212) 463-0742. Irregular.

ASSOCIATIONS, PROFESSIONAL SOCIETIES, ADVOCACY AND SUPPORT GROUPS

Alcoholics Anonymous (AA). General Service Office Board, P.O. Box 459, Grand Central Station, New York, NY 10163. Phone: (212) 686-1100.

American College of Obstetricians and Gynecologists (ACOG). 409 12th St. S.W., Washington, DC 20024-2188. Phone: (202) 638-5577.

March of Dimes Birth Defects Foundation (MDBDF). 1275 Mamaroneck Ave., White Plains, NY 10605. Phone: (914) 428-7100. Fax: (914) 428-8203.

National Council on Alcoholism and Drug Dependence, Inc.. 12 W. 21st St., New York, NY 10010. Phone: (212) 206-6770.

BIBLIOGRAPHIES

Bibliography and Research Guide on Alcohol and other Drugs for Social Work Educators. National Clearinghouse for Alcohol and Drug Information, Dept. PP, P.O. Box 2345, Rockville, MD 20852.

Fetal Alcohol Syndrome. National Technical Information Service, 5285 Port Royal Rd., Springfield, VA 22161. Phone: (703) 487-4650. Fax: (703) 321-8547. May 1978-July 1989 PB90-857996/CBY.

CD ROM DATABASES

PsycLit. SilverPlatter Information, Inc., River Ridge Office Park, 100 River Ridge Rd., Norwood, MA 02062. Phone: (617) 769-2599. Fax: (617) 769-8763. Quarterly.

SCISEARCH. Institute for Scientific Information, 3501 Market St., Philadelphia, PA 19104. Phone: (215) 386-0100. Fax: (215) 386-6362.

ENCYCLOPEDIAS, DICTIONARIES, WORD BOOKS

Encyclopedia of Alcoholism. Robert O'Brien, Morris Evans, Glen Chafetz (eds.). Facts on File, Inc., 460 Park Ave. S., New York, NY 10016-7382. Phone: (212) 683-2244. Fax: (212) 683-3633. 1991.

JOURNALS

Alcholism and Addiction. IPG, 4949 Commerce Parkway, Cleveland, OH 44128. Phone: (800) 342-6237.

American Journal of Obstetrics and Gynecology. Mosby-Year Book, 11830 Westline Industrial Drive, St. Louis, MO 63146. Phone: (800) 325-4177. Fax: (314) 432-1380. Monthly.

Developmental Genetics. John Wiley & Sons, Inc., 605 Third Ave., New York, NY 10158-0012. Phone: (212) 850-6000. Fax: (212) 850-6088. Bimonthly.

Journal of Substance Abuse Treatment. Pergamon Press, 660 White Plains Rd., Tarrytown, NY 10591-5153. Phone: (914) 592-7700. Fax: (914) 592-3625. 6/year.

Pediatrics. American Academy of Pediatrics, 141 Northwest Point Rd., Elk Grove Village, IL 60009-0927. Phone: (708) 228-5005. Fax: (708) 228-5097. Monthly.

ONLINE DATABASES

EMBASE. Elsevier Science Publishing Co., Inc., P.O. Box 882, Madison Square Station, New York, NY 10159-2101. Phone: (212) 989-5800. Fax: (212) 633-3990.

ETOH (Alcohol and Alcohol Programs Science Database). National Institute on Alcohol Abuse and Alcoholism, 1400 Eye St. N.W., Ste. 600, Washington, DC 20005. Phone: (202) 842-7600.

MEDLINE. National Library of Medicine, 8600 Rockville Pike, Bethesda, MD 20894. Phone: (800) 638-8480.

PsycInfo. SilverPlatter Information, Inc., River Ridge Office Park, 100 River Ridge Rd., Norwood, MA 02062. Phone: (617) 769-2599. Fax: (617) 769-8763. Quarterly.

SciSearch. Institute for Scientific Information, 3501 Market St., Philadelphia, PA 19104. Phone: (215) 386-0100. Fax: (215) 386-6362.

POPULAR WORKS AND PATIENT EDUCATION

The Broken Cord. Michael Dorris. HarperCollins Publishers, Inc., 10 E. 53rd St., New York, NY 10022-5299. Phone: (800) 242-7737. 1990.

Facts About Drinking. Gail G. Milgram. Consumer Reports Books, 9180 LeSaint Dr., Fairfield, OH 45014. Phone: (513) 860-1178. 1989.

True Selves: Twelve-Step Recovery from Codependency. Roseann Lloyd, Merle A. Fossum. HarperCollins Publishers, 10 E. 53rd St., New York, NY 10022-5299. Phone: (800) 242-7737. 1991.

The Twelve Steps of Alcoholics Anonymous. Karen Elliot. HarperCollins Pubs., Inc., 10 E. 53rd St., New York, NY 10022-5299. Phone: (212) 207-7000. Fax: (800) 242-7737. 1987.

RESEARCH CENTERS, INSTITUTES, CLEARINGHOUSES

Center of Alcohol Studies. Rutgers University. Busch Campus, Smithers Hall, Piscataway, NJ 08855-0969. Phone: (908) 932-2190. Fax: (908) 932-5944.

Hazelden Foundation. Box 176, Center City, MN 55012-0176. Phone: (800) 328-9000.

National Clearinghouse for Alcohol and Drug Information (NCADI). P.O. Box 2345, Rockville, MD 20852. Phone: (301) 468-2600.

FETAL DEVELOPMENT

See also: BIRTH DEFECTS; PERINATOLOGY

ABSTRACTING, INDEXING, AND CURRENT AWARENESS PUBLICATIONS

Current Contents/Clinical Medicine. Institute for Scientific Information, 3501 Market St., Philadelphia, PA 19104. Phone: (800) 523-1850. Fax: (215) 386-6362. Weekly.

Excerpta Medica. Section 7: Pediatrics and Pediatric Surgery. Elsevier Science Publishing Co., Inc., P.O. Box 882, Madison Square Station, New York, NY 10159-2101. Phone: (212) 989-5800. Fax: (212) 633-3990. 24/year.

Index Medicus. U.S. National Library of Medicine, 8600 Rockville Pike, Bethesda, MD 20894. Phone: (800) 638-8480. Monthly.

Research Alert: Fetal Medicine. Institute for Scientific Information, 3501 Market St., Philadelphia, PA 19104. Phone: (800) 523-1850. Fax: (215) 386-6362. Weekly.

Science Citation Index. Institute for Scientific Information, 3501 Market St., Philadelphia, PA 19104. Phone: (800) 523-1850. Fax: (215) 386-6362. Bimonthly.

ANNUALS AND REVIEWS

Fetal Medicine Review. Cambridge University Press, 40 W. 20th St., New York, NY 10011. Phone: (800) 431-1580. Semiannual.

CD-ROM DATABASES

Critical Concepts of Fetal Monitoring. Blood. Williams & Wilkins, 428 East Preston St., Baltimore, MD 21202. Phone: (800) 638-0672. Fax: (800) 447-8438. 1990.

SCISEARCH. Institute for Scientific Information, 3501 Market St., Philadelphia, PA 19104. Phone: (215) 386-0100. Fax: (215) 386-6362.

ENCYCLOPEDIAS, DICTIONARIES, WORD BOOKS

Birth Defects Encyclopedia. Mary Louise Buyse (ed.). Mosby-Year Book, 11830 Westline Industrial Drive, St. Louis, MO 63146. Phone: (800) 325-4177. Fax: (314) 432-1380. 1990.

HANDBOOKS, GUIDES, MANUALS, ATLASES

Chromosome Anomalies and Prenatal Development: An Atlas. Dorothy Warburton, Julianne Byrne, Nina Canki. Oxford University Press, 200 Madison Ave., New York, NY 10016. Phone: (212) 679-7300. 1991.

Manual of Fetal Assessment. M.J. Whittle, J.P. Neilson. Butterworth-Heinemann, 80 Montvale Ave., Stoneham, MA 02180. Phone: (617) 438-8464. Fax: (617) 279-4851. 1991.

JOURNALS

Biology of the Neonate. S. Karger Publishers, Inc., 26 W. Avon Rd., P.O. Box 529, Farmington, CT 06085. Phone: (203) 675-7834. Fax: (203) 675-7302.

Early Human Development. Elsevier Science Publishing Co., Inc., P.O. Box 882, Madison Square Station, New York, NY 10159-2101. Phone: (212) 989-5800. Fax: (212) 633-3990. 12/year.

Journal of Genetic Counseling. Human Sciences Press, 233 Spring St., New York, NY 10013-1578. Phone: (800) 221-9369. Fax: (212) 807-1047. Quarterly.

Journal of Perinatal Medicine. Walter de Gruyter and Co., Genthiner Str. 17, W-1000 Berlin 30, Germany. Phone: 030 26005-251.

Journal of Perinatology. Appleton & Lange, 25 Van Zant St., East Norwalk, CT 06855. Phone: (800) 423-1359. Fax: (203) 854-9486. Quarterly.

Seminars in Perinatology. W.B. Saunders Co., The Curtis Center, Independence Sqare W., Philadelphia, PA 19106-3399. Phone: (215) 238-7800.

ONLINE DATABASES

EMBASE. Elsevier Science Publishing Co., Inc., P.O. Box 882, Madison Square Station, New York, NY 10159-2101. Phone: (212) 989-5800. Fax: (212) 633-3990.

MEDLINE. National Library of Medicine, 8600 Rockville Pike, Bethesda, MD 20894. Phone: (800) 638-8480.

SciSearch. Institute for Scientific Information, 3501 Market St., Philadelphia, PA 19104. Phone: (215) 386-0100. Fax: (215) 386-6362.

TEXTBOOKS AND MONOGRAPHS

Abnormal Fetal Growth. Divon. Elsevier Science Publishing Co., Inc., P.O. Box 882, Madison Square Station, New York, NY 10159-2101. Phone: (212) 989-5800. Fax: (212) 633-3990. 1991.

Assessment and Care of the Fetus: Physiological, Clinical, and Medicolegal Principles. Robert D. Eden, Frank H. Boehm. Appleton & Lange, 25 Van Zant St., East Norwalk, CT 06855. Phone: (800) 423-1359. Fax: (203) 854-9486. 1990.

Catalog of Prenatally Diagnosed Conditions. David D. Weaver. Johns Hopkins University Press, 701 W. 40th St., Suite 275, Baltimore, MD 21211-2190. Phone: (800) 537-5487. Fax: (410) 516-6998. Second edition 1992.

Developmental Pathology of the Embryo and Fetus. James E. Dimmick, Dagmar K. Kalousek (eds.). J.B. Lippincott Co., 227 E. Washington Square, Philadelphia, PA 19106-3780. Phone: (215) 238-4200. Fax: (215) 238-4227. 1992.

Fetal Echocardiography. Rudy E. Sabbagha, Samuel Gidding, Janette Strasburger. Appleton & Lange, 25 Van Zant St., East Norwalk, CT 06855. Phone: (800) 423-1359. Fax: (203) 854-9486. 1991.

Fetal Heart Rate Monitoring. Freeman. Williams & Wilkins, 428 East Preston St., Baltimore, MD 21202. Phone: (800) 638-0672. Fax: (800) 447-8438. Second edition 1991.

Fetal Monitoring: Physiology and Techniques of Antenatal and Intrapartum Assessment. John A.D. Spencer (ed.). F.A. Davis Co., 1915 Arch St., Philadelphia, PA 19103. Phone: (800) 523-4049. Fax: (215) 568-5065. 1989.

The Fetal and Neonatal Brain Stem: Developmental and Clinical Issues. M.A. Hanson (ed.). Cambridge University Press, 40 W. 20th St., New York, NY 10011. Phone: (800) 431-1580. 1991.

Fetal and Neonatal Cardiology. Walker A. Long. W.B. Saunders Co., The Curtis Center, Independence Square W., Philadelphia, PA 19106-3399. Phone: (215) 238-7800. 1990.

Fetal Neural Development and Adult Schizophrenia. Sarnoff A. Mednick, Tyrone D. Cannon, Christopher E. Barr. Cambridge University Press, 40 W. 20th St., New York, NY 10011. Phone: (800) 431-1580. 1991.

Fetus and Neonate: Physiology and Clinical Applications. Mark Hanson, John Spencer, Charles Rodeck. Cambridge University Press, 40 W. 20th St., New York, NY 10011. Phone: (800) 431-1580. 1992.

Infectious Diseases of the Fetus and Newborn Infant. Jack Remington, Jerome Klein. W.B. Saunders Co., The Curtis Center, Independence Sqare W., Philadelphia, PA 19106-3399. Phone: (215) 238-7800. Third Edition 1990.

Introduction to Fetal Medicine. M.J. Whittle, R.J. Morrow. Butterworth-Heinemann, 80 Montvale Ave., Stoneham, MA 02180. Phone: (617) 438-8464. Fax: (617) 279-4851. 1991.

Maternal, Fetal, and Neonatal Physiology: A Clinical Perspective. Susan Tucker Blackburn, Donna Lee Loper. W.B. Saunders Co., The Curtis Center, Independence Sqare W., Philadelphia, PA 19106-3399. Phone: (215) 238-7800. 1992.

Medicine of the Fetus and Mother. Reece. J.B. Lippincott Co., 227 E. Washington Square, Philadelphia, PA 19106-3780. Phone: (215) 238-4200. Fax: (215) 238-4227. 1992.

More Exercises in Fetal Monitoring. Barry S. Schifrin. Mosby-Year Book, 11830 Westline Industrial Drive, St. Louis, MO 63146. Phone: (800) 325-4177. Fax: (314) 432-1380. 1992.

Neonatal and Perinatal Medicine: Diseases of the Fetus and Infant. Avory Fanaroff, Richard Martin. Mosby-Year Book, 11830 Westline Industrial Drive, St. Louis, MO 63146. Phone: (800) 325-4177. Fax: (314) 432-1380. 5th edition, 1992.

The Unborn Patient: Prenatal Diagnosis and Treatment. Michael R. Harrison, Mitchell S. Golbus, Roy A. Filly. W.B. Saunders Co., The Curtis Center, Independence Square W., Philadelphia, PA 19106-3399. Phone: (215) 238-7800. Second edition 1991.

FIBROCYSTIC BREAST DISEASE

See: GYNECOLOGIC DISORDERS

FIRST AID

See: EMERGENCY MEDICINE

FLU

See: INFECTIOUS DISEASES

FOOD ADDITIVES

ABSTRACTING, INDEXING, AND CURRENT AWARENESS PUBLICATIONS

BIOSIS/CAS Selects: Nutrition & Immunology. BIOSIS, 2100 Arch St., Philadelphia, PA 19103-1399. Phone: (215) 587-4800. Fax: (215) 587-2016. Biweekly.

CA Selects: Food Toxicity. Chemical Abstracts Service, 2540 Olentangy River Rd., P.O. Box 3012, Columbus, OH 43210-0012. Phone: (800) 848-6538. #094.

CA Selects: Nutritional Aspects of Cancer. Chemical Abstracts Service, 2540 Olentangy River Road, P.O. Box 3012, Columbus, OH 43210-0012. Phone: (800) 848-6538. Biweekly.

Excerpta Medica. Section 52: Toxicology. Elsevier Science Publishing Co., Inc., P.O. Box 882, Madison Square Station, New York, NY 10159-2101. Phone: (212) 989-5800. Fax: (212) 633-3990. 20/year.

General Science Index. H.W. Wilson Co., 950 University Ave., Bronx, NY 10452. Phone: (800) 367-6770.

Toxicology Abstracts. Cambridge Scientific Abstracts, 7200 Wisconsin Ave., Bethesda, MD 20814-4823. Phone: (800) 843-7751. Fax: (301) 961-6720. Monthly.

HANDBOOKS, GUIDES, MANUALS, ATLASES

Food Additives Handbook. Richard J. Lewis. Thomson Publishing Co., 115 Fifth Ave., New York, NY 10003. Phone: (800) 926-2665. 1989.

Food Additives Tables. M. Fondu, H. Zegers de Beyl, G. Bronkers and others (eds.). Elsevier Science Publishing Co., Inc., P.O. Box 882, Madison Square Station, New York, NY 10159-2101. Phone: (212) 989-5800. Fax: (212) 633-3990. Second edition 1989.

JOURNALS

FDA Consumer. U.S. Government Printing Office, Superintendent of Documents, P.O. Box 371954, Pittsburgh, PA 15250-7954. Phone: (202) 783-3238. Fax: (202) 512-2250. Monthly.

Food and Chemical Toxicology. Pergamon Press, 660 White Plains Rd., Tarrytown, NY 10591-5153. Phone: (914) 592-7700. Fax: (914) 592-3625.

POPULAR WORKS AND PATIENT EDUCATION

A Consumer's Dictionary to Food Additives. Ruth Winter. Random House, Inc., 201 E. 50th St., New York, NY 10022. Phone: (800) 726-0600. Third edition 1989.

Food Additives: A Source Guide. Gordon Press Publishers, P.O. Box 459, Bowling Green Sta., New York, NY 10004. Phone: (718) 624-8419. 1991.

Food Pharmacy Guide to Good Eating. Jean Carper. Bantam Books, Inc., 666 Fifth Ave., New York, NY 10103. Phone: (800) 223-6834. 1992.

In Bad Taste: The MSG Syndrome. George R. Schwartz. Viking Penguin, 375 Hudson St., New York, NY 10014-3657. Phone: (800) 331-4624. 1990.

Prevention Magazine's Complete Nutrition Reference Handbook: Over 1,000 Foods and Meals Analyzed and Rated for Health Effect. Mark Bricklin. Rodale Press, Inc., 33 E. Minor St., Emmaus, PA 18098. Phone: (800) 527-8200. Fax: (215) 967-6263. 1992.

RESEARCH CENTERS, INSTITUTES, CLEARINGHOUSES

Food and Nutrition Information Center (FNIC). Department of Agriculture, National Agricultural Library, Rm. 304, 10301 Baltimore Blvd., Beltsville, MD 20705. Phone: (301) 344-3719.

Human Nutrition Information Service (HNIS). Department of Agriculture, 6505 Belcrest Rd., West Hyattsville, MD 20782. Phone: (301) 436-7725.

TEXTBOOKS AND MONOGRAPHS

Extra Pharmacopeia. J. Reynolds, W. Martindale. Pharmaceutical Press, Rittenhouse Book Distributors, 511 Feheley Dr., King of Prussia, PA 19406. Phone: (800) 345-6425. 29th edition 1989.

FOOD ALLERGIES

See also: ALLERGIES

ABSTRACTING, INDEXING, AND CURRENT AWARENESS PUBLICATIONS

Biological Abstracts. BIOSIS, 2100 Arch St., Philadelphia, PA 19103-1399. Phone: (800) 523-4800. Fax: (215) 587-2016.

Excerpta Medica. Section 52: Toxicology. Elsevier Science Publishing Co., Inc., P.O. Box 882, Madison Square Station, New York, NY 10159-2101. Phone: (212) 989-5800. Fax: (212) 633-3990. 20/year.

Index Medicus. U.S. National Library of Medicine, 8600 Rockville Pike, Bethesda, MD 20894. Phone: (800) 638-8480. Monthly.

Science Citation Index. Institute for Scientific Information, 3501 Market St., Philadelphia, PA 19104. Phone: (800) 523-1850. Fax: (215) 386-6362. Bimonthly.

BIBLIOGRAPHIES

Nutri-Topics: Food Allergy, Sensitivity and Intolerance. Food and Nutrition Center, National Agricultural Library, 10301 Baltimore Blvd., Beltsville, MD 20705.

CD-ROM DATABASES

Biological Abstracts on Compact Disc. BIOSIS, 2100 Arch St., Philadelphia, PA 19103-1399. Phone: (800) 523-4800. Fax: (215) 587-2016. Quarterly.

SCISEARCH. Institute for Scientific Information, 3501 Market St., Philadelphia, PA 19104. Phone: (215) 386-0100. Fax: (215) 386-6362.

DIRECTORIES

Directory of Certified Allergists/Immunologists. American Board of Medical Specialties, 1 Rotary Center, Suite 805, Evanston, IL 60201. Phone: (708) 491-9091. Biennial.

JOURNALS

Food and Chemical Toxicology. Pergamon Press, 660 White Plains Rd., Tarrytown, NY 10591-5153. Phone: (914) 592-7700. Fax: (914) 592-3625.

Journal of Allergy and Clinical Immunology. Mosby-Year Book, 11830 Westline Industrial Drive, St. Louis, MO 63146. Phone: (800) 325-4177. Fax: (314) 432-1380. Monthly.

ONLINE DATABASES

BIOSIS Previews. BIOSIS, 2100 Arch St., Philadelphia, PA 19103-1399. Phone: (800) 523-4800. Fax: (215) 587-2016.

EMBASE. Elsevier Science Publishing Co., Inc., P.O. Box 882, Madison Square Station, New York, NY 10159-2101. Phone: (212) 989-5800. Fax: (212) 633-3990.

MEDLINE. National Library of Medicine, 8600 Rockville Pike, Bethesda, MD 20894. Phone: (800) 638-8480.

SciSearch. Institute for Scientific Information, 3501 Market St., Philadelphia, PA 19104. Phone: (215) 386-0100. Fax: (215) 386-6362.

POPULAR WORKS AND PATIENT EDUCATION

Allergies. Edward Edelson. Chelsea House Pubs., 95 Madison Ave., New York, NY 10016. Phone: (212) 683-4400. 1989.

Your Child's Food Allergies: Detecting & Treating Hyperactivity, Congestion, Irritability and Other Symptoms Caused by Common Food Allergies. Jane McNicol. John Wiley & Sons, Inc., 605 Third Ave., New York, NY 10158-0012. Phone: (212) 850-6000. Fax: (212) 850-6088. 1992.

TEXTBOOKS AND MONOGRAPHS

Food Allergy. Metcalfe. Blackwell Scientific Publications, Inc., 3 Cambridge Ctr., Cambridge, MA 02142. Phone: (800) 759-6102. 1991.

FOOD POISONING

See also: POISONING

ABSTRACTING, INDEXING, AND CURRENT AWARENESS PUBLICATIONS

Excerpta Medica. Section 49: Forensic Science Abstracts. Elsevier Science Publishing Co., Inc., P.O. Box 882, Madison Square Station, New York, NY 10159-2101. Phone: (212) 989-5800. Fax: (212) 633-3990. 6/year.

Index Medicus. U.S. National Library of Medicine, 8600 Rockville Pike, Bethesda, MD 20894. Phone: (800) 638-8480. Monthly.

Science Citation Index. Institute for Scientific Information, 3501 Market St., Philadelphia, PA 19104. Phone: (800) 523-1850. Fax: (215) 386-6362. Bimonthly.

Toxicology Abstracts. Cambridge Scientific Abstracts, 7200 Wisconsin Ave., Bethesda, MD 20814-4823. Phone: (800) 843-7751. Fax: (301) 961-6720. Monthly.

BIBLIOGRAPHIES

Food Poisoning and Food Borne Disease. National Technical Information Service, 5285 Port Royal Rd., Springfield, VA 22161. Phone: (703) 487-4650. Fax: (703) 321-8547. Jan. 1978-May 1989 PB89-863286/CBY.

CD-ROM DATABASES

Morbidity Mortality Weekly Report. MEP, 124 Mt. Auburn St., Cambridge, MA 02138. Phone: (800) 342-1338. Fax: (617) 868-7738. Annual.

SCISEARCH. Institute for Scientific Information, 3501 Market St., Philadelphia, PA 19104. Phone: (215) 386-0100. Fax: (215) 386-6362.

JOURNALS

FDA Consumer. U.S. Government Printing Office, Superintendent of Documents, P.O. Box 371954, Pittsburgh,

PA 15250-7954. Phone: (202) 783-3238. Fax: (202) 512-2250. Monthly.

Journal of Toxicology: Clinical Toxicology. Marcel Dekker, Inc., 270 Madison Ave., New York, NY 10016. Phone: (800) 228-1160.

Morbidity and Mortality Weekly Report. Massachusetts Medical Society, 1440 Main St., Waltham, MA 02154-1649. Phone: (617) 893-3800. Fax: (617) 893-0413. Weekly.

ONLINE DATABASES

EMBASE. Elsevier Science Publishing Co., Inc., P.O. Box 882, Madison Square Station, New York, NY 10159-2101. Phone: (212) 989-5800. Fax: (212) 633-3990.

MEDLINE. National Library of Medicine, 8600 Rockville Pike, Bethesda, MD 20894. Phone: (800) 638-8480.

SciSearch. Institute for Scientific Information, 3501 Market St., Philadelphia, PA 19104. Phone: (215) 386-0100. Fax: (215) 386-6362.

RESEARCH CENTERS, INSTITUTES, CLEARINGHOUSES

Food Safety and Inspection Service. U.S. Department of Agriculture, 14th & Independence Ave. S.W., Washington, DC 20250. Phone: (202) 447-8217.

STANDARDS AND STATISTICS SOURCES

Botulinum Toxin. Consensus Statement. NIH Consensus Development Conference. November 12-14, 1990. National Institutes of Health, Office of Medical Applications of Research, Federal Bldg., Rm. 618, Bethesda, MD 20892. 1990.

TEXTBOOKS AND MONOGRAPHS

Food Contamination from Environmental Sources. Jerome O. Nriagu, Milagros Simmons (eds.). John Wiley & Sons, Inc., 605 Third Ave., New York, NY 10158-0012. Phone: (212) 850-6000. Fax: (212) 850-6088. 1990.

Salmonella. Rufus K. Guthrie. CRC Press, Inc., 2000 Corporate Blvd. N.W., Boca Raton, FL 33431. Phone: (407) 994-0555. Fax: (407) 997-0949. 1992.

Seafood Safety. Committee on Evaluation of the Safety of Fishery Products. National Academy Press, 2101 Constitution Ave., NW, Washington, DC 20418. Phone: (800) 642-6242. 1991.

FOOT DISORDERS

See also: PODIATRY

ABSTRACTING, INDEXING, AND CURRENT AWARENESS PUBLICATIONS

Index Medicus. U.S. National Library of Medicine, 8600 Rockville Pike, Bethesda, MD 20894. Phone: (800) 638-8480. Monthly.

ANNUALS AND REVIEWS

Clinics in Podiatric Medicine and Surgery. W.B. Saunders Co., The Curtis Center, Independence Square W., Philadelphia, PA 19106-3399. Phone: (215) 238-7800. Quarterly.

Year Book of Podiatric Medicine and Surgery. Mosby-Year Book, 11830 Westline Industrial Drive, St. Louis, MO 63146. Phone: (800) 325-4177. Fax: (314) 432-1380. Annual.

ASSOCIATIONS, PROFESSIONAL SOCIETIES, ADVOCACY AND SUPPORT GROUPS

American Association of Foot Specialists. P.O. Box 54, Union City, NJ 07087. Phone: (201) 688-1616.

American Podiatric Medical Association (APMA). 9312 Old Georgetown Rd., Bethesda, MD 20814. Phone: (301) 571-9200. Fax: (301) 530-2752.

HANDBOOKS, GUIDES, MANUALS, ATLASES

A Color Atlas of the Foot in Clinical Diagnosis. Mosby-Year Book, 11830 Westline Industrial Drive, St. Louis, MO 63146. Phone: (800) 325-4177. Fax: (314) 432-1380. 1992.

Manual of Ankle and Foot Arthroscopy. Richard O. Lundeen. Churchill Livingstone Inc., 650 Avenue of the Americas, New York, NY 10011. Phone: (212) 819-5400. Fax: (212) 302-6598. 1991.

Manual of Digital Surgery of the Foot. Michael S. Downey, D. Scot Malay. Churchill Livingstone Inc., 650 Avenue of the Americas, New York, NY 10011. Phone: (212) 819-5400. Fax: (212) 302-6598. 1991.

JOURNALS

The Foot. Churchill Livingstone Inc., 650 Avenue of the Americas, New York, NY 10011. Phone: (212) 819-5400. Fax: (212) 302-6598. Quarterly.

NEWSLETTERS

The Podiatrist's Patient Newsletter. Doctor's Press, Inc., Pitney Rd., P.O. Box 11177, Lancaster, PA 17605. Phone: (800) 233-0196. Quarterly.

ONLINE DATABASES

EMBASE. Elsevier Science Publishing Co., Inc., P.O. Box 882, Madison Square Station, New York, NY 10159-2101. Phone: (212) 989-5800. Fax: (212) 633-3990.

MEDLINE. National Library of Medicine, 8600 Rockville Pike, Bethesda, MD 20894. Phone: (800) 638-8480.

SciSearch. Institute for Scientific Information, 3501 Market St., Philadelphia, PA 19104. Phone: (215) 386-0100. Fax: (215) 386-6362.

POPULAR WORKS AND PATIENT EDUCATION

The Complete Foot Book: First Aid for Your Feet. Donald S. Pritt, Morton Walker. Avery Publishing Group, Inc., 120 Old Broadway, Garden City Park, NY 11040. Phone: (800) 548-5757. 1991.

The Doctor's Sore Foot Book. Daniel M. McGann, L.R. Robinson. William Morrow & Company, Inc., 1350 Ave. of the Americas, New York, NY 10019. Phone: (800) 237-0657. 1991.

The Foot Book: Relief for Overused, Abused and Ailing Feet. Glenn Copeland. John Wiley & Sons, Inc., 605 Third Ave., New York, NY 10158-0012. Phone: (212) 850-6000. Fax: (212) 850-6088. 1992.

TEXTBOOKS AND MONOGRAPHS

Current Therapy in Foot and Ankle Surgery. Mark Myerson. Mosby-Year Book, 11830 Westline Industrial Drive, St. Louis, MO 63146. Phone: (800) 325-4177. Fax: (314) 432-1380. 1993.

Disorders of the Foot and Ankle: Medical and Surgical Management. Melvin Jahss. W.B. Saunders Co., The Curtis Center, Independence Sqare W., Philadelphia, PA 19106-3399. Phone: (215) 238-7800. 1991.

Surgery of the Foot and Ankle. Roger A. Mann, Michael Coughlin. Mosby-Year Book, 11830 Westline Industrial Drive, St. Louis, MO 63146. Phone: (800) 325-4177. Fax: (314) 432-1380. 6th edition, 1992.

FORENSIC MEDICINE

ABSTRACTING, INDEXING, AND CURRENT AWARENESS PUBLICATIONS

Current Contents/Clinical Medicine. Institute for Scientific Information, 3501 Market St., Philadelphia, PA 19104. Phone: (800) 523-1850. Fax: (215) 386-6362. Weekly.

Excerpta Medica. Section 1: Anatomy, Anthropology, Embryology & Histology. Elsevier Science Publishing Co., Inc., P.O. Box 882, Madison Square Station, New York, NY 10159-2101. Phone: (212) 989-5800. Fax: (212) 633-3990. 16/year.

Excerpta Medica. Section 49: Forensic Science Abstracts. Elsevier Science Publishing Co., Inc., P.O. Box 882, Madison Square Station, New York, NY 10159-2101. Phone: (212) 989-5800. Fax: (212) 633-3990. 6/year.

Index Medicus. U.S. National Library of Medicine, 8600 Rockville Pike, Bethesda, MD 20894. Phone: (800) 638-8480. Monthly.

Science Citation Index. Institute for Scientific Information, 3501 Market St., Philadelphia, PA 19104. Phone: (800) 523-1850. Fax: (215) 386-6362. Bimonthly.

ASSOCIATIONS, PROFESSIONAL SOCIETIES, ADVOCACY AND SUPPORT GROUPS

American Academy of Forensic Sciences. Box 669, Colorado Springs, CO 80901. Phone: (719) 636-1100. Fax: (719) 636-1993.

American Association of Physical Anthropologists. c/o Dr. Joyce E. Sirianni, Dept. of Anthropology, 380-MFAC, SUNY-Buffalo, Buffalo, NY 14261.

American Board of Forensic Anthropology (ABFA). c/o Michael Finnegan, Ph.D., Kansas State University, Osteology Laboratory, 204 Walters Hall, Manhattan, KS 66506. Phone: (913) 532-6865. Fax: (913) 532-7114.

American Board of Forensic Psychiatry (ABFP). 819 Park Ave., Baltimore, MD 21201. Phone: (301) 539-0379.

American Board of Forensic Psychology. Park Plaza, 128 N. Craig St., Pittsburgh, PA 15213. Phone: (412) 681-3000. Fax: (412) 681-1478.

International Reference Organization in Forensic Medicine and Sciences (INFORM). P.O. Box 8282, Wichita, KS 67208. Phone: (316) 685-7612.

Society for Medical Anthropology. 1703 New Hampshire Ave. N.W., Washington, DC 20009. Phone: (202) 232-8800.

CD-ROM DATABASES

SCISEARCH. Institute for Scientific Information, 3501 Market St., Philadelphia, PA 19104. Phone: (215) 386-0100. Fax: (215) 386-6362.

DIRECTORIES

American Academy of Forensic Psychology-Directory of Diplomates. American Board of Forensic Psychology, Park Plaza, 128 N. Craig St., Pittsburgh, PA 15213. Phone: (412) 681-3000. Fax: (412) 681-1478. Biennial.

American Academy of Forensic Sciences-Membership Directory. American Academy of Forensic Sciences, Box 669, Colorado Springs, CO 80901. Phone: (719) 636-1100. Fax: (719) 636-1993.

Directory of Medical Specialists. Marquis Who's Who, 3002 Glenview Rd., Wilmette, IL 60091. Phone: (800) 621-9669. Fax: (708) 441-2264. Biennial.

Directory of Physicians in the United States. American Medical Association, 515 North State St., Chicago, IL 60610. Phone: (312) 464-0183. Fax: (312) 464-5834. Biennial.

Forensic Services Directory. National Forensic Center, 17 Temple Terrace, Lawrenceville, NJ 08648. Phone: (800) 526-5177. Fax: (609) 883-7622. Annual.

HANDBOOKS, GUIDES, MANUALS, ATLASES

Medical Anthropology: A Handbook of Theory and Method. Thomas M. Johnson, Carolyn F. Sargent (eds.). Greenwood Publishing Group, Inc., 88 Post Rd. W., P.O. Box 5007, Westport, CT 06881. Phone: (203) 226-3571. 1990.

JOURNALS

American Journal of Forensic Medicine and Pathology. Raven Press, 1185 Avenue of the Americas, New York, NY 10036. Phone: (212) 930-9500. Fax: (212) 869-3495. Quarterly.

American Journal of Forensic Psychiatry. Edward Miller, 26701 Quail Creek, No. 295, Laguna Hills, CA 92656. Phone: (714) 831-0236. Quarterly.

Forensic Reports. Taylor & Francis Inc., 1900 Frost Rd., Suite 101, Bristol, PA 19007-1598. Phone: (800) 821-8312. Fax: (215) 785-5515. Quarterly.

Forensic Science International. Elsevier Science Publishing Co., Inc., P.O. Box 882, Madison Square Station, New York, NY 10159-2101. Phone: (212) 989-5800. Fax: (212) 633-3990. 12/year.

Journal of Forensic Sciences. American Society for Testing and Materials, 1916 Race St., Philadelphia, PA 19103. Phone: (215) 299-5400. Fax: (215) 977-9679. Bimonthly.

Medical Anthropology. Gordon & Breach Science Publishers, P.O. Box 786, Cooper Station, New York, NY 10276. Phone: (212) 206-8900. Quarterly.

Medical Anthropology Quarterly. American Anthropological Association, 1703 New Hampshire Ave. N.W., Washington, DC 20009. Phone: (202) 232-8800. Quarterly.

ONLINE DATABASES

EMBASE. Elsevier Science Publishing Co., Inc., P.O. Box 882, Madison Square Station, New York, NY 10159-2101. Phone: (212) 989-5800. Fax: (212) 633-3990.

MEDLINE. National Library of Medicine, 8600 Rockville Pike, Bethesda, MD 20894. Phone: (800) 638-8480.

SciSearch. Institute for Scientific Information, 3501 Market St., Philadelphia, PA 19104. Phone: (215) 386-0100. Fax: (215) 386-6362.

RESEARCH CENTERS, INSTITUTES, CLEARINGHOUSES

Armed Forces Institute of Pathology. Washington, DC 20306.

International Reference Organization in Forensic Medicine and Sciences-Library and Reference Center. Box 8282, Wichita, KS 67208. Phone: (316) 685-7612.

TEXTBOOKS AND MONOGRAPHS

Encounters with Biomedicine: Case Studies in Medical Anthropology. Hans A. Baer (ed.). Gordon & Breach Science Publishers, P.O. Box 786, Cooper Station, New York, NY 10276. Phone: (212) 206-8900. 1987.

Forensic Pathology. Knight. Oxford University Press, 200 Madison Ave., New York, NY 10016. Phone: (212) 679-7300. 1991.

Introduction to Forensic Sciences. William G. Eckert. CRC Press, Inc., 2000 Corporate Blvd. N.W., Boca Raton, FL 33431. Phone: (407) 994-0555. Fax: (407) 997-0949. Second edition 1992.

Lecture Notes on Forensic Medicine. D.J. Dee. Blackwell Scientific Publications, Inc., 3 Cambridge Ctr., Cambridge, MA 02142. Phone: (800) 759-6102. Fifth edition 1989.

Legal Issues in Anesthesia Practice. William H.L. Dornette (ed.). F.A. Davis Co., 1915 Arch St., Philadelphia, PA 19103. Phone: (800) 523-4049. Fax: (215) 568-5065. 1991.

FRACTURES

See also: ORTHOPEDICS

ABSTRACTING, INDEXING, AND CURRENT AWARENESS PUBLICATIONS

Current Contents/Clinical Medicine. Institute for Scientific Information, 3501 Market St., Philadelphia, PA 19104. Phone: (800) 523-1850. Fax: (215) 386-6362. Weekly.

Excerpta Medica. Section 33: Orthopedic Surgery. Elsevier Science Publishing Co., Inc., P.O. Box 882, Madison Square Station, New York, NY 10159-2101. Phone: (212) 989-5800. Fax: (212) 633-3990. 10/year.

Index Medicus. U.S. National Library of Medicine, 8600 Rockville Pike, Bethesda, MD 20894. Phone: (800) 638-8480. Monthly.

Science Citation Index. Institute for Scientific Information, 3501 Market St., Philadelphia, PA 19104. Phone: (800) 523-1850. Fax: (215) 386-6362. Bimonthly.

ANNUALS AND REVIEWS

Advances in Orthopaedic Surgery. Data Trace Medical Publishers, Inc., P.O. Box 1239, Brooklandville, MD 21022. Phone: (410) 494-4994. Fax: (410) 494-0515. Bimonthly.

Current Opinion in Orthopaedics. Current Science Ltd., 20 N. Third St., Philadelphia, PA 19106-2199. Phone: (800) 552-5866. Fax: (215) 574-2270. Bimonthly.

Year Book of Orthopedics. Mosby-Year Book, 11830 Westline Industrial Drive, St. Louis, MO 63146. Phone: (800) 325-4177. Fax: (314) 432-1380. Annual.

ASSOCIATIONS, PROFESSIONAL SOCIETIES, ADVOCACY AND SUPPORT GROUPS

American Academy of Orthopedic Surgeons (AAOS). 222 S. Prospect Ave., Park Ridge, IL 60068-4058. Phone: (708) 823-7186. Fax: (708) 823-8125.

American Fracture Association. P.O. Box 668, Bloomington, IL 61701. Phone: (309) 663-6272.

CD-ROM DATABASES

Ortholine. Aries Systems Corporation, One Dundee Park, Andover, MA 01810. Phone: (508) 475-7200. Fax: (508) 474-8860. Monthly or quarterly.

SCISEARCH. Institute for Scientific Information, 3501 Market St., Philadelphia, PA 19104. Phone: (215) 386-0100. Fax: (215) 386-6362.

ENCYCLOPEDIAS, DICTIONARIES, WORD BOOKS

Handbook of Orthopedic Terminology. Kilcoyne. CRC Press, Inc., 2000 Corporate Blvd. N.W., Boca Raton, FL 33431. Phone: (407) 994-0555. Fax: (407) 997-0949. 1991.

Orthopedic Word Book. Thomas J. Cittadine. Springhouse Publishing Co., 1111 Bethlehem Pike, Spring House, PA 19477. Phone: (800) 331-3170. Fax: (215) 646-8716. 1992.

Orthopedic Words. Stedman. Williams & Wilkins, 428 East Preston St., Baltimore, MD 21202. Phone: (800) 638-0672. Fax: (800) 447-8438. 1992.

HANDBOOKS, GUIDES, MANUALS, ATLASES

The Fracture Classification Manual. Roman B. Gustilo. Mosby-Year Book, 11830 Westline Industrial Drive, St. Louis, MO 63146. Phone: (800) 325-4177. Fax: (314) 432-1380. 1991.

JOURNALS

Journal of Bone and Joint Surgery: American Volume. Journal of Bone and Joint Surgery, Inc., 10 Shattuck St., Boston, MA 02115. Phone: (617) 734-2835. 10/year.

Journal of Orthopaedic and Sports Physical Therapy. Williams & Wilkins, 428 E. Preston St., Baltimore, MD 21202. Phone: (800) 638-0672. Fax: (800) 447-8438. Monthly.

TEXTBOOKS AND MONOGRAPHS

Current Orthopaedic Practice. Philip Yeoman, Daniel M. Spangler (eds.). Butterworth-Heinemann, 80 Montvale Ave., Stoneham, MA 02180. Phone: (617) 438-8464. Fax: (617) 279-4851. 1991.

Fractures. Charles A. Rockwood, and others. J.B. Lippincott Co., 227 E. Washington Square, Philadelphia, PA 19106-3780. Phone: (215) 238-4200. Fax: (215) 238-4227. Three volumes, 1991.

Hip Arthroplasty. Harlan C. Amstutz (ed.). Churchill Livingstone Inc., 650 Avenue of the Americas, New York, NY 10011. Phone: (212) 819-5400. Fax: (212) 302-6598. 1991.

Practical Fracture Treatment. McRae. Churchill Livingstone Inc., 650 Ave. of the Americas, New York, NY 10011. Phone: (212) 819-5400. Fax: (212) 302-6598. Second edition 1989.

Practical Orthopedics. Lonnie R. Mercier, Fred J. Pettid, Dean F. Tamisea, et. al.. Mosby-Year Book, 11830 Westline Industrial Drive, St. Louis, MO 63146. Phone: (800) 325-4177. Fax: (314) 432-1380. Third edition 1991.

Techniques in Fracture Fixation. Bray. Raven Press, 1185 Ave. of the Americas, New York, NY 10036. Phone: (212) 930-9500. Fax: (212) 869-3495. 1992.

FROSTBITE

See: WOUNDS AND INJURIES

FUNGAL DISEASES

See also: INFECTIOUS DISEASES

ABSTRACTING, INDEXING, AND CURRENT AWARENESS PUBLICATIONS

BIOSIS/CAS Selects: Antifungal Agents. BIOSIS, 2100 Arch St., Philadelphia, PA 19103-1399. Phone: (215) 587-4800. Fax: (215) 587-2016. Biweekly.

CA Selects: Antifungal & Antimycotic Agents. Chemical Abstracts Service, 2540 Olentangy River Road, P.O. Box 3012, Columbus, OH 43210-0012. Phone: (800) 848-6538. Biweekly.

CAB Abstracts. C.A.B. International, 845 N. Park Ave., Tucson, AZ 85719. Phone: (800) 528-4841.

Current Contents/Clinical Medicine. Institute for Scientific Information, 3501 Market St., Philadelphia, PA 19104. Phone: (800) 523-1850. Fax: (215) 386-6362. Weekly.

Excerpta Medica. Section 4: Microbiology, Mycology, Parasitology and Virology. Elsevier Science Publishers, P.O. Box 882, Madison Square Station, New York, NY 10159-2101. Phone: (212) 633-3950. Fax: (212) 633-3990. 32/year.

Index Medicus. U.S. National Library of Medicine, 8600 Rockville Pike, Bethesda, MD 20894. Phone: (800) 638-8480. Monthly.

Microbiology Abstracts. Section C: Algology, Mycology & Protozoology. Cambridge Scientific Abstracts, 7200 Wisconsin Ave., Bethesda, MD 20814-4823. Phone: (800) 843-7751. Fax: (301) 961-6720. Monthly.

Research Alert: Antifungal Agents. Institute for Scientific Information, 3501 Market St., Philadelphia, PA 19104. Phone: (800) 523-1850. Fax: (215) 386-6362. Weekly.

Science Citation Index. Institute for Scientific Information, 3501 Market St., Philadelphia, PA 19104. Phone: (800) 523-1850. Fax: (215) 386-6362. Bimonthly.

ANNUALS AND REVIEWS

Infectious Disease Clinics. W.B. Saunders Co., The Curtis Center, Independence Square W., Philadelphia, PA 19106-3399. Phone: (215) 238-7800. Quarterly.

Review of Medical and Veterinary Mycology. C.A.B. International, 845 N. Park Ave., Tucson, AZ 85719. Phone: (800) 528-4841. Quarterly.

ASSOCIATIONS, PROFESSIONAL SOCIETIES, ADVOCACY AND SUPPORT GROUPS

Infectious Diseases Society of America (IDSA). Yale University School of Medicine, 333 Cedar St., 201 LCI, New Haven, CT 06510-8056. Phone: (203) 785-4141.

Medical Mycological Society of the Americas. Dept. of Microbiology, Methodist Hospital, 305 W. Colorado, Dallas, TX 75208. Phone: (214) 944-8247.

BIBLIOGRAPHIES

Candidiasis: Detection, Diagnosis, Therapy, and Treatment. National Technical Information Service, 5285 Port Royal Rd., Springfield, VA 22161. Phone: (703) 487-4650. Fax: (703) 321-8547. Jan. 1978-May 1989 PB89-862288/CBY.

CD-ROM DATABASES

CABCD (CAB Abstracts on CD-ROM). C.A.B. International, 845 N. Park Ave., Tucson, AZ 85719. Phone: (800) 528-4841.

Infectious Diseases MEDLINE. MEP, 124 Mt. Auburn St., Cambridge, MA 02138. Phone: (800) 342-1338. Fax: (617) 868-7738. Quarterly.

SCISEARCH. Institute for Scientific Information, 3501 Market St., Philadelphia, PA 19104. Phone: (215) 386-0100. Fax: (215) 386-6362.

HANDBOOKS, GUIDES, MANUALS, ATLASES

Chemotherapy of Fungal Diseases. J.F. Ryley (ed.). Springer-Verlag New York Inc., 175 Fifth Ave., New York, NY 10010. Phone: (212) 460-1500. Fax: (212) 473-6272. Handbook of Experimental Pharmacology Series Volume 96 1990.

JOURNALS

Journal of Infection. Academic Press, Inc., 1250 Sixth Ave., San Diego, CA 92101-4311. Phone: (619) 699-6345. Fax: (619) 699-6715.

Journal of Infectious Diseases. University of Chicago Press, P.O. Box 37005, Chicago, IL 60637. Phone: (312) 753-3347. Fax: (312) 753-0811. Monthly.

ONLINE DATABASES

EMBASE. Elsevier Science Publishing Co., Inc., P.O. Box 882, Madison Square Station, New York, NY 10159-2101. Phone: (212) 989-5800. Fax: (212) 633-3990.

MEDLINE. National Library of Medicine, 8600 Rockville Pike, Bethesda, MD 20894. Phone: (800) 638-8480.

SciSearch. Institute for Scientific Information, 3501 Market St., Philadelphia, PA 19104. Phone: (215) 386-0100. Fax: (215) 386-6362.

RESEARCH CENTERS, INSTITUTES, CLEARINGHOUSES

Infectious Diseases Research Laboratories. Ohio State University. 410 W. 10th Ave., Columbus, OH 43210. Phone: (614) 293-8732. Fax: (614) 293-4556.

TEXTBOOKS AND MONOGRAPHS

Diagnosis and Therapy of Systemic Fungal Infections. Kenneth Holmberg, Richard D. Meyer. Raven Press, 1185 Ave. of the Americas, New York, NY 10036. Phone: (212) 930-9500. Fax: (212) 869-3495. 1989.

Fungal Infection in the Compromised Patient. D.W. Warnock, M.D. Richardson (eds.). John Wiley & Sons, Inc., 605 Third Ave., New York, NY 10158-0012. Phone: (212) 850-6000. Fax: (212) 850-6088. Second edition 1991.

Mycoses in AIDS Patients. Hugo Vanden Bossche, Donald W.R. Mackenzie, et al.. Plenum Publishing Co., 233 Spring St., New York, NY 10013-1578. Phone: (212) 620-8000. Fax: (212) 463-0742. 1990.

Pathogenic Yeasts and Yeast Infections. Esther Segal, Gerald L. Baum. CRC Press, Inc., 2000 Corporate Blvd. N.W., Boca Raton, FL 33431. Phone: (407) 994-0555. Fax: (407) 997-0949. 1992.

G

GALL BLADDER DISEASES

See: BILIARY DISORDERS

GALL BLADDER SURGERY

See: GASTROINTESTINAL SURGERY

GALLSTONES

See: BILIARY DISORDERS

GAMBLING

ABSTRACTING, INDEXING, AND CURRENT AWARENESS PUBLICATIONS

Psychological Abstracts. American Psychological Association, 1200 17th St. NW, Washington, DC 20036. Phone: (202) 955-7600. Monthly.

ASSOCIATIONS, PROFESSIONAL SOCIETIES, ADVOCACY AND SUPPORT GROUPS

Gam-Anon International Service Office. P.O. Box 157, Whitestone, NY 11357. Phone: (718) 352-1671.

Gamblers Anonymous. 3255 Wilshire Blvd. # 610, Los Angeles, CA 90010. Phone: (213) 386-8789.

National Council on Problem Gambling. 445 W. 59th St., Rm. 1521, New York, NY 10019. Phone: (800) 522-4700.

CD-ROM DATABASES

Excerpta Medica CD: Psychiatry. SilverPlatter Information, Inc., River Ridge Office Park, 100 River Ridge Rd., Norwood, MA 02062. Phone: (617) 769-2599. Fax: (617) 769-8763. Quarterly.

PsycLit. SilverPlatter Information, Inc., River Ridge Office Park, 100 River Ridge Rd., Norwood, MA 02062. Phone: (617) 769-2599. Fax: (617) 769-8763. Quarterly.

JOURNALS

American Journal of Psychiatry. American Psychiatric Press, Inc., 1400 K St. NW, Washington, DC 20005. Phone: (202) 682-6268. Fax: (202) 789-2648. Monthly.

NEWSLETTERS

Addictions Alert. American Health Consultants, Department C1290, P.O. Box 740060, Atlanta, GA 30374. Phone: (800) 559-1032. Monthly.

ONLINE DATABASES

PsycInfo. SilverPlatter Information, Inc., River Ridge Office Park, 100 River Ridge Rd., Norwood, MA 02062. Phone: (617) 769-2599. Fax: (617) 769-8763. Quarterly.

GASTRIC ULCERS

See: ULCERS

GASTRITIS

See: GASTROINTESTINAL DISORDERS

GASTROENTEROLOGY

See also: GASTROINTESTINAL DISORDERS; GASTROINTESTINAL SURGERY

ABSTRACTING, INDEXING, AND CURRENT AWARENESS PUBLICATIONS

Core Journals in Gastroenterology. Elsevier Science Publishing Co., Inc., P.O. Box 882, Madison Square Station, New York, NY 10159-2101. Phone: (212) 989-5800. Fax: (212) 633-3990. 11/year.

Excerpta Medica. Section 48: Gastroenterology. Elsevier Science Publishing Co., Inc., P.O. Box 882, Madison Square Station, New York, NY 10159-2101. Phone: (212) 989-5800. Fax: (212) 633-3990. 20/year.

Index Medicus. U.S. National Library of Medicine, 8600 Rockville Pike, Bethesda, MD 20894. Phone: (800) 638-8480. Monthly.

Science Citation Index. Institute for Scientific Information, 3501 Market St., Philadelphia, PA 19104. Phone: (800) 523-1850. Fax: (215) 386-6362. Bimonthly.

ANNUALS AND REVIEWS

Annual of Gastrointestinal Endoscopy. Current Science Group, 20 N. Third St., Philadelphia, PA 19106-2199. Phone: (800) 552-5866. Fax: (215) 574-2270. Annual.

Current Gastroenterology. Mosby-Year Book, 11830 Westline Industrial Drive, St. Louis, MO 63146. Phone: (800) 325-4177. Fax: (314) 432-1380. Annual.

Current Opinion in Gastroenterology. Current Science Group, 20 N. Third St., Philadelphia, PA 19106-2199. Phone: (800) 552-5866. Fax: (215) 574-2270. Bimonthly.

Gastroenterology Annual. Elsevier Science Publishing Co., Inc., P.O. Box 882, Madison Square Station, New York, NY 10159-2101. Phone: (212) 989-5800. Fax: (212) 633-3990. Annual.

Gastroenterology Clinics. W.B. Saunders Co., The Curtis Center, Independence Square W., Philadelphia, PA 19106-3399. Phone: (215) 238-7800. Quarterly.

ASSOCIATIONS, PROFESSIONAL SOCIETIES, ADVOCACY AND SUPPORT GROUPS

American College of Gastroenterology (ACG). 4222 King St., Alexandria, VA 22302. Phone: (703) 549-4440.

American Gastroenterological Association (AGA). 6900 Grove Rd., Thorofare, NJ 08086. Phone: (609) 848-9218. Fax: (609) 853-5991.

American Society for Gastrointestinal Endoscopy (ASGE). 13 Elm St., P.O. Box 1565, Manchester, MA 01944. Phone: (508) 526-8330.

Digestive Disease National Coalition (DDNC). 711 Second St. NE, Suite 200, Washington, DC 20002. Phone: (202) 544-7497.

National Foundation for Ileitis and Colitis (NFIC). 444 Park Ave. S., 11th Fl., New York, NY 10016-7374. Phone: (800) 343-3637. Fax: (212) 779-4098.

North American Society for Pediatric Gastroenterology. c/o Judith Sondheimer, Children's Hospital, 1056 E. 19th Ave., Denver, CO 80218. Phone: (303) 861-6669.

Society of American Gastrointestinal Endoscopic Surgeons (SAGES). 1271 Stoner Ave., Suite 409, Los Angeles, CA 90025. Phone: (213) 479-3249.

CD-ROM DATABASES

Excerpta Medica CD: Gastroenterology. SilverPlatter Information, Inc., River Ridge Office Park, 100 River Ridge Rd., Norwood, MA 02062. Phone: (617) 769-2599. Fax: (617) 769-8763. Quarterly.

Gastroenterology and Hepatology MEDLINE. MEP, 124 Mt. Auburn St., Cambridge, MA 02138. Phone: (800) 342-1338. Fax: (617) 868-7738. Quarterly.

SCISEARCH. Institute for Scientific Information, 3501 Market St., Philadelphia, PA 19104. Phone: (215) 386-0100. Fax: (215) 386-6362.

DIRECTORIES

Directory of Medical Specialists. Marquis Who's Who, 3002 Glenview Rd., Wilmette, IL 60091. Phone: (800) 621-9669. Fax: (708) 441-2264. Biennial.

Directory of Physicians in the United States. American Medical Association, 515 North State St., Chicago, IL 60610. Phone: (312) 464-0183. Fax: (312) 464-5834. Biennial.

ENCYCLOPEDIAS, DICTIONARIES, WORD BOOKS

Gastrointestinal Words. Stedman. Williams & Wilkins, 428 East Preston St., Baltimore, MD 21202. Phone: (800) 638-0672. Fax: (800) 447-8438. 1992.

HANDBOOKS, GUIDES, MANUALS, ATLASES

Atlas of Clinical Gastroenterology. J.J. Misiewicz, C.I. Bartram. Lea & Febiger, 428 E. Preston St., Baltimore, MD 21202. Phone: (800) 638-0672. Fax: (800) 447-8438. 1987.

Gastrointestinal Pathology: An Atlas and Text. Cecilia M. Fenoglio-Preiser, and others. Raven Press, 1185 Avenue of the Americas, New York, NY 10036. Phone: (212) 930-9500. Fax: (212) 869-3495. 1989.

Manual of Gastroenterology. Gregory Eastwood, Canan Avunduk. Little, Brown and Company, 34 Beacon St., Boston, MA 02108. Phone: (617) 227-0730. 1988.

JOURNALS

American Journal of Gastroenterology. Williams & Wilkins, 428 E. Preston St., Baltimore, MD 21202. Phone: (800) 638-0672. Fax: (800) 447-8438. Monthly.

Digestive Diseases and Sciences. Plenum Publishing Co., 233 Spring St., New York, NY 10013-1578. Phone: (212) 620-8000. Fax: (212) 463-0742. Monthly.

European Journal of Gastroenterology & Hepatology. Current Science Group, 20 N. Third St., Philadelphia, PA 19106-2199. Phone: (800) 552-5866. Fax: (215) 574-2270. Monthly.

Gastrointestinal Endoscopy. Mosby-Year Book, 11830 Westline Industrial Drive, St. Louis, MO 63146. Phone: (800) 325-4177. Fax: (314) 432-1380. Bimonthly.

Gut. BMJ Publishing Group, BMA House, Tavistock Square, London WC1H 9JR, England. Phone: 071-383 6244/6638. Fax: 071-383 6662. Monthly.

Journal of Clinical Gastroenterology. Raven Press, 1185 Avenue of the Americas, New York, NY 10036. Phone: (212) 930-9500. Fax: (212) 869-3495. Bimonthly.

ONLINE DATABASES

EMBASE. Elsevier Science Publishing Co., Inc., P.O. Box 882, Madison Square Station, New York, NY 10159-2101. Phone: (212) 989-5800. Fax: (212) 633-3990.

MEDLINE. National Library of Medicine, 8600 Rockville Pike, Bethesda, MD 20894. Phone: (800) 638-8480.

SciSearch. Institute for Scientific Information, 3501 Market St., Philadelphia, PA 19104. Phone: (215) 386-0100. Fax: (215) 386-6362.

POPULAR WORKS AND PATIENT EDUCATION

Complete Book of Better Digestion: A Gut-Level Guide to Gastric Relief. Michael Oppenheim. Rodale Press, Inc., 33 E. Minor St., Emmaus, PA 18098. Phone: (800) 527-8200. Fax: (215) 967-6263. 1990.

Eating Right for a Bad Gut: The Complete Nutritional Guide to Illeitis, Colitis, Crohn's Disease & Irritable Bowel Syndrome. James Scala. NAL/Dutton, 375 Hudson St., New York, NY 10014-3657. Phone: (212) 366-2000. 1990.

Gastrointestinal Health: A Self-Help Nutritional Program to Prevent, Alleviate, or Cure the Symptoms of Irritable Bowel Syndrome, Ulcers, Heartburn,. Steven R. Peikin. HarperCollins Pubs., Inc., 10 E. 53rd St., New York, NY 10022-5299. Phone: (212) 207-7000. Fax: (800) 242-7737. 1991.

Gut Reactions: Understanding Symptoms of the Digestive Tract. W.G. Thompson. Plenum Publishing Co., 233 Spring St., New York, NY 10013-1578. Phone: (323) 620-8000. Fax: (212) 463-0742. 1989.

RESEARCH CENTERS, INSTITUTES, CLEARINGHOUSES

National Digestive Diseases Information Clearinghouse (NDDIC). P.O. Box NDDIC, Bethesda, MD 20892. Phone: (301) 468-6344.

TEXTBOOKS AND MONOGRAPHS

Clinical Gastroenterology. Edgar Achkar, Richard G. Farmer, Bertram Fleshler. Lea & Febiger, 428 E. Preston St., Baltimore, MD 21202. Phone: (800) 638-0672. Fax: (800) 447-8438. 1992.

The Development of American Gastroenterology. Joseph B. Kirsner. Raven Press, 1185 Avenue of the Americas, New York, NY 10036. Phone: (212) 930-9500. Fax: (212) 869-3495. 1990.

Gastrointestinal Disease: Pathophysiology, Diagnosis, Management. Marvin H. Sleisenger, John. S. Fordtran. W.B. Saunders Co., The Curtis Center, Independence Square W., Philadelphia, PA 19106-3399. Phone: (215) 238-7800. Fourth edition. Two volumes. 1989.

Modern Concepts in Gastroenterology. E. Shaffer, A. Thompson (eds.). Plenum Publishing Co., 233 Spring St., New York, NY 10013-1578. Phone: (323) 620-8000. Fax: (212) 463-0742 Volume 2. 1989. Topics in Gastroenterology Series.

Textbook of Gastroenterology and Nutrition in Infancy. Emanuel Lebenthal (ed.). Raven Press, 1185 Avenue of the Americas, New York, NY 10036. Phone: (212) 930-9500. Fax: (212) 869-3495. Second edition 1989.

GASTROINTESTINAL DISORDERS

ABSTRACTING, INDEXING, AND CURRENT AWARENESS PUBLICATIONS

Biological Abstracts. BIOSIS, 2100 Arch St., Philadelphia, PA 19103-1399. Phone: (800) 523-4800. Fax: (215) 587-2016.

Core Journals in Gastroenterology. Elsevier Science Publishing Co., Inc., P.O. Box 882, Madison Square Station, New York, NY 10159-2101. Phone: (212) 989-5800. Fax: (212) 633-3990. 11/year.

Current Contents/Clinical Medicine. Institute for Scientific Information, 3501 Market St., Philadelphia, PA 19104. Phone: (800) 523-1850. Fax: (215) 386-6362. Weekly.

Excerpta Medica. Section 48: Gastroenterology. Elsevier Science Publishing Co., Inc., P.O. Box 882, Madison Square Station, New York, NY 10159-2101. Phone: (212) 989-5800. Fax: (212) 633-3990. 20/year.

Index Medicus. U.S. National Library of Medicine, 8600 Rockville Pike, Bethesda, MD 20894. Phone: (800) 638-8480. Monthly.

Research Alert: Gastroenterology-Diseases. Institute for Scientific Information, 3501 Market St., Philadelphia, PA 19104. Phone: (800) 523-1850. Fax: (215) 386-6362. Weekly.

Science Citation Index. Institute for Scientific Information, 3501 Market St., Philadelphia, PA 19104. Phone: (800) 523-1850. Fax: (215) 386-6362. Bimonthly.

ANNUALS AND REVIEWS

Advances in Gastrointestinal Radiology. Mosby-Year Book, 11830 Westline Industrial Drive, St. Louis, MO 63146. Phone: (800) 325-4177. Fax: (314) 432-1380. Annual.

Annual of Gastrointestinal Endoscopy. Current Science Group, 20 N. Third St., Philadelphia, PA 19106-2199. Phone: (800) 552-5866. Fax: (215) 574-2270. Annual.

Current Gastroenterology. Mosby-Year Book, 11830 Westline Industrial Drive, St. Louis, MO 63146. Phone: (800) 325-4177. Fax: (314) 432-1380. Annual.

Current Opinion in Gastroenterology. Current Science Group, 20 N. Third St., Philadelphia, PA 19106-2199. Phone: (800) 552-5866. Fax: (215) 574-2270. Bimonthly.

Frontiers of Gastrointestinal Research. S. Karger Publishers, Inc., 26 West Avon Rd., P.O. Box 529, Farmington, CT 06085. Phone: (203) 675-7834. Fax: (203) 675-7302. Irregular.

Gastroenterology Annual. Elsevier Science Publishing Co., Inc., P.O. Box 882, Madison Square Station, New York, NY 10159-2101. Phone: (212) 989-5800. Fax: (212) 633-3990. Annual.

Gastroenterology Clinics. W.B. Saunders Co., The Curtis Center, Independence Square W., Philadelphia, PA 19106-3399. Phone: (215) 238-7800. Quarterly.

Gastrointestinal Endoscopy Clinics of North America. W.B. Saunders Co., The Curtis Center, Independence Square W., Philadelphia, PA 19106-3399. Phone: (215) 238-7800. Quarterly.

Year Book of Digestive Diseases. Mosby-Year Book, 11830 Westline Industrial Drive, St. Louis, MO 63146. Phone: (800) 325-4177. Fax: (314) 432-1380. Annual.

ASSOCIATIONS, PROFESSIONAL SOCIETIES, ADVOCACY AND SUPPORT GROUPS

American College of Gastroenterology (ACG). 4222 King St., Alexandria, VA 22302. Phone: (703) 549-4440.

American Gastroenterological Association (AGA). 6900 Grove Rd., Thorofare, NJ 08086. Phone: (609) 848-9218. Fax: (609) 853-5991.

American Society for Gastrointestinal Endoscopy (ASGE). 13 Elm St., P.O. Box 1565, Manchester, MA 01944. Phone: (508) 526-8330.

Celiac Sprue Association/USA, Inc.. P.O. Box 31700, Omaha, NE 68131-0700. Phone: (402) 558-0600.

Crohn's & Colitis Foundation of America, Inc.. 444 Park Ave. S., 11th Flr., New York, NY 10016-7374. Phone: (800) 343-3637.

Digestive Disease National Coalition (DDNC). 711 Second St. NE, Suite 200, Washington, DC 20002. Phone: (202) 544-7497.

National Foundation for Ileitis and Colitis (NFIC). 444 Park Ave. S., 11th Fl., New York, NY 10016-7374. Phone: (800) 343-3637. Fax: (212) 779-4098.

Society of American Gastrointestinal Endoscopic Surgeons (SAGES). 1271 Stoner Ave., Suite 409, Los Angeles, CA 90025. Phone: (213) 479-3249.

BIBLIOGRAPHIES

Gastrointestinal Bacteria: Campylobacter Pylori. National Technical Information Service, 5285 Port Royal Rd., Springfield, VA 22161. Phone: (703) 487-4650. Fax: (703) 321-8547. Jan. 1978 - Dec. 1988. NTIS order no.: PB89-854152/CBY.

Gastrointestinal Ulcers. National Technical Information Service, 5285 Port Royal Rd., Springfield, VA 22161. Phone: (703) 487-4650. Fax: (703) 321-8547. Feb. 1979 - Aug. 1989. NTIS order no.: PB90-851015/CBY.

CD-ROM DATABASES

Abdominal Pain. Hoffer. Williams & Wilkins, 428 East Preston St., Baltimore, MD 21202. Phone: (800) 638-0672. Fax: (800) 447-8438. 1987.

Biological Abstracts on Compact Disc. BIOSIS, 2100 Arch St., Philadelphia, PA 19103-1399. Phone: (800) 523-4800. Fax: (215) 587-2016. Quarterly.

Excerpta Medica CD: Gastroenterology. SilverPlatter Information, Inc., River Ridge Office Park, 100 River Ridge Rd., Norwood, MA 02062. Phone: (617) 769-2599. Fax: (617) 769-8763. Quarterly.

Gastroenterology and Hepatology MEDLINE. MEP, 124 Mt. Auburn St., Cambridge, MA 02138. Phone: (800) 342-1338. Fax: (617) 868-7738. Quarterly.

SCISEARCH. Institute for Scientific Information, 3501 Market St., Philadelphia, PA 19104. Phone: (215) 386-0100. Fax: (215) 386-6362.

DIRECTORIES

Directory of Digestive Diseases Organizations. National Digestive Diseases Information Clearinghouse, P.O. Box NDDIC, Bethesda, MD 20892. Phone: (301) 468-6344. Biennial.

ENCYCLOPEDIAS, DICTIONARIES, WORD BOOKS

Gastrointestinal Words. Stedman. Williams & Wilkins, 428 East Preston St., Baltimore, MD 21202. Phone: (800) 638-0672. Fax: (800) 447-8438. 1992.

HANDBOOKS, GUIDES, MANUALS, ATLASES

Atlas of Gastroenterology. Yamada. J.B. Lippincott Co., 227 E. Washington Square, Philadelphia, PA 19106-3780. Phone: (215) 238-4200. Fax: (215) 238-4227. 1992.

A Color Atlas of Gastrointestinal Endoscopy. K.F.R. Schiller and others. W.B. Saunders Co., The Curtis Center, Independence Sqare W., Philadelphia, PA 19106-3399. Phone: (215) 238-7800. 1987.

Color Atlas of Gastrointestinal Pathology. Basil C. Morson. W.B. Saunders Co., The Curtis Center, Independence Square W., Philadelphia, PA 19106-3399. Phone: (215) 238-7800. 1988.

Gastrointestinal Pathology: An Atlas and Text. Cecilia M. Fenoglio-Preiser, and others. Raven Press, 1185 Avenue of the Americas, New York, NY 10036. Phone: (212) 930-9500. Fax: (212) 869-3495. 1989.

Handbook of Gastrointestinal Drug Therapy. Van Ness. Little, Brown and Co., 34 Beacon St., Boston, MA 02108. Phone: (617) 227-0730. Fax: (617) 227-0790. 1989.

JOURNALS

American Journal of Gastroenterology. Williams & Wilkins, 428 E. Preston St., Baltimore, MD 21202. Phone: (800) 638-0672. Fax: (800) 447-8438. Monthly.

Contemporary Gastroenterology. Medical Economics, Five Paragon Dr., Montvale, NJ 07645-1742. Phone: (800) 222-3045. Fax: (201) 573-4956. 6/year.

Digestion. S. Karger Publishers, Inc., 26 W. Avon Rd., P.O. Box 529, Farmington, CT 06085. Phone: (203) 675-7834. Fax: (203) 675-7302.

Digestive Diseases and Sciences. Plenum Publishing Co., 233 Spring St., New York, NY 10013-1578. Phone: (212) 620-8000. Fax: (212) 463-0742. Monthly.

Diseases of the Colon and Rectum. Williams & Wilkins, 428 E. Preston St., Baltimore, MD 21202. Phone: (800) 638-0672. Fax: (800) 447-8438. Monthly.

European Journal of Gastroenterology & Hepatology. Current Science Group, 20 N. Third St., Philadelphia, PA 19106-2199. Phone: (800) 552-5866. Fax: (215) 574-2270. Monthly.

Gastroenterology. W.B. Saunders Co., The Curtis Center, Independence Sqare W., Philadelphia, PA 19106-3399. Phone: (215) 238-7800.

Gastrointestinal Endoscopy. Mosby-Year Book, 11830 Westline Industrial Drive, St. Louis, MO 63146. Phone: (800) 325-4177. Fax: (314) 432-1380. Bimonthly.

Gut. BMJ Publishing Group, BMA House, Tavistock Square, London WC1H 9JR, England. Phone: 071-383 6244/6638. Fax: 071-383 6662. Monthly.

International Journal of Colorectal Disease. Springer-Verlag New York Inc., 175 Fifth Ave., New York, NY 10010. Phone: (212) 460-1500. Fax: (212) 473-6272. 4/year.

Journal of Clinical Gastroenterology. Raven Press, 1185 Avenue of the Americas, New York, NY 10036. Phone: (212) 930-9500. Fax: (212) 869-3495. Bimonthly.

Journal of ET Nursing. Mosby-Year Book, 11830 Westline Industrial Drive, St. Louis, MO 63146. Phone: (800) 325-4177. Fax: (314) 432-1380. Bimonthly.

Journal of Hepatology. Elsevier Science Publishing Co., Inc., P.O. Box 882, Madison Square Station, New York, NY 10159-2101. Phone: (212) 989-5800. Fax: (212) 633-3990. 6/year.

Journal of Pediatric Gastroenterology and Nutrition. Raven Press, 1185 Ave. of the Americas, New York, NY 10036. Phone: (212) 930-9500. Fax: (212) 869-3495.

NEWSLETTERS

IBD News. National Foundation for Ileitis & Colitis, Inc., 444 Park Ave., S., New York, NY 10016-7374. Phone: (800) 343-3637. Fax: (212) 779-4098. 3/year.

ONLINE DATABASES

BIOSIS Previews. BIOSIS, 2100 Arch St., Philadelphia, PA 19103-1399. Phone: (800) 523-4800. Fax: (215) 587-2016.

Combined Health Information Database (CHID). U.S. National Institutes of Health, P.O. Box NDIC, Bethesda, MD 20892. Phone: (301) 496-2162. Fax: (301) 770-5164. Quarterly.

EMBASE. Elsevier Science Publishing Co., Inc., P.O. Box 882, Madison Square Station, New York, NY 10159-2101. Phone: (212) 989-5800. Fax: (212) 633-3990.

MEDLINE. National Library of Medicine, 8600 Rockville Pike, Bethesda, MD 20894. Phone: (800) 638-8480.

SciSearch. Institute for Scientific Information, 3501 Market St., Philadelphia, PA 19104. Phone: (215) 386-0100. Fax: (215) 386-6362.

POPULAR WORKS AND PATIENT EDUCATION

Complete Book of Better Digestion: A Gut-Level Guide to Gastric Relief. Michael Oppenheim. Rodale Press, Inc., 33 E. Minor St., Emmaus, PA 18098. Phone: (800) 527-8200. Fax: (215) 967-6263. 1990.

Eating Right for a Bad Gut: The Complete Nutritional Guide to Illeitis, Colitis, Crohn's Disease & Irritable Bowel Syndrome. James Scala. NAL/Dutton, 375 Hudson St., New York, NY 10014-3657. Phone: (212) 366-2000. 1990.

Gastrointestinal Health: A Self-Help Nutritional Program to Prevent, Alleviate, or Cure the Symptoms of Irritable Bowel Syndrome, Ulcers, Heartburn,. Steven R. Peikin. HarperCollins Pubs., Inc., 10 E. 53rd St., New York, NY 10022-5299. Phone: (212) 207-7000. Fax: (800) 242-7737. 1991.

Gut Reactions: Understanding Symptoms of the Digestive Tract. W.G. Thompson. Plenum Publishing Co., 233 Spring St., New York, NY 10013-1578. Phone: (323) 620-8000. Fax: (212) 463-0742. 1989.

The Hemmorrhoid Book. Sidney E. Wanderman, Betty Rothbart, and others. Consumer Reports Books, 101 Truman Ave., Yonkers, NY 10703. Phone: (914) 378-2000. 1991.

The IBD Nutrition Book. Jan K. Greenwood. John Wiley & Sons, Inc., 605 Third Ave., New York, NY 10158-0012. Phone: (212) 850-6000. Fax: (212) 850-6088. 1992.

IBD: The Complete Guide to Managing Inflammatory Bowel Disease. Jon H. Zonderman, Ronald Vender. John Wiley & Sons, Inc., 605 Third Ave., New York, NY 10158-0012. Phone: (212) 850-6000. Fax: (212) 850-6088. 1992.

Irritable Bowel Syndrome and Diverticulosis: A Self-Help Plan. Shirley Trickett. HarperCollins Pubs., Inc., 10 E. 53rd St., New York, NY 10022-5299. Phone: (212) 207-7000. 1992.

Treating IBD: A Patient's Guide to the Medical and Surgical Management of Inflammatory Bowel Disease. Lawrence J. Brand, Penny Steiner-Grossman (eds.). Raven Press, 1185 Avenue of the Americas, New York, NY 10036. Phone: (212) 930-9500. Fax: (212) 869-3495. 1989.

The Wellness Book of I.B.S.: How to Achieve Relief from Irritable Bowel Syndrome and Live a Symptom-Free Life. Deralee Scanlon, Barbara C. Becnel. St. Martin's Press, 175 Fifth Ave., New York, NY 10010. Phone: (212) 674-5151. 1991.

RESEARCH CENTERS, INSTITUTES, CLEARINGHOUSES

Gastrointestinal Research Group. University of Calgary. Health Sciences Centre, 3330 Hospital Dr. N.W., Calgary, AB, Canada T2N 1N4. Phone: (403) 220-4539. Fax: (403) 270-3353.

National Digestive Diseases Information Clearinghouse (NDDIC). P.O. Box NDDIC, Bethesda, MD 20892. Phone: (301) 468-6344.

TEXTBOOKS AND MONOGRAPHS

Advanced Therapeutic Endoscopy. Jamie S. Barkin, Cesar A. O'Phelan (eds.). Raven Press, 1185 Avenue of the Americas, New York, NY 10036. Phone: (212) 930-9500. Fax: (212) 869-3495. 1990.

Constipation in Childhood. Grahm Claden, Ulfur Agnarsson. Oxford University Press, 200 Madison Ave., New York, NY 10016. Phone: (212) 679-7300. 1991.

Diarrhea. Michael Gracey. CRC Press, Inc., 2000 Corporate Blvd. N.W., Boca Raton, FL 33431. Phone: (407) 994-0555. Fax: (407) 997-0949. 1991.

Disorders of the Pancreas: Current Issues in Diagnosis and Management. Gerard P. Burns, Simmy Bank. McGraw-Hill, Inc., Health Professions Division, 1221 Avenue of the Americas, 28th Floor, New York, NY 10020. Phone: (212) 512-4228. 1992.

Flexible Sigmoidoscopy: Techniques and Utilization. Melvin Schapiro, Glen A. Lehman (eds.). Williams & Wilkins, 428 E. Preston St., Baltimore, MD 21202. Phone: (800) 638-0672. Fax: (800) 447-8438. 1990.

Fundamentals of Gastroenterology. Lawrie W. Powell, Douglas W. Piper. McGraw-Hill, Inc., Health Professions Division, 1221 Avenue of the Americas, 28th Floor, New York, NY 10020. Phone: (212) 512-4228. Fifth edition 1991.

Gastritis. Robert A. Kozol. CRC Press, Inc., 2000 Corporate Blvd. N.W., Boca Raton, FL 33431. Phone: (407) 994-0555. Fax: (407) 997-0949. 1992.

Gastrointestinal Disease: Pathophysiology, Diagnosis, Management. Marvin H. Sleisenger, John. S. Fordtran. W.B. Saunders Co., The Curtis Center, Independence Square W., Philadelphia, PA 19106-3399. Phone: (215) 238-7800. Fourth edition. Two volumes. 1989.

Gastrointestinal Emergencies. Mark B. Taylor. Williams & Wilkins, 428 E. Preston St., Baltimore, MD 21202. Phone: (800) 638-0672. Fax: (800) 447-8438. 1991.

Gastrointestinal Radiology: A Concise Text. B. Plavsic, A. Robinson, R.B. Jeffrey. McGraw-Hill, Inc., Health Professions Division, 1221 Avenue of the Americas, 28th Floor, New York, NY 10020. Phone: (212) 512-4228. 1992.

Inflammatory Bowel Disease. Joseph B. Kirsner, Roy G. Shorter (eds.). Lea & Febiger, 428 E. Preston St., Baltimore, MD 21202. Phone: (800) 638-0672. Fax: (800) 447-8438. Third edition 1988.

Inflammatory Bowel Diseases. R.N. Allan, M.R.B. Keighley, J. Alexander-Williams, et. al.. Churchill Livingstone Inc., 650 Avenue of the Americas, New York, NY 10011. Phone: (212) 819-5400. Fax: (212) 302-6598. Second edition 1990.

Management of Inflammatory Bowel Disease. Korelitz. Mosby-Year Book, 11830 Westline Industrial Drive, St. Louis, MO 63146. Phone: (800) 325-4177. Fax: (314) 432-1380. 1992.

Nausea and Vomiting: Recent Research and Clinical Advances. John Kucharczyk, David J. Stewart, Alan Miller. CRC Press, Inc., 2000 Corporate Blvd. N.W., Boca Raton, FL 33431. Phone: (407) 994-0555. Fax: (407) 997-0949. 1992.

Patient Care in Colorectal Surgery. David E. Beck, David P. Welling. Little, Brown and Company, 34 Beacon St., Boston, MA 02108. Phone: (617) 227-0730. 1991.

Pediatric Gastrointestinal Disease: Pathophysiology, Diagnosis, Management. Allan W. Walker, and others. Mosby-Year Book, 11830 Westline Industrial Drive, St. Louis, MO 63146. Phone: (800) 325-4177. Fax: (314) 432-1380. Two volumes 1991.

Practical Gastrointestinal Endoscopy. Peter B. Cotton, Christopher B. Williams. Mosby-Year Book, 11830 Westline Industrial Drive, St. Louis, MO 63146. Phone: (800) 325-4177. Fax: (314) 432-1380. Third edition 1990.

Shackelford's Surgery of the Alimentary Tract. George D. Zuidema (ed.). W.B. Saunders Co., The Curtis Center, Independence Square W., Philadelphia, PA 19106-3399. Phone: (215) 238-7800. Third edition Five volumes 1991.

Stomach. Gustavsoon. Churchill Livingstone Inc., 650 Ave. of the Americas, New York, NY 10011. Phone: (212) 819-5400. Fax: (212) 302-6598. 1992.

Ulcerative Colitis. Colm A. O'Morain. CRC Press, Inc., 2000 Corporate Blvd. N.W., Boca Raton, FL 33431. Phone: (407) 994-0555. Fax: (407) 997-0949. 1991.

GASTROINTESTINAL SURGERY

ABSTRACTING, INDEXING, AND CURRENT AWARENESS PUBLICATIONS

Current Contents/Clinical Medicine. Institute for Scientific Information, 3501 Market St., Philadelphia, PA 19104. Phone: (800) 523-1850. Fax: (215) 386-6362. Weekly.

Excerpta Medica. Section 48: Gastroenterology. Elsevier Science Publishing Co., Inc., P.O. Box 882, Madison Square Station, New York, NY 10159-2101. Phone: (212) 989-5800. Fax: (212) 633-3990. 20/year.

Index Medicus. U.S. National Library of Medicine, 8600 Rockville Pike, Bethesda, MD 20894. Phone: (800) 638-8480. Monthly.

Science Citation Index. Institute for Scientific Information, 3501 Market St., Philadelphia, PA 19104. Phone: (800) 523-1850. Fax: (215) 386-6362. Bimonthly.

ANNUALS AND REVIEWS

Annual of Gastrointestinal Endoscopy. Current Science Group, 20 N. Third St., Philadelphia, PA 19106-2199. Phone: (800) 552-5866. Fax: (215) 574-2270. Annual.

Current Gastroenterology. Mosby-Year Book, 11830 Westline Industrial Drive, St. Louis, MO 63146. Phone: (800) 325-4177. Fax: (314) 432-1380. Annual.

Current Opinion in Gastroenterology. Current Science Group, 20 N. Third St., Philadelphia, PA 19106-2199. Phone: (800) 552-5866. Fax: (215) 574-2270. Bimonthly.

Gastroenterology Annual. Elsevier Science Publishing Co., Inc., P.O. Box 882, Madison Square Station, New York, NY 10159-2101. Phone: (212) 989-5800. Fax: (212) 633-3990. Annual.

Gastroenterology Clinics. W.B. Saunders Co., The Curtis Center, Independence Square W., Philadelphia, PA 19106-3399. Phone: (215) 238-7800. Quarterly.

Gastrointestinal Endoscopy Clinics of North America. W.B. Saunders Co., The Curtis Center, Independence Square W., Philadelphia, PA 19106-3399. Phone: (215) 238-7800. Quarterly.

Year Book of Digestive Diseases. Mosby-Year Book, 11830 Westline Industrial Drive, St. Louis, MO 63146. Phone: (800) 325-4177. Fax: (314) 432-1380. Annual.

ASSOCIATIONS, PROFESSIONAL SOCIETIES, ADVOCACY AND SUPPORT GROUPS

American College of Gastroenterology (ACG). 4222 King St., Alexandria, VA 22302. Phone: (703) 549-4440.

American Gastroenterological Association (AGA). 6900 Grove Rd., Thorofare, NJ 08086. Phone: (609) 848-9218. Fax: (609) 853-5991.

American Society for Gastrointestinal Endoscopy (ASGE). 13 Elm St., P.O. Box 1565, Manchester, MA 01944. Phone: (508) 526-8330.

National Foundation for Ileitis and Colitis (NFIC). 444 Park Ave. S., 11th Fl., New York, NY 10016-7374. Phone: (800) 343-3637. Fax: (212) 779-4098.

Society of American Gastrointestinal Endoscopic Surgeons (SAGES). 1271 Stoner Ave., Suite 409, Los Angeles, CA 90025. Phone: (213) 479-3249.

CD-ROM DATABASES

Excerpta Medica CD: Gastroenterology. SilverPlatter Information, Inc., River Ridge Office Park, 100 River Ridge Rd., Norwood, MA 02062. Phone: (617) 769-2599. Fax: (617) 769-8763. Quarterly.

Gastroenterology and Hepatology MEDLINE. MEP, 124 Mt. Auburn St., Cambridge, MA 02138. Phone: (800) 342-1338. Fax: (617) 868-7738. Quarterly.

SCISEARCH. Institute for Scientific Information, 3501 Market St., Philadelphia, PA 19104. Phone: (215) 386-0100. Fax: (215) 386-6362.

ENCYCLOPEDIAS, DICTIONARIES, WORD BOOKS

Gastrointestinal Words. Stedman. Williams & Wilkins, 428 East Preston St., Baltimore, MD 21202. Phone: (800) 638-0672. Fax: (800) 447-8438. 1992.

HANDBOOKS, GUIDES, MANUALS, ATLASES

Atlas of Esophageal Surgery. David B. Skinner. Churchill Livingstone Inc., 650 Avenue of the Americas, New York, NY 10011. Phone: (212) 819-5400. Fax: (212) 302-6598. 1991.

Atlas of Gastric Surgery. Michael Zinner. Churchill Livingstone Inc., 650 Avenue of the Americas, New York, NY 10011. Phone: (212) 819-5400. Fax: (212) 302-6598. 1991.

Atlas of Hernia Surgery. George E. Wantz. Raven Press, 1185 Avenue of the Americas, New York, NY 10036. Phone: (212) 930-9500. Fax: (212) 869-3495. 1991.

Atlas of Operative Surgery: Gallbladder, Bile Ducts, Pancreas. K. Kremer, W. Lierse, W. Platzer, and others. Thieme Medical Publishers, Inc., 381 Park Ave. S., New York, NY 10016. Phone: (212) 683-5088. Fax: (212) 779-9020. 1991.

Gastrointestinal Pathology: An Atlas and Text. Cecilia M. Fenoglio-Preiser, and others. Raven Press, 1185 Avenue of the Americas, New York, NY 10036. Phone: (212) 930-9500. Fax: (212) 869-3495. 1989.

JOURNALS

American Journal of Gastroenterology. Williams & Wilkins, 428 E. Preston St., Baltimore, MD 21202. Phone: (800) 638-0672. Fax: (800) 447-8438. Monthly.

American Journal of Surgery. Reed Publishing USA, 249 W. 17th St., New York, NY 10011. Phone: (212) 645-0067. Fax: (212) 242-6987. Monthly.

American Surgeon. J.B. Lippincott Company, 227 E. Washington Square, Philadelphia, PA 19106-3780. Phone: (215) 238-4200. Fax: (215) 238-4227. Monthly.

Annals of Surgery. J.B. Lippincott Company, 227 E. Washington Square, Philadelphia, PA 19106-3780. Phone: (215) 238-4200. Fax: (215) 238-4227. Monthly.

British Journal of Surgery. Butterworth-Heinemann, 80 Montvale Ave., Stoneham, MA 02180. Phone: (617) 438-8464. Fax: (617) 279-4851. Monthly Monthly.

Diseases of the Colon and Rectum. Williams & Wilkins, 428 E. Preston St., Baltimore, MD 21202. Phone: (800) 638-0672. Fax: (800) 447-8438. Monthly.

Gastrointestinal Endoscopy. Mosby-Year Book, 11830 Westline Industrial Drive, St. Louis, MO 63146. Phone: (800) 325-4177. Fax: (314) 432-1380. Bimonthly.

Surgical Clinics of North America. W.B. Saunders Co., The Curtis Center, Independence Sq. W., Philadelphia, PA 19106-3399. Phone: (215) 238-7800. Bimonthly.

ONLINE DATABASES

EMBASE. Elsevier Science Publishing Co., Inc., P.O. Box 882, Madison Square Station, New York, NY 10159-2101. Phone: (212) 989-5800. Fax: (212) 633-3990.

MEDLINE. National Library of Medicine, 8600 Rockville Pike, Bethesda, MD 20894. Phone: (800) 638-8480.

SciSearch. Institute for Scientific Information, 3501 Market St., Philadelphia, PA 19104. Phone: (215) 386-0100. Fax: (215) 386-6362.

POPULAR WORKS AND PATIENT EDUCATION

Complete Book of Better Digestion: A Gut-Level Guide to Gastric Relief. Michael Oppenheim. Rodale Press, Inc., 33 E. Minor St., Emmaus, PA 18098. Phone: (800) 527-8200. Fax: (215) 967-6263. 1990.

Eating Right for a Bad Gut: The Complete Nutritional Guide to Illeitis, Colitis, Crohn's Disease & Irritable Bowel Syndrome. James Scala. NAL/Dutton, 375 Hudson St., New York, NY 10014-3657. Phone: (212) 366-2000. 1990.

Gastrointestinal Health: A Self-Help Nutritional Program to Prevent, Alleviate, or Cure the Symptoms of Irritable Bowel Syndrome, Ulcers, Heartburn,. Steven R. Peikin. HarperCollins Pubs., Inc., 10 E. 53rd St., New York, NY 10022-5299. Phone: (212) 207-7000. Fax: (800) 242-7737. 1991.

Gut Reactions: Understanding Symptoms of the Digestive Tract. W.G. Thompson. Plenum Publishing Co., 233 Spring St., New York, NY 10013-1578. Phone: (323) 620-8000. Fax: (212) 463-0742. 1989.

RESEARCH CENTERS, INSTITUTES, CLEARINGHOUSES

National Digestive Diseases Information Clearinghouse (NDDIC). P.O. Box NDDIC, Bethesda, MD 20892. Phone: (301) 468-6344.

STANDARDS AND STATISTICS SOURCES

Gastrointestinal Surgery for Severe Obesity. Consensus Statement. NIH Consensus Development Conference. March 25-27, 1991. National Institutes of Health, Office of Medical Applications of Research, Federal Bldg., Rm. 618, Bethesda, MD 20892. 1990.

TEXTBOOKS AND MONOGRAPHS

Advanced Therapeutic Endoscopy. Jamie S. Barkin, Cesar A. O'Phelan (eds.). Raven Press, 1185 Avenue of the Americas, New York, NY 10036. Phone: (212) 930-9500. Fax: (212) 869-3495. 1990.

Colon and Rectal Surgery. Marvin L. Corman. J.B. Lippincott Co., 227 East Washington Square, Philadelphia, PA 19106-3780. Phone: (215) 238-4200. Fax: (215) 238-4227. Third edition 1992.

Decision Making in Gastrointestinal Surgery. Larry C. Carey, Edwin C. Ellision. Mosby-Year Book, 11830 Westline Industrial Drive, St. Louis, MO 63146. Phone: (800) 325-4177. Fax: (314) 432-1380. 1991.

Flexible Sigmoidoscopy: Techniques and Utilization. Melvin Schapiro, Glen A. Lehman (eds.). Williams & Wilkins, 428 E. Preston St., Baltimore, MD 21202. Phone: (800) 638-0672. Fax: (800) 447-8438. 1990.

Gastrointestinal Emergencies. Mark B. Taylor. Williams & Wilkins, 428 E. Preston St., Baltimore, MD 21202. Phone: (800) 638-0672. Fax: (800) 447-8438. 1991.

An Introduction to Gastrointestinal Endoscopy. J. Baillie, W. Hogan. Butterworth-Heinemann, 80 Montvale Ave., Stoneham, MA 02180. Phone: (617) 438-8464. Fax: (617) 279-4851. 1991.

Lasers in Gastroenterology. Ell Riemann. Thieme Medical Publishers, Inc., 381 Park Ave. S., New York, NY 10016. Phone: (212) 683-5088. 1989.

Lithotripsy and Related Techniques for Gallstone Treatment. Paumgartner. Mosby-Year Book, 11830 Westline Industrial Drive, St. Louis, MO 63146. Phone: (800) 325-4177. Fax: (314) 432-1380. 1991.

Patient Care in Colorectal Surgery. David E. Beck, David P. Welling. Little, Brown and Company, 34 Beacon St., Boston, MA 02108. Phone: (617) 227-0730. 1991.

Practical Gastrointestinal Endoscopy. Peter B. Cotton, Christopher B. Williams. Mosby-Year Book, 11830 Westline Industrial Drive, St. Louis, MO 63146. Phone: (800) 325-4177. Fax: (314) 432-1380. Third edition 1990.

Reoperative Gastrointestinal Surgery. Thomas T. White, Michael W. Mulholland. Appleton & Lange, 25 Van Zant St., East Norwalk, CT 06855. Phone: (800) 423-1359. Fax: (203) 854-9486. 1989.

Shackelford's Surgery of the Alimentary Tract. George D. Zuidema (ed.). W.B. Saunders Co., The Curtis Center, Independence Square W., Philadelphia, PA 19106-3399. Phone: (215) 238-7800. Third edition Five volumes 1991.

Stomach. Gustavsoon. Churchill Livingstone Inc., 650 Ave. of the Americas, New York, NY 10011. Phone: (212) 819-5400. Fax: (212) 302-6598. 1992.

Surgical Treatment of Digestive Disease. Frank G. Moody, Larry C. Carey, R. Scott Jones, and others. Mosby-Year Book, 11830 Westline Industrial Drive, St. Louis, MO 63146. Phone: (800) 325-4177. Fax: (314) 432-1380. Second edition 1990.

GENDER IDENTITY

See: SEXUAL DISORDERS

GENERAL MEDICINE

ABSTRACTING, INDEXING, AND CURRENT AWARENESS PUBLICATIONS

Abridged Index Medicus. U.S. National Library of Medicine, 8600 Rockville Pike, Bethesda, MD 20894. Phone: (800) 638-8480. Monthly.

Cumulated Index Medicus. U.S. National Library of Medicine, 8600 Rockville Pike, Bethesda, MD 20894. Phone: (800) 638-8480. Annual.

Current Contents/Clinical Medicine. Institute for Scientific Information, 3501 Market St., Philadelphia, PA 19104. Phone: (800) 523-1850. Fax: (215) 386-6362. Weekly.

The Edell Health Letter. Hippocrates, Inc., 475 Gate Five Rd., Ste. 100, Sausalito, CA 94965. Bimonthly.

Excerpta Medica. Section 6: Internal Medicine. Elsevier Science Publishers, P.O. Box 882, Madison Square Station,

New York, NY 10159-2101. Phone: (212) 633-3950. Fax: (212) 633-3990. 24/year.

Medical Abstracts Newsletter. Communi-T Publications, P.O. Box 2170, Teaneck, NJ 07666. Phone: (201) 836-5030. Monthly.

MEDOC: Index to U.S. Government Publications in the Medical and Health Sciences. Spencer S. Eccles Health Sciences Library, University of Utah, Bldg. 589, Salt Lake City, UT 84112. Phone: (801) 581-5268. Quarterly.

National Library of Medicine Audiovisuals Catalog. U.S. National Library of Medicine, 8600 Rockville Pike, Bethesda, MD 20894. Phone: (800) 638-8480. Quarterly.

National Library of Medicine Current Catalog. U.S. National Library of Medicine, 8600 Rockville Pike, Bethesda, MD 20894. Phone: (800) 638-8480. Quarterly.

PDR Journal Abstracts. Medical Economics, Five Paragon Dr., Montvale, NJ 07645-1742. Phone: (800) 222-3045. Fax: (201) 573-4956. Annual.

Reference Update. Research Information Systems, Inc., Camino Corporate Ctr., 2355 Camino Vida Roble, Carlsbad, CA 92009-1572. Phone: (800) 722-1227. Fax: (619) 438-5573. Weekly.

Science Citation Index. Institute for Scientific Information, 3501 Market St., Philadelphia, PA 19104. Phone: (800) 523-1850. Fax: (215) 386-6362. Bimonthly.

ANNUALS AND REVIEWS

Annual Review of Medicine. Annual Reviews Inc., 4139 El Camino Way, P.O. Box 10139, Palo Alto, CA 94303-0897. Phone: (415) 493-4400. Fax: (415) 855-9815. Annual.

Medical Clinics. W.B. Saunders Co., The Curtis Center, Independence Square W., Philadelphia, PA 19106-3399. Phone: (215) 238-7800. Bimonthly.

ASSOCIATIONS, PROFESSIONAL SOCIETIES, ADVOCACY AND SUPPORT GROUPS

American Council on Science and Health. 1995 Broadway, 16th Flr., New York, NY 10023-5860. Phone: (212) 362-7044. Fax: (212) 362-4919.

American Health Foundation (AHF). 320 E. 43rd St., New York, NY 10017. Phone: (212) 953-1900. Fax: (212) 687-2339.

American Medical Association (AMA). 515 N. State St., Chicago, IL 60610. Phone: (312) 464-5000. Fax: (312) 645-4184.

Canadian Medical Association. 1867 Alta Vista Dr., Box 8650, Ottawa, ON, Canada K1G 0G8. Phone: (613) 731-9331. Fax: (913) 731-0937.

National Medical Association (NMA). 1012 10th St. N.W., Washington, DC 20001. Phone: (202) 347-1895.

Royal College of Physicians and Surgeons of Canada. 74 Stanley, Ottawa, ON, Canada K1M 1P4.

BIBLIOGRAPHIES

Core Collection of Medical Books and Journals 1992. Howard Hague, Michael Jackson. Medical Information Working Party,

Henry Hochland, Haigh and Hochland Ltd., The Precinct Ctr., Oxford Rd., Manchester M13 9QA, England. 1992.

Health Information Resources in the Federal Government. OOPHP National Health Information Ctr., Office of Disease Prevention and Health Promotion, Public Health Service, 330 C St. S.W., Rm. 2132, Washington, DC 20201. Phone: (800) 336-4797. Fax: (301) 565-5112. Irregular.

Information Sources in the Medical Sciences. Leslie Morton, Shane Godbolt (eds.). R.R. Bowker Co., 245 W. 17th St., New York, NY 10011. Phone: (800) 521-8110. Fourth edition 1992.

Medical and Health Care Books and Serials in Print. R.R. Bowker Co., 245 W. 17th St., New York, NY 10011. Phone: (800) 521-8110. Fax: (908) 665-6688. Annual.

CD-ROM DATABASES

1993 PDR Library on CD-ROM. Medical Economics, Five Paragon Dr., Montvale, NJ 07645-1742. Phone: (800) 232-7379. Fax: (201) 573-4956. 1993.

American Family Physician. CMC ReSearch, Inc., 7150 S.W. Hampton, Suite C-120, Portland, OR 97223. Phone: (800) 262-7668. Fax: (503) 639-1796. Annual.

Annals of Internal Medicine. MEP, 124 Mt. Auburn St., Cambridge, MA 02138. Phone: (800) 342-1338. Fax: (617) 868-7738. Semiannual.

Bibliomed. Healthcare Information Services, Inc., 2235 American River Dr., Suite 307, Sacramento, CA 95825. Phone: (800) 468-1128. Fax: (916) 648-8078. Quarterly.

British Medical Journal. MEP, 124 Mt. Auburn St., Cambridge, MA 02138. Phone: (800) 342-1338. Fax: (617) 868-7738. Annual.

Health Reference Center. Information Access Company, 362 Lakeside Dr., Foster City, CA 94404. Phone: (800) 227-8431. Monthly.

Internal Medicine '92. Macmillan New Media, 124 Mt. Auburn St., Cambridge, MA 02138. Phone: (800) 342-1338. 1992.

Journal of the American Medical Association. Macmillan New Media, 124 Mt. Auburn St., Cambridge, MA 02138. Weekly.

MAXX: Maximum Access to Diagnosis and Therapy. Little, Brown and Company, 34 Beacon St., Boston, MA 02108. Phone: (617) 227-0730. The Electronic Library of Medicine.

MEDLINE. Cambridge Scientific Abstracts, 7200 Wisconsin Ave., Bethesda, MD 20814-4823. Phone: (800) 843-7751. Fax: (301) 961-6720. Monthly.

Medline Express. SilverPlatter Information, Inc., River Ridge Office Park, 100 River Ridge Rd., Norwood, MA 02062. Phone: (617) 769-2599. Fax: (617) 769-8763. Bimonthly.

MEDLINE Knowledge Finder. Aries Systems Corporation, One Dundee Park, Andover, MA 01810. Phone: (508) 475-7200. Fax: (508) 474-8860. Quarterly.

Medline Professional. SilverPlatter Information, Inc., River Ridge Office Park, 100 River Ridge Rd., Norwood, MA 02062. Phone: (617) 769-2599. Fax: (617) 769-8763. Bimonthly.

Merck Manual TextStack. Keyboard Publishing, Inc., Ste. 111, 482 Norristown Rd., Blue Bell, PA 19422. Phone: (800) 945-4551. Fax: (215) 832-0945.

New England Journal of Medicine. CMC ReSearch, Inc., 7150 S.W. Hampton, Suite C-120, Portland, OR 97223. Phone: (800) 262-7668. Fax: (503) 639-1796. 3/year.

The New England Journal of Medicine on CD-ROM. MEP, 124 Mt. Auburn St., Cambridge, MA 02138. Phone: (800) 342-1338. Fax: (617) 868-7738. Semiannual.

Oxford Textbook of Medicine. Oxford University Press, 200 Madison Ave., New York, NY 10016. Phone: (212) 679-7300. Irregular.

The Physician's MEDLINE. MEP, 124 Mt. Auburn St., Cambridge, MA 02138. Phone: (800) 342-1338. Fax: (617) 868-7738. Quarterly.

Scientific American Medicine CONSULT. Scientific American, Inc., 415 Madison Ave., New York, NY 10017. Phone: (212) 754-0550. Fax: (212) 980-3062. Quarterly.

SCISEARCH. Institute for Scientific Information, 3501 Market St., Philadelphia, PA 19104. Phone: (215) 386-0100. Fax: (215) 386-6362.

Year Books on Disc. CMC ReSearch, Inc., 7150 S.W. Hampton, Suite C-120, Portland, OR 97223. Phone: (800) 262-7668. Fax: (503) 639-1796. Annual includes Year Books of Cardiology, Dermatology, Diagnostic Radiology, Drug Therapy, Emergency Medicine, Family Practice, Medicine, Neurology and Neurosurgery, Obstetrics and Gynecology, Oncology, Pediatrics, and Psychiatry and Applied Mental Health.

DIRECTORIES

Directory of Physicians in the United States. American Medical Association, 515 North State St., Chicago, IL 60610. Phone: (312) 464-0183. Fax: (312) 464-5834. Biennial.

Foundation Directory. The Foundation Center, 79 Fifth Ave., New York, NY 10003. Phone: (212) 620-4230.

Health and Medical Care Directory. Yellow Pages of America, Inc., 719 Main St., Niagara Falls, NY 14301. Phone: (800) 387-4209. Annual.

Medical and Health Information Directory. Karen Backus (ed.). Gale Research, Inc., 835 Penobscot Bldg., Detroit, MI 48226-4094. Phone: (800) 877-4253. Fax: (313) 961-6083. Fifth edition Three volumes 1990.

ENCYCLOPEDIAS, DICTIONARIES, WORD BOOKS

The American Medical Association Encyclopedia of Medicine. Random House, Inc., 201 E. 50th St., New York, NY 10022. Phone: (800) 726-0600. 1989.

Black's Medical Dictionary. Gordon Macpherson (ed.). Barnes & Noble Books, 4270 Boston Way, Lanham, MD 20706. Phone: (800) 462-6420. 37th edition 1992.

Churchill's Illustrated Medical Dictionary. Churchill Livingstone Inc., 650 Ave. of the Americas, New York, NY 10011. Phone: (212) 819-5400. Fax: (212) 302-6598. 1989.

Dictionary of Medical Syndromes. S. Magalini and others. J.B. Lippincott Co., 227 E. Washington Square, Philadelphia, PA

19106-3780. Phone: (215) 238-4200. Fax: (215) 238-4227. Third edition 1990.

The Dictionary of Modern Medicine. J.C. Segen. The Parthenon Publishing Group, Inc., 120 Mill Rd., Park Ridge, NJ 07656. Phone: (201) 391-6796. 1992.

Encyclopedia of Health. Chelsea House Publishers, 95 Madison Ave., New York, NY 10016. Phone: (800) 848-2665. Irregular.

Melloni's Illustrated Medical Dictionary. Dox. Williams & Wilkins, 428 East Preston St., Baltimore, MD 21202. Phone: (800) 638-0672. Fax: (800) 447-8438. Second edition 1985.

The Mosby Medical Encyclopedia. Viking Penguin, 375 Hudson St., New York, NY 10014-3657. Phone: (800) 331-4624. Revised edition 1992.

Mosby's Medical, Nursing, and Allied Health Dictionary. Kenneth N. Anderson, Lois Anderson, Walter D. Glanze (eds.). Mosby-Year Book, 11830 Westline Industrial Dr., St. Louis, MO 63146. Phone: (800) 325-4177. Fax: (314) 432-1380. Third edition 1990.

Taber's Cyclopedic Medical Dictionary. Clayton L. Thomas (ed.). F.A. Davis Co., 1915 Arch St., Philadelphia, PA 19103. Phone: (800) 523-4049. Fax: (215) 568-5065. Seventeenth edition 1993.

HANDBOOKS, GUIDES, MANUALS, ATLASES

A Color Atlas of Clinical Medicine. C.D. Forbes, W.F. Jackson. Mosby-Year Book, 11830 Westline Industrial Drive, St. Louis, MO 63146. Phone: (800) 325-4177. Fax: (314) 432-1380. 1992.

Merck Manual of Diagnosis and Therapy. Robert Berkow (ed.). Merck & Co., Inc., P.O. Box 2000, Rahway, NJ 07065. Phone: (201) 855-4558. 16th edition. 1992.

Physicians' Guide to Rare Diseases. Jess G. Thoene (ed.). Dowden Publishing Co., Inc., 110 Summit Ave., Montvale, NJ 07645. Phone: (201) 391-9100. Fax: (301) 391-2778. 1992.

Random House Personal Medical Handbook: First Aid Away from Home. Paula Dranov. Random House, Inc., 201 E. 50th St., New York, NY 10022. Phone: (800) 726-0600. 1990.

JOURNALS

American Journal of Medicine. Reed Publishing USA, 249 W. 17th St., New York, NY 10011. Phone: (212) 645-0067. Fax: (212) 242-6987. Monthly.

Annals of Internal Medicine. American College of Physicians, Independence Mall W., Sixth St. at Race, Philadelphia, PA 19106-1572. Phone: (800) 523-1546. Fax: (215) 351-2594. Semimonthly.

BMJ. BMJ Publishing Group, BMA House, Tavistock Square, London WC1H 9JR, England. Phone: 071-383 6244/6638. Fax: 071-383 6662. Weekly.

Disease-A-Month. Mosby-Year Book, 11830 Westline Industrial Drive, St. Louis, MO 63146. Phone: (800) 325-4177. Fax: (314) 432-1380. Monthly.

Journal of the American Medical Association. American Medical Association, 515 North State St., Chicago, IL 60610. Phone: (312) 464-0183. Fax: (312) 464-5834. Weekly.

Journal of Clinical Investigation. Rockefeller University Press, 222 E. 70th St., New York, NY 10021. Phone: (212) 570-8572. Fax: (212) 570-7944. Monthly.

The Journal of NIH Research. Journal of NIH Research, 2101 L St. NW, Suite 207, Washington, DC 20037. Phone: (202) 785-5333. Fax: (202) 872-7738. Monthly.

Journal of the Royal Society of Medicine. Royal Society of Medicine Services Ltd., 1 Wimpole St., London W1M 8AE, England. Phone: 071-408 2119. Fax: 071-355 3198. Monthly.

Lancet. Williams & Wilkins, 428 East Preston St., Baltimore, MD 21202. Phone: (800) 638-0672. Fax: (800) 447-8438. Weekly.

The New England Journal of Medicine. Massachusetts Medical Society, 1440 Main St., Waltham, MA 02154-1649. Phone: (617) 893-3800. Fax: (617) 893-0413. Weekly.

Patient Care. Medical Economics, Five Paragon Dr., Montvale, NJ 07645-1742. Phone: (800) 222-3045. Fax: (201) 573-4956. Semimonthly.

Western Journal of Medicine. California Medical Association, P.O. Box 7602, San Francisco, CA 94120-7602. Phone: (415) 882-5179. Fax: (415) 882-5116. Monthly.

Year Book of Medicine. Mosby-Year Book, 11830 Westline Industrial Drive, St. Louis, MO 63146. Phone: (800) 325-4177. Fax: (314) 432-1380. Annual.

NEWSLETTERS

American Medical News. American Medical Association, 515 North State St., Chicago, IL 60610. Phone: (312) 464-0183. Fax: (312) 464-5834. Weekly.

Consumer Reports on Health. Consumer Reports, P.O. Box 52148, Boulder, CO 80322. Monthly.

Harvard Family Health Letter. Harvard Medical School Publications Group, 164 Longwood Ave., Boston, MA 02115. Monthly.

The Harvard Health Letter. Dept. of Continuing Education. Harvard Medical School, 164 Longwood Ave., 4th Flr., Boston, MA 02115. Phone: (617) 432-1485. Fax: (617) 432-1506. Monthly.

Health Facts. Center for Medical Consumers, 237 Thompson St., New York, NY 10012. Phone: (212) 674-7105. Monthly.

Health Letter. Public Citizen Health Research Group, 2000 P St. N.W., Ste. 700, Washington, DC 20036. Phone: (202) 872-0320. Monthly.

Health News. Faculty of Medicine. University of Toronto, Medical Sciences Bldg., Toronto, ON, Canada M5S 1A8. Phone: (416) 948-5411. Fax: (416) 978-4552. Bimonthly.

Health & You. Health Ink Co., One Executive Dr., Moorestown, NJ 08057. Quarterly.

Healthline. Mosby-Year Book, 11830 Westline Industrial Drive, St. Louis, MO 63146. Phone: (800) 325-4177. Fax: (314) 432-1380. Monthly.

Johns Hopkins Medical Letter: Health After 50. Medletter Associates, Inc., P.O. Box 359179, Palm Coast, FL 32137. Monthly.

Journal Watch. Massachusetts Medical Society, 1440 Main St., Waltham, MA 02154-1649. Phone: (617) 893-3800. Fax: (617) 893-0413. Semimonthly.

Mayo Clinic Health Letter. Mayo Foundation for Medical Education and Research, 200 First St. N.W., Rochester, MN 55905. Phone: (507) 284-4587. Fax: (507) 284-5410. Monthly.

Medical Update. Medical Society. Medical Education and Research Foundation. Benjamin Franklin Literary & Medical Society, P.O. Box 567, Indianapolis, IN 46206. Phone: (317) 636-8881. Fax: (317) 637-0126. !MO.

Men's Health Newsletter. Rodale Press, Inc., 33 E. Minor St., Emmaus, PA 18098. Phone: (800) 527-8200. Fax: (215) 967-6263. Monthly.

Tufts University Diet & Nutrition Letter. Tufts University, 203 Harrison Ave., Boston, MA 02111. Phone: (800) 274-7581. Monthly.

University of California, Berkeley Wellness Letter. Health Letter Associates, Box 412, Prince St. Sta., New York, NY 10003-0007. Phone: (212) 505-2255. Fax: (212) 505-5462. Monthly.

The University of Texas Lifetime Health Letter. Health Science Center. University of Texas, 1100 Holcombe Blvd., P.O. Box 20036, Houston, TX 77225. Phone: (800) 274-6377. Monthly.

ONLINE DATABASES

Comprehensive Core Medical Library (CCML). BRS Information Technologies, 8000 Westpark Dr., Mc Lean, VA 22102. Phone: (800) 289-4277. Fax: (703) 893-4632. Weekly.

Foundation Directory. The Foundation Center, 79 Fifth Ave., New York, NY 10003. Phone: (212) 620-4230.

Foundation Grants Index. The Foundation Center, 79 Fifth Ave., New York, NY 10003. Phone: (212) 620-4230. Bimonthly.

MEDIS. Mead Data Central, P.O. Box 1830, Dayton, OH 45401. Phone: (800) 227-4908.

The New England Journal of Medicine. Massachusetts Medical Society, Medical Publishing Group, 1440 Main St., Waltham, MA 02254. Phone: (617) 893-4610. Weekly.

The Online Journal of Current Clinical Trials. American Association for the Advancement of Science, 1333 H St. N.W., Rm. 1155, Washington, DC 20005. Phone: (202) 326-6446.

Postgraduate Medicine. McGraw-Hill Inc., 11 West 19th St., New York, NY 10011. Phone: (212) 337-5001. Fax: (212) 337-4092. Monthly.

POPULAR WORKS AND PATIENT EDUCATION

The American Medical Association Family Medical Guide. Random House, Inc., 201 E. 50th St., New York, NY 10022. Phone: (800) 726-0600. Sixth edition 1987.

The Columbia University College of Physicians and Surgeons Complete Home Medical Guide. Genell Subak-Sharpe (ed.). Random House, Inc., 201 E. 50th St., New York, NY 10022. Phone: (800) 726-0600. 1989 Revised edition 1989.

The Consumer's Guide to Common Illnesses. Ruth Lever. Simon & Schuster, 1230 Ave. of the Americas, New York, NY 10020. Phone: (800) 223-2348. Fax: (800) 284-0735. 1992.

International Travel Health Guide. Stuart R. Rose. Travel Medicine, Inc., 351 Pleasant St., No. 312, Northampton, MA 01060. Phone: (413) 584-0381. Annual.

The Johns Hopkins Medical Handbook. Random House, Inc., 201 E. 50th St., New York, NY 10022. Phone: (800) 726-0600. 1992.

Mayo Clinic Family Health Book. David E. Larson (ed.). William Morrow & Company, Inc., 1350 Ave. of the Americas, New York, NY 10019. Phone: (800) 237-0657. 1991.

New Good Housekeeping Family Health and Medical Guide. Hearst Corporation, 60 E. 42nd St., New York, NY 10165. Phone: (212) 297-9680. Fax: (415) 588-6867. Revised edition 1988.

The World Book Rush-Presbyterian St. Luke's Medical Center Medical Encyclopedia. World Book, Inc., 525 W. Monroe, 20th Flr., Chicago, IL 60661. Phone: (800) 621-8202. 1991.

RESEARCH CENTERS, INSTITUTES, CLEARINGHOUSES

Howard Hughes Medical Institute. 6701 Rockledge Dr., Bethesda, MD 20817. Phone: (301) 571-0200. Fax: (301) 571-0309.

National Health Information Center. Office of Disease Prevention and Health Promotion, P.O. Box 1133, Washington, DC 20013-1133. Phone: (800) 336-4797.

The Pew Charitable Trusts. Three Parkway, Ste. 501, Philadelphia, PA 19102-1305. Phone: (215) 568-3330.

The Proctor and Gamble Foundation. P.O. Box 599, Cincinnati, OH 45201. Phone: (513) 983-3913.

Robert Wood Johnson Foundation. P.O. Box 2316, Princeton, NJ 08543-2316. Phone: (609) 452-8701.

W.K. Kellogg Foundation. 400 North Ave., Battle Creek, MI 49017-3398. Phone: (616) 968-1611.

TEXTBOOKS AND MONOGRAPHS

Cecil Textbook of Medicine. J.B. Wyngaarden, L.H. Smith. W.B. Saunders Co., The Curtis Center, Independence Square W., Philadelphia, PA 19106-3399. Phone: (215) 238-7800. 18th edition 1988.

Conn's Current Therapy. W.B. Saunders Co., The Curtis Center, Independence Square W., Philadelphia, PA 19106-3399. Phone: (215) 238-7800. Annual.

Davidson's Principles and Practice of Medicine. I. Bouchier, C. Edwards. Churchill Livingstone Inc., 650 Ave. of the Americas, New York, NY 10011. Phone: (212) 819-5400. Fax: (212) 302-6598. 16th edition 1991.

Harrison's Principles of Internal Medicine. Jean D. Wilson, Eugene Braunwald, Kurt J. Isselbacher, et. al.. McGraw-Hill, Inc., Health Professions Division, 1221 Avenue of the Americas, 28th Floor, New York, NY 10020. Phone: (212) 512-4228. 12th edition 1991.

Oxford Companion to Medicine. Sir J. Walton, P.B. Beeson. Oxford University Press, 200 Madison Ave., New York, NY 10016. Phone: (212) 679-7300. Two volumes 1986.

Oxford Textbook of Medicine. D.J. Weatherall, J.G.G. Ledingham, D.A. Warrell. Oxford University Press, 200

Madison Ave., New York, NY 10016. Phone: (212) 679-7300. Fax: (212) 725-2972. Second edition 1987.

Scientific American Medicine. Scientific American, 415 Madison Ave., New York, NY 10017. Phone: (800) 545-0554. Monthly.

GENERAL PRACTICE

See: FAMILY MEDICINE

GENES

See: GENETICS

GENETIC COUNSELING

See: GENETICS

GENETIC DISEASES

See also: TAY-SACHS DISEASE

ABSTRACTING, INDEXING, AND CURRENT AWARENESS PUBLICATIONS

Current Contents/Clinical Medicine. Institute for Scientific Information, 3501 Market St., Philadelphia, PA 19104. Phone: (800) 523-1850. Fax: (215) 386-6362. Weekly.

Current Contents/Life Sciences. Institute for Scientific Information, 3501 Market St., Philadelphia, PA 19104. Phone: (215) 386-0100. Fax: (215) 386-6362.

Excerpta Medica. Section 22: Human Genetics. Elsevier Science Publishers, P.O. Box 882, Madison Square Station, New York, NY 10159-2101. Phone: (212) 633-3950. Fax: (212) 633-3990. 24/year.

Index Medicus. U.S. National Library of Medicine, 8600 Rockville Pike, Bethesda, MD 20894. Phone: (800) 638-8480. Monthly.

Research Alert: Gene Therapy. Institute for Scientific Information, 3501 Market St., Philadelphia, PA 19104. Phone: (800) 523-1850. Fax: (215) 386-6362. Weekly.

ANNUALS AND REVIEWS

Annual Review of Genetics. Annual Reviews Inc., 4139 El Camino Way, P.O. Box 10139, Palo Alto, CA 94303-0897. Phone: (415) 493-4400. Fax: (415) 855-9815. Annual.

ASSOCIATIONS, PROFESSIONAL SOCIETIES, ADVOCACY AND SUPPORT GROUPS

Alliance of Genetic Support Groups. 35 Wisconsin Circle, Suite 440, Chevy Chase, MD 20815. Phone: (800) 336-4363.

March of Dimes Birth Defects Foundation (MDBDF). 1275 Mamaroneck Ave., White Plains, NY 10605. Phone: (914) 428-7100. Fax: (914) 428-8203.

National Foundation for Jewish Genetic Diseases (NFJGD). 250 Park Ave., Ste. 1000, New York, NY 10017. Phone: (212) 371-1030.

National Marfan Foundation (NMF). 382 Main St., Port Washington, NY 11050. Phone: (516) 883-8712.

CD-ROM DATABASES

Biotechnology Citation Index. Institute for Scientific Information, 3501 Market St., Philadelphia, PA 19104. Phone: (215) 386-0100. Fax: (215) 386-6362. Bimonthly.

ENCYCLOPEDIAS, DICTIONARIES, WORD BOOKS

Birth Defects Encyclopedia. Mary Louise Buyse (ed.). Mosby-Year Book, 11830 Westline Industrial Drive, St. Louis, MO 63146. Phone: (800) 325-4177. Fax: (314) 432-1380. 1990.

Encyclopedia of Genetic Disorders and Birth Defects. Mark D. Ludman, James Wynbrandt. Facts on File, Inc., 460 Park Ave. S., New York, NY 10016-7382. Phone: (212) 683-2244. Fax: (212) 683-3633. 1991.

Glossary of Genetics. Rieger. Springer-Verlag New York Inc., 175 Fifth Ave., New York, NY 10010. Phone: (212) 460-1500. Fax: (212) 473-6272. Fifth edition 1991.

JOURNALS

American Journal of Human Genetics. University of Chicago Press, P.O. Box 37005, Chicago, IL 60637. Phone: (312) 753-3347. Fax: (312) 753-0811. Monthly.

Clinical Genetics. Munksgaard International Publishers Ltd., P.O. Box 2148, DK-1016 Copenhagen K, Denmark. Phone: 33- 127030. Fax: 33- 129387.

Human Gene Therapy. Mary Ann Liebert, Inc., 1651 Third Ave., New York, NY 10128. Phone: (212) 289-2300. Fax: (212) 289-4697. Bimonthly.

Journal of Genetic Counseling. Human Sciences Press, 233 Spring St., New York, NY 10013-1578. Phone: (800) 221-9369. Fax: (212) 807-1047. Quarterly.

Journal of Medical Genetics. BMJ Publishing Group, BMA House, Tavistock Square, London WC1H 9JR, England. Phone: 071-383 6244/6638. Fax: 071-383 6662. Monthly.

Mutation Research. Elsevier Science Publishing Co., Inc., P.O. Box 882, Madison Square Station, New York, NY 10159-2101. Phone: (212) 989-5800. Fax: (212) 633-3990. 60/year.

Psychiatric Genetics. Rapid Communications of Oxford Ltd., The Old Malthouse, Paradise St., Oxford OX1 1LD, England. Phone: 44-865-790447. Fax: 44-865-244012. 4/year.

NEWSLETTERS

National Tay-Sachs & Allied Diseases Association-Breakthrough. National Tay-Sachs & Allied Diseases Association, Inc., 385 Elliot St., Newton, MA 02164. Phone: (617) 964-5508. 2/year.

ONLINE DATABASES

CSA Life Sciences Collection. Cambridge Scientific Abstracts, 7200 Wisconsin Ave., Bethesda, MD 20814-4823. Phone: (800) 843-7751. Fax: (301) 961-6720.

EMBASE. Elsevier Science Publishing Co., Inc., P.O. Box 882, Madison Square Station, New York, NY 10159-2101. Phone: (212) 989-5800. Fax: (212) 633-3990.

MEDLINE. National Library of Medicine, 8600 Rockville Pike, Bethesda, MD 20894. Phone: (800) 638-8480.

SciSearch. Institute for Scientific Information, 3501 Market St., Philadelphia, PA 19104. Phone: (215) 386-0100. Fax: (215) 386-6362.

RESEARCH CENTERS, INSTITUTES, CLEARINGHOUSES

Birth Defects and Genetic Disorders Unit. T311 General Hospital, University of Iowa, Iowa City, IA 52242. Phone: (319) 353-6687.

Center for Human Genetics. Firehouse Hill, Bar Harbor, ME 04609. Phone: (207) 288-5815.

Division of Human Genetics. University of California, Irvine. UCI Medical Center, 101 The City Dr., Orange, CA 92668. Phone: (714) 634-5791.

Human Genetics Center. Indiana University. School of Medicine, 975 W. Walnut St., Indianapolis, IN 46202-5251. Phone: (317) 274-2241. Fax: (317) 274-2387.

Medical Genetics Group. Alberta Children's Hospital Research Centre, 1820 Richmond Rd. SW, Calgary, AB, Canada T2T 5C7. Phone: (403) 229-7373.

TEXTBOOKS AND MONOGRAPHS

Gene Transfer and Gene Therapy. Arthur L. Beaudet, Richard Mulligan, Inder M. Verma (eds.). John Wiley & Sons, Inc., 605 Third Ave., New York, NY 10158-0012. Phone: (212) 850-6000. Fax: (212) 850-6088. 1989.

Genetics in Obstetrics and Gynecology. Joe Leigh Simpson, Mitchell S. Golbus. W.B. Saunders Co., The Curtis Center, Independence Sqare W., Philadelphia, PA 19106-3399. Phone: (215) 238-7800. 2nd edition, 1992.

Maternal Genetic Disease. Mark I. Evans, Mark Johnson, Arie Drugan, Nelson Isada. Appleton & Lange, 25 Van Zant St., East Norwalk, CT 06855. Phone: (800) 423-1359. Fax: (203) 854-9486. 1991.

Therapy for Genetic Disease. Theodore Friedmann. Oxford University Press, 200 Madison Ave., New York, NY 10016. Phone: (212) 679-7300. 1991.

Treatment of Genetic Diseases. Robert J. Desnick (ed.). Churchill Livingstone Inc., 650 Avenue of the Americas, New York, NY 10011. Phone: (212) 819-5400. Fax: (212) 302-6598. 1991.

GENETIC ENGINEERING

See: BIOTECHNOLOGY

GENETICS

See also: BIRTH DEFECTS

ABSTRACTING, INDEXING, AND CURRENT AWARENESS PUBLICATIONS

Biological Abstracts. BIOSIS, 2100 Arch St., Philadelphia, PA 19103-1399. Phone: (800) 523-4800. Fax: (215) 587-2016.

BIOSIS/CAS Selects: Bacterial & Viral Genetics. BIOSIS, 2100 Arch St., Philadelphia, PA 19103-1399. Phone: (215) 587-4800. Fax: (215) 587-2016. Biweekly.

CAS BioTech Updates: DNA Formation & Repair. Chemical Abstracts Service, 2540 Olentangy River Road, P.O. Box 3012, Columbus, OH 43210-0012. Phone: (800) 848-6538. Biweekly.

CAS BioTech Updates: DNA & RNA Probes. Chemical Abstracts Service, 2540 Olentangy River Road, P.O. Box 3012, Columbus, OH 43210-0012. Phone: (800) 848-6538. Biweekly.

CAS BioTech Updates: Genetic Engineering. Chemical Abstracts Service, 2540 Olentangy River Road, P.O. Box 3012, Columbus, OH 43210-0012. Phone: (800) 848-6538. Biweekly.

Current Contents/Life Sciences. Institute for Scientific Information, 3501 Market St., Philadelphia, PA 19104. Phone: (215) 386-0100. Fax: (215) 386-6362.

Excerpta Medica, Section 22: Human Genetics. Elsevier Science Publishers, P.O. Box 882, Madison Square Station, New York, NY 10159-2101. Phone: (212) 633-3950. Fax: (212) 633-3990. 24/year.

Genetics Abstracts. Cambridge Scientific Abstracts, 7200 Wisconsin Ave., Bethesda, MD 20814-4823. Phone: (800) 843-7751. Fax: (301) 961-6720. Monthly.

Human Genome Abstracts. Cambridge Scientific Abstracts, 7200 Wisconsin Ave., Bethesda, MD 20814-4823. Phone: (800) 843-7751. Fax: (301) 961-6720. Bimonthly.

Index Medicus. U.S. National Library of Medicine, 8600 Rockville Pike, Bethesda, MD 20894. Phone: (800) 638-8480. Monthly.

Research Alert: Genetics-Human. Institute for Scientific Information, 3501 Market St., Philadelphia, PA 19104. Phone: (800) 523-1850. Fax: (215) 386-6362. Weekly.

Science Citation Index. Institute for Scientific Information, 3501 Market St., Philadelphia, PA 19104. Phone: (800) 523-1850. Fax: (215) 386-6362. Bimonthly.

ANNUALS AND REVIEWS

Advances in Genetics. Academic Press, Inc., 1250 Sixth Ave., San Diego, CA 92101-4311. Phone: (619) 699-6345. Fax: (619) 699-6715.

Advances in Human Genetics. Plenum Publishing Co., 233 Spring St., New York, NY 10013-1578. Phone: (212) 620-800. Fax: (212) 463-0742.

Annual Review of Genetics. Annual Reviews Inc., 4139 El Camino Way, P.O. Box 10139, Palo Alto, CA 94303-0897. Phone: (415) 493-4400. Fax: (415) 855-9815. Annual.

ASSOCIATIONS, PROFESSIONAL SOCIETIES, ADVOCACY AND SUPPORT GROUPS

American Society of Human Genetics. 9650 Rockville Pike, Bethesda, MD 20814. Phone: (301) 571-1825.

March of Dimes Birth Defects Foundation (MDBDF). 1275 Mamaroneck Ave., White Plains, NY 10605. Phone: (914) 428-7100. Fax: (914) 428-8203.

National Down Syndrome Society. 141 Fifth Ave., New York, NY 10010. Phone: (800) 221-4602.

National Genetics Foundation (NGF). 180 W. 58th St., New York, NY 10019. Phone: (212) 245-7443.

CD-ROM DATABASES

Biological Abstracts on Compact Disc. BIOSIS, 2100 Arch St., Philadelphia, PA 19103-1399. Phone: (800) 523-4800. Fax: (215) 587-2016. Quarterly.

CD-Gene. Hitachi America, Ltd., 2000 Sierra Point Pkwy., Brisbane, CA 94005-1819. Phone: (415) 589-8300. Semiannual.

SCISEARCH. Institute for Scientific Information, 3501 Market St., Philadelphia, PA 19104. Phone: (215) 386-0100. Fax: (215) 386-6362.

ENCYCLOPEDIAS, DICTIONARIES, WORD BOOKS

Birth Defects Encyclopedia. Mary Louise Buyse (ed.). Mosby-Year Book, 11830 Westline Industrial Drive, St. Louis, MO 63146. Phone: (800) 325-4177. Fax: (314) 432-1380. 1990.

Glossary of Genetics. Rieger. Springer-Verlag New York Inc., 175 Fifth Ave., New York, NY 10010. Phone: (212) 460-1500. Fax: (212) 473-6272. Fifth edition 1991.

HANDBOOKS, GUIDES, MANUALS, ATLASES

Chromosome Anomalies and Prenatal Development: An Atlas. Dorothy Warburton, Julianne Byrne, Nina Canki. Oxford University Press, 200 Madison Ave., New York, NY 10016. Phone: (212) 679-7300. 1991.

A Colour Atlas of Clinical Genetics. M. Baraitser. Sheridan House, Inc., 145 Palisade St., Dobbs Ferry, NY 10522. Phone: (914) 693-2410. 1988.

Human Chromosomes: A Manual of Basic Techniques. Ram S. Verma, Arvind Babu. McGraw-Hill, Inc., Health Professions Division, 1221 Avenue of the Americas, 28th Floor, New York, NY 10020. Phone: (212) 512-4228. 1989.

Merck Manual of Diagnosis and Therapy. Robert Berkow (ed.). Merck & Co., Inc., P.O. Box 2000, Rahway, NJ 07065. Phone: (201) 855-4558. 16th edition. 1992.

JOURNALS

American Journal of Human Genetics. University of Chicago Press, P.O. Box 37005, Chicago, IL 60637. Phone: (312) 753-3347. Fax: (312) 753-0811. Monthly.

American Journal of Medical Genetics. John Wiley & Sons, Inc., 605 Third Ave., New York, NY 10158-0012. Phone: (212) 850-6000. Fax: (212) 850-6088. 16/year.

Chromosome Research. Rapid Communications of Oxford Ltd., The Old Malthouse, Paradise St., Oxford OX1 1LD, England. Phone: 44-865-790447. Fax: 44-865-244012. 4/year.

Current Genetics. Springer-Verlag New York Inc., 175 Fifth Ave., New York, NY 10010. Phone: (212) 460-1500. Fax: (212) 473-6272.

Developmental Genetics. John Wiley & Sons, Inc., 605 Third Ave., New York, NY 10158-0012. Phone: (212) 850-6000. Fax: (212) 850-6088. Bimonthly.

Gene. Elsevier Science Publishing Co., Inc., P.O. Box 882, Madison Square Station, New York, NY 10159-2101. Phone: (212) 989-5800. Fax: (212) 633-3990. 26/year.

Genetic Analysis: Techniques and Applications. Elsevier Science Publishing Co., Inc., P.O. Box 882, Madison Square Station, New York, NY 10159-2101. Phone: (212) 989-5800. Fax: (212) 633-3990. 6/year.

Genetics. Waverly Press, 428 E. Preston St., Baltimore, MD 21202. Phone: (800) 638-0672. Fax: (800) 447-8438. Monthly.

Human Gene Therapy. Mary Ann Liebert, Inc., 1651 Third Ave., New York, NY 10128. Phone: (212) 289-2300. Fax: (212) 289-4697. Bimonthly.

Human Genetics. Springer-Verlag New York Inc., 175 Fifth Ave., New York, NY 10010. Phone: (212) 460-1500. Fax: (212) 473-6272.

Journal of Genetic Counseling. Human Sciences Press, 233 Spring St., New York, NY 10013-1578. Phone: (800) 221-9369. Fax: (212) 807-1047. Quarterly.

Journal of Medical Genetics. BMJ Publishing Group, BMA House, Tavistock Square, London WC1H 9JR, England. Phone: 071-383 6244/6638. Fax: 071-383 6662. Monthly.

Trends in Genetics. Elsevier Science Publishing Co., Inc., P.O. Box 882, Madison Square Station, New York, NY 10159-2101. Phone: (212) 989-5800. Fax: (212) 633-3990. 12 + 1/year.

ONLINE DATABASES

BIOSIS Previews. BIOSIS, 2100 Arch St., Philadelphia, PA 19103-1399. Phone: (800) 523-4800. Fax: (215) 587-2016.

CSA Life Sciences Collection. Cambridge Scientific Abstracts, 7200 Wisconsin Ave., Bethesda, MD 20814-4823. Phone: (800) 843-7751. Fax: (301) 961-6720.

EMBASE. Elsevier Science Publishing Co., Inc., P.O. Box 882, Madison Square Station, New York, NY 10159-2101. Phone: (212) 989-5800. Fax: (212) 633-3990.

GenBank (Genetic Sequence Databank). IntelliGenetics, Inc., 700 E. El Camino Real, Mountain View, CA 94040. Phone: (415) 962-7300. Fax: (415) 962-7302. Quarterly.

MEDLINE. National Library of Medicine, 8600 Rockville Pike, Bethesda, MD 20894. Phone: (800) 638-8480.

SciSearch. Institute for Scientific Information, 3501 Market St., Philadelphia, PA 19104. Phone: (215) 386-0100. Fax: (215) 386-6362.

POPULAR WORKS AND PATIENT EDUCATION

The Family Genetic Sourcebook. Benjamin A. Pierce. John Wiley & Sons, Inc., 605 Third Ave., New York, NY 10158-0012. Phone: (212) 850-6000. Fax: (212) 850-6088. 1990.

Genome: The Story of Our Astounding Attempt to Map All the Genes in the Human Body. Jerry E. Bishop. Simon & Schuster, Inc., 1230 Ave. of the Americas, New York, NY 10020. Phone: (212) 698-7000. 1992.

RESEARCH CENTERS, INSTITUTES, CLEARINGHOUSES

Beckman Research Institute. City of Hope. 1450 E. Duarte Rd., Duarte, CA 91010. Phone: (818) 357-9711.

Birth Defects and Genetic Disorders Unit. T311 General Hospital, University of Iowa, Iowa City, IA 52242. Phone: (319) 353-6687.

Boston Biomedical Research Institute. 20 Staniford St., Boston, MA 02114. Phone: (617) 742-2010.

Center for Demographic and Population Genetics. University of Texas Health Science Center at Houston. P.O. Box 20334, Houston, TX 77225. Phone: (713) 792-4680. Fax: (713) 794-1601.

Center for Human Genetics. Firehouse Hill, Bar Harbor, ME 04609. Phone: (207) 288-5815.

Coriell Institute for Medical Research (Camden). 401 Haddon Ave., Camden, NJ 08103. Phone: (609) 966-7377. Fax: (609) 964-0254.

Developmental Biology Center. Case Western Reserve University. 2109 Adelbert Rd., Cleveland, OH 44106-4901. Phone: (216) 368-3484. Fax: (216) 368-4335.

Division of Human Genetics. University of California, Irvine. UCI Medical Center, 101 The City Dr., Orange, CA 92668. Phone: (714) 634-5791.

General Clinical Research Center at Harbor-UCLA Medical Center. 1000 W. Carson St., Torrance, CA 90509. Phone: (213) 533-2503. Fax: (213) 320-6515.

Genetics Section of Pediatrics. Louisiana State University. Medical Center, 1501 Kings Hwy., Shreveport, LA 71130. Phone: (318) 674-6088.

Human Genetics Center. Indiana University. School of Medicine, 975 W. Walnut St., Indianapolis, IN 46202-5251. Phone: (317) 274-2241. Fax: (317) 274-2387.

Huntington's Disease Diagnostic and Referral Center. Hahnemann University. 1427 Vine St., 1st Floor, Philadelphia, PA 19102. Phone: (215) 246-5010.

Jackson Laboratory. Bar Harbor, ME 04609. Phone: (207) 288-3371. Fax: (207) 288-5079.

Laboratory of Genetics. University of Wisconsin-Madison. 445 Henry Mall, Madison, WI 53705. Phone: (608) 262-3112. Fax: (608) 262-2976.

Laboratory of Medical Genetics. University of Alabama at Birmingham. University Station, Birmingham, AL 35294. Phone: (205) 934-4973. Fax: (205) 934-1078.

Medical Genetics Group. Alberta Children's Hospital Research Centre, 1820 Richmond Rd. SW, Calgary, AB, Canada T2T 5C7. Phone: (403) 229-7373.

Southwest Biomedical Research Institute. 6401 E. Thomas Rd., Scottsdale, AZ 85251. Phone: (602) 945-4363. Fax: (602) 947-8220.

TEXTBOOKS AND MONOGRAPHS

Elements of Medical Genetics. Emergy. Churchill Livingstone Inc., 650 Ave. of the Americas, New York, NY 10011. Phone: (212) 819-5400. Fax: (212) 302-6598. Eighth edition 1992.

Essential Medical Genetics. J.M. Connor, M.A. Ferguson-Smith. Blackwell Scientific Publications, Inc., 3 Cambridge Ctr., Cambridge, MA 02142. Phone: (800) 759-6102. Third edition 1990.

Heredity and Ability: How Genetics Affects Your Child and What You Can Do About It. Charles M. Strom. Plenum Publishing Co., 233 Spring St., New York, NY 10013-1578. Phone: (212) 620-8000. Fax: (212) 463-0742. 1990.

Introduction to Human Biochemical and Molecular Genetics. A. Beaudet, M. Brown, D. Frederickson, and others. McGraw-Hill, Inc., Health Professions Division, 1221 Avenue of the Americas, 28th Floor, New York, NY 10020. Phone: (212) 512-4228. 1990.

Introduction to Risk Calculation in Genetic Counseling. Young. Oxford University Press, 200 Madison Ave., New York, NY 10016. Phone: (212) 679-7300. 1991.

Medical Genetics. J.J. Nora, F.C. Fraser. Williams & Wilkins, 428 East Preston St., Baltimore, MD 21202. Phone: (800) 638-0672. Fax: (800) 447-8438. Third edition 1989.

New Genetics and Clinical Practice. D.J. Weatherall. Oxford University Press, 200 Madison Ave., New York, NY 10016. Phone: (212) 679-7300. Third edition 1991.

Prenatal Diagnosis of Congenital Abnormalities. Romero. Appleton & Lange, 25 Van Zant St., East Norwalk, CT 06855. Phone: (800) 423-1359. Fax: (203) 854-9486. 1988.

Principles of Medical Genetics. Thomas D. Gelehrter, Francis S. Collins. Williams & Wilkins, 428 East Preston St., Baltimore, MD 21202. Phone: (800) 638-0672. Fax: (800) 447-8438. 1990.

Principles and Practice of Medical Genetics. ALan E.H. Emery, David J. Rimoin (eds.). Churchill Livingstone Inc., 650 Avenue of the Americas, New York, NY 10011. Phone: (212) 819-5400. Fax: (212) 302-6598. Second edition. Two volumes. 1990.

Thompson and Thompson Genetics in Medicine. Margaret W. Thompson, Roderick R. McInnes. W.B. Saunders Co., The Curtis Center, Independence Square W., Philadelphia, PA 19106-3399. Phone: (215) 238-7800. Fifth edition 1991.

GENITAL CANCER

See: PROSTATE CANCER; TESTICULAR CANCER; UROLOGY

GENITOURINARY SURGERY

See: UROLOGIC DISORDERS; UROLOGY

GERIATRICS

ABSTRACTING, INDEXING, AND CURRENT AWARENESS PUBLICATIONS

Current Contents/Clinical Medicine. Institute for Scientific Information, 3501 Market St., Philadelphia, PA 19104. Phone: (800) 523-1850. Fax: (215) 386-6362. Weekly.

Current Literature on Aging. National Council on the Aging, 600 Maryland Ave. S.W., Washington, DC 20024. Phone: (202) 749-1200.

Excerpta Medica. Section 20: Gerontology and Geriatrics. Elsevier Science Publishers, P.O. Box 882, Madison Square Station, New York, NY 10159-2101. Phone: (212) 633-3950. Fax: (212) 633-3990. 8/year.

Index Medicus. U.S. National Library of Medicine, 8600 Rockville Pike, Bethesda, MD 20894. Phone: (800) 638-8480. Monthly.

Research Alert: Aging/Geriatrics. Institute for Scientific Information, 3501 Market St., Philadelphia, PA 19104. Phone: (800) 523-1850. Fax: (215) 386-6362. Weekly.

Science Citation Index. Institute for Scientific Information, 3501 Market St., Philadelphia, PA 19104. Phone: (800) 523-1850. Fax: (215) 386-6362. Bimonthly.

Senior Health Digest. CD Publications, 8204 Fenton St., Silver Spring, MD 20910.

ANNUALS AND REVIEWS

Annual Review of Gerontology and Geriatrics. Springer Publishing Co., Inc., 536 Broadway, 11th Floor, New York, NY 10012. Phone: (212) 431-4370.

Clinics in Geriatric Medicine. W.B. Saunders Co., The Curtis Center, Independence Square W., Philadelphia, PA 19106-3399. Phone: (215) 238-7800. Quarterly.

Contemporary Geriatric Medicine. Plenum Publishing Co., 233 Spring St., New York, NY 10013-1578. Phone: (212) 620-8000. Fax: (212) 463-0742. Irregular.

In Development New Medicines for Older Americans. Pharmaceutical Manufacturers Association, 1100 15th St. N.W., Washington, DC 20005. Phone: (202) 835-3400. Annual.

Year Book of Geriatrics and Gerontology. Mosby-Year Book, 11830 Westline Industrial Drive, St. Louis, MO 63146. Phone: (800) 325-4177. Fax: (314) 432-1380. Annual.

ASSOCIATIONS, PROFESSIONAL SOCIETIES, ADVOCACY AND SUPPORT GROUPS

American Geriatrics Society (AGS). 770 Lexington Ave., Ste. 400, New York, NY 10021. Phone: (212) 308-1414. Fax: (212) 832-8646.

National Geriatrics Society. 212 W. Wisconsin Ave., 3rd Fl., Milwaukee, WI 53203. Phone: (414) 272-4130.

BIBLIOGRAPHIES

Fundamentals of Geriatrics for Health Care Professionals: An Annotated Bibliography. Joddi L. Teitelman, Iris A. Parham (eds.). Greenwood Publishing Group, Inc., 88 Post Rd. W., P.O. Box 5007, Westport, CT 06881. Phone: (203) 226-3571. 1990.

CD-ROM DATABASES

SCISEARCH. Institute for Scientific Information, 3501 Market St., Philadelphia, PA 19104. Phone: (215) 386-0100. Fax: (215) 386-6362.

DIRECTORIES

Directory of Medical Specialists. Marquis Who's Who, 3002 Glenview Rd., Wilmette, IL 60091. Phone: (800) 621-9669. Fax: (708) 441-2264. Biennial.

Directory of Physicians in the United States. American Medical Association, 515 North State St., Chicago, IL 60610. Phone: (312) 464-0183. Fax: (312) 464-5834. Biennial.

HANDBOOKS, GUIDES, MANUALS, ATLASES

Clinical Manual of Geriatrics. Lonergan. Appleton & Lange, 25 Van Zant St., East Norwalk, CT 06855. Phone: (800) 423-1359. Fax: (203) 854-9486. 1992.

Color Atlas of Geriatric Medicine. Asif Kamal, J.C. Brocklehurst. Mosby-Year Book, 11830 Westline Industrial Drive, St. Louis, MO 63146. Phone: (800) 325-4177. Fax: (314) 432-1380. Second edition 1991.

Geriatric Pharmacology. Rubin Bressler, Michael Katz. McGraw-Hill, Inc., Health Professions Division, 1221 Avenue of the Americas, 28th Floor, New York, NY 10020. Phone: (212) 512-4228. 1992.

Handbook of Prescribing Medications for Geriatric Patients. Ahronheim. Little, Brown and Co., 34 Beacon St., Boston, MA 02108. Phone: (617) 227-0730. Fax: (617) 227-0790. 1992.

Merck Manual of Geriatrics. Merck & Co., Inc., P.O. Box 2000, Rahway, NJ 07065. Phone: (201) 855-4558. Irregular.

JOURNALS

American Journal of Geriatric Psychiatry. American Psychiatric Press, Inc., 1400 K St. NW, Washington, DC 20005. Phone: (202) 682-6268. Fax: (202) 789-2648. Quarterly.

Archives of Gerontology and Geriatrics. Elsevier Science Publishing Co., Inc., P.O. Box 882, Madison Square Station, New York, NY 10159-2101. Phone: (212) 989-5800. Fax: (212) 633-3990. 6/year.

Geriatric Nephrology and Urology. Kluwer Academic Publishers, P.O. Box 358, Accord Station, Hingham, MA 02018-0358. Phone: (617) 871-6600. Fax: (617) 871-6528. 3/year.

Geriatric Nursing. Mosby-Year Book, 11830 Westline Industrial Drive, St. Louis, MO 63146. Phone: (800) 325-4177. Fax: (314) 432-1380. Bimonthly.

Geriatrics: Medicine for Midlife and Beyond. Edgell Communications, 7500 Old Oak Blvd., Cleveland, OH 44130. Phone: (216) 826-2839. Fax: (216) 891-2726. Monthly.

International Journal of Geriatic Psychiatry. John Wiley & Sons, Inc., 605 Third Ave., New York, NY 10158-0012. Phone: (212) 850-6000. Fax: (212) 850-6088. Monthly.

Journal of the American Geriatrics Society. Williams & Wilkins, 428 E. Preston St., Baltimore, MD 21202. Phone: (800) 638-0672. Fax: (800) 447-8438. Monthly.

Journal of Geriatric Psychiatry and Neurology. Mosby-Year Book, 11830 Westline Industrial Drive, St. Louis, MO 63146. Phone: (800) 325-4177. Fax: (314) 432-1380. Quarterly.

Journal of The American Geriatrics Society. Elsevier Science Publishing Co., Inc., P.O. Box 882, Madison Square Station, New York, NY 10159-2101. Phone: (212) 989-5800. Fax: (212) 633-3990. Monthly.

NEWSLETTERS

American Geriatrics Society-Newsletter. American Geriatrics Society, 770 Lexington Ave., Ste. 400, New York, NY 10021. Phone: (212) 308-1414. Bimonthly.

ONLINE DATABASES

AgeLine. American Association of Retired Persons, 601 E. St. NW, Washington, DC 20049. Phone: (202) 434-6231. Bimonthly.

EMBASE. Elsevier Science Publishing Co., Inc., P.O. Box 882, Madison Square Station, New York, NY 10159-2101. Phone: (212) 989-5800. Fax. (212) 633-3990.

MEDLINE. National Library of Medicine, 8600 Rockville Pike, Bethesda, MD 20894. Phone: (800) 638-8480.

SciSearch. Institute for Scientific Information, 3501 Market St., Philadelphia, PA 19104. Phone: (215) 386-0100. Fax: (215) 386-6362.

POPULAR WORKS AND PATIENT EDUCATION

Complete Guide to Symptoms, Illness and Surgery for People over Fifty. H. Winter Griffith. Putnam Publishing Group, 200 Madison Ave., New York, NY 10016. Phone: (800) 631-8571. 1992.

The Johns Hopkins Medical Handbook. Random House, Inc., 201 E. 50th St., New York, NY 10022. Phone: (800) 726-0600. 1992.

The Pill Book for Senior Citizens. Harold M. Silverman. Bantam Books, Inc., 666 Fifth Ave., New York, NY 10103. Phone: (800) 223-6834. 1989.

RESEARCH CENTERS, INSTITUTES, CLEARINGHOUSES

Center for Aging. University of Alabama at Birmingham. Community Health Service Bldg., Room 118, 933 S. 19th St., Birmingham, AL 35294. Phone: (205) 934-3260. Fax: (205) 934-7239.

Center for Geriatrics, Gerontology, and Long-Term Care. Columbia University. 100 Haven Ave., Tower 3-29F, New York, NY 10032. Phone: (212) 781-0600.

Center for Gerontology and Health Care Research. Brown University. Box G, Providence, RI 02912. Phone: (401) 863-3490. Fax: (401) 863-3489.

Center on Health and Aging. Atlanta University. 223 James P. Brawley Dr. S.W., Atlanta, GA 30313. Phone: (404) 653-8610.

Center for Study of Aging and Human Development. Duke University Medical Ctr., Box 3003, Durham, NC 27710. Phone: (919) 684-2248. Fax: (919) 684-8569.

Dallas Geriatric Research Institute. 2525 Centerville Rd., Dallas, TX 75228. Phone: (214) 327-4503.

Edward and Esther Polisher Research Institute. Philadelphia Geriatric Center. 5301 Old York Rd., Philadelphia, PA 19141. Phone: (215) 456-2000. Fax: (215) 456-2017.

Health Services Research Center. University of North Carolina at Chapel Hill. Chase Hall, CB 7490, Chapel Hill, NC 27599-7490. Phone: (919) 966-5011. Fax: (919) 966-5764.

National Eldercare Institute on Health Promotion. 601 E St. N.W., 5th Flr., Washington, DC 20049. Phone: (202) 434-2200. Fax: (202) 434-6474.

University Center on Aging and Health. Case Western Reserve University. 2009 Adelbert Rd., Cleveland, OH 44106. Phone: (216) 368-2692. Fax: (216) 368-6389.

TEXTBOOKS AND MONOGRAPHS

Aging: Health Care Challenge. Lewis. F.A. Davis Co., 1915 Arch St., Philadelphia, PA 19103. Phone: (800) 523-4049. Fax: (215) 568-5065. Second edition 1990.

The Challenge of Geriatric Medicine. Bernard Isaacs. Oxford University Press, 200 Madison Ave., New York, NY 10016. Phone: (212) 679-7300. 1992.

The Clinical Neurology of Old Age. R. Tallis. John Wiley & Sons, Inc., 605 Third Ave., New York, NY 10158-0012. Phone: (212) 850-6000. Fax: (212) 850-6088. 1989.

Essentials of Clinical Geriatrics. Robert L. Kane, Joseph G. Ouslander, Itamar B. Abrass. McGraw-Hill Inc., 11 West 19th St., New York, NY 10011. Phone: (212) 337-5001. Fax: (212) 337-4092. Second edition 1989.

Geriatric Emergency Medicine. Gideon Bosker, George Schwartz, Jeffrey S. Jones, et. al.. Mosby-Year Book, 11830 Westline Industrial Drive, St. Louis, MO 63146. Phone: (800) 325-4177. Fax: (314) 432-1380. 1990.

Geriatric Medicine. Robert W. Schrier. W.B. Saunders Co., The Curtis Center, Independence Square W., Philadelphia, PA 19106-3399. Phone: (215) 238-7800. 1990.

Geriatric Nutrition. Chernoff. Aspen Publishers, Inc., 200 Orchard Ridge Dr., Gaithersburg, MD 20878. Phone: (800) 638-8437. 1991.

Geriatrics: A Textbook. Pietro de Nicola. John Wiley & Sons, Inc., 605 Third Ave., New York, NY 10158-0012. Phone: (212) 850-6000. Fax: (212) 850-6088. 1991.

Geriatrics for the Internist. Rothschild. Mosby-Year Book, 11830 Westline Industrial Drive, St. Louis, MO 63146. Phone: (800) 325-4177. Fax: (314) 432-1380. 1990.

Oxford Textbook of Geriatric Medicine. Evans. Oxford University Press, 200 Madison Ave., New York, NY 10016. Phone: (212) 679-7300. 1992.

Primary Care Geriatrics: A Case-Based Approach. Richard J. Ham, Philip D. Sloane. Mosby-Year Book, 11830 Westline

Industrial Drive, St. Louis, MO 63146. Phone: (800) 325-4177. Fax: (314) 432-1380. Second edition 1992.

Principles of Geriatric Medicine and Gerontology. William R. Hazzard, Reubin Andreas, Edwin L. Bierman, et. al.. McGraw-Hill, Inc., Health Professions Division, 1221 Avenue of the Americas, 28th Floor, New York, NY 10020. Phone: (212) 512-4228. Second edition 1990.

Principles and Practice of Geriatric Medicine. Pathy. John Wiley & Sons, Inc., 605 Third Ave., New York, NY 10158-0012. Phone: (212) 850-6000. Fax: (212) 850-6088. Second edition 1992.

Textbook of Geriatric Medicine and Gerontology. Chernoff. Churchill Livingstone Inc., 650 Ave. of the Americas, New York, NY 10011. Phone: (212) 819-5400. Fax: (212) 302-6598. Fourth edition 1992.

GERMAN MEASLES

See: INFECTIOUS DISEASES

GERONTOLOGY

ABSTRACTING, INDEXING, AND CURRENT AWARENESS PUBLICATIONS

Abstracts in Social Gerontology: Current Literature on Aging. Sage Publications, Inc., 2455 Teller Road, P.O. Box 5084, Newbury Park, CA 91320. Phone: (805) 499-0721. Fax: (805) 499-0871. Quarterly.

Biological Abstracts. BIOSIS, 2100 Arch St., Philadelphia, PA 19103-1399. Phone: (800) 523-4800. Fax: (215) 587-2016.

Current Literature on Aging. National Council on the Aging, 600 Maryland Ave. S.W., Washington, DC 20024. Phone: (202) 749-1200.

Excerpta Medica. Section 20: Gerontology and Geriatrics. Elsevier Science Publishers, P.O. Box 882, Madison Square Station, New York, NY 10159-2101. Phone: (212) 633-3950. Fax: (212) 633-3990. 8/year.

Gerontological Abstracts. University Information Services, Inc., University of Michigan, 5212 School of Dentistry, Ann Arbor, MI 48109-1078. Phone: (313) 764-1555. Bimonthly.

Index to Periodical Literature on Aging. Lorraine Publications, 2162 Chene, Detroit, MI 48207. Phone: (313) 834-4570. Biennial.

New Literature on Old Age. Center for Policy on Ageing, 25/31 Ironmonger Row, London EC1V 3QP, England. 6/year.

ANNUALS AND REVIEWS

Annual Review of Gerontology and Geriatrics. Springer Publishing Co., Inc., 536 Broadway, 11th Floor, New York, NY 10012. Phone: (212) 431-4370.

Reviews in Clinical Gerontology. Cambridge University Press, 40 W. 20th St., New York, NY 10011. Phone: (800) 431-1580. Quarterly.

Year Book of Geriatrics and Gerontology. Mosby-Year Book, 11830 Westline Industrial Drive, St. Louis, MO 63146. Phone: (800) 325-4177. Fax: (314) 432-1380. Annual.

ASSOCIATIONS, PROFESSIONAL SOCIETIES, ADVOCACY AND SUPPORT GROUPS

American Aging Association (AGE). 600 S. 42nd St., Omaha, NE 68198-4635. Phone: (402) 559-4416. Fax: (402) 559-5844.

American Association of Retired Persons. 1909 K St. N.W., Washington, DC 20049. Phone: (202) 872-4700.

Canadian Association on Gerontology. 1565 Carling Ave., Suite 110, Ottawa, ON, Canada K1Z 8R1.

Gerontological Society of America (GSA). 1275 K St. N.W., Ste. 350, Washington, DC 20005. Phone: (202) 842-1275.

Gray Panthers. 1424 16th St. N.W., Suite 602, Washington, DC 20036.

International Association of Gerontology. c/o Dr. Ewald Busse, Duke University Medical Center, Durham, NC 27710. Phone: (919) 684-3416.

National Alliance of Senior Citizens. 2525 Wilson Blvd., Arlington, VA 22201. Phone: (703) 528-4380.

National Council on Aging. 600 Maryland Ave. S.W., W. Wing 100, Washington, DC 20024. Phone: (202) 479-1200.

National Council of Senior Citizens. 925 15th St. N.W., Washington, DC 20005.

CD-ROM DATABASES

Biological Abstracts on Compact Disc. BIOSIS, 2100 Arch St., Philadelphia, PA 19103-1399. Phone: (800) 523-4800. Fax: (215) 587-2016. Quarterly.

HANDBOOKS, GUIDES, MANUALS, ATLASES

Clinical Manual of Geriatrics. Lonergan. Appleton & Lange, 25 Van Zant St., East Norwalk, CT 06855. Phone: (800) 423-1359. Fax: (203) 854-9486. 1992.

Merck Manual of Geriatrics. Merck & Co., Inc., P.O. Box 2000, Rahway, NJ 07065. Phone: (201) 855-4558. Irregular.

JOURNALS

Age and Aging. Oxford University Press, 200 Madison Ave., New York, NY 10016. Phone: (212) 679-7300. Bimonthly.

Archives of Gerontology and Geriatrics. Elsevier Science Publishing Co., Inc., P.O. Box 882, Madison Square Station, New York, NY 10159-2101. Phone: (212) 989-5800. Fax: (212) 633-3990. 6/year.

The Gerontologist. Gerontological Society of America, 1275 K St. N.W., Ste. 250, Washington, DC 20005-4006. Phone: (202) 842-1275. Bimonthly.

Journal of Cross-Cultural Gerontology. Kluwer Academic Publishers, P.O. Box 358, Accord Station, Hingham, MA 02018-0358. Phone: (617) 871-6600. Fax: (617) 871-6528. 4/year.

Journal of Gerontological Nursing. SLACK Inc., 6900 Grove Rd., Thorofare, NJ 08086-9447. Phone: (800) 257-8290. Fax: (609) 853-5991. Monthly.

Journals of Gerontology. Gerontological Society of America, 1275 K St. N.W., Ste. 250, Washington, DC 20005-4006. Phone: (202) 842-1275. Bimonthly.

ONLINE DATABASES

AgeLine. American Association of Retired Persons, 601 E. St. NW, Washington, DC 20049. Phone: (202) 434-6231. Bimonthly.

BIOSIS Previews. BIOSIS, 2100 Arch St., Philadelphia, PA 19103-1399. Phone: (800) 523-4800. Fax: (215) 587-2016.

RESEARCH CENTERS, INSTITUTES, CLEARINGHOUSES

Center on Aging. University of Maryland. College Park, MD 20742. Phone: (301) 405-2469. Fax: (301) 314-9167.

Center for Geriatrics, Gerontology, and Long-Term Care. Columbia University. 100 Haven Ave., Tower 3-29F, New York, NY 10032. Phone: (212) 781-0600.

Center for Gerontological Studies. University of Florida. 3357 Turlington Hall, Gainesville, FL 32611. Phone: (904) 392-2116. Fax: (904) 392-3584.

Center for Gerontology and Health Care Research. Brown University. Box G, Providence, RI 02912. Phone: (401) 863-3490. Fax: (401) 863-3489.

Edward and Esther Polisher Research Institute. Philadelphia Geriatric Center. 5301 Old York Rd., Philadelphia, PA 19141. Phone: (215) 456-2000. Fax: (215) 456-2017.

Ethel Percy Andrus Gerontology Center. University of Southern California. University Park, MC 0191, Los Angeles, CA 90089-0191. Phone: (213) 740-6060. Fax: (213) 740-8241.

Gerontology Center. Boston University. Medical Campus, Boston, MA 02118. Phone: (617) 638-8383. Fax: (617) 638-8387.

Gerontology Center. Pennsylvania State University. S-210 Henderson Bldg., University Park, PA 16802. Phone: (814) 865-1710.

Gerontology Center. University of Georgia. 100 Candler Hall, Athens, GA 30602. Phone: (404) 542-3954. Fax: (404) 542-4805.

Gerontology Center. University of Illinois at Chicago. 2121 W. Taylor St., M/C 922, Chicago, IL 60612. Phone: (312) 996-6310.

Gerontology Institute. University of Massachusetts at Boston. Downtown Center, Boston, MA 02125. Phone: (617) 287-7300.

Institute on Aging. Temple University. University Services Bldg., 1601 N. Broad St., Philadelphia, PA 19122. Phone: (215) 787-6970.

Institute of Gerontology. University of Michigan. 300 N. Ingalis, Ann Arbor, MI 48109-2007. Phone: (313) 764-3493. Fax: (313) 936-2116.

Institute of Gerontology. Wayne State University. 226 Knapp Bldg., 71-C E. Ferry, Detroit, MI 48202. Phone: (313) 577-2297. Fax: (313) 577-4864.

National Institute on Aging Information Center. NIH Bldg. 31, Rm. 5C-35, 9000 Rockville Pike, Bethesda, MD 20892. Phone: (301) 496-1752. Fax: (301) 589-3014.

Policy Center on Aging. Brandeis University. Heller Graduate School, Waltham, MA 02254. Phone: (617) 736-3874. Fax: (617) 736-3881.

Sanders-Brown Center on Aging. University of Kentucky. 101 Sanders-Brown Bldg., Lexington, KY 40536. Phone: (606) 233-6040. Fax: (606) 258-2866.

TEXTBOOKS AND MONOGRAPHS

Aging: Health Care Challenge. Lewis. F.A. Davis Co., 1915 Arch St., Philadelphia, PA 19103. Phone: (800) 523-4049. Fax: (215) 568-5065. Second edition 1990.

Essentials of Clinical Geriatrics. Robert L. Kane, Joseph G. Ouslander, Itamar B. Abrass. McGraw-Hill Inc., 11 West 19th St., New York, NY 10011. Phone: (212) 337-5001. Fax: (212) 337-4092. Second edition 1989.

Geriatric Medicine. Katz. Churchill Livingstone Inc., 650 Ave. of the Americas, New York, NY 10011. Phone: (212) 819-5400. Fax: (212) 302-6598. 1991.

Management and Care of the Elderly: Psychosocial Perspectives. Mary S. Harper (ed.). Sage Publications, Inc., 2455 Teller Road, P.O. Box 5084, Newbury Park, CA 91320. Phone: (805) 499-0721. Fax: (805) 499-0871. 1991.

Oxford Textbook of Geriatric Medicine. Evans. Oxford University Press, 200 Madison Ave., New York, NY 10016. Phone: (212) 679-7300. 1992.

Principles of Geriatric Medicine and Gerontology. William R. Hazzard, Reubin Andreas, Edwin L. Bierman, et. al.. McGraw-Hill, Inc., Health Professions Division, 1221 Avenue of the Americas, 28th Floor, New York, NY 10020. Phone: (212) 512-4228. Second edition 1990.

Principles and Practice of Geriatric Medicine. Pathy. John Wiley & Sons, Inc., 605 Third Ave., New York, NY 10158-0012. Phone: (212) 850-6000. Fax: (212) 850-6088. Second edition 1992.

Textbook of Geriatric Medicine and Gerontology. Chernoff. Churchill Livingstone Inc., 650 Ave. of the Americas, New York, NY 10011. Phone: (212) 819-5400. Fax: (212) 302-6598. Fourth edition 1992.

GINGIVAL DISEASES

See: PERIODONTICS

GINGIVECTOMY

See: ORAL SURGERY

GINGIVOPLASTY

See: ORAL SURGERY

GLAUCOMA

See also: EYE DISEASES; EYE SURGERY;
VISION DISORDERS

ABSTRACTING, INDEXING, AND CURRENT AWARENESS PUBLICATIONS

Core Journals in Ophthalmology. Elsevier Science Publishing Co., Inc., P.O. Box 882, Madison Square Station, New York, NY 10159-2101. Phone: (212) 989-5800. Fax: (212) 633-3990. 11/year.

Current Contents/Clinical Medicine. Institute for Scientific Information, 3501 Market St., Philadelphia, PA 19104. Phone: (800) 523-1850. Fax: (215) 386-6362. Weekly.

Excerpta Medica. Section 12: Ophthalmology. Elsevier Science Publishing Co., Inc., P.O. Box 882, Madison Square Station, New York, NY 10159-2101. Phone: (212) 989-5800. Fax: (212) 633-3990. 16/year.

Index Medicus. U.S. National Library of Medicine, 8600 Rockville Pike, Bethesda, MD 20894. Phone: (800) 638-8480. Monthly.

Ophthalmic Literature. Institute of Ophthalmology, Judd St., London WC1H 9QS, England. 7/year.

Research Alert: Glaucoma, Diabetic Retinopathy & Related Diseases. Institute for Scientific Information, 3501 Market St., Philadelphia, PA 19104. Phone: (800) 523-1850. Fax: (215) 386-6362. Weekly.

Science Citation Index. Institute for Scientific Information, 3501 Market St., Philadelphia, PA 19104. Phone: (800) 523-1850. Fax: (215) 386-6362. Bimonthly.

ANNUALS AND REVIEWS

Year Book of Ophthalmology. Mosby-Year Book, 11830 Westline Industrial Drive, St. Louis, MO 63146. Phone: (800) 325-4177. Fax: (314) 432-1380. Annual.

ASSOCIATIONS, PROFESSIONAL SOCIETIES, ADVOCACY AND SUPPORT GROUPS

American Academy of Ophthalmology (AAO). 655 Beach St., San Francisco, CA 94109. Phone: (415) 561-8500. Fax: (415) 561-8533.

American Society of Contemporary Ophthalmology (ASCO). 233 E. Erie St., St. 710, Chicago, IL 60611. Phone: (312) 951-1400.

Foundation for Glaucoma Research (FGR). 490 Post St., Ste. 830, San Francisco, CA 94102. Phone: (415) 986-3162. Fax: (415) 986-3763.

International Glaucoma Congress (IGC). 233 E. Erie St., Ste. 710, Chicago, IL 60611. Phone: (312) 951-1400.

National Society to Prevent Blindness. 500 E. Remington Rd., Schaumburg, IL 60173. Phone: (800) 331-2020.

CD-ROM DATABASES

SCISEARCH. Institute for Scientific Information, 3501 Market St., Philadelphia, PA 19104. Phone: (215) 386-0100. Fax: (215) 386-6362.

HANDBOOKS, GUIDES, MANUALS, ATLASES

Glaucoma: A Colour Manual of Diagnosis and Treatment. Jack J. Kanski, James McAllister. Butterworth-Heinemann, 80 Montvale Ave., Stoneham, MA 02180. Phone: (617) 438-8464. Fax: (617) 279-4851. 1989.

NEWSLETTERS

Gleams. Foundation for Glaucoma Research, 490 Post St., Ste. 830, San Francisco, CA 94102. Phone: (800) 245-3005. Quarterly.

ONLINE DATABASES

Combined Health Information Database (CHID). U.S. National Institutes of Health, P.O. Box NDIC, Bethesda, MD 20892. Phone: (301) 496-2162. Fax: (301) 770-5164. Quarterly.

EMBASE. Elsevier Science Publishing Co.; Inc., P.O. Box 882, Madison Square Station, New York, NY 10159-2101. Phone: (212) 989-5800. Fax: (212) 633-3990.

MEDLINE. National Library of Medicine, 8600 Rockville Pike, Bethesda, MD 20894. Phone: (800) 638-8480.

SciSearch. Institute for Scientific Information, 3501 Market St., Philadelphia, PA 19104. Phone: (215) 386-0100. Fax: (215) 386-6362.

RESEARCH CENTERS, INSTITUTES, CLEARINGHOUSES

Hermann Eye Center. University of Texas Health Science Center at Houston. Dept. of Ophthalmology, 6411 Fannin St., Houston, TX 77030. Phone: (713) 797-1777.

Wilmer Ophthalmological Institute. Johns Hopkins University. 601 N. Broadway, Baltimore, MD 21205. Phone: (301) 955-6846. Fax: (301) 955-0675.

W.K. Kellogg Eye Center. University of Michigan. 1000 Wall St., Ann Arbor, MI 48105-1994. Phone: (313) 763-1415. Fax: (313) 936-2340.

TEXTBOOKS AND MONOGRAPHS

Applied Pharmacology of Glaucoma. Stephen M. Drance, Michael Vanbuskirk, Arthur H. Neufeld. Williams & Wilkins, 428 East Preston St., Baltimore, MD 21202. Phone: (800) 638-0672. Fax: (800) 447-8438. 1991.

Becker and Shaffer's Diagnosis and Therapy of the Glaucomas. Hoskins. Mosby-Year Book, 11830 Westline Industrial Drive, St. Louis, MO 63146. Phone: (800) 325-4177. Fax: (314) 432-1380. Sixth edition 1989.

Clinical Practice of Glaucoma. William C. Stewart. SLACK Inc., 6900 Grove Rd., Thorofare, NJ 08086-9447. Phone: (800) 257-8290. Fax: (609) 853-5991. 1990.

Complications of Glaucoma Therapy. Mark B. Sherwood, George L. Spaeth (eds.). SLACK Inc., 6900 Grove Rd., Thorofare, NJ 08086-9447. Phone: (800) 257-8290. Fax: (609) 853-5991. 1990.

Glaucoma. Ritch. Mosby-Year Book, 11830 Westline Industrial Drive, St. Louis, MO 63146. Phone: (800) 325-4177. Fax: (314) 432-1380. Two volumes 1989.

Glaucoma Surgery. Obstbaum. Appleton & Lange, 25 Van Zant St., East Norwalk, CT 06855. Phone: (800) 423-1359. Fax: (203) 854-9486. 1991.

The Glaucomas. Robert Ritch, and others. Mosby-Year Book, 11830 Westline Industrial Drive, St. Louis, MO 63146. Phone: (800) 325-4177. Fax: (314) 432-1380. 1991.

The Physician's Guide to Cataracts, Glaucoma and Other Eye Problems. John Eden. Consumer Reports Books, 9180 LeSaint Dr., Fairfield, OH 45014. Phone: (513) 860-1178. 1992.

Textbook of Glaucoma. M. Bruce Shields. Williams & Wilkins, 428 East Preston St., Baltimore, MD 21202. Phone: (800) 638-0672. Fax: (800) 447-8438. Third edition 1991.

Will's Treatment of Eye Disease. Friedberg. J.B. Lippincott Co., 227 E. Washington Square, Philadelphia, PA 19106-3780. Phone: (215) 238-4200. Fax: (215) 238-4227. 1990.

GOITER

See: THYROID DISEASES

GONORRHEA

See: SEXUALLY TRANSMITTED DISEASES

GRANTS

See: RESEARCH SUPPORT

GROUP PRACTICE

See: PRACTICE MANAGEMENT

GROWTH HORMONE DEFICIENCY

See: ENDOCRINE DISORDERS

GUM DISEASES

See: PERIODONTICS

GUNSHOT WOUNDS

See: WOUNDS AND INJURIES

GYNECOLOGIC CANCER

See: BREAST CANCER; OVARIAN CANCER; UTERINE CANCER

GYNECOLOGIC DISORDERS

See also: HYSTERECTOMY; OBSTETRICS AND GYNECOLOGY

ABSTRACTING, INDEXING, AND CURRENT AWARENESS PUBLICATIONS

Core Journals in Obstetrics and Gynecology. Elsevier Science Publishing Co., Inc., P.O. Box 882, Madison Square Station, New York, NY 10159-2101. Phone: (212) 989-5800. Fax: (212) 633-3990. 11/year.

Current Contents/Clinical Medicine. Institute for Scientific Information, 3501 Market St., Philadelphia, PA 19104. Phone: (800) 523-1850. Fax: (215) 386-6362. Weekly.

Excerpta Medica. Section 10: Obstetrics and Gynecology. Elsevier Science Publishing Co., Inc., P.O. Box 882, Madison Square Station, New York, NY 10159-2101. Phone: (212) 989-5800. Fax: (212) 633-3990. 20/year.

Index Medicus. U.S. National Library of Medicine, 8600 Rockville Pike, Bethesda, MD 20894. Phone: (800) 638-8480. Monthly.

ANNUALS AND REVIEWS

Breast Diseases: A Year Book Quarterly. Mosby-Year Book, 11830 Westline Industrial Drive, St. Louis, MO 63146. Phone: (800) 325-4177. Fax: (314) 432-1380. Quarterly.

Contributions to Gynecology and Obstetrics. S. Karger Publishers, Inc., 26 West Avon Rd., P.O. Box 529, Farmington, CT 06085. Phone: (203) 675-7834. Fax: (203) 675-7302. Irregular.

Current Concepts in Endometriosis. Dev. R. Chada, Veasy C. Buttram (eds.). John Wiley & Sons, Inc., 605 Third Ave., New York, NY 10158-0012. Phone: (212) 850-6000. Fax: (212) 850-6088. 1989.

In Development New Medicines for Women. Pharmaceutical Manufacturers Association, 1100 15th St. N.W., Washington, DC 20005. Phone: (202) 835-3400. Annual.

Obstetrics and Gynecology Clinics. W.B. Saunders Co., The Curtis Center, Independence Square W., Philadelphia, PA 19106-3399. Phone: (215) 238-7800. Quarterly.

Year Book of Obstetrics and Gynecology. Mosby-Year Book, 11830 Westline Industrial Drive, St. Louis, MO 63146. Phone: (800) 325-4177. Fax: (314) 432-1380. Annual.

ASSOCIATIONS, PROFESSIONAL SOCIETIES, ADVOCACY AND SUPPORT GROUPS

American Association of Gynecological Laparoscopists (AAGL). 13021 E. Florence Ave., Santa Fe Springs, CA 90670. Phone: (213) 946-8774.

American College of Obstetricians and Gynecologists (ACOG). 409 12th St. S.W., Washington, DC 20024-2188. Phone: (202) 638-5577.

American Gynecological and Obstetrical Society (AGOS). 601 Elmwood Ave., P.O. Box 668, Rochester, NY 14642. Phone: (716) 275-5201.

The Campaign for Women's Health. 666 11th St. N.W., Ste. 700, Washington, DC 20001. Phone: (202) 783-6686.

Endometriosis Association (EA). 8585 N. 76th Pl., Milwaukee, WI 53223. Phone: (414) 355-2200.

International Women's Health Coalition (IWHC). 24 E. 21st St., 5th Flr., New York, NY 10010. Phone: (212) 979-8500.

National Women's Health Network (NWHN). 1325 G St. N.W., Washington, DC 20005. Phone: (202) 347-1140. Fax: (202) 347-1168.

BIBLIOGRAPHIES

Toxic Shock Syndrome. National Technical Information Service, 5285 Port Royal Rd., Springfield, VA 22161. Phone: (703) 487-4650. Fax: (703) 321-8547. June 1979-July 1989 PB90-858655/CBY.

CD-ROM DATABASES

Excerpta Medica CD: Obstetrics & Gynecology. SilverPlatter Information, Inc., River Ridge Office Park, 100 River Ridge Rd., Norwood, MA 02062. Phone: (617) 769-2599. Fax: (617) 769-8763. Quarterly.

OBGLine. Aries Systems Corporation, One Dundee Park, Andover, MA 01810. Phone: (508) 475-7200. Fax: (508) 474-8860. Monthly or quarterly.

Obstetrics and Gynecology MEDLINE. MEP, 124 Mt. Auburn St., Cambridge, MA 02138. Phone: (800) 342-1338. Fax: (617) 868-7738. Quarterly.

DIRECTORIES

Directory of Physicians in the United States. American Medical Association, 515 North State St., Chicago, IL 60610. Phone: (312) 464-0183. Fax: (312) 464-5834. Biennial.

ENCYCLOPEDIAS, DICTIONARIES, WORD BOOKS

Obstetric and Gynecologic Word Book. Helen E. Littrell. Springhouse Publishing Co., 1111 Bethlehem Pike, Spring House, PA 19477. Phone: (800) 331-3170. Fax: (215) 646-8716. 1992.

Obstetric and Gynecological Words. Stedman. Williams & Wilkins, 428 East Preston St., Baltimore, MD 21202. Phone: (800) 638-0672. Fax: (800) 447-8438. 1992.

HANDBOOKS, GUIDES, MANUALS, ATLASES

Atlas of Breast Disease. Volker Barth, Klaus Prechtel. Mosby-Year Book, 11830 Westline Industrial Drive, St. Louis, MO 63146. Phone: (800) 325-4177. Fax: (314) 432-1380. Second edition 1991.

Atlas of Gynecologic Histopathology: A Concise Review. Debra S. Heller, Martin L. Stone. Little, Brown and Company, 34 Beacon St., Boston, MA 02108. Phone: (617) 227-0730. 1992.

Clinical Atlas of Gynecology. Evers. Mosby-Year Book, 11830 Westline Industrial Drive, St. Louis, MO 63146. Phone: (800) 325-4177. Fax: (314) 432-1380. 1990.

Colposcopy: Text and Atlas. Burke. Appleton & Lange, 25 Van Zant St., East Norwalk, CT 06855. Phone: (800) 423-1359. Fax: (203) 854-9486. 1991.

Gynecology on Call. Thomas G. Stovall, Robert L. Summitt Jr., Charles Beckman. McGraw-Hill, Inc., 1221 Avenue of the

Americas, 28th Floor, New York, NY 10020. Phone: (212) 512-4228. Second edition 1992.

Handbook of Gynecology and Obstetrics. Brown. Appleton & Lange, 25 Van Zant St., East Norwalk, CT 06855. Phone: (800) 423-1359. Fax: (203) 854-9486. 1992.

Manual of Outpatient Gynecology. Carol Havens, Nancy Sullivan, Patty Tilton. Little, Brown and Company, 34 Beacon St., Boston, MA 02108. Phone: (617) 227-0730. Second edition 1991.

OB-GYN Secrets: Questions You Will Be Asked...On Rounds, In the Clinic, In the OR, On Oral Exams. Helen M. Frederickson, Louise Wilkins-Haug. Mosby-Year Book, 11830 Westline Industrial Drive, St. Louis, MO 63146. Phone: (800) 325-4177. Fax: (314) 432-1380. 1991.

A Text and Atlas of Integrated Colposcopy. Malcolm C. Anderson, J.A. Jordan, A.R. Morse, F. Sharp. Mosby-Year Book, 11830 Westline Industrial Drive, St. Louis, MO 63146. Phone: (800) 325-4177. Fax: (314) 432-1380. 1991.

Zuspan and Quilligan's Manual of Obstetrics and Gynecology. Jay D. Iams, Frederick P. Zuspan, Edward J. Quilligan. Mosby-Year Book, 11830 Westline Industrial Drive, St. Louis, MO 63146. Phone: (800) 325-4177. Fax: (314) 432-1380. Second edition 1990.

JOURNALS

Clinical Practice of Gynecology. Elsevier Science Publishing Co., Inc., P.O. Box 882, Madison Square Station, New York, NY 10159-2101. Phone: (212) 989-5800. Fax: (212) 633-3990.

International Journal of Gynecological Pathology. Raven Press, 1185 Ave. of the Americas, New York, NY 10036. Phone: (212) 930-9500. Fax: (212) 869-3495.

International Journal of Gynecology and Obstetrics. Elsevier Science Publishing Co., Inc., P.O. Box 882, Madison Square Station, New York, NY 10159-2101. Phone: (212) 989-5800. Fax: (212) 633-3990. 12/year.

Journal of Gynecologic Surgery. Mary Ann Liebert, Inc., 1651 Third Ave., New York, NY 10128. Phone: (212) 289-2300. Fax: (212) 289-4697. Quarterly.

Journal of Women's Health. Mary Ann Liebert, Inc., 1651 Third Ave., New York, NY 10128. Phone: (212) 289-2300. Fax: (212) 289-4697. Quarterly.

NEWSLETTERS

ACOG Newsletter. American College of Obstetricians and Gynecologists, 409 12th St. S.W., Washington, DC 20024-2188. Phone: (202) 638-5577. Monthly.

Endometriosis Association Newsletter. U.S.-Canadian Endometriosis Association, 8585 N. 76th Place, Milwaukee, WI 53223. Phone: (800) 992-3636. Bimonthly.

A Friend Indeed: For Women in the Prime of Life. A Friend Indeed Publications, Inc., Box 515, Place du Parc Sta., Montreal, PQ, Canada H2W 2P1. Phone: (514) 843-5730. 10/yr..

National Women's Health Network-Network News. National Women's Health Network, 1325 G St. N.W., Washington, DC 20005. Phone: (202) 347-1140. Bimonthly.

OB/GYN Clinical Alert. American Health Consultants, Department C1290, P.O. Box 740060, Atlanta, GA 30374. Phone: (800) 559-1032. Fax: (404) 352-1971. Monthly.

Second Opinion and CDRR News. The Coalition for the Medical Rights of Women, 2845 24th St., San Francisco, CA 94110. Monthly.

ONLINE DATABASES

CANCERLIT. U.S. National Cancer Institute, International Cancer Information Center, Building 82, Room 102, Bethesda, MD 20892. Phone: (301) 496-7403. Fax: (301) 480-8105. Monthly.

EMBASE. Elsevier Science Publishing Co., Inc., P.O. Box 882, Madison Square Station, New York, NY 10159-2101. Phone: (212) 989-5800. Fax: (212) 633-3990.

MEDLINE. National Library of Medicine, 8600 Rockville Pike, Bethesda, MD 20894. Phone: (800) 638-8480.

Physician Data Query (PDQ) Cancer Information File. U.S. National Cancer Institute, International Cancer Information Center, Building 82, Room 102, Bethesda, MD 20892. Phone: (301) 496-7403. Fax: (301) 480-8105. Monthly.

Physician Data Query (PDQ) Directory File. U.S. National Cancer Institute, International Cancer Information Center, Building 82, Room 102, Bethesda, MD 20892. Phone: (301) 496-7403. Fax: (301) 480-8105. Monthly.

Physician Data Query (PDQ) Protocol File. U.S. National Cancer Institute, International Cancer Information Center, Building 82, Room 102, Bethesda, MD 20892. Phone: (301) 496-7403. Fax: (301) 480-8105. Monthly.

SciSearch. Institute for Scientific Information, 3501 Market St., Philadelphia, PA 19104. Phone: (215) 386-0100. Fax: (215) 386-6362.

POPULAR WORKS AND PATIENT EDUCATION

Every Woman's Medical Handbook. Marie Stoppard. Ballantine Books, Inc., 201 E. 50th St., New York, NY 10022. Phone: (800) 733-3000. 1991.

The New A-to-Z of Women's Health. Christine Ammer. Facts on File, Inc., 460 Park Ave. S., New York, NY 10016-7382. Phone: (212) 683-2244. Fax: (212) 683-3633. Revised edition.

The New Our Bodies, Ourselves: The Updated and Expanded Edition. The Boston Women's Health Book Collective. Simon & Schuster, 1230 Ave. of the Americas, New York, NY 10020. Phone: (800) 223-2348. Fax: (800) 284-0735. 1992.

Take This Book to the Gynecologist with You: Consumer's Guide to Women's Health. Gale Malesky. Addison-Wesley Publishing Co., Rte. 128, Reading, MA 01867. Phone: (800) 447-2226. 1991.

When a Woman's Body Says No to Sex: Understanding and Overcoming Vaginismus. Linda Valina. Viking Penguin, 375 Hudson St., New York, NY 10014-3657. Phone: (800) 331-4624. 1992.

The Woman's Guide to Good Health. Mary J. Gray, Florence Haseltine, and others. Consumer Reports Books, 101 Truman Ave., Yonkers, NY 10703. Phone: (914) 378-2000. 1991.

Women Talk about Gynecological Surgery: From Diagnosis to Recovery. Amy Gross, Dee Ito. HarperCollins Pubs., Inc., 10 E. 53rd St., New York, NY 10022-5299. Phone: (212) 207-7000. Fax: (800) 242-7737. 1992.

Women's Health Alert: What Most Doctors Won't Tell You About. Sidney M. Wolfe. Addison-Wesley Publishing Co., Rte. 128, Reading, MA 01867. Phone: (800) 447-2226. 1990.

TEXTBOOKS AND MONOGRAPHS

Basic and Advanced Laser Surgery in Gynecology. Michael S. Baggish. Appleton & Lange, 25 Van Zant St., East Norwalk, CT 06855. Phone: (800) 423-1359. Fax: (203) 854-9486. Second edition 1991.

The Breast: Comprehensive Management of Benign and Malignant Diseases. Kirby I. Bland, Edward M. Copeland III. W.B. Saunders Co., The Curtis Center, Independence Square W., Philadelphia, PA 19106-3399. Phone: (215) 238-7800. 1991.

Clinical Gynecologic Oncology. Philip J. DiSaia, William T. Creasman. Mosby-Year Book, 11830 Westline Industrial Drive, St. Louis, MO 63146. Phone: (800) 325-4177. Fax: (314) 432-1380. Fourth edition 1992.

Comprehensive Gynecology. Arthur L. Herbert, and others. Mosby-Year Book, 11830 Westline Industrial Drive, St. Louis, MO 63146. Phone: (800) 325-4177. Fax: (314) 432-1380. 2nd edition, 1991.

Computers in Obstetrics and Gynecology. K.J. Dalton, T. Chard (eds.). Elsevier Science Publishing Co., Inc., P.O. Box 882, Madison Square Station, New York, NY 10159-2101. Phone: (212) 989-5800. Fax: (212) 633-3990. 1990.

Contraception and Mechanisms of Endometrial Bleeding. C. D'Arcangues, I.S. Fraser, J.R. Newton, V. Odlind (eds.). Cambridge University Press, 40 W. 20th St., New York, NY 10011. Phone: (800) 431-1580. 1990.

Current Obstetric and Gynecologic Diagnosis and Treatment. Martin L. Pernoll. Appleton & Lange, 25 Van Zant St., East Norwalk, CT 06855. Phone: (800) 423-1359. Fax: (203) 854-9486. Seventh Edition 1991.

Diseases of the Vulva. Jean Hewitt, Monique Pelisse, Bernard Paniel. McGraw-Hill, Inc., Health Professions Division, 1221 Avenue of the Americas, 28th Floor, New York, NY 10020. Phone: (212) 512-4228. 1991.

Green's Gynecology: Essentials of Clinical Practice. Daniel L. Clarke-Pearson, M. Yusoff Dawood. Little, Brown and Co., 34 Beacon St., Boston, MA 02108. Phone: (617) 227-0730. Fourth edition 1990.

Gynecologic Surgery. David H Nichols. Mosby-Year Book, 11830 Westline Industrial Drive, St. Louis, MO 63146. Phone: (800) 325-4177. Fax: (314) 432-1380. 1992.

Gynecology: Principles and Practice. Zev Rosenwaks, Fred Benjamin, Martin L. Stone, et. al.. McGraw-Hill, Inc., Health Professions Division, 1221 Avenue of the Americas, 28th Floor, New York, NY 10020. Phone: (212) 512-4228. Second edition 1992.

Infections of the Female Genital Tract. Richard L. Sweet. Williams & Wilkins, 428 East Preston St., Baltimore, MD 21202. Phone: (800) 638-0672. Fax: (800) 447-8438. Second edition 1990.

Kistner's Gynecology: Principles and Practice. Kenneth J. Ryan, and others (eds.). Mosby-Year Book, 11830 Westline Industrial Drive, St. Louis, MO 63146. Phone: (800) 325-4177. Fax: (314) 432-1380. Fifth edition 1990.

Laser Surgery in Gynecology and Obstetrics. William R. Keye Jr.. Mosby-Year Book, 11830 Westline Industrial Drive, St. Louis, MO 63146. Phone: (800) 325-4177. Fax: (314) 432-1380. 1990.

Lasers in Gynecology. McLaughlin. J.B. Lippincott Co., 227 E. Washington Square, Philadelphia, PA 19106-3780. Phone: (215) 238-4200. Fax: (215) 238-4227. 1991.

Novak's Textbook of Gynecolgy. Howard W. Wentz III, Anne Colston, Burnett, Lonnie Jones. Williams & Wilkins, 428 East Preston St., Baltimore, MD 21202. Phone: (800) 638-0672. Fax: (800) 447-8438. Eleventh edition 1988.

Office Gynecology. Morton A. Stenchever. Mosby-Year Book, 11830 Westline Industrial Drive, St. Louis, MO 63146. Phone: (800) 325-4177. Fax: (314) 432-1380. 1991.

Pathology for Gynaecologists. Fox. Williams & Wilkins, 428 East Preston St., Baltimore, MD 21202. Phone: (800) 638-0672. Fax: (800) 447-8438. Second edition 1991.

Re-Operative Gynecologic Surgery. David H. Nichols. Mosby-Year Book, 11830 Westline Industrial Drive, St. Louis, MO 63146. Phone: (800) 325-4177. Fax: (314) 432-1380. 1991.

TeLinde's Operative Gynecology. John D. Thompson, John A. Rock. J.B. Lippincott Co., 227 East Washington Square, Philadelphia, PA 19106-3780. Phone: (215) 238-4200. Fax: (215) 238-4227. Seventh edition 1991.

Textbook of Breast Disease. John H. Isaacs. Mosby-Year Book, 11830 Westline Industrial Drive, St. Louis, MO 63146. Phone: (800) 325-4177. Fax: (314) 432-1380. 1992.

Toxic Shock Syndrome. Merlin S. Bergdoll, P. Joan Chesne. CRC Press, Inc., 2000 Corporate Blvd. N.W., Boca Raton, FL 33431. Phone: (407) 994-0555. Fax: (407) 997-0949. 1990.

Transvaginal Ultrasound. Nyberg. Mosby-Year Book, 11830 Westline Industrial Drive, St. Louis, MO 63146. Phone: (800) 325-4177. Fax: (314) 432-1380. Second edition 1992.

GYNECOLOGY

See: GYNECOLOGIC DISORDERS; OBSTETRICS AND GYNECOLOGY

H

HALLUCINATIONS

See: PSYCHIATRIC DISORDERS

HAND SURGERY

See also: ORTHOPEDICS; PLASTIC AND
COSMETIC SURGERY

ABSTRACTING, INDEXING, AND CURRENT AWARENESS PUBLICATIONS

Current Contents/Clinical Medicine. Institute for Scientific Information, 3501 Market St., Philadelphia, PA 19104. Phone: (800) 523-1850. Fax: (215) 386-6362. Weekly.

Excerpta Medica. Section 33: Orthopedic Surgery. Elsevier Science Publishing Co., Inc., P.O. Box 882, Madison Square Station, New York, NY 10159-2101. Phone: (212) 989-5800. Fax: (212) 633-3990. 10/year.

Index Medicus. U.S. National Library of Medicine, 8600 Rockville Pike, Bethesda, MD 20894. Phone: (800) 638-8480. Monthly.

Science Citation Index. Institute for Scientific Information, 3501 Market St., Philadelphia, PA 19104. Phone: (800) 523-1850. Fax: (215) 386-6362. Bimonthly.

ANNUALS AND REVIEWS

Current Opinion in Orthopaedics. Current Science Ltd., 20 N. Third St., Philadelphia, PA 19106-2199. Phone: (800) 552-5866. Fax: (215) 574-2270. Bimonthly.

Year Book of Hand Surgery. Mosby-Year Book, 11830 Westline Industrial Drive, St. Louis, MO 63146. Phone: (800) 325-4177. Fax: (314) 432-1380. Annual.

ASSOCIATIONS, PROFESSIONAL SOCIETIES, ADVOCACY AND SUPPORT GROUPS

American Society for Surgery of the Hand. 3025 S. Parker Rd., Suite 65, Aurora, CO 80014. Phone: (303) 755-4588.

CD-ROM DATABASES

SCISEARCH. Institute for Scientific Information, 3501 Market St., Philadelphia, PA 19104. Phone: (215) 386-0100. Fax: (215) 386-6362.

DIRECTORIES

Directory of Certified Orthopaedic Surgeons. American Board of Medical Specialties, 1 Rotary Center, Suite 805, Evanston, IL 60201. Phone: (708) 491-9091. Biennial.

ENCYCLOPEDIAS, DICTIONARIES, WORD BOOKS

Orthopedic Word Book. Thomas J. Cittadine. Springhouse Publishing Co., 1111 Bethlehem Pike, Spring House, PA 19477. Phone: (800) 331-3170. Fax: (215) 646-8716. 1992.

HANDBOOKS, GUIDES, MANUALS, ATLASES

Atlas of Surgical Anatomy of the Hand. Zancolli. Churchill Livingstone Inc., 650 Ave. of the Americas, New York, NY 10011. Phone: (212) 819-5400. Fax: (212) 302-6598. 1992.

Wrist Arthroscopy: A Text and Atlas. A. Leo Osterman, Robert Temill. Mosby-Year Book, 11830 Westline Industrial Drive, St. Louis, MO 63146. Phone: (800) 325-4177. Fax: (314) 432-1380. 1992.

JOURNALS

Hand Clinics. W.B. Saunders Co., The Curtis Center, Independence Sqare W., Philadelphia, PA 19106-3399. Phone: (215) 238-7800.

Journal of Bone and Joint Surgery: American Volume. Journal of Bone and Joint Surgery, Inc., 10 Shattuck St., Boston, MA 02115. Phone: (617) 734-2835. 10/year.

The Journal of Hand Surgery (American Volume). Mosby-Year Book, 11830 Westline Industrial Drive, St. Louis, MO 63146. Phone: (800) 325-4177. Fax: (314) 432-1380. Bimonthly.

ONLINE DATABASES

EMBASE. Elsevier Science Publishing Co., Inc., P.O. Box 882, Madison Square Station, New York, NY 10159-2101. Phone: (212) 989-5800. Fax: (212) 633-3990.

MEDLINE. National Library of Medicine, 8600 Rockville Pike, Bethesda, MD 20894. Phone: (800) 638-8480.

SciSearch. Institute for Scientific Information, 3501 Market St., Philadelphia, PA 19104. Phone: (215) 386-0100. Fax: (215) 386-6362.

TEXTBOOKS AND MONOGRAPHS

Flynn's Hand Surgery. Jupiter. Williams & Wilkins, 428 East Preston St., Baltimore, MD 21202. Phone: (800) 638-0672. Fax: (800) 447-8438. Fourth edition 1992.

The Hand Book. Ariyan. McGraw-Hill Inc., 11 West 19th St., New York, NY 10011. Phone: (212) 337-5001. Fax: (212) 337-4092. 1989.

Hand Rehabilitation. Clark. Churchill Livingstone Inc., 650 Ave. of the Americas, New York, NY 10011. Phone: (212) 819-5400. Fax: (212) 302-6598. 1992.

Hand Surgery: General Aspects, Elective Surgery. H. Nigst, and others. Thieme Medical Publishers, Inc., 381 Park Ave. S., New York, NY 10016. Phone: (212) 683-5088. Fax: (212) 779-9020. 1988.

Operative Hand Surgery. Green. Churchill Livingstone Inc., 650 Ave. of the Americas, New York, NY 10011. Phone: (212) 819-5400. Fax: (212) 302-6598. Second edition. Three volumes. 1988.

Rehabilitation of the Hand. Hunter. Mosby-Year Book, 11830 Westline Industrial Drive, St. Louis, MO 63146. Phone: (800) 325-4177. Fax: (314) 432-1380. Third edition 1990.

Technical Tips for Hand Surgery. Morton Kasdon, and others. Mosby-Year Book, 11830 Westline Industrial Drive, St. Louis, MO 63146. Phone: (800) 325-4177. Fax: (314) 432-1380. 1992.

HANDICAPPED

ABSTRACTING, INDEXING, AND CURRENT AWARENESS PUBLICATIONS

ERIC. Educational Resources Information Center, U.S. Dept. of Education, 555 New Jersey Ave. N.W., Washington, DC 20208. Phone: (800) 424-1616.

Excerpta Medica. Section 19: Rehabilitation and Physical Medicine. Elsevier Science Publishing Co., Inc., P.O. Box 882, Madison Square Station, New York, NY 10159-2101. Phone: (212) 989-5800. Fax: (212) 633-3990. 8/year.

Rehabilitative Index. The British Library, Boston Spa, Wetherby, W. Yorkshire LS23 7BQ, England. Phone: 0937 546611.

ASSOCIATIONS, PROFESSIONAL SOCIETIES, ADVOCACY AND SUPPORT GROUPS

American Association for Rehabilitation Therapy. P.O. Box 93, North Little Rock, AR 72116.

Canadian Rehabilitation Council for the Disabled. 45 Sheppard Ave. E., Suite 801, Toronto, ON, Canada M4J 3R8. Phone: (416) 250-7490. Fax: (416) 229-1371.

Disabled American Veterans. 3725 Alexandria Pike, Cold Spring, KY 41076. Phone: (606) 441-7300.

BIBLIOGRAPHIES

Library Resources for the Blind and Physically Handicapped. National Library Service for the Blind and Physically Handicapped, Library of Congress, 1291 Taylor St. N.W., Washington, DC 20542. Phone: (800) 424-8567. Fax: (202) 707-0712. Annual.

Nutri-Topics: Nutrition and the Handicapped. Food and Nutrition Center, National Agricultural Library, 10301 Baltimore Blvd., Beltsville, MD 20705.

DIRECTORIES

Directory of National Information Sources on Handicapping Conditions and Related Services. Office of Special Education and Rehabilitative Services, National Institute of Disability and Rehabilitation Research, Dept. of Education, Washington, DC 20202. Phone: (202) 732-1202. Fax: (202) 732-5015. Irregular.

Directory of Organizations Serving People with Disabilities. Commission on Accreditation of Rehabilitation Facilities, 101 N. Wilmot Rd., Ste. 500, Tucson, AZ 85711. Phone: (602) 748-1212. Annual.

JOURNALS

American Journal of Occupational Therapy. American Occupational Therapy Association, 1383 Piccard Dr., P.O. Box 1725, Rockville, MD 20849-1725. Phone: (301) 948-9626. Fax: (301) 948-5512. Monthly.

International Journal of Rehabilitation Research. Heidelberger Verlagsantalt in Druckerei GmbH, Edition Schindele, Hans-Bunte-Str. 18, D-6900 Heidelberg, Germany.

International Rehabilitation Review. Rehabilitation International, 25 E. 21st St., New York, NY 10010.

Journal of Visual Impairment and Blindness. AER, 206 N. Washington St., Alexandria, VA 22314.

Sexuality and Disability. Plenum Publishing Co., 233 Spring St., New York, NY 10013-1578. Phone: (212) 620-8000. Fax: (212) 463-0742. Quarterly.

NEWSLETTERS

Paraplegia News. Paralyzed Veterans of America, 801 18th St. N.W., Washington, DC 20006. Monthly.

ONLINE DATABASES

ABLEDATA. Newington Children's Hospital, Adaptive Equipment Center, 181 E. Cedar St., Newington, CT 06111. Phone: (800) 344-5405. Monthly.

POPULAR WORKS AND PATIENT EDUCATION

A Reader's Guide for Parents of Children with Mental, Physical, or Emotional Disabilities. Cory Moore. Woodbine House, 5615 Fishers Ln., Rockville, MD 20852. Phone: (800) 843-7323. Third edition 1990.

RESEARCH CENTERS, INSTITUTES, CLEARINGHOUSES

Clearinghouse on Disability Information. Office of Special Education and Rehabilitative Services, Switzer Bldg., Rm. 3132, 330 C St. S.W., Washington, DC 20202-2524. Phone: (202) 205-8240. Fax: (202) 205-9252.

Developmental Center for Handicapped Persons. UMC 68, Utah State University, Logan, UT 84322-6800. Phone: (801) 750-1981. Fax: (801) 750-2044.

Disability Rights Center. 1616 P St. N.W., Suite 435, Washington, DC 20036. Phone: (202) 328-5198.

National Information Center for Children and Youth with Handicaps. P.O. Box 1492, Washington, DC 20013. Phone: (703) 522-3332.

National Library Service for the Blind and Physically Handicapped (NLS). Library of Congress, 1291 Taylor St. N.W., Washington, DC 20542. Phone: (800) 424-8567.

National Rehabilitation Information Center (NARIC). 8455 Colesville Rd., Ste. 935, Silver Spring, MD 20910. Phone: (800) 34N-ARIC.

Rehabilitation Research and Development Center. Edward Hines Jr. V.A. Hospital, P.O. Box 20, Hines, IL 60141. Phone: (708) 216-2240.

TEXTBOOKS AND MONOGRAPHS

Activities with Developmentally Disabled Elderly and Older Adults. M. Jean Keller (ed.). Haworth Press, 10 Alice Street, Binghamton, NY 13904-1580. Phone: (800) 342-9678. Fax: (607) 722-1424. 1991.

Disability and Dependency. L. Barton. Taylor & Francis Inc., 1900 Frost Rd., Suite 101, Bristol, PA 19007-1598. Phone: (800) 821-8312. Fax: (215) 785-5515. 1989.

Disabling Diseases. D. Frank. Butterworth-Heinemann, 80 Montvale Ave., Stoneham, MA 02180. Phone: (617) 438-8464. Fax: (617) 279-4851. 1989.

HANSEN'S DISEASE

ABSTRACTING, INDEXING, AND CURRENT AWARENESS PUBLICATIONS

Current Contents/Clinical Medicine. Institute for Scientific Information, 3501 Market St., Philadelphia, PA 19104. Phone: (800) 523-1850. Fax: (215) 386-6362. Weekly.

Index Medicus. U.S. National Library of Medicine, 8600 Rockville Pike, Bethesda, MD 20894. Phone: (800) 638-8480. Monthly.

ASSOCIATIONS, PROFESSIONAL SOCIETIES, ADVOCACY AND SUPPORT GROUPS

American Leprosy Missions (ALM). 120 Broadus Ave., Greenville, SC 29601. Phone: (201) 794-8650.

Damien Dutton Society for Leprosy. 616 Bedford Ave., Bellmore, NY 11710. Phone: (516) 221-5829.

International Christian Leprosy Mission. 6917 S.W. Oak Dr., Portland, OR 97223.

International Federation of Anti-Leprosy Associations. 234 Blythe Rd., London W14 0HJ, England.

Leonard Wood Memorial American Leprosy Foundation. 11600 Nebel St., Rockville, MD 20852. Phone: (301) 984-1336.

Lepra. Fairfax House, Causton Rd., Colchester, Essex C01 1PU, England.

JOURNALS

International Journal of Leprosy and Other Mycobacterial Diseases. American Leprosy Missions, 1 ALM Way, Greenville, SC 29601. Phone: (803) 271-7040. Fax: (803) 271-7062. Quarterly.

ONLINE DATABASES

EMBASE. Elsevier Science Publishing Co., Inc., P.O. Box 882, Madison Square Station, New York, NY 10159-2101. Phone: (212) 989-5800. Fax: (212) 633-3990.

MEDLINE. National Library of Medicine, 8600 Rockville Pike, Bethesda, MD 20894. Phone: (800) 638-8480.

SciSearch. Institute for Scientific Information, 3501 Market St., Philadelphia, PA 19104. Phone: (215) 386-0100. Fax: (215) 386-6362.

RESEARCH CENTERS, INSTITUTES, CLEARINGHOUSES

Gillis W. Long Hansen's Disease Center. U.S. Public Health Service, Carville, LA 70721. Phone: (504) 642-7771.

TEXTBOOKS AND MONOGRAPHS

Leprosy. A.D.M. Bryceson, R.E. Pfaltzgraff. Churchill Livingstone Inc., 650 Ave. of the Americas, New York, NY 10011. Phone: (212) 819-5400. Fax: (212) 302-6598. Third edition 1990.

Leprosy, Racism and Public Health: Social Policy in Chronic Disease Control. Zachary Gussow. Westview Publishing Co., 5500 Central Ave., Boulder, CO 80301. Phone: (303) 444-3541. 1989.

HAY FEVER

See: ALLERGIES

HAZARDOUS WASTE

See: ENVIRONMENTAL POLLUTANTS; INDUSTRIAL TOXICOLOGY

HEAD AND NECK CANCER

See also: CANCER

ABSTRACTING, INDEXING, AND CURRENT AWARENESS PUBLICATIONS

Current Contents/Clinical Medicine. Institute for Scientific Information, 3501 Market St., Philadelphia, PA 19104. Phone: (800) 523-1850. Fax: (215) 386-6362. Weekly.

Excerpta Medica. Section 16: Cancer. Elsevier Science Publishing Co., Inc., P.O. Box 882, Madison Square Station, New York, NY 10159-2101. Phone: (212) 989-5800. Fax: (212) 633-3990. 32/year.

ICRDB Cancergram: Neoplasia of the Head and Neck--Diagnosis, Treatment. U.S. Government Printing Office, Superintendent of Documents, P.O. Box 371954, Pittsburgh, PA 15250-7954. Phone: (202) 783-3238. Fax: (202) 512-2250. Monthly.

Index Medicus. U.S. National Library of Medicine, 8600 Rockville Pike, Bethesda, MD 20894. Phone: (800) 638-8480. Monthly.

Science Citation Index. Institute for Scientific Information, 3501 Market St., Philadelphia, PA 19104. Phone: (800) 523-1850. Fax: (215) 386-6362. Bimonthly.

Statistical Reference Index. Congressional Information Service, 4520 East-West Hwy., Bethesda, MD 20814. Phone: (800) 639-8380. 1980-Present Monthly.

ANNUALS AND REVIEWS

In Development New Medicines for Older Americans. 1991 Annual Survey. More Medicines in Testing for Cancer Than for Any Other Disease of Aging. Pharmaceutical Manufacturers Association, 1100 15th St. N.W., Washington, DC 20005. Phone: (202) 835-3400. 1991.

ASSOCIATIONS, PROFESSIONAL SOCIETIES, ADVOCACY AND SUPPORT GROUPS

American Cancer Society (ACS). 1599 Clifton Rd. N.E., Atlanta, GA 30329. Phone: (404) 320-3333.

National Foundation for Cancer Research (NFCR). 7315 Wisconsin Ave., Ste. 332W, Bethesda, MD 20814. Phone: (800) 321-2875. Fax: (301) 654-5824.

CD-ROM DATABASES

OncoDisc. J.B. Lippincott Co., 227 East Washington Square, Philadelphia, PA 19106-3780. Phone: (215) 238-4200. Fax: (215) 238-4227. Bimonthly.

SCISEARCH. Institute for Scientific Information, 3501 Market St., Philadelphia, PA 19104. Phone: (215) 386-0100. Fax: (215) 386-6362.

ENCYCLOPEDIAS, DICTIONARIES, WORD BOOKS

Oncology Words. Stedman. Williams & Wilkins, 428 East Preston St., Baltimore, MD 21202. Phone: (800) 638-0672. Fax: (800) 447-8438. 1992.

JOURNALS

American Journal of Clinical Oncology. Raven Press, 1185 Ave. of the Americas, New York, NY 10036. Phone: (212) 930-9500. Fax: (212) 869-3495. Bimonthly.

Cancer Causes and Control. Rapid Communications of Oxford Ltd., The Old Malthouse, Paradise St., Oxford OX1 1LD, England. Phone: 44-865-790447. Fax: 44-865-244012. 6/year.

Journal of Clinical Oncology. W.B. Saunders Co., The Curtis Center, Independence Square W., Philadelphia, PA 19106-3399. Phone: (215) 238-7800. Monthly.

Journal of the National Cancer Institute. Superintendent of Documents, P.O. Box 371954, Pittsburgh, PA 15250-7954. Fax: (202) 512-2233. Semimonthly.

ONLINE DATABASES

CANCERLIT. U.S. National Cancer Institute, International Cancer Information Center, Building 82, Room 102, Bethesda, MD 20892. Phone: (301) 496-7403. Fax: (301) 480-8105. Monthly.

Clinical Protocols. U.S. National Cancer Institute, International Cancer Information Center, Building 82, Room 102, Bethesda, MD 20892. Phone: (301) 496-7403. Fax: (301) 480-8105.

EMBASE. Elsevier Science Publishing Co., Inc., P.O. Box 882, Madison Square Station, New York, NY 10159-2101. Phone: (212) 989-5800. Fax: (212) 633-3990.

MEDLINE. National Library of Medicine, 8600 Rockville Pike, Bethesda, MD 20894. Phone: (800) 638-8480.

Physician Data Query (PDQ) Cancer Information File. U.S. National Cancer Institute, International Cancer Information Center, Building 82, Room 102, Bethesda, MD 20892. Phone: (301) 496-7403. Fax: (301) 480-8105. Monthly.

Physician Data Query (PDQ) Directory File. U.S. National Cancer Institute, International Cancer Information Center, Building 82, Room 102, Bethesda, MD 20892. Phone: (301) 496-7403. Fax: (301) 480-8105. Monthly.

Physician Data Query (PDQ) Protocol File. U.S. National Cancer Institute, International Cancer Information Center, Building 82, Room 102, Bethesda, MD 20892. Phone: (301) 496-7403. Fax: (301) 480-8105. Monthly.

SciSearch. Institute for Scientific Information, 3501 Market St., Philadelphia, PA 19104. Phone: (215) 386-0100. Fax: (215) 386-6362.

POPULAR WORKS AND PATIENT EDUCATION

Cancervive: The Challenge of Life After Cancer. Susan Nessim, Judith Ellis. Houghton Mifflin Co., 1 Beacon St., Boston, MA 02108. Phone: (800) 225-3362. 1991.

Everyone's Guide to Cancer Therapy: How Cancer is Diagnosed, Treated, and Managed on a Day to Day Basis. Malin Dollinger, Ernest H. Rosenbaum, Greg Cable. Andrews & McMeel, 4900 Main St., Kansas City, MO 64112. Phone: (800) 826-4216. 1991.

RESEARCH CENTERS, INSTITUTES, CLEARINGHOUSES

Cancer Information Service (CIS). Office of Cancer Communications, National Cancer Institute, Bldg. 31, Rm. 10A24, 9000 Rockville Pike, Bethesda, MD 20892. Phone: (800) 4CA-NCER.

TEXTBOOKS AND MONOGRAPHS

Adenoid Cystic Cancer of the Head and Neck. J. Conley, J.D. Casler. Thieme Medical Publishers, Inc., 381 Park Ave. S., New York, NY 10016. Phone: (212) 683-5088. Fax: (212) 779-9020. 1991.

Cancer: Principles and Practice of Oncology. Vincent T. DeVita. J.B. Lippincott Co., 227 E. Washington Square, Philadelphia, PA 19106-3780. Phone: (215) 238-4200. Fax: (215) 238-4227. 1989 3rd edtion.

Head and Neck Oncology for the General Surgeon. Paul E. Preece, and others. Mosby-Year Book, 11830 Westline Industrial Drive, St. Louis, MO 63146. Phone: (800) 325-4177. Fax: (314) 432-1380. 1991.

Melanoma of the Head and Neck. John Conley. Thieme Medical Publishers, Inc., 381 Park Ave. S., New York, NY 10016. Phone: (212) 683-5088. Fax: (212) 779-9020. 1990.

HEAD AND NECK SURGERY

See: OTOLARYNGOLOGY - HEAD AND NECK SURGERY

HEAD INJURIES

See: WOUNDS AND INJURIES

HEADACHE

See also: PAIN

ABSTRACTING, INDEXING, AND CURRENT AWARENESS PUBLICATIONS

Current Contents/Clinical Medicine. Institute for Scientific Information, 3501 Market St., Philadelphia, PA 19104. Phone: (800) 523-1850. Fax: (215) 386-6362. Weekly.

Excerpta Medica. Section 8: Neurology and Neurosurgery. Elsevier Science Publishers, P.O. Box 882, Madison Square Station, New York, NY 10159-2101. Phone: (212) 633-3950. Fax: (212) 633-3990. 32/year.

Index Medicus. U.S. National Library of Medicine, 8600 Rockville Pike, Bethesda, MD 20894. Phone: (800) 638-8480. Monthly.

Science Citation Index. Institute for Scientific Information, 3501 Market St., Philadelphia, PA 19104. Phone: (800) 523-1850. Fax: (215) 386-6362. Bimonthly.

ASSOCIATIONS, PROFESSIONAL SOCIETIES, ADVOCACY AND SUPPORT GROUPS

American Association for the Study of Headache (AASH). 875 Kings Hwy., Ste. 200, Woodbury, NJ 08096. Phone: (609) 845-0322. Fax: (609) 853-0411.

American Council for Headache Education. 875 King's Highway, Deptford, NJ 08096. Phone: (800) 255-2243.

National Headache Foundation. 5252 N. Western Ave., Chicago, IL 60625. Phone: (312) 878-7715. Fax: (312) 878-2782.

CD-ROM DATABASES

Excerpta Medica CD: Neurosciences. SilverPlatter Information, Inc., River Ridge Office Park, 100 River Ridge Rd., Norwood, MA 02062. Phone: (617) 769-2599. Fax: (617) 769-8763. Quarterly.

SCISEARCH. Institute for Scientific Information, 3501 Market St., Philadelphia, PA 19104. Phone: (215) 386-0100. Fax: (215) 386-6362.

JOURNALS

Headache. American Association for the Study of Headache, 875 Kings Hwy., Ste. 200, Woodbury, NJ 08096. Phone: (609) 845-0322.

Headache Quarterly. International Universities Press, Inc., 59 Boston Post Rd., P.O. Box 1524, Madison, CT 06443-1524. Phone: (203) 245-4000. Quarterly.

Pain and Headache. S. Karger Publishers, Inc., 26 West Avon Rd., P.O. Box 529, Farmington, CT 06085. Phone: (203) 675-7834. Fax: (203) 675-7302. Irregular.

NEWSLETTERS

National Headache Foundation-Newsletter. National Headache Foundation, 5252 N. Western Ave., Chicago, IL 60625. Phone: (312) 878-8815. Quarterly.

ONLINE DATABASES

EMBASE. Elsevier Science Publishing Co., Inc., P.O. Box 882, Madison Square Station, New York, NY 10159-2101. Phone: (212) 989-5800. Fax: (212) 633-3990.

MEDLINE. National Library of Medicine, 8600 Rockville Pike, Bethesda, MD 20894. Phone: (800) 638-8480.

SciSearch. Institute for Scientific Information, 3501 Market St., Philadelphia, PA 19104. Phone: (215) 386-0100. Fax: (215) 386-6362.

POPULAR WORKS AND PATIENT EDUCATION

Defeating Pain: The War Against a Silent Epidemic. Patrick D. Wall, Mervyn Jones. Plenum Publishing Co., 233 Spring St., New York, NY 10013-1578. Phone: (212) 620-8000. Fax: (212) 463-0742. 1991.

Headache: A Special Report. HMS Health Publications Group, P.O. Box 380, Boston, MA 02117. 1991.

The Headache Book. Symour Solomon, Steven Fraccaro. Consumer Reports Books, 9180 LeSaint Dr., Fairfield, OH 43014. Phone: (513) 860-1178. 1991.

Headache Relief. Alan Rapoport, Fred Sheftell. Simon & Schuster, 1230 Ave. of the Americas, New York, NY 10020. Phone: (800) 223-2348. Fax: (800) 284-0735. 1990.

Overcoming Migraine. Betsy Wykoff. Station Hill Press, Station Hill Road, Barrytown, NY 12507. Phone: (914) 758-5840.

RESEARCH CENTERS, INSTITUTES, CLEARINGHOUSES

Baltimore Headache Institute. 11 E. Chase St., Baltimore, MD 21202. Phone: (301) 547-0200.

TEXTBOOKS AND MONOGRAPHS

Headache and Facial Pain: Diagnosis and Management. Alan L. Jacobson, William C. Donlon. Raven Press, 1185 Avenue of the Americas, New York, NY 10036. Phone: (212) 930-9500. Fax: (212) 869-3495. 1990.

Migraine Headache Prevention and Management. Seymour Diamond. Marcel Dekker, Inc., 270 Madison Ave., New York, NY 10016. Phone: (800) 228-1160. 1990.

Migraine and Other Headaches. M.D. Ferrari, X. Lataske. Parthenon Publishing Group, Inc., 120 Mill Rd., Park Ridge, NJ 07656. Phone: (201) 391-6796. 1989.

Practicing Physician's Approach to Headache. Seymour Diamond. Williams & Wilkins, 428 East Preston St., Baltimore, MD 21202. Phone: (800) 638-0672. Fax: (800) 447-8438. Fifth edition 1992.

HEALTH ASSESSMENT

See: DIAGNOSIS

HEALTH CARE ADMINISTRATION

See also: HEALTH MAINTENANCE ORGANIZATIONS; HOSPITALS; NURSING HOMES

ABSTRACTING, INDEXING, AND CURRENT AWARENESS PUBLICATIONS

Excerpta Medica. Section 36: Health Policy, Economics and Management. Elsevier Science Publishers, P.O. Box 882, Madison Square Station, New York, NY 10159-2101. Phone: (212) 633-3950. Fax: (212) 633-3990. 6/year.

Hospital Literature Index. American Hospital Association, 840 N. Lake Shore Dr., Chicago, IL 60611. Phone: (800) 242-2626. Fax: (312) 280-6015. Quarterly.

Index Medicus. U.S. National Library of Medicine, 8600 Rockville Pike, Bethesda, MD 20894. Phone: (800) 638-8480. Monthly.

MEDOC: Index to U.S. Government Publications in the Medical and Health Sciences. Spencer S. Eccles Health Sciences Library, University of Utah, Bldg. 589, Salt Lake City, UT 84112. Phone: (801) 581-5268. Quarterly.

ANNUALS AND REVIEWS

Year Book of Health Care Management. Mosby-Year Book, 11830 Westline Industrial Drive, St. Louis, MO 63146. Phone: (800) 325-4177. Fax: (314) 432-1380. Annual.

ASSOCIATIONS, PROFESSIONAL SOCIETIES, ADVOCACY AND SUPPORT GROUPS

American College of Health Care Administrators (ACHCA). 325 S. Patrick St., Alexandria, VA 22314. Phone: (703) 549-5822. Fax: (703) 739-7901.

American College of Healthcare Executives (ACHE). 840 N. Lake Shore Dr., Ste. 1103W, Chicago, IL 60611. Phone: (312) 943-0544.

American College of Physician Executives (ACPE). 4890 W. Kennedy Blvd., Ste. 200, Tampa, FL 33609. Phone: (813) 287-2000. Fax: (813) 287-8993.

American Health Planning Association. 1110 Vermont Ave. N.W., Washington, DC 20005. Phone: (202) 861-1200.

American Hospital Association (AHA). 840 N. Lake Shore Dr., Chicago, IL 60611. Phone: (312) 280-6000. Fax: (312) 280-5979.

American Osteopathic Hospital Association (AOHA). 1454 Duke St., Alexandria, VA 22314. Phone: (703) 684-7700.

Healthcare Information and Management Systems Society (HIMSS). 840 N. Lake Shore Dr., Chicago, IL 60611. Phone: (312) 280-6147. Fax: (312) 280-4152.

International Society of Health Care Executives. 6416 Bardera Hwy., San Antonio, TX 78238. Phone: (512) 647-5039.

CD-ROM DATABASES

CD Plus/Health. CD Plus, 333 7th Ave., 6th Floor, New York, NY 10001. Phone: (212) 563-3006. Monthly.

Health Planning & Administration/EBSCO-CD. EBSCO Publishing, P.O. Box 325, Topsfield, MA 01983. Phone: (800) 221-1826. Fax: (508) 887-3923. Quarterly.

HealthPlan-CD. SilverPlatter Information, Inc., River Ridge Office Park, 100 River Ridge Rd., Norwood, MA 02062. Phone: (617) 769-2599. Fax: (617) 769-8763. Quarterly.

DIRECTORIES

American College of Health Care Executives Directory. American College of Health Care Executives, 840 N. Lakeshore Dr., Chicago, IL 60611. Phone: (312) 943-3791.

Medical and Health Information Directory. Karen Backus (ed.). Gale Research, Inc., 835 Penobscot Bldg., Detroit, MI 48226-4094. Phone: (800) 877-4253. Fax: (313) 961-6083. Fifth edition Three volumes 1990.

Medical & Healthcare Marketplace Guide. MLR Biomedical Information Services, 2 World Trade Ctr., 18th Flr., New York, NY 10048. Phone: (212) 227-1200. Eighth edition 1992.

ENCYCLOPEDIAS, DICTIONARIES, WORD BOOKS

Facts on File Dictionary of Health Care Management. Joseph C. Rhea, and others. Facts On File, Inc., 460 Park Ave. S., New York, NY 10016-7382. Phone: (800) 322-8755. Fax: (212) 683-3633. 1988.

Health Care Terms. Vergil N. Slee, Debora A. Slee. Tringa Press, P.O. Box 8181, St. Paul, MN 55108. Second edition 1991.

HANDBOOKS, GUIDES, MANUALS, ATLASES

Handbook of Health Care Human Resources Management. Norman Metzger (ed.). Aspen Publishers, Inc., 200 Orchard Ridge Dr., Gaithersburg, MD 20878. Phone: (800) 638-8437. Second edition 1990.

Handbook of Medical Staff Management. Cindy A. Orsund-Gassiot, Sharon S. Lindsey (eds.). Aspen Publishers, Inc., 200 Orchard Ridge Dr., Gaithersburg, MD 20878. Phone: (800) 638-8437. 1990.

JOURNALS

Frontiers of Health Services Management. Health Administration Press, 1021 E. Huron St., Ann Arbor, MI 48104-9990. Phone: (313) 764-1380. Fax: (313) 763-1105. Quarterly.

Health Care Information Management. Health Care Information and Management Systems Society, 840 N. Lakeshore Dr., Chicago, IL 60657. Phone: (312) 280-6148.

Health Care Management Review. Aspen Publishers, Inc., 200 Orchard Ridge Dr., Gaithersburg, MD 20878. Phone: (800) 638-8437.

Health Care Strategic Management. Business World, 730 N. LaSalle St., Chicago, IL 60610. Phone: (800) 521-7210.

Hospital & Health Services Administration. Health Administration Press, 1021 E. Huron St., Ann Arbor, MI 48104-9990. Phone: (313) 764-1380. Fax: (313) 763-1105. Quarterly.

Hospitals. American Hospital Publishing, Inc., 211 E. Chicago Ave., Ste. 700, Chicago, IL 60611. Phone: (312) 440-6800. Semimonthly.

Medical Care Review. Health Administration Press, 1021 E. Huron St., Ann Arbor, MI 48104-9990. Phone: (313) 764-1380. Fax: (313) 763-1105. Quarterly.

NEWSLETTERS

Hospital Administration Newsletter. National Research Bureau, Inc., 424 N. Third St., Burlington, IA 52601. Phone: (319) 752-5415. Fax: (319) 752-3421. Monthly.

ONLINE DATABASES

EMBASE. Elsevier Science Publishing Co., Inc., P.O. Box 882, Madison Square Station, New York, NY 10159-2101. Phone: (212) 989-5800. Fax: (212) 633-3990.

Health Planning and Administration. U.S. National Library of Medicine, MEDLARS Management Section, 8600 Rockville Pike, Bethesda, MD 20894. Phone: (800) 638-8480. Monthly.

MEDLINE. National Library of Medicine, 8600 Rockville Pike, Bethesda, MD 20894. Phone: (800) 638-8480.

SciSearch. Institute for Scientific Information, 3501 Market St., Philadelphia, PA 19104. Phone: (215) 386-0100. Fax: (215) 386-6362.

RESEARCH CENTERS, INSTITUTES, CLEARINGHOUSES

Agency for Health Care Policy and Research Publications Clearinghouse. P.O. Box 8547, Silver Spring, MD 20907. Phone: (800) 358-9295.

Cecil G. Sheps Center for Health Services Research. University of North Carolina at Chapel Hill. Chase Hall, CB 7490, Chapel Hill, NC 27599-7490. Phone: (919) 966-5011. Fax: (919) 966-5764.

Center for Health Management Studies. Rush University. 202 Academic Facility, 1753 W. Harrison St., Chicago, IL 60612. Phone: (312) 942-5402.

Health Services Research and Development Center. Johns Hopkins University. 624 N. Broadway, Baltimore, MD 21205. Phone: (301) 955-6562. Fax: (301) 955-0470.

Health Systems Management Center. Case Western Reserve University. 312 Wickenden Bldg., Cleveland, OH 44106. Phone: (216) 368-2143.

Health Systems Management Group. Yale University. 12 Prospect Place, P.O. Box 1A, New Haven, CT 06520. Phone: (203) 432-5996.

TEXTBOOKS AND MONOGRAPHS

Basic Accounting and Budgeting for Hospitals. Pelfrey. Delmar Publishers, Inc., 2 Computer Dr. W., Albany, NY 12205. Phone: (800) 347-7707. 1988.

Budgeting for Hospital Resource Management. Truman H. Esmond Jr.. American Hospital Association, 840 N. Lake Shore Dr., Chicago, IL 60611. Phone: (800) 242-2626. Fax: (312) 280-6015. 1990.

Effective Hospital-Physician Relationships. Stephen M. Shortell. Health Administration Press, 1021 E. Huron St., Ann Arbor, MI 48104-9990. Phone: (313) 764-1380. Fax: (313) 763-1105. 1990.

Essentials of Hospital Risk Management. Barbara J. Youngberg (ed.). Aspen Publishers, Inc., 200 Orchard Ridge Dr., Gaithersburg, MD 20878. Phone: (800) 638-8437. 1990.

Fiscal Management of Healthcare Institutions. Robert W. Broyles, Michael D. Rosko. Williams & Wilkins, 428 East Preston St., Baltimore, MD 21202. Phone: (800) 638-0672. Fax: (800) 447-8438. 1990.

Health Care Administration: Principles and Practice. Lawrence F. Wolper, Jesus J. Pena (eds.). Aspen Publishers, Inc., 200 Orchard Ridge Dr., Gaithersburg, MD 20878. Phone: (800) 638-8437. 1987.

Health Services Management: Readings and Commentary. Anthony R. Kovner, Duncan Neuhauser (eds.). Health Administration Press, 1021 E. Huron St., Ann Arbor, MI 48104-9990. Phone: (313) 764-1380. Fax: (313) 763-1105. Fourth edition 1990.

Hospital Structure and Performance. Ann B. Flood, Richard W. Scott. Johns Hopkins University Press, 701 W. 40th St., Suite 275, Baltimore, MD 21211-2190. Phone: (800) 537-5487. Fax: (410) 516-6998. 1987.

Introduction to Health Planning. Philip N. Reeves Jr., Russell C. Coile. Information Resources Press, 1110 N. Glebe Rd., Ste. 550, Arlington, VA 22201. Phone: (703) 558-8270. Fax: (703) 558-4979. 1990.

Introduction to Managed Care: Health Maintenance Organizations, Preferred Provider Organizations, and Competitive Medical Plans. Robert G. Shouldice. Information Resources Press, 1110 N. Glebe Rd., Ste. 550, Arlington, VA 22201. Phone: (703) 558-8270. Fax: (703) 558-4979. 1991.

Management of Hospitals and Health Services: Strategic Issues and Performances. Rockwell Schulz, Aeton C. Johnson. Mosby-Year Book, 11830 Westline Industrial Drive, St. Louis, MO 63146. Phone: (800) 325-4177. Fax: (314) 432-1380. Third edition 1990.

Management Problems in Health Care. G. Fandel (ed.). Springer-Verlag New York Inc., 175 Fifth Ave., New York, NY 10010. Phone: (212) 460-1500. Fax: (212) 473-6272. 1988.

Managing Computers in Health Care: A Guide for Professionals. John Abbott Worthley, Philip DiSalvio. Health Administration Press, 1021 E. Huron St., Ann Arbor, MI 48104-9990. Phone: (313) 764-1380. Fax: (313) 763-1105. 1989.

The New Medicine: Reshaping Medical Practice and Health Care Management. Russell C. Coile Jr.. Aspen Publishers, Inc., 200 Orchard Ridge Dr., Gaithersburg, MD 20878. Phone: (800) 638-8437. 1989.

Strategic Management of Hospitals and Health Care Facilities. Carl C. Pegels, Kenneth A. Rogers. Aspen Publishers, Inc., 200 Orchard Ridge Dr., Gaithersburg, MD 20878. Phone: (800) 638-8437. 1988.

HEALTH CARE FINANCING

See also: DIAGNOSTIC RELATED GROUPS

ABSTRACTING, INDEXING, AND CURRENT AWARENESS PUBLICATIONS

Abstract Newsletter: Health Care. U.S. National Technical Information Service, 5285 Port Royal Rd., Springfield, VA 22161. Phone: (703) 487-4929. Fax: (703) 321-8199. Weekly.

Cumulative Index to Nursing and Allied Health Literature. Glendale Adventist Medical Center, P.O. Box 871, Glendale, CA 91209. Phone: (818) 409-8005. Bimonthly.

Excerpta Medica. Section 36: Health Policy, Economics and Management. Elsevier Science Publishers, P.O. Box 882, Madison Square Station, New York, NY 10159-2101. Phone: (212) 633-3950. Fax: (212) 633-3990. 6/year.

Hospital Literature Index. American Hospital Association, 840 N. Lake Shore Dr., Chicago, IL 60611. Phone: (800) 242-2626. Fax: (312) 280-6015. Quarterly.

Index Medicus. U.S. National Library of Medicine, 8600 Rockville Pike, Bethesda, MD 20894. Phone: (800) 638-8480. Monthly.

MEDOC: Index to U.S. Government Publications in the Medical and Health Sciences. Spencer S. Eccles Health Sciences Library, University of Utah, Bldg. 589, Salt Lake City, UT 84112. Phone: (801) 581-5268. Quarterly.

ASSOCIATIONS, PROFESSIONAL SOCIETIES, ADVOCACY AND SUPPORT GROUPS

The Center for National Program Studies. 1493 Cambridge St., Cambridge, MA 02139. Phone: (617) 661-1064.

Healthcare Financial Management Association (HFMA). Two Westbrook Corporate Ctr., Ste. 700, Westchester, IL 60154. Phone: (708) 531-9600. Fax: (708) 531-0032.

CD-ROM DATABASES

CD Plus/Health. CD Plus, 333 7th Ave., 6th Floor, New York, NY 10001. Phone: (212) 563-3006. Monthly.

Health Planning & Administration/EBSCO-CD. EBSCO Publishing, P.O. Box 325, Topsfield, MA 01983. Phone: (800) 221-1826. Fax: (508) 887-3923. Quarterly.

HealthPlan-CD. SilverPlatter Information, Inc., River Ridge Office Park, 100 River Ridge Rd., Norwood, MA 02062. Phone: (617) 769-2599. Fax: (617) 769-8763. Quarterly.

HFCA --On CD-ROM. FD Inc., 600 New Hampshire Ave. NW, Suite 355, Washington, DC 20037. Phone: (800) 332-6623. Fax: (202) 337-0457. Monthly.

Nursing and Allied Health (CINAHL) on CD-ROM. CINAHL, 1509 Wilson Terrace, P.O. Box 871, Glendale, CA 91209-0871. Phone: (818) 409-8005.

DIRECTORIES

Medical & Healthcare Marketplace Guide. MLR Biomedical Information Services, 2 World Trade Ctr., 18th Flr., New York, NY 10048. Phone: (212) 227-1200. Eighth edition 1992.

ENCYCLOPEDIAS, DICTIONARIES, WORD BOOKS

Facts on File Dictionary of Health Care Management. Joseph C. Rhea, and others. Facts On File, Inc., 460 Park Ave. S., New York, NY 10016-7382. Phone: (800) 322-8755. Fax: (212) 683-3633. 1988.

Health Care Terms. Vergil N. Slee, Debora A. Slee. Tringa Press, P.O. Box 8181, St. Paul, MN 55108. Second edition 1991.

JOURNALS

Health Care Financing Administration Manuals. U.S. National Technical Information Service, 5285 Port Royal Rd., Springfield, VA 22161. Phone: (703) 487-4650. Fax: (703) 321-8547.

Health Care Financing Review. Health Care Financing Administration, Oak Meadows Building, 6325 Security Blvd., Baltimore, MD 21207. Phone: (301) 966-6573.

Hospital Cost Management and Accounting. Aspen Publishers, Inc., 200 Orchard Ridge Dr., Gaithersburg, MD 20878. Phone: (800) 638-8437.

Hospitals. American Hospital Publishing, Inc., 211 E. Chicago Ave., Ste. 700, Chicago, IL 60611. Phone: (312) 440-6800. Semimonthly.

Journal of Health Care Marketing. American Marketing Association, 250 S. Wacker Dr., Suite 200, Chicago, IL 60606-5819. Phone: (312) 648-0536. Fax: (312) 993-7542. Quarterly.

Topics in Health Care Financing. Aspen Publishers, Inc., 200 Orchard Ridge Dr., Gaithersburg, MD 20878. Phone: (800) 638-8437.

NEWSLETTERS

American Medical News. American Medical Association, 515 North State St., Chicago, IL 60610. Phone: (312) 464-0183. Fax: (312) 464-5834. Weekly.

Physician's Payment Update. American Health Consultants, Department C1290, P.O. Box 740060, Atlanta, GA 30374. Phone: (800) 559-1032. Fax: (404) 352-1971. Monthly.

ONLINE DATABASES

EMBASE. Elsevier Science Publishing Co., Inc., P.O. Box 882, Madison Square Station, New York, NY 10159-2101. Phone: (212) 989-5800. Fax: (212) 633-3990.

Health Planning and Administration. U.S. National Library of Medicine, MEDLARS Management Section, 8600 Rockville Pike, Bethesda, MD 20894. Phone: (800) 638-8480. Monthly.

MEDLINE. National Library of Medicine, 8600 Rockville Pike, Bethesda, MD 20894. Phone: (800) 638-8480.

Nursing and Allied Health (CINAHL). CINAHL, 1509 Wilson Terrace, P.O. Box 871, Glendale, CA 91209-0871. Phone: (818) 409-8005.

SciSearch. Institute for Scientific Information, 3501 Market St., Philadelphia, PA 19104. Phone: (215) 386-0100. Fax: (215) 386-6362.

POPULAR WORKS AND PATIENT EDUCATION

Marketplace Medicine: The Rise of the For-Profit Hospital Chains. Dave Lindorff. Bantam Books, Inc., 666 Fifth Ave., New York, NY 10103. Phone: (800) 223-6834. 1992.

RESEARCH CENTERS, INSTITUTES, CLEARINGHOUSES

Agency for Health Care Policy and Research Publications Clearinghouse. P.O. Box 8547, Silver Spring, MD 20907. Phone: (800) 358-9295.

Cecil G. Sheps Center for Health Services Research. University of North Carolina at Chapel Hill. Chase Hall, CB 7490, Chapel Hill, NC 27599-7490. Phone: (919) 966-5011. Fax: (919) 966-5764.

Center for Health Management Studies. Rush University. 202 Academic Facility, 1753 W. Harrison St., Chicago, IL 60612. Phone: (312) 942-5402.

Health Care Financing Administration Research Center. University of Minnesota. Division of Health Services Research and Policy, 420 Delaware St. S.E., Box 729, Minneapolis, MN 55455-0392. Phone: (612) 624-5669. Fax: (612) 624-2196.

Health Systems Management Center. Case Western Reserve University. 312 Wickenden Bldg., Cleveland, OH 44106. Phone: (216) 368-2143.

Health Systems Management Group. Yale University. 12 Prospect Place, P.O. Box 1A, New Haven, CT 06520. Phone: (203) 432-5996.

Johns Hopkins University Center for Hospital Finance and Management. 624 N. Broadway, Rm. 300, Baltimore, MD 21205. Phone: (301) 955-2300.

Leonard Davis Institute of Health Economics. University of Pennsylvania. 3641 Locust Walk, Philadelphia, PA 19104-6218. Phone: (215) 898-4752. Fax: (215) 898-0229.

Pittsburgh Research Institute. 5th Ave. Pl., Ste. 1711, Pittsburgh, PA 15222. Phone: (412) 255-7824. Fax: (412) 255-8159.

STANDARDS AND STATISTICS SOURCES

HCFA Statistics. Health Care Financing Administration, Oak Meadows Building, 6325 Security Blvd., Baltimore, MD 21207. Phone: (301) 966-6573. Annual.

Health Care Financing Program Statistics: Medicare and Medicaid Data Book. Health Care Financing Administration, Oak Meadows Building, 6325 Security Blvd., Baltimore, MD 21207. Phone: (301) 966-6573. Biennial.

TEXTBOOKS AND MONOGRAPHS

Driving Down Health Care Costs: Strategies and Solutions. William S. Custer, Carson E. Beadle, Catherine D. Bennett, et. al.. Panel Publishers, Inc., 36 W. 44th St., New York, NY 10109-0247. Phone: (800) 457-9222. 1992.

The Financial Management of Hospitals. Howard J. Berman, Lewis E. Weeks, Steven F. Kukla. Health Administration Press, 1021 E. Huron St., Ann Arbor, MI 48104-9990. Phone: (313) 764-1380. Fax: (313) 763-1105. Seventh edition 1990.

Fiscal Management of Healthcare Institutions. Robert W. Broyles, Michael D. Rosko. Williams & Wilkins, 428 East

Preston St., Baltimore, MD 21202. Phone: (800) 638-0672. Fax: (800) 447-8438. 1990.

Health Care Administration: Principles and Practice. Lawrence F. Wolper, Jesus J. Pena (eds.). Aspen Publishers, Inc., 200 Orchard Ridge Dr., Gaithersburg, MD 20878. Phone: (800) 638-8437. 1987.

The Medical Cost-Containment Crisis: Fears, Opinions, and Facts. Jack D. McCue (ed.). Health Administration Press, 1021 E. Huron St., Ann Arbor, MI 48104-9990. Phone: (313) 764-1380. Fax: (313) 763-1105. 1989.

HEALTH CARE FRAUD AND QUACKERY

ABSTRACTING, INDEXING, AND CURRENT AWARENESS PUBLICATIONS

Consumer Health and Nutrition Index. Alan Rees. Oryx Press, 4041 N. Central, Suite 700, Phoenix, AZ 85012. Phone: (800) 279-6799. Fax: (800) 279-4663. Quarterly.

Index Medicus. U.S. National Library of Medicine, 8600 Rockville Pike, Bethesda, MD 20894. Phone: (800) 638-8480. Monthly.

ASSOCIATIONS, PROFESSIONAL SOCIETIES, ADVOCACY AND SUPPORT GROUPS

American Association of Retired Persons. 1909 K St. N.W., Washington, DC 20049. Phone: (202) 872-4700.

American Medical Association (AMA). 515 N. State St., Chicago, IL 60610. Phone: (312) 464-5000. Fax: (312) 645-4184.

Arthritis Foundation (AF). 1314 Spring St. N.W., Atlanta, GA 30309. Phone: (404) 872-2100. Fax: (404) 872-0457.

National Council Against Health Fraud. P.O. Box 1276, Loma Linda, CA 92354. Phone: (714) 824-4690.

BIBLIOGRAPHIES

The Guide to the American Medical Association Historical Health Fraud and Alternative Medicine Collection. American Medical Association, 515 North State St., Chicago, IL 60610. Phone: (312) 464-0183. Fax: (312) 464-5834. 1992.

JOURNALS

FDA Consumer. U.S. Government Printing Office, Superintendent of Documents, P.O. Box 371954, Pittsburgh, PA 15250-7954. Phone: (202) 783-3238. Fax: (202) 512-2250. Monthly.

Journal of the American Quack Association. Roy Kupsinel, P.O. Box 550, Oviedo, FL 32765.

NEWSLETTERS

Consumer Reports on Health. Consumer Reports, P.O. Box 52148, Boulder, CO 80322. Monthly.

NCAHF Newsletter. National Council Against Health Fraud, Inc., P.O. Box 1276, Loma Linda, CA 92354. Bimonthly.

ONLINE DATABASES

EMBASE. Elsevier Science Publishing Co., Inc., P.O. Box 882, Madison Square Station, New York, NY 10159-2101. Phone: (212) 989-5800. Fax: (212) 633-3990.

MEDLINE. National Library of Medicine, 8600 Rockville Pike, Bethesda, MD 20894. Phone: (800) 638-8480.

SciSearch. Institute for Scientific Information, 3501 Market St., Philadelphia, PA 19104. Phone: (215) 386-0100. Fax: (215) 386-6362.

POPULAR WORKS AND PATIENT EDUCATION

Health Schemes, Scams, and Frauds. Stephen Barrett. Consumer Reports Books, 101 Truman Ave., Yonkers, NY 10703. Phone: (914) 378-2000. 1990.

RESEARCH CENTERS, INSTITUTES, CLEARINGHOUSES

Food and Drug Administration. 5600 Fishers Lane, Rockville, MD 20857. Phone: (301) 443-2410.

HEALTH EDUCATION

ABSTRACTING, INDEXING, AND CURRENT AWARENESS PUBLICATIONS

Consumer Health and Nutrition Index. Alan Rees. Oryx Press, 4041 N. Central, Suite 700, Phoenix, AZ 85012. Phone: (800) 279-6799. Fax: (800) 279-4663. Quarterly.

Cumulative Index to Nursing and Allied Health Literature. Glendale Adventist Medical Center, P.O. Box 871, Glendale, CA 91209. Phone: (818) 409-8005. Bimonthly.

Health Education Index. B. Edsall & Co., Ltd., Greater London House, Hampstead Rd., London NW1, England. 2/year.

Medical Abstracts Newsletter. Communi-T Publications, P.O. Box 2170, Teaneck, NJ 07666. Phone: (201) 836-5030. Monthly.

ANNUALS AND REVIEWS

Advances in Health Education. AMS Press, 56 E. 13th St., New York, NY 10003. Phone: (212) 777-4700. Annual.

ASSOCIATIONS, PROFESSIONAL SOCIETIES, ADVOCACY AND SUPPORT GROUPS

American School Health Association (ASHA). 7263 State Rte. 43, P.O. Box 708, Kent, OH 44240. Phone: (216) 678-1601. Fax: (216) 678-4526.

Association for the Advancement of Health Education (AAHE). 1900 Association Dr., Reston, VA 22091. Phone: (703) 476-3437.

Association of American Medical Colleges. One Dupont Circle N.W., Suite 200, Washington, DC 20036. Phone: (202) 828-0400.

Educational Commission for Foreign Medical Graduates. 3624 Market St., Philadelphia, PA 19104. Phone: (215) 386-5900.

Liaison Committee on Medical Education. Association of American Medical Colleges, One Dupont Circle N.W., Washington, DC 20036. Phone: (202) 828-0670.

National Association of Health Career Schools. 9570 W. Pied Blvd., Los Angeles, CA 90035. Phone: (213) 553-8626.

National Center for Health Education (NCHE). 30 E. 29th St., 3rd Flr., New York, NY 10016. Phone: (212) 689-1886. Fax: (212) 689-1728.

Wellness Councils of America. 1823 Harney St., Ste. 201, Omaha, NE 68102. Phone: (402) 444-1711.

BIBLIOGRAPHIES

Sex Education: A Bibliography of Educational Materials for Children, Adolescents, and Their Families. American Academy of Pediatrics, 141 Northwest Point Blvd., P.O. Box 927, Elk Grove Village, IL 60009-0927. Phone: (800) 433-9016. Fax: (708) 228-1281. Annual.

CD-ROM DATABASES

Family Doctor. CMC ReSearch, Inc., 7150 S.W. Hampton, Suite C-120, Portland, OR 97223. Phone: (800) 262-7668. Fax: (503) 639-1796. Irregular.

Nursing and Allied Health (CINAHL) on CD-ROM. CINAHL, 1509 Wilson Terrace, P.O. Box 871, Glendale, CA 91209-0871. Phone: (818) 409-8005.

Personal Medical Library CD-ROM. EBSCO Publishing, P.O. Box 325, Topsfield, MA 01983. Phone: (800) 221-1826. Fax: (508) 887-3923.

DIRECTORIES

National Healthlines Directory. Louanne Marinos. Information Resources Press, 1110 N. Glebe Rd., Ste. 550, Arlington, VA 22201. Phone: (703) 558-8270. Fax: (703) 558-4979. 1992.

JOURNALS

Health Education Journal. Royal Society of Medicine Services Ltd., 1 Wimpole St., London W1M 8AE, England. Phone: 071-408 2119. Fax: 071-355 3198. Quarterly.

Health Education Quarterly. John Wiley & Sons, Inc., 605 Third Ave., New York, NY 10158-0012. Phone: (212) 850-6000. Fax: (212) 850-6088. Quarterly.

Health Values: The Journal of Health Behavior, Education & Promotion. PNG Publications, P.O. Box 4593, Star City, WV 26504-4593. Phone: (304) 293-4699. Fax: (304) 293-4693. Bimonthly.

NEWSLETTERS

Allied Health Education Newsletter. American Medical Association, 515 North State St., Chicago, IL 60610. Phone: (312) 464-0183. Fax: (312) 464-5834. Bimonthly.

ONLINE DATABASES

Combined Health Information Database (CHID). U.S. National Institutes of Health, P.O. Box NDIC, Bethesda, MD 20892. Phone: (301) 496-2162. Fax: (301) 770-5164. Quarterly.

Health Periodicals Database. Information Access Company, 362 Lakeside Dr., Foster City, CA 94404. Phone: (800) 227-8431. Weekly.

Nursing and Allied Health (CINAHL). CINAHL, 1509 Wilson Terrace, P.O. Box 871, Glendale, CA 91209-0871. Phone: (818) 409-8005.

RESEARCH CENTERS, INSTITUTES, CLEARINGHOUSES

Tel-Med, Inc.. 925 S. Mt. Vernon, Colton, CA 92324. Phone: (714) 825-6034.

TEXTBOOKS AND MONOGRAPHS

Locating Resources for Healthy People 2000 Health Promotion Projects. Public Health Service, Office of Disease Prevention and Health Promotion, Washington, DC 20201. 1991.

HEALTH INSURANCE

See also: DIAGNOSTIC RELATED GROUPS; LONG TERM CARE; MEDICARE AND MEDICAID

ABSTRACTING, INDEXING, AND CURRENT AWARENESS PUBLICATIONS

Cumulative Index to Nursing and Allied Health Literature. Glendale Adventist Medical Center, P.O. Box 871, Glendale, CA 91209. Phone: (818) 409-8005. Bimonthly.

Excerpta Medica. Section 36: Health Policy, Economics and Management. Elsevier Science Publishers, P.O. Box 882, Madison Square Station, New York, NY 10159-2101. Phone: (212) 633-3950. Fax: (212) 633-3990. 6/year.

Index Medicus. U.S. National Library of Medicine, 8600 Rockville Pike, Bethesda, MD 20894. Phone: (800) 638-8480. Monthly.

MEDOC: Index to U.S. Government Publications in the Medical and Health Sciences. Spencer S. Eccles Health Sciences Library, University of Utah, Bldg. 589, Salt Lake City, UT 84112. Phone: (801) 581-5268. Quarterly.

ASSOCIATIONS, PROFESSIONAL SOCIETIES, ADVOCACY AND SUPPORT GROUPS

American Association of Retired Persons. 1909 K St. N.W., Washington, DC 20049. Phone: (202) 872-4700.

Blue Cross and Blue Shield Association (BCBSA). 676 N. St. Clair St., Chicago, IL 60611. Phone: (312) 440-6000. Fax: (312) 440-6609.

The Center for National Program Studies. 1493 Cambridge St., Cambridge, MA 02139. Phone: (617) 661-1064.

Health Care Financing Administration. Oak Meadows Building, 6325 Security Blvd., Baltimore, MD 21207. Phone: (301) 966-6573.

Health Insurance Association of America. 1025 Connecticut Ave. N.W., Washington, DC 20036. Phone: (202) 223-7780.

CD-ROM DATABASES

Health Planning & Administration/EBSCO-CD. EBSCO Publishing, P.O. Box 325, Topsfield, MA 01983. Phone: (800) 221-1826. Fax: (508) 887-3923. Quarterly.

ENCYCLOPEDIAS, DICTIONARIES, WORD BOOKS

Facts on File Dictionary of Health Care Management. Joseph C. Rhea, and others. Facts On File, Inc., 460 Park Ave. S., New York, NY 10016-7382. Phone: (800) 322-8755. Fax: (212) 683-3633. 1988.

JOURNALS

Health Care Financing Review. Health Care Financing Administration, Oak Meadows Building, 6325 Security Blvd., Baltimore, MD 21207. Phone: (301) 966-6573.

Social Security Bulletin. U.S. Government Printing Office, Superintendent of Documents, P.O. Box 371954, Pittsburgh, PA 15250-7954. Phone: (202) 783-3238. Fax: (202) 512-2250. Monthly.

NEWSLETTERS

Parent Care Advisor. American Health Consultants, P.O. Box 71266, Chicago, IL 60691-9987. Phone: (800) 688-2421. Monthly.

ONLINE DATABASES

EMBASE. Elsevier Science Publishing Co., Inc., P.O. Box 882, Madison Square Station, New York, NY 10159-2101. Phone: (212) 989-5800. Fax: (212) 633-3990.

MEDLINE. National Library of Medicine, 8600 Rockville Pike, Bethesda, MD 20894. Phone: (800) 638-8480.

SciSearch. Institute for Scientific Information, 3501 Market St., Philadelphia, PA 19104. Phone: (215) 386-0100. Fax: (215) 386-6362.

POPULAR WORKS AND PATIENT EDUCATION

Avoiding the Medicaid Trap. Armond D. Budish. Avon Books, 1350 Ave. of the Americas, 2nd Flr., New York, NY 10019. Phone: (800) 238-0658. 1991.

A Guide for Senior Citizens: Social Security, Medicare, Legal & Tax Assistance Including an Address and Phone Number Directory. Gordon Press Publishers, P.O. Box 459, Bowling Green Sta., New York, NY 10004. Phone: (718) 624-8419. 1991.

Keys to Understanding Medicare. Jim Gaffney. Barron's Educational Series, Inc., P.O. Box 8040, 250 Wireless Blvd., Hauppauge, NY 11788. Phone: (516) 434-3311. Fax: (516) 434-3723. 1991.

Mastering the Medicare Maze: An Essential Guide to Benefits, Appeals and Medigap Insurance. Betsy Abramson, Jeffrey Spitzer-Resnick, Margie Groom, and others. Center for Public Representation, Inc., 121 S. Pinckney St., Madison, WI 53703-1999. Phone: (608) 251-4008. 1991.

Medicare Made Easy: Everything You Need to Know to Make Medicare Work for You. Charles B. Inlander. Addison-Wesley Publishing Co., Rte. 128, Reading, MA 01867. Phone: (800) 447-2226. Revised edition 1991.

Medicare/Medigap: The Essential Guide for Older Americans and Their Families. Carl Oshiro, Harry Snyder. Consumer Reports Books, 9180 LeSaint Dr., Fairfield, OH 45014. Phone: (513) 860-1178. 1990.

STANDARDS AND STATISTICS SOURCES

The Medicare and Medicaid Data Book. U.S. Health Care Financing Administration, 200 Independence Ave. S.W., Baltimore, MD 21218. Phone: (202) 245-6113. Annual.

National Medical Expenditure Survey: A Profile of Uninsured Americans: Research Findings 1. P.F. Short, A. Monheit, K. Beauregard. National Ctr. for Health Servs. Research and Health Care Technology Assessment, 5600 Fishers Lane, Room 18-05, Rockville, MD 20857. Phone: (301) 443-5650. 1989.

National Medical Expenditure Survey: Estimates of the Uninsured Population, Calendar Year 1987: Data Summary 2. P.F. Short. National Ctr. for Health Servs. Research and Health Care Technology Assessment, 5600 Fishers Lane, Room 18-05, Rockville, MD 20857. Phone: (301) 443-5650. 1990.

Source Book of Health Insurance Data. Health Insurance Association of America, 1025 Connecticut Ave. N.W., Washington, DC 20036. Phone: (202) 223-7780. Annual.

TEXTBOOKS AND MONOGRAPHS

Driving Down Health Care Costs: Strategies and Solutions. William S. Custer, Carson E. Beadle, Catherine D. Bennett, et. al.. Panel Publishers, Inc., 36 W. 44th St., New York, NY 10109-0247. Phone: (800) 457-9222. 1992.

Health Insurance in Practice: International Variations in Financing, Benefits, and Problems. William A. Glaser. Jossey-Bass Inc., 350 Sansome St., San Francisco, CA 94104. Phone: (415) 433-1740. 1991.

The Medical Cost-Containment Crisis: Fears, Opinions, and Facts. Jack D. McCue (ed.). Health Administration Press, 1021 E. Huron St., Ann Arbor, MI 48104-9990. Phone: (313) 764-1380. Fax: (313) 763-1105. 1989.

Medicare and Medigaps: A Guide to Retirement Health Insurance. Susan Hellman, Leonard H. Hellman. Sage Publications, Inc., 2455 Teller Road, P.O. Box 5084, Newbury Park, CA 91320. Phone: (805) 499-0721. Fax: (805) 499-0871. 1991.

Too Poor to be Sick: Access to Medical Care for the Uninsured. Patricia A. Butler. American Public Health Association, 1015 15th St. N.W., Washington, DC 20005. Phone: (202) 789-5600. Fax: (202) 789-5661. 1988.

Understanding Medical Insurance: A Step-by-Step Guide. JoAnn C. Rowell. Medical Economics, Five Paragon Dr., Montvale, NJ 07645-1742. Phone: (800) 222-3045. Fax: (201) 573-4956. 1990.

HEALTH LEGISLATION

See: HEALTH POLICY

HEALTH MAINTENANCE ORGANIZATIONS

See also: HEALTH CARE ADMINISTRATION

ABSTRACTING, INDEXING, AND CURRENT AWARENESS PUBLICATIONS

Cumulative Index to Nursing and Allied Health Literature. Glendale Adventist Medical Center, P.O. Box 871, Glendale, CA 91209. Phone: (818) 409-8005. Bimonthly.

Excerpta Medica. Section 36: Health Policy, Economics and Management. Elsevier Science Publishers, P.O. Box 882, Madison Square Station, New York, NY 10159-2101. Phone: (212) 633-3950. Fax: (212) 633-3990. 6/year.

Hospital Literature Index. American Hospital Association, 840 N. Lake Shore Dr., Chicago, IL 60611. Phone: (800) 242-2626. Fax: (312) 280-6015. Quarterly.

MEDOC: Index to U.S. Government Publications in the Medical and Health Sciences. Spencer S. Eccles Health Sciences Library, University of Utah, Bldg. 589, Salt Lake City, UT 84112. Phone: (801) 581-5268. Quarterly.

CD-ROM DATABASES

Health Planning & Administration/EBSCO-CD. EBSCO Publishing, P.O. Box 325, Topsfield, MA 01983. Phone: (800) 221-1826. Fax: (508) 887-3923. Quarterly.

HealthPlan-CD. SilverPlatter Information, Inc., River Ridge Office Park, 100 River Ridge Rd., Norwood, MA 02062. Phone: (617) 769-2599. Fax: (617) 769-8763. Quarterly.

HFCA --On CD-ROM. FD Inc., 600 New Hampshire Ave. NW, Suite 355, Washington, DC 20037. Phone: (800) 332-6623. Fax: (202) 337-0457. Monthly.

Nursing and Allied Health (CINAHL) on CD-ROM. CINAHL, 1509 Wilson Terrace, P.O. Box 871, Glendale, CA 91209-0871. Phone: (818) 409-8005.

DIRECTORIES

Blue Book Digest of HMOs. National Association of Employers on Health Care Action, 240 Crandon Blvd., Ste. 110, P.O. Box 220, Key Biscayne, FL 33149. Phone: (305) 361-2810. Fax: (305) 361-2842. Annual.

HMO/PPO Directory. Medical Economics, Five Paragon Dr., Montvale, NJ 07645-1742. Phone: (800) 222-3045. Fax: (201) 573-4956. Annual.

Medical and Health Information Directory. Karen Backus (ed.). Gale Research, Inc., 835 Penobscot Bldg., Detroit, MI 48226-4094. Phone: (800) 877-4253. Fax: (313) 961-6083. Fifth edition Three volumes 1990.

ENCYCLOPEDIAS, DICTIONARIES, WORD BOOKS

Facts on File Dictionary of Health Care Management. Joseph C. Rhea, and others. Facts On File, Inc., 460 Park Ave. S., New York, NY 10016-7382. Phone: (800) 322-8755. Fax: (212) 683-3633. 1988.

Health Care Terms. Vergil N. Slee, Debora A. Slee. Tringa Press, P.O. Box 8181, St. Paul, MN 55108. Second edition 1991.

JOURNALS

HMO Magazine. Group Health Association of America, 1129 20th St. N.W., Washington, DC 20036. Phone: (202) 778-3247.

Topics in Health Care Financing. Aspen Publishers, Inc., 200 Orchard Ridge Dr., Gaithersburg, MD 20878. Phone: (800) 638-8437.

ONLINE DATABASES

EMBASE. Elsevier Science Publishing Co., Inc., P.O. Box 882, Madison Square Station, New York, NY 10159-2101. Phone: (212) 989-5800. Fax: (212) 633-3990.

Health Planning and Administration. U.S. National Library of Medicine, MEDLARS Management Section, 8600 Rockville Pike, Bethesda, MD 20894. Phone: (800) 638-8480. Monthly.

MEDLINE. National Library of Medicine, 8600 Rockville Pike, Bethesda, MD 20894. Phone: (800) 638-8480.

Nursing and Allied Health (CINAHL). CINAHL, 1509 Wilson Terrace, P.O. Box 871, Glendale, CA 91209-0871. Phone: (818) 409-8005.

SciSearch. Institute for Scientific Information, 3501 Market St., Philadelphia, PA 19104. Phone: (215) 386-0100. Fax: (215) 386-6362.

RESEARCH CENTERS, INSTITUTES, CLEARINGHOUSES

Agency for Health Care Policy and Research Publications Clearinghouse. P.O. Box 8547, Silver Spring, MD 20907. Phone: (800) 358-9295.

TEXTBOOKS AND MONOGRAPHS

Introduction to Managed Care: Health Maintenance Organizations, Preferred Provider Organizations, and Competitive Medical Plans. Robert G. Shouldice. Information Resources Press, 1110 N. Glebe Rd., Ste. 550, Arlington, VA 22201. Phone: (703) 558-8270. Fax: (703) 558-4979. 1991.

HEALTH POLICY

ABSTRACTING, INDEXING, AND CURRENT AWARENESS PUBLICATIONS

Abstract Newsletter: Health Care. U.S. National Technical Information Service, 5285 Port Royal Rd., Springfield, VA 22161. Phone: (703) 487-4929. Fax: (703) 321-8199. Weekly.

BIOSIS/CAS Selects: Food & Drug Legislation. BIOSIS, 2100 Arch St., Philadelphia, PA 19103-1399. Phone: (215) 587-4800. Fax: (215) 587-2016. Biweekly.

Excerpta Medica. Section 36: Health Policy, Economics and Management. Elsevier Science Publishers, P.O. Box 882, Madison Square Station, New York, NY 10159-2101. Phone: (212) 633-3950. Fax: (212) 633-3990. 6/year.

Hospital Literature Index. American Hospital Association, 840 N. Lake Shore Dr., Chicago, IL 60611. Phone: (800) 242-2626. Fax: (312) 280-6015. Quarterly.

Index Medicus. U.S. National Library of Medicine, 8600 Rockville Pike, Bethesda, MD 20894. Phone: (800) 638-8480. Monthly.

MEDOC: Index to U.S. Government Publications in the Medical and Health Sciences. Spencer S. Eccles Health Sciences Library, University of Utah, Bldg. 589, Salt Lake City, UT 84112. Phone: (801) 581-5268. Quarterly.

ASSOCIATIONS, PROFESSIONAL SOCIETIES, ADVOCACY AND SUPPORT GROUPS

American Association of Retired Persons. 1909 K St. N.W., Washington, DC 20049. Phone: (202) 872-4700.

American Health Planning Association. 1110 Vermont Ave. N.W., Washington, DC 20005. Phone: (202) 861-1200.

The Center for National Program Studies. 1493 Cambridge St., Cambridge, MA 02139. Phone: (617) 661-1064.

Health Policy Advisory Center. 17 Murray St., New York, NY 10007. Phone: (212) 267-8890.

Public Citizen Health Research Group (PCHRG). 2000 P St. N.W., Ste. 700, Washington, DC 20036. Phone: (202) 872-0320.

CD-ROM DATABASES

American Journal of Public Health. MEP, 124 Mt. Auburn St., Cambridge, MA 02138. Phone: (800) 342-1338. Fax: (617) 868-7738. Annual.

CD Plus/Health. CD Plus, 333 7th Ave., 6th Floor, New York, NY 10001. Phone: (212) 563-3006. Monthly.

Health Planning & Administration/EBSCO-CD. EBSCO Publishing, P.O. Box 325, Topsfield, MA 01983. Phone: (800) 221-1826. Fax: (508) 887-3923. Quarterly.

HealthPlan-CD. SilverPlatter Information, Inc., River Ridge Office Park, 100 River Ridge Rd., Norwood, MA 02062. Phone: (617) 769-2599. Fax: (617) 769-8763. Quarterly.

DIRECTORIES

National Health Directory. Aspen Publishers, Inc., 200 Orchard Ridge Dr., Gaithersburg, MD 20878. Phone: (301) 417-7500. Annual.

ENCYCLOPEDIAS, DICTIONARIES, WORD BOOKS

Health Care Terms. Vergil N. Slee, Debora A. Slee. Tringa Press, P.O. Box 8181, St. Paul, MN 55108. Second edition 1991.

JOURNALS

Health Affairs. People-to-People Foundation, Project Hope, Millwood, VA 22646. Phone: (703) 837-2100.

Health Policy. Elsevier Science Publishing Co., Inc., P.O. Box 882, Madison Square Station, New York, NY 10159-2101. Phone: (212) 989-5800. Fax: (212) 633-3990. 9/year.

Journal of Health and Social Policy. Haworth Press, 10 Alice St., Binghamton, NY 13904-1580. Phone: (803) 429-6784. Fax: (607) 722-1424.

The Milbank Quarterly. Cambridge University Press, 40 W. 20th St., New York, NY 10011. Phone: (800) 431-1580. Quarterly.

NEWSLETTERS

American Medical News. American Medical Association, 515 North State St., Chicago, IL 60610. Phone: (312) 464-0183. Fax: (312) 464-5834. Weekly.

Bigel Institute for Health Policy-Newsletter. Bigel Institute for Health Policy. Brandeis University, Heller Graduate School, 415 South St., Waltham, MA 02254. Semiannual.

ONLINE DATABASES

EMBASE. Elsevier Science Publishing Co., Inc., P.O. Box 882, Madison Square Station, New York, NY 10159-2101. Phone: (212) 989-5800. Fax: (212) 633-3990.

Health Planning and Administration. U.S. National Library of Medicine, MEDLARS Management Section, 8600 Rockville Pike, Bethesda, MD 20894. Phone: (800) 638-8480. Monthly.

MEDLINE. National Library of Medicine, 8600 Rockville Pike, Bethesda, MD 20894. Phone: (800) 638-8480.

SciSearch. Institute for Scientific Information, 3501 Market St., Philadelphia, PA 19104. Phone: (215) 386-0100. Fax: (215) 386-6362.

POPULAR WORKS AND PATIENT EDUCATION

America's Health Care Revolution: Who Lives? Who Dies? Who Pays?. Joseph A. Califano Jr.. Simon & Schuster, Inc., 1230 Ave. of the Americas, New York, NY 10020. Phone: (212) 698-7000. 1989.

RESEARCH CENTERS, INSTITUTES, CLEARINGHOUSES

Agency for Health Care Policy and Research Clearinghouse. P.O. Box 8547, Silver Spring, MD 20907-8547. Phone: (800) 358-9295. Fax: (301) 589-3014.

Agency for Health Care Policy and Research Publications Clearinghouse. P.O. Box 8547, Silver Spring, MD 20907. Phone: (800) 358-9295.

American Medical Association Center for Health Policy Research. 515 N. State St., Chicago, IL 60610. Phone: (312) 464-5022. Fax: (312) 464-4184.

Bigel Institute for Health Policy. Brandeis University. Heller Graduate School, 415 South St., Waltham, MA 02254-9110. Phone: (617) 736-3900. Fax: (617) 736-3905.

Center for Health Research. 1315 N. Kaiser Center Dr., Portland, OR 97227-1042. Phone: (503) 335-2400. Fax: (503) 335-2424.

Center for Health Services and Policy Research. Northwestern University. 629 Noyes St., Evanston, IL 60208-4170. Phone: (708) 491-5643. Fax: (708) 491-2202.

Division of Health Policy Research and Education. Harvard University. 25 Shattuck St., Parcel B, 1st Floor, Boston, MA 02115. Phone: (617) 432-1325. Fax: (617) 432-0173.

Health Policy Institute. Boston University. 53 Bay State Rd., Boston, MA 02215. Phone: (617) 353-4520.

Health Policy Institute. University of Texas Health Science Center at Houston. Room 11.160, P.O. Box 20036, Houston, TX 77225. Phone: (713) 792-4975. Fax: (713) 792-4986.

Institute for Health and Aging. University of California, San Francisco. School of Nursing, San Francisco, CA 94143-0612. Phone: (415) 476-3236. Fax: (415) 476-1253.

Institute for Health Policy Studies. University of California, San Francisco. 1388 Sutter St., 11th Floor, San Francisco, CA 94109. Phone: (415) 476-4921.

Policy Information Center (PIC). Department of Health and Human Services, HHH Building, Rm. 438-F, 200 Independence Ave. S.W., Washington, DC 20201. Phone: (202) 245-6445.

RAND Corporation. 1700 Main St., P.O. Box 2138, Santa Monica, CA 90407-2138. Phone: (213) 393-0411. Fax: (213) 393-4818.

HEALTH PROMOTION

See also: CORPORATE FITNESS

ABSTRACTING, INDEXING, AND CURRENT AWARENESS PUBLICATIONS

Consumer Health and Nutrition Index. Alan Rees. Oryx Press, 4041 N. Central, Suite 700, Phoenix, AZ 85012. Phone: (800) 279-6799. Fax: (800) 279-4663. Quarterly.

Cumulative Index to Nursing and Allied Health Literature. Glendale Adventist Medical Center, P.O. Box 871, Glendale, CA 91209. Phone: (818) 409-8005. Bimonthly.

Health Education Index. B. Edsall & Co., Ltd., Greater London House, Hampstead Rd., London NW1, England. 2/year.

MEDOC: Index to U.S. Government Publications in the Medical and Health Sciences. Spencer S. Eccles Health Sciences Library, University of Utah, Bldg. 589, Salt Lake City, UT 84112. Phone: (801) 581-5268. Quarterly.

ANNUALS AND REVIEWS

Advances in Health Education. AMS Press, 56 E. 13th St., New York, NY 10003. Phone: (212) 777-4700. Annual.

ASSOCIATIONS, PROFESSIONAL SOCIETIES, ADVOCACY AND SUPPORT GROUPS

Association for Fitness in Business, Inc.. 310 N. Alabama, Suite A100, Indianapolis, IN 46204. Phone: (317) 636-6621.

The Health Promotion Resource Center. Morehouse School of Medicine, 720 Westview Dr. S.W., Atlanta, GA 30310. Phone: (404) 752-1622.

Wellness Councils of America. 1823 Harney St., Ste. 201, Omaha, NE 68102. Phone: (402) 444-1711.

CD-ROM DATABASES

Nursing and Allied Health (CINAHL) on CD-ROM. CINAHL, 1509 Wilson Terrace, P.O. Box 871, Glendale, CA 91209-0871. Phone: (818) 409-8005.

JOURNALS

American Journal of Health Promotion. American Journal of Health Promotion, 1812 S. Rouchester # 200, Rochester Hills, MI 48307. Phone: (313) 650-9600.

Health Values: The Journal of Health Behavior, Education & Promotion. PNG Publications, P.O. Box 4593, Star City, WV 26504-4593. Phone: (304) 293-4699. Fax: (304) 293-4693. Bimonthly.

NEWSLETTERS

Employee Health and Fitness. American Health Consultants, Department C1290, P.O. Box 740060, Atlanta, GA 30374. Phone: (800) 559-1032. Monthly.

Executive Good Health Report. Executive Good Health Report, P.O. Box 8800, Chapel Hill, NC 27515.

Health Promotion Practitioner. HES, 802 E. Ashman, P.O. Box 1335, Midland, MI 48640-1335. Phone: (800) 326-2317. Fax: (517) 839-0025. Monthly.

Healthy People 2000: Statistics and Surveillance. U.S. Dept. of Health and Human Services. U.S. Govt. Printing Office, Superintendent of Documents, Washington, DC 20402-9325. Phone: (202) 783-3238. Quarterly.

University of California, Berkeley Wellness Letter. Health Letter Associates, Box 412, Prince St. Sta., New York, NY 10003-0007. Phone: (212) 505-2255. Fax: (212) 505-5462. Monthly.

ONLINE DATABASES

Combined Health Information Database (CHID). U.S. National Institutes of Health, P.O. Box NDIC, Bethesda, MD 20892. Phone: (301) 496-2162. Fax: (301) 770-5164. Quarterly.

EMBASE. Elsevier Science Publishing Co., Inc., P.O. Box 882, Madison Square Station, New York, NY 10159-2101. Phone: (212) 989-5800. Fax: (212) 633-3990.

MEDLINE. National Library of Medicine, 8600 Rockville Pike, Bethesda, MD 20894. Phone: (800) 638-8480.

Nursing and Allied Health (CINAHL). CINAHL, 1509 Wilson Terrace, P.O. Box 871, Glendale, CA 91209-0871. Phone: (818) 409-8005.

SciSearch. Institute for Scientific Information, 3501 Market St., Philadelphia, PA 19104. Phone: (215) 386-0100. Fax: (215) 386-6362.

POPULAR WORKS AND PATIENT EDUCATION

Wellness Encyclopedia: The Comprehensive Family Resource. Houghton Mifflin Co., 1 Beacon St., Boston, MA 02108. Phone: (800) 225-3362. 1992.

RESEARCH CENTERS, INSTITUTES, CLEARINGHOUSES

American Institute for Preventive Medicine. 244450 Evergreen Road, Southfield, MI 48075. Phone: (313) 971-6077.

Center for Health Promotion Research and Development. P.O. Box 20186, University of Texas, Houston, TX 77225. Phone: (713) 792-8540.

National Center for Health Promotion. 3920 Varsity Dr., Ann Arbor, MI 48108. Phone: (313) 971-6077.

National Eldercare Institute on Health Promotion. 601 E St. N.W., 5th Flr., Washington, DC 20049. Phone: (202) 434-2200. Fax: (202) 434-6474.

National Resource Center for Worksite Health Promotion. 777 N. Capitol St. N.E., Ste. 800, Washington, DC 20002. Phone: (202) 408-9320.

Office of Health Promotion Research. University of Vermont. 235 Rowell Bldg., Burlington, VT 05405. Phone: (802) 656-4187. Fax: (802) 656-8826.

TEXTBOOKS AND MONOGRAPHS

Connections for Health. Kathleen Mullen, and others. Brown and Benchmark Publishers, 2460 Kerper Blvd., Dubuque, IA 52001. 3rd edition.

Driving Down Health Care Costs: Strategies and Solutions. William S. Custer, Carson E. Beadle, Catherine D. Bennett, et. al.. Panel Publishers, Inc., 36 W. 44th St., New York, NY 10109-0247. Phone: (800) 457-9222. 1992.

Healthy People 2000: National Health Promotion and Disease Prevention Objectives. U.S. Dept. of Health and Human Services. U.S. Government Printing Office, Superintendent of Documents, P.O. Box 371954, Pittsburgh, PA 15250-7954. Phone: (202) 783-3238. Fax: (202) 512-2250. 1991.

Locating Resources for Healthy People 2000 Health Promotion Projects. Public Health Service, Office of Disease Prevention and Health Promotion, Washington, DC 20201. 1991.

HEARING AIDS

See: DEAFNESS

HEARING DISORDERS

See also: AUDIOLOGY; DEAFNESS; TINNITUS

ABSTRACTING, INDEXING, AND CURRENT AWARENESS PUBLICATIONS

Current Contents/Clinical Medicine. Institute for Scientific Information, 3501 Market St., Philadelphia, PA 19104. Phone: (800) 523-1850. Fax: (215) 386-6362. Weekly.

Excerpta Medica. Section 11: Otorhinolaryngology. Elsevier Science Publishing Co., Inc., P.O. Box 882, Madison Square Station, New York, NY 10159-2101. Phone: (212) 989-5800. Fax: (212) 633-3990. 16/year.

Index Medicus. U.S. National Library of Medicine, 8600 Rockville Pike, Bethesda, MD 20894. Phone: (800) 638-8480. Monthly.

Science Citation Index. Institute for Scientific Information, 3501 Market St., Philadelphia, PA 19104. Phone: (800) 523-1850. Fax: (215) 386-6362. Bimonthly.

ASSOCIATIONS, PROFESSIONAL SOCIETIES, ADVOCACY AND SUPPORT GROUPS

Alexander Graham Bell Association for the Deaf (AGBAD). 3417 Volta Pl. N.W., Washington, DC 20007. Phone: (202) 337-5220.

American Hearing Research Foundation. 55 E. Washington St., Suite 2022, Chicago, IL 60602. Phone: (312) 726-9670.

American Tinnitus Association (ATA). P.O. Box 5, Portland, OR 97207. Phone: (503) 248-9985.

Deafness Research Foundation (DRF). 9 E. 38th St., 7th Flr., New York, NY 10016. Phone: (800) 535-3323. Fax: (212) 779-2125.

Helen Keller National Center for Deaf-Blind Youths and Adults (HKNC). 111 Middle Neck Rd., Sands Point, NY 11050. Phone: (516) 944-8900. Fax: (516) 944-7302.

National Hearing Aid Society. 20361 Middlebelt Rd., Livonia, MI 48152. Phone: (800) 521-5247.

National Hearing Aid Society (NHAS). 20361 Middlebelt Rd., Livonia, MI 48152. Phone: (313) 478-2610. Fax: (313) 478-4520.

National Hearing Association. 711 Enterprise Dr., Suite 101, Oak Brook, IL 60521.

CD-ROM DATABASES

SCISEARCH. Institute for Scientific Information, 3501 Market St., Philadelphia, PA 19104. Phone: (215) 386-0100. Fax: (215) 386-6362.

ENCYCLOPEDIAS, DICTIONARIES, WORD BOOKS

Encyclopedia of Deafness and Hearing Disorders. Carol Turkington, Allen Sussman. Facts on File, Inc., 460 Park Ave. S., New York, NY 10016-7382. Phone: (212) 683-2244. Fax: (212) 683-3633. 1992.

JOURNALS

Audiology. S. Karger Publishers, Inc., 26 W. Avon Rd., P.O. Box 529, Farmington, CT 06085. Phone: (203) 675-7834. Fax: (203) 675-7302.

British Journal of Audiology. Academic Press, Inc., 1250 Sixth Ave., San Diego, CA 92101-4311. Phone: (619) 699-6345. Fax: (619) 699-6715.

Ear and Hearing. Williams & Wilkins, 428 E. Preston St., Baltimore, MD 21202. Phone: (800) 638-0672. Fax: (800) 447-8438. Bimonthly.

Hearing Journal. Laux Company, 63 Great Rd., Maynard, MA 01754. Phone: (617) 897-5552.

Hearing Research. Elsevier Science Publishing Co., Inc., P.O. Box 882, Madison Square Station, New York, NY 10159-2101. Phone: (212) 989-5800. Fax: (212) 633-3990. 16/year.

Seminars in Hearing. Thieme Medical Publishers, Inc., 381 Park Ave. S., New York, NY 10016. Phone: (212) 683-5088. Fax: (212) 779-9020. Quarterly.

NEWSLETTERS

American Hearing Research Foundation Newsletter. American Hearing Research Foundation, 55 E. Washington St., Ste. 2022, Chicago, IL 60602. Quarterly.

ONLINE DATABASES

EMBASE. Elsevier Science Publishing Co., Inc., P.O. Box 882, Madison Square Station, New York, NY 10159-2101. Phone: (212) 989-5800. Fax: (212) 633-3990.

MEDLINE. National Library of Medicine, 8600 Rockville Pike, Bethesda, MD 20894. Phone: (800) 638-8480.

SciSearch. Institute for Scientific Information, 3501 Market St., Philadelphia, PA 19104. Phone: (215) 386-0100. Fax: (215) 386-6362.

POPULAR WORKS AND PATIENT EDUCATION

Living with Tinnitus. David W. Rees, Simon D. Smith. St. Martin's Press, 175 Fifth Ave., New York, NY 10010. Phone: (212) 674-5151. 1992.

Living Well with Hearing Loss: A Guide for the Hearing Impaired and Their Families. Debbie Huning. John Wiley & Sons, Inc., 605 Third Ave., New York, NY 10158-0012. Phone: (212) 850-6000. Fax: (212) 850-6088. 1992.

RESEARCH CENTERS, INSTITUTES, CLEARINGHOUSES

Child Study Centre. University of Ottawa. School of Psychology, 120 University Priv., Ottawa, ON, Canada K1N 6N5. Phone: (613) 564-2249. Fax: (613) 564-7898.

Eaton-Peabody Laboratory of Auditory Physiology. Massachusetts Eye and Ear Infirmary, 243 Charles St., Boston, MA 02114. Phone: (617) 573-3745. Fax: (617) 720-4408.

Gallaudet Research Institute. Gallaudet University. 800 Florida Ave. NE, Washington, DC 20002. Phone: (202) 651-5400.

House Ear Institute. 2100 W. 3rd St., 5th Fl., Los Angeles, CA 90057. Phone: (213) 483-4431. Fax: (213) 413-6739.

Kresge Hearing Research Institute. University of Michigan. 1301 E. Ann St., Room 5032, Ann Arbor, MI 48109-0506. Phone: (313) 764-8111. Fax: (313) 764-0014.

National Information Center on Deafness (NICD). Gallaudet University, 800 Florida Ave. N.E., Washington, DC 20002-3625. Phone: (202) 651-5051. Fax: (202) 651-5463.

National Institute on Deafness and Other Communications Disorders. NIH Bldg. 31, 9000 Rockville Pike, Bethesda, MD 20892. Phone: (301) 496-7243.

Self-Help for Hard of Hearing People. 7800 Wisconsin Ave., Bethesda, MD 20814. Phone: (301) 657-2248.

STANDARDS AND STATISTICS SOURCES

Noise and Hearing Loss. Consensus Statement. NIH Consensus Development Conference. January 22-24, 1990. National Institutes of Health, Office of Medical Applications of Research, Federal Bldg., Rm. 618, Bethesda, MD 20892. 1990.

TEXTBOOKS AND MONOGRAPHS

Hearing: An Introduction to Psychological and Physical. Marcel Dekker, Inc., 270 Madison Ave., New York, NY 10016. Phone: (800) 228-1160.

Noise-Induced Hearing Loss. Dancer. Mosby-Year Book, 11830 Westline Industrial Drive, St. Louis, MO 63146. Phone: (800) 325-4177. Fax: (314) 432-1380. 1992.

HEARING TESTS

See: HEARING DISORDERS

HEART ATTACK

See: HEART DISEASES

HEART DISEASES

See also: ARRHYTHMIA; ATHEROSCLEROSIS;
CARDIOLOGY; CARDIOVASCULAR
SURGERY; VASCULAR DISEASES

ABSTRACTING, INDEXING, AND CURRENT AWARENESS PUBLICATIONS

Biological Abstracts. BIOSIS, 2100 Arch St., Philadelphia, PA 19103-1399. Phone: (800) 523-4800. Fax: (215) 587-2016.

BIOSIS/CAS Selects: Antiarrhythmic Drugs. BIOSIS, 2100 Arch St., Philadelphia, PA 19103-1399. Phone: (215) 587-4800. Fax: (215) 587-2016. Biweekly.

CA Selects: Atherosclerosis & Heart Disease. Chemical Abstracts Service, 2540 Olentangy River Road, P.O. Box 3012, Columbus, OH 43210-0012. Phone: (800) 848-6538. Biweekly.

CA Selects: Calcium Channel Blockers. Chemical Abstracts Service, 2540 Olentangy River Road, P.O. Box 3012, Columbus, OH 43210-0012. Phone: (800) 848-6538. Biweekly.

Core Journals in Cardiology. Elsevier Science Publishing Co., Inc., P.O. Box 882, Madison Square Station, New York, NY 10159-2101. Phone: (212) 989-5800. Fax: (212) 633-3990. 11/year.

Current Contents/Clinical Medicine. Institute for Scientific Information, 3501 Market St., Philadelphia, PA 19104. Phone: (800) 523-1850. Fax: (215) 386-6362. Weekly.

Current Contents/Life Sciences. Institute for Scientific Information, 3501 Market St., Philadelphia, PA 19104. Phone: (215) 386-0100. Fax: (215) 386-6362.

Excerpta Medica. Section 18: Cardiovascular Disease and Cardiovascular Surgery. Elsevier Science Publishing Co., Inc., P.O. Box 882, Madison Square Station, New York, NY 10159-2101. Phone: (212) 989-5800. Fax: (212) 633-3990. 24/year.

Index Medicus. U.S. National Library of Medicine, 8600 Rockville Pike, Bethesda, MD 20894. Phone: (800) 638-8480. Monthly.

Research Alert: Angina Pectoris/Antianginal Drugs. Institute for Scientific Information, 3501 Market St., Philadelphia, PA 19104. Phone: (800) 523-1850. Fax: (215) 386-6362. Weekly.

Research Alert: Antiarrhythmial Drugs. Institute for Scientific Information, 3501 Market St., Philadelphia, PA 19104. Phone: (800) 523-1850. Fax: (215) 386-6362. Weekly.

Research Alert: Cardiovascular Diseases-Coronary Disease & Myocardial Infarction. Institute for Scientific Information, 3501 Market St., Philadelphia, PA 19104. Phone: (800) 523-1850. Fax: (215) 386-6362. Weekly.

Research Alert: Cardiovascular Diseases-Interventional Cardiology. Institute for Scientific Information, 3501 Market St., Philadelphia, PA 19104. Phone: (800) 523-1850. Fax: (215) 386-6362. Weekly.

Research Alert: Cardiovascular Research & Regulation. Institute for Scientific Information, 3501 Market St.,
Philadelphia, PA 19104. Phone: (800) 523-1850. Fax: (215) 386-6362. Weekly.

Science Citation Index. Institute for Scientific Information, 3501 Market St., Philadelphia, PA 19104. Phone: (800) 523-1850. Fax: (215) 386-6362. Bimonthly.

ANNUALS AND REVIEWS

Acute Myocardial Infarction. Bernard Gersh, Shahbudin H. Rahimtoola (eds.). Elsevier Science Publishing Co., Inc., P.O. Box 882, Madison Square Station, New York, NY 10159-2101. Phone: (212) 989-5800. Fax: (212) 633-3990. 1991.

Cardiology. Butterworth-Heinemann, 80 Montvale Ave., Stoneham, MA 02180. Phone: (617) 438-8464. Fax: (617) 279-4851. Annual.

Cardiology Clinics. W.B. Saunders Co., The Curtis Center, Independence Square W., Philadelphia, PA 19106-3399. Phone: (215) 238-7800. Quarterly.

Cardiovascular Clinics. F.A. Davis Co., 1915 Arch St., Philadelphia, PA 19103. Phone: (800) 523-4049. 3/year.

Current Opinion in Cardiology. Current Science Group, 20 N. Third St., Philadelphia, PA 19106-2199. Phone: (800) 552-5866. Fax: (215) 574-2270. Bimonthly.

Current Problems in Cardiology. Mosby-Year Book, 11830 Westline Industrial Drive, St. Louis, MO 63146. Phone: (800) 325-4177. Fax: (314) 432-1380. Monthly.

In Development New Medicines for Older Americans. 1991 Annual Survey. 93 Cardiovascular, Cerebrovascular Medicines in Testing for Top Causes of Death. Pharmaceutical Manufacturers Association, 1100 15th St. N.W., Washington, DC 20005. Phone: (202) 835-3400. 1991.

Progress in Cardiology. Lea & Febiger, 428 East Preston St., Baltimore, MD 21202. Phone: (800) 638-0672. Fax: (800) 447-8438. Semiannual.

Year Book of Cardiology. Mosby-Year Book, 11830 Westline Industrial Drive, St. Louis, MO 63146. Phone: (800) 325-4177. Fax: (314) 432-1380. Annual.

ASSOCIATIONS, PROFESSIONAL SOCIETIES, ADVOCACY AND SUPPORT GROUPS

American College of Cardiology (ACC). 9111 Old Georgetown Rd., Bethesda, MD 20814. Phone: (800) 253-4636. Fax: (301) 897-9745.

American Heart Association (AHA). 7320 Greenville Ave., Dallas, TX 75231. Phone: (214) 373-6300.

American Society of Echocardiography (ASE). 4101 Lake Boone Trail, Suite 201, Raleigh, NC 27607. Phone: (919) 787-5181.

Association of Black Cardiologists (ABC). 2300 Garrison Blvd., Suite 150, Baltimore, MD 21216. Phone: (301) 945-2525.

Coronary Club (CC). 9500 Euclid Ave., Cleveland, OH 44106. Phone: (216) 444-3690.

International Society for Cardiovascular Surgery (ICVS). 13 Elm St., P.O. Box 1565, Manchester, MA 01944. Phone: (508) 526-8330. Fax: (508) 526-4018.

Michael E. DeBakey International Surgical Society (MEDISS). 1 Baylor Plaza, Dept. of Surgery, Houston, TX 77030. Phone: (713) 798-4557.

BIBLIOGRAPHIES

Childhood Obesity and Cardiovascular Disease. Food and Nutrition Center, National Agricultural Library, 10301 Baltimore Blvd., Beltsville, MD 20705. January 1985 - May 1990.

Nutri-Topics: Nutrition and Cardiovascular Disease. Food and Nutrition Center, National Agricultural Library, 10301 Baltimore Blvd., Beltsville, MD 20705.

Streptokinase: An Agent Used to Dissolve Blood Clots. National Technical Information Service, 5285 Port Royal Rd., Springfield, VA 22161. Phone: (703) 487-4650. Fax: (703) 321-8547. Jan. 1978-Jan. 1989 PB89-855522/CBY.

Tissue Plasminogen Activator (TP-A): An Agent Used to Dissolve Blood Clots. National Technical Information Service, 5285 Port Royal Rd., Springfield, VA 22161. Phone: (703) 487-4650. Fax: (703) 321-8547. Jan. 1978-Jan. 1989 PB89-855407/CBY.

Tissue Plasminogen Activator (TP-A) and Streptokinase: Thrombolytic Drugs Market. National Technical Information Service, 5285 Port Royal Rd., Springfield, VA 22161. Phone: (703) 487-4650. Fax: (703) 321-8547. Jan. 1985 - Jan. 1989. NTIS order no.: PB89-855506/CBY.

CD-ROM DATABASES

Bibliomed Cardiology Disc. Healthcare Information Services, Inc., 2235 American River Dr., Suite 307, Sacramento, CA 95825. Phone: (800) 468-1128. Fax: (916) 648-8078. Quarterly.

Biological Abstracts on Compact Disc. BIOSIS, 2100 Arch St., Philadelphia, PA 19103-1399. Phone: (800) 523-4800. Fax: (215) 587-2016. Quarterly.

Cardiology MEDLINE. MEP, 124 Mt. Auburn St., Cambridge, MA 02138. Phone: (800) 342-1338. Fax: (617) 868-7738. Quarterly.

CardLine. Aries Systems Corporation, One Dundee Park, Andover, MA 01810. Phone: (508) 475-7200. Fax: (508) 474-8860. Monthly or quarterly.

Chest Pain. Hoffer. Williams & Wilkins, 428 East Preston St., Baltimore, MD 21202. Phone: (800) 638-0672. Fax: (800) 447-8438. 1987.

Excerpta Medica CD: Cardiology. SilverPlatter Information, Inc., River Ridge Office Park, 100 River Ridge Rd., Norwood, MA 02062. Phone: (617) 769-2599. Fax: (617) 769-8763. Quarterly.

Heartlab. Bergeron. Williams & Wilkins, 428 East Preston St., Baltimore, MD 21202. Phone: (800) 638-0672. Fax: (800) 447-8438. 1991.

Hyperlipidemia. Hoffer. Williams & Wilkins, 428 East Preston St., Baltimore, MD 21202. Phone: (800) 638-0672. Fax: (800) 447-8438. 1992.

Morbidity Mortality Weekly Report. MEP, 124 Mt. Auburn St., Cambridge, MA 02138. Phone: (800) 342-1338. Fax: (617) 868-7738. Annual.

SCISEARCH. Institute for Scientific Information, 3501 Market St., Philadelphia, PA 19104. Phone: (215) 386-0100. Fax: (215) 386-6362.

Year Books on Disc. CMC ReSearch, Inc., 7150 S.W. Hampton, Suite C-120, Portland, OR 97223. Phone: (800) 262-7668. Fax: (503) 639-1796. Annual includes Year Books of Cardiology, Dermatology, Diagnostic Radiology, Drug Therapy, Emergency Medicine, Family Practice, Medicine, Neurology and Neurosurgery, Obstetrics and Gynecology, Oncology, Pediatrics, and Psychiatry and Applied Mental Health.

ENCYCLOPEDIAS, DICTIONARIES, WORD BOOKS

Cardiology Words. Stedman. Williams & Wilkins, 428 East Preston St., Baltimore, MD 21202. Phone: (800) 638-0672. Fax: (800) 447-8438. 1992.

Cardiovascular and Pulmonary Word Book. Helen E. Littrell. Springhouse Publishing Co., 1111 Bethlehem Pike, Spring House, PA 19477. Phone: (800) 331-3170. Fax: (215) 646-8716. 1992.

Clinician's Illustrated Dictionary of Cardiology. R.H. Anderson, P.J. Oldershaw, R. Dawson, E. Rowland. Science Press Ltd., 20 N. Third St., Philadelphia, PA 19106-2199. Phone: (800) 552-5866. Fax: (215) 574-2270. Second edition 1991.

HANDBOOKS, GUIDES, MANUALS, ATLASES

Cardiology Drug Facts. Ezra A. Amsterdam, Jonathan Abrams, Dale Berg, and others. J.B. Lippincott Co., 227 E. Washington Square, Philadelphia, PA 19106-3780. Phone: (215) 238-4200. Fax: (215) 238-4227. 1990.

Color Atlas of Heart Disease: Pathological, Clinical and Investigatory Features. George C. Sutton, Kim Fox. J.B. Lippincott Co., 227 E. Washington Square, Philadelphia, PA 19106-3780. Phone: (215) 238-4200. Fax: (215) 238-4227. 1990.

Handbook of Cardiac Drugs. Ralph Purdy, Robert Boucek. Little, Brown and Co., 34 Beacon St., Boston, MA 02108. Phone: (617) 227-0730. Fax: (617) 227-0790. 1988.

The Heart: Companion Handbook. Robert C. Schlant, J. Willis Hurst. McGraw-Hill, Inc., 1221 Avenue of the Americas, 28th Floor, New York, NY 10020. Phone: (212) 512-4228. Seventh edition 1990.

Manual of Cardiovascular Diagnosis and Therapy. Joseph S. Alpert, James M. Rippe. Little, Brown and Co., 34 Beacon St., Boston, MA 02108. Phone: (617) 227-0730. Third edition 1988.

Manual of Clinical Problems in Cardiology. L. David Hillis, Peter J. Wells, Michael D. Winniford (eds.). Little, Brown and Co., 34 Beacon St., Boston, MA 02108. Phone: (617) 227-0730. Fourth edition 1992.

Manual of Coronary Care. Joseph S. Alpert, Gary S. Francis. Little, Brown and Co., 34 Beacon St., Boston, MA 02108. Phone: (617) 227-0730. Fourth edition 1987.

Random House Personal Medical Handbook: For People with Heart Disease. Paula Dranov. Random House, Inc., 201 E. 50th St., New York, NY 10022. Phone: (800) 726-0600. 1990.

JOURNALS

American Heart Journal. Mosby-Year Book, 11830 Westline Industrial Drive, St. Louis, MO 63146. Phone: (800) 325-4177. Fax: (314) 432-1380. Monthly.

American Journal of Cardiology. Reed Publising USA, 249 W. 17th St., New York, NY 10011. Phone: (212) 645-0067. Fax: (212) 242-6987. 22/year.

British Heart Journal. BMJ Publishing Group, BMA House, Tavistock Square, London WC1H 9JR, England. Phone: 071383 6244/6638. Fax: 071383 6662. Monthly.

Cardiology. S. Karger Publishers, Inc., 26 W. Avon Rd., P.O. Box 529, Farmington, CT 06085. Phone: (203) 675-7834. Fax: (203) 675-7302. Bimonthly.

Cardiology in the Elderly. Current Science Group, 20 North Third St., Philadelphia, PA 19106-2199. Phone: (215) 574-2266. Fax: (215) 574-2270. Bimonthly.

Cardiology in Review. Williams & Wilkins, 428 E. Preston St., Baltimore, MD 21202. Phone: (800) 638-0672. Fax: (800) 447-8438. 6/year.

Cardiovascular Research. BMJ Publishing Group, BMA House, Tavistock Square, London WC1H 9JR, England. Phone: 071-383 6244/6638. Fax: 071-383 6662. Monthly.

Catheterization and Cardiovascular Diagnosis. John Wiley & Sons, Inc., 605 Third Ave., New York, NY 10158-0012. Phone: (212) 850-6000. Fax: (212) 850-6088. Monthly.

Circulation. American Heart Association, 7320 Greenville Ave., Dallas, TX 75231-4599. Phone: (214) 706-1310. Fax: (214) 691-2704. Monthly.

Circulation Research. American Heart Association, 7320 Greenville Ave., Dallas, TX 75231. Phone: (214) 706-1310. Fax: (214) 691-6342. Monthly.

Coronary Artery Disease. Current Science Group, 20 N. Third St., Philadelphia, PA 19106-2199. Phone: (215) 574-2266. Fax: (215) 574-2270. Monthly.

European Heart Journal. Academic Press, Inc., 1250 Sixth Ave., San Diego, CA 92101-4311. Phone: (619) 699-6345. Fax: (619) 699-6715. Monthly.

International Journal of Cardiology. Elsevier Science Publishing Co., Inc., P.O. Box 882, Madison Square Station, New York, NY 10159-2101. Phone: (212) 989-5800. Fax: (212) 633-3990. 12/year.

Journal of the American College of Cardiology. Elsevier Science Publishing Co., Inc., P.O. Box 882, Madison Square Station, New York, NY 10159-2101. Phone: (212) 989-5800. Fax: (212) 633-3990. Monthly.

Journal of Thoracic and Cardiovascular Surgery. Mosby-Year Book, 11830 Westline Industrial Drive, St. Louis, MO 63146. Phone: (800) 325-4177. Fax: (314) 432-1380. Monthly.

Morbidity and Mortality Weekly Report. Massachusetts Medical Society, 1440 Main St., Waltham, MA 02154-1649. Phone: (617) 893-3800. Fax: (617) 893-0413. Weekly.

Trends in Cardiovascular Medicine. Elsevier Science Publishing Co., Inc., P.O. Box 882, Madison Square Station, New York, NY 10159-2101. Phone: (212) 989-5800. Fax: (212) 633-3990. 6/year.

NEWSLETTERS

Cardiac Alert. Phillips Publishing, Inc., 7811 Montrose Rd., Potomac, MD 20854. Phone: (800) 722-9000. Fax: (301) 897-9745. Monthly.

Cardiology. American College of Cardiology, 9111 Old Georgetown Rd., Bethesda, MD 20814. Phone: (800) 253-4636. Fax: (301) 897-9745. Monthly.

Clinical Cardiology Alert. American Health Consultants, Department C1290, P.O. Box 740060, Atlanta, GA 30374. Phone: (800) 559-1032. Fax: (404) 352-1971. Monthly.

Harvard Heart Letter. Harvard Medical School Publications Group, 164 Longwood Ave., Boston, MA 02115. Monthly.

ONLINE DATABASES

BIOSIS Previews. BIOSIS, 2100 Arch St., Philadelphia, PA 19103-1399. Phone: (800) 523-4800. Fax: (215) 587-2016.

EMBASE. Elsevier Science Publishing Co., Inc., P.O. Box 882, Madison Square Station, New York, NY 10159-2101. Phone: (212) 989-5800. Fax: (212) 633-3990.

MEDIS. Mead Data Central, P.O. Box 1830, Dayton, OH 45401. Phone: (800) 227-4908.

MEDLINE. National Library of Medicine, 8600 Rockville Pike, Bethesda, MD 20894. Phone: (800) 638-8480.

SciSearch. Institute for Scientific Information, 3501 Market St., Philadelphia, PA 19104. Phone: (215) 386-0100. Fax: (215) 386-6362.

POPULAR WORKS AND PATIENT EDUCATION

The 8-Week Cholesterol Cure: How to Lower Your Blood Cholesterol by Up to 40 Percent Without Drugs or Deprivation. Robert E. Kowalski. HarperCollins Publishers., Inc., 10 E. 53rd St., New York, NY 10022-5299. Phone: (212) 207-7000. Fax: (800) 242-7737. Revised edition 1990.

American Heart Association Cookbook. Ballantine Books, 201 E. 50th St., New York, NY 10022. Phone: (800) 733-3000.

Cholesterol & Children: A Parent's Guide to Giving Children a Future Free of Heart Disease. Robert E. Kowalski. HarperCollins Publishers, Inc., 10 E. 53rd St., New York, NY 10022-5299. Phone: (800) 242-7737. 1989.

The Cooper Clinic Cardiac Rehabilitation Program: Featuring the Unique Heart Points System. Neil F. Gordon, Larry W. Gibbons. Pocket Books, Inc., 1230 Ave. of the Americas, New York, NY 10020. Phone: (800) 223-2348. Fax: (800) 284-0735. 1990.

Coronary Heart Disease: The Facts. Desmond Julian, Claire Marley. Oxford University Press, 200 Madison Ave., New York, NY 10016. Phone: (212) 679-7300. Fax: (212) 725-2972. Second edition 1991.

Dr. Dean Ornish's Program for Reversing Heart Disease Without Drugs or Surgery. Dean Ornish. Ballantine Books, Inc., 201 E. 50th St., New York, NY 10022. Phone: (800) 726-0600. 1992.

Eight Steps to a Healthy Heart: The Complete Guide to Recovering from Heart Attack, Bypass Surgery, and Heart Disease. Robert E. Kowalski. Warner Books, Inc., 666 Fifth

Ave., 9th Flr., New York, NY 10103. Phone: (212) 484-2900. 1992.

The Handbook of Heart Drugs: A Consumer's Guide to Safe and Effective Use. Martin Goldman. Holt, Rinehart & Winston, 115 W. 18th St., New York, NY 10011. Phone: (800) 488-5233. 1992.

The Heart Attack Handbook. Joseph S. Alpert. Consumer Reports Books, 9180 LeSaint Dr., Fairfield, OH 45014. Phone: (513) 860-1178. 1993.

Living with Angina: A Practical Guide to Dealing with Coronary Disease and Your Doctor. James A. Pantano. HarperCollins Pubs., Inc., 10 E. 53rd St., New York, NY 10022-5299. Phone: (212) 207-7000. Fax: (800) 242-7737. 1991.

Yale University School of Medicine Heart Book. Barry L. Zaret, Lawrence S. Cohen, Marvin Moser, and others. William Morrow & Company, Inc., 1350 Ave. of the Americas, New York, NY 10019. Phone: (800) 237-0657. 1992.

RESEARCH CENTERS, INSTITUTES, CLEARINGHOUSES

Alabama Congenital Heart Disease Diagnosis and Treatment Center. University of Alabama at Birmingham. Department of Surgery, University Station, Birmingham, AL 35294. Phone: (205) 934-2344.

Arizona Heart Institute. 2632 N. 20th St., Phoenix, AZ 85006. Phone: (602) 266-2200.

Cardiovascular Research Group. University of Calgary. Faculty of Medicine, 1663 Health Sciences Center, 3390 Hospital Dr. NW, Calgary, AB, Canada T2N 4N1. Phone: (403) 220-4521. Fax: (403) 270-0313.

Cardiovascular Research and Training Center. University of Alabama at Birmingham. THT Room 311, Birmingham, AL 35294. Phone: (205) 934-3624. Fax: (205) 934-5596.

Cleveland Clinic Foundation Research Institute. 9500 Euclid Ave., Cleveland, OH 44195-5210. Phone: (216) 444-3900. Fax: (216) 444-3279.

DeBakey Heart Center. Baylor College of Medicine. Texas Medical Center, 1 Baylor Plaza, Houston, TX 77030. Phone: (701) 797-9353. Fax: (713) 793-1192.

Division of Cardiology. University of Michigan. University Hospital, Ann Arbor, MI 48109. Phone: (313) 936-5255.

Framingham Heart Study. 5 Thurber St., Framingham, MA 01701. Phone: (508) 872-4386.

Heart Institute. University of Ottawa. Ottawa Civic Hospital, 1053 Carling Ave., Ottawa, ON, Canada K1V 4E9. Phone: (613) 725-4794. Fax: (613) 729-3937.

Heart and Vascular Institute. Henry Ford Hospital, 2799 W. Grand Blvd., Detroit, MI 48202. Phone: (313) 876-2695. Fax: (313) 876-2687.

High Blood Pressure Information Center (HBPIC). 4733 Bethesda Ave., Suite 530, Bethesda, MD 20814-4820. Phone: (301) 951-3260.

Hope Heart Institute. 528 18th Ave., Seattle, WA 98122. Phone: (206) 320-2001. Fax: (206) 328-0355.

Ischemic Heart Disease Specialized Center of Research. Johns Hopkins University. Johns Hopkins Hospital, 600 Wolfe, Baltimore, MD 21205. Phone: (301) 955-6023.

National Center for Cardiovascular Health. Louisiana State University. 1542 Tulane Ave., New Orleans, LA 70112. Phone: (504) 568-5845. Fax: (504) 568-2127.

National Heart, Lung, and Blood Institute Education Programs Information Center. 4733 Bethesda Ave., Ste. 530, Bethesda, MD 20814. Phone: (301) 951-3260.

Specialized Center of Research in Coronary Heart Disease. University of California, San Diego. Dept. of Medicine, M-013B, La Jolla, CA 92093. Phone: (619) 534-3347.

Specialized Center of Research in Ischemic Heart Disease. Duke University. Department of Medicine, Division of Cardiology, Box 3845, Durham, NC 27710. Phone: (919) 681-5392.

Texas Heart Institute. P.O. Box 20345, Houston, TX 77225-0345. Phone: (713) 791-3709. Fax: (713) 791-3089.

STANDARDS AND STATISTICS SOURCES

National Heart, Lung, and Blood Institute Fact Book. National Heart, Lung, and Blood Institute, NIH Bldg. 31, 9000 Rockville Pike, Bethesda, MD 20892. Phone: (301) 496-5166. Annual.

TEXTBOOKS AND MONOGRAPHS

Cardiac Catheterization, Angiography, and Intervention. Willam Grossman, Donald S. Baim (eds.). Lea & Febiger, 428 E. Preston St., Baltimore, MD 21202. Phone: (800) 638-0672. Fax: (800) 447-8438. Fourth edition 1991.

Cardiology. William W. Parmley, Kanu Chatterjee (eds.). J.B. Lippincott Co., 227 E. Washington Square, Philadelphia, PA 19106-3780. Phone: (215) 238-4200. Fax: (215) 238-4227. Two volumes 1991.

Cardiovascular Disease: Prevention and Treatment. Penny M. Kris-Etherton (ed.). American Dietetic Association, 216 W. Jackson Blvd., Suite 800, Chicago, IL 60606-6995. Phone: (312) 899-0040. 1990.

Cardiovascular Diseases: Genetics, Epidemiology and Prevention. James J. Nora, Kare Berg, Audrey Hart Nora. Oxford University Press, 200 Madison Ave., New York, NY 10016. Phone: (212) 679-7300. 1991.

Clinical Cardiology. Maurice Sokolow, and others. Appleton & Lange, 25 Van Zant Street, East Norwalk, CT 06855. Phone: (800) 423-1359. Fax: (203) 854-9486. Fifth edition 1990.

Current Management of Arrhythmias. Leonard N. Horowitz. Mosby-Year Book, 11830 Westline Industrial Drive, St. Louis, MO 63146. Phone: (800) 325-4177. Fax: (314) 432-1380. 1990.

Current Therapy in Cardiovascular Disease. J. Willis Hurst. Mosby-Year Book, 11830 Westline Industrial Drive, St. Louis, MO 63146. Phone: (800) 325-4177. Fax: (314) 432-1380. Third edition 1991.

Essentials of Clinical Cardiology. Emmanuel Goldberger. J.B. Lippincott Co., 227 E. Washington Square, Philadelphia, PA 19106-3780. Phone: (215) 238-4200. Fax: (215) 238-4227. 1990.

Fetal, Neonatal, and Infant Cardiac Disease. James H. Moller, William A. Neal (eds.). Appleton & Lange, 25 Van Zant Street, East Norwalk, CT 06855. Phone: (800) 423-1359. Fax: (203) 854-9486. 1990.

The Heart. J. Willis Hurst, Robert C. Schlant, et. al.. McGraw-Hill, Inc., Health Professions Division, 1221 Avenue of the Americas, 28th Floor, New York, NY 10020. Phone: (212) 512-4228. Seventh edition 1990.

Heart Disease: A Textbook of Cardiovascular Medicine. Eugene Braunwald (ed.). W.B. Saunders Co., The Curtis Center, Independence Square W., Philadelphia, PA 19106-3399. Phone: (215) 238-7800. Third edition. Two volumes. 1988.

The Heart: Physiology and Metabolism. Lionel H. Opie. Raven Press, 1185 Avenue of the Americas, New York, NY 10036. Phone: (212) 930-9500. Fax: (212) 869-3495. Second edition 1991.

Hypertension: Pathophysiology, Diagnosis, and Management. John H. Laragh, Barry M. Brenner (eds.). Raven Press, 1185 Avenue of the Americas, New York, NY 10036. Phone: (212) 930-9500. Fax: (212) 869-3495. Two volumes 1990.

Introduction to Clinical Cardiology. C. Richard Conti. Raven Press, 1185 Avenue of the Americas, New York, NY 10036. Phone: (212) 930-9500. Fax: (212) 869-3495. 1991.

Pediatric Arrhythmias: Electrophysiology and Pacing. Paul C. Gillette, Arthur Garson Jr.. W.B. Saunders Co., The Curtis Center, Independence Square W., Philadelphia, PA 19106-3399. Phone: (215) 238-7800. 1990.

The Practice of Cardiology: The Medical and Surgical Cardiac Units at the Massachusetts General Hospital. Kim A. Eagle, and others (eds.). Little, Brown and Company, 34 Beacon St., Boston, MA 02108. Phone: (617) 227-0730. Second edition. Two volumes. 1989.

Principles of Cardiac Arrhythmias. Edward K. Chung. Williams & Wilkins, 428 E. Preston St., Baltimore, MD 21202. Phone: (800) 638-0672. Fax: (800) 447-8438. Fourth edition 1989.

The Science and Practice of Pediatric Cardiology. Arthur Garson Jr., J. Timothy Bricker, Dan G. McNamara. Williams & Wilkins, 428 East Preston St., Baltimore, MD 21202. Phone: (800) 638-0672. Fax: (800) 447-8438. Three volumes 1990.

Textbook of Interventional Cardiology. Eric J. Topol (ed.). W.B. Saunders Co., The Curtis Center, Independence Square W., Philadelphia, PA 19106-3399. Phone: (215) 238-7800. 1990.

HEART SURGERY

See: CARDIOVASCULAR SURGERY

HEART TRANSPLANTATION

See: TRANSPLANTATION

HEIMLICH MANEUVER

See: EMERGENCY MEDICINE

HEMATOLOGIC DISORDERS

See also: HEMATOLOGY; HEMOPHILIA; LEUKEMIA; SICKLE CELL ANEMIA

ABSTRACTING, INDEXING, AND CURRENT AWARENESS PUBLICATIONS

Current Contents/Clinical Medicine. Institute for Scientific Information, 3501 Market St., Philadelphia, PA 19104. Phone: (800) 523-1850. Fax: (215) 386-6362. Weekly.

Current Contents/Life Sciences. Institute for Scientific Information, 3501 Market St., Philadelphia, PA 19104. Phone: (215) 386-0100. Fax: (215) 386-6362.

Excerpta Medica. Section 25: Hematology. Elsevier Science Publishers, P.O. Box 882, Madison Square Station, New York, NY 10159-2101. Phone: (212) 633-3950. Fax: (212) 633-3990. 24/year.

Index Medicus. U.S. National Library of Medicine, 8600 Rockville Pike, Bethesda, MD 20894. Phone: (800) 638-8480. Monthly.

Research Alert: Blood Coagulation Factors & Hemorrhagic Disorders. Institute for Scientific Information, 3501 Market St., Philadelphia, PA 19104. Phone: (800) 523-1850. Fax: (215) 386-6362. Weekly.

Research Alert: Hematology-Hemoglobinpathies, Sickle Cell Anemia & Thalassemia. Institute for Scientific Information, 3501 Market St., Philadelphia, PA 19104. Phone: (800) 523-1850. Fax: (215) 386-6362. Weekly.

ANNUALS AND REVIEWS

Contemporary Hematology/Oncology. Plenum Publishing Co., 233 Spring St., New York, NY 10013-1578. Phone: (212) 620-8000. Fax: (212) 463-0742. Irregular.

Current Studies in Hematology and Blood Transfusion. S. Karger Publishers, Inc., 26 West Avon Rd., P.O. Box 529, Farmington, CT 06085. Phone: (203) 675-7834. Fax: (203) 675-7302. Irregular.

Hematology/Oncology Clinics. W.B. Saunders Co., The Curtis Center, Independence Square W., Philadelphia, PA 19106-3399. Phone: (215) 238-7800. Bimonthly.

ASSOCIATIONS, PROFESSIONAL SOCIETIES, ADVOCACY AND SUPPORT GROUPS

Leukemia Society of America (LSA). 733 Third Ave., New York, NY 10017. Phone: (212) 573-8484. Fax: (212) 972-5776.

CD-ROM DATABASES

Anemia. Hoffer. Williams & Wilkins, 428 East Preston St., Baltimore, MD 21202. Phone: (800) 638-0672. Fax: (800) 447-8438. 1988.

HANDBOOKS, GUIDES, MANUALS, ATLASES

Atlas of Haematology. George A. McDonald, Bruce Cruickshank, James Paul. Churchill Livingstone Inc., 650 Ave. of the Americas, New York, NY 10011. Phone: (212) 819-5400. Fax: (212) 302-6598. Fifth edition 1989.

Manual of Clinical Hematology. Mazza. Little, Brown and Co., 34 Beacon St., Boston, MA 02108. Phone: (617) 227-0730. 1988.

Red Cell Manual. Robert S. Hillman, Clement A. Finch. F.A. Davis Co., 1915 Arch St., Philadelphia, PA 19103. Phone: (800) 523-4049. Fax: (215) 568-5065. Sixth edition 1992.

JOURNALS

Acta Hematologica. S. Karger Publishers, Inc., 26 W. Avon Rd., P.O. Box 529, Farmington, CT 06085. Phone: (203) 675-7834. Fax: (203) 675-7302.

Blood. W.B. Saunders Co., The Curtis Center, Independence Sqare W., Philadelphia, PA 19106-3399. Phone: (215) 238-7800.

Blood Coagulation and Fibrinolysis. Rapid Communications of Oxford Ltd., The Old Malthouse, Paradise St., Oxford OX1 1LD, England. Phone: 44-865-790447. Fax: 44-865-244012. 6/year.

British Journal of Hematology. Blackwell Scientific Publications, Inc., 3 Cambridge Center, Cambridge, MA 02142. Phone: (800) 759-6102.

Clincal and Laboratory Haematology. Blackwell Scientific Publications, Inc., 3 Cambridge Center, Cambridge, MA 02142. Phone: (800) 759-6102.

Hemoglobin. Marcel Dekker, Inc., 270 Madison Ave., New York, NY 10016. Phone: (800) 228-1160.

ONLINE DATABASES

EMBASE. Elsevier Science Publishing Co., Inc., P.O. Box 882, Madison Square Station, New York, NY 10159-2101. Phone: (212) 989-5800. Fax: (212) 633-3990.

MEDLINE. National Library of Medicine, 8600 Rockville Pike, Bethesda, MD 20894. Phone: (800) 638-8480.

SciSearch. Institute for Scientific Information, 3501 Market St., Philadelphia, PA 19104. Phone: (215) 386-0100. Fax: (215) 386-6362.

RESEARCH CENTERS, INSTITUTES, CLEARINGHOUSES

Blood Research Institute. Blood Center of Southeastern Wisconsin. 1701 W. Wisconsin Ave., Milwaukee, WI 53233. Phone: (414) 933-5000.

Cardeza Foundation for Hematologic Research. Thomas Jefferson University. 1015 Walnut St., Philadelphia, PA 19107. Phone: (215) 955-7786.

Center for Blood Research. 800 Huntington Ave., Boston, MA 02115. Phone: (617) 731-6470.

Center for Thrombosis and Hemostasis. University of North Carolina at Chapel Hill. Campus Box 7015, UNC-CH School of Medicine, Chapel Hill, NC 27599-7015. Phone: (919) 966-3704. Fax: (919) 966-6012.

Comprehensive Sickle Cell Center. 560 Lenox Ave., Columbia University, New York, NY 10037. Phone: (212) 491-8074.

Foundation for Blood Research. P.O. Box 190, Scarborough, ME 04074. Phone: (207) 883-4131. Fax: (207) 883-1527.

Hematology Research Laboratory. University of Southern California. 2025 Zonal Ave., Los Angeles, CA 90033. Phone: (213) 224-6412. Fax: (213) 224-6687.

Sol Sherry Thrombosis Research Center. Temple University. 3400 N. Broad St., Philadelphia, PA 19140. Phone: (215) 221-4665. Fax: (215) 221-2783.

TEXTBOOKS AND MONOGRAPHS

Blood: Principles and Practice of Hematology. Robert I. Handin, Samuel E. Lux, Thomas P. Stossel. J.B. Lippincott Co., 227 East Washington Square, Philadelphia, PA 19106-3780. Phone: (215) 238-4200. Fax: (215) 238-4227. 1991.

Clinical Hematology and Principles of Hemostasis. Denise Harmening (ed.). F.A. Davis Co., 1915 Arch St., Philadelphia, PA 19103. Phone: (800) 523-4049. Fax: (215) 568-5065. Second edition 1992.

Disorders of Heomstasis. Oscar D. Ratnoff, Charles D. Forbes. W.B. Saunders Co., The Curtis Center, Independence Square W., Philadelphia, PA 19106-3399. Phone: (215) 238-7800. Second edition 1991.

Wintrobe's Clinical Hematology. G. Richard Lee, Thomas C. Bithell, John Foerster, and others. Williams & Wilkins, 428 E. Preston St., Baltimore, MD 21202. Phone: (800) 638-0672. Fax: (800) 447-8438. Ninth edition. Two volumes. 1992.

HEMATOLOGY

See also: HEMATOLOGIC DISORDERS; TRANSFUSIONS

ABSTRACTING, INDEXING, AND CURRENT AWARENESS PUBLICATIONS

CA Selects: Blood Coagulation. Chemical Abstracts Service, 2540 Olentangy River Road, P.O. Box 3012, Columbus, OH 43210-0012. Phone: (800) 848-6538. Biweekly.

Chemical Abstracts. Chemical Abstracts Service, 2540 Olentangy River Rd., P.O. Box 3012, Columbus, OH 43210-0012. Phone: (800) 848-6538.

Current Contents/Life Sciences. Institute for Scientific Information, 3501 Market St., Philadelphia, PA 19104. Phone: (215) 386-0100. Fax: (215) 386-6362.

Excerpta Medica. Section 25: Hematology. Elsevier Science Publishers, P.O. Box 882, Madison Square Station, New York, NY 10159-2101. Phone: (212) 633-3950. Fax: (212) 633-3990. 24/year.

Index Medicus. U.S. National Library of Medicine, 8600 Rockville Pike, Bethesda, MD 20894. Phone: (800) 638-8480. Monthly.

Science Citation Index. Institute for Scientific Information, 3501 Market St., Philadelphia, PA 19104. Phone: (800) 523-1850. Fax: (215) 386-6362. Bimonthly.

ANNUALS AND REVIEWS

Contemporary Hematology/Oncology. Plenum Publishing Co., 233 Spring St., New York, NY 10013-1578. Phone: (212) 620-8000. Fax: (212) 463-0742. Irregular.

Year Book of Hematology. Mosby-Year Book, 11830 Westline Industrial Drive, St. Louis, MO 63146. Phone: (800) 325-4177. Fax: (314) 432-1380. Annual.

ASSOCIATIONS, PROFESSIONAL SOCIETIES, ADVOCACY AND SUPPORT GROUPS

American Society of Hematology (ASH). 6900 Grove Rd., Thorofare, NJ 08086. Phone: (609) 845-0003. Fax: (609) 853-5991.

Cooley's Anemia Foundation (CAF). 105 E. 22nd St., Ste. 911, New York, NY 10010. Phone: (212) 598-0911.

Society for the Study of Blood. 13 Elm St., Manchester, MA 01944. Phone: (508) 526-8330.

CD-ROM DATABASES

SCISEARCH. Institute for Scientific Information, 3501 Market St., Philadelphia, PA 19104. Phone: (215) 386-0100. Fax: (215) 386-6362.

DIRECTORIES

Directory of Medical Specialists. Marquis Who's Who, 3002 Glenview Rd., Wilmette, IL 60091. Phone: (800) 621-9669. Fax: (708) 441-2264. Biennial.

Directory of Physicians in the United States. American Medical Association, 515 North State St., Chicago, IL 60610. Phone: (312) 464-0183. Fax: (312) 464-5834. Biennial.

ENCYCLOPEDIAS, DICTIONARIES, WORD BOOKS

A Word Book in Oncology and Hematology: With Special Reference to AIDS. Sheila D. Sloane. Mosby-Year Book, 11830 Westline Industrial Drive, St. Louis, MO 63146. Phone: (800) 325-4177. Fax: (314) 432-1380. 1992.

HANDBOOKS, GUIDES, MANUALS, ATLASES

Atlas of Haematology. George A. McDonald, Bruce Cruickshank, James Paul. Churchill Livingstone Inc., 650 Ave. of the Americas, New York, NY 10011. Phone: (212) 819-5400. Fax: (212) 302-6598. Fifth edition 1989.

Blood: Atlas and Sourcebook of Hematology. Carola T. Kapff, James H. Jandl. Little, Brown and Company, 34 Beacon St., Boston, MA 02108. Phone: (617) 227-0730. Second edition 1992.

Manual of Clinical Hematology. Mazza. Little, Brown and Co., 34 Beacon St., Boston, MA 02108. Phone: (617) 227-0730. 1988.

Practical Haematology. Sir John V. Dacie, S.M. Lewis (eds.). Churchill Livingstone Inc., 650 Avenue of the Americas, New York, NY 10011. Phone: (212) 819-5400. Fax: (212) 302-6598. Seventh edition 1991.

JOURNALS

American Journal of Hematology. John Wiley & Sons, Inc., 605 Third Ave., New York, NY 10158-0012. Phone: (212) 850-6000. Fax: (212) 850-6088. 12/year.

Blood Coagulation and Fibrinolysis. Rapid Communications of Oxford Ltd., The Old Malthouse, Paradise St., Oxford OX1 1LD, England. Phone: 44-865-790447. Fax: 44-865-244012. 6/year.

Blood Reviews. Churchill Livingstone Inc., 650 Avenue of the Americas, New York, NY 10011. Phone: (212) 819-5400. Fax: (212) 302-6598. Quarterly.

International Journal of Hematology. Elsevier Science Publishing Co., Inc., P.O. Box 882, Madison Square Station, New York, NY 10159-2101. Phone: (212) 989-5800. Fax: (212) 633-3990. 6/year.

ONLINE DATABASES

CA File (Chemical Abstracts File). Chemical Abstracts Service, 2540 Olentangy River Rd., P.O. Box 3012, Columbus, OH 43210-0012. Phone: (800) 848-6538.

Combined Health Information Database (CHID). U.S. National Institutes of Health, P.O. Box NDIC, Bethesda, MD 20892. Phone: (301) 496-2162. Fax: (301) 770-5164. Quarterly.

EMBASE. Elsevier Science Publishing Co., Inc., P.O. Box 882, Madison Square Station, New York, NY 10159-2101. Phone: (212) 989-5800. Fax: (212) 633-3990.

MEDLINE. National Library of Medicine, 8600 Rockville Pike, Bethesda, MD 20894. Phone: (800) 638-8480.

SciSearch. Institute for Scientific Information, 3501 Market St., Philadelphia, PA 19104. Phone: (215) 386-0100. Fax: (215) 386-6362.

RESEARCH CENTERS, INSTITUTES, CLEARINGHOUSES

Blood Research Institute. Blood Center of Southeastern Wisconsin. 1701 W. Wisconsin Ave., Milwaukee, WI 53233. Phone: (414) 933-5000

Cardeza Foundation for Hematologic Research. Thomas Jefferson University. 1015 Walnut St., Philadelphia, PA 19107. Phone: (215) 955-7786.

Center for Blood Research. 800 Huntington Ave., Boston, MA 02115. Phone: (617) 731-6470.

Center for Thrombosis and Hemostasis. University of North Carolina at Chapel Hill. Campus Box 7015, UNC-CH School of Medicine, Chapel Hill, NC 27599-7015. Phone: (919) 966-3704. Fax: (919) 966-6012.

Foundation for Blood Research. P.O. Box 190, Scarborough, ME 04074. Phone: (207) 883-4131. Fax: (207) 883-1527.

Hematology Research Laboratory. University of Southern California. 2025 Zonal Ave., Los Angeles, CA 90033. Phone: (213) 224-6412. Fax: (213) 224-6687.

Sol Sherry Thrombosis Research Center. Temple University. 3400 N. Broad St., Philadelphia, PA 19140. Phone: (215) 221-4665. Fax: (215) 221-2783.

TEXTBOOKS AND MONOGRAPHS

Blood Diseases of Infancy and Childhood. Denis R. Miller, Robert L. Baehner. Mosby-Year Book, 11830 Westline Industrial Drive, St. Louis, MO 63146. Phone: (800) 325-4177. Fax: (314) 432-1380. Sixth edition 1990.

Blood: Principles and Practice of Hematology. Robert I. Handin, Samuel E. Lux, Thomas P. Stossel. J.B. Lippincott Co., 227 East Washington Square, Philadelphia, PA 19106-3780. Phone: (215) 238-4200. Fax: (215) 238-4227. 1991.

Clinical Guide to Bleeding and Thrombotic Disorders. WIlliam E. Hathaway, Scott H. Goodnight Jr.. McGraw-Hill, Inc., Health Professions Division, 1221 Avenue of the Americas, 28th Floor, New York, NY 10020. Phone: (212) 512-4228. 1992.

Clinical Haematology. R.D. Eastham, R. Slade. Butterworth-Heinemann, 80 Montvale Ave., Stoneham, MA 02180. Phone: (617) 438-8464. Fax: (617) 279-4851. Seventh edition 1991.

Clinical Hematology and Principles of Hemostasis. Denise Harmening (ed.). F.A. Davis Co., 1915 Arch St., Philadelphia, PA 19103. Phone: (800) 523-4049. Fax: (215) 568-5065. Second edition 1992.

Clinical Hematology: Principles, Procedures, Correlations. Cheryl A. Lotspeich-Steininger and others (eds.). J.B. Lippincott Co., 227 E. Washington Square, Philadelphia, PA 19106-3780. Phone: (215) 238-4200. Fax: (215) 238-4227. 1992.

Current Therapy in Hematology. Michael Brain, Paul Carbone. Mosby-Year Book, 11830 Westline Industrial Drive, St. Louis, MO 63146. Phone: (800) 325-4177. Fax: (314) 432-1380. 4th edition, 1991.

Hematology. William J. Williams, Ernest Erslev, Allan J. Beutler, et. al.. McGraw-Hill, Inc., Health Professions Division, 1221 Avenue of the Americas, 28th Floor, New York, NY 10020. Phone: (212) 512-4228. Fourth edition 1990.

Hematology: A Combined Theoretical and Technical Approach. Arthur Simmons. W.B. Saunders Co., The Curtis Center, Independence Square W., Philadelphia, PA 19106-3399. Phone: (215) 238-7800. 1989.

Hematology: Basic Principles and Practice. Ronald Hoffman, Edward J. Benz Jr., Sanford J. Shattil. Churchill Livingstone Inc., 650 Avenue of the Americas, New York, NY 10011. Phone: (212) 819-5400. Fax: (212) 302-6598. 1991.

Hematology of Infancy and Childhood. David G. Nathan, Frank A. Oski. W.B. Saunders Co., The Curtis Center, Independence Square W., Philadelphia, PA 19106-3399. Phone: (215) 238-7800. Fourth edition. Two volumes. 1991.

Hematology: Principles and Procedures. Barbara A. Brown. Williams & Wilkins, 428 East Preston St., Baltimore, MD 21202. Phone: (800) 638-0672. Fax: (800) 447-8438. 1988.

Iron and Human Disease. R.B. Lauffer. CRC Press, Inc., 2000 Corporate Blvd. N.W., Boca Raton, FL 33431. Phone: (407) 994-0555. Fax: (407) 997-0949. 1992.

Medical Laboratory Haematology. Roger Hall, Bob Malia. Butterworth-Heinemann, 80 Montvale Ave., Stoneham, MA 02180. Phone: (617) 438-8464. Fax: (617) 279-4851. Second edition 1991.

Wintrobe's Clinical Hematology. G. Richard Lee, Thomas C. Bithell, John Foerster, and others. Williams & Wilkins, 428 E. Preston St., Baltimore, MD 21202. Phone: (800) 638-0672. Fax: (800) 447-8438. Ninth edition. Two volumes. 1992.

HEMODIALYSIS

See: KIDNEY DIALYSIS

HEMOPHILIA

See also: HEMATOLOGIC DISORDERS

ABSTRACTING, INDEXING, AND CURRENT AWARENESS PUBLICATIONS

Current Contents/Clinical Medicine. Institute for Scientific Information, 3501 Market St., Philadelphia, PA 19104. Phone: (800) 523-1850. Fax: (215) 386-6362. Weekly.

Index Medicus. U.S. National Library of Medicine, 8600 Rockville Pike, Bethesda, MD 20894. Phone: (800) 638-8480. Monthly.

Research Alert: Hemophilia. Institute for Scientific Information, 3501 Market St., Philadelphia, PA 19104. Phone: (800) 523-1850. Fax: (215) 386-6362. Weekly.

Science Citation Index. Institute for Scientific Information, 3501 Market St., Philadelphia, PA 19104. Phone: (800) 523-1850. Fax: (215) 386-6362. Bimonthly.

ANNUALS AND REVIEWS

Recent Advances in Hemophilia Care. Carol K. Kasper (ed.). John Wiley & Sons, Inc., 605 Third Ave., New York, NY 10158-0012. Phone: (212) 850-6000. Fax: (212) 850-6088. 1989.

ASSOCIATIONS, PROFESSIONAL SOCIETIES, ADVOCACY AND SUPPORT GROUPS

National Hemophilia Foundation (NHF). 110 Green St., Rm. 406, New York, NY 10012. Phone: (212) 219-8180. Fax: (212) 966-9247.

CD-ROM DATABASES

Bleeding Disorders. Edward R. Hoffer. Williams & Wilkins, 428 East Preston St., Baltimore, MD 21202. Phone: (800) 638-0672. Fax: (800) 447-8438. 1987.

SCISEARCH. Institute for Scientific Information, 3501 Market St., Philadelphia, PA 19104. Phone: (215) 386-0100. Fax: (215) 386-6362.

JOURNALS

American Journal of Hematology. John Wiley & Sons, Inc., 605 Third Ave., New York, NY 10158-0012. Phone: (212) 850-6000. Fax: (212) 850-6088. 12/year.

Blood. W.B. Saunders Co., The Curtis Center, Independence Sqare W., Philadelphia, PA 19106-3399. Phone: (215) 238-7800.

Blood Coagulation and Fibrinolysis. Rapid Communications of Oxford Ltd., The Old Malthouse, Paradise St., Oxford OX1 1LD, England. Phone: 44-865-790447. Fax: 44-865-244012. 6/year.

NEWSLETTERS

Hemophilia Newsnotes. National Hemophilia Foundation, 110 Green St., Rm. 406, New York, NY 10012. Phone: (212) 219-8180. Fax: (212) 966-9247. Quarterly.

ONLINE DATABASES

EMBASE. Elsevier Science Publishing Co., Inc., P.O. Box 882, Madison Square Station, New York, NY 10159-2101. Phone: (212) 989-5800. Fax: (212) 633-3990.

MEDLINE. National Library of Medicine, 8600 Rockville Pike, Bethesda, MD 20894. Phone: (800) 638-8480.

SciSearch. Institute for Scientific Information, 3501 Market St., Philadelphia, PA 19104. Phone: (215) 386-0100. Fax: (215) 386-6362.

RESEARCH CENTERS, INSTITUTES, CLEARINGHOUSES

Center for Blood Research. 800 Huntington Ave., Boston, MA 02115. Phone: (617) 731-6470.

TEXTBOOKS AND MONOGRAPHS

Blood Diseases of Infancy and Childhood. Denis R. Miller, Robert L. Baehner. Mosby-Year Book, 11830 Westline Industrial Drive, St. Louis, MO 63146. Phone: (800) 325-4177. Fax: (314) 432-1380. Sixth edition 1990.

Hemophilia in the Child and Adult. Margaret W. Hilgartner, Carl E. Pochedly. Raven Press, 1185 Avenue of the Americas, New York, NY 10036. Phone: (212) 930-9500. Fax: (212) 869-3495. Third edition 1989.

Wintrobe's Clinical Hematology. G. Richard Lee, Thomas C. Bithell, John Foerster, and others. Williams & Wilkins, 428 E. Preston St., Baltimore, MD 21202. Phone: (800) 638-0672. Fax: (800) 447-8438. Ninth edition. Two volumes. 1992.

HEMORRHOIDS

See: GASTROINTESTINAL DISORDERS

HEPATIC DISEASES

See: HEPATITIS; LIVER DISEASES

HEPATITIS

ABSTRACTING, INDEXING, AND CURRENT AWARENESS PUBLICATIONS

Core Journals in Gastroenterology. Elsevier Science Publishing Co., Inc., P.O. Box 882, Madison Square Station, New York, NY 10159-2101. Phone: (212) 989-5800. Fax: (212) 633-3990. 11/year.

Current Contents/Clinical Medicine. Institute for Scientific Information, 3501 Market St., Philadelphia, PA 19104. Phone: (800) 523-1850. Fax: (215) 386-6362. Weekly.

Current Contents/Life Sciences. Institute for Scientific Information, 3501 Market St., Philadelphia, PA 19104. Phone: (215) 386-0100. Fax: (215) 386-6362.

Excerpta Medica. Section 48: Gastroenterology. Elsevier Science Publishing Co., Inc., P.O. Box 882, Madison Square Station, New York, NY 10159-2101. Phone: (212) 989-5800. Fax: (212) 633-3990. 20/year.

Index Medicus. U.S. National Library of Medicine, 8600 Rockville Pike, Bethesda, MD 20894. Phone: (800) 638-8480. Monthly.

Research Alert: Hepatitis. Institute for Scientific Information, 3501 Market St., Philadelphia, PA 19104. Phone: (800) 523-1850. Fax: (215) 386-6362. Weekly.

Science Citation Index. Institute for Scientific Information, 3501 Market St., Philadelphia, PA 19104. Phone: (800) 523-1850. Fax: (215) 386-6362. Bimonthly.

ANNUALS AND REVIEWS

Current Gastroenterology. Mosby-Year Book, 11830 Westline Industrial Drive, St. Louis, MO 63146. Phone: (800) 325-4177. Fax: (314) 432-1380. Annual.

Current Hepatology. Mosby-Year Book, 11830 Westline Industrial Drive, St. Louis, MO 63146. Phone: (800) 325-4177. Fax: (314) 432-1380. Annual.

Current Opinion in Gastroenterology. Current Science Group, 20 N. Third St., Philadelphia, PA 19106-2199. Phone: (800) 552-5866. Fax: (215) 574-2270. Bimonthly.

Frontiers of Gastrointestinal Research. S. Karger Publishers, Inc., 26 West Avon Rd., P.O. Box 529, Farmington, CT 06085. Phone: (203) 675-7834. Fax: (203) 675-7302. Irregular.

Gastroenterology Annual. Elsevier Science Publishing Co., Inc., P.O. Box 882, Madison Square Station, New York, NY 10159-2101. Phone: (212) 989-5800. Fax: (212) 633-3990. Annual.

Gastroenterology Clinics. W.B. Saunders Co., The Curtis Center, Independence Square W., Philadelphia, PA 19106-3399. Phone: (215) 238-7800. Quarterly.

ASSOCIATIONS, PROFESSIONAL SOCIETIES, ADVOCACY AND SUPPORT GROUPS

American Association for the Study of Liver Diseases (AASLD). 6900 Grove Rd., Thorofare, NJ 08086. Phone: (800) 257-8290. Fax: (609) 853-5991.

American Hepatitis Association (AHA). 133 E. 58th St., New York, NY 10022. Phone: (212) 753-8068.

American Liver Foundation (ALF). 1425 Pompton Ave., Cedar Grove, NJ 07009. Phone: (201) 256-2550. Fax: (201) 661-4027.

Children's Liver Foundation (CLF). 14245 Ventura Blvd., Ste. 201, Sherman Oaks, CA 91423. Phone: (800) 526-1593.

International Hepato-Biliary-Pancreatic Association (IHBPA). c/o A.R. Moossa, University of California, San Diego, Dept. of Surgery, 225 W. Dickenson St., San Diego, CA 92103. Phone: (619) 543-5860.

BIBLIOGRAPHIES

Hepatitis B Prevention: A Resouce Guide 1990. National Digestive Diseases Information Clearinghouse, P.O. Box NDDIC, Bethesda, MD 20892. Phone: (301) 468-6344. 1990 NIH Pub. No. 90-494.

Hepatitis: Treatment and Therapy. National Technical Information Service, 5285 Port Royal Rd., Springfield, VA 22161. Phone: (703) 487-4650. Fax: (703) 321-8547. Jan. 1978-May 1989 PB89-863260/CBY.

Hepatitis Vaccine Development and Marketing Aspects. National Technical Information Service, 5285 Port Royal Rd., Springfield, VA 22161. Phone: (703) 487-4650. Fax: (703) 321-8547. Jan. 1985-May 1989.

Hepatitis Vaccines and Immunization. National Technical Information Service, 5285 Port Royal Rd., Springfield, VA 22161. Phone: (703) 487-4650. Fax: (703) 321-8547. Jan. 1978-May 1989 PB89-862841/CBY.

CD-ROM DATABASES

Annals of Internal Medicine. MEP, 124 Mt. Auburn St., Cambridge, MA 02138. Phone: (800) 342-1338. Fax: (617) 868-7738. Semiannual.

Excerpta Medica CD: Gastroenterology. SilverPlatter Information, Inc., River Ridge Office Park, 100 River Ridge Rd., Norwood, MA 02062. Phone: (617) 769-2599. Fax: (617) 769-8763. Quarterly.

New England Journal of Medicine. CMC ReSearch, Inc., 7150 S.W. Hampton, Suite C-120, Portland, OR 97223. Phone: (800) 262-7668. Fax: (503) 639-1796. 3/year.

The New England Journal of Medicine on CD-ROM. MEP, 124 Mt. Auburn St., Cambridge, MA 02138. Phone: (800) 342-1338. Fax: (617) 868-7738. Semiannual.

SCISEARCH. Institute for Scientific Information, 3501 Market St., Philadelphia, PA 19104. Phone: (215) 386-0100. Fax: (215) 386-6362.

Viral Hepatitis Compact Library. MEP, 124 Mt. Auburn St., Cambridge, MA 02138. Phone: (800) 342-1338. Fax: (617) 868-7738. Annual.

JOURNALS

American Journal of Gastroenterology. Williams & Wilkins, 428 E. Preston St., Baltimore, MD 21202. Phone: (800) 638-0672. Fax: (800) 447-8438. Monthly.

American Journal of Infection Control. Mosby-Year Book, 11830 Westline Industrial Drive, St. Louis, MO 63146. Phone: (800) 325-4177. Fax: (314) 432-1380. Bimonthly.

Annals of Internal Medicine. American College of Physicians, Independence Mall W., Sixth St. at Race, Philadelphia, PA 19106-1572. Phone: (800) 523-1546. Fax: (215) 351-2594. Semimonthly.

Hepatology. Mosby-Year Book, 11830 Westline Industrial Drive, St. Louis, MO 63146. Phone: (800) 325-4177. Fax: (314) 432-1380. Monthly.

Infection Control and Hospital Epidemiology. SLACK Inc., 6900 Grove Rd., Thorofare, NJ 08086-9447. Phone: (800) 257-8290. Fax: (609) 853-5991.

Journal of Infectious Diseases. University of Chicago Press, P.O. Box 37005, Chicago, IL 60637. Phone: (312) 753-3347. Fax: (312) 753-0811. Monthly.

Journal of Virology. American Society for Microbiology, 1325 Massachusetts Ave. N.W., Washington, DC 20005. Phone: (202) 737-3600. Monthly.

Lancet. Williams & Wilkins, 428 East Preston St., Baltimore, MD 21202. Phone: (800) 638-0672. Fax: (800) 447-8438. Weekly.

The New England Journal of Medicine. Massachusetts Medical Society, 1440 Main St., Waltham, MA 02154-1649. Phone: (617) 893-3800. Fax: (617) 893-0413. Weekly.

Seminars in Hematology. W.B. Saunders Co., The Curtis Center, Independence Sqare W., Philadelphia, PA 19106-3399. Phone: (215) 238-7800.

Seminars in Liver Disease. Thieme Medical Publishers, Inc., 381 Park Ave. S., New York, NY 10016. Phone: (212) 683-5088. Fax: (212) 779-9020. Quarterly.

Virology. Academic Press, Inc., 1250 Sixth Ave., San Diego, CA 92101-4311. Phone: (619) 699-6345. Fax: (619) 699-6715. Monthly.

ONLINE DATABASES

EMBASE. Elsevier Science Publishing Co., Inc., P.O. Box 882, Madison Square Station, New York, NY 10159-2101. Phone: (212) 989-5800. Fax: (212) 633-3990.

MEDLINE. National Library of Medicine, 8600 Rockville Pike, Bethesda, MD 20894. Phone: (800) 638-8480.

SciSearch. Institute for Scientific Information, 3501 Market St., Philadelphia, PA 19104. Phone: (215) 386-0100. Fax: (215) 386-6362.

POPULAR WORKS AND PATIENT EDUCATION

CDC Hepatitis Hotline. Centers for Disease Control, 1600 Clifton Rd. N.E., Atlanta, GA 30333. Phone: (404) 488-4698.

Hepatitis B Prevention. Centers for Disease Control, 1600 Clifton Rd. N.E., Atlanta, GA 30333. Phone: (404) 488-4698.

Hepatitis B: What Parents Need to Know. American Academy of Pediatrics, 141 Northwest Point Blvd., P.O. Box 927, Elk Grove Village, IL 60009-0927. Phone: (708) 228-5005.

RESEARCH CENTERS, INSTITUTES, CLEARINGHOUSES

Hepatitis Branch. Centers for Disease Control, 1600 Clifton Rd. N.E., Atlanta, GA 30333. Phone: (404) 488-4698.

National Digestive Diseases Information Clearinghouse (NDDIC). P.O. Box NDDIC, Bethesda, MD 20892. Phone: (301) 468-6344.

STANDARDS AND STATISTICS SOURCES

Hepatitis Surveillance Report No. 53. Centers for Disease Control, 1600 Clifton Rd. N.E., Atlanta, GA 30333. Phone: (404) 488-4698. Dec. 1990.

TEXTBOOKS AND MONOGRAPHS

Complications of Chronic Liver Disease. Rector. Mosby-Year Book, 11830 Westline Industrial Drive, St. Louis, MO 63146. Phone: (800) 325-4177. Fax: (314) 432-1380. 1992.

Diseases of the Liver. Leon Schiff, Eugenee R. Schiff. J.B. Lippincott Co., 227 E. Washington Square, Philadelphia, PA 19106-3780. Phone: (215) 238-4200. Fax: (215) 238-4227. Sixth edition 1987.

Diseases of the Liver and Biliary System. Sherlock. Blackwell Scientific Publications, Inc., 3 Cambridge Ctr., Cambridge, MA 02142. Phone: (800) 759-6102. Ninth edition 1992.

Hepatitis A. Ian D. Gust, Stephen M. Feinstone (eds.). CRC Press, Inc., 2000 Corporate Blvd. N.W., Boca Raton, FL 33431. Phone: (407) 994-0555. Fax: (407) 997-0949. 1988.

Hepatology: A Textbook of Liver Disease. David Zakim, Thomas D. Boyer. W.B. Saunders Co., The Curtis Center, Independence Square W., Philadelphia, PA 19106-3399. Phone: (215) 238-7800. Second edition 1990.

The Liver and Biliary System. Gitnick. Mosby-Year Book, 11830 Westline Industrial Drive, St. Louis, MO 63146. Phone: (800) 325-4177. Fax: (314) 432-1380. 1991.

Liver Diseases. Leavy. Mosby-Year Book, 11830 Westline Industrial Drive, St. Louis, MO 63146. Phone: (800) 325-4177. Fax: (314) 432-1380. 1991.

Liver Function. Derek Cramp, Ewart Carson (eds.). Routledge, Chapman & Hall, Inc., 29 W. 35th St., New York, NY 10001-2291. Phone: (212) 244-3336. 1990.

Modern Concepts of Acute and Chronic Hepatitis. G. Gitnick (ed.). Plenum Publishing Co., 233 Spring St., New York, NY 10013-1578. Phone: (212) 620-8000. Fax: (212) 463-0742. 1989.

Progress in Liver Diseases. Hans Popper, Fenton Schaffner (eds.). W.B. Saunders Co., The Curtis Center, Independence Square W., Philadelphia, PA 19106-3399. Phone: (215) 238-7800. Irregular.

Textbook of Liver and Biliary Surgery. William C. Meyers, R. Scott Jones. J.B. Lippincott Co., 227 E. Washington Square, Philadelphia, PA 19106-3780. Phone: (215) 238-4200. Fax: (215) 238-4227. 1990.

Viral Hepatitis. F. Blaine Hollinger, William S. Robinson, Robert Purcell. Raven Press, 1185 Avenue of the Americas, New York, NY 10036. Phone: (212) 930-9500. Fax: (212) 869-3495. Second edition 1991.

Viral Hepatitis and Liver Disease. Arie J. Zuckerman (ed.). John Wiley & Sons, Inc., 605 Third Ave., New York, NY 10158-0012. Phone: (212) 850-6000. Fax: (212) 850-6088. 1988.

Wright's Liver and Biliary Disease. G.H. Millward-Sadler, M. Arthur. W.B. Saunders Co., The Curtis Center, Independence Square W., Philadelphia, PA 19106-3399. Phone: (215) 238-7800. Third edition 1991.

HERBAL MEDICINE

See also: ALTERNATIVE MEDICINE

ABSTRACTING, INDEXING, AND CURRENT AWARENESS PUBLICATIONS

Complementary Medicine Index. Medical Information Service, British Library, Boston Spa, Wetherby, W. Yorkshire LS23 7BQ, England. Phone: 0937-546039. Fax: 0937-546236. Monthly.

Consumer Health and Nutrition Index. Alan Rees. Oryx Press, 4041 N. Central, Suite 700, Phoenix, AZ 85012. Phone: (800) 279-6799. Fax: (800) 279-4663. Quarterly.

Index Medicus. U.S. National Library of Medicine, 8600 Rockville Pike, Bethesda, MD 20894. Phone: (800) 638-8480. Monthly.

ASSOCIATIONS, PROFESSIONAL SOCIETIES, ADVOCACY AND SUPPORT GROUPS

The American Botanical Council. P.O. Box 201660, Austin, TX 78720.

Dr. Edward Bach Healing Society. 655 Merrick Rd., Lynbrook, NY 11563. Phone: (516) 593-2206.

Herb Research Foundation. 1007 Pearl St., Boulder, CO 80302. Phone: (303) 449-2265.

HANDBOOKS, GUIDES, MANUALS, ATLASES

CRC Handbook of Medicinal Herbs. James A. Duke (ed.). CRC Press, Inc., 2000 Corporate Blvd. N.W., Boca Raton, FL 33431. Phone: (407) 994-0555. Fax: (407) 997-0949. 1985.

Handbook of Complementary Medicine. S. Fulder. Oxford University Press, 200 Madison Ave., New York, NY 10016. Phone: (212) 679-7300. 2nd edition 1988.

JOURNALS

Alternative Medicine. V.S.P. International Science Publishers, P.O. Box 346, 3700 AH, Zeist, Netherlands. Phone: 03404-51902. Fax: 03404-58620. Quarterly.

East West: The Journal of Natural Health and Living. East West Journal, Inc., 17 Station St., P.O. Box 1200, Brookline, MA 02146. Monthly.

Planta Medica. Thieme Medical Publishers, Inc., 381 Park Ave. S., New York, NY 10016. Phone: (212) 683-5088. Fax: (212) 779-9020. Bimonthly.

NEWSLETTERS

Alternatives. Mountain Home Publishing, P.O.Box 829, Ingram, TX 78025. Phone: (800) 527-3044. Monthly.

American Herb Association Quarterly Newsletter. American Herb Association, P.O. Box 353, Rescue, CA 95672. Phone: (916) 626-5046. Quarterly.

Edward Bach Healing Society-Newsletter. Edward Bach Healing Society, 644 Merrick Rd., Lynbrook, NY 11563-2332. Phone: (516) 825-1677. 4/year.

ONLINE DATABASES

EMBASE. Elsevier Science Publishing Co., Inc., P.O. Box 882, Madison Square Station, New York, NY 10159-2101. Phone: (212) 989-5800. Fax: (212) 633-3990.

MEDLINE. National Library of Medicine, 8600 Rockville Pike, Bethesda, MD 20894. Phone: (800) 638-8480.

SciSearch. Institute for Scientific Information, 3501 Market St., Philadelphia, PA 19104. Phone: (215) 386-0100. Fax: (215) 386-6362.

POPULAR WORKS AND PATIENT EDUCATION

Alternatives in Healing. Simon Mills, Steven Finando. Penguin USA, 375 Hudson St., New York, NY 10014-3657. Phone: (800) 331-4624.

Doctor's Book of Home Remedies. Prevention Magazine Staff. Rodale Press, Inc., 33 E. Minor St., Emmaus, PA 18098. Phone: (800) 527-8200. Fax: (215) 967-6263. 1990.

Earl Mindell's Herb Bible. Earl Mindell. Simon & Schuster, Inc., 1230 Ave. of the Americas, New York, NY 10020. Phone: (800) 223-2348. Fax: (800) 284-0735. 1992.

The Encyclopedia of Alternative Health Care. Kristin G. Olsen. Simon & Schuster, Inc., 1230 Ave. of the Americas, New York, NY 10020. Phone: (212) 698-7000. 1990.

Healing Herbs. Michael Castleman. St. Martin's Press, 175 Fifth Ave., New York, NY 10010. Phone: (212) 674-5151. 1991.

The Natural Healing and Nutrition Annual. Mark Bricklin, Sharon Stocker (eds.). Rodale Press, Inc., 33 E. Minor St., Emmaus, PA 18098. Phone: (800) 527-8200. Fax: (215) 967-6263. Annual.

The Nutrition Desk Reference. Robert H. Garrison. Keats Publishing, Inc., P.O. Box 876, New Canaan, CT 06840. Phone: (203) 966-8721. Revised edition 1990.

TEXTBOOKS AND MONOGRAPHS

Conservation of Medicinal Plants. Olayiwola Akerele, Vernon Heywood, Hugh Synge (eds.). Cambridge University Press, 40 W. 20th St., New York, NY 10011. Phone: (800) 431-1580. 1991.

Healing Power of Herbs. Murray. St. Martin's Press, 175 Fifth Ave., New York, NY 10010. Phone: (212) 674-5151. 1992.

HEREDITARY DISORDERS

See: BIRTH DEFECTS; GENETIC DISEASES

HERPES SIMPLEX

See: HERPESVIRUS INFECTIONS

HERPES ZOSTER

See: HERPESVIRUS INFECTIONS

HERPESVIRUS INFECTIONS

See also: SEXUALLY TRANSMITTED DISEASES

ABSTRACTING, INDEXING, AND CURRENT AWARENESS PUBLICATIONS

Current Contents/Clinical Medicine. Institute for Scientific Information, 3501 Market St., Philadelphia, PA 19104. Phone: (800) 523-1850. Fax: (215) 386-6362. Weekly.

Excerpta Medica. Section 13: Dermatology and Venereology. Elsevier Science Publishing Co., Inc., P.O. Box 882, Madison Square Station, New York, NY 10159-2101. Phone: (212) 989-5800. Fax: (212) 633-3990. 16/year.

Index Medicus. U.S. National Library of Medicine, 8600 Rockville Pike, Bethesda, MD 20894. Phone: (800) 638-8480. Monthly.

Science Citation Index. Institute for Scientific Information, 3501 Market St., Philadelphia, PA 19104. Phone: (800) 523-1850. Fax: (215) 386-6362. Bimonthly.

ASSOCIATIONS, PROFESSIONAL SOCIETIES, ADVOCACY AND SUPPORT GROUPS

American Social Health Association (ASHA). P.O. Box 13827, Research Triangle Park, NC 27709. Phone: (919) 361-8400. Fax: (919) 361-8425.

CD-ROM DATABASES

SCISEARCH. Institute for Scientific Information, 3501 Market St., Philadelphia, PA 19104. Phone: (215) 386-0100. Fax: (215) 386-6362.

HANDBOOKS, GUIDES, MANUALS, ATLASES

Color Atlas of Sexually Transmitted Diseases. Anthony Wisdom. Mosby-Year Book, 11830 Westline Industrial Drive, St. Louis, MO 63146. Phone: (800) 325-4177. Fax: (314) 432-1380. 1990.

ONLINE DATABASES

EMBASE. Elsevier Science Publishing Co., Inc., P.O. Box 882, Madison Square Station, New York, NY 10159-2101. Phone: (212) 989-5800. Fax: (212) 633-3990.

MEDLINE. National Library of Medicine, 8600 Rockville Pike, Bethesda, MD 20894. Phone: (800) 638-8480.

SciSearch. Institute for Scientific Information, 3501 Market St., Philadelphia, PA 19104. Phone: (215) 386-0100. Fax: (215) 386-6362.

POPULAR WORKS AND PATIENT EDUCATION

Shingles. Thomas Carl Thomsen. Cross River Press, P.O. Box 473, Cross River, NY 10518. Phone: (914) 763-8030. 1990.

TEXTBOOKS AND MONOGRAPHS

Herpesvirus Transcription and Its Regulation. Edward K. Wagner. CRC Press, Inc., 2000 Corporate Blvd. N.W., Boca Raton, FL 33431. Phone: (407) 994-0555. Fax: (407) 997-0949. 1991.

Sexually Transmitted Diseases. King K. Holmes, Per-Anders Mardh, P. Frederick, et. al.. McGraw-Hill, Inc., Health Professions Division, 1221 Avenue of the Americas, 28th Floor, New York, NY 10020. Phone: (212) 512-4228. Second edition 1990.

HIGH BLOOD PRESSURE

See: HYPERTENSION

HISTORY OF MEDICINE

ABSTRACTING, INDEXING, AND CURRENT AWARENESS PUBLICATIONS

Index Medicus. U.S. National Library of Medicine, 8600 Rockville Pike, Bethesda, MD 20894. Phone: (800) 638-8480. Monthly.

ASSOCIATIONS, PROFESSIONAL SOCIETIES, ADVOCACY AND SUPPORT GROUPS

American Academy of the History of Dentistry. 211 E. Chicago Ave., Chicago, IL 60611. Phone: (312) 440-2500.

Association of Libraries in the History of the Health Sciences. c/o Mr. Glen Jenkins, Allen Memorial Library, 1100 Euclid Ave., Cleveland, OH 44106. Phone: (216) 368-3649.

BIBLIOGRAPHIES

Bibliography of the History of Medicine. U.S. National Library of Medicine, 8600 Rockville Pike, Bethesda, MD 20894. Phone: (800) 638-8480. Annual.

Current Work in the History of Medicine. BMJ Publishing Group, BMA House, Tavistock Square, London WC1H 9JR, England. Phone: 071-383 6244/6638. Fax: 071-383 6662. Quarterly.

Morton's Medical Bibliography. Jeremy M. Norman (ed.). Scolar Press, Old Post Road, Brookfield, VT 05036. Phone: (800) 535-9544. Fax: (802) 276-3837. Fifth edition, 1991.

ENCYCLOPEDIAS, DICTIONARIES, WORD BOOKS

Biographical Dictionary of Medicine. Jessica Bendiner Elmer. Facts on File, Inc., 460 Park Ave. S., New York, NY 10016-7382. Phone: (212) 683-2244. Fax: (212) 683-3633. 1990.

JOURNALS

Journal of Medical Biography. Royal Society of Medicine, 1 Wimpole St., London W1M 8AE, England. Phone: 071-408 2119. Fax: 071-355 3198. Quarterly.

Medical History. BMJ Publishing Group, BMA House, Tavistock Square, London WC1H 9JR, England. Phone: 071-383 6244/6638. Fax: 071-383 6662. Quarterly.

ONLINE DATABASES

EMBASE. Elsevier Science Publishing Co., Inc., P.O. Box 882, Madison Square Station, New York, NY 10159-2101. Phone: (212) 989-5800. Fax: (212) 633-3990.

HISTLINE. U.S. National Library of Medicine, MEDLARS Management Section, 8600 Rockville Pike, Bethesda, MD 20894. Phone: (800) 638-8480. Monthly.

MEDLINE. National Library of Medicine, 8600 Rockville Pike, Bethesda, MD 20894. Phone: (800) 638-8480.

SciSearch. Institute for Scientific Information, 3501 Market St., Philadelphia, PA 19104. Phone: (215) 386-0100. Fax: (215) 386-6362.

POPULAR WORKS AND PATIENT EDUCATION

History of Medicine. Magner (ed.). Marcel Dekker, Inc., 270 Madison Ave., New York, NY 10016. Phone: (800) 228-1160. 1992.

Medicine's Great Journey: One Hundred Years of Healing. Rick Smolan, Philip Moffitt, Richard Flaste. Little, Brown and Co., 34 Beacon St., Boston, MA 02108. Phone: (617) 227-0730. Fax: (617) 227-0790.

RESEARCH CENTERS, INSTITUTES, CLEARINGHOUSES

Laboratory of the History of Medicine and Science. 1230 York Ave., Rockefeller University, New York, NY 10021. Phone: (212) 570-8616.

TEXTBOOKS AND MONOGRAPHS

Cambridge History of Medicine. Cambridge University Press, 40 W. 20th St., New York, NY 10011. Phone: (800) 431-1580. Irregular.

The Cambridge World History of Human Disease. Kenneth F. Kiple (ed.). Cambridge University Press, 40 W. 20th St., New York, NY 10011. Phone: (800) 431-1580. 1992.

Explaining Epidemic and Other Studies in the History of Medicine. Charles Rosenberg. Cambridge University Press, 40 W. 20th St., New York, NY 10011. Phone: (800) 431-1580. 1992.

Oxford Companion to Medicine. Sir J. Walton, P.B. Beeson. Oxford University Press, 200 Madison Ave., New York, NY 10016. Phone: (212) 679-7300. Two volumes 1986.

HMOS

See: HEALTH MAINTENANCE ORGANIZATIONS

HODGKIN'S DISEASE

See: LYMPHOMAS

HOLISTIC MEDICINE

See also: ALTERNATIVE MEDICINE

ABSTRACTING, INDEXING, AND CURRENT AWARENESS PUBLICATIONS

Complementary Medicine Index. Medical Information Service, British Library, Boston Spa, Wetherby, W. Yorkshire LS23 7BQ, England. Phone: 0937-546039. Fax: 0937-546236. Monthly.

Consumer Health and Nutrition Index. Alan Rees. Oryx Press, 4041 N. Central, Suite 700, Phoenix, AZ 85012. Phone: (800) 279-6799. Fax: (800) 279-4663. Quarterly.

Index Medicus. U.S. National Library of Medicine, 8600 Rockville Pike, Bethesda, MD 20894. Phone: (800) 638-8480. Monthly.

ASSOCIATIONS, PROFESSIONAL SOCIETIES, ADVOCACY AND SUPPORT GROUPS

American Holistic Medical Association (AHMA). 4101 Lake Boone Tr., Ste. 201, Raleigh, NC 27607. Phone: (919) 787-5146. Fax: (919) 787-4916.

Association for Holistic Health. P.O. Box 1122, Del Mar, CA 92014. Phone: (619) 535-0101.

Holistic Dental Association. c/o Dr. Paul Plowman, 4801 Richmond Sq., Oklahoma City, OK 73118. Phone: (405) 840-5600.

International Association of Holistic Health Practitioners. 3419 Thom Blvd., Las Vegas, NV 89130. Phone: (702) 873-4542.

DIRECTORIES

American Holistic Medical Association-Directory of Members. American Holistic Medical Association, 4101 Lake Boone Tr., Ste. 201, Raleigh, NC 27607. Phone: (919) 787-5146. Fax: (919) 787-4916. Annual.

Holistic Practioners Directory. American Business Directories, Inc., 5711 S. 86th Circle, Omaha, NE 68127. Phone: (402) 593-4600. Fax: (402) 331-1505. Annual.

JOURNALS

Alternative Medicine. V.S.P. International Science Publishers, P.O. Box 346, 3700 AH, Zeist, Netherlands. Phone: 03404-51902. Fax: 03404-58620. Quarterly.

East West: The Journal of Natural Health and Living. East West Journal, Inc., 17 Station St., P.O. Box 1200, Brookline, MA 02146. Monthly.

Journal of Holistic Nursing. American Holistic Nurses Association, 4101 Lake Boone Tr., Ste. 201, Raleigh, NC 27607. Phone: (919) 787-5181. Fax: (919) 787-4916. Annual.

NEWSLETTERS

Holistic Medicine. American Holistic Medical Association, 4101 Lake Boone Trail, Ste. 201, Raleigh, NC 27607. Phone: (919) 787-5146. Fax: (919) 787-4916. Bimonthly.

ONLINE DATABASES

EMBASE. Elsevier Science Publishing Co., Inc., P.O. Box 882, Madison Square Station, New York, NY 10159-2101. Phone: (212) 989-5800. Fax: (212) 633-3990.

MEDLINE. National Library of Medicine, 8600 Rockville Pike, Bethesda, MD 20894. Phone: (800) 638-8480.

SciSearch. Institute for Scientific Information, 3501 Market St., Philadelphia, PA 19104. Phone: (215) 386-0100. Fax: (215) 386-6362.

TEXTBOOKS AND MONOGRAPHS

Holistic Health Promotion: A Guide for Practice. Barbara M. Dossey, and others. Aspen Publishers, Inc., 200 Orchard Ridge Dr., Gaithersburg, MD 20878. Phone: (800) 638-8437. 1989.

Tibetan Medicine: And Other Holistic Health-Care. Tom Dummer. Viking Penguin, 375 Hudson St., New York, NY 10014-3657. Phone: (800) 331-4624. 1989.

HOME HEALTH CARE

ABSTRACTING, INDEXING, AND CURRENT AWARENESS PUBLICATIONS

Cumulative Index to Nursing and Allied Health Literature. Glendale Adventist Medical Center, P.O. Box 871, Glendale, CA 91209. Phone: (818) 409-8005. Bimonthly.

Hospital Literature Index. American Hospital Association, 840 N. Lake Shore Dr., Chicago, IL 60611. Phone: (800) 242-2626. Fax: (312) 280-6015. Quarterly.

Index Medicus. U.S. National Library of Medicine, 8600 Rockville Pike, Bethesda, MD 20894. Phone: (800) 638-8480. Monthly.

International Nursing Index. American Journal of Nursing Co., 555 W. 57th St., New York, NY 10019. Phone: (212) 582-8820. Quarterly.

ASSOCIATIONS, PROFESSIONAL SOCIETIES, ADVOCACY AND SUPPORT GROUPS

American Association for Continuity of Care. 1101 Connecticut Ave. N.W., Washington, DC 20036. Phone: (202) 857-1194.

Division of Ambulatory Care and Health Promotion (DACHP). American Hospital Association, 840 N. Lake Shore Dr., Chicago, IL 60611. Phone: (312) 280-6461. Fax: (312) 280-5979.

Foundation for Hospice and Homecare (FHH). 519 C St. NE, Stanton Park, Washington, DC 20002. Phone: (202) 547-6586.

National Association for Home Care (NAHC). 519 C St. N.E., Stanton Park, Washington, DC 20002. Phone: (202) 547-7424. Fax: (202) 547-3540.

CD-ROM DATABASES

Nursing and Allied Health (CINAHL) on CD-ROM. CINAHL, 1509 Wilson Terrace, P.O. Box 871, Glendale, CA 91209-0871. Phone: (818) 409-8005.

DIRECTORIES

Home Health Care and Hospice Directory. National Association of Home Care, 519 C St. NE, Washington, DC 20002. Phone: (202) 547-7424. Fax: (202) 547-3540. Annual.

National Home Care and Hospice Directory. National Association of Home Care, 519 C St. N.E., Washington, DC 20002. Phone: (202) 547-7424. Fax: (202) 547-3540. Annual.

HANDBOOKS, GUIDES, MANUALS, ATLASES

Home Care: A Technical Manual for the Professional. Rovinski Zastocki. W.B. Saunders Co., The Curtis Center, Independence Square W., Philadelphia, PA 19106-3399. Phone: (215) 238-7800. 1989.

Home Health Nursing Manual: Procedures and Documentation. Sunny Sutton. Williams & Wilkins, 428 East Preston St., Baltimore, MD 21202. Phone: (800) 638-0672. Fax: (800) 447-8438. 1988.

The Home Rehabilitation Program Guide. Paul A. Roggow, Debra K. Berg, Michael D. Lewis. SLACK Inc., 6900 Grove Rd., Thorofare, NJ 08086-9447. Phone: (800) 257-8290. Fax: (609) 853-5991. 1990.

NEWSLETTERS

Hospital Home Health. American Health Consultants, Department C1290, P.O. Box 740060, Atlanta, GA 30374. Phone: (800) 559-1032. Monthly.

Parent Care Advisor. American Health Consultants, P.O. Box 71266, Chicago, IL 60691-9987. Phone: (800) 688-2421. Monthly.

ONLINE DATABASES

EMBASE. Elsevier Science Publishing Co., Inc., P.O. Box 882, Madison Square Station, New York, NY 10159-2101. Phone: (212) 989-5800. Fax: (212) 633-3990.

MEDLINE. National Library of Medicine, 8600 Rockville Pike, Bethesda, MD 20894. Phone: (800) 638-8480.

Nursing and Allied Health (CINAHL). CINAHL, 1509 Wilson Terrace, P.O. Box 871, Glendale, CA 91209-0871. Phone: (818) 409-8005.

SciSearch. Institute for Scientific Information, 3501 Market St., Philadelphia, PA 19104. Phone: (215) 386-0100. Fax: (215) 386-6362.

POPULAR WORKS AND PATIENT EDUCATION

Dying at Home: A Family Guide for Caregiving. Andrea Sankar. Johns Hopkins University Press, 701 W. 40th St., Suite 275, Baltimore, MD 21211-2190. Phone: (800) 537-5487. 1991.

Home Health Care Options: A Guide for Older Persons and Concerned Families. Connie Zuckerman, Nacy Neveloff Dubler, Bart Collopy (eds.). Plenum Publishing Co., 233 Spring St., New York, NY 10013-1578. Phone: (212) 620-8000. Fax: (212) 463-0742. 1990.

Taking Care of Caregivers: For Families and Others Who Care for People with Alzheimer's Disease and Other Forms of Dementia. D. Jeanne Roberts. Bull Publishing Co., 110 Gilbert Ave., Menlo Park, CA 94025. Phone: (800) 676-2855. 1991.

When Your Parents Need You: A Caregiver's Guide. Rita Robinson. Borgo Press, P.O. Box 2845, San Bernardino, CA 92406-2845. Phone: (909) 884-5813. Fax: (909) 888-4942. 1990.

TEXTBOOKS AND MONOGRAPHS

Being a Homemaker/Home Health Aide. Elana D. Zucker. Prentice Hall, 113 Sylvan Ave., Rt. 9W, Prentice Hall Bldg., Englewood Cliffs, NJ 07632. Phone: (201) 767-5937. 1991.

Client Teaching Guides for Home Health Care. Donna Meyers. Aspen Publishers, Inc., 200 Orchard Ridge Dr., Gaithersburg, MD 20878. Phone: (800) 638-8437. 1989.

Home Care Nursing: An Orientation to Practice. Carolyn Humphrey, Paula Milone-Nuzzo. Appleton & Lange, 25 Van Zant St., East Norwalk, CT 06855. Phone: (800) 423-1359. Fax: (203) 854-9486. 1990.

Home Health Care Management. Lazelle Emminizer Benefield. Prentice Hall, 113 Sylvan Ave., Rt. 9W, Prentice Hall Bldg., Englewood Cliffs, NJ 07632. Phone: (201) 767-5937. 1988.

Home Health Care Nursing. Ida Martinson, Ann Widmer. W.B. Saunders Co., The Curtis Center, Independence Sqare W., Philadelphia, PA 19106-3399. Phone: (215) 238-7800. 1989.

Home Health Care Nursing: Concepts and Practice. Keating, Kelman. J.B. Lippincott Co., 227 E. Washington Square, Philadelphia, PA 19106-3780. Phone: (215) 238-4200. Fax: (215) 238-4227. 1988.

Quality Assurance Policies and Procedures for Health Care. Judith Bulau. Aspen Publishers, Inc., 200 Orchard Ridge Dr., Gaithersburg, MD 20878. Phone: (800) 638-8437. 1989.

HOMEOPATHY

See also: ALTERNATIVE MEDICINE

ABSTRACTING, INDEXING, AND CURRENT AWARENESS PUBLICATIONS

Complementary Medicine Index. Medical Information Service, British Library, Boston Spa, Wetherby, W. Yorkshire LS23 7BQ, England. Phone: 0937-546039. Fax: 0937-546236. Monthly.

Consumer Health and Nutrition Index. Alan Rees. Oryx Press, 4041 N. Central, Suite 700, Phoenix, AZ 85012. Phone: (800) 279-6799. Fax: (800) 279-4663. Quarterly.

Index Medicus. U.S. National Library of Medicine, 8600 Rockville Pike, Bethesda, MD 20894. Phone: (800) 638-8480. Monthly.

ASSOCIATIONS, PROFESSIONAL SOCIETIES, ADVOCACY AND SUPPORT GROUPS

American Foundation for Homeopathy. 706 Edgewood Rd., San Mateo, CA 94402. Phone: (415) 342-0815.

American Institute of Homeopathy. 1500 Massachusetts Ave., Suite 41, Washington, DC 20005. Phone: (202) 223-6182.

National Center for Homeopathy (NCH). 801 N. Fairfax St., Ste. 306, Alexandria, VA 22314. Phone: (703) 548-7790.

DIRECTORIES

Directory of United States Homeopathic Practitioners. National Center for Homeopathy, 1500 Massachusetts Ave. N.W., Ste. 42, Washington, DC 20005. Phone: (202) 223-6182. Biennial.

HANDBOOKS, GUIDES, MANUALS, ATLASES

Handbook of Complementary Medicine. S. Fulder. Oxford University Press, 200 Madison Ave., New York, NY 10016. Phone: (212) 679-7300. 2nd edition 1988.

JOURNALS

Alternative Medicine. V.S.P. International Science Publishers, P.O. Box 346, 3700 AH, Zeist, Netherlands. Phone: 03404-51902. Fax: 03404-58620. Quarterly.

British Homeopathic Journal. Royal London Homeopathic Hospital, Faculty of Homeopathy, Great Ormond St., London WC1N 3HR, England. Phone: 01-837-8833. Quarterly.

East West: The Journal of Natural Health and Living. East West Journal, Inc., 17 Station St., P.O. Box 1200, Brookline, MA 02146. Monthly.

Homeopath. Society of Homeopaths, 2 Artizan Rd., Northampton NN1 4HU, England.

Homeopathy. British Homeopathic Association, 27a Devonshire St., London W1N 1RJ, England. Bimonthly.

Journal of the American Institute of Homeopathy. American Institute of Homeopathy, 1500 Massachusetts Ave. N.W., Washington, DC 20005. Phone: (800) 848-5777. Quarterly.

NEWSLETTERS

Homeopathy Today. National Center for Homeopathy, 1500 Massachusetts Ave. N.W., No. 41, Washington, DC 20005. Phone: (202) 223-6182. Monthly.

ONLINE DATABASES

EMBASE. Elsevier Science Publishing Co., Inc., P.O. Box 882, Madison Square Station, New York, NY 10159-2101. Phone: (212) 989-5800. Fax: (212) 633-3990.

MEDLINE. National Library of Medicine, 8600 Rockville Pike, Bethesda, MD 20894. Phone: (800) 638-8480.

SciSearch. Institute for Scientific Information, 3501 Market St., Philadelphia, PA 19104. Phone: (215) 386-0100. Fax: (215) 386-6362.

POPULAR WORKS AND PATIENT EDUCATION

The Encyclopedia of Alternative Health Care. Kristin G. Olsen. Simon & Schuster, Inc., 1230 Ave. of the Americas, New York, NY 10020. Phone: (212) 698-7000. 1990.

The Natural Healing and Nutrition Annual. Mark Bricklin, Sharon Stocker (eds.). Rodale Press, Inc., 33 E. Minor St., Emmaus, PA 18098. Phone: (800) 527-8200. Fax: (215) 967-6263. Annual.

The Nutrition Desk Reference. Robert H. Garrison. Keats Publishing, Inc., P.O. Box 876, New Canaan, CT 06840. Phone: (203) 966-8721. Revised edition 1990.

RESEARCH CENTERS, INSTITUTES, CLEARINGHOUSES

Hahnemanian Research Center. 2232 Southeast Bristol, No. 102, Santa Ana Heights, CA 92707. Phone: (714) 852-9038.

Homeopathic Educational Service. 2124 Kittredge St., Berkeley, CA 94704. Phone: (415) 653-9270.

TEXTBOOKS AND MONOGRAPHS

Homeopathy: Medicine for the 21st Century. Dana Ullman. North Atlantic Books, 2800 Woolsey St., Berkeley, CA 94705. Phone: (415) 652-5309.

HOMOSEXUALITY

ABSTRACTING, INDEXING, AND CURRENT AWARENESS PUBLICATIONS

General Science Index. H.W. Wilson Co., 950 University Ave., Bronx, NY 10452. Phone: (800) 367-6770.

Psychological Abstracts. American Psychological Association, 1200 17th St. NW, Washington, DC 20036. Phone: (202) 955-7600. Monthly.

ASSOCIATIONS, PROFESSIONAL SOCIETIES, ADVOCACY AND SUPPORT GROUPS

Gay Medical Association. BM/GMA, London WC1N 3XX, England.

Gay Men's Health Crisis. 129 W. 20th St., New York, NY 10011. Phone: (212) 807-6664. Fax: (212) 337-3656.

National Lesbian and Gay Health Foundation. P.O. Box 65472, Washington, DC 20035. Phone: (202) 797-3708.

Society for the Pscyhological Study of Lesbian and Gay Issues (SPSLGI). c/o American Psychological Association, 1200 17th St. N.W., Washington, DC 20036. Phone: (202) 955-7727.

CD-ROM DATABASES

PsycLit. SilverPlatter Information, Inc., River Ridge Office Park, 100 River Ridge Rd., Norwood, MA 02062. Phone: (617) 769-2599. Fax: (617) 769-8763. Quarterly.

JOURNALS

Journal of Homosexuality. Haworth Press, 10 Alice St., Binghamton, NY 13904-1580. Phone: (803) 429-6784. Fax: (607) 722-1424.

Journal of Sex Research. Society for the Scientific Study of Sex, Box 208, Mount Vernon, IA 52314. Phone: (319) 895-8407.

ONLINE DATABASES

Human Sexuality. Clinical Communications, Inc., 132 Hutchin Hill, Shady, NY 12409. Phone: (914) 679-2217. Weekly to biweekly.

PsycInfo. SilverPlatter Information, Inc., River Ridge Office Park, 100 River Ridge Rd., Norwood, MA 02062. Phone: (617) 769-2599. Fax: (617) 769-8763. Quarterly.

HORMONES

See also: ENDOCRINOLOGY

ABSTRACTING, INDEXING, AND CURRENT AWARENESS PUBLICATIONS

BIOSIS/CAS Selects: Hormones & Gene Expression. BIOSIS, 2100 Arch St., Philadelphia, PA 19103-1399. Phone: (215) 587-4800. Fax: (215) 587-2016. Biweekly.

CA Selects: Steroids (Biochemical Aspects). Chemical Abstracts Service, 2540 Olentangy River Road, P.O. Box 3012, Columbus, OH 43210-0012. Phone: (800) 848-6538. Biweekly.

CA Selects: Steroids (Chemical Aspects). Chemical Abstracts Service, 2540 Olentangy River Road, P.O. Box 3012, Columbus, OH 43210-0012. Phone: (800) 848-6538. Biweekly.

Current Contents/Life Sciences. Institute for Scientific Information, 3501 Market St., Philadelphia, PA 19104. Phone: (215) 386-0100. Fax: (215) 386-6362.

Endocrinology Abstracts. Cambridge Scientific Abstracts, 7200 Wisconsin Ave., Bethesda, MD 20814-4823. Phone: (800) 843-7751. Fax: (301) 961-6720. Monthly.

Excerpta Medica. Section 3: Endocrinology. Elsevier Science Publishing Co., Inc., P.O. Box 882, Madison Square Station, New York, NY 10159-2101. Phone: (212) 989-5800. Fax: (212) 633-3990. 24/year.

Index Medicus. U.S. National Library of Medicine, 8600 Rockville Pike, Bethesda, MD 20894. Phone: (800) 638-8480. Monthly.

Research Alert: Hormones-Protein & Peptide. Institute for Scientific Information, 3501 Market St., Philadelphia, PA 19104. Phone: (800) 523-1850. Fax: (215) 386-6362. Weekly.

Research Alert: Hormones-Steroid. Institute for Scientific Information, 3501 Market St., Philadelphia, PA 19104. Phone: (800) 523-1850. Fax: (215) 386-6362. Weekly.

Science Citation Index. Institute for Scientific Information, 3501 Market St., Philadelphia, PA 19104. Phone: (800) 523-1850. Fax: (215) 386-6362. Bimonthly.

ANNUALS AND REVIEWS

Advances in Endocrinology and Metabolism. Mosby-Year Book, 11830 Westline Industrial Drive, St. Louis, MO 63146. Phone: (800) 325-4177. Fax: (314) 432-1380. Annual.

Progress in Reproductive Biology and Medicine. S. Karger Publishers, Inc., 26 West Avon Rd., P.O. Box 529, Farmington, CT 06085. Phone: (203) 675-7834. Fax: (203) 675-7302. Irregular.

Year Book of Endocrinology. Mosby-Year Book, 11830 Westline Industrial Drive, St. Louis, MO 63146. Phone: (800) 325-4177. Fax: (314) 432-1380. Annual.

ASSOCIATIONS, PROFESSIONAL SOCIETIES, ADVOCACY AND SUPPORT GROUPS

DES Action, U.S.A.. Long Island Jewish Medical Ctr., New Hyde Park, NY 11040. Phone: (516) 775-3450.

Endocrine Society (ES). 9650 Rockville Pike, Bethesda, MD 20814. Phone: (301) 571-1802.

CD-ROM DATABASES

SCISEARCH. Institute for Scientific Information, 3501 Market St., Philadelphia, PA 19104. Phone: (215) 386-0100. Fax: (215) 386-6362.

HANDBOOKS, GUIDES, MANUALS, ATLASES

Handbook of Clinical Endocrinology. Fitzgerald. Appleton & Lange, 25 Van Zant St., East Norwalk, CT 06855. Phone: (800) 423-1359. Fax: (203) 854-9486. Second edition 1992.

Handbook of Diabetes. Williams. Blackwell Scientific Publications, Inc., 3 Cambridge Ctr., Cambridge, MA 02142. Phone: (800) 759-6102. 1992.

Handbook of Drug Therapy in Reproductive Endocrinology. Rivlin. Little, Brown and Co., 34 Beacon St., Boston, MA 02108. Phone: (617) 227-0730. Fax: (617) 227-0790. 1990.

JOURNALS

Hormone and Metabolic Research. Thieme Medical Publishers, Inc., 381 Park Ave. S., New York, NY 10016. Phone: (212) 683-5088. Fax: (212) 779-9020. Monthly.

Hormone Research. S. Karger Publishers, Inc., 26 W. Avon Rd., P.O. Box 529, Farmington, CT 06085. Phone: (203) 675-7834. Fax: (203) 675-7302.

Hormones and Behavior. Academic Press, Inc., 1250 Sixth Ave., San Diego, CA 92101-4311. Phone: (619) 699-6345. Fax: (619) 699-6715.

Journal of Clinical Endocrinology & Metabolism. Williams & Wilkins, 428 E. Preston St., Baltimore, MD 21202. Phone: (800) 638-0672. Fax: (900) 447-8438. Monthly.

Steroids: Structure, Function, and Regulation. Butterworth-Heinemann, 80 Montvale Ave., Stoneham, MA 02180. Phone: (617) 438-8464. Fax: (617) 279-4851. Monthly.

NEWSLETTERS

Menopause News. Menopause News, 2074 Union St., San Francisco, CA 94123. 6/year.

ONLINE DATABASES

CSA Life Sciences Collection. Cambridge Scientific Abstracts, 7200 Wisconsin Ave., Bethesda, MD 20814-4823. Phone: (800) 843-7751. Fax: (301) 961-6720.

EMBASE. Elsevier Science Publishing Co., Inc., P.O. Box 882, Madison Square Station, New York, NY 10159-2101. Phone: (212) 989-5800. Fax: (212) 633-3990.

MEDLINE. National Library of Medicine, 8600 Rockville Pike, Bethesda, MD 20894. Phone: (800) 638-8480.

SciSearch. Institute for Scientific Information, 3501 Market St., Philadelphia, PA 19104. Phone: (215) 386-0100. Fax: (215) 386-6362.

POPULAR WORKS AND PATIENT EDUCATION

Estrogen: A Complete Guide to Reversing the Effects of Menopause Using Hormone Replacement Therapy. Lila Nachtigall, Joan R. Heilman. HarperCollins Pubs., Inc., 10 E. 53rd St., New York, NY 10022-5299. Phone: (212) 207-7000. Fax: (800) 242-7737. Revised edition 1991.

Hormones, Hot Flashes & Mood Swings: Living Through the Ups & Downs of Menopause. Clark Gillespie. HarperCollins Pubs., Inc., 10 E. 53rd St., New York, NY 10022-5299. Phone: (212) 207-7000. Fax: (800) 242-7737. 1989.

Managing Your Menopause. Wulf H. Utian. Prentice Hall, 113 Sylvan Ave., Rt. 9W, Prentice Hall Bldg., Englewood Cliffs, NJ 07632. Phone: (201) 767-5937. 1991.

TEXTBOOKS AND MONOGRAPHS

Clinical Pediatric Endocrinology. Hung. Mosby-Year Book, 11830 Westline Industrial Drive, St. Louis, MO 63146. Phone: (800) 325-4177. Fax: (314) 432-1380. 1992.

Endocrinology and Metabolism. Philip Felig, John D. Baxter, Lawrence A. Frohman. McGraw-Hill, Inc., Health Professions Division, 1221 Avenue of the Americas, 28th Floor, New York, NY 10020. Phone: (212) 512-4228. Third edition 1992.

Practical Approach to Pediatric Endocrinology. Bacon. Mosby-Year Book, 11830 Westline Industrial Drive, St. Louis, MO 63146. Phone: (800) 325-4177. Fax: (314) 432-1380. Third edition 1990.

Principles and Practice of Endocrinology and Metabolism. Kenneth L. Becker, John P. Bilezikian, William J Bremner. J.B. Lippincott Co., 227 East Washington Square, Philadelphia, PA 19106-3780. Phone: (215) 238-4200. Fax: (215) 238-4227. 1990.

Steroid and Non-Steroid Hormones: Their Assays and Applications. D. Kilshaw, K. Morris. Butterworth-Heinemann, 80 Montvale Ave., Stoneham, MA 02180. Phone: (617) 438-8464. Fax: (617) 279-4851. 1991.

Textbook of Diabetes. Pickup. Blackwell Scientific Publications, Inc., 3 Cambridge Ctr., Cambridge, MA 02142. Phone: (800) 759-6102. Two volumes 1991.

HOSPICES

See also: TERMINAL CARE

ABSTRACTING, INDEXING, AND CURRENT AWARENESS PUBLICATIONS

Hospital Literature Index. American Hospital Association, 840 N. Lake Shore Dr., Chicago, IL 60611. Phone: (800) 242-2626. Fax: (312) 280-6015. Quarterly.

Index Medicus. U.S. National Library of Medicine, 8600 Rockville Pike, Bethesda, MD 20894. Phone: (800) 638-8480. Monthly.

MEDOC: Index to U.S. Government Publications in the Medical and Health Sciences. Spencer S. Eccles Health Sciences Library, University of Utah, Bldg. 589, Salt Lake City, UT 84112. Phone: (801) 581-5268. Quarterly.

Palliative Care Index. Medical Information Service, British Library, Boston Spa, Wetherby, W. Yorkshire LS23 7BQ, England. Phone: 0937-546039. Fax: 0937-546236. Monthly.

ASSOCIATIONS, PROFESSIONAL SOCIETIES, ADVOCACY AND SUPPORT GROUPS

Children's Hospice International. 1101 King St., No. 131, Alexandria, VA 22314. Phone: (703) 684-0330.

Foundation for Hospice and Homecare (FHH). 519 C St. NE, Stanton Park, Washington, DC 20002. Phone: (202) 547-6586.

Hospice Association of America (HAA). 519 C St. NE, Stanton Park, Washington, DC 20002. Phone: (202) 546-4759. Fax: (202) 547-3540.

Hospice Education Institute (HEI). 5 Essex Sq., Ste. 3-B, P.O. Box 713, Essex, CT 06426. Phone: (203) 767-1620. Fax: (203) 767-2746.

National Hospice Organization (NHO). 1901 N. Moore St., Ste. 901, Arlington, VA 22209. Phone: (703) 243-5900. Fax: (703) 525-5762.

DIRECTORIES

Guide to the Nation's Hospices. National Hospice Organization, 1901 N. Moore St., Ste. 901, Arlington, VA 22209. Phone: (703) 243-5900. Fax: (703) 525-5762. Annual.

Home Health Care and Hospice Directory. National Association of Home Care, 519 C St. NE, Washington, DC 20002. Phone: (202) 547-7424. Fax: (202) 547-3540. Annual.

Hospices Directory. American Business Directories, Inc., 5711 S. 86th Circle, Omaha, NE 68127. Phone: (402) 593-4600. Fax: (402) 331-1505. Annual.

National Home Care and Hospice Directory. National Association of Home Care, 519 C St. N.E., Washington, DC 20002. Phone: (202) 547-7424. Fax: (202) 547-3540. Annual.

JOURNALS

American Journal of Hospice Care. Prime National Publishing, 470 Boston Post Rd., Weston, MA 02193. Phone: (617) 899-2702.

American Journal of Nursing. American Journal of Nursing Co., 555 W. 57th St., New York, NY 10019. Phone: (212) 582-8820. Monthly.

Archives of Disease in Childhood. BMJ Publishing Group, BMA House, Tavistock Square, London WC1H 9JR, England. Phone: 071-383 6244/6638. Fax: 071-383 6662. Monthly.

Archives of Internal Medicine. American Medical Association, 515 North State St., Chicago, IL 60610. Phone: (312) 464-0183. Fax: (312) 464-5834. Monthly.

BMJ. BMJ Publishing Group, BMA House, Tavistock Square, London WC1H 9JR, England. Phone: 071-383 6244/6638. Fax: 071-383 6662. Weekly.

Cancer. J.B. Lippincott Co., 227 East Washington Square, Philadelphia, PA 19106-3780. Phone: (215) 238-4200. Fax: (215) 238-4227. Semimonthly.

Geriatrics: Medicine for Midlife and Beyond. Edgell Communications, 7500 Old Oak Blvd., Cleveland, OH 44130. Phone: (216) 826-2839. Fax: (216) 891-2726. Monthly.

Hospice Journal. Haworth Press, 10 Alice Street, Binghamton, NY 13904-1580. Phone: (800) 429-6784. Fax: (607) 722-1424. Quarterly.

NEWSLETTERS

Hospice Letter. Health Resources Publishing, Brinley Professional Plaza, 3100 Hwy. 138, Wall, NJ 07719-1442. Phone: (201) 681-1133. Monthly.

Hospice Newsletter. Sovereign Hospitaller Order of Saint John, Villa Anneslie, 529 Dunkirk Rd., Baltimore, MD 21212. Phone: (301) 377-4352. Annual.

NHO Hospice News. National Hospice Organization, 1901 N. Moore St., Ste. 901, Arlington, VA 22209. Phone: (703) 243-5900. Fax: (703) 525-5762. Monthly.

ONLINE DATABASES

EMBASE. Elsevier Science Publishing Co., Inc., P.O. Box 882, Madison Square Station, New York, NY 10159-2101. Phone: (212) 989-5800. Fax: (212) 633-3990.

Health Planning and Administration. U.S. National Library of Medicine, MEDLARS Management Section, 8600 Rockville Pike, Bethesda, MD 20894. Phone: (800) 638-8480. Monthly.

MEDLINE. National Library of Medicine, 8600 Rockville Pike, Bethesda, MD 20894. Phone: (800) 638-8480.

SciSearch. Institute for Scientific Information, 3501 Market St., Philadelphia, PA 19104. Phone: (215) 386-0100. Fax: (215) 386-6362.

POPULAR WORKS AND PATIENT EDUCATION

Among Friends: Hospice Care for the Person with AIDS. Robert W. Buckingham. Prometheus Books, 700 E. Amherst St., Buffalo, NY 14215. Phone: (800) 421-0351. 1992.

The Complete Guide to Hospice Care. Larry Beresford. Little, Brown and Co., 34 Beacon St., Boston, MA 02108. Phone: (617) 227-0730. Fax: (617) 227-0790. 1992.

The Hospice Movement: A Better Way of Caring for the Dying. Sandol Stoddard. Random House, Inc., 201 E. 50th St., New York, NY 10022. Phone: (800) 726-0600. Expanded edition 1991.

In the Light of Dying: THe Journals of a Hospice Volunteer. Joan L. Taylor. Continuum Publishing Co., 370 Lexington Ave., New York, NY 10017. Phone: (212) 532-3650. 1983.

When a Loved One Is Ill: How to Take Better Care of Your Loved One, Your Family and Yourself. Leonard Felder. Viking Penguin, 375 Hudson St., New York, NY 10014-3657. Phone: (800) 331-4624. 1990.

STANDARDS AND STATISTICS SOURCES

Hospice Standards Manual. Joint Commission on Accreditation of Healthcare Organizations, Dept. of Publications, 1 Renaissance Blvd., OakBrook Terrace, IL 60181. Phone: (708) 916-5600.

TEXTBOOKS AND MONOGRAPHS

AIDS and the Hospice Community. Madalon O'Rawe, Amenta Claire Tehan (eds.). Haworth Press, 10 Alice Street, Binghamton, NY 13904-1580. Phone: (800) 342-9678. Fax: (607) 722-1424. 1991.

Hospice Care Systems: Structure, Process, Costs and Outcome. Vincent Mor. Springer Publishing Co., Inc., 536 Broadway, 11th Floor, New York, NY 10012. Phone: (212) 431-4370. 1987.

The Hospice Experiment. Vincent Mor and others. Johns Hopkins University Press, 701 W. 40th St., Suite 275, Baltimore, MD 21211-2190. Phone: (800) 537-5487. Fax: (410) 516-6998. 1988.

The Nature, Characteristics, and Processes of Hospice Care Delivery in the United States. Joint Commission on Accreditation of Healthcare Organizations, Dept. of Publications, 1 Renaissance Blvd., OakBrook Terrace, IL 60181. Phone: (708) 916-5600. Two volumes.

Notes on Symptom Control in Hospice and Palliative Care. Peter Kaye. Hospice Education Institute, P.O. Box 713, Essex, CT 06426. Phone: (203) 767-1620. 1990.

HOSPITAL ADMINISTRATION

See: HEALTH CARE ADMINISTRATION;
HOSPITALS

HOSPITAL MORTALITY RATES

See: HOSPITALS

HOSPITALS

See also: HEALTH CARE ADMINISTRATION

ABSTRACTING, INDEXING, AND CURRENT AWARENESS PUBLICATIONS

Cumulative Index to Nursing and Allied Health Literature. Glendale Adventist Medical Center, P.O. Box 871, Glendale, CA 91209. Phone: (818) 409-8005. Bimonthly.

Hospital Literature Index. American Hospital Association, 840 N. Lake Shore Dr., Chicago, IL 60611. Phone: (800) 242-2626. Fax: (312) 280-6015. Quarterly.

Index Medicus. U.S. National Library of Medicine, 8600 Rockville Pike, Bethesda, MD 20894. Phone: (800) 638-8480. Monthly.

Research Alert: Infections-Hospital Associated. Institute for Scientific Information, 3501 Market St., Philadelphia, PA 19104. Phone: (800) 523-1850. Fax: (215) 386-6362. Weekly.

ASSOCIATIONS, PROFESSIONAL SOCIETIES, ADVOCACY AND SUPPORT GROUPS

American Hospital Association (AHA). 840 N. Lake Shore Dr., Chicago, IL 60611. Phone: (312) 280-6000. Fax: (312) 280-5979.

American Osteopathic Hospital Association (AOHA). 1454 Duke St., Alexandria, VA 22314. Phone: (703) 684-7700.

Canadian Hospital Association. 17 York St., Ste. 100, Ottawa, ON, Canada K1N 9J6. Phone: (613) 238-8005. Fax: (613) 238-6924.

Catholic Health Association of the United States (CHA). 4455 Woodson Rd., St. Louis, MO 63134-0889. Phone: (314) 427-2500. Fax: (314) 427-0029.

Joint Commission on Accreditation of Healthcare Organizations (JCAHO). One Renaissance Blvd., Oakbrook Terrace, IL 60181. Phone: (708) 916-5600.

CD-ROM DATABASES

Health Planning & Administration/EBSCO-CD. EBSCO Publishing, P.O. Box 325, Topsfield, MA 01983. Phone: (800) 221-1826. Fax: (508) 887-3923. Quarterly.

Morbidity Mortality Weekly Report. MEP, 124 Mt. Auburn St., Cambridge, MA 02138. Phone: (800) 342-1338. Fax: (617) 868-7738. Annual.

Nursing and Allied Health (CINAHL) on CD-ROM. CINAHL, 1509 Wilson Terrace, P.O. Box 871, Glendale, CA 91209-0871. Phone: (818) 409-8005.

DIRECTORIES

Buyers Guide for the Health Care Industry. American Hospital Association, 840 N. Lake Shore Dr., Chicago, IL 60611. Phone: (800) 242-2626. Fax: (312) 280-6015. Annual.

Canadian Hospital Directory. Canadian Hospital Association, 17 York St., Ste. 100, Ottawa, ON, Canada K1N 9J6. Phone: (613) 238-8005. Fax: (613) 238-6924. Annual.

Directory of Health Care Professionals. American Hospital Association, 840 N. Lake Shore Dr., Chicago, IL 60611. Phone: (800) 242-2626. Fax: (312) 280-6015. Annual.

Directory of Hospital Personnel. Medical Economics, Five Paragon Dr., Montvale, NJ 07645-1742. Phone: (800) 222-3045. Fax: (201) 573-4956. Annual.

Directory of U.S. Hospitals. Health Care Investment Analysts, Inc., 300 E. Lombard St., Baltimore, MD 21202. Phone: (410) 576-9600. Fax: (410) 783-0575. First edition 1991.

Health and Medical Care Directory. Yellow Pages of America, Inc., 719 Main St., Niagara Falls, NY 14301. Phone: (800) 387-4209. Annual.

ENCYCLOPEDIAS, DICTIONARIES, WORD BOOKS

Facts on File Dictionary of Health Care Management. Joseph C. Rhea, and others. Facts On File, Inc., 460 Park Ave. S., New York, NY 10016-7382. Phone: (800) 322-8755. Fax: (212) 683-3633. 1988.

Health Care Terms. Vergil N. Slee, Debora A. Slee. Tringa Press, P.O. Box 8181, St. Paul, MN 55108. Second edition 1991.

JOURNALS

Hospital & Health Services Administration. Health Administration Press, 1021 E. Huron St., Ann Arbor, MI 48104-9990. Phone: (313) 764-1380. Fax: (313) 763-1105. Quarterly.

Hospital Infection Control. American Health Consultants, P.O. Box 71266, Chicago, IL 60691. Phone: (800) 688-2421. Fax: (404) 352-1971.

Hospitals. American Hospital Publishing, Inc., 211 E. Chicago Ave., Ste. 700, Chicago, IL 60611. Phone: (312) 440-6800. Semimonthly.

NEWSLETTERS

Hospital Administration Newsletter. National Research Bureau, Inc., 424 N. Third St., Burlington, IA 52601. Phone: (319) 752-5415. Fax: (319) 752-3421. Monthly.

Hospital Peer Review. American Health Consultants, P.O. Box 71266, Chicago, IL 60691. Phone: (800) 688-2421. Fax: (404) 352-1971.

Hospital Risk Management. American Health Consultants, Department C1290, P.O. Box 740060, Atlanta, GA 30374. Phone: (800) 559-1032. Monthly.

ONLINE DATABASES

EMBASE. Elsevier Science Publishing Co., Inc., P.O. Box 882, Madison Square Station, New York, NY 10159-2101. Phone: (212) 989-5800. Fax: (212) 633-3990.

Health Planning and Administration. U.S. National Library of Medicine, MEDLARS Management Section, 8600 Rockville Pike, Bethesda, MD 20894. Phone: (800) 638-8480. Monthly.

Hospital Database. Urban Decision Systems, Inc., 2040 Armacost Ave., P.O. Box 25953, Los Angeles, CA 90025. Phone: (800) 633-9568. Fax: (213) 826-0933. Irregular.

MEDIS. Mead Data Central, P.O. Box 1830, Dayton, OH 45401. Phone: (800) 227-4908.

MEDLINE. National Library of Medicine, 8600 Rockville Pike, Bethesda, MD 20894. Phone: (800) 638-8480.

Nursing and Allied Health (CINAHL). CINAHL, 1509 Wilson Terrace, P.O. Box 871, Glendale, CA 91209-0871. Phone: (818) 409-8005.

SciSearch. Institute for Scientific Information, 3501 Market St., Philadelphia, PA 19104. Phone: (215) 386-0100. Fax: (215) 386-6362.

POPULAR WORKS AND PATIENT EDUCATION

Best Medicine: Your Essential Guide to Finding Top Doctors, Hospitals and Treatments. Robert Arnot. Addison-Wesley Publishing Co., Rte. 128, Reading, MA 01867. Phone: (800) 447-2226. 1992.

Consumers' Guide to Hospitals. Consumers Checkbook, 806 15th St. N.W., Ste. 925, Washington, DC 20005. Phone: (202) 347-9612. 1988.

The Great White Lie: How America's Hospitals Betray Our Trust and Endanger Our Lives. Walt Bogdanich. Simon & Schuster, Inc., 1230 Ave. of the Americas, New York, NY 10020. Phone: (212) 698-7000. 1991.

Marketplace Medicine: The Rise of the For-Profit Hospital Chains. Dave Lindorff. Bantam Books, Inc., 666 Fifth Ave., New York, NY 10103. Phone: (800) 223-6834. 1992.

So Your Doctor Recommended Surgery. John Lewis. Holt, Rinehart & Winston, 115 W. 18th St., New York, NY 10011. Phone: (800) 488-5233. 1992.

Take This Book to the Hospital with You: A Consumer Guide to Surviving Your Hospital Stay. Charles B. Inlander, Ed. Weiner. Random House, Inc., 201 E. 50th St., New York, NY 10022. Phone: (800) 726-0600. 1991.

RESEARCH CENTERS, INSTITUTES, CLEARINGHOUSES

Agency for Health Care Policy and Research Publications Clearinghouse. P.O. Box 8547, Silver Spring, MD 20907. Phone: (800) 358-9295.

Connecticut Hospital Research and Education Foundation, Inc.. P.O. Box 90, 110 Barnes Rd., Wallingford, CT 06492. Phone: (203) 265-7611.

Hospital Research and Educational Trust. 840 N. Lake Shore Dr., Chicago, IL 60611. Phone: (312) 280-6000. Fax: (312) 280-6450.

Johns Hopkins University Center for Hospital Finance and Management. 624 N. Broadway, Rm. 300, Baltimore, MD 21205. Phone: (301) 955-2300.

STANDARDS AND STATISTICS SOURCES

1989 Summary: National Hospital Discharge Summary. National Center for Health Statistics, 6525 Belcrest Rd., Rm. 1064, Hyattsville, MD 20782. Phone: (301) 436-8500. PHS 91-1250. 1991.

Accreditation Manual for Hospitals. Joint Commission on Accreditation of Healthcare Organizations, Dept. of

Publications, 1 Renaissance Blvd., OakBrook Terrace, IL 60181. Phone: (708) 916-5600. Two volumes. Annual.

AHA Hospital Statistics. American Hospital Association, 840 N. Lake Shore Dr., Chicago, IL 60611. Phone: (800) 242-2626. Fax: (312) 280-6015. Annual.

American Hospital Association Guide to the Health Care Field. American Hospital Association, 840 N. Lake Shore Dr., Chicago, IL 60611. Phone: (800) 242-2626. Fax: (312) 280-6015. Annual.

American Hospital Association Hospital Statistics. American Hospital Association, 840 N. Lake Shore Dr., Chicago, IL 60611-2431. Phone: (800) 242-2626. Annual.

The Comparative Performance of U.S. Hospitals: The Sourcebook. Health Care Investment Analysts, Inc., 300 E. Lombard St., Baltimore, MD 21202. Phone: (410) 576-9600. Fax: (410) 783-0575. Annual.

Detailed Diagnoses and Procedures, National Hospital Discharge Survey, 1988. National Center for Health Statistics, 6525 Belcrest Rd., Rm. 1064, Hyattsville, MD 20782. Phone: (301) 436-8500. PHS 91-1768 1991.

Detailed Diagnoses and Procedures, National Hospital Discharge Survey, 1989. National Center for Health Statistics, 6525 Belcrest Rd., Rm. 1064, Hyattsville, MD 20782. Phone: (301) 436-8500. PHS 91-1769 1991.

Hospital Statistics: Data from the AHA Annual Survey. American Hospital Association, 840 N. Lake Shore Dr., Chicago, IL 60611. Phone: (312) 280-6000. Fax: (312) 280-5979. Annual.

Length of Stay, by Diagnosis and Operation. HCIA Inc., P.O. Box 303, Ann Arbor, MI 48106-0303. Annual.

Medicare Hospital Mortality Information. Health Care Financing Administration, Oak Meadows Building, 6325 Security Blvd., Baltimore, MD 21207. Phone: (301) 966-6573. Annual.

National Hospital Discharge Survey: Annual Summary, 1988. National Center for Health Statistics, 6525 Belcrest Rd., Rm. 1064, Hyattsville, MD 20782. Phone: (301) 436-8500. PHS 91-1767 1991.

Vital and Health Statistics. Series 13. Data on Health Resources Utilization. National Center for Health Statistics, 6525 Belcrest Rd., Rm. 1064, Hyattsville, MD 20782. Phone: (301) 436-8500. Irregular.

TEXTBOOKS AND MONOGRAPHS

Basic Accounting and Budgeting for Hospitals. Pelfrey. Delmar Publishers, Inc., 2 Computer Dr. W., Albany, NY 12205. Phone: (800) 347-7707. 1988.

Budgeting for Hospital Resource Management. Truman H. Esmond Jr.. American Hospital Association, 840 N. Lake Shore Dr., Chicago, IL 60611. Phone: (800) 242-2626. Fax: (312) 280-6015. 1990.

The Financial Management of Hospitals. Howard J. Berman, Lewis E. Weeks, Steven F. Kukla. Health Administration Press, 1021 E. Huron St., Ann Arbor, MI 48104-9990. Phone: (313) 764-1380. Fax: (313) 763-1105. Seventh edition 1990.

Hospital Administration for Middle Management: A Practical Approach. Stanley J. Malsky. Warren H. Green, Inc., 8536

Olive Blvd., St. Louis, MO 63132. Phone: (800) 537-0655. 1991.

Hospital Infections. John V. Bennett, Philip Brachman (eds.). Little, Brown and Company, 34 Beacon St., Boston, MA 02108. Phone: (617) 227-0730. Third edition 1992.

Hospital Organization and Management: Text and Readings. Kurt Darr and others. Health Professions Press, P.O. Box 10624, Baltimore, MD 21285-0624. Phone: (301) 337-9585. Fourth edition 1990.

Hospital Structure and Performance. Ann B. Flood, Richard W. Scott. Johns Hopkins University Press, 701 W. 40th St., Suite 275, Baltimore, MD 21211-2190. Phone: (800) 537-5487. Fax: (410) 516-6998. 1987.

Introduction to Managed Care: Health Maintenance Organizations, Preferred Provider Organizations, and Competitive Medical Plans. Robert G. Shouldice. Information Resources Press, 1110 N. Glebe Rd., Ste. 550, Arlington, VA 22201. Phone: (703) 558-8270. Fax: (703) 558-4979. 1991.

Management of Hospitals and Health Services: Strategic Issues and Performances. Rockwell Schulz, Aeton C. Johnson. Mosby-Year Book, 11830 Westline Industrial Drive, St. Louis, MO 63146. Phone: (800) 325-4177. Fax: (314) 432-1380. Third edition 1990.

Strategic Management of Hospitals and Health Care Facilities. Carl C. Pegels, Kenneth A. Rogers. Aspen Publishers, Inc., 200 Orchard Ridge Dr., Gaithersburg, MD 20878. Phone: (800) 638-8437. 1988.

HUMAN IMMUNODEFICIENCY VIRUS

See also: AIDS; IMMUNOLOGIC DISORDERS

ABSTRACTING, INDEXING, AND CURRENT AWARENESS PUBLICATIONS

CA Selects: AIDS & Related Immunodeficiencies. Chemical Abstracts Service, 2540 Olentangy River Road, P.O. Box 3012, Columbus, OH 43210-0012. Phone: (800) 848-6538. Biweekly.

Current Contents/Clinical Medicine. Institute for Scientific Information, 3501 Market St., Philadelphia, PA 19104. Phone: (800) 523-1850. Fax: (215) 386-6362. Weekly.

Current Contents/Life Sciences. Institute for Scientific Information, 3501 Market St., Philadelphia, PA 19104. Phone: (215) 386-0100. Fax: (215) 386-6362.

Excerpta Medica. Section 26: Immunology, Serology and Transplantation. Elsevier Science Publishing Co., Inc., P.O. Box 882, Madison Square Station, New York, NY 10159-2101. Phone: (212) 989-5800. Fax: (212) 633-3990. 32/year.

Index Medicus. U.S. National Library of Medicine, 8600 Rockville Pike, Bethesda, MD 20894. Phone: (800) 638-8480. Monthly.

MEDOC: Index to U.S. Government Publications in the Medical and Health Sciences. Spencer S. Eccles Health Sciences Library, University of Utah, Bldg. 589, Salt Lake City, UT 84112. Phone: (801) 581-5268. Quarterly.

Science Citation Index. Institute for Scientific Information, 3501 Market St., Philadelphia, PA 19104. Phone: (800) 523-1850. Fax: (215) 386-6362. Bimonthly.

ASSOCIATIONS, PROFESSIONAL SOCIETIES, ADVOCACY AND SUPPORT GROUPS

National Association of People with AIDS. 2025 I St. N.W., Washington, DC 20006. Phone: (202) 429-2856.

People with AIDS Health Group. 150 W. 20th St., New York, NY 10010.

BIBLIOGRAPHIES

AIDS Information Sourcebook. H. Robert Malinovsky, Gerald J. Perry (eds.). Oryx Press, 4041 N. Central, Suite 700, Phoenix, AZ 85012. Phone: (800) 279-ORYX. Fax: (800) 279-4663. 3rd edition,1991.

CD-ROM DATABASES

Biotechnology Citation Index. Institute for Scientific Information, 3501 Market St., Philadelphia, PA 19104. Phone: (215) 386-0100. Fax: (215) 386-6362. Bimonthly.

Excerpta Medica CD: Immunology & AIDS. SilverPlatter Information, Inc., River Ridge Office Park, 100 River Ridge Rd., Norwood, MA 02062. Phone: (617) 769-2599. Fax: (617) 769-8763. Quarterly.

Morbidity Mortality Weekly Report. MEP, 124 Mt. Auburn St., Cambridge, MA 02138. Phone: (800) 342-1338. Fax: (617) 868-7738. Annual.

SCISEARCH. Institute for Scientific Information, 3501 Market St., Philadelphia, PA 19104. Phone: (215) 386-0100. Fax: (215) 386-6362.

HANDBOOKS, GUIDES, MANUALS, ATLASES

The AIDS Benefits Handbook. T. McCormack. Yale University Press, 302 Temple St., New Haven, CT 06520. Phone: (203) 432-0940. 1990.

The Handbook of Immunopharmacology. Academic Press, Inc., 1250 Sixth Ave., San Diego, CA 92101-4311. Phone: (619) 699-6345. Fax: (619) 699-6715. Irregular.

Manual of Allergy and Immunology: Diagnosis and Therapy. Gleen J. Lawlor Jr., Thomas J. Fischer. Little, Brown and Co., 34 Beacon St., Boston, MA 02108. Phone: (617) 227-0730. Second edition 1988.

JOURNALS

AIDS Education & Prevention: An Interdisciplinary Journal. Guilford Publications, Inc., 72 Spring St., New York, NY 10012. Phone: (800) 365-7006. Fax: (212) 966-6708. Quarterly.

AIDS Research and Human Retroviruses. Mary Ann Liebert, Inc., 1651 Third Ave., New York, NY 10128. Phone: (212) 289-2300. Fax: (212) 289-4697. Monthly.

International Journal of STD and AIDS. Royal Society of Medicine Services Ltd., 1 Wimpole St., London W1M 8AE, England. Phone: 071-408 2119. Fax: 071-355 3198. Bimonthly.

Journal of Acquired Immune Deficiency Syndromes. Raven Press, 1185 Avenue of the Americas, New York, NY 10036. Phone: (212) 930-9500. Fax: (212) 869-3495. Monthly.

Journal of Infectious Diseases. University of Chicago Press, P.O. Box 37005, Chicago, IL 60637. Phone: (312) 753-3347. Fax: (312) 753-0811. Monthly.

Morbidity and Mortality Weekly Report. Massachusetts Medical Society, 1440 Main St., Waltham, MA 02154-1649. Phone: (617) 893-3800. Fax: (617) 893-0413. Weekly.

NEWSLETTERS

AIDS Alert. American Health Consultants, Department C1290, P.O. Box 740060, Atlanta, GA 30374. Phone: (800) 559-1032. Monthly.

AIDS Clinical Care. Massachusetts Medical Society, 1440 Main St., Waltham, MA 02154-1649. Phone: (617) 893-3800. Fax: (617) 893-0413. Monthly.

The AIDS Letter. Royal Society of Medicine Services Ltd., 1 Wimpole St., London W1M 8AE, England. Phone: 071-408 2119. Fax: 071-355 3198. Bimonthly.

BETA: The Bulletin of Experimental Treatments for AIDS. San Francisco AIDS Foundation, P.O. Box 2189, Berkeley, CA 94702-0189. Phone: (800) 327-9893. Fax: (415) 549-4342. Quarterly.

Common Sense about AIDS. American Health Consultants, P.O. Box 71266, Chicago, IL 60691-9987. Phone: (800) 688-2421.

ONLINE DATABASES

AIDSDRUGS. AIDS Clinical Trials Information Service, P.O. Box 6421, Rockville, MD 20850. Phone: (800) 874-2572. Monthly.

AIDSLINE. Division. U.S. National Library of Medicine, Specialized Information Services Division, 8600 Rockville Pike, Bethesda, MD 20894. Phone: (301) 496-6531. Weekly.

EMBASE. Elsevier Science Publishing Co., Inc., P.O. Box 882, Madison Square Station, New York, NY 10159-2101. Phone: (212) 989-5800. Fax: (212) 633-3990.

MEDLINE. National Library of Medicine, 8600 Rockville Pike, Bethesda, MD 20894. Phone: (800) 638-8480.

SciSearch. Institute for Scientific Information, 3501 Market St., Philadelphia, PA 19104. Phone: (215) 386-0100. Fax: (215) 386-6362.

POPULAR WORKS AND PATIENT EDUCATION

39 Development AIDS Medicines: Drugs and Vaccines. Pharmaceutical Manufacturers Association, 1100 15th St. N.W., Washington, DC 20005. Phone: (202) 835-3400. Annual.

The Essential HIV Treatment Fact Book. Laura Pinsky, Paul Harding Douglas, Craig Metroka. Pocket Books, Inc., 1230 Ave. of the Americas, New York, NY 10020. Phone: (800) 223-2348. Fax: (800) 284-0735. 1992.

The Guide to Living with HIV Infection: Developed at the Johns Hopkins AIDS Clinic. John G. Bartlett, Ann K. Finkbeiner. Johns Hopkins University Press, 701 W. 40th St., Suite 275, Baltimore, MD 21211-2190. Phone: (800) 537-5487. Fax: (410) 516-6998. 1991.

The HIV Test: What You Need to Know to Make an Informed Decision. Marc Vargo. Pocket Books, Inc., 1230 Ave. of the Americas, New York, NY 10020. Phone: (800) 223-2348. Fax: (800) 284-0735. 1992.

RESEARCH CENTERS, INSTITUTES, CLEARINGHOUSES

Center for HIV Education and Research. University of South Florida. 13301 Bruce B. Downs Blvd., Tampa, FL 33612-3899. Phone: (813) 974-4430.

TEXTBOOKS AND MONOGRAPHS

AIDS. Aggleton. Taylor & Francis Inc., 1900 Frost Rd., Suite 101, Bristol, PA 19007-1598. Phone: (800) 821-8312. Fax: (215) 785-5515. 1991.

AIDS and Alcohol/Drug Abuse: Psychosocial Research. Dennis G. Fisher (ed.). Haworth Press, 10 Alice Street, Binghamton, NY 13904-1580. Phone: (800) 342-9678. Fax: (607) 722-1424. 1991.

AIDS and HIV Diseases. Luc Montagnier. Mosby-Year Book, 11830 Westline Industrial Drive, St. Louis, MO 63146. Phone: (800) 325-4177. Fax: (314) 432-1380. 1990.

AIDS and the Hospice Community. Madalon O'Rawe, Amenta Claire Tehan (eds.). Haworth Press, 10 Alice Street, Binghamton, NY 13904-1580. Phone: (800) 342-9678. Fax: (607) 722-1424. 1991.

The AIDS Knowledge Base. P.T. Cohen, Merle A. Sande, Paul A. Volberding (eds.). Massachusetts Medical Society, 1440 Main St., Waltham, MA 02154-1649. Phone: (617) 893-3800. Fax: (617) 893-0413. 1992.

AIDS and Other Manifestations of HIV Infection. G. Wormser (ed.). Noyes Publications, Mill Rd. at Grand Ave., Park Ridge, NJ 07656. Phone: (201) 391-8484. 1987.

Cocaine, AIDS and Intravenous Drug Use. Samuel R. Friedman, Douglas S. Lipton (eds.). Haworth Press, 10 Alice Street, Binghamton, NY 13904-1580. Phone: (800) 3HA-WORTH. Fax: (607) 722-1424. 1991.

Fundamental Immunology. Robert M. Coleman and others. William C. Brown Communications, Inc., 2460 Kerper Blvd., Dubuque, IA 52001. Phone: (800) 338-5578. 1989.

The Human Retroviruses. Robert C. Gallo, Gilbert Jay (eds.). Academic Press, Inc., 1250 Sixth Ave., San Diego, CA 92101-4311. Phone: (619) 699-6345. Fax: (619) 699-6715. 1991.

Living and Dying with AIDS. Ahmed. Plenum Publishing Co., 233 Spring St., New York, NY 10013-1578. Phone: (212) 620-8000. Fax: (212) 463-0742. 1992.

The Medical Management of AIDS. Merle A. Sande, Paul A. Volberding. W.B. Saunders Co., The Curtis Center, Independence Square W., Philadelphia, PA 19106-3399. Phone: (215) 238-7800. Second edition 1991.

HUNTINGTON CHOREA

ABSTRACTING, INDEXING, AND CURRENT AWARENESS PUBLICATIONS

Current Contents/Clinical Medicine. Institute for Scientific Information, 3501 Market St., Philadelphia, PA 19104. Phone: (800) 523-1850. Fax: (215) 386-6362. Weekly.

Excerpta Medica. Section 22: Human Genetics. Elsevier Science Publishers, P.O. Box 882, Madison Square Station, New York, NY 10159-2101. Phone: (212) 633-3950. Fax: (212) 633-3990. 24/year.

Science Citation Index. Institute for Scientific Information, 3501 Market St., Philadelphia, PA 19104. Phone: (800) 523-1850. Fax: (215) 386-6362. Bimonthly.

ASSOCIATIONS, PROFESSIONAL SOCIETIES, ADVOCACY AND SUPPORT GROUPS

Association to Combat Huntington's Chorea (ACHC). 34A Station Rd., Hickley, Leics. LE10 1AP, England.

Hereditary Disease Foundation. 1427 7th St., Suite 2, Santa Monica, CA 90401. Phone: (213) 458-4183.

Huntington's Disease Society of America (HDSA). 140 W. 22nd St., 6th Fl., New York, NY 10011-2420. Phone: (212) 242-1968. Fax: (212) 243-2443.

CD-ROM DATABASES

SCISEARCH. Institute for Scientific Information, 3501 Market St., Philadelphia, PA 19104. Phone: (215) 386-0100. Fax: (215) 386-6362.

JOURNALS

American Journal of Human Genetics. University of Chicago Press, P.O. Box 37005, Chicago, IL 60637. Phone: (312) 753-3347. Fax: (312) 753-0811. Monthly.

Annals of Neurology. Little, Brown and Co., 34 Beacon St., Boston, MA 02108. Phone: (617) 227-0730. Fax: (617) 227-0790. Monthly.

Dementia. S. Karger Publishers, Inc., 26 West Avon Rd., P.O. Box 529, Farmington, CT 06085. Phone: (203) 675-7834. Fax: (203) 675-7302. Bimonthly.

Journal of Genetic Counseling. Human Sciences Press, 233 Spring St., New York, NY 10013-1578. Phone: (800) 221-9369. Fax: (212) 807-1047. Quarterly.

Journal of Medical Ethics. BMJ Publishing Group, BMA House, Tavistock Square, London WC1H 9JR, England. Phone: 071-383 6244/6638. Fax: 071-383 6662. Quarterly.

Journal of Neurology, Neurosurgery & Psychiatry. BMJ Publishing Group, BMA House, Tavistock Square, London WC1H 9JR, England. Phone: 071-383 6244/6638. Fax: 071-383 6662. Monthly.

Lancet. Williams & Wilkins, 428 East Preston St., Baltimore, MD 21202. Phone: (800) 638-0672. Fax: (800) 447-8438. Weekly.

Neurology. Edgell Communications, 7500 Old Oak Blvd., Cleveland, OH 44130. Phone: (216) 826-2839. Fax: (216) 891-2726. Monthly.

NEWSLETTERS

Marker. Huntington's Disease Society of America, 140 W. 22nd St., New York, NY 10011. Phone: (212) 242-1968.

ONLINE DATABASES

EMBASE. Elsevier Science Publishing Co., Inc., P.O. Box 882, Madison Square Station, New York, NY 10159-2101. Phone: (212) 989-5800. Fax: (212) 633-3990.

MEDLINE. National Library of Medicine, 8600 Rockville Pike, Bethesda, MD 20894. Phone: (800) 638-8480.

SciSearch. Institute for Scientific Information, 3501 Market St., Philadelphia, PA 19104. Phone: (215) 386-0100. Fax: (215) 386-6362.

RESEARCH CENTERS, INSTITUTES, CLEARINGHOUSES

Birth Defects and Genetic Disorders Unit. T311 General Hospital, University of Iowa, Iowa City, IA 52242. Phone: (319) 353-6687.

Huntington's Disease Diagnostic and Referral Center. Hahnemann University. 1427 Vine St., 1st Floor, Philadelphia, PA 19102. Phone: (215) 246-5010.

TEXTBOOKS AND MONOGRAPHS

Huntington's Disease: A Disorder of Families. Susan E. Folstein. Johns Hopkins University Press, 701 W. 40th St., Suite 275, Baltimore, MD 21211-2190. Phone: (800) 537-5487. Fax: (410) 516-6998. 1989.

Treatment of Genetic Diseases. Robert J. Desnick (ed.). Churchill Livingstone Inc., 650 Avenue of the Americas, New York, NY 10011. Phone: (212) 819-5400. Fax: (212) 302-6598. 1991.

HYPERACTIVITY

See also: ATTENTION DEFICIT DISORDER

ABSTRACTING, INDEXING, AND CURRENT AWARENESS PUBLICATIONS

Index Medicus. U.S. National Library of Medicine, 8600 Rockville Pike, Bethesda, MD 20894. Phone: (800) 638-8480. Monthly.

Science Citation Index. Institute for Scientific Information, 3501 Market St., Philadelphia, PA 19104. Phone: (800) 523-1850. Fax: (215) 386-6362. Bimonthly.

ASSOCIATIONS, PROFESSIONAL SOCIETIES, ADVOCACY AND SUPPORT GROUPS

American Academy of Pediatrics (AAP). 141 Northwest Point Blvd., P.O. Box 927, Elk Grove Village, IL 60009-0927. Phone: (708) 228-5005. Fax: (708) 228-5097.

Attention-Deficit Disorder Association (ADDA). 8091 S. Ireland Way, Aurora, CO 80016. Phone: (303) 690-7548.

CHADD (Children with Attention Deficit Disorders). 1859 North Pine Island Rd., Suite 185, Plantation, FL 33322. Phone: (305) 587-3700.

Feingold Foundation of the United States. P.O. Box 6550, Alexandria, VA 22306. Phone: (703) 768-3287.

CD-ROM DATABASES

SCISEARCH. Institute for Scientific Information, 3501 Market St., Philadelphia, PA 19104. Phone: (215) 386-0100. Fax: (215) 386-6362.

HANDBOOKS, GUIDES, MANUALS, ATLASES

Attention-Deficit Hyperactivity Disorder: A Clinical Guide to Diagnosis and Treatment. Larry B. Silver. American Psychiatric Press, Inc., 1400 K St. NW, Washington, DC 20005. Phone: (202) 682-6268. Fax: (202) 789-2648. 1991.

JOURNALS

American Academy of Child and Adolescent Psychiatry Journal. Williams & Wilkins, 428 East Preston St., Baltimore, MD 21202. Phone: (800) 638-0672. Fax: (800) 447-8438.

Clinical Pediatrics. J.B. Lippincott Co., 227 E. Washington Square, Philadelphia, PA 19106-3780. Phone: (215) 238-4200. Fax: (215) 238-4227.

Journal of Pediatrics. Mosby-Year Book, 11830 Westline Industrial Drive, St. Louis, MO 63146. Phone: (800) 325-4177. Fax: (314) 432-1380. Monthly.

ONLINE DATABASES

EMBASE. Elsevier Science Publishing Co., Inc., P.O. Box 882, Madison Square Station, New York, NY 10159-2101. Phone: (212) 989-5800. Fax: (212) 633-3990.

MEDLINE. National Library of Medicine, 8600 Rockville Pike, Bethesda, MD 20894. Phone: (800) 638-8480.

PsycInfo. SilverPlatter Information, Inc., River Ridge Office Park, 100 River Ridge Rd., Norwood, MA 02062. Phone: (617) 769-2599. Fax: (617) 769-8763. Quarterly.

SciSearch. Institute for Scientific Information, 3501 Market St., Philadelphia, PA 19104. Phone: (215) 386-0100. Fax: (215) 386-6362.

POPULAR WORKS AND PATIENT EDUCATION

The ADD Hyperactivity Workbook for Parents, Teachers, and Kids. H.C. Parker. Impact Publications, 1859 North Pine Island Rd., Suite 185, Plantation, FL 33322. Phone: (305) 587-3700.

Dr. Larry Silver's Advice to Parents on Attention-Deficit Hyperactivity Disorder. Larry B. Silver. American Psychiatric Press, Inc., 1400 K St. NW, Washington, DC 20005. Phone: (202) 682-6268. Fax: (202) 789-2648. 1992.

Help for the Hyperactive Child.. William G. Crook. Professional Books/Future Health, Inc., P.O. Box 3246, Jackson, TN 38301. Phone: (901) 423-5400. 1991.

Helping Your Hyperactive Child: From Effective Treatments and Developing Discipline and Self-Esteem to Helping Your Family Adjust. John F. Taylor. Prima Publishing, P.O. Box 1260, Rocklin, CA 95677-1260. Phone: (916) 786-0426. 1990.

Parent's Guide to Attention Deficit Disorders. Lisa J. Bain. Doubleday & Co., Inc., 666 Fifth Ave., New York, NY 10103. Phone: (800) 223-6834. 1991.

Your Hyperactive Child: A Parent's Guide to Coping with Attention Deficit Disorder. B.D. Ingersoll. Bantam Doubleday

Dell, 666 Fifth Ave., New York, NY 10103. Phone: (800) 223-6834. 1988.

RESEARCH CENTERS, INSTITUTES, CLEARINGHOUSES

Carrier Foundation Division of Research. P.O. Box 147, Belle Mead, NJ 08502. Phone: (908) 281-1000.

Child Behavior Research Unit. State University of New York Health Center at Brooklyn. 450 Clarkson Ave., Box 1195, Brooklyn, NY 11203. Phone: (718) 245-2326.

HYPERGLYCEMIA

See: DIABETES

HYPERLIPIDEMIA

See: ATHEROSCLEROSIS; NUTRITIONAL DISORDERS

HYPERTENSION

ABSTRACTING, INDEXING, AND CURRENT AWARENESS PUBLICATIONS

CA Selects: Hypertension & Antihypertensives. Chemical Abstracts Service, 2540 Olentangy River Road, P.O. Box 3012, Columbus, OH 43210-0012. Phone: (800) 848-6538. Biweekly.

Core Journals in Cardiology. Elsevier Science Publishing Co., Inc., P.O. Box 882, Madison Square Station, New York, NY 10159-2101. Phone: (212) 989-5800. Fax: (212) 633-3990. 11/year.

Current Contents/Clinical Medicine. Institute for Scientific Information, 3501 Market St., Philadelphia, PA 19104. Phone: (800) 523-1850. Fax: (215) 386-6362. Weekly.

Current Literature in Nephrology, Hypertension and Transplantation. Current Literature Publications, Inc., 1513 E St., Bellingham, WA 98225. Phone: (206) 671-6664. Monthly.

Excerpta Medica. Section 18: Cardiovascular Disease and Cardiovascular Surgery. Elsevier Science Publishing Co., Inc., P.O. Box 882, Madison Square Station, New York, NY 10159-2101. Phone: (212) 989-5800. Fax: (212) 633-3990. 24/year.

Index Medicus. U.S. National Library of Medicine, 8600 Rockville Pike, Bethesda, MD 20894. Phone: (800) 638-8480. Monthly.

Research Alert: Antihypertensive Agents. Institute for Scientific Information, 3501 Market St., Philadelphia, PA 19104. Phone: (800) 523-1850. Fax: (215) 386-6362. Weekly.

Research Alert: Cardiovascular Diseases-Hypertension. Institute for Scientific Information, 3501 Market St., Philadelphia, PA 19104. Phone: (800) 523-1850. Fax: (215) 386-6362. Weekly.

Science Citation Index. Institute for Scientific Information, 3501 Market St., Philadelphia, PA 19104. Phone: (800) 523-1850. Fax: (215) 386-6362. Bimonthly.

ASSOCIATIONS, PROFESSIONAL SOCIETIES, ADVOCACY AND SUPPORT GROUPS

American Heart Association (AHA). 7320 Greenville Ave., Dallas, TX 75231. Phone: (214) 373-6300.

Citizens for the Treatment of High Blood Pressure - Public Action on Cholest erol (CTHBP). 7200 Wisconsin Ave., Ste. 1002, Bethesda, MD 20814. Phone: (301) 907-7790.

Clinical Research Institute of Montreal. 110 Pine Ave. W., Montreal, PQ, Canada H2W 1R7. Phone: (514) 987-5500. Fax: (514) 987-5679.

International Society of Hypertension. c/o Dr. J.H. Laragh, Hypertension Center, New York Hospital, Cornell Medical Center, New York, NY 10021. Phone: (212) 472-5454.

National Hypertension Association (NHA). 324 E. 30th St., New York, NY 10016. Phone: (212) 889-3557.

National Institute of Hypertension Studies - Institute of Hypertension School of Research (NIHS). 13217 Livernois, Detroit, MI 48238. Phone: (313) 931-3427.

BIBLIOGRAPHIES

Hypertension: Cause and Treatment. National Technical Information Service, 5285 Port Royal Rd., Springfield, VA 22161. Phone: (703) 487-4650. Fax: (703) 321-8547. Jan. 1978-Jun. 1988 PB88-866165/CBY.

Hypertension: Therapies and Prevention. National Technical Information Service, 5285 Port Royal Rd., Springfield, VA 22161. Phone: (703) 487-4650. Fax: (703) 321-8547. Jan. 1970-Jun. 1988 PB88-86795/CBY.

CD-ROM DATABASES

Excerpta Medica CD: Cardiology. SilverPlatter Information, Inc., River Ridge Office Park, 100 River Ridge Rd., Norwood, MA 02062. Phone: (617) 769-2599. Fax: (617) 769-8763. Quarterly.

Hypertension Management. Hoffer. Williams & Wilkins, 428 East Preston St., Baltimore, MD 21202. Phone: (800) 638-0672. Fax: (800) 447-8438. 1989.

SCISEARCH. Institute for Scientific Information, 3501 Market St., Philadelphia, PA 19104. Phone: (215) 386-0100. Fax: (215) 386-6362.

DIRECTORIES

International Society of Hypertension-Membership Directory. International Society of Hypertension, c/o Dr. P.A. van Zwieten, Departments of Pharmacotherapy and Cardiology, Academic Medical Centre and Academic Hospital, University of Amsterdam, Meiberg dreef 15, NL-1105 AZ Amsterdam, Netherlands. Phone: 20-5664977.

HANDBOOKS, GUIDES, MANUALS, ATLASES

An Atlas of Hypertension. P.F. Semple, G.B.M. Lindop. The Parthenon Publishing Group, Inc., 120 Mill Rd., Park Ridge, NJ 07656. Phone: (201) 391-6796. 1992.

Clinical Atlas of Hypertension. J.D. Swales, P.S. Sever, Sir Stanley Peart. J.B. Lippincott Co., 227 East Washington Square, Philadelphia, PA 19106-3780. Phone: (215) 238-4200. Fax: (215) 238-4227. 1991.

A Color Atlas of Hypertension. Leonard M. Shapiro, Maurice B. Buchalter. Mosby-Year Book, 11830 Westline Industrial Drive, St. Louis, MO 63146. Phone: (800) 325-4177. Fax: (314) 432-1380. Second edition 1991.

JOURNALS

American Heart Journal. Mosby-Year Book, 11830 Westline Industrial Drive, St. Louis, MO 63146. Phone: (800) 325-4177. Fax: (314) 432-1380. Monthly.

American Journal of Cardiology. Reed Publishing USA, 249 W. 17th St., New York, NY 10011. Phone: (212) 645-0067. Fax: (212) 242-6987. 22/year.

American Journal of Hypertension. Elsevier Science Publishing Co., Inc., P.O. Box 882, Madison Square Station, New York, NY 10159-2101. Phone: (212) 989-5800. Fax: (212) 633-3990. Monthly.

British Heart Journal. BMJ Publishing Group, BMA House, Tavistock Square, London WC1H 9JR, England. Phone: 071383 6244/6638. Fax: 071383 6662. Monthly.

Circulation. American Heart Association, 7320 Greenville Ave., Dallas, TX 75231-4599. Phone: (214) 706-1310. Fax: (214) 691-2704. Monthly.

Hypertension. American Heart Association, 7320 Greenville Ave., Dallas, TX 75231. Phone: (214) 706-1310. Fax: (214) 691-6342. Monthly.

Journal of the American College of Cardiology. Elsevier Science Publishing Co., Inc., P.O. Box 882, Madison Square Station, New York, NY 10159-2101. Phone: (212) 989-5800. Fax: (212) 633-3990. Monthly.

Journal of Hypertension. Current Science Group, 20 N. Third St., Philadelphia, PA 19106-2199. Phone: (800) 552-5866. Fax: (215) 574-2270. Monthly.

ONLINE DATABASES

Combined Health Information Database (CHID). U.S. National Institutes of Health, P.O. Box NDIC, Bethesda, MD 20892. Phone: (301) 496-2162. Fax: (301) 770-5164. Quarterly.

EMBASE. Elsevier Science Publishing Co., Inc., P.O. Box 882, Madison Square Station, New York, NY 10159-2101. Phone: (212) 989-5800. Fax: (212) 633-3990.

MEDLINE. National Library of Medicine, 8600 Rockville Pike, Bethesda, MD 20894. Phone: (800) 638-8480.

SciSearch. Institute for Scientific Information, 3501 Market St., Philadelphia, PA 19104. Phone: (215) 386-0100. Fax: (215) 386-6362.

POPULAR WORKS AND PATIENT EDUCATION

About Your High Blood Pressure Medicines. United States Pharmacopeial Convention, Inc., 12601 Twinbrook Parkway, Rockville, MD 20852. Phone: (800) 227-8772. Fax: (301) 816-8148. Fourth edition 1992.

Blood Pressure: Questions You Have, Answeres You Need. Ed Weiner. People's Medical Society, 462 Walnut St., Allentown, PA 18102. Phone: (215) 770-1670. 1992.

Complete Guide to Living with High Blood Pressure. Michael K. Rees. Prentice Hall, 113 Sylvan Ave., Rt. 9W, Prentice Hall

Bldg., Englewood Cliffs, NJ 07632. Phone: (201) 767-5937. 1988.

Coping with High Blood Pressure. Sandy Sorrentino, Carl Hansman. Dembner Books, 80 Eight Ave., New York, NY 10011. Phone: (212) 924-2525. 1990.

The H.A.R.T. Program - Hypertension Autonomic Relaxation Treatment: A Comprehensive Guide to Lowering Your Blood Pressure without Drugs Based on Research. Ariel Kerman, Richard Trubo. HarperCollins Pubs., Inc., 10 E. 53rd St., New York, NY 10022. Phone: (212) 207-7000. 1992.

Hypertension: How to Work with Your Doctor and Take Charge of Your Health. Mike Samuels, Nancy Samuels. Simon and Schuster, 1230 Ave. of the Americas, New York, NY 10020. Phone: (800) 223-2348. Fax: (800) 284-0735. 1991.

Yale University School of Medicine Heart Book. Barry L. Zaret, Lawrence S. Cohen, Marvin Moser, and others. William Morrow & Company, Inc., 1350 Ave. of the Americas, New York, NY 10019. Phone: (800) 237-0657. 1992.

RESEARCH CENTERS, INSTITUTES, CLEARINGHOUSES

Cleveland Clinic Foundation Research Institute. 9500 Euclid Ave., Cleveland, OH 44195-5210. Phone: (216) 444-3900. Fax: (216) 444-3279.

DeBakey Heart Center. Baylor College of Medicine. Texas Medical Center, 1 Baylor Plaza, Houston, TX 77030. Phone: (701) 797-9353. Fax: (713) 793-1192.

Division of Hypertension. University of Michigan. 3918 Taubman Center, Ann Arbor, MI 48109-0356. Phone: (313) 936-4790.

Framingham Heart Study. 5 Thurber St., Framingham, MA 01701. Phone: (508) 872-4386.

Hypertension/Atherosclerosis Unit. University of Virginia. Medical Center, Box 146, Charlottesville, VA 22908. Phone: (804) 924-2765. Fax: (804) 924-2581.

Hypertension Research Center. Indiana University. 421 Clinical Bldg., 541 Clinical Dr., Indianapolis, IN 46223. Phone: (317) 274-8153.

National Heart, Lung, and Blood Institute. 4733 Bethesda Ave., Ste. 530, Bethesda, MD 20814. Phone: (301) 951-3260.

National Heart, Lung, and Blood Institute Education Programs Information Center. 4733 Bethesda Ave., Ste. 530, Bethesda, MD 20814. Phone: (301) 951-3260.

Specialized Center for Research in Hypertension. University of Alabama at Birmingham. Zeigler Research Bldg., 703 S. 19th St., Birmingham, AL 35294. Phone: (205) 934-2580. Fax: (205) 934-0424.

Specialized Center of Research in Hypertension. Vanderbilt University. Garland Ave., Nashville, TN 37232. Phone: (615) 322-3353. Fax: (615) 322-4349.

Whitaker Cardiovascular Institute. Boston University. 80 E. Concord St., Boston, MA 02118. Phone: (917) 638-4018. Fax: (617) 638-5258.

TEXTBOOKS AND MONOGRAPHS

Clinical Hypertension. Norman Kaplan, Ellin Lieberman. Williams & Wilkins, 428 E. Preston St., Baltimore, MD 21202.

Phone: (800) 638-0672. Fax: (800) 447-8438. Fifth edition 1990.

Personality, Elevated Blood Pressure, and Essential Hypertension. Ernest H. Johnson, and others (eds.). Taylor & Francis Inc., 1900 Frost Rd., Suite 101, Bristol, PA 19007-1598. Phone: (800) 821-8312. Fax: (215) 785-5515. 1991.

Working Group Report on Management of Patients with Hypertension and High Blood Cholesterol. National Heart, Lung, and Blood Institute, 4733 Bethesda Ave., Ste. 530, Bethesda, MD 20814. Phone: (301) 951-3260. NIH Pub. No. 90-2361 1990.

HYPERTHYROIDISM

See: THYROID DISEASES

HYPNOSIS

ABSTRACTING, INDEXING, AND CURRENT AWARENESS PUBLICATIONS

Index Medicus. U.S. National Library of Medicine, 8600 Rockville Pike, Bethesda, MD 20894. Phone: (800) 638-8480. Monthly.

Psychological Abstracts. American Psychological Association, 1200 17th St. NW, Washington, DC 20036. Phone: (202) 955-7600. Monthly.

ASSOCIATIONS, PROFESSIONAL SOCIETIES, ADVOCACY AND SUPPORT GROUPS

American Association of Professional Hypnotherapists (AAPH). P.O. Box 731, Mc Lean, VA 22101. Phone: (703) 448-9623.

American Guild of Hypnotherapists. 7117 Farnham St., Omaha, NE 68132. Phone: (402) 397-1500.

American Society of Clinical Hypnosis (ASCH). 2200 E. Devon Ave., Ste. 291, Des Plaines, IL 60018-4501. Phone: (708) 297-3317. Fax: (708) 297-7309.

Society for Clinical and Experimental Hypnosis. 128-A Kings Park Dr., Liverpool, NY 13090.

CD-ROM DATABASES

PsycLit. SilverPlatter Information, Inc., River Ridge Office Park, 100 River Ridge Rd., Norwood, MA 02062. Phone: (617) 769-2599. Fax: (617) 769-8763. Quarterly.

DIRECTORIES

American Society of Clinical Hypnosis-Membership Directory. 2200 E. Devon Ave., Ste. 291, Des Plaines, IL 60018-4501. Phone: (708) 297-3317. Fax: (708) 297-7309. Biennial.

JOURNALS

American Journal of Clinical Hypnosis. American Society of Clinical Hypnosis, 2250 E. Devon, Ste. 336, Des Plaines, IL 60018. Phone: (708) 297-3317. Quarterly.

Contemporary Hypnosis. Whurr Publishers, Contemporary Hypnosis, P.O. Box 1897, Lawrence, KS 66044-8897. Phone: (913) 843-1221. Fax: (913) 843-1274. 3/year.

International Journal of Clinical and Experimental Hypnosis. Society for Clinical and Experimental Hypnosis, 128-A Kings Park Dr., Liverpool, NY 13090.

NEWSLETTERS

American Society of Clinical Hypnosis-Newsletter. American Society of Clinical Hypnosis, 2250 E. Devon St., Ste. 336, Des Plaines, IL 60018. Phone: (708) 297-3317. 6/year.

Hypnotherapy in Review. Academy of Scientific Hypnotherapy, P.O. Box 12041, San Diego, CA 92112-3041. Phone: (619) 427-6225. Irregular.

Hypnotherapy Today. American Association of Professional Hypnotherapists, P.O. Box 731, Mc Lean, VA 22101. Phone: (703) 448-9623. 4/year.

ONLINE DATABASES

EMBASE. Elsevier Science Publishing Co., Inc., P.O. Box 882, Madison Square Station, New York, NY 10159-2101. Phone: (212) 989-5800. Fax: (212) 633-3990.

MEDLINE. National Library of Medicine, 8600 Rockville Pike, Bethesda, MD 20894. Phone: (800) 638-8480.

PsycInfo. SilverPlatter Information, Inc., River Ridge Office Park, 100 River Ridge Rd., Norwood, MA 02062. Phone: (617) 769-2599. Fax: (617) 769-8763. Quarterly.

SciSearch. Institute for Scientific Information, 3501 Market St., Philadelphia, PA 19104. Phone: (215) 386-0100. Fax: (215) 386-6362.

RESEARCH CENTERS, INSTITUTES, CLEARINGHOUSES

American Board of Psychological Hypnosis. International University School of Medicine, 791 Union Dr., Indianapolis, IN 46223.

Institute for Research in Hypnosis and Psychotherapy. 1991 Broadway No. 1803, New York, NY 10023. Phone: (212) 874-5290.

Pain Center. University of Alabama at Birmingham. UAB Medical Center, 1813 6th Ave., Birmingham, AL 35233. Phone: (205) 934-6174.

TEXTBOOKS AND MONOGRAPHS

Hypnosis and Hypnotherapy in Children. Karen Olness, G. Gail Gardner. W.B. Saunders Co., The Curtis Center, Independence Sqare W., Philadelphia, PA 19106-3399. Phone: (215) 238-7800. 1988.

HYPOGLYCEMIA

See: DIABETES

HYPOTHYROIDISM

See: THYROID DISEASES

HYSTERECTOMY

See also: GYNECOLOGIC DISORDERS;
OBSTETRICS AND GYNECOLOGY

ABSTRACTING, INDEXING, AND CURRENT AWARENESS PUBLICATIONS

Core Journals in Obstetrics and Gynecology. Elsevier Science Publishing Co., Inc., P.O. Box 882, Madison Square Station, New York, NY 10159-2101. Phone: (212) 989-5800. Fax: (212) 633-3990. 11/year.

Cumulative Index to Nursing and Allied Health Literature. Glendale Adventist Medical Center, P.O. Box 871, Glendale, CA 91209. Phone: (818) 409-8005. Bimonthly.

Current Contents/Clinical Medicine. Institute for Scientific Information, 3501 Market St., Philadelphia, PA 19104. Phone: (800) 523-1850. Fax: (215) 386-6362. Weekly.

Excerpta Medica. Section 10: Obstetrics and Gynecology. Elsevier Science Publishing Co., Inc., P.O. Box 882, Madison Square Station, New York, NY 10159-2101. Phone: (212) 989-5800. Fax: (212) 633-3990. 20/year.

Index Medicus. U.S. National Library of Medicine, 8600 Rockville Pike, Bethesda, MD 20894. Phone: (800) 638-8480. Monthly.

Science Citation Index. Institute for Scientific Information, 3501 Market St., Philadelphia, PA 19104. Phone: (800) 523-1850. Fax: (215) 386-6362. Bimonthly.

ASSOCIATIONS, PROFESSIONAL SOCIETIES, ADVOCACY AND SUPPORT GROUPS

American College of Obstetricians and Gynecologists (ACOG). 409 12th St. S.W., Washington, DC 20024-2188. Phone: (202) 638-5577.

The Campaign for Women's Health. 666 11th St. N.W., Ste. 700, Washington, DC 20001. Phone: (202) 783-6686.

HERS (Hysterectomy Education Resources and Services) Foundation. 422 Bryn Mawr Ave., Bala Cynwyd, PA 19004. Phone: (215) 667-7757.

CD-ROM DATABASES

Excerpta Medica CD: Obstetrics & Gynecology. SilverPlatter Information, Inc., River Ridge Office Park, 100 River Ridge Rd., Norwood, MA 02062. Phone: (617) 769-2599. Fax: (617) 769-8763. Quarterly.

Nursing and Allied Health (CINAHL) on CD-ROM. CINAHL, 1509 Wilson Terrace, P.O. Box 871, Glendale, CA 91209-0871. Phone: (818) 409-8005.

SCISEARCH. Institute for Scientific Information, 3501 Market St., Philadelphia, PA 19104. Phone: (215) 386-0100. Fax: (215) 386-6362.

ENCYCLOPEDIAS, DICTIONARIES, WORD BOOKS

Obstetric and Gynecological Words. Stedman. Williams & Wilkins, 428 East Preston St., Baltimore, MD 21202. Phone: (800) 638-0672. Fax: (800) 447-8438. 1992.

JOURNALS

American Journal of Obstetrics and Gynecology. Mosby-Year Book, 11830 Westline Industrial Drive, St. Louis, MO 63146. Phone: (800) 325-4177. Fax: (314) 432-1380. Monthly.

Journal of Women's Health. Mary Ann Liebert, Inc., 1651 Third Ave., New York, NY 10128. Phone: (212) 289-2300. Fax: (212) 289-4697. Quarterly.

NEWSLETTERS

ACOG Newsletter. American College of Obstetricians and Gynecologists, 409 12th St. S.W., Washington, DC 20024-2188. Phone: (202) 638-5577. Monthly.

HERS Newsletter. Hysterectomy Educational Resources and Services Foundation, 422 Bryn Mawr Ave., Bala Cynwyd, PA 19004. Phone: (215) 667-7757. Quarterly.

National Women's Health Network-Network News. National Women's Health Network, 1325 G St. N.W., Washington, DC 20005. Phone: (202) 347-1140. Bimonthly.

ONLINE DATABASES

Nursing and Allied Health (CINAHL). CINAHL, 1509 Wilson Terrace, P.O. Box 871, Glendale, CA 91209-0871. Phone: (818) 409-8005.

POPULAR WORKS AND PATIENT EDUCATION

Every Woman's Medical Handbook. Marie Stoppard. Ballantine Books, Inc., 201 E. 50th St., New York, NY 10022. Phone: (800) 733-3000. 1991.

Hysterectomy: Before & After: A Comprehensive Guide to Preventing, Preparing for, and Maximizing Health After Hysterectomy. Winnifred B. Cutler. HarperCollins Pubs., Inc., 10 E. 53rd St., New York, NY 10022-5299. Phone: (212) 207-7000. Fax: (800) 242-7737. 1990.

Hysterectomy - Before and After: A Comprehensive Guide to Preventing, Preparing for, and Maximizing Health after Hysterectomy - With Essential Information. Winnifred B. Cutler. HarperCollins Pubs., Inc., 10 E. 53rd St., New York, NY 10022-5299. Phone: (212) 207-7000. Fax: (800) 242-7737. 1990.

The New Our Bodies, Ourselves: The Updated and Expanded Edition. The Boston Women's Health Book Collective. Simon & Schuster, 1230 Ave. of the Americas, New York, NY 10020. Phone: (800) 223-2348. Fax: (800) 284-0735. 1992.

The No-Hysterectomy Option: Your Body-Your Choice. Herbert A. Goldfarb, Judith Greif. John Wiley & Sons, Inc., 605 Third Ave., New York, NY 10158-0012. Phone: (212) 850-6000. Fax: (212) 850-6088. 1990.

No More Hysterectomies. Vickie G. Hufnagel, Susan K. Golant. Viking Penguin, 375 Hudson St., New York, NY 10014-3657. Phone: (800) 331-4624. 1989.

Recovering from a Hysterectomy. Harris. HarperCollins Pubs., Inc., 10 E. 53rd St., New York, NY 10022-5299. Phone: (212) 207-7000. Fax: (800) 242-7737. 1992.

Well-Informed Patient's Guide to Hysterectomy. Kathryn Cox. Bantam Doubleday Dell, 666 Fifth Ave., New York, NY 10103. Phone: (800) 223-6834. 1991.

I

ILEOSTOMY

See: COLORECTAL SURGERY

IMMUNIZATION

ABSTRACTING, INDEXING, AND CURRENT AWARENESS PUBLICATIONS

Current Contents/Clinical Medicine. Institute for Scientific Information, 3501 Market St., Philadelphia, PA 19104. Phone: (800) 523-1850. Fax: (215) 386-6362. Weekly.

Current Contents/Life Sciences. Institute for Scientific Information, 3501 Market St., Philadelphia, PA 19104. Phone: (215) 386-0100. Fax: (215) 386-6362.

Index Medicus. U.S. National Library of Medicine, 8600 Rockville Pike, Bethesda, MD 20894. Phone: (800) 638-8480. Monthly.

Science Citation Index. Institute for Scientific Information, 3501 Market St., Philadelphia, PA 19104. Phone: (800) 523-1850. Fax: (215) 386-6362. Bimonthly.

ANNUALS AND REVIEWS

In Development New Medicines for Children. Pharmaceutical Manufacturers Association, 1100 15th St. N.W., Washington, DC 20005. Phone: (202) 835-3400. Quarterly.

Progress in Vaccinology. Springer-Verlag New York Inc., 175 Fifth Ave., New York, NY 10010. Phone: (212) 460-1500. Fax: (212) 473-6272. Irregular.

Year Book of Infectious Diseases. Mosby-Year Book, 11830 Westline Industrial Drive, St. Louis, MO 63146. Phone: (800) 325-4177. Fax: (314) 432-1380. Annual.

BIBLIOGRAPHIES

Infectious Disease Vaccines. National Technical Information Service, 5285 Port Royal Rd., Springfield, VA 22161. Phone: (703) 487-4650. Fax: (703) 321-8547. Jan. 1970-Feb. 1988 PB88-858691/CBY.

Vaccination and Immunization: Side Effects and Safety. National Technical Information Service, 5285 Port Royal Rd., Springfield, VA 22161. Phone: (703) 487-4650. Fax: (703) 321-8547. Jan. 1978-Apr. 1989 PB89-859755/CBY.

CD-ROM DATABASES

Infectious Diseases MEDLINE. MEP, 124 Mt. Auburn St., Cambridge, MA 02138. Phone: (800) 342-1338. Fax: (617) 868-7738. Quarterly.

SCISEARCH. Institute for Scientific Information, 3501 Market St., Philadelphia, PA 19104. Phone: (215) 386-0100. Fax: (215) 386-6362.

HANDBOOKS, GUIDES, MANUALS, ATLASES

The Handbook of Immunopharmacology. Academic Press, Inc., 1250 Sixth Ave., San Diego, CA 92101-4311. Phone: (619) 699-6345. Fax: (619) 699-6715. Irregular.

Immunizing Children (Practical Guide for General Practice). Sue Sefi, Aidan Macfarlane. Oxford University Press, 200 Madison Ave., New York, NY 10016. Phone: (212) 679-7300. 1989.

International Travel and Health: Vaccination Requirements and Health Advice. World Health Organization, Ave. Appia, CH-1211, Geneva 27, Switzerland.

JOURNALS

Infection and Immunity. American Society for Microbiology, 1325 Massachusetts Ave. NW, Washington, DC 20005-4171. Phone: (202) 737-3600. Fax: (202) 737-0368. Monthly.

Vaccine: Production and Use of Human and Veterinary Vaccines. Butterworth-Heinemann, 80 Montvale Ave., Stoneham, MA 02180. Phone: (617) 438-8464. Fax: (617) 279-4851. 14/year.

Vaccine Research. Mary Ann Liebert, Inc., 1651 Third Ave., New York, NY 10128. Phone: (212) 289-2300. Fax: (212) 289-4697. Quarterly.

ONLINE DATABASES

EMBASE. Elsevier Science Publishing Co., Inc., P.O. Box 882, Madison Square Station, New York, NY 10159-2101. Phone: (212) 989-5800. Fax: (212) 633-3990.

MEDLINE. National Library of Medicine, 8600 Rockville Pike, Bethesda, MD 20894. Phone: (800) 638-8480.

SciSearch. Institute for Scientific Information, 3501 Market St., Philadelphia, PA 19104. Phone: (215) 386-0100. Fax: (215) 386-6362.

POPULAR WORKS AND PATIENT EDUCATION

39 Development AIDS Medicines: Drugs and Vaccines. Pharmaceutical Manufacturers Association, 1100 15th St.

N.W., Washington, DC 20005. Phone: (202) 835-3400. Annual.

Immunization Decision: A Guide for Parents. Randall Neustaedter. North Atlantic Books, 2800 Woolsey St., Berkeley, CA 94705. Phone: (415) 652-5309.

RESEARCH CENTERS, INSTITUTES, CLEARINGHOUSES

Center for Immunization Research. Johns Hopkins University. School of Hygiene & Public Health, Hampton House 125, 624 N. Broadway, Baltimore, MD 21205. Phone: (301) 955-4376. Fax: (301) 955-2791.

STANDARDS AND STATISTICS SOURCES

Immunization: Survey of Recent Research. Centers for Disease Control, 1600 Clifton Rd. N.E., Atlanta, GA 30333. Phone: (404) 488-4698. Annual.

TEXTBOOKS AND MONOGRAPHS

Immunization in Practice: A Guide for Health Workers Who Give Vaccines. World Health Organization. Oxford University Press, 200 Madison Ave., New York, NY 10016. Phone: (212) 679-7300. 1989.

Vaccines and Immunotherapy. S.J. Cryz. McGraw-Hill, Inc., Health Professions Division, 1221 Avenue of the Americas, 28th Floor, New York, NY 10020. Phone: (212) 512-4228. 1991.

IMMUNOLOGIC DISORDERS

See also: AIDS; HUMAN
IMMUNODEFICIENCY VIRUS

ABSTRACTING, INDEXING, AND CURRENT AWARENESS PUBLICATIONS

Current Contents/Life Sciences. Institute for Scientific Information, 3501 Market St., Philadelphia, PA 19104. Phone: (215) 386-0100. Fax: (215) 386-6362.

Excerpta Medica. Section 26: Immunology, Serology and Transplantation. Elsevier Science Publishing Co., Inc., P.O. Box 882, Madison Square Station, New York, NY 10159-2101. Phone: (212) 989-5800. Fax: (212) 633-3990. 32/year.

Immunology Abstracts. Cambridge Scientific Abstracts, 7200 Wisconsin Ave., Bethesda, MD 20814-4823. Phone: (800) 843-7751. Fax: (301) 961-6720. Monthly.

Index Medicus. U.S. National Library of Medicine, 8600 Rockville Pike, Bethesda, MD 20894. Phone: (800) 638-8480. Monthly.

ANNUALS AND REVIEWS

Advances in Immunology. Academic Press, Inc., 1250 Sixth Ave., San Diego, CA 92101-4311. Phone: (619) 699-6345. Fax: (619) 699-6715. Irregular.

Annual Review of Immunology. Annual Reviews Inc., 4139 El Camino Way, P.O. Box 10139, Palo Alto, CA 94303-0897. Phone: (415) 493-4400. Fax: (415) 855-9815. Annual.

Contemporary Topics in Immunobiology. Plenum Publishing Co., 233 Spring St., New York, NY 10013-1578. Phone: (212) 620-8000. Fax: (212) 463-0742. Irregular.

Contributions to Microbiology and Immunology. S. Karger Publishers, Inc., 26 West Avon Rd., P.O. Box 529, Farmington, CT 06085. Phone: (203) 675-7834. Fax: (203) 675-7302. Irregular.

Critical Reviews in Immunology. CRC Press, Inc., 2000 Corporate Blvd. N.W., Boca Raton, FL 33431. Phone: (407) 994-0555. Fax: (407) 997-0949. Quarterly.

Current Advances in Immunology. Pergamon Press, 660 White Plains Rd., Tarrytown, NY 10591-5153. Phone: (914) 592-7700. Fax: (914) 592-3625.

Current Topics in Microbiology and Immunology. Springer-Verlag New York, Inc., 175 Fifth Ave., New York, NY 10010. Phone: (212) 460-1500. Fax: (212) 473-6272. Irregular.

Developments in Immunology. Elsevier Science Publishing Co., Inc., P.O. Box 882, Madison Square Station, New York, NY 10159-2101. Phone: (212) 989-5800. Fax: (212) 633-3990. Irregular.

Immunological Reviews. Munksgaard International Publishers Ltd., P.O. Box 2148, DK-1016, Copenhagen K, Denmark. Phone: 33-127030. Fax: 33-129387. Bimonthly.

Immunology and Allergy Clinics. W.B. Saunders Co., The Curtis Center, Independence Square W., Philadelphia, PA 19106-3399. Phone: (215) 238-7800. Quarterly.

The Year in Immunology. S. Karger Publishers, Inc., 26 West Avon Rd., P.O. Box 529, Farmington, CT 06085. Phone: (203) 675-7834. Fax: (203) 675-7302. Annual.

CD-ROM DATABASES

CSA Life Sciences Collection. Cambridge Scientific Abstracts, 7200 Wisconsin Ave., Bethesda, MD 20814-4823. Phone: (800) 843-7751. Fax: (301) 961-6720.

DIRECTORIES

American Academy of Allergy & Immunology-Membership Directory. American Academy of Allergy & Immunology, 611 E. Wells St., Milwaukee, WI 53202. Phone: (414) 272-6071. Fax: (414) 276-3349. Biennial.

Directory of Certified Allergists/Immunologists. American Board of Medical Specialties, 1 Rotary Center, Suite 805, Evanston, IL 60201. Phone: (708) 491-9091. Biennial.

ENCYCLOPEDIAS, DICTIONARIES, WORD BOOKS

Dictionary of Immunology. F. Rosen and others (eds.). Macmillan Publishing Co., 866 Third Ave., New York, NY 10011. Phone: (800) 257-5755. 1988.

HANDBOOKS, GUIDES, MANUALS, ATLASES

The Handbook of Immunopharmacology. Academic Press, Inc., 1250 Sixth Ave., San Diego, CA 92101-4311. Phone: (619) 699-6345. Fax: (619) 699-6715. Irregular.

Manual of Allergy and Immunology: Diagnosis and Therapy. Gleen J. Lawlor Jr., Thomas J. Fischer. Little, Brown and Co., 34 Beacon St., Boston, MA 02108. Phone: (617) 227-0730. Second edition 1988.

JOURNALS

Cellular Immunology. Academic Press, Inc., 1250 Sixth Ave., San Diego, CA 92101-4311. Phone: (619) 699-6345. Fax: (619) 699-6715. 14/year.

Clinical and Experimental Immunology. Blackwell Scientific Publications Ltd., Osney Mead, Oxon. OX2 OEL, England. Phone: 0865-240201. Fax: 0865-721205. Monthly.

Immunologic Research. S. Karger Publishers, Inc., 26 West Avon Rd., P.O. Box 529, Farmington, CT 06085. Phone: (203) 675-7834. Fax: (203) 675-7302. Quarterly.

Immunological Investigations. Marcel Dekker, Inc., 270 Madison Ave., New York, NY 10016. Phone: (800) 228-1160. 8/year.

Immunology. Blackwell Scientific Publications, Inc., 3 Cambridge Ctr., Cambridge, MA 02142. Phone: (800) 759-6102. Monthly.

Immunology and Infectious Diseases. Rapid Communications of Oxford Ltd., The Old Malthouse, Paradise St., Oxford OX1 1LD, England. Phone: 44-865-790447. Fax: 44-865-244012. 4/year.

Immunopharmacology. Elsevier Science Publishing Co., Inc., P.O. Box 882, Madison Square Station, New York, NY 10159-2101. Phone: (212) 989-5800. Fax: (212) 633-3990. 6/year.

Journal of Allergy and Clinical Immunology. Mosby-Year Book, 11830 Westline Industrial Drive, St. Louis, MO 63146. Phone: (800) 325-4177. Fax: (314) 432-1380. Monthly.

Journal of Immunological Methods. Elsevier Science Publishing Co., Inc., P.O. Box 882, Madison Square Station, New York, NY 10159-2101. Phone: (212) 989-5800. Fax: (212) 633-3990. 20/year.

Journal of Immunology. Williams & Wilkins, 428 E. Preston St., Baltimore, MD 21202. Phone: (800) 638-0672. Fax: (800) 447-8438. Semimonthly.

ONLINE DATABASES

CSA Life Sciences Collection. Cambridge Scientific Abstracts, 7200 Wisconsin Ave., Bethesda, MD 20814-4823. Phone: (800) 843-7751. Fax: (301) 961-6720.

EMBASE. Elsevier Science Publishing Co., Inc., P.O. Box 882, Madison Square Station, New York, NY 10159-2101. Phone: (212) 989-5800. Fax: (212) 633-3990.

Journal of Allergy and Clinical Immunology. Mosby-Year Book, 11830 Westline Industrial Drive, St. Louis, MO 63146. Phone: (800) 325-4177. Fax: (314) 432-1380.

MEDLINE. National Library of Medicine, 8600 Rockville Pike, Bethesda, MD 20894. Phone: (800) 638-8480.

SciSearch. Institute for Scientific Information, 3501 Market St., Philadelphia, PA 19104. Phone: (215) 386-0100. Fax: (215) 386-6362.

POPULAR WORKS AND PATIENT EDUCATION

The Essential HIV Treatment Fact Book. Laura Pinsky, Paul Harding Douglas, Craig Metroka. Pocket Books, Inc., 1230 Ave. of the Americas, New York, NY 10020. Phone: (800) 223-2348. Fax: (800) 284-0735. 1992.

The HIV Test: What You Need to Know to Make an Informed Decision. Marc Vargo. Pocket Books, Inc., 1230 Ave. of the Americas, New York, NY 10020. Phone: (800) 223-2348. Fax: (800) 284-0735. 1992.

RESEARCH CENTERS, INSTITUTES, CLEARINGHOUSES

Beirne Carter Center for Immunology Research. University of Virginia. Health Sciences Center, Box MR-4-4012, Charlotte, NC 28226. Phone: (804) 924-1155. Fax: (804) 924-1155.

Division of Rheumatology and Immunology. University of Southern California. 2011 Zonal Ave., HMR 711, Los Angeles, CA 90033. Phone: (213) 342-1946. Fax: (213) 342-2874.

TEXTBOOKS AND MONOGRAPHS

Advanced Immunology. Male. Raven Press, 1185 Ave. of the Americas, New York, NY 10036. Phone: (212) 930-9500. Fax: (212) 869-3495. Second edition 1991.

The AIDS Knowledge Base. P.T. Cohen, Merle A. Sande, Paul A. Volberding (eds.). Massachusetts Medical Society, 1440 Main St., Waltham, MA 02154-1649. Phone: (617) 893-3800. Fax: (617) 893-0413. 1992.

AIDS and Other Manifestations of HIV Infection. G. Wormser (ed.). Noyes Publications, Mill Rd. at Grand Ave., Park Ridge, NJ 07656. Phone: (201) 391-8484. 1987.

Basic and Clinical Immunology. Daniel P. Stites, Abba T. Terr. Appleton & Lange, 25 Van Zant St., East Norwalk, CT 06855. Phone: (800) 423-1359. Fax: (203) 854-9486. Seventh edition 1990.

Basic Human Immunology. Stites, Terr (eds.). Appleton & Lange, 25 Van Zant St., East Norwalk, CT 06855. Phone: (800) 423-1359. Fax: (203) 854-9486. 1991.

Clinical Immunology. Jonathan Brostoff, Glenis K. Scadding, David K. Male, et. al.. J.B. Lippincott Co., 227 East Washington Square, Philadelphia, PA 19106-3780. Phone: (215) 238-4200. Fax: (215) 238-4227. 1991.

Clinical Immunology: A Practical Approach. H.C. Gooi, H. Chapel (eds.). Oxford University Press, 200 Madison Ave., New York, NY 10016. Phone: (212) 679-7300. 1990.

Current Therapy in Allergy, Immunology and Rheumatology. Lawrence M. Lichtenstein, Anthony Fauci. Mosby-Year Book, 11830 Westline Industrial Drive, St. Louis, MO 63146. Phone: (800) 325-4177. Fax: (314) 432-1380. Fourth edition 1991.

Fundamental Immunology. Robert M. Coleman and others. William C. Brown Communications, Inc., 2460 Kerper Blvd., Dubuque, IA 52001. Phone: (800) 338-5578. 1989.

Fundamentals of Immunolgy and Allergy. Richard F. Lockey. W.B. Saunders Co., The Curtis Center, Independence Square W., Philadelphia, PA 19106-3399. Phone: (215) 238-7800. 1987.

Immunologic Disorders in Infants and Children. E. Richard Stiehm. W.B. Saunders Co., The Curtis Center, Independence Square W., Philadelphia, PA 19106-3399. Phone: (215) 238-7800. Third edition 1989.

Immunology. Male. Raven Press, 1185 Ave. of the Americas, New York, NY 10036. Phone: (212) 930-9500. Fax: (212) 869-3495. Second edition 1991.

The Medical Management of AIDS. Merle A. Sande, Paul A. Volberding. W.B. Saunders Co., The Curtis Center, Independence Square W., Philadelphia, PA 19106-3399. Phone: (215) 238-7800. Second edition 1991.

IMMUNOLOGY

See also: ALLERGIES; AUTOIMMUNE
DISEASES

ABSTRACTING, INDEXING, AND CURRENT AWARENESS PUBLICATIONS

Biological Abstracts. BIOSIS, 2100 Arch St., Philadelphia, PA 19103-1399. Phone: (800) 523-4800. Fax: (215) 587-2016.

BIOSIS/CAS Selects: Cancer Immunology. BIOSIS, 2100 Arch St., Philadelphia, PA 19103-1399. Phone: (215) 587-4800. Fax: (215) 587-2016. Biweekly.

BIOSIS/CAS Selects: Nutrition & Immunology. BIOSIS, 2100 Arch St., Philadelphia, PA 19103-1399. Phone: (215) 587-4800. Fax: (215) 587-2016. Biweekly.

Current Contents/Life Sciences. Institute for Scientific Information, 3501 Market St., Philadelphia, PA 19104. Phone: (215) 386-0100. Fax: (215) 386-6362.

Excerpta Medica. Section 26: Immunology, Serology and Transplantation. Elsevier Science Publishing Co., Inc., P.O. Box 882, Madison Square Station, New York, NY 10159-2101. Phone: (212) 989-5800. Fax: (212) 633-3990. 32/year.

ICRDB Cancergram: Clinical Cancer Immunology and Biological Therapy. U.S. Government Printing Office, Superintendent of Documents, P.O. Box 371954, Pittsburgh, PA 15250-7954. Phone: (202) 783-3238. Fax: (202) 512-2250. Monthly.

Immunology Abstracts. Cambridge Scientific Abstracts, 7200 Wisconsin Ave., Bethesda, MD 20814-4823. Phone: (800) 843-7751. Fax: (301) 961-6720. Monthly.

Index Medicus. U.S. National Library of Medicine, 8600 Rockville Pike, Bethesda, MD 20894. Phone: (800) 638-8480. Monthly.

Research Alert: Cancer Immunology & Immunotherapy. Institute for Scientific Information, 3501 Market St., Philadelphia, PA 19104. Phone: (800) 523-1850. Fax: (215) 386-6362. Weekly.

Research Alert: Immunology-Antibodies/Immunoglobulins. Institute for Scientific Information, 3501 Market St., Philadelphia, PA 19104. Phone: (800) 523-1850. Fax: (215) 386-6362. Weekly.

Research Alert: Immunology-Cell Mediated. Institute for Scientific Information, 3501 Market St., Philadelphia, PA 19104. Phone: (800) 523-1850. Fax: (215) 386-6362. Weekly.

Research Alert: Immunology-Complement, Opsonins. Institute for Scientific Information, 3501 Market St., Philadelphia, PA 19104. Phone: (800) 523-1850. Fax: (215) 386-6362. Weekly.

Research Alert: Immunology-Macrophages/Monocytes. Institute for Scientific Information, 3501 Market St., Philadelphia, PA 19104. Phone: (800) 523-1850. Fax: (215) 386-6362. Weekly.

Research Alert: Immunopathology-Autoimmune Disease. Institute for Scientific Information, 3501 Market St., Philadelphia, PA 19104. Phone: (800) 523-1850. Fax: (215) 386-6362. Weekly.

Research Alert: T-Cell Research. Institute for Scientific Information, 3501 Market St., Philadelphia, PA 19104. Phone: (800) 523-1850. Fax: (215) 386-6362. Weekly.

Science Citation Index. Institute for Scientific Information, 3501 Market St., Philadelphia, PA 19104. Phone: (800) 523-1850. Fax: (215) 386-6362. Bimonthly.

ANNUALS AND REVIEWS

Advances in Immunology. Academic Press, Inc., 1250 Sixth Ave., San Diego, CA 92101-4311. Phone: (619) 699-6345. Fax: (619) 699-6715. Irregular.

Annual Review of Immunology. Annual Reviews Inc., 4139 El Camino Way, P.O. Box 10139, Palo Alto, CA 94303-0897. Phone: (415) 493-4400. Fax: (415) 855-9815. Annual.

Cambridge Reviews in Clinical Immunology. Cambridge University Press, 40 W. 20th St., New York, NY 10011. Phone: (800) 431-1580. Irregular.

Contemporary Topics in Immunobiology. Plenum Publishing Co., 233 Spring St., New York, NY 10013-1578. Phone: (212) 620-8000. Fax: (212) 463-0742. Irregular.

Contemporary Topics in Molecular Immunology. Plenum Publishing Co., 233 Spring St., New York, NY 10013-1578. Phone: (212) 620-8000. Fax: (212) 463-0742. Irregular.

Critical Reviews in Immunology. CRC Press, Inc., 2000 Corporate Blvd. N.W., Boca Raton, FL 33431. Phone: (407) 994-0555. Fax: (407) 997-0949. Quarterly.

Current Opinion in Immunology. Current Science Group, 20 N. Third St., Philadelphia, PA 19106-2199. Phone: (800) 552-5866. Fax: (215) 574-2270. Bimonthly.

Current Topics in Microbiology and Immunology. Springer-Verlag New York, Inc., 175 Fifth Ave., New York, NY 10010. Phone: (212) 460-1500. Fax: (212) 473-6272. Irregular.

Developments in Immunology. Elsevier Science Publishing Co., Inc., P.O. Box 882, Madison Square Station, New York, NY 10159-2101. Phone: (212) 989-5800. Fax: (212) 633-3990. Irregular.

Immunological Reviews. Munksgaard International Publishers Ltd., P.O. Box 2148, DK-1016, Copenhagen K, Denmark. Phone: 33-127030. Fax: 33-129387. Bimonthly.

Immunology and Allergy Clinics. W.B. Saunders Co., The Curtis Center, Independence Square W., Philadelphia, PA 19106-3399. Phone: (215) 238-7800. Quarterly.

The Year in Immunology. S. Karger Publishers, Inc., 26 West Avon Rd., P.O. Box 529, Farmington, CT 06085. Phone: (203) 675-7834. Fax: (203) 675-7302. Annual.

ASSOCIATIONS, PROFESSIONAL SOCIETIES, ADVOCACY AND SUPPORT GROUPS

American Association of Immunologists (AAI). 9650 Rockville Pike, Bethesda, MD 20814. Phone: (301) 530-7178. Fax: (301) 571-1816.

American Board of Allergy and Immunology (ABAI). University City Science Ctr., 3624 Market St., Philadelphia, PA 19104. Phone: (215) 349-9466.

American College of Allergy and Immunology (AACIA). 800 E. Northwest Hwy., Ste. 1080, Palatine, IL 60067. Phone: (312) 255-0380.

Canadian Society for Immunology. c/o Dept. of Immunology, University of Manitoba, 730 William Ave., Winnipeg, MB, Canada R3E 0W3. Phone: (204) 788-6509. Fax: (204) 722-7924.

CD-ROM DATABASES

Biological Abstracts on Compact Disc. BIOSIS, 2100 Arch St., Philadelphia, PA 19103-1399. Phone: (800) 523-4800. Fax: (215) 587-2016. Quarterly.

Biotechnology Citation Index. Institute for Scientific Information, 3501 Market St., Philadelphia, PA 19104. Phone: (215) 386-0100. Fax: (215) 386-6362. Bimonthly.

CSA Life Sciences Collection. Cambridge Scientific Abstracts, 7200 Wisconsin Ave., Bethesda, MD 20814-4823. Phone: (800) 843-7751. Fax: (301) 961-6720.

Excerpta Medica CD: Immunology & AIDS. SilverPlatter Information, Inc., River Ridge Office Park, 100 River Ridge Rd., Norwood, MA 02062. Phone: (617) 769-2599. Fax: (617) 769-8763. Quarterly.

SCISEARCH. Institute for Scientific Information, 3501 Market St., Philadelphia, PA 19104. Phone: (215) 386-0100. Fax: (215) 386-6362.

DIRECTORIES

American Academy of Allergy & Immunology-Membership Directory. American Academy of Allergy & Immunology, 611 E. Wells St., Milwaukee, WI 53202. Phone: (414) 272-6071. Fax: (414) 276-3349. Biennial.

Directory of Certified Allergists/Immunologists. American Board of Medical Specialties, 1 Rotary Center, Suite 805, Evanston, IL 60201. Phone: (708) 491-9091. Biennial.

Directory of Medical Specialists. Marquis Who's Who, 3002 Glenview Rd., Wilmette, IL 60091. Phone: (800) 621-9669. Fax: (708) 441-2264. Biennial.

Directory of Physicians in the United States. American Medical Association, 515 North State St., Chicago, IL 60610. Phone: (312) 464-0183. Fax: (312) 464-5834. Biennial.

ENCYCLOPEDIAS, DICTIONARIES, WORD BOOKS

Dictionary of Immunology. F. Rosen and others (eds.). Macmillan Publishing Co., 866 Third Ave., New York, NY 10011. Phone: (800) 257-5755. 1988.

Encyclopedia of Immunology. Ivan Delves, Peter J. Roitt (eds.). Academic Press, Inc., 1250 Sixth Ave., San Diego, CA 92101-4311. Phone: (619) 699-6345. Fax: (619) 699-6715. Three volumes 1992.

Immunologic and AIDS Word Book. Helen E. Littrell. Springhouse Publishing Co., 1111 Bethlehem Pike, Spring House, PA 19477. Phone: (800) 331-3170. Fax: (215) 646-8716. 1992.

HANDBOOKS, GUIDES, MANUALS, ATLASES

The Handbook of Immunopharmacology. Academic Press, Inc., 1250 Sixth Ave., San Diego, CA 92101-4311. Phone: (619) 699-6345. Fax: (619) 699-6715. Irregular.

Manual of Allergy and Immunology: Diagnosis and Therapy. Gleen J. Lawlor Jr., Thomas J. Fischer. Little, Brown and Co., 34 Beacon St., Boston, MA 02108. Phone: (617) 227-0730. Second edition 1988.

JOURNALS

Cellular Immunology. Academic Press, Inc., 1250 Sixth Ave., San Diego, CA 92101-4311. Phone: (619) 699-6345. Fax: (619) 699-6715. 14/year.

Clinical and Experimental Immunology. Blackwell Scientific Publications Ltd., Osney Mead, Oxon. OX2 OEL, England. Phone: 0865-240201. Fax: 0865-721205. Monthly.

FEMS Mircobiology Immunology. Elsevier Science Publishing Co., Inc., P.O. Box 882, Madison Square Station, New York, NY 10159-2101. Phone: (212) 989-5800. Fax: (212) 633-3990. 6/year.

Human Immunology. Elsevier Science Publishing Co., Inc., P.O. Box 882, Madison Square Station, New York, NY 10159-2101. Phone: (212) 989-5800. Fax: (212) 633-3990. 12/year.

Immunologic Research. S. Karger Publishers, Inc., 26 West Avon Rd., P.O. Box 529, Farmington, CT 06085. Phone: (203) 675-7834. Fax: (203) 675-7302. Quarterly.

Immunological Investigations. Marcel Dekker, Inc., 270 Madison Ave., New York, NY 10016. Phone: (800) 228-1160. 8/year.

Immunology. Blackwell Scientific Publications, Inc., 3 Cambridge Ctr., Cambridge, MA 02142. Phone: (800) 759-6102. Monthly.

Immunology Letters. Elsevier Science Publishing Co., Inc., P.O. Box 882, Madison Square Station, New York, NY 10159-2101. Phone: (212) 989-5800. Fax: (212) 633-3990. 15/year.

Immunology Today. Elsevier Science Publishing Co., Inc., P.O. Box 882, Madison Square Station, New York, NY 10159-2101. Phone: (212) 989-5800. Fax: (212) 633-3990. Monthly.

Immunopharmacology. Elsevier Science Publishing Co., Inc., P.O. Box 882, Madison Square Station, New York, NY 10159-2101. Phone: (212) 989-5800. Fax: (212) 633-3990. 6/year.

Infection and Immunity. American Society for Microbiology, 1325 Massachusetts Ave. NW, Washington, DC 20005-4171. Phone: (202) 737-3600. Fax: (202) 737-0368. Monthly.

Journal of Allergy and Clinical Immunology. Mosby-Year Book, 11830 Westline Industrial Drive, St. Louis, MO 63146. Phone: (800) 325-4177. Fax: (314) 432-1380. Monthly.

Journal of Clinical Immunology. Plenum Publishing Co., 233 Spring St., New York, NY 10013-1578. Phone: (212) 620-8000. Fax: (212) 463-0742. Bimonthly.

Journal of Immunological Methods. Elsevier Science Publishing Co., Inc., P.O. Box 882, Madison Square Station, New York, NY 10159-2101. Phone: (212) 989-5800. Fax: (212) 633-3990. 20/year.

Journal of Immunology. Williams & Wilkins, 428 E. Preston St., Baltimore, MD 21202. Phone: (800) 638-0672. Fax: (800) 447-8438. Semimonthly.

Journal of Neuroimmunology. Elsevier Science Publishing Co., Inc., P.O. Box 882, Madison Square Station, New York, NY 10159-2101. Phone: (212) 989-5800. Fax: (212) 633-3990. 18/year.

Mediators of Inflammation. Rapid Communications of Oxford Ltd., The Old Malthouse, Paradise St., Oxford OX1 1LD, England. Phone: 44-865-790447. Fax: 44-865-244012. 6/year.

Research in Immunology. Elsevier Science Publishing Co., Inc., P.O. Box 882, Madison Square Station, New York, NY 10159-2101. Phone: (212) 989-5800. Fax: (212) 633-3990. 9/year.

Viral Immunology. Mary Ann Liebert, Inc., 1651 Third Ave., New York, NY 10128. Phone: (212) 289-2300. Fax: (212) 289-4697. Quarterly.

NEWSLETTERS

American Academy of Allergy and Immunology-News and Notes. American Academy of Allergy and Immunology, 611 E. Wells St., Milwaukee, WI 53202. Phone: (414) 272-6071. Quarterly.

Clinical Immunology Newsletter. Elsevier Science Publishing Co., Inc., P.O. Box 882, Madison Square Station, New York, NY 10159-2101. Phone: (212) 989-5800. Fax: (212) 633-3990. 12/year.

ONLINE DATABASES

BIOSIS Previews. BIOSIS, 2100 Arch St., Philadelphia, PA 19103-1399. Phone: (800) 523-4800. Fax: (215) 587-2016.

CSA Life Sciences Collection. Cambridge Scientific Abstracts, 7200 Wisconsin Ave., Bethesda, MD 20814-4823. Phone: (800) 843-7751. Fax: (301) 961-6720.

EMBASE. Elsevier Science Publishing Co., Inc., P.O. Box 882, Madison Square Station, New York, NY 10159-2101. Phone: (212) 989-5800. Fax: (212) 633-3990.

Journal of Allergy and Clinical Immunology. Mosby-Year Book, 11830 Westline Industrial Drive, St. Louis, MO 63146. Phone: (800) 325-4177. Fax: (314) 432-1380.

MEDLINE. National Library of Medicine, 8600 Rockville Pike, Bethesda, MD 20894. Phone: (800) 638-8480.

SciSearch. Institute for Scientific Information, 3501 Market St., Philadelphia, PA 19104. Phone: (215) 386-0100. Fax: (215) 386-6362.

RESEARCH CENTERS, INSTITUTES, CLEARINGHOUSES

Allergy Disease Research Laboratory. Mayo Clinic and Foundation. 200 First St. SW, Rochester, MN 55905. Phone: (507) 284-2789. Fax: (507) 284-1637.

Allergy & Immunology Center. University of Colorado. Division of Immunology, 4200 E. 9th Ave., CB 164, Denver, CO 80262. Phone: (303) 270-7601.

Arthritis Center. University of Missouri-Columbia. MA427 Health Sciences Center, 1 Hospital Dr., Columbia, MO 65212. Phone: (314) 882-8738. Fax: (314) 884-3996.

Center for Allergy and Immunological Disorders. Baylor College of Medicine. 1 Baylor Plaza, Houston, TX 77030. Phone: (713) 791-4219.

Center for Interdisciplinary Research in Immunology and Diseases at UCLA. UCLA School of Medicine, 12-262 Factor Bldg., Los Angeles, CA 90024. Phone: (213) 825-1510. Fax: (213) 206-3865.

Center for Multidisciplinary Research in Immunology and DIseases at UCLA. UCLA School of Medicine, 12-262 Factor Bldg., Los Angeles, CA 90024. Phone: (213) 825-1510. Fax: (213) 206-3865.

Department of Immunology. University of Toronto. Medical Sciences Bldg., Toronto, ON, Canada M5S 1A8. Phone: (416) 978-6382. Fax: (416) 978-1938.

Fred Hutchinson Cancer Research Center. 1124 Columbia St., Seattle, WA 98104. Phone: (206) 467-5000. Fax: (206) 467-5268.

Immunobiology Research Group. University of Montreal. 2900 Blvd. Edouard-Montpetit, C.P. 6128, Succursale "A", Montreal, PQ, Canada H3C 3J7. Phone: (514) 343-6273. Fax: (514) 343-5701.

Immunology Research Program. Duke University. Medical Center, Box 3010, Durham, NC 27710. Phone: (919) 684-4119. Fax: (919) 684-8982.

Laboratory of Immunology. Rockefeller University. 1230 York Ave., New York, NY 10021-6399. Phone: (212) 570-8000.

Mary Imogene Bassett Medical Research Institute. 1 Atwell Rd., Cooperstown, NY 13326. Phone: (607) 547-3045. Fax: (607) 547-3061.

Max Samter Institute of Allergy and Clinical Immunology. Grant Hospital of Chicago, 550 W. Webster, Chicago, IL 60614. Phone: (312) 883-3655.

National Jewish Center for Immunology and Respiratory Medicine. 1400 Jackson St., Denver, CO 80206. Phone: (303) 388-4461.

Scripps Research Institute. 10666 N. Torrey Pines Rd., La Jolla, CA 92037. Phone: (619) 554-8265. Fax: (619) 554-9899.

TEXTBOOKS AND MONOGRAPHS

Advanced Immunology. Male. Raven Press, 1185 Ave. of the Americas, New York, NY 10036. Phone: (212) 930-9500. Fax: (212) 869-3495. Second edition 1991.

Basic and Clinical Immunology. Daniel P. Stites, Abba T. Terr. Appleton & Lange, 25 Van Zant St., East Norwalk, CT 06855. Phone: (800) 423-1359. Fax: (203) 854-9486. Seventh edition 1990.

Basic and Clinical Immunology: An Integrated Approach. L.H. Sigal, Y. Ron. McGraw-Hill, Inc., Health Professions Division, 1221 Avenue of the Americas, 28th Floor, New York, NY 10020. Phone: (212) 512-4228. 1992.

Basic Human Immunology. Stites, Terr (eds.). Appleton & Lange, 25 Van Zant St., East Norwalk, CT 06855. Phone: (800) 423-1359. Fax: (203) 854-9486. 1991.

Clinical Immunology. Jonathan Brostoff, Glenis K. Scadding, David K. Male, et. al.. J.B. Lippincott Co., 227 East

Washington Square, Philadelphia, PA 19106-3780. Phone: (215) 238-4200. Fax: (215) 238-4227. 1991.

Clinical Immunology: A Practical Approach. H.C. Gooi, H. Chapel (eds.). Oxford University Press, 200 Madison Ave., New York, NY 10016. Phone: (212) 679-7300. 1990.

Essential Immunology. Roitt. Blackwell Scientific Publications, Inc., 3 Cambridge Ctr., Cambridge, MA 02142. Phone: (800) 759-6102. Seventh edition 1992.

The Experimental Foundations of Modern Immunology. William P. Clark. John Wiley & Sons, Inc., 605 Third Ave., New York, NY 10158-0012. Phone: (212) 850-6000. Fax: (212) 850-6088. Fourth edition 1992.

Fundamental Immunology. William E. Paul. Raven Press, 1185 Avenue of the Americas, New York, NY 10036. Phone: (212) 930-9500. Fax: (212) 869-3495. Second edition 1989.

Fundamentals of Immunolgy and Allergy. Richard F. Lockey. W.B. Saunders Co., The Curtis Center, Independence Square W., Philadelphia, PA 19106-3399. Phone: (215) 238-7800. 1987.

Fundamentals of Immunology. O.G. Bier and others (eds.). Springer-Verlag New York Inc., 175 Fifth Ave., New York, NY 10010. Phone: (212) 460-1500. Fax: (212) 473-6272. Second edition 1986.

The Immune System: Evolutionary Principles Guide Our Understanding of This Complex Biological Defense System. Rodney E. Langman. Academic Press, Inc., 1250 Sixth Ave., San Diego, CA 92101-4311. Phone: (619) 699-6345. Fax: (619) 699-6715. 1989.

Immunology. Jan Klein. Blackwell Scientific Publications, Inc., 3 Cambridge Ctr., Cambridge, MA 02142. Phone: (800) 759-6102. 1990.

Immunology and Serology in Laboratory Medicine. Mary Louise Turgeon. Mosby-Year Book, 11830 Westline Industrial Drive, St. Louis, MO 63146. Phone: (800) 325-4177. Fax: (314) 432-1380. 1990.

Medical Immunology: Text and Review. James T. Barrett. F.A. Davis Co., 1915 Arch St., Philadelphia, PA 19103. Phone: (800) 523-4049. Fax: (215) 568-5065. 1991.

Medical Microbiology and Immunology. Levinson. Appleton & Lange, 25 Van Zant St., East Norwalk, CT 06855. Phone: (800) 423-1359. Fax: (203) 854-9486. Second edition 1992.

Textbook of Immunology. James T. Barrett. Mosby-Year Book, 11830 Westline Industrial Drive, St. Louis, MO 63146. Phone: (800) 325-4177. Fax: (314) 432-1380. 1987.

IMMUNOSUPPRESSION

See: TRANSPLANTATION

IMMUNOTHERAPY

See: IMMUNOLOGY

IMPETIGO

See: DERMATOLOGIC DISEASES

IMPOTENCE

See: SEXUAL DISORDERS

IN VITRO FERTILIZATION

See also: INFERTILITY

ABSTRACTING, INDEXING, AND CURRENT AWARENESS PUBLICATIONS

Current Contents/Clinical Medicine. Institute for Scientific Information, 3501 Market St., Philadelphia, PA 19104. Phone: (800) 523-1850. Fax: (215) 386-6362. Weekly.

Current Contents/Life Sciences. Institute for Scientific Information, 3501 Market St., Philadelphia, PA 19104. Phone: (215) 386-0100. Fax: (215) 386-6362.

Index Medicus. U.S. National Library of Medicine, 8600 Rockville Pike, Bethesda, MD 20894. Phone: (800) 638-8480. Monthly.

Research Alert: Reproductive Endocrinology. Institute for Scientific Information, 3501 Market St., Philadelphia, PA 19104. Phone: (800) 523-1850. Fax: (215) 386-6362. Weekly.

Science Citation Index. Institute for Scientific Information, 3501 Market St., Philadelphia, PA 19104. Phone: (800) 523-1850. Fax: (215) 386-6362. Bimonthly.

ANNUALS AND REVIEWS

Reproductive Medicine Review. Cambridge University Press, 40 W. 20th St., New York, NY 10011. Phone: (800) 431-1580. Semiannual.

ASSOCIATIONS, PROFESSIONAL SOCIETIES, ADVOCACY AND SUPPORT GROUPS

American Fertility Society (AFS). 2140 11th Ave. S., Ste. 200, Birmingham, AL 35205-2800. Phone: (205) 933-8494. Fax: (205) 930-9904.

Fertility Research Foundation (FRF). 1430 Second Ave., Ste. 103, New York, NY 10021. Phone: (212) 744-5500.

CD-ROM DATABASES

SCISEARCH. Institute for Scientific Information, 3501 Market St., Philadelphia, PA 19104. Phone: (215) 386-0100. Fax: (215) 386-6362.

DIRECTORIES

Infertility: Medical and Social Choices. Office of Technology Assesment, 600 Pennsylvania Ave. S.E., Washington, DC 20510. Phone: (202) 224-3827. Fax: (202) 275-0019. 1988.

HANDBOOKS, GUIDES, MANUALS, ATLASES

CRC Handbook of In Vitro Fertilization. Alan Trounson, David K. Gardner. CRC Press, Inc., 2000 Corporate Blvd.

N.W., Boca Raton, FL 33431. Phone: (407) 994-0555. Fax: (407) 997-0949. 1992.

The Johns Hopkins Handbook of In Vitro Fertilization and Assisted Reproductive Technologies. Marian D. Damewood (ed.). Little, Brown and Company, 34 Beacon St., Boston, MA 02108. Phone: (617) 227-0730. 1990.

JOURNALS

Archives of Andrology. Taylor & Francis Inc., 1900 Frost Rd., Suite 101, Bristol, PA 19007-1598. Phone: (800) 821-8312. Fax: (215) 785-5515. Bimonthly.

Fertility and Sterility. American Fertility Society, 2140 11th Ave., Suite 200, Birmingham, AL 35205-2800. Phone: (205) 933-8494. Fax: (205) 930-9904. Monthly.

In Vitro Cellular and Developmental Biology. Tissue Culture Association, 1910 Montgomery Village Ave., No. 300, Gaithersburg, MD 20879.

Journal of Andrology. J.B. Lippincott Co., 227 East Washington Square, Philadelphia, PA 19106-3780. Phone: (215) 238-4200. Fax: (215) 238-4227. Bimonthly.

Journal of In Vitro Fertilization and Embryo Transfer. Plenum Publishing Co., 233 Spring St., New York, NY 10013-1578. Phone: (212) 620-8000. Fax: (212) 463-0742. Bimonthly.

Seminars in Reproductive Endocrinology. Thieme Medical Publishers, Inc., 381 Park Ave. S., New York, NY 10016. Phone: (212) 683-5088. Fax: (212) 779-9020. Quarterly.

ONLINE DATABASES

EMBASE. Elsevier Science Publishing Co., Inc., P.O. Box 882, Madison Square Station, New York, NY 10159-2101. Phone: (212) 989-5800. Fax: (212) 633-3990.

MEDLINE. National Library of Medicine, 8600 Rockville Pike, Bethesda, MD 20894. Phone: (800) 638-8480.

POPLINE. U.S. National Library of Medicine, MEDLARS Management Section, 8600 Rockville Pike, Bethesda, MD 20894. Phone: (800) 638-8480. Monthly.

SciSearch. Institute for Scientific Information, 3501 Market St., Philadelphia, PA 19104. Phone: (215) 386-0100. Fax: (215) 386-6362.

POPULAR WORKS AND PATIENT EDUCATION

A Couple's Guide to Fertility: How New Medical Advances Can Help You Have a Baby. Berger. Doubleday & Co., Inc., 666 Fifth Ave., New York, NY 10103. Phone: (800) 223-6834. 1989.

How to Get Pregnant with the New Technology. Sherman J. Silber. Warner Books, Inc., 666 Fifth Ave., 9th Flr., New York, NY 10103. Phone: (212) 484-2900. 1991.

RESEARCH CENTERS, INSTITUTES, CLEARINGHOUSES

Howard and Georgeanne Jones Institute for Reproductive Medicine. 855 W. Brambleton Ave., Norfolk, VA 23510. Phone: (804) 446-5628.

Laboratory of Human Reproduction and Reproductive Biology. Harvard University. Harvard Medical School, 45 Shattuck, Boston, MA 02115. Phone: (617) 432-2038. Fax: (617) 566-7980.

TEXTBOOKS AND MONOGRAPHS

Assisted Human Reproductive Technology. E.S.E. Hafez (ed.). Taylor & Francis Inc., 1900 Frost Rd., Suite 101, Bristol, PA 19007-1598. Phone: (800) 821-8312. Fax: (215) 785-5515. 1991.

A Textbook of In Vitro Fertilization. P.R. Brindsen, P.A. Rainsbury (eds.). The Parthenon Publishing Group, Inc., 120 Mill Rd., Park Ridge, NJ 07656. Phone: (201) 391-6796. 1992.

INCEST

ABSTRACTING, INDEXING, AND CURRENT AWARENESS PUBLICATIONS

Psychological Abstracts. American Psychological Association, 1200 17th St. NW, Washington, DC 20036. Phone: (202) 955-7600. Monthly.

ASSOCIATIONS, PROFESSIONAL SOCIETIES, ADVOCACY AND SUPPORT GROUPS

Families of Sex Offenders Anonymous. 208 W. Walk, West Haven, CT 06516. Phone: (207) 931-0015.

National Center for Prevention of Child Abuse. 1033 N. Fairfax St., Alexandria, VA 22314. Phone: (703) 739-0321.

CD-ROM DATABASES

PsycLit. SilverPlatter Information, Inc., River Ridge Office Park, 100 River Ridge Rd., Norwood, MA 02062. Phone: (617) 769-2599. Fax: (617) 769-8763. Quarterly.

JOURNALS

Journal of the American Academy of Child and Adolescent Psychiatry. Williams & Wilkins, 428 East Preston St., Baltimore, MD 21202. Phone: (800) 638-0672. Fax: (800) 447-8438.

ONLINE DATABASES

PsycInfo. SilverPlatter Information, Inc., River Ridge Office Park, 100 River Ridge Rd., Norwood, MA 02062. Phone: (617) 769-2599. Fax: (617) 769-8763. Quarterly.

POPULAR WORKS AND PATIENT EDUCATION

Allies in Healing: When the Person You Love Was Sexually Abused as a Child, a Support Book for Partners. Laura Davis. HarperCollins Pubs., Inc., 10 E. 53rd St., New York, NY 10022-5299. Phone: (212) 207-7000. 1991.

Secret Survivors: Uncovering Incest and Its After Effects. E. Sue Blume. John Wiley & Sons, Inc., 605 Third Ave., New York, NY 10158-0012. Phone: (212) 850-6000. Fax: (212) 850-6088. 1990.

RESEARCH CENTERS, INSTITUTES, CLEARINGHOUSES

Clearinghouse on Child Abuse and Neglect Information. P.O. Box 1182, Washington, DC 20013. Phone: (703) 821-2086.

TEXTBOOKS AND MONOGRAPHS

Incest-Related Syndromes of Adult Psychopathology. Richard P. Kluft (ed.). American Psychiatric Press, Inc., 1400 K St. NW, Washington, DC 20005. Phone: (202) 682-6268. Fax: (202) 789-2648. 1990.

INCONTINENCE

See: UROLOGIC DISORDERS

INDUSTRIAL TOXICOLOGY

See also: OCCUPATIONAL HEALTH AND
SAFETY; TOXICOLOGY

ABSTRACTING, INDEXING, AND CURRENT AWARENESS PUBLICATIONS

CA Selects: Chemical Hazards, Health, & Safety. Chemical Abstracts Service, 2540 Olentangy River Road, P.O. Box 3012, Columbus, OH 43210-0012. Phone: (800) 848-6538. Biweekly.

Excerpta Medica. Section 35: Occupational Health and Industrial Medicine. Elsevier Science Publishing Co., Inc., P.O. Box 882, Madison Square Station, New York, NY 10159-2101. Phone: (212) 989-5800. Fax: (212) 633-3990. 16/year.

Excerpta Medica. Section 52: Toxicology. Elsevier Science Publishing Co., Inc., P.O. Box 882, Madison Square Station, New York, NY 10159-2101. Phone: (212) 989-5800. Fax: (212) 633-3990. 20/year.

Science Citation Index. Institute for Scientific Information, 3501 Market St., Philadelphia, PA 19104. Phone: (800) 523-1850. Fax: (215) 386-6362. Bimonthly.

Toxicology Abstracts. Cambridge Scientific Abstracts, 7200 Wisconsin Ave., Bethesda, MD 20814-4823. Phone: (800) 843-7751. Fax: (301) 961-6720. Monthly.

ANNUALS AND REVIEWS

Reviews of Environmental Contamination and Toxicology. Ware. Springer-Verlag New York, Inc., 175 Fifth Ave., New York, NY 10010. Phone: (212) 460-1500. Fax: (212) 473-6272. 1991.

Year Book of Toxicology. CRC Press, Inc., 2000 Corporate Blvd. N.W., Boca Raton, FL 33431. Phone: (407) 994-0555. Fax: (407) 997-0949. Annual.

ASSOCIATIONS, PROFESSIONAL SOCIETIES, ADVOCACY AND SUPPORT GROUPS

American College of Toxicology. 9650 Rockville Pike, Bethesda, MD 20814. Phone: (301) 571-1840.

American Industrial Health Council. 1330 Connecticut Ave. N.W., Washington, DC 20036. Phone: (202) 659-0060.

Chemical Industry Institute of Technology. P.O. Box 12137, Research Triangle Park, NC 27709. Phone: (919) 541-2070.

Society of Toxicology. 1133 15th St. N.W., No. 1000, Washington, DC 20005. Phone: (202) 293-5935.

Toxicology Forum. 1575 I St. N.W., No. 800, Washington, DC 20005. Phone: (202) 659-0030.

CD-ROM DATABASES

PolTox. Cambridge Scientific Abstracts, 7200 Wisconsin Ave., Bethesda, MD 20814-4823. Phone: (800) 843-7751. Fax: (301) 961-6720. Quarterly.

SCISEARCH. Institute for Scientific Information, 3501 Market St., Philadelphia, PA 19104. Phone: (215) 386-0100. Fax: (215) 386-6362.

TOXLINE. SilverPlatter Information, Inc., River Ridge Office Park, 100 River Ridge Rd., Norwood, MA 02062. Phone: (617) 769-2599. Fax: (617) 769-8763. Quarterly.

TOXLINE Plus. SilverPlatter Information, Inc., River Ridge Office Park, 100 River Ridge Rd., Norwood, MA 02062. Phone: (617) 769-2599. Fax: (617) 769-8763. Quarterly.

HANDBOOKS, GUIDES, MANUALS, ATLASES

Handbook of Medical Toxicology. Peter Viccellio (ed.). Little, Brown and Company, 34 Beacon St., Boston, MA 02108. Phone: (617) 227-0730. 1992.

JOURNALS

British Journal of Industrial Medicine. BMJ Publishing Group, BMA House, Tavistock Square, London WC1H 9JR, England. Phone: 071-383-6244. Fax: 071-383-6662.

Fundamental and Applied Technology. Academic Press, Inc., 1250 Sixth Ave., San Diego, CA 92101-4311. Phone: (619) 699-6345. Fax: (619) 699-6715.

Human and Experimental Toxicology. Macmillan Publishing Co., 866 Third Ave., New York, NY 10011. Phone: (800) 257-5755.

Journal of Applied Toxicology. John Wiley & Sons, Inc., 605 Third Ave., New York, NY 10158-0012. Phone: (212) 850-6000. Fax: (212) 850-6088. Bimonthly.

Journal of Toxicology and Environmental Health. Taylor & Francis Inc., 1900 Frost Rd., Suite 101, Bristol, PA 19007-1598. Phone: (800) 821-8312. Fax: (215) 785-5515. Monthly.

ONLINE DATABASES

TOXLINE. U.S. National Library of Medicine, Toxicology Information Program, 8600 Rockville Pike, Bethesda, MD 20894. Phone: (800) 638-8480. Monthly.

INDUSTRIAL WASTE

See: ENVIRONMENTAL POLLUTANTS

INFANT MORTALITY

See: VITAL STATISTICS

INFECTION CONTROL

ABSTRACTING, INDEXING, AND CURRENT AWARENESS PUBLICATIONS

Cumulative Index to Nursing and Allied Health Literature. Glendale Adventist Medical Center, P.O. Box 871, Glendale, CA 91209. Phone: (818) 409-8005. Bimonthly.

Excerpta Medica. Section 6: Internal Medicine. Elsevier Science Publishers, P.O. Box 882, Madison Square Station, New York, NY 10159-2101. Phone: (212) 633-3950. Fax: (212) 633-3990. 24/year.

Hospital Literature Index. American Hospital Association, 840 N. Lake Shore Dr., Chicago, IL 60611. Phone: (800) 242-2626. Fax: (312) 280-6015. Quarterly.

Research Alert: Infections-Hospital Associated. Institute for Scientific Information, 3501 Market St., Philadelphia, PA 19104. Phone: (800) 523-1850. Fax: (215) 386-6362. Weekly.

ASSOCIATIONS, PROFESSIONAL SOCIETIES, ADVOCACY AND SUPPORT GROUPS

Association for Practioners in Infection Control (APIC). 505 E. Hawley St., Mundelein, IL 60060. Phone: (708) 949-6052. Fax: (312) 566-7282.

CD-ROM DATABASES

Morbidity Mortality Weekly Report. MEP, 124 Mt. Auburn St., Cambridge, MA 02138. Phone: (800) 342-1338. Fax: (617) 868-7738. Annual.

Nursing and Allied Health (CINAHL) on CD-ROM. CINAHL, 1509 Wilson Terrace, P.O. Box 871, Glendale, CA 91209-0871. Phone: (818) 409-8005.

JOURNALS

American Journal of Infection Control. Mosby-Year Book, 11830 Westline Industrial Drive, St. Louis, MO 63146. Phone: (800) 325-4177. Fax: (314) 432-1380. Bimonthly.

Hospital Infection Control. American Health Consultants, P.O. Box 71266, Chicago, IL 60691. Phone: (800) 688-2421. Fax: (404) 352-1971.

Infection Control and Hospital Epidemiology. SLACK Inc., 6900 Grove Rd., Thorofare, NJ 08086-9447. Phone: (800) 257-8290. Fax: (609) 853-5991.

Infection and Immunity. American Society for Microbiology, 1325 Massachusetts Ave. NW, Washington, DC 20005-4171. Phone: (202) 737-3600. Fax: (202) 737-0368. Monthly.

Journal of Hospital Infection. Academic Press, Inc., 1250 Sixth Ave., San Diego, CA 92101-4311. Phone: (619) 699-6345. Fax: (619) 699-6715.

Journal of Infection. Academic Press, Inc., 1250 Sixth Ave., San Diego, CA 92101-4311. Phone: (619) 699-6345. Fax: (619) 699-6715.

Morbidity and Mortality Weekly Report. Massachusetts Medical Society, 1440 Main St., Waltham, MA 02154-1649. Phone: (617) 893-3800. Fax: (617) 893-0413. Weekly.

ONLINE DATABASES

EMBASE. Elsevier Science Publishing Co., Inc., P.O. Box 882, Madison Square Station, New York, NY 10159-2101. Phone: (212) 989-5800. Fax: (212) 633-3990.

MEDLINE. National Library of Medicine, 8600 Rockville Pike, Bethesda, MD 20894. Phone: (800) 638-8480.

Nursing and Allied Health (CINAHL). CINAHL, 1509 Wilson Terrace, P.O. Box 871, Glendale, CA 91209-0871. Phone: (818) 409-8005.

SciSearch. Institute for Scientific Information, 3501 Market St., Philadelphia, PA 19104. Phone: (215) 386-0100. Fax: (215) 386-6362.

TEXTBOOKS AND MONOGRAPHS

Infection Control: Dilemmas and Practical Solutions. K.R. Cundy, and others. Plenum Publishing Co., 233 Spring St., New York, NY 10013-1578. Phone: (212) 620-800. Fax: (212) 463-0742. 1990.

Infection Control in Intensive Care Units by Selective Decontamination. H.K Saene, and others. Springer-Verlag New York Inc., 175 Fifth Ave., New York, NY 10010. Phone: (212) 460-1500. Fax: (212) 473-6272. 1989.

Principles and Practice of Disinfection, Preservation, and Sterilization. Russell. Blackwell Scientific Publications, Inc., 3 Cambridge Ctr., Cambridge, MA 02142. Phone: (800) 759-6102. Second edition 1992.

INFECTIOUS DISEASES

See also: ANTIBIOTICS; FUNGAL DISEASES; VIRAL DISEASES

ABSTRACTING, INDEXING, AND CURRENT AWARENESS PUBLICATIONS

Abstracts on Hygiene and Communicable Diseases. Bureau of Hygiene and Tropical Diseases, Keppel St., London WC1E 7HT, England. Monthly.

Current Contents/Clinical Medicine. Institute for Scientific Information, 3501 Market St., Philadelphia, PA 19104. Phone: (800) 523-1850. Fax: (215) 386-6362. Weekly.

Current Contents/Life Sciences. Institute for Scientific Information, 3501 Market St., Philadelphia, PA 19104. Phone: (215) 386-0100. Fax: (215) 386-6362.

Hospital Literature Index. American Hospital Association, 840 N. Lake Shore Dr., Chicago, IL 60611. Phone: (800) 242-2626. Fax: (312) 280-6015. Quarterly.

Index Medicus. U.S. National Library of Medicine, 8600 Rockville Pike, Bethesda, MD 20894. Phone: (800) 638-8480. Monthly.

Research Alert: Infections Diseases-Viral. Institute for Scientific Information, 3501 Market St., Philadelphia, PA 19104. Phone: (800) 523-1850. Fax: (215) 386-6362. Weekly.

Science Citation Index. Institute for Scientific Information, 3501 Market St., Philadelphia, PA 19104. Phone: (800) 523-1850. Fax: (215) 386-6362. Bimonthly.

ANNUALS AND REVIEWS

Current Clinical Topics in Infectious Diseases. Blackwell Scientific Publications, Inc., 3 Cambridge Ctr., Cambridge, MA 02142. Phone: (800) 759-6102. Irregular.

Current Opinion in Infectious Diseases. Current Science Ltd., 20 N. Third St., Philadelphia, PA 19106-2199. Phone: (800) 552-5866. Fax: (215) 574-2270. Bimonthly.

Infectious Disease Clinics. W.B. Saunders Co., The Curtis Center, Independence Square W., Philadelphia, PA 19106-3399. Phone: (215) 238-7800. Quarterly.

Year Book of Infectious Diseases. Mosby-Year Book, 11830 Westline Industrial Drive, St. Louis, MO 63146. Phone: (800) 325-4177. Fax: (314) 432-1380. Annual.

ASSOCIATIONS, PROFESSIONAL SOCIETIES, ADVOCACY AND SUPPORT GROUPS

Association for Practioners in Infection Control (APIC). 505 E. Hawley St., Mundelein, IL 60060. Phone: (708) 949-6052. Fax: (312) 566-7282.

Infectious Diseases Society of America (IDSA). Yale University School of Medicine, 333 Cedar St., 201 LCI, New Haven, CT 06510-8056. Phone: (203) 785-4141.

National Foundation for Infectious Diseases. 4733 Bethesda Ave., No. 750, Bethesda, MD 20814. Phone: (301) 656-0003.

BIBLIOGRAPHIES

Infectious Disease Vaccines. National Technical Information Service, 5285 Port Royal Rd., Springfield, VA 22161. Phone: (703) 487-4650. Fax: (703) 321-8547. Jan. 1970-Feb. 1988 PB88-858691/CBY.

CD-ROM DATABASES

Infectious Diseases MEDLINE. MEP, 124 Mt. Auburn St., Cambridge, MA 02138. Phone: (800) 342-1338. Fax: (617) 868-7738. Quarterly.

Internal Medicine '92. Macmillan New Media, 124 Mt. Auburn St., Cambridge, MA 02138. Phone: (800) 342-1338. 1992.

Morbidity Mortality Weekly Report. MEP, 124 Mt. Auburn St., Cambridge, MA 02138. Phone: (800) 342-1338. Fax: (617) 868-7738. Annual.

Pediatric Infectious Disease Journal. CMC ReSearch, Inc., 7150 S.W. Hampton, Suite C-120, Portland, OR 97223. Phone: (800) 262-7668. Fax: (503) 639-1796. Annual.

SCISEARCH. Institute for Scientific Information, 3501 Market St., Philadelphia, PA 19104. Phone: (215) 386-0100. Fax: (215) 386-6362.

DIRECTORIES

Directory of Medical Specialists. Marquis Who's Who, 3002 Glenview Rd., Wilmette, IL 60091. Phone: (800) 621-9669. Fax: (708) 441-2264. Biennial.

Directory of Physicians in the United States. American Medical Association, 515 North State St., Chicago, IL 60610. Phone: (312) 464-0183. Fax: (312) 464-5834. Biennial.

ENCYCLOPEDIAS, DICTIONARIES, WORD BOOKS

Professional Guide to Diseases. Springhouse Publishing Co., 1111 Bethlehem Pike, Spring House, PA 19477. Phone: (800) 331-3170. Fax: (215) 646-8716. Fourth edition 1992.

HANDBOOKS, GUIDES, MANUALS, ATLASES

Atlas of Infectious Disease. Edmond. Mosby-Year Book, 11830 Westline Industrial Drive, St. Louis, MO 63146. Phone: (800) 325-4177. Fax: (314) 432-1380. Second edition 1987.

A Color Atlas of Pediatric Infectious Diseases. C.A. Hart. Mosby-Year Book, 11830 Westline Industrial Drive, St. Louis, MO 63146. Phone: (800) 325-4177. Fax: (314) 432-1380. 1992.

Control of Communicable Diseases in Man. Abram S. Benenson (ed.). American Public Health Association, 1015 15th St. N.W., Washington, DC 20005. Phone: (202) 789-5600. Fax: (202) 789-5661. 15th edition 1990.

Manual of Antibiotics and Infectious Disease. Conte. Williams & Wilkins, 428 East Preston St., Baltimore, MD 21202. Phone: (800) 638-0672. Fax: (800) 447-8438. Seventh edition 1992.

Pocketbook of Infectious Disease Therapy. Bartlett. Williams & Wilkins, 428 East Preston St., Baltimore, MD 21202. Phone: (800) 638-0672. Fax: (800) 447-8438. 1991.

JOURNALS

American Journal of Infection Control. Mosby-Year Book, 11830 Westline Industrial Drive, St. Louis, MO 63146. Phone: (800) 325-4177. Fax: (314) 432-1380. Bimonthly.

Clinical Infectious Diseases. University of Chicago Press, P.O. Box 37005, Chicago, IL 60637. Phone: (312) 753-3347. Fax: (312) 753-0811. Monthly.

Diagnostic Microbiology and Infectious Disease. Elsevier Science Publishing Co., Inc., P.O. Box 882, Madison Square Station, New York, NY 10159-2101. Phone: (212) 989-5800. Fax: (212) 633-3990. 8/year.

Immunology and Infectious Diseases. Rapid Communications of Oxford Ltd., The Old Malthouse, Paradise St., Oxford OX1 1LD, England. Phone: 44-865-790447. Fax: 44-865-244012. 4/year.

Infection Control and Hospital Epidemiology. SLACK Inc., 6900 Grove Rd., Thorofare, NJ 08086-9447. Phone: (800) 257-8290. Fax: (609) 853-5991.

Infection and Immunity. American Society for Microbiology, 1325 Massachusetts Ave. NW, Washington, DC 20005-4171. Phone: (202) 737-3600. Fax: (202) 737-0368. Monthly.

Infectious Diseases in Clinical Practice. Williams & Wilkins, 428 E. Preston St., Baltimore, MD 21202. Phone: (800) 638-0672. Fax: (800) 447-8438. Bimonthly.

Journal of Hospital Infection. Academic Press, Inc., 1250 Sixth Ave., San Diego, CA 92101-4311. Phone: (619) 699-6345. Fax: (619) 699-6715.

Journal of Infection. Academic Press, Inc., 1250 Sixth Ave., San Diego, CA 92101-4311. Phone: (619) 699-6345. Fax: (619) 699-6715.

Journal of Infectious Diseases. University of Chicago Press, P.O. Box 37005, Chicago, IL 60637. Phone: (312) 753-3347. Fax: (312) 753-0811. Monthly.

Journal of Wildlife Diseases. Wildlife Diseases Association, 224 S.E. 16th St., Ames, IA 50010. Phone: (515) 233-1931.

Morbidity and Mortality Weekly Report. Massachusetts Medical Society, 1440 Main St., Waltham, MA 02154-1649. Phone: (617) 893-3800. Fax: (617) 893-0413. Weekly.

The Pediatric Infectious Disease Journal. Williams & Wilkins, 428 E. Preston St., Baltimore, MD 21202. Phone: (800) 638-0672. Fax: (800) 447-8438. Monthly.

Review of Infectious Diseases. Infectious Diseases Society of America, 5720 S. Woodlawn Ave., Chicago, IL 60637. Phone: (312) 753-3347.

NEWSLETTERS

Infectious Disease Alert. American Health Consultants, Department C1290, P.O. Box 740060, Atlanta, GA 30374. Phone: (800) 559-1032. Fax: (404) 352-1971. Semimonthly.

Infectious Diseases Newsletter. Elsevier Science Publishing Co., Inc., P.O. Box 882, Madison Square Station, New York, NY 10159-2101. Phone: (212) 989-5800. Fax: (212) 633-3990. 12/year.

Morbidity and Mortality Weekly Report. Centers for Disease Control, 1600 Clifton Rd. N.E., Atlanta, GA 30333. Phone: (404) 488-4698.

ONLINE DATABASES

EMBASE. Elsevier Science Publishing Co., Inc., P.O. Box 882, Madison Square Station, New York, NY 10159-2101. Phone: (212) 989-5800. Fax: (212) 633-3990.

MEDLINE. National Library of Medicine, 8600 Rockville Pike, Bethesda, MD 20894. Phone: (800) 638-8480.

SciSearch. Institute for Scientific Information, 3501 Market St., Philadelphia, PA 19104. Phone: (215) 386-0100. Fax: (215) 386-6362.

RESEARCH CENTERS, INSTITUTES, CLEARINGHOUSES

Division of Geographic Medicine. Case Western Reserve University. School of Medicine, 2109 Adelbert Rd., Cleveland, OH 44106. Phone: (216) 368-4818. Fax: (216) 368-4825.

Division of Infectious Diseases. University of Maryland. Medical School Teaching Facility, 10 S. Pine St., Baltimore, MD 21201. Phone: (301) 328-7560. Fax: (301) 328-8700.

Hastings Foundation Infectious Disease Research Laboratories. University of Southern California. LAC-USC Medical Center, General Research Laboratory Bldg., Rm. 2G24, Los Angeles, CA 90033. Phone: (213) 226-3825.

Infectious Disease Research Group. University of Calgary. 3330 Hospital Dr. N.W., Calgary, AB, Canada T2N 4N1. Phone: (403) 220-6037. Fax: (403) 283-8814.

Infectious Diseases Research Laboratories. Ohio State University. 410 W. 10th Ave., Columbus, OH 43210. Phone: (614) 293-8732. Fax: (614) 293-4556.

National Institute of Allergy and Infectious Diseases. NIH Bldg. 31, Rm. 7A-32, 9000 Rockville Pike, Bethesda, MD 20892. Phone: (301) 496-5717.

STANDARDS AND STATISTICS SOURCES

Incidence and Impact of Selected Infectious Diseases in Childhood. National Center for Health Statistics, 6525 Belcrest Rd., Rm. 1064, Hyattsville, MD 20782. Phone: (301) 436-8500. PHS 91-1508 1991.

National Institue of Allergy and Infectious Diseases Profile. National Institute of Allergy and Infectious Diseases, Building 31, Room 7A32, 9000 Rockville Pike, Bethesda, MD 20892. Phone: (301) 496-5717. Annual.

Summary of Notifiable Diseases, U.S.. Centers for Disease Control, 1600 Clifton Rd. N.E., Atlanta, GA 30333. Phone: (404) 488-4698. Annual.

TEXTBOOKS AND MONOGRAPHS

Bacterial Infections of Humans: Epidemiology and Control. Alfred S. Evans, Philip S. Brachman (eds.). Plenum Publishing Co., 233 Spring St., New York, NY 10013-1578. Phone: (212) 620-8000. Fax: (212) 463-0742. Second edition 1991.

The Biologic and Clinical Basis of Infectious Diseases. Stanford Shulman, and others. W.B. Saunders Co., The Curtis Center, Independence Sqare W., Philadelphia, PA 19106-3399. Phone: (215) 238-7800. 4th edition, 1992.

Enteric Infection: Mechanisms, Manifestations, and Management. M.J.G. Farthing, G.T. Keusch. Raven Press, 1185 Avenue of the Americas, New York, NY 10036. Phone: (212) 930-9500. Fax: (212) 869-3495. 1989.

Fever: basic Mechanisms and Management. Philip A. Mackowiak (ed.). Raven Press, 1185 Avenue of the Americas, New York, NY 10036. Phone: (212) 930-9500. Fax: (212) 869-3495. 1991.

Infectious Diseases. Farrar. Raven Press, 1185 Ave. of the Americas, New York, NY 10036. Phone: (212) 930-9500. Fax: (212) 869-3495. 1992.

Infectious Diseases of Children. Saul Krugman, Samuel L. Katz, Anne A. Gershon, et. al.. Mosby-Year Book, 11830 Westline Industrial Drive, St. Louis, MO 63146. Phone: (800) 325-4177. Fax: (314) 432-1380. Ninth edition 1992.

Infectious Diseases of the Fetus and Newborn Infant. Jack Remington, Jerome Klein. W.B. Saunders Co., The Curtis Center, Independence Sqare W., Philadelphia, PA 19106-3399. Phone: (215) 238-7800. Third Edition 1990.

Infectious Diseases in Medicine and Surgery. Sherwood L. Gorbach, John Bartlett, Neil R. Blacklow. W.B. Saunders Co., The Curtis Center, Independence Square W., Philadelphia, PA 19106-3399. Phone: (215) 238-7800. 1991.

Pathology of Infectious Diseases. Von Lichtenberg. Raven Press, 1185 Ave. of the Americas, New York, NY 10036. Phone: (212) 930-9500. Fax: (212) 869-3495. 1991.

Post-Polio Syndrome. Theodore L. Munstat. Butterworth-Heinemann, 80 Montvale Ave., Stoneham, MA 02180. Phone: (617) 438-8464. Fax: (617) 279-4851. 1991.

Principles and Practice of Infectious Diseases. Gerald L. Mandell, R. Gordon Douglas Jr., John Bennett. Churchill Livingstone Inc., 650 Avenue of the Americas, New York, NY 10011. Phone: (212) 819-5400. Fax: (212) 302-6598. Third edition 1989.

Report of the Committee on Infections Diseases. American Academy of Pediatrics, 141 Northwest Point Blvd., P.O. Box 927, Elk Grove Village, IL 60009-0927. Phone: (800) 433-9016. Fax: (708) 228-1281. 22nd edition 1991.

Textbook of Pediatric Infectious Diseases. Ralph D. Feigin, James D. Cherry. W.B. Saunders Co., The Curtis Center, Independence Square W., Philadelphia, PA 19106-3399. Phone: (215) 238-7800. Second edition. Two volumes. 1987.

Understanding Infectious Disease. Paul D. Ellner, Harold C. Neu. Mosby-Year Book, 11830 Westline Industrial Drive, St. Louis, MO 63146. Phone: (800) 325-4177. Fax: (314) 432-1380. 1992.

World Guide to Infections: Diseases, Distribution, Diagnosis. Mary E. Wilson. Oxford University Press, 200 Madison Ave., New York, NY 10016. Phone: (212) 679-7300. 1991.

INFERTILITY

See also: IN VITRO FERTILIZATION; REPRODUCTION

ABSTRACTING, INDEXING, AND CURRENT AWARENESS PUBLICATIONS

Current Contents/Clinical Medicine. Institute for Scientific Information, 3501 Market St., Philadelphia, PA 19104. Phone: (800) 523-1850. Fax: (215) 386-6362. Weekly.

Current Contents/Life Sciences. Institute for Scientific Information, 3501 Market St., Philadelphia, PA 19104. Phone: (215) 386-0100. Fax: (215) 386-6362.

Index Medicus. U.S. National Library of Medicine, 8600 Rockville Pike, Bethesda, MD 20894. Phone: (800) 638-8480. Monthly.

Latest Literature in Family Planning. Family Planning Information Service, 27-35 Mortimer St., London W1N 7RJ, England. Bimonthly.

Research Alert: Fertility & Sterility. Institute for Scientific Information, 3501 Market St., Philadelphia, PA 19104. Phone: (800) 523-1850. Fax: (215) 386-6362. Weekly.

Research Alert: Infertility. Institute for Scientific Information, 3501 Market St., Philadelphia, PA 19104. Phone: (800) 523-1850. Fax: (215) 386-6362. Weekly.

Science Citation Index. Institute for Scientific Information, 3501 Market St., Philadelphia, PA 19104. Phone: (800) 523-1850. Fax: (215) 386-6362. Bimonthly.

ANNUALS AND REVIEWS

Advances in Human Fertility and Reproductive Endocrinology. Raven Press, 1185 Ave. of the Americas, New York, NY 10036. Phone: (212) 930-9500. Fax: (212) 869-3495.

Assisted Reproduction Reviews. Williams & Wilkins, 428 E. Preston St., Baltimore, MD 21202. Phone: (800) 638-0672. Fax: (800) 447-8438. Quarterly.

Infertility and Reproductive Medicine Clinics of North America. W.B. Saunders Co., The Curtis Center, Independence Square W., Philadelphia, PA 19106-3399. Phone: (215) 238-7800. Quarterly.

Reproductive Medicine Review. Cambridge University Press, 40 W. 20th St., New York, NY 10011. Phone: (800) 431-1580. Semiannual.

Year Book of Infertility. Mosby-Year Book, 11830 Westline Industrial Drive, St. Louis, MO 63146. Phone: (800) 325-4177. Fax: (314) 432-1380. Annual.

ASSOCIATIONS, PROFESSIONAL SOCIETIES, ADVOCACY AND SUPPORT GROUPS

American Fertility Society (AFS). 2140 11th Ave. S., Ste. 200, Birmingham, AL 35205-2800. Phone: (205) 933-8494. Fax: (205) 930-9904.

Fertility Research Foundation (FRF). 1430 Second Ave., Ste. 103, New York, NY 10021. Phone: (212) 744-5500.

Resolve Inc.. Five Water St., Arlington, MA 02174. Phone: (617) 643-2424.

BIBLIOGRAPHIES

Infertility in Men. National Technical Information Service, 5285 Port Royal Rd., Springfield, VA 22161. Phone: (703) 487-4650. Fax: (703) 321-8547. Jan. 1978-Jan. 1988 PB88-855465/CBY.

Infertility in Women. National Technical Information Service, 5285 Port Royal Rd., Springfield, VA 22161. Phone: (703) 487-4650. Fax: (703) 321-8547. Jan. 1978-Dec. 1987.

CD-ROM DATABASES

SCISEARCH. Institute for Scientific Information, 3501 Market St., Philadelphia, PA 19104. Phone: (215) 386-0100. Fax: (215) 386-6362.

DIRECTORIES

Infertility: Medical and Social Choices. Office of Technology Assesment, 600 Pennsylvania Ave. S.E., Washington, DC 20510. Phone: (202) 224-3827. Fax: (202) 275-0019. 1988.

HANDBOOKS, GUIDES, MANUALS, ATLASES

CRC Handbook of the Laboratory Diagnosis and Treatment of Infertility. Brooks A. Keel, Bobby W. Webster (eds.). CRC Press, Inc., 2000 Corporate Blvd. N.W., Boca Raton, FL 33431. Phone: (407) 994-0555. Fax: (407) 997-0949. 1990.

Infertility: A Clinician's Guide to Diagnosis and Treatment. Melvin L. Taymor. Plenum Publishing Co., 233 Spring St., New York, NY 10013-1578. Phone: (212) 620-8000. Fax: (212) 463-0742. 1990.

The Johns Hopkins Handbook of In Vitro Fertilization and Assisted Reproductive Technologies. Marian D. Damewood (ed.). Little, Brown and Company, 34 Beacon St., Boston, MA 02108. Phone: (617) 227-0730. 1990.

JOURNALS

Archives of Andrology. Taylor & Francis Inc., 1900 Frost Rd., Suite 101, Bristol, PA 19007-1598. Phone: (800) 821-8312. Fax: (215) 785-5515. Bimonthly.

Fertility and Sterility. American Fertility Society, 2140 11th Ave., Suite 200, Birmingham, AL 35205-2800. Phone: (205) 933-8494. Fax: (205) 930-9904. Monthly.

Infertility. Taylor & Francis Inc., 1900 Frost Rd., Suite 101, Bristol, PA 19007-1598. Phone: (800) 821-8312. Fax: (215) 785-5515. Quarterly.

International Journal of Fertility. MSP International, 347 Fifth Ave., No. 706, New York, NY 10016. Phone: (212) 532-9166.

Journal of Reproduction and Fertility. Journals of Reproduction and Fertility Ltd., 22 Newmarket Rd., Cambridge CB5 8DT, England. Phone: 0223-351809. Fax: 0223-359754. Bimonthly.

Journal of Reproductive Medicine. Journal of Reproductive Medicine, Inc., P.O. Drawer 12425, 8342 Olive Blvd., St. Louis, MO 63132. Phone: (314) 991-4440. Fax: (314) 991-4654. Monthly.

ONLINE DATABASES

EMBASE. Elsevier Science Publishing Co., Inc., P.O. Box 882, Madison Square Station, New York, NY 10159-2101. Phone: (212) 989-5800. Fax: (212) 633-3990.

MEDLINE. National Library of Medicine, 8600 Rockville Pike, Bethesda, MD 20894. Phone: (800) 638-8480.

POPLINE. U.S. National Library of Medicine, MEDLARS Management Section, 8600 Rockville Pike, Bethesda, MD 20894. Phone: (800) 638-8480. Monthly.

SciSearch. Institute for Scientific Information, 3501 Market St., Philadelphia, PA 19104. Phone: (215) 386-0100. Fax: (215) 386-6362.

POPULAR WORKS AND PATIENT EDUCATION

Conquering Infertility: A Guide for Couples. Stephen L. Corson. Prentice Hall, 113 Sylvan Ave., Rt. 9W, Prentice Hall Bldg., Englewood Cliffs, NJ 07632. Phone: (201) 767-5937. Revised edition 1991.

A Couple's Guide to Fertility: How New Medical Advances Can Help You Have a Baby. Berger. Doubleday & Co., Inc., 666 Fifth Ave., New York, NY 10103. Phone: (800) 223-6834. 1989.

Getting Pregnant: A Guide for the Infertile Couple. D. Llewellyn-Jones. Bantam Doubleday Dell, 666 Fifth Ave., New York, NY 10103. Phone: (800) 223-6834. 1991.

How to Get Pregnant with the New Technology. Sherman J. Silber. Warner Books, Inc., 666 Fifth Ave., 9th Flr., New York, NY 10103. Phone: (212) 484-2900. 1991.

Surviving Infertility: A Compassionate Guide Through the Emotional Crisis of Infertility. Linda P. Salzer. HarperCollins Pubs., Inc., 10 E. 53rd St., New York, NY 10022-5299. Phone: (212) 207-7000. Fax: (800) 242-7737. Revised edition 1991.

RESEARCH CENTERS, INSTITUTES, CLEARINGHOUSES

Alan Guttmacher Institute. 111 5th Ave., New York, NY 10003. Phone: (212) 254-5656. Fax: (212) 254-9891.

Center for Population and Family Health. Columbia University. Level B-3, 60 Haven Ave., New York, NY 10032. Phone: (212) 305-6960. Fax: (212) 305-7024.

Center for Reproductive Sciences. Columbia University. 630 W. 168th St., New York, NY 10032. Phone: (212) 305-4178. Fax: (212) 305-3869.

Howard and Georgeanne Jones Institute for Reproductive Medicine. 855 W. Brambleton Ave., Norfolk, VA 23510. Phone: (804) 446-5628.

Kinsey Institute for Research in Sex, Gender, and Reproduction, Inc.. Morrison Hall, 3rd. Fl., Bloomington, IN 47405. Phone: (812) 855-7686. Fax: (812) 855-8277.

Laboratory of Human Reproduction and Reproductive Biology. Harvard University. Harvard Medical School, 45 Shattuck, Boston, MA 02115. Phone: (617) 432-2038. Fax: (617) 566-7980.

Male Reproduction and Microsurgery Unit. Cornell University. Infertility Clinic, Division of Urology, 525 E. 68th. St., Rm. 900, New York, NY 10021. Phone: (615) 576-2866.

UCLA Population Research Center. Harbor-UCLA Medical Center, Walter Martin Research Bldg. RB-1, 1124 W. Carson St., Torrance, CA 90509. Phone: (310) 212-1867. Fax: (310) 320-6515.

TEXTBOOKS AND MONOGRAPHS

Clinical Gynecological Endocrinology and Infertility. Leon Speroff, and others. Williams & Wilkins, 428 East Preston St., Baltimore, MD 21202. Phone: (800) 638-0672. Fax: (800) 447-8438. 4th edition, 1988.

Infertility: A Comprehensive Text. Machelle Seibel. Appleton & Lange, 25 Van Zant St., East Norwalk, CT 06855. Phone: (800) 423-1359. Fax: (203) 854-9486. 1990.

Infertility: A Practical Guide for the Physician. Hammond. Blackwell Scientific Publications, Inc., 3 Cambridge Ctr., Cambridge, MA 02142. Phone: (800) 759-6102. Third edition 1992.

Infertility in the Male. Lipshultz. Mosby-Year Book, 11830 Westline Industrial Drive, St. Louis, MO 63146. Phone: (800) 325-4177. Fax: (314) 432-1380. Second edition 1991.

Infertility Surgery. John J. Stangel. Appleton & Lange, 25 Van Zant St., East Norwalk, CT 06855. Phone: (800) 423-1359. Fax: (203) 854-9486. 1990.

Pathology of Infertility. Ivan Damjanov. Mosby-Year Book, 11830 Westline Industrial Drive, St. Louis, MO 63146. Phone: (800) 325-4177. Fax: (314) 432-1380. 1992.

Pathology of Reproductive Failure. Kraus. Williams & Wilkins, 428 East Preston St., Baltimore, MD 21202. Phone: (800) 638-0672. Fax: (800) 447-8438. 1991.

INFLAMMATORY BOWEL DISEASE

See: GASTROINTESTINAL DISORDERS

INFLUENZA

See: INFECTIOUS DISEASES

INFORMED CONSENT

See also: MEDICAL CONSUMERISM

ABSTRACTING, INDEXING, AND CURRENT AWARENESS PUBLICATIONS

Cumulative Index to Nursing and Allied Health Literature. Glendale Adventist Medical Center, P.O. Box 871, Glendale, CA 91209. Phone: (818) 409-8005. Bimonthly.

Hospital Literature Index. American Hospital Association, 840 N. Lake Shore Dr., Chicago, IL 60611. Phone: (800) 242-2626. Fax: (312) 280-6015. Quarterly.

Index Medicus. U.S. National Library of Medicine, 8600 Rockville Pike, Bethesda, MD 20894. Phone: (800) 638-8480. Monthly.

ASSOCIATIONS, PROFESSIONAL SOCIETIES, ADVOCACY AND SUPPORT GROUPS

American Civil Liberties Union. 132 W. 43rd St., New York, NY 10036.

The Campaign for Women's Health. 666 11th St. N.W., Ste. 700, Washington, DC 20001. Phone: (202) 783-6686.

Public Citizen Health Research Group (PCHRG). 2000 P St. N.W., Ste. 700, Washington, DC 20036. Phone: (202) 872-0320.

CD-ROM DATABASES

Nursing and Allied Health (CINAHL) on CD-ROM. CINAHL, 1509 Wilson Terrace, P.O. Box 871, Glendale, CA 91209-0871. Phone: (818) 409-8005.

NEWSLETTERS

Health Facts. Center for Medical Consumers, 237 Thompson St., New York, NY 10012. Phone: (212) 674-7105. Monthly.

ONLINE DATABASES

EMBASE. Elsevier Science Publishing Co., Inc., P.O. Box 882, Madison Square Station, New York, NY 10159-2101. Phone: (212) 989-5800. Fax: (212) 633-3990.

MEDLINE. National Library of Medicine, 8600 Rockville Pike, Bethesda, MD 20894. Phone: (800) 638-8480.

Nursing and Allied Health (CINAHL). CINAHL, 1509 Wilson Terrace, P.O. Box 871, Glendale, CA 91209-0871. Phone: (818) 409-8005.

SciSearch. Institute for Scientific Information, 3501 Market St., Philadelphia, PA 19104. Phone: (215) 386-0100. Fax: (215) 386-6362.

POPULAR WORKS AND PATIENT EDUCATION

150 Ways to Be a Savvy Medical Consumer. Charles B. Inlander. People's Medical Society, 462 Walnut St., Allentown, PA 18102. Phone: (215) 770-1670. 1992.

Best Medicine: Your Essential Guide to Finding Top Doctors, Hospitals and Treatments. Robert Arnot. Addison-Wesley Publishing Co., Rte. 128, Reading, MA 01867. Phone: (800) 447-2226. 1992.

Medicine on Trial: The Appalling Story of Medical Ineptitude and the Arrogance that Overlooks It. Charles B. Inlander, Lowell S. Levin, Ed Weiner. Random House, Inc., 201 E. 50th St., New York, NY 10022. Phone: (800) 726-0600. 1990.

Personal Health Reporter. Alan Rees, Charlene Wiley. Gale Research, Inc., 835 Penobscot Bldg., Detroit, MI 48226-4094. Phone: (800) 877-GALE. Fax: (313) 961-6083. 1992.

The Rights of Patients: The Basic ACLU Guide to Patient Rights. George J. Annas. Southern Illinois University Press, P.O. Box 3697, Carbondale, IL 62902-3697. Phone: (618) 453-2281. 1989.

RESEARCH CENTERS, INSTITUTES, CLEARINGHOUSES

Center for Medical Consumers and Health Care Information (CMC). 237 Thompson St., New York, NY 10012. Phone: (212) 674-7105. Fax: (212) 674-7100.

TEXTBOOKS AND MONOGRAPHS

Consent to Treatment: A Practical Guide. Fay A. Rozovsky. Little, Brown and Company, 34 Beacon St., Boston, MA 02108. Phone: (617) 227-0730. Second edition 1989.

Patient Compliance in Medical Practice and Clinical Trials. Joyce A. Cramer, Bert Spilker. Raven Press, 1185 Avenue of the Americas, New York, NY 10036. Phone: (212) 930-9500. Fax: (212) 869-3495. 1991.

INJURIES

See: WOUNDS AND INJURIES

INSOMNIA

See: SLEEP DISORDERS

INSTRUMENTATION

See: MEDICAL DEVICES AND INSTRUMENTATION

INSULIN

See: DIABETES

INSURANCE

See: HEALTH INSURANCE

INTENSIVE CARE

See also: NEONATOLOGY

ABSTRACTING, INDEXING, AND CURRENT AWARENESS PUBLICATIONS

Current Contents/Clinical Medicine. Institute for Scientific Information, 3501 Market St., Philadelphia, PA 19104. Phone: (800) 523-1850. Fax: (215) 386-6362. Weekly.

Index Medicus. U.S. National Library of Medicine, 8600 Rockville Pike, Bethesda, MD 20894. Phone: (800) 638-8480. Monthly.

Science Citation Index. Institute for Scientific Information, 3501 Market St., Philadelphia, PA 19104. Phone: (800) 523-1850. Fax: (215) 386-6362. Bimonthly.

CD-ROM DATABASES

Basic Life Support. Hoffer. Williams & Wilkins, 428 East Preston St., Baltimore, MD 21202. Phone: (800) 638-0672. Fax: (800) 447-8438. 1989.

Critical Care MEDLINE. MEP, 124 Mt. Auburn St., Cambridge, MA 02138. Phone: (800) 342-1338. Fax: (617) 868-7738. Quarterly.

SCISEARCH. Institute for Scientific Information, 3501 Market St., Philadelphia, PA 19104. Phone: (215) 386-0100. Fax: (215) 386-6362.

HANDBOOKS, GUIDES, MANUALS, ATLASES

Handbook of Pediatric Intensive Care. Mark C. Rogers (ed.). Williams & Wilkins, 428 East Preston St., Baltimore, MD 21202. Phone: (800) 638-0672. Fax: (800) 447-8438. 1989.

Handbook of Surgical Intensive Care. Lyerly. Mosby-Year Book, 11830 Westline Industrial Drive, St. Louis, MO 63146. Phone: (800) 325-4177. Fax: (314) 432-1380. Third edition 1992.

Intensive Care Manual. E.D. Teik. Butterworth-Heinemann, 80 Montvale Ave., Stoneham, MA 02180. Phone: (617) 438-8464. Fax: (617) 279-4851. 1990.

Manual of Intensive Care Medicine. Rippe. Little, Brown and Co., 34 Beacon St., Boston, MA 02108. Phone: (617) 227-0730. Fax: (617) 227-0790. Second edition 1989.

Neonatal Intensive Care Handbook. Goetzman. Mosby-Year Book, 11830 Westline Industrial Drive, St. Louis, MO 63146. Phone: (800) 325-4177. Fax: (314) 432-1380. Second edition 1991.

JOURNALS

Care of the Critically Ill. Mosby-Year Book, 11830 Westline Industrial Drive, St. Louis, MO 63146. Phone: (800) 325-4177. Fax: (314) 432-1380. Bimonthly.

Intensive Care Medicine. Springer-Verlag New York Inc., 175 Fifth Ave., New York, NY 10010. Phone: (212) 460-1500. Fax: (212) 473-6272.

Intensive Care Nursing. Churchill Livingstone Inc., 650 Avenue of the Americas, New York, NY 10011. Phone: (212) 819-5400. Fax: (212) 302-6598. Quarterly.

Intensive Care World. King and Wirth Publishing Co., Hillside, Arnolds Lane, Hinxworth, Baldock, Herts. SG7 5HR, England. Phone: 44-46274-2580. Fax: 44-46274-2986. Quarterly.

ONLINE DATABASES

EMBASE. Elsevier Science Publishing Co., Inc., P.O. Box 882, Madison Square Station, New York, NY 10159-2101. Phone: (212) 989-5800. Fax: (212) 633-3990.

MEDLINE. National Library of Medicine, 8600 Rockville Pike, Bethesda, MD 20894. Phone: (800) 638-8480.

SciSearch. Institute for Scientific Information, 3501 Market St., Philadelphia, PA 19104. Phone: (215) 386-0100. Fax: (215) 386-6362.

RESEARCH CENTERS, INSTITUTES, CLEARINGHOUSES

Institute of Critical Care Medicine. 1975 Zonal Ave., KAM 307B, Los Angeles, CA 90033. Phone: (213) 225-9633.

TEXTBOOKS AND MONOGRAPHS

Current Therapy in Critical Care Medicine. Joseph E. Parrillo. Mosby-Year Book, 11830 Westline Industrial Drive, St. Louis, MO 63146. Phone: (800) 325-4177. Fax: (314) 432-1380. 1991.

Essentials of Pediatric Intensive Care. Levin. Quality Publications, P.O. Box 1060, Abilene, TX 79604. Phone: (800) 359-7708. 1990.

Intensive Care Medicine. James M. Rippe, Richard S. Irwin, Joseph S. Alpert, et. al.. Little, Brown and Company, 34 Beacon St., Boston, MA 02108. Phone: (617) 227-0730. Second edition 1991.

Surgical Intensive Care. Phillip S. Barie, G. Tom Shires (eds.). Little, Brown and Company, 34 Beacon St., Boston, MA 02108. Phone: (617) 227-0730. 1992.

Textbook of Pediatric Intensive Care. Rogers. Williams & Wilkins, 428 East Preston St., Baltimore, MD 21202. Phone: (800) 638-0672. Fax: (800) 447-8438. Two volumes. Second edition. 1992.

Total Parenteral Nutrition. Josef E. Fischer. Little, Brown and Company, 34 Beacon St., Boston, MA 02108. Phone: (617) 227-0730. Second edition 1991.

Trauma: Anesthesia and Intensive Care. levon M. Capan, Sanford Miller, Herman Turndorf (eds.). J.B. Lippincott Co., 227 East Washington Square, Philadelphia, PA 19106-3780. Phone: (215) 238-4200. Fax: (215) 238-4227. 1991.

INTERFERON

ABSTRACTING, INDEXING, AND CURRENT AWARENESS PUBLICATIONS

BIOSIS/CAS Selects: Interferon. BIOSIS, 2100 Arch St., Philadelphia, PA 19103-1399. Phone: (215) 587-4800. Fax: (215) 587-2016. Biweekly.

Current Contents/Life Sciences. Institute for Scientific Information, 3501 Market St., Philadelphia, PA 19104. Phone: (215) 386-0100. Fax: (215) 386-6362.

Excerpta Medica. Section 26: Immunology, Serology and Transplantation. Elsevier Science Publishing Co., Inc., P.O. Box 882, Madison Square Station, New York, NY 10159-2101. Phone: (212) 989-5800. Fax: (212) 633-3990. 32/year.

Excerpta Medica. Section 47: Virology. Elsevier Science Publishing Co., Inc., P.O. Box 882, Madison Square Station, New York, NY 10159-2101. Phone: (212) 989-5800. Fax: (212) 633-3990.

General Science Index. H.W. Wilson Co., 950 University Ave., Bronx, NY 10452. Phone: (800) 367-6770.

Hospital Literature Index. American Hospital Association, 840 N. Lake Shore Dr., Chicago, IL 60611. Phone: (800) 242-2626. Fax: (312) 280-6015. Quarterly.

Index Medicus. U.S. National Library of Medicine, 8600 Rockville Pike, Bethesda, MD 20894. Phone: (800) 638-8480. Monthly.

Research Alert: Interferon & Interferon Inducers. Institute for Scientific Information, 3501 Market St., Philadelphia, PA 19104. Phone: (800) 523-1850. Fax: (215) 386-6362. Weekly.

Science Citation Index. Institute for Scientific Information, 3501 Market St., Philadelphia, PA 19104. Phone: (800) 523-1850. Fax: (215) 386-6362. Bimonthly.

ASSOCIATIONS, PROFESSIONAL SOCIETIES, ADVOCACY AND SUPPORT GROUPS

Interferon Foundation (IF). 1 Shell Plaza, Ste. 3990, 910 Louisiana St., Houston, TX 77002. Phone: (713) 224-8224.

BIBLIOGRAPHIES

Interferon. National Technical Information Service, 5285 Port Royal Rd., Springfield, VA 22161. Phone: (703) 487-4650. Fax: (703) 321-8547. Mar. 1974-Nov. 1989 PB90-857590/CBY.

CD-ROM DATABASES

SCISEARCH. Institute for Scientific Information, 3501 Market St., Philadelphia, PA 19104. Phone: (215) 386-0100. Fax: (215) 386-6362.

JOURNALS

Interferon. Academic Press, Inc., 1250 Sixth Ave., San Diego, CA 92101-4311. Phone: (619) 699-6345. Fax: (619) 699-6715.

Journal of Immunology. Williams & Wilkins, 428 E. Preston St., Baltimore, MD 21202. Phone: (800) 638-0672. Fax: (800) 447-8438. Semimonthly.

Journal of Interferon Research. Mary Ann Liebert, Inc., 1651 Third Ave., New York, NY 10128. Phone: (212) 289-2300. Fax: (212) 289-4697. Bimonthly.

ONLINE DATABASES

EMBASE. Elsevier Science Publishing Co., Inc., P.O. Box 882, Madison Square Station, New York, NY 10159-2101. Phone: (212) 989-5800. Fax: (212) 633-3990.

MEDLINE. National Library of Medicine, 8600 Rockville Pike, Bethesda, MD 20894. Phone: (800) 638-8480.

SciSearch. Institute for Scientific Information, 3501 Market St., Philadelphia, PA 19104. Phone: (215) 386-0100. Fax: (215) 386-6362.

TEXTBOOKS AND MONOGRAPHS

Interferons and Other Regulatory Cytokines. Edward De Maeyer, Jacqueline De Maeyer-Guignard. John Wiley & Sons, Inc., 605 Third Ave., New York, NY 10158-0012. Phone: (212) 850-6000. Fax: (212) 850-6088. 1988.

INTERNAL MEDICINE

ABSTRACTING, INDEXING, AND CURRENT AWARENESS PUBLICATIONS

Current Contents/Clinical Medicine. Institute for Scientific Information, 3501 Market St., Philadelphia, PA 19104. Phone: (800) 523-1850. Fax: (215) 386-6362. Weekly.

The Edell Health Letter. Hippocrates, Inc., 475 Gate Five Rd., Ste. 100, Sausalito, CA 94965. Bimonthly.

Excerpta Medica. Section 6: Internal Medicine. Elsevier Science Publishers, P.O. Box 882, Madison Square Station, New York, NY 10159-2101. Phone: (212) 633-3950. Fax: (212) 633-3990. 24/year.

Index Medicus. U.S. National Library of Medicine, 8600 Rockville Pike, Bethesda, MD 20894. Phone: (800) 638-8480. Monthly.

Medical Abstracts Newsletter. Communi-T Publications, P.O. Box 2170, Teaneck, NJ 07666. Phone: (201) 836-5030. Monthly.

PDR Journal Abstracts. Medical Economics, Five Paragon Dr., Montvale, NJ 07645-1742. Phone: (800) 222-3045. Fax: (201) 573-4956. Annual.

Reference Update. Research Information Systems, Inc., Camino Corporate Ctr., 2355 Camino Vida Roble, Carlsbad, CA 92009-1572. Phone: (800) 722-1227. Fax: (619) 438-5573. Weekly.

Science Citation Index. Institute for Scientific Information, 3501 Market St., Philadelphia, PA 19104. Phone: (800) 523-1850. Fax: (215) 386-6362. Bimonthly.

ANNUALS AND REVIEWS

Advances in Internal Medicine. Mosby-Year Book, 11830 Westline Industrial Drive, St. Louis, MO 63146. Phone: (800) 325-4177. Fax: (314) 432-1380. Annual.

Annual Review of Medicine. Annual Reviews Inc., 4139 El Camino Way, P.O. Box 10139, Palo Alto, CA 94303-0897. Phone: (415) 493-4400. Fax: (415) 855-9815. Annual.

Contemporary Internal Medicine. Plenum Publishing Co., 233 Spring St., New York, NY 10013-1578. Phone: (212) 620-8000. Fax: (212) 463-0742. Irregular.

Contemporary Management in Internal Medicine. Churchill Livingstone Inc., 650 Avenue of the Americas, New York, NY 10011. Phone: (212) 819-5400. Fax: (212) 302-6598. 6/year.

Current Medical Diagnosis and Treatment. Appleton & Lange, 25 Van Zant St., East Norwalk, CT 06855. Phone: (800) 423-1359. Fax: (203) 854-9486. Annual.

Medical Clinics. W.B. Saunders Co., The Curtis Center, Independence Square W., Philadelphia, PA 19106-3399. Phone: (215) 238-7800. Bimonthly.

Primary Care: Clinics in Office Practice. W.B. Saunders Co., The Curtis Center, Independence Square W., Philadelphia, PA 19106-3399. Phone: (215) 238-7800. Quarterly.

ASSOCIATIONS, PROFESSIONAL SOCIETIES, ADVOCACY AND SUPPORT GROUPS

American Board of Internal Medicine (ABIM). 3624 Market St., Philadelphia, PA 19104. Phone: (215) 243-1500.

American College of Physicians (ACP). Independence Mall W., 6th St. at Race, Philadelphia, PA 19106. Phone: (215) 351-2400.

American Medical Association (AMA). 515 N. State St., Chicago, IL 60610. Phone: (312) 464-5000. Fax: (312) 645-4184.

American Society of Internal Medicine (ASIM). 1101 Vermont Ave. N.W., Ste. 500, Washington, DC 20005-3457. Phone: (202) 289-1700. Fax: (202) 682-8659.

Canadian Medical Association. 1867 Alta Vista Dr., Box 8650, Ottawa, ON, Canada K1G 0G8. Phone: (613) 731-9331. Fax: (913) 731-0937.

Royal College of Physicians and Surgeons of Canada. 74 Stanley, Ottawa, ON, Canada K1M 1P4.

BIBLIOGRAPHIES

Core Collection of Medical Books and Journals 1992. Howard Hague, Michael Jackson. Medical Information Working Party, Henry Hochland, Haigh and Hochland Ltd., The Precinct Ctr., Oxford Rd., Manchester M13 9QA, England. 1992.

Medical and Health Care Books and Serials in Print. R.R. Bowker Co., 245 W. 17th St., New York, NY 10011. Phone: (800) 521-8110. Fax: (908) 665-6688. Annual.

CD-ROM DATABASES

1993 PDR Library on CD-ROM. Medical Economics, Five Paragon Dr., Montvale, NJ 07645-1742. Phone: (800) 232-7379. Fax: (201) 573-4956. 1993.

American Family Physician. CMC ReSearch, Inc., 7150 S.W. Hampton, Suite C-120, Portland, OR 97223. Phone: (800) 262-7668. Fax: (503) 639-1796. Annual.

Annals of Internal Medicine. MEP, 124 Mt. Auburn St., Cambridge, MA 02138. Phone: (800) 342-1338. Fax: (617) 868-7738. Semiannual.

British Medical Journal. MEP, 124 Mt. Auburn St., Cambridge, MA 02138. Phone: (800) 342-1338. Fax: (617) 868-7738. Annual.

Directory of Physicians in the United States. American Medical Association, 515 North State St., Chicago, IL 60610. Phone: (312) 464-0183. Fax: (312) 464-5834. Annual.

Family Practice MEDLINE. MEP, 124 Mt. Auburn St., Cambridge, MA 02138. Phone: (800) 342-1338. Fax: (617) 868-7738. Quarterly.

Health Reference Center. Information Access Company, 362 Lakeside Dr., Foster City, CA 94404. Phone: (800) 227-8431. Monthly.

Internal Medicine '92. Macmillan New Media, 124 Mt. Auburn St., Cambridge, MA 02138. Phone: (800) 342-1338. 1992.

Journal of the American Medical Association. Macmillan New Media, 124 Mt. Auburn St., Cambridge, MA 02138. Weekly.

MAXX: Maximum Access to Diagnosis and Therapy. Little, Brown and Company, 34 Beacon St., Boston, MA 02108. Phone: (617) 227-0730. The Electronic Library of Medicine.

New England Journal of Medicine. CMC ReSearch, Inc., 7150 S.W. Hampton, Suite C-120, Portland, OR 97223. Phone: (800) 262-7668. Fax: (503) 639-1796. 3/year.

The New England Journal of Medicine on CD-ROM. MEP, 124 Mt. Auburn St., Cambridge, MA 02138. Phone: (800) 342-1338. Fax: (617) 868-7738. Semiannual.

Oxford Textbook of Medicine. Oxford University Press, 200 Madison Ave., New York, NY 10016. Phone: (212) 679-7300. Irregular.

PDR on CD-ROM. Medical Economics, Five Paragon Dr., Montvale, NJ 07645-1742. Phone: (800) 222-3045. Fax: (201) 573-4956. 3/year.

The Physician's MEDLINE. MEP, 124 Mt. Auburn St., Cambridge, MA 02138. Phone: (800) 342-1338. Fax: (617) 868-7738. Quarterly.

Scientific American Medicine CONSULT. Scientific American, Inc., 415 Madison Ave., New York, NY 10017. Phone: (212) 754-0550. Fax: (212) 980-3062. Quarterly.

SCISEARCH. Institute for Scientific Information, 3501 Market St., Philadelphia, PA 19104. Phone: (215) 386-0100. Fax: (215) 386-6362.

Year Books on Disc. CMC ReSearch, Inc., 7150 S.W. Hampton, Suite C-120, Portland, OR 97223. Phone: (800) 262-7668. Fax: (503) 639-1796. Annual includes Year Books of Cardiology, Dermatology, Diagnostic Radiology, Drug Therapy, Emergency Medicine, Family Practice, Medicine, Neurology and Neurosurgery, Obstetrics and Gynecology, Oncology, Pediatrics, and Psychiatry and Applied Mental Health.

DIRECTORIES

Directory of Certified Internists. American Board of Medical Specialties, 1 Rotary Center, Suite 805, Evanston, IL 60201. Phone: (708) 491-9091. Biennial.

Directory of Medical Specialists. Marquis Who's Who, 3002 Glenview Rd., Wilmette, IL 60091. Phone: (800) 621-9669. Fax: (708) 441-2264. Biennial.

Directory of Physicians in the United States. American Medical Association, 515 North State St., Chicago, IL 60610. Phone: (312) 464-0183. Fax: (312) 464-5834. Biennial.

ENCYCLOPEDIAS, DICTIONARIES, WORD BOOKS

The American Medical Association Encyclopedia of Medicine. Random House, Inc., 201 E. 50th St., New York, NY 10022. Phone: (800) 726-0600. 1989.

Churchill's Illustrated Medical Dictionary. Churchill Livingstone Inc., 650 Ave. of the Americas, New York, NY 10011. Phone: (212) 819-5400. Fax: (212) 302-6598. 1989.

Dictionary of Medical Syndromes. S. Magalini and others. J.B. Lippincott Co., 227 E. Washington Square, Philadelphia, PA 19106-3780. Phone: (215) 238-4200. Fax: (215) 238-4227. Third edition 1990.

Dictionary of Modern Medicine. Segen. The Parthenon Publishing Group, Inc., 120 Mill Rd., Park Ridge, NJ 07656. Phone: (201) 391-6796. 1992.

English-Spanish/Spanish-English Medical Dictionary. Glenn T. Rogers. McGraw-Hill, Inc., Health Professions Division, 1221 Avenue of the Americas, 28th Floor, New York, NY 10020. Phone: (212) 512-4228. 1992.

Melloni's Illustrated Medical Dictionary. Dox. Williams & Wilkins, 428 East Preston St., Baltimore, MD 21202. Phone: (800) 638-0672. Fax: (800) 447-8438. Second edition 1985.

The Mosby Medical Encyclopedia. Viking Penguin, 375 Hudson St., New York, NY 10014-3657. Phone: (800) 331-4624. Revised edition 1992.

Mosby's Medical, Nursing, and Allied Health Dictionary. Kenneth N. Anderson, Lois Anderson, Walter D. Glanze (eds.). Mosby-Year Book, 11830 Westline Industrial Dr., St. Louis, MO 63146. Phone: (800) 325-4177. Fax: (314) 432-1380. Third edition 1990.

Professional Guide to Diseases. Springhouse Publishing Co., 1111 Bethlehem Pike, Spring House, PA 19477. Phone: (800) 331-3170. Fax: (215) 646-8716. Fourth edition 1992.

HANDBOOKS, GUIDES, MANUALS, ATLASES

Guide to Clinical Trials. Bert Spilker. Raven Press, 1185 Avenue of the Americas, New York, NY 10036. Phone: (212) 930-9500. Fax: (212) 869-3495. 1991.

Internal Medicine: Diagnosis and Therapy. Jay H. Stein. Appleton & Lange, 25 Van Zant St., East Norwalk, CT 06855. Phone: (800) 423-1359. Fax: (203) 854-9486. Second edition 1990.

Manual of Clinical Problems in Internal Medicine. Jerry L. Spivak, H. Verdun Barnes. Little, Brown and Co., 34 Beacon St., Boston, MA 02108. Phone: (617) 227-0730. Fax: (617) 227-0790. 1990.

Merck Manual of Diagnosis and Therapy. Robert Berkow (ed.). Merck & Co., Inc., P.O. Box 2000, Rahway, NJ 07065. Phone: (201) 855-4558. 16th edition. 1992.

Oxford Handbook of Clinical Medicine. R.A. Hope, J.M. Longmore, P.A.H. Moss, A.N. Warrens. Oxford University Press, 200 Madison Ave., New York, NY 10016. Phone: (212) 679-7300. Second Edition 1989.

Random House Personal Medical Handbook: First Aid Away from Home. Paula Dranov. Random House, Inc., 201 E. 50th St., New York, NY 10022. Phone: (800) 726-0600. 1990.

Rush Internal Medicine Handbook. Bone. Mosby-Year Book, 11830 Westline Industrial Drive, St. Louis, MO 63146. Phone: (800) 325-4177. Fax: (314) 432-1380. 1990.

JOURNALS

Annals of Internal Medicine. American College of Physicians, Independence Mall W., Sixth St. at Race, Philadelphia, PA 19106-1572. Phone: (800) 523-1546. Fax: (215) 351-2594. Semimonthly.

Archives of Internal Medicine. American Medical Association, 515 North State St., Chicago, IL 60610. Phone: (312) 464-0183. Fax: (312) 464-5834. Monthly.

BMJ. BMJ Publishing Group, BMA House, Tavistock Square, London WC1H 9JR, England. Phone: 071-383 6244/6638. Fax: 071-383 6662. Weekly.

Disease-A-Month. Mosby-Year Book, 11830 Westline Industrial Drive, St. Louis, MO 63146. Phone: (800) 325-4177. Fax: (314) 432-1380. Monthly.

IM-Internal Medicine for the Specialist. Medical Economics, Five Paragon Dr., Montvale, NJ 07645-1742. Phone: (800) 222-3045. Fax: (201) 573-4956. Monthly.

Journal of the American Medical Association. American Medical Association, 515 North State St., Chicago, IL 60610. Phone: (312) 464-0183. Fax: (312) 464-5834. Weekly.

Journal of Clinical Investigation. Rockefeller University Press, 222 E. 70th St., New York, NY 10021. Phone: (212) 570-8572. Fax: (212) 570-7944. Monthly.

Journal of Osteopathic Sports Medicine. American Osteopathic Academy of Sports Medicine, P.O. Box 623, Middleton, WI 53562-0623.

Journal of the Royal Society of Medicine. Royal Society of Medicine Services Ltd., 1 Wimpole St., London W1M 8AE, England. Phone: 071-408 2119. Fax: 071-355 3198. Monthly.

Lancet. Williams & Wilkins, 428 East Preston St., Baltimore, MD 21202. Phone: (800) 638-0672. Fax: (800) 447-8438. Weekly.

Medicine. Williams & Wilkins, 428 E. Preston St., Baltimore, MD 21202. Phone: (800) 638-0672. Fax: (800) 447-8438. Bimonthly.

The New England Journal of Medicine. Massachusetts Medical Society, 1440 Main St., Waltham, MA 02154-1649. Phone: (617) 893-3800. Fax: (617) 893-0413. Weekly.

Patient Care. Medical Economics, Five Paragon Dr., Montvale, NJ 07645-1742. Phone: (800) 222-3045. Fax: (201) 573-4956. Semimonthly.

Western Journal of Medicine. California Medical Association, P.O. Box 7602, San Francisco, CA 94120-7602. Phone: (415) 882-5179. Fax: (415) 882-5116. Monthly.

NEWSLETTERS

Consumer Reports on Health. Consumer Reports, P.O. Box 52148, Boulder, CO 80322. Monthly.

Harvard Family Health Letter. Harvard Medical School Publications Group, 164 Longwood Ave., Boston, MA 02115. Monthly.

The Harvard Health Letter. Dept. of Continuing Education. Harvard Medical School, 164 Longwood Ave., 4th Flr., Boston, MA 02115. Phone: (617) 432-1485. Fax: (617) 432-1506. Monthly.

Harvard Heart Letter. Harvard Medical School Publications Group, 164 Longwood Ave., Boston, MA 02115. Monthly.

Health News. Faculty of Medicine. University of Toronto, Medical Sciences Bldg., Toronto, ON, Canada M5S 1A8. Phone: (416) 948-5411. Fax: (416) 978-4552. Bimonthly.

Health & You. Health Ink Co., One Executive Dr., Moorestown, NJ 08057. Quarterly.

Healthline. Mosby-Year Book, 11830 Westline Industrial Drive, St. Louis, MO 63146. Phone: (800) 325-4177. Fax: (314) 432-1380. Monthly.

Internal Medicine Alert. American Health Consultants, Department C1290, P.O. Box 740060, Atlanta, GA 30374. Phone: (800) 559-1032. Fax: (404) 352-1971. Semimonthly.

Johns Hopkins Medical Letter: Health After 50. Medletter Associates, Inc., P.O. Box 359179, Palm Coast, FL 32137. Monthly.

Mayo Clinic Health Letter. Mayo Foundation for Medical Education and Research, 200 First St. N.W., Rochester, MN 55905. Phone: (507) 284-4587. Fax: (507) 284-5410. Monthly.

Medical Update. Medical Society. Medical Education and Research Foundation. Benjamin Franklin Literary & Medical Society, P.O. Box 567, Indianapolis, IN 46206. Phone: (317) 636-8881. Fax: (317) 637-0126. !MO.

Men's Health Newsletter. Rodale Press, Inc., 33 E. Minor St., Emmaus, PA 18098. Phone: (800) 527-8200. Fax: (215) 967-6263. Monthly.

University of California, Berkeley Wellness Letter. Health Letter Associates, Box 412, Prince St. Sta., New York, NY 10003-0007. Phone: (212) 505-2255. Fax: (212) 505-5462. Monthly.

The University of Texas Lifetime Health Letter. Health Science Center. University of Texas, 1100 Holcombe Blvd., P.O. Box 20036, Houston, TX 77225. Phone: (800) 274-6377. Monthly.

ONLINE DATABASES

Comprehensive Core Medical Library (CCML). BRS Information Technologies, 8000 Westpark Dr., Mc Lean, VA 22102. Phone: (800) 289-4277. Fax: (703) 893-4632. Weekly.

EMBASE. Elsevier Science Publishing Co., Inc., P.O. Box 882, Madison Square Station, New York, NY 10159-2101. Phone: (212) 989-5800. Fax: (212) 633-3990.

MEDIS. Mead Data Central, P.O. Box 1830, Dayton, OH 45401. Phone: (800) 227-4908.

MEDLINE. National Library of Medicine, 8600 Rockville Pike, Bethesda, MD 20894. Phone: (800) 638-8480.

The New England Journal of Medicine. Massachusetts Medical Society, Medical Publishing Group, 1440 Main St., Waltham, MA 02254. Phone: (617) 893-4610. Weekly.

The Online Journal of Current Clinical Trials. American Association for the Advancement of Science, 1333 H St. N.W., Rm. 1155, Washington, DC 20005. Phone: (202) 326-6446.

Postgraduate Medicine. McGraw-Hill Inc., 11 West 19th St., New York, NY 10011. Phone: (212) 337-5001. Fax: (212) 337-4092. Monthly.

SciSearch. Institute for Scientific Information, 3501 Market St., Philadelphia, PA 19104. Phone: (215) 386-0100. Fax: (215) 386-6362.

POPULAR WORKS AND PATIENT EDUCATION

The American Medical Association Family Medical Guide. Random House, Inc., 201 E. 50th St., New York, NY 10022. Phone: (800) 726-0600. Sixth edition 1987.

The Columbia University College of Physicians and Surgeons Complete Home Medical Guide. Genell Subak-Sharpe (ed.). Random House, Inc., 201 E. 50th St., New York, NY 10022. Phone: (800) 726-0600. 1989 Revised edition 1989.

Complete Guide to Symptoms, Illness and Surgery for People over Fifty. H. Winter Griffith. Putnam Publishing Group, 200 Madison Ave., New York, NY 10016. Phone: (800) 631-8571. 1992.

A Doctor's Guide to the Best Medical Care: A Practical, No-Nonsense Evaluation of Your Treatment Options for Over 100 Conditions and Diseases. Michael Oppenheim. Rodale Press, Inc., 33 E. Minor St., Emmaus, PA 18098. Phone: (800) 527-8200. Fax: (215) 967-6263. 1992.

Mayo Clinic Family Health Book. David E. Larson (ed.). William Morrow & Company, Inc., 1350 Ave. of the Americas, New York, NY 10019. Phone: (800) 237-0657. 1991.

New Good Housekeeping Family Health and Medical Guide. Hearst Corporation, 60 E. 42nd St., New York, NY 10165. Phone: (212) 297-9680. Fax: (415) 588-6867. Revised edition 1988.

TEXTBOOKS AND MONOGRAPHS

Cecil Textbook of Medicine. J.B. Wyngaarden, L.H. Smith. W.B. Saunders Co., The Curtis Center, Independence Square W., Philadelphia, PA 19106-3399. Phone: (215) 238-7800. 18th edition 1988.

Conn's Current Therapy. W.B. Saunders Co., The Curtis Center, Independence Square W., Philadelphia, PA 19106-3399. Phone: (215) 238-7800. Annual.

Current Diagnosis 8. Rex Conn (ed.). Williams & Wilkins, 428 East Preston St., Baltimore, MD 21202. Phone: (800) 638-0672. Fax: (800) 447-8438. 1991.

Davidson's Principles and Practice of Medicine. I. Bouchier, C. Edwards. Churchill Livingstone Inc., 650 Ave. of the Americas, New York, NY 10011. Phone: (212) 819-5400. Fax: (212) 302-6598. 16th edition 1991.

Harrison's Principles of Internal Medicine. Jean D. Wilson, Eugene Braunwald, Kurt J. Isselbacher, et. al.. McGraw-Hill, Inc., Health Professions Division, 1221 Avenue of the Americas, 28th Floor, New York, NY 10020. Phone: (212) 512-4228. 12th edition 1991.

Medicine. Mark C. Fishman, Andrew R. Hoffman, Richard D. Klausner (eds.). J.B. Lippincott Co., 227 East Washington Square, Philadelphia, PA 19106-3780. Phone: (215) 238-4200. Fax: (215) 238-4227. Third edition 1991.

Oxford Companion to Medicine. Sir J. Walton, P.B. Beeson. Oxford University Press, 200 Madison Ave., New York, NY 10016. Phone: (212) 679-7300. Two volumes 1986.

Oxford Textbook of Medicine. D.J. Weatherall, J.G.G. Ledingham, D.A. Warrell. Oxford University Press, 200 Madison Ave., New York, NY 10016. Phone: (212) 679-7300. Fax: (212) 725-2972. Second edition 1987.

The Principles and Practice of Medicine. A. Harvey And Others. Appleton & Lange, 25 Van Zant St., East Norwalk, CT 06855. Phone: (800) 423-1359. Fax: (203) 854-9486. 1988.

Scientific American Medicine. Scientific American, 415 Madison Ave., New York, NY 10017. Phone: (800) 545-0554. Monthly.

Textbook of Internal Medicine. William N. Kelley (ed.). J.B. Lippincott Co., 227 East Washington Square, Philadelphia, PA 19106-3780. Phone: (215) 238-4200. Fax: (215) 238-4227. Second edition 1991.

INTESTINAL DISEASES

See: GASTROINTESTINAL DISORDERS

INTRAUTERINE DEVICE

See: CONTRACEPTION

IRON DEFICIENCY ANEMIA

See: HEMATOLOGY

IUD

See: CONTRACEPTION

J

JAUNDICE

See: LIVER DISEASES

JOINT DISEASES

See: BONE AND JOINT DISEASES

**JUVENILE RHEUMATOID
ARTHRITIS**

See: ARTHRITIS

K

KAPOSI'S SARCOMA

See: AIDS

KERATITIS

See: EYE DISEASES

KIDNEY CANCER

See: CANCER; KIDNEY DISEASES

KIDNEY DIALYSIS

ABSTRACTING, INDEXING, AND CURRENT AWARENESS PUBLICATIONS

Current Contents/Clinical Medicine. Institute for Scientific Information, 3501 Market St., Philadelphia, PA 19104. Phone: (800) 523 1850. Fax: (215) 386-6362. Weekly.

Index Medicus. U.S. National Library of Medicine, 8600 Rockville Pike, Bethesda, MD 20894. Phone: (800) 638-8480. Monthly.

Science Citation Index. Institute for Scientific Information, 3501 Market St., Philadelphia, PA 19104. Phone: (800) 523-1850. Fax: (215) 386-6362. Bimonthly.

ANNUALS AND REVIEWS

Advances in Nephrology. Mosby-Year Book, 11830 Westline Industrial Drive, St. Louis, MO 63146. Phone: (800) 325-4177. Fax: (314) 432-1380.

Seminars in Dialysis. Waverly Press, 428 E. Preston St., Baltimore, MD 21202. Phone: (800) 638-0672. Fax: (800) 447-8438. Quarterly.

ASSOCIATIONS, PROFESSIONAL SOCIETIES, ADVOCACY AND SUPPORT GROUPS

American Association of Kidney Patients. 1 Davis Blvd., Tampa, FL 33606. Phone: (813) 251-0725.

American Council on Transplantation. 700 N. Fairfax St., No. 505, Alexandria, VA 22314. Phone: (703) 836-4301.

American Kidney Fund (AKF). 6110 Executive Blvd., Ste. 1010, Rockville, MD 20852. Phone: (301) 881-3052. Fax: (301) 881-0898.

International Society for Peritoneal Dialysis (ISPD). Georgetown University Medical Ctr., 3800 Reservoir Rd. N.W., Ste. F6003-PHC, Washington, DC 20007. Phone: (202) 784-3662. Fax: (202) 687-2808.

National Kidney Foundation (NKF). 30 E. 33rd St., Ste. 1100, New York, NY 10016. Phone: (212) 889-2210. Fax: (212) 689-9261.

CD-ROM DATABASES

SCISEARCH. Institute for Scientific Information, 3501 Market St., Philadelphia, PA 19104. Phone: (215) 386-0100. Fax: (215) 386-6362.

DIRECTORIES

National Listing of Providers Furnishing Kidney Dialysis and Transplant Services. Health Care Financing Administration, Oak Meadows Building, 6325 Security Blvd., Baltimore, MD 21207. Phone: (301) 966-6573. Annual.

HANDBOOKS, GUIDES, MANUALS, ATLASES

Handbook of Dialysis. John T. Daugirdas, Todd S. Ing (eds.). Little, Brown and Company, 34 Beacon St., Boston, MA 02108. Phone: (617) 227-0730. Second edition 1992.

JOURNALS

American Journal of Kidney Diseases. W.B. Saunders Co., The Curtis Center, Independence Sqare W., Philadelphia, PA 19106-3399. Phone: (215) 238-7800.

American Journal of Nephrology. S. Karger Publishers, Inc., 26 W. Avon Rd., P.O. Box 529, Farmington, CT 06085. Phone: (203) 675-7834. Fax: (203) 675-7302.

Nephrology, Dialysis and Transplantation. Springer-Verlag New York Inc., 175 Fifth Ave., New York, NY 10010. Phone: (212) 460-1500. Fax: (212) 473-6272.

Renal Transplantation and Dialysis. Sheffield University Biomedical Information Service, University of Sheffield, Sheffield, S. Yorkshire SI0 2TN, England.

NEWSLETTERS

Transplant Action. American Council on Transplantation, 700 N. Fairfax St., No. 505, Alexandria, VA 22314. Phone: (703) 836-4301.

ONLINE DATABASES

EMBASE. Elsevier Science Publishing Co., Inc., P.O. Box 882, Madison Square Station, New York, NY 10159-2101. Phone: (212) 989-5800. Fax: (212) 633-3990.

MEDLINE. National Library of Medicine, 8600 Rockville Pike, Bethesda, MD 20894. Phone: (800) 638-8480.

SciSearch. Institute for Scientific Information, 3501 Market St., Philadelphia, PA 19104. Phone: (215) 386-0100. Fax: (215) 386-6362.

POPULAR WORKS AND PATIENT EDUCATION

A Patient's Guide to Dialysis and Transplantation. Roger Gabriel. Kluwer Academic Publishers, P.O. Box 358, Accord Station, Hingham, MA 02018-0358. Phone: (617) 871-6600. Fax: (617) 871-6528. 1990.

RESEARCH CENTERS, INSTITUTES, CLEARINGHOUSES

National Kidney and Urologic Diseases Information Clearinghouse (NKUDIC). P.O. Box NKUDIC, 9000 Rockville Pike, Bethesda, MD 20892. Phone: (301) 468-6345.

TEXTBOOKS AND MONOGRAPHS

Ambulatory Periotoneal Dialysis. Morrell M. Avram, Carmelo Giordana (eds.). Plenum Publishing Co., 233 Spring St., New York, NY 10013-1578. Phone: (212) 620-8000. Fax: (212) 463-0742. 1990.

Clinical Dialysis. Nissenson. Appleton & Lange, 25 Van Zant St., East Norwalk, CT 06855. Phone: (800) 423-1359. Fax: (203) 854-9486. Second edition 1990.

Ethical Problems in Dialysis and Transplantation. Carl M. Kjellstrand, John B. Dossetor (eds.). Kluwer Academic Publishers, P.O. Box 358, Accord Station, Hingham, MA 02018-0358. Phone: (617) 871-6600. Fax: (617) 871-6528. 1992.

Introducation to Dialysis. Martin G. Cogan, Patricia Schoenfeld (eds.). Churchill Livingstone Inc., 650 Avenue of the Americas, New York, NY 10011. Phone: (212) 819-5400. Fax: (212) 302-6598. Second edition 1991.

KIDNEY DISEASES

See also: UROLOGIC DISORDERS

ABSTRACTING, INDEXING, AND CURRENT AWARENESS PUBLICATIONS

Current Contents/Clinical Medicine. Institute for Scientific Information, 3501 Market St., Philadelphia, PA 19104. Phone: (800) 523-1850. Fax: (215) 386-6362. Weekly.

Current Literature in Nephrology, Hypertension and Transplantation. Current Literature Publications, Inc., 1513 E St., Bellingham, WA 98225. Phone: (206) 671-6664. Monthly.

Excerpta Medica. Section 28: Urology and Nephrology. Elsevier Science Publishing Co., Inc., P.O. Box 882, Madison Square Station, New York, NY 10159-2101. Phone: (212) 989-5800. Fax: (212) 633-3990. 20/year.

Index Medicus. U.S. National Library of Medicine, 8600 Rockville Pike, Bethesda, MD 20894. Phone: (800) 638-8480. Monthly.

Research Alert: Nephrology-Clinical. Institute for Scientific Information, 3501 Market St., Philadelphia, PA 19104. Phone: (800) 523-1850. Fax: (215) 386-6362. Weekly.

Science Citation Index. Institute for Scientific Information, 3501 Market St., Philadelphia, PA 19104. Phone: (800) 523-1850. Fax: (215) 386-6362. Bimonthly.

ANNUALS AND REVIEWS

Advances in Nephrology. Mosby-Year Book, 11830 Westline Industrial Drive, St. Louis, MO 63146. Phone: (800) 325-4177. Fax: (314) 432-1380.

Advances in Urology. Mosby-Year Book, 11830 Westline Industrial Drive, St. Louis, MO 63146. Phone: (800) 325-4177. Fax: (314) 432-1380. Annual.

Contemporary Issues in Nephrology. Churchill Livingstone Inc., 650 Avenue of the Americas, New York, NY 10011. Phone: (212) 819-5400. Fax: (212) 302-6598. Irregular.

Contemporary Nephrology. Plenum Publishing Co., 233 Spring St., New York, NY 10013-1578. Phone: (212) 620-8000. Fax: (212) 463-0742. Irregular.

Contributions to Nephrology. S. Karger Publishers, Inc., 26 West Avon Rd., P.O. Box 529, Farmington, CT 06085. Phone: (203) 675-7834. Fax: (203) 675-7302. Irregular.

Current Nephrology. Mosby-Year Book, 11830 Westline Industrial Drive, St. Louis, MO 63146. Phone: (800) 325-4177. Fax: (314) 432-1380.

Year Book of Nephrology. Mosby-Year Book, 11830 Westline Industrial Drive, St. Louis, MO 63146. Phone: (800) 325-4177. Fax: (314) 432-1380. Annual.

Year Book of Urology. Mosby-Year Book, 11830 Westline Industrial Drive, St. Louis, MO 63146. Phone: (800) 325-4177. Fax: (314) 432-1380. Annual.

ASSOCIATIONS, PROFESSIONAL SOCIETIES, ADVOCACY AND SUPPORT GROUPS

American Association of Kidney Patients. 1 Davis Blvd., Tampa, FL 33606. Phone: (813) 251-0725.

American Kidney Fund (AKF). 6110 Executive Blvd., Ste. 1010, Rockville, MD 20852. Phone: (301) 881-3052. Fax: (301) 881-0898.

American Society of Nephrology (ASN). 1101 Connecticut Ave. N.W., Ste. 700, Washington, DC 20036. Phone: (202) 857-1190. Fax: (202) 223-4579.

National Kidney Foundation (NKF). 30 E. 33rd St., Ste. 1100, New York, NY 10016. Phone: (212) 889-2210. Fax: (212) 689-9261.

BIBLIOGRAPHIES

Searches on File: Topics in Kidney and Urologic Diseases. Renal Nutrition. National Kidney and Urologic Diseases Information Clearinghouse, P.O. Box NKUDIC, 9000 Rockville Pike, Bethesda, MD 20892. Phone: (301) 468-6345.

Searches on File: Topics in Kidney and Urologic Diseases. Urinary Stones Patient Materials. National Kidney and Urologic Diseases Information Clearinghouse, P.O. Box NKUDIC, 9000 Rockville Pike, Bethesda, MD 20892. Phone: (301) 468-6345.

CD-ROM DATABASES

Renal Tumors of Children. CMC ReSearch, Inc., 7150 S.W. Hampton, Suite C-120, Portland, OR 97223. Phone: (800) 262-7668. Fax: (503) 639-1796. Irregular.

SCISEARCH. Institute for Scientific Information, 3501 Market St., Philadelphia, PA 19104. Phone: (215) 386-0100. Fax: (215) 386-6362.

DIRECTORIES

Directory of Certified Urologists. American Board of Medical Specialties, 1 Rotary Center, Suite 805, Evanston, IL 60201. Phone: (708) 491-9091. Biennial.

Directory of Medical Specialists. Marquis Who's Who, 3002 Glenview Rd., Wilmette, IL 60091. Phone: (800) 621-9669. Fax: (708) 441-2264. Biennial.

Directory of Physicians in the United States. American Medical Association, 515 North State St., Chicago, IL 60610. Phone: (312) 464-0183. Fax: (312) 464-5834. Biennial.

Nephrology Resource Directory. Virgil Smimow Associates, 8501 Burdette Rd., P.O. Box 34425, Bethesda, MD 20827. Phone: (301) 469-7933. Fax: (301) 469-6532. Irregular.

HANDBOOKS, GUIDES, MANUALS, ATLASES

Handbook of Drug Therapy in Liver and Kidney Disease. Schrier. Little, Brown and Co., 34 Beacon St., Boston, MA 02108. Phone: (617) 227-0730. Fax: (617) 227-0790. 1991.

Handbook of Nephrology. Gower. Blackwell Scientific Publications, Inc., 3 Cambridge Ctr., Cambridge, MA 02142. Phone: (800) 759-6102. Second edition 1991.

Manual of Clinical Problems in Nephrology. Rose. Little, Brown and Co., 34 Beacon St., Boston, MA 02108. Phone: (617) 227-0730. Fax: (617) 227-0790. 1988.

Manual of Nephrology: Diagnosis and Therapy. Robert W. Schrier (ed.). Little, Brown and Company, 34 Beacon St., Boston, MA 02108. Phone: (617) 227-0730. Third edition 1990.

JOURNALS

American Journal of Kidney Diseases. W.B. Saunders Co., The Curtis Center, Independence Sqare W., Philadelphia, PA 19106-3399. Phone: (215) 238-7800.

Journal of the American Society of Nephrology. Williams & Wilkins, 428 E. Preston St., Baltimore, MD 21202. Phone: (800) 638-0672. Fax: (800) 447-8438. Monthly.

Kidney. National Kidney Foundation, 30 E. 33rd St., New York, NY 10016. Phone: (212) 889-2210.

Nephron. S. Karger Publishers, Inc., 26 W. Avon Rd., P.O. Box 529, Farmington, CT 06085. Phone: (203) 675-7834. Fax: (203) 675-7302.

Seminars in Nephrology. W.B. Saunders Co., The Curtis Center, Independence Sqare W., Philadelphia, PA 19106-3399. Phone: (215) 238-7800.

Urologic Nursing. Mosby-Year Book, 11830 Westline Industrial Drive, St. Louis, MO 63146. Phone: (800) 325-4177. Fax: (314) 432-1380. Quarterly.

NEWSLETTERS

Torchbearer Newsletter. American Kidney Foundation, 6110 Executive Blvd., Rockville, MD 20852-3903. Phone: (800) 638-8294.

ONLINE DATABASES

Combined Health Information Database (CHID). U.S. National Institutes of Health, P.O. Box NDIC, Bethesda, MD 20892. Phone: (301) 496-2162. Fax: (301) 770-5164. Quarterly.

EMBASE. Elsevier Science Publishing Co., Inc., P.O. Box 882, Madison Square Station, New York, NY 10159-2101. Phone: (212) 989-5800. Fax: (212) 633-3990.

MEDLINE. National Library of Medicine, 8600 Rockville Pike, Bethesda, MD 20894. Phone: (800) 638-8480.

SciSearch. Institute for Scientific Information, 3501 Market St., Philadelphia, PA 19104. Phone: (215) 386-0100. Fax: (215) 386-6362.

RESEARCH CENTERS, INSTITUTES, CLEARINGHOUSES

Division of Nephrology. University of Southern California. 2025 Zonal Ave., Los Angeles, CA 90033. Phone: (213) 226-7307. Fax: (213) 226-3958.

Kidney Disease Program. University of Louisville. 500 S. Floyd St., Louisville, KY 40292. Phone: (502) 588-5757. Fax: (502) 588-7643.

National Kidney and Urologic Diseases Information Clearinghouse (NKUDIC). P.O. Box NKUDIC, 9000 Rockville Pike, Bethesda, MD 20892. Phone: (301) 468-6345.

Nephrology Research Program. University of Rochester. 601 Elmwood, Rochester, NY 14642. Phone: (716) 275-4517. Fax: (716) 442-9201.

Nephrology Research and Training Center. University of Alabama at Birmingham. UAB Sta., Birmingham, AL 35294. Phone: (205) 934-3585. Fax: (205) 934-1879.

Polycystic Kidney Research Foundation. 922 Walnut St., Kansas City, MO 64106. Phone: (816) 421-1869.

STANDARDS AND STATISTICS SOURCES

End Stage Renal Disease: Health Care Financing Research Report. Health Care Financing Administration, Oak Meadows Building, 6325 Security Blvd., Baltimore, MD 21207. Phone: (301) 966-6573. Annual.

TEXTBOOKS AND MONOGRAPHS

Clinical Management of Renal Transplantation. Mary G. McGeown (ed.). Kluwer Academic Publishers, P.O. Box 358, Accord Station, Hingham, MA 02018-0358. Phone: (617) 871-6600. Fax: (617) 871-6528. 1992.

Clinical Nephrology in Medical Practice. Becker. Blackwell Scientific Publications, Inc., 3 Cambridge Ctr., Cambridge, MA 02142. Phone: (800) 759-6102. 1992.

Diseases of the Kidney. Robert W. Schrier, Carl W. Gottschalk (eds.). Little, Brown and Company, 34 Beacon St., Boston, MA 02108. Phone: (617) 227-0730. Fifth edition 1992.

The Kidney: Physiology and Pathophysiology. Donald W. Seldin, Gerhard Giebisch. Raven Press, 1185 Avenue of the Americas, New York, NY 10036. Phone: (212) 930-9500. Fax: (212) 869-3495. Second edition. Two volumes. 1991.

The Kidney: Structure and Function. Adalbert Bohle, Hermine V. Gartner, Hans G. Laberke, et. al.. John Wiley & Sons, Inc., 605 Third Ave., New York, NY 10158-0012. Phone: (212) 850-6000. Fax: (212) 850-6088. 1989.

New Therapeutic Strategies in Nephrology. Andreucci. Kluwer Academic Publishers, P.O. Box 358, Accord Station, Hingham, MA 02018-0358. Phone: (617) 871-6600. Fax: (617) 871-6528. 1991.

Oxford Textbook of Clinical Nephrology. J. Stewart Cameron, Alex M. Davison, Jean-Pierr Grunfeld. Oxford University Press, 200 Madison Ave., New York, NY 10016. Phone: (212) 679-7300. Fax: (212) 725-2972. Three volumes 1992.

Pathology of the Kidney. Robert H. Heptinstall. Little, Brown and Co., 34 Beacon St., Boston, MA 02108. Phone: (617) 227-0730. Fax: (617) 227-0790. Fourth edition 1992.

Pediatric Kidney Disease. Chester M. Edelmann Jr. (ed.). Little, Brown and Company, 34 Beacon St., Boston, MA 02108. Phone: (617) 227-0730. Second edition 1992.

Principles and Practice of Nephrology. Jacobson. Mosby-Year Book, 11830 Westline Industrial Drive, St. Louis, MO 63146. Phone: (800) 325-4177. Fax: (314) 432-1380. 1991.

Renal and Electrolyte Disorders. Robert W. Schrier. Little, Brown and Company, 34 Beacon St., Boston, MA 02108. Phone: (617) 227-0730. 1992.

Renal Physiology. Arthur J. Vander. McGraw-Hill, Inc., 1221 Avenue of the Americas, 28th Floor, New York, NY 10020. Phone: (212) 512-4228. Fourth edition 1991.

Shock Wave Lithotripsy 2: Urinary and Biliary Lithotripsy. James E. Lingeman, Daniel M. Newman (eds.). Plenum Publishing Co., 233 Spring St., New York, NY 10013-1578. Phone: (212) 620-8000. Fax: (212) 463-0742. 1989.

Textbook of Nephrology. Massry. Williams & Wilkins, 428 East Preston St., Baltimore, MD 21202. Phone: (800) 638-0672. Fax: (800) 447-8438. Second edition 1989.

Therapy of Renal Diseases and Related Disorders. Suki. Kluwer Academic Publishers, P.O. Box 358, Accord Station, Hingham, MA 02018-0358. Phone: (617) 871-6600. Fax: (617) 871-6528. Second edition 1991.

KIDNEY STONES

See: KIDNEY DISEASES; UROLOGIC DISORDERS; UROLOGY

KIDNEY TRANSPLANTATION

See: TRANSPLANTATION

KNEE SURGERY

See also: ARTHROSCOPY; ORTHOPEDICS

ABSTRACTING, INDEXING, AND CURRENT AWARENESS PUBLICATIONS

Current Contents/Clinical Medicine. Institute for Scientific Information, 3501 Market St., Philadelphia, PA 19104. Phone: (800) 523-1850. Fax: (215) 386-6362. Weekly.

Excerpta Medica. Section 33: Orthopedic Surgery. Elsevier Science Publishing Co., Inc., P.O. Box 882, Madison Square Station, New York, NY 10159-2101. Phone: (212) 989-5800. Fax: (212) 633-3990. 10/year.

Index Medicus. U.S. National Library of Medicine, 8600 Rockville Pike, Bethesda, MD 20894. Phone: (800) 638-8480. Monthly.

Science Citation Index. Institute for Scientific Information, 3501 Market St., Philadelphia, PA 19104. Phone: (800) 523-1850. Fax: (215) 386-6362. Bimonthly.

ANNUALS AND REVIEWS

Current Opinion in Orthopaedics. Current Science Ltd., 20 N. Third St., Philadelphia, PA 19106-2199. Phone: (800) 552-5866. Fax: (215) 574-2270. Bimonthly.

ASSOCIATIONS, PROFESSIONAL SOCIETIES, ADVOCACY AND SUPPORT GROUPS

American Academy of Orthopedic Surgeons (AAOS). 222 S. Prospect Ave., Park Ridge, IL 60068-4058. Phone: (708) 823-7186. Fax: (708) 823-8125.

American Orthopaedic Society for Sports Medicine (AOSSM). 2250 E. Devon Ave., Ste. 115, Des Plaines, IL 60018. Phone: (708) 836-7000. Fax: (708) 803-8653.

Arthroscopy Association of North America (AANA). 2250 E. Devon Ave., Ste. 101, Des Plaines, IL 60018. Phone: (708) 299-9444. Fax: (708) 299-4913.

International Society of the Knee. 70 W. Hubbard, No. 202, Chicago, IL 60610. Phone: (312) 644-2623.

CD-ROM DATABASES

Ortholine. Aries Systems Corporation, One Dundee Park, Andover, MA 01810. Phone: (508) 475-7200. Fax: (508) 474-8860. Monthly or quarterly.

SCISEARCH. Institute for Scientific Information, 3501 Market St., Philadelphia, PA 19104. Phone: (215) 386-0100. Fax: (215) 386-6362.

DIRECTORIES

Directory of Certified Orthopaedic Surgeons. American Board of Medical Specialties, 1 Rotary Center, Suite 805, Evanston, IL 60201. Phone: (708) 491-9091. Biennial.

ENCYCLOPEDIAS, DICTIONARIES, WORD BOOKS

Handbook of Orthopedic Terminology. Kilcoyne. CRC Press, Inc., 2000 Corporate Blvd. N.W., Boca Raton, FL 33431. Phone: (407) 994-0555. Fax: (407) 997-0949. 1991.

Orthopedic Word Book. Thomas J. Cittadine. Springhouse Publishing Co., 1111 Bethlehem Pike, Spring House, PA 19477. Phone: (800) 331-3170. Fax: (215) 646-8716. 1992.

Orthopedic Words. Stedman. Williams & Wilkins, 428 East Preston St., Baltimore, MD 21202. Phone: (800) 638-0672. Fax: (800) 447-8438. 1992.

JOURNALS

The American Journal of Knee Surgery. SLACK Inc., 6900 Grove Rd., Thorofare, NJ 08086-9447. Phone: (800) 257-8290. Fax: (609) 853-5991. Quarterly.

American Journal of Sports Medicine. American Orthopedic Society for Sports Medicine, P.O. Box 9517, Columbus, GA 31995. Phone: (404) 576-3340.

Archives of Orthopaedic and Traumatic Surgery. Springer-Verlag New York Inc., 175 Fifth Ave., New York, NY 10010. Phone: (212) 460-1500. Fax: (212) 473-6272.

Arthroscopy. Raven Press, 1185 Avenue of the Americas, New York, NY 10036. Phone: (212) 930-9500. Fax: (212) 869-3495. Quarterly.

Clinical Orthopedics and Related Research. J.B. Lippincott Co., 227 E. Washington Square, Philadelphia, PA 19106-3780. Phone: (215) 238-4200. Fax: (215) 238-4227.

Journal of Bone and Joint Surgery: American Volume. Journal of Bone and Joint Surgery, Inc., 10 Shattuck St., Boston, MA 02115. Phone: (617) 734-2835. 10/year.

ONLINE DATABASES

EMBASE. Elsevier Science Publishing Co., Inc., P.O. Box 882, Madison Square Station, New York, NY 10159-2101. Phone: (212) 989-5800. Fax: (212) 633-3990.

MEDLINE. National Library of Medicine, 8600 Rockville Pike, Bethesda, MD 20894. Phone: (800) 638-8480.

SciSearch. Institute for Scientific Information, 3501 Market St., Philadelphia, PA 19104. Phone: (215) 386-0100. Fax: (215) 386-6362.

RESEARCH CENTERS, INSTITUTES, CLEARINGHOUSES

Hospital for Special Surgery. 535 E. 70th St., New York, NY 10021. Phone: (212) 606-1412.

Massachusetts General Hospital. 55 Front St., Boston, MA 02114.

TEXTBOOKS AND MONOGRAPHS

Arthroscopic Surgery. Terry Whipple. J.B. Lippincott Co., 227 E. Washington Square, Philadelphia, PA 19106-3780. Phone: (215) 238-4200. Fax: (215) 238-4227. 1992.

Arthroscopy of the Knee. R. Aigner, J. Gillquist. Thieme Medical Publishers, Inc., 381 Park Ave. S., New York, NY 10016. Phone: (212) 683-5088. Fax: (212) 779-9020. 1991.

Arthroscopy Surgery. Orrin Sherman, Jeffrey Minkoff. Williams & Wilkins, 428 East Preston St., Baltimore, MD 21202. Phone: (800) 638-0672. Fax: (800) 447-8438. 1990.

Articular Cartilage and Knee Joint Function: Basic Science and Arthroscopy. J. Whit Ewing. Raven Press, 1185 Avenue of the Americas, New York, NY 10036. Phone: (212) 930-9500. Fax: (212) 869-3495. 1990.

Diagnostic and Operative Arthroscopy of the Knee Joint. W. Glinz. Hugrefe and Huber, P.O. Box 51, Lewiston, NY 14092. Phone: (716) 282-1610. 2nd edition.

Illustrated Guide to the Knee. Tria. Churchill Livingstone Inc., 650 Ave. of the Americas, New York, NY 10011. Phone: (212) 819-5400. Fax: (212) 302-6598. 1992.

Knee Ligament Rehabilitation. Robert P. Engle (ed.). Churchill Livingstone Inc., 650 Avenue of the Americas, New York, NY 10011. Phone: (212) 819-5400. Fax: (212) 302-6598. 1991.

Knee Ligaments: Structure, Function, Injury, and Repair. Dale M. Daniel, Wayne H. Akeson, John J. O'Connor. Raven Press, 1185 Avenue of the Americas, New York, NY 10036. Phone: (212) 930-9500. Fax: (212) 869-3495. 1990.

Knee Pain and Disability. Cailliet. F.A. Davis Co., 1915 Arch St., Philadelphia, PA 19103. Phone: (800) 523-4049. Fax: (215) 568-5065. Third edition 1991.

L

LABOR

See: CHILDBIRTH

LABORATORY ANIMALS

See: ANIMALS, LABORATORY

LABORATORY MEDICINE

See also: DIAGNOSIS; MEDICAL
TECHNOLOGY

ABSTRACTING, INDEXING, AND CURRENT AWARENESS PUBLICATIONS

Cumulative Index to Nursing and Allied Health Literature. Glendale Adventist Medical Center, P.O. Box 871, Glendale, CA 91209. Phone: (818) 409-8005. Bimonthly.

Current Contents/Life Sciences. Institute for Scientific Information, 3501 Market St., Philadelphia, PA 19104. Phone: (215) 386-0100. Fax: (215) 386-6362.

Excerpta Medica. Section 5: General Pathology and Pathological Anatomy. Elsevier Science Publishers, P.O. Box 882, Madison Square Station, New York, NY 10159-2101. Phone: (212) 633-3950. Fax: (212) 633-3990. 24/year.

Index Medicus. U.S. National Library of Medicine, 8600 Rockville Pike, Bethesda, MD 20894. Phone: (800) 638-8480. Monthly.

Science Citation Index. Institute for Scientific Information, 3501 Market St., Philadelphia, PA 19104. Phone: (800) 523-1850. Fax: (215) 386-6362. Bimonthly.

ANNUALS AND REVIEWS

Advances in Pathology and Laboratory Medicine. Mosby-Year Book, 11830 Westline Industrial Drive, St. Louis, MO 63146. Phone: (800) 325-4177. Fax: (314) 432-1380. Annual.

Clinics in Laboratory Medicine. W.B. Saunders Co., The Curtis Center, Independence Square W., Philadelphia, PA 19106-3399. Phone: (215) 238-7800. Quarterly.

Critical Reviews in Clinical Laboratory Sciences. CRC Press, Inc., 2000 Corporate Blvd. N.W., Boca Raton, FL 33431. Phone: (407) 994-0555. Fax: (407) 997-0949. Quarterly.

ASSOCIATIONS, PROFESSIONAL SOCIETIES, ADVOCACY AND SUPPORT GROUPS

American Association for Clinical Chemistry. 1725 K St. N.W., Washington, DC 20006. Phone: (202) 857-0717.

Association of Clinical Scientists. Dept. of Laboratory Medicine, University of Connecticut School of Medicine, Farmington, CT 06032. Phone: (203) 679-2328.

Canadian Society of Laboratory Technologists. P.O. Box 2830, Hamilton, ON, Canada L8N 3N5. Phone: (416) 528-8642. Fax: (416) 528-4968.

Clinical Laboratory Management Association (CLMA). 195 W. Lancaster Ave., Paoli, PA 19301. Phone: (215) 647-8970. Fax: (215) 889-9731.

CD ROM DATABASES

Medlabl. Goldberg. Oxford University Press, 200 Madison Ave., New York, NY 10016. Phone: (212) 679-7300. 1990.

Nursing and Allied Health (CINAHL) on CD-ROM. CINAHL, 1509 Wilson Terrace, P.O. Box 871, Glendale, CA 91209-0871. Phone: (818) 409-8005.

SCISEARCH. Institute for Scientific Information, 3501 Market St., Philadelphia, PA 19104. Phone: (215) 386-0100. Fax: (215) 386-6362.

ENCYCLOPEDIAS, DICTIONARIES, WORD BOOKS

Clinical Laboratory Word Book. Barbara De Lorenzo. Springhouse Publishing Co., 1111 Bethlehem Pike, Spring House, PA 19477. Phone: (800) 331-3170. Fax: (215) 646-8716. 1992.

HANDBOOKS, GUIDES, MANUALS, ATLASES

Clinical Guide to Laboratory Tests. Norbert W. Tietz (ed.). W.B. Saunders Co., The Curtis Center, Independence Square W., Philadelphia, PA 19106-3399. Phone: (215) 238-7800. Second edition 1990.

Clinical Laboratory Tests: Values and Implications. Springhouse Publishing Co., 1111 Bethlehem Pike, Spring House, PA 19477. Phone: (800) 331-3170. Fax: (215) 646-8716. 1991.

CLR/Clinical Laboratory Reference. Medical Economics, Five Paragon Dr., Montvale, NJ 07645-1742. Phone: (800) 222-3045. Fax: (201) 573-4956. Annual.

Drug-Test Interactions Handbook. Jack G. Salway. Raven Press, 1185 Avenue of the Americas, New York, NY 10036. Phone: (212) 930-9500. Fax: (212) 869-3495. 1990.

Handbook of Laboratory Health and Safety Measures. Pal. Kluwer Academic Publishers, P.O. Box 358, Accord Station, Hingham, MA 02018-0358. Phone: (617) 871-6600. Fax: (617) 871-6528. Second edition 1990.

Interpretation of Diagnostic Tests. Jacques Wallach. Little, Brown and Company, 34 Beacon St., Boston, MA 02108. Phone: (617) 227-0730. Fifth edition 1992.

Laboratory Test Handbook. David S. Jacobs, Bernard L. Kasten Jr., Wayne R. DeMott. Williams & Wilkins, 428 E. Preston St., Baltimore, MD 21202. Phone: (800) 638-0672. Fax: (800) 447-8438. Second edition 19990.

A Manual of Laboratory and Diagnostic Tests. Frances Fischbach. J.B. Lippincott Co., 227 East Washington Square, Philadelphia, PA 19106-3780. Phone: (215) 238-4200. Fax: (215) 238-4227. 1992.

JOURNALS

Annals of Clinical and Laboratory Science. Institute for Clinical Science, 1833 Delancey Place, Philadelphia, PA 19103. Phone: (215) 922-6554.

Archives of Pathology & Laboratory Medicine. American Medical Association, 515 North State St., Chicago, IL 60610. Phone: (312) 464-0183. Fax: (312) 464-5834. Monthly.

The Journal of Laboratory and Clinical Medicine. Mosby-Year Book, 11830 Westline Industrial Drive, St. Louis, MO 63146. Phone: (800) 325-4177. Fax: (314) 432-1380. Monthly.

Laboratory Investigation. Williams & Wilkins, 428 E. Preston St., Baltimore, MD 21202. Phone: (800) 638-0672. Fax: (800) 447-8438. Monthly.

Stain Technology. Williams & Wilkins, 428 East Preston St., Baltimore, MD 21202. Phone: (800) 638-0672. Fax: (800) 447-8438.

ONLINE DATABASES

EMBASE. Elsevier Science Publishing Co., Inc., P.O. Box 882, Madison Square Station, New York, NY 10159-2101. Phone: (212) 989-5800. Fax: (212) 633-3990.

MEDLINE. National Library of Medicine, 8600 Rockville Pike, Bethesda, MD 20894. Phone: (800) 638-8480.

Nursing and Allied Health (CINAHL). CINAHL, 1509 Wilson Terrace, P.O. Box 871, Glendale, CA 91209-0871. Phone: (818) 409-8005.

SciSearch. Institute for Scientific Information, 3501 Market St., Philadelphia, PA 19104. Phone: (215) 386-0100. Fax: (215) 386-6362.

POPULAR WORKS AND PATIENT EDUCATION

Complete Guide to Medical Tests. Griffith H. Winter. Fisher Books, P.O. Box 38040, Tucson, AZ 85740-8040. Phone: (602) 292-9080. 1988.

Patient's Guide to Medical Tests. Cathy Pickney. Facts on File, Inc., 460 Park Ave. S., New York, NY 10016-7382. Phone: (212) 683-2244. Fax: (212) 683-3633. Third edition 1987.

TEXTBOOKS AND MONOGRAPHS

Antibiotics in Laboratory Medicine. Lorian. Williams & Wilkins, 428 East Preston St., Baltimore, MD 21202. Phone: (800) 638-0672. Fax: (800) 447-8438. Third edition 1991.

Basic Technniques in Clinical Laboratory Science. Jean Linne, Karen Ringsted. Mosby-Year Book, 11830 Westline Industrial Drive, St. Louis, MO 63146. Phone: (800) 325-4177. Fax: (314) 432-1380. 3rd edition, 1991.

Clinical Diagnosis & Management by Laboratory Methods. Hohn Bernard Henry (ed.). W.B. Saunders Co., The Curtis Center, Independence Square W., Philadelphia, PA 19106-3399. Phone: (215) 238-7800. 18th edition 1991.

Clinical Laboratory Medicine. Tilton. Mosby-Year Book, 11830 Westline Industrial Drive, St. Louis, MO 63146. Phone: (800) 325-4177. Fax: (314) 432-1380. 1992.

Clinical Laboratory Medicine: Clinical Application of Laboratory Data. Richard Ravel. Mosby-Year Book, 11830 Westline Industrial Drive, St. Louis, MO 63146. Phone: (800) 325-4177. Fax: (314) 432-1380. Fifth edition 1989.

Immunology and Serology in Laboratory Medicine. Mary Louise Turgeon. Mosby-Year Book, 11830 Westline Industrial Drive, St. Louis, MO 63146. Phone: (800) 325-4177. Fax: (314) 432-1380. 1990.

An Introduction to Clinical Laboratory Sciences. Jeanne Clere, and others. Mosby-Year Book, 11830 Westline Industrial Drive, St. Louis, MO 63146. Phone: (800) 325-4177. Fax: (314) 432-1380. 1992.

Laboratory Medicine: Test Selection and Interpretation. Joan H. Howanitz, Peter J. Howanitz, Joanne Cornbleet, et. al.. Churchill Livingstone Inc., 650 Avenue of the Americas, New York, NY 10011. Phone: (212) 819-5400. Fax: (212) 302-6598. 1991.

Medical Laboratory Haematology. Roger Hall, Bob Malia. Butterworth-Heinemann, 80 Montvale Ave., Stoneham, MA 02180. Phone: (617) 438-8464. Fax: (617) 279-4851. Second edition 1991.

Widmann's Clinical Interpretation of Laboratory Tests. Ronald A. Sacher, Richard A. McPherson, Joseph M. Caompos. F.A. Davis Co., 1915 Arch St., Philadelphia, PA 19103. Phone: (800) 523-4049. Fax: (215) 568-5065. 10th edition, 1991.

LABORATORY TESTS

See: LABORATORY MEDICINE

LACTOSE INTOLERANCE

See: GASTROINTESTINAL DISORDERS

LAPAROSCOPY

See: DIAGNOSIS; ENDOSCOPY

LARYNGEAL DISEASES

See: OTOLARYNGOLOGY

LASER SURGERY

See also: EYE SURGERY; SURGERY

ABSTRACTING, INDEXING, AND CURRENT AWARENESS PUBLICATIONS

Current Contents/Clinical Medicine. Institute for Scientific Information, 3501 Market St., Philadelphia, PA 19104. Phone: (800) 523-1850. Fax: (215) 386-6362. Weekly.

Excerpta Medica. Section 9: Surgery. Elsevier Science Publishing Co., Inc., P.O. Box 882, Madison Square Station, New York, NY 10159-2101. Phone: (212) 989-5800. Fax: (212) 633-3990. 24/year.

Index Medicus. U.S. National Library of Medicine, 8600 Rockville Pike, Bethesda, MD 20894. Phone: (800) 638-8480. Monthly.

Lasers in Medicine. Elsevier Science Publishing Co., Inc., P.O. Box 882, Madison Square Station, New York, NY 10159-2101. Phone: (212) 989-5800. Fax: (212) 633-3990. 12/year.

Research Alert: Laser Applications in Medicine. Institute for Scientific Information, 3501 Market St., Philadelphia, PA 19104. Phone: (800) 523-1850. Fax: (215) 386-6362. Weekly

Science Citation Index. Institute for Scientific Information, 3501 Market St., Philadelphia, PA 19104. Phone: (800) 523-1850. Fax: (215) 386-6362. Bimonthly.

ANNUALS AND REVIEWS

Advances in Surgery. Mosby-Year Book, 11830 Westline Industrial Drive, St. Louis, MO 63146. Phone: (800) 325-4177. Fax: (314) 432-1380. Annual.

ASSOCIATIONS, PROFESSIONAL SOCIETIES, ADVOCACY AND SUPPORT GROUPS

American Society for Laser Medicine and Surgery (ASLMS). 2404 Stewart Sq., Wausau, WI 54401. Phone: (715) 845-9283. Fax: (715) 848-2493.

BIBLIOGRAPHIES

Laser Eye Surgery. National Technical Information Service, 5285 Port Royal Rd., Springfield, VA 22161. Phone: (703) 487-4650. Fax: (703) 321-8547. Jan. 1975-Apr. 1989 PB89-859763/CBY.

CD-ROM DATABASES

SCISEARCH. Institute for Scientific Information, 3501 Market St., Philadelphia, PA 19104. Phone: (215) 386-0100. Fax: (215) 386-6362.

HANDBOOKS, GUIDES, MANUALS, ATLASES

Atlas of Cutaneous Laser Surgery. David B. Apfelberg. Raven Press, 1185 Avenue of the Americas, New York, NY 10036. Phone: (212) 930-9500. Fax: (212) 869-3495. 1991.

Illustrated Cutaneous Laser Surgery: A Practitioner's Atlas. Jeffrey S. Dover, Kenneth A. Arndt, Roy Geronemus, and others. Appleton & Lange, 25 Van Zant St., East Norwalk, CT 06855. Phone: (800) 423-1359. Fax: (203) 854-9486. 1990.

JOURNALS

Journal of Clinical Laser Medicine & Surgery. Mary Ann Liebert, Inc., 1651 Third Ave., New York, NY 10128. Phone: (212) 289-2300. Fax: (212) 289-4697. Bimonthly.

Lasers in Surgery and Medicine. John Wiley & Sons, Inc., 605 Third Ave., New York, NY 10158-0012. Phone: (212) 850-6000. Fax: (212) 850-6088. Bimonthly + Supplement 3.

NEWSLETTERS

Clinical Laser Monthly. American Health Consultants, Department C1290, P.O. Box 740060, Atlanta, GA 30374. Phone: (800) 559-1032. Fax: (404) 352-1971. Monthly.

ONLINE DATABASES

EMBASE. Elsevier Science Publishing Co., Inc., P.O. Box 882, Madison Square Station, New York, NY 10159-2101. Phone: (212) 989-5800. Fax: (212) 633-3990.

MEDLINE. National Library of Medicine, 8600 Rockville Pike, Bethesda, MD 20894. Phone: (800) 638-8480.

SciSearch. Institute for Scientific Information, 3501 Market St., Philadelphia, PA 19104. Phone: (215) 386-0100. Fax: (215) 386-6362.

POPULAR WORKS AND PATIENT EDUCATION

Cataract Surgery: Before and After. Robert I. Johnson. SLACK Inc., 6900 Grove Rd., Thorofare, NJ 08086-9447. Phone: (800) 257-8290. Fax: (609) 853-5991. Two volumes 1989.

RESEARCH CENTERS, INSTITUTES, CLEARINGHOUSES

Institute for Applied Laser Surgery. 2 Bala Plaza, Suite IL-17, Bala Cynwyd, PA 19004. Phone: (215) 667-4080.

Institute for Laser Medicine. 4200 E. 9th Ave., Box B210, Denver, CO 80262. Phone: (303) 394-8641.

TEXTBOOKS AND MONOGRAPHS

Basic and Advanced Laser Surgery in Gynecology. Michael S. Baggish. Appleton & Lange, 25 Van Zant St., East Norwalk, CT 06855. Phone: (800) 423-1359. Fax: (203) 854-9486. Second edition 1991.

Current Surgical Diagnosis and Treatment. L.W. Way. Appleton & Lange, 25 Van Zant St., East Norwalk, CT 06855. Phone: (800) 423-1359. Fax: (203) 854-9486. Ninth edition 1990.

Laser Surgery in Gynecology and Obstetrics. William R. Keye Jr.. Mosby-Year Book, 11830 Westline Industrial Drive, St. Louis, MO 63146. Phone: (800) 325-4177. Fax: (314) 432-1380. 1990.

Laser Surgery in Ophthalmology. Weingeist. Appleton & Lange, 25 Van Zant St., East Norwalk, CT 06855. Phone: (800) 423-1359. Fax: (203) 854-9486. 1992.

Lasers in General Surgery. Stephen N. Joffe (ed.). Williams & Wilkins, 428 E. Preston St., Baltimore, MD 21202. Phone: (800) 638-0672. Fax: (800) 447-8438. 1989.

Lasers in Gynecology. McLaughlin. J.B. Lippincott Co., 227 E. Washington Square, Philadelphia, PA 19106-3780. Phone: (215) 238-4200. Fax: (215) 238-4227. 1991.

Lasers: The Perioperative Challenge. Kay Ball. Mosby-Year Book, 11830 Westline Industrial Drive, St. Louis, MO 63146. Phone: (800) 325-4177. Fax: (314) 432-1380. 1990.

Lasers in Urologic Surgery. Joseph Smith, and others. Mosby-Year Book, 11830 Westline Industrial Drive, St. Louis, MO 63146. Phone: (800) 325-4177. Fax: (314) 432-1380. 1989.

Ophthalmic Lasers. Wayne F. March (ed.). SLACK Inc., 6900 Grove Rd., Thorofare, NJ 08086-9447. Phone: (800) 257-8290. Fax: (609) 853-5991. Second edition 1990.

Therapeutic Application of Lasers. P.B. Boulos, S.G. Brown (eds.). Butterworth-Heinemann, 80 Montvale Ave., Stoneham, MA 02180. Phone: (617) 438-8464. Fax: (617) 279-4851. 1991.

LAXATIVES

See: GASTROINTESTINAL DISORDERS

LEAD POISONING

See also: POISONING

ABSTRACTING, INDEXING, AND CURRENT AWARENESS PUBLICATIONS

Excerpta Medica. Section 5: General Pathology and Pathological Anatomy. Elsevier Science Publishers, P.O. Box 882, Madison Square Station, New York, NY 10159-2101. Phone: (212) 633-3950. Fax: (212) 633-3990. 24/year.

Excerpta Medica. Section 52: Toxicology. Elsevier Science Publishing Co., Inc., P.O. Box 882, Madison Square Station, New York, NY 10159-2101. Phone: (212) 989-5800. Fax: (212) 633-3990. 20/year.

Index Medicus. U.S. National Library of Medicine, 8600 Rockville Pike, Bethesda, MD 20894. Phone: (800) 638-8480. Monthly.

Toxicology Abstracts. Cambridge Scientific Abstracts, 7200 Wisconsin Ave., Bethesda, MD 20814-4823. Phone: (800) 843-7751. Fax: (301) 961-6720. Monthly.

ASSOCIATIONS, PROFESSIONAL SOCIETIES, ADVOCACY AND SUPPORT GROUPS

Alliance to End Childhood Lead Poisoning. 600 Pennsylvania Ave. S.E., Ste. 100, Washington, DC 20003.

American Association of Poison Control Centers. c/o Dr. Ted Tong, Arizona Poison & Drug Information Center, 1501 N. Campbell, Tucson, AZ 85725. Phone: (602) 626-1587.

BIBLIOGRAPHIES

Childhood Lead Exposure Hazards. National Technical Information Service, 5285 Port Royal Rd., Springfield, VA 22161. Phone: (703) 487-4650. Fax: (703) 321-8547. Jan. 1978 to Feb. 1989. PB89-858070/CBY.

Lead Exposure: Public and Occupational Health Hazards. National Technical Information Service, 5285 Port Royal Rd., Springfield, VA 22161. Phone: (703) 487-4650. Fax: (703) 321-8547. Jan. 1978 to Apr. 1989. PB89-860928/CBY.

Lead Poisoning: A Selected Bibliography. Robert W. Locerby. Vance Bibliographies, P.O. Box 229, 112 N. Charter St., Monticello, IL 61856. Phone: (217) 762-3831. 1988.

CD-ROM DATABASES

American Journal of Public Health. MEP, 124 Mt. Auburn St., Cambridge, MA 02138. Phone: (800) 342-1338. Fax: (617) 868-7738. Annual.

Journal of the American Medical Association. Macmillan New Media, 124 Mt. Auburn St., Cambridge, MA 02138. Weekly.

Morbidity Mortality Weekly Report. MEP, 124 Mt. Auburn St., Cambridge, MA 02138. Phone: (800) 342-1338. Fax: (617) 868-7738. Annual.

PolTox. Cambridge Scientific Abstracts, 7200 Wisconsin Ave., Bethesda, MD 20814-4823. Phone: (800) 843-7751. Fax: (301) 961-6720. Quarterly.

TOXLINE. SilverPlatter Information, Inc., River Ridge Office Park, 100 River Ridge Rd., Norwood, MA 02062. Phone: (617) 769-2599. Fax: (617) 769-8763. Quarterly.

TOXLINE Plus. SilverPlatter Information, Inc., River Ridge Office Park, 100 River Ridge Rd., Norwood, MA 02062. Phone: (617) 769-2599. Fax: (617) 769-8763. Quarterly.

ENCYCLOPEDIAS, DICTIONARIES, WORD BOOKS

Lead: Occupational Health Hazards. National Technical Information Service, 5285 Port Royal Rd., Springfield, VA 22161. Phone: (703) 487-4650. Fax: (703) 321-8547. Jan. 1970 to Apr. 1989. PB89-860191/CBY.

JOURNALS

American Journal of Diseases of Children. American Medical Association, 515 North State St., Chicago, IL 60610. Phone: (312) 464-0183. Fax: (312) 464-5834. Monthly.

American Journal of Public Health. American Public Health Association, 1015 15th St. NW, Washington, DC 20005. Phone: (202) 789-5666. Monthly.

Archives of Environmental Health. Heldref Publications, 4000 Albemarle St. N.W., Washington, DC 20016. Phone: (202) 362-6445. Bimonthly.

Journal of Pediatrics. Mosby-Year Book, 11830 Westline Industrial Drive, St. Louis, MO 63146. Phone: (800) 325-4177. Fax: (314) 432-1380. Monthly.

Journal of Toxicology and Environmental Health. Taylor & Francis Inc., 1900 Frost Rd., Suite 101, Bristol, PA 19007-1598. Phone: (800) 821-8312. Fax: (215) 785-5515. Monthly.

Morbidity and Mortality Weekly Report. Massachusetts Medical Society, 1440 Main St., Waltham, MA 02154-1649. Phone: (617) 893-3800. Fax: (617) 893-0413. Weekly.

Pediatrics. American Academy of Pediatrics, 141 Northwest Point Rd., Elk Grove Village, IL 60009-0927. Phone: (708) 228-5005. Fax: (708) 228-5097. Monthly.

Toxicology. Elsevier Science Publishing Co., Inc., P.O. Box 882, Madison Square Station, New York, NY 10159-2101. Phone: (212) 989-5800. Fax: (212) 633-3990. 6/year.

ONLINE DATABASES

EMBASE. Elsevier Science Publishing Co., Inc., P.O. Box 882, Madison Square Station, New York, NY 10159-2101. Phone: (212) 989-5800. Fax: (212) 633-3990.

MEDLINE. National Library of Medicine, 8600 Rockville Pike, Bethesda, MD 20894. Phone: (800) 638-8480.

SciSearch. Institute for Scientific Information, 3501 Market St., Philadelphia, PA 19104. Phone: (215) 386-0100. Fax: (215) 386-6362.

TOXLINE. U.S. National Library of Medicine, Toxicology Information Program, 8600 Rockville Pike, Bethesda, MD 20894. Phone: (800) 638-8480. Monthly.

TEXTBOOKS AND MONOGRAPHS

Dietary and Environmental Lead: Human Health Effects. K.R. Mahaffey (ed.). Elsevier Science Publishing Co., Inc., P.O. Box 882, Madison Square Station, New York, NY 10159-2101. Phone: (212) 989-5800. Fax: (212) 633-3990. 1985.

Exposure of Infants and Children to Lead: Working Document for the 30th Meeting of the Joint FAO-WHO Expert Committee on Food Additives Held in Rome, Italy. A. Oskarsson. UNIPUB, 4611-F Assembly Dr., Lanham, MD 20706-4391. Phone: (800) 274-4888. 1989.

Human Lead Exposure. Herbert L. Needleman. CRC Press, Inc., 2000 Corporate Blvd. N.W., Boca Raton, FL 33431. Phone: (407) 994-0555. Fax: (407) 997-0949. 1992.

Lead Exposure and Child Development: An International Assessment. M. Smith (ed.). Kluwer Academic Publishers, P.O. Box 358, Accord Station, Hingham, MA 02018-0358. Phone: (617) 871-6600. Fax: (617) 871-6528. 1989.

Principles and Practice of Clinical Toxicology. Gossel. Raven Press, 1185 Ave. of the Americas, New York, NY 10036. Phone: (212) 930-9500. Fax: (212) 869-3495. Second edition 1990.

LEGIONNAIRE'S DISEASE

See: RESPIRATORY TRACT INFECTIONS

LEGISLATION

See: HEALTH POLICY

LEPROSY

See: HANSEN'S DISEASE

LEUKEMIA

See also: CANCER; HEMATOLOGIC
DISORDERS

ABSTRACTING, INDEXING, AND CURRENT AWARENESS PUBLICATIONS

Current Contents/Clinical Medicine. Institute for Scientific Information, 3501 Market St., Philadelphia, PA 19104. Phone: (800) 523-1850. Fax: (215) 386-6362. Weekly.

Excerpta Medica. Section 16: Cancer. Elsevier Science Publishing Co., Inc., P.O. Box 882, Madison Square Station, New York, NY 10159-2101. Phone: (212) 989-5800. Fax: (212) 633-3990. 32/year.

ICRDB Cancergram: Leukemia and Multiple Myeloma-- Diagnosis, Treatment. U.S. Government Printing Office, Superintendent of Documents, P.O. Box 371954, Pittsburgh, PA 15250-7954. Phone: (202) 783-3238. Fax: (202) 512-2250. Monthly.

Index Medicus. U.S. National Library of Medicine, 8600 Rockville Pike, Bethesda, MD 20894. Phone: (800) 638-8480. Monthly.

Science Citation Index. Institute for Scientific Information, 3501 Market St., Philadelphia, PA 19104. Phone: (800) 523-1850. Fax: (215) 386-6362. Bimonthly.

ANNUALS AND REVIEWS

In Development New Medicines for Older Americans. 1991 Annual Survey. More Medicines in Testing for Cancer Than for Any Other Disease of Aging. Pharmaceutical Manufacturers Association, 1100 15th St. N.W., Washington, DC 20005. Phone: (202) 835-3400. 1991.

ASSOCIATIONS, PROFESSIONAL SOCIETIES, ADVOCACY AND SUPPORT GROUPS

American Cancer Society (ACS). 1599 Clifton Rd. N.E., Atlanta, GA 30329. Phone: (404) 320-3333.

Leukemia Society of America (LSA). 733 Third Ave., New York, NY 10017. Phone: (212) 573-8484. Fax: (212) 972-5776.

BIBLIOGRAPHIES

Bone Marrow Transplantation as Treatment for Leukemia. National Technical Information Service, 5285 Port Royal Rd., Springfield, VA 22161. Phone: (703) 487-4650. Fax: (703) 321-8547. Jan. 1978-Jul. 1989 PB89-866552/CBY.

Lymphocytic and Lymphoblastic Leukemias: Chromosome Aberrations. National Technical Information Service, 5285 Port Royal Rd., Springfield, VA 22161. Phone: (703) 487-4650. Fax: (703) 321-8547. Jan. 1978-Jan. 1989 PB89-854988/CBY.

Myelogeneous Leukemias and Nonlymphocytic Leukemias: Chromosomal Aberrations. National Technical Information Service, 5285 Port Royal Rd., Springfield, VA 22161. Phone: (703) 487-4650. Fax: (703) 321-8547. Jan. 1978-Jan. 1989 PB89-854966/CBY.

CD-ROM DATABASES

OncoDisc. J.B. Lippincott Co., 227 East Washington Square, Philadelphia, PA 19106-3780. Phone: (215) 238-4200. Fax: (215) 238-4227. Bimonthly.

SCISEARCH. Institute for Scientific Information, 3501 Market St., Philadelphia, PA 19104. Phone: (215) 386-0100. Fax: (215) 386-6362.

DIRECTORIES

Directory of Medical Specialists. Marquis Who's Who, 3002 Glenview Rd., Wilmette, IL 60091. Phone: (800) 621-9669. Fax: (708) 441-2264. Biennial.

Directory of Physicians in the United States. American Medical Association, 515 North State St., Chicago, IL 60610. Phone: (312) 464-0183. Fax: (312) 464-5834. Biennial.

ENCYCLOPEDIAS, DICTIONARIES, WORD BOOKS

Oncology Words. Stedman. Williams & Wilkins, 428 East Preston St., Baltimore, MD 21202. Phone: (800) 638-0672. Fax: (800) 447-8438. 1992.

A Word Book in Oncology and Hematology: With Special Reference to AIDS. Sheila B. Sloane. Mosby-Year Book, 11830 Westline Industrial Drive, St. Louis, MO 63146. Phone: (800) 325-4177. Fax: (314) 432-1380. 1992.

JOURNALS

Blood. W.B. Saunders Co., The Curtis Center, Independence Sqare W., Philadelphia, PA 19106-3399. Phone: (215) 238-7800.

Cancer Causes and Control. Rapid Communications of Oxford Ltd., The Old Malthouse, Paradise St., Oxford OX1 1LD, England. Phone: 44-865-790447. Fax: 44-865-244012. 6/year.

Journal of the National Cancer Institute. Superintendent of Documents, P.O. Box 371954, Pittsburgh, PA 15250-7954. Fax: (202) 512-2233. Semimonthly.

Leukemia & Lymphoma. Harwood Academic Publishers, P.O. Box 768, Cooper Station, New York, NY 10276. Phone: (800) 545-8398. Fax: (212) 654-2549. Monthly.

NEWSLETTERS

Leukemia Society of America-Society News. Leukemia Society of America, Inc., 733 Third Ave., New York, NY 10017. Phone: (800) 284-4271. Fax: (212) 972-5776. Bimonthly.

ONLINE DATABASES

Clinical Protocols. U.S. National Cancer Institute, International Cancer Information Center, Building 82, Room 102, Bethesda, MD 20892. Phone: (301) 496-7403. Fax: (301) 480-8105.

EMBASE. Elsevier Science Publishing Co., Inc., P.O. Box 882, Madison Square Station, New York, NY 10159-2101. Phone: (212) 989-5800. Fax: (212) 633-3990.

MEDLINE. National Library of Medicine, 8600 Rockville Pike, Bethesda, MD 20894. Phone: (800) 638-8480.

Physician Data Query (PDQ) Cancer Information File. U.S. National Cancer Institute, International Cancer Information Center, Building 82, Room 102, Bethesda, MD 20892. Phone: (301) 496-7403. Fax: (301) 480-8105. Monthly.

Physician Data Query (PDQ) Directory File. U.S. National Cancer Institute, International Cancer Information Center,

Building 82, Room 102, Bethesda, MD 20892. Phone: (301) 496-7403. Fax: (301) 480-8105. Monthly.

Physician Data Query (PDQ) Protocol File. U.S. National Cancer Institute, International Cancer Information Center, Building 82, Room 102, Bethesda, MD 20892. Phone: (301) 496-7403. Fax: (301) 480-8105. Monthly.

SciSearch. Institute for Scientific Information, 3501 Market St., Philadelphia, PA 19104. Phone: (215) 386-0100. Fax: (215) 386-6362.

POPULAR WORKS AND PATIENT EDUCATION

Cancervive: The Challenge of Life After Cancer. Susan Nessim, Judith Ellis. Houghton Mifflin Co., 1 Beacon St., Boston, MA 02108. Phone: (800) 225-3362. 1991.

Everyone's Guide to Cancer Therapy: How Cancer is Diagnosed, Treated, and Managed on a Day to Day Basis. Malin Dollinger, Ernest H. Rosenbaum, Greg Cable. Andrews & McMeel, 4900 Main St., Kansas City, MO 64112. Phone: (800) 826-4216. 1991.

RESEARCH CENTERS, INSTITUTES, CLEARINGHOUSES

Cancer Information Service (CIS). Office of Cancer Communications, National Cancer Institute, Bldg. 31, Rm. 10A24, 9000 Rockville Pike, Bethesda, MD 20892. Phone: (800) 4CA-NCER.

Cancer and Leukemia Group B. Dana Farber Cancer Institute, 303 Brylston St., Brookline, MA 02146. Phone: (617) 732-3670.

Comparative Leukemia Unit. University of Pennsylvania, New Bolton Center, 382 West Street Road, Kennett Square, PA 19348. Phone: (215) 444-5800.

National Marrow Donor Program. 3433 Broadway St. N.E., Minneapolis, MN 55417. Phone: (800) 654-1247.

TEXTBOOKS AND MONOGRAPHS

Acute Myelogenous Leukemia: Progress and Controversies (UCLA Symposia on Molecular and Cellular Biology). Robert P. Gale (ed.). John Wiley & Sons, Inc., 605 Third Ave., New York, NY 10158-0012. Phone: (212) 850-6000. Fax: (212) 850-6088. 1990.

Cancer: Principles and Practice of Oncology. Vincent T. DeVita. J.B. Lippincott Co., 227 E. Washington Square, Philadelphia, PA 19106-3780. Phone: (215) 238-4200. Fax: (215) 238-4227. 1989 3rd edtion.

Childhood Leukemia. Kobayashi. Kluwer Academic Publishers, P.O. Box 358, Accord Station, Hingham, MA 02018-0358. Phone: (617) 871-6600. Fax: (617) 871-6528. 1991.

Current Therapy in Hematology. Michael Brain, Paul Carbone. Mosby-Year Book, 11830 Westline Industrial Drive, St. Louis, MO 63146. Phone: (800) 325-4177. Fax: (314) 432-1380. 4th edition, 1991.

Leukemia. Edward Henderson, T. Andrew. W.B. Saunders Co., The Curtis Center, Independence Sqare W., Philadelphia, PA 19106-3399. Phone: (215) 238-7800. 1990.

The Lymphoid Leukaemias. D. Catovsky, R. Foa. Butterworth-Heinemann, 80 Montvale Ave., Stoneham, MA 02180. Phone: (617) 438-8464. Fax: (617) 279-4851. 1990.

LIBRARIES, MEDICAL

See: MEDICAL LIBRARIES

LICE

See: PARASITIC DISEASES

LIFE EXPECTANCY

See: VITAL STATISTICS

LIPOSUCTION

See: PLASTIC AND COSMETIC SURGERY

LIVER CANCER

ABSTRACTING, INDEXING, AND CURRENT AWARENESS PUBLICATIONS

Current Contents/Clinical Medicine. Institute for Scientific Information, 3501 Market St., Philadelphia, PA 19104. Phone: (800) 523-1850. Fax: (215) 386-6362. Weekly.

Excerpta Medica. Section 16: Cancer. Elsevier Science Publishing Co., Inc., P.O. Box 882, Madison Square Station, New York, NY 10159-2101. Phone: (212) 989-5800. Fax: (212) 633-3990. 32/year.

Index Medicus. U.S. National Library of Medicine, 8600 Rockville Pike, Bethesda, MD 20894. Phone: (800) 638-8480. Monthly.

Science Citation Index. Institute for Scientific Information, 3501 Market St., Philadelphia, PA 19104. Phone: (800) 523-1850. Fax: (215) 386-6362. Bimonthly.

ASSOCIATIONS, PROFESSIONAL SOCIETIES, ADVOCACY AND SUPPORT GROUPS

American Cancer Society (ACS). 1599 Clifton Rd. N.E., Atlanta, GA 30329. Phone: (404) 320-3333.

CD-ROM DATABASES

SCISEARCH. Institute for Scientific Information, 3501 Market St., Philadelphia, PA 19104. Phone: (215) 386-0100. Fax: (215) 386-6362.

ENCYCLOPEDIAS, DICTIONARIES, WORD BOOKS

Cardiovascular and Pulmonary Word Book. Helen E. Littrell. Springhouse Publishing Co., 1111 Bethlehem Pike, Spring House, PA 19477. Phone: (800) 331-3170. Fax: (215) 646-8716. 1992.

JOURNALS

CA - A Cancer Journal for Clinicians. J.B. Lippincott Co., 227 E. Washington Square, Philadelphia, PA 19106-3780. Phone: (215) 238-4200. Fax: (215) 238-4227. Bimonthly.

Journal of the National Cancer Institute. Superintendent of Documents, P.O. Box 371954, Pittsburgh, PA 15250-7954. Fax: (202) 512-2233. Semimonthly.

Journal of Surgical Oncology. John Wiley & Sons, Inc., 605 Third Ave., New York, NY 10158-0012. Phone: (212) 850-6000. Fax: (212) 850-6088. Monthly.

ONLINE DATABASES

EMBASE. Elsevier Science Publishing Co., Inc., P.O. Box 882, Madison Square Station, New York, NY 10159-2101. Phone: (212) 989-5800. Fax: (212) 633-3990.

MEDLINE. National Library of Medicine, 8600 Rockville Pike, Bethesda, MD 20894. Phone: (800) 638-8480.

Physician Data Query (PDQ) Cancer Information File. U.S. National Cancer Institute, International Cancer Information Center, Building 82, Room 102, Bethesda, MD 20892. Phone: (301) 496-7403. Fax: (301) 480-8105. Monthly.

Physician Data Query (PDQ) Directory File. U.S. National Cancer Institute, International Cancer Information Center, Building 82, Room 102, Bethesda, MD 20892. Phone: (301) 496-7403. Fax: (301) 480-8105. Monthly.

Physician Data Query (PDQ) Protocol File. U.S. National Cancer Institute, International Cancer Information Center, Building 82, Room 102, Bethesda, MD 20892. Phone: (301) 496-7403. Fax: (301) 480-8105. Monthly.

SciSearch. Institute for Scientific Information, 3501 Market St., Philadelphia, PA 19104. Phone: (215) 386-0100. Fax: (215) 386-6362.

POPULAR WORKS AND PATIENT EDUCATION

Everyone's Guide to Cancer Therapy: How Cancer is Diagnosed, Treated, and Managed on a Day to Day Basis. Malin Dollinger, Ernest H. Rosenbaum, Greg Cable. Andrews & McMeel, 4900 Main St., Kansas City, MO 64112. Phone: (800) 826-4216. 1991.

RESEARCH CENTERS, INSTITUTES, CLEARINGHOUSES

Cancer Information Service (CIS). Office of Cancer Communications, National Cancer Institute, Bldg. 31, Rm. 10A24, 9000 Rockville Pike, Bethesda, MD 20892. Phone: (800) 4CA-NCER.

TEXTBOOKS AND MONOGRAPHS

Early Detection and Treatment of Liver Cancer. Kunio Okuda, Takayoshi Tobe, Tomoyuki Kitagawa (eds.). Taylor & Francis Inc., 1900 Frost Rd., Suite 101, Bristol, PA 19007-1598. Phone: (800) 821-8312. Fax: (215) 785-5515. 1991.

Liver Cell Carcinoma. P. Bannasch, and others (eds.). Kluwer Academic Publishers, P.O. Box 358, Accord Station, Hingham, MA 02018-0358. Phone: (617) 871-6600. Fax: (617) 871-6528. 1989.

LIVER DISEASES

See also: BILIARY DISORDERS

ABSTRACTING, INDEXING, AND CURRENT AWARENESS PUBLICATIONS

Core Journals in Gastroenterology. Elsevier Science Publishing Co., Inc., P.O. Box 882, Madison Square Station, New York, NY 10159-2101. Phone: (212) 989-5800. Fax: (212) 633-3990. 11/year.

Current Contents/Clinical Medicine. Institute for Scientific Information, 3501 Market St., Philadelphia, PA 19104. Phone: (800) 523-1850. Fax: (215) 386-6362. Weekly.

Excerpta Medica. Section 48: Gastroenterology. Elsevier Science Publishing Co., Inc., P.O. Box 882, Madison Square Station, New York, NY 10159-2101. Phone: (212) 989-5800. Fax: (212) 633-3990. 20/year.

Index Medicus. U.S. National Library of Medicine, 8600 Rockville Pike, Bethesda, MD 20894. Phone: (800) 638-8480. Monthly.

Science Citation Index. Institute for Scientific Information, 3501 Market St., Philadelphia, PA 19104. Phone: (800) 523-1850. Fax: (215) 386-6362. Bimonthly.

ANNUALS AND REVIEWS

Annual of Gastrointestinal Endoscopy. Current Science Group, 20 N. Third St., Philadelphia, PA 19106-2199. Phone: (800) 552-5866. Fax: (215) 574-2270. Annual.

Current Gastroenterology. Mosby-Year Book, 11830 Westline Industrial Drive, St. Louis, MO 63146. Phone: (800) 325-4177. Fax: (314) 432-1380. Annual.

Current Opinion in Gastroenterology. Current Science Group, 20 N. Third St., Philadelphia, PA 19106-2199. Phone: (800) 552-5866. Fax: (215) 574-2270. Bimonthly.

Frontiers of Gastrointestinal Research. S. Karger Publishers, Inc., 26 West Avon Rd., P.O. Box 529, Farmington, CT 06085. Phone: (203) 675-7834. Fax: (203) 675-7302. Irregular.

Gastroenterology Annual. Elsevier Science Publishing Co., Inc., P.O. Box 882, Madison Square Station, New York, NY 10159-2101. Phone: (212) 989-5800. Fax: (212) 633-3990. Annual.

Gastroenterology Clinics. W.B. Saunders Co., The Curtis Center, Independence Square W., Philadelphia, PA 19106-3399. Phone: (215) 238-7800. Quarterly.

ASSOCIATIONS, PROFESSIONAL SOCIETIES, ADVOCACY AND SUPPORT GROUPS

American Association for the Study of Liver Diseases (AASLD). 6900 Grove Rd., Thorofare, NJ 08086. Phone: (800) 257-8290. Fax: (609) 853-5991.

American Liver Foundation (ALF). 1425 Pompton Ave., Cedar Grove, NJ 07009. Phone: (201) 256-2550. Fax: (201) 661-4027.

Children's Liver Foundation (CLF). 14245 Ventura Blvd., Ste. 201, Sherman Oaks, CA 91423. Phone: (800) 526-1593.

International Hepato-Biliary-Pancreatic Association (IHBPA). c/o A.R. Moossa, University of California, San Diego, Dept. of Surgery, 225 W. Dickenson St., San Diego, CA 92103. Phone: (619) 543-5860.

Pediatric Liver Research Foundation (PLRF). 342 Lincoln Ave., Cherry Hill, NJ 08002. Phone: (609) 663-2609.

Wilson's Disease Association. P.O. Box 75324, Washington, DC 20013. Phone: (703) 636-3003.

CD-ROM DATABASES

Excerpta Medica CD: Gastroenterology. SilverPlatter Information, Inc., River Ridge Office Park, 100 River Ridge Rd., Norwood, MA 02062. Phone: (617) 769-2599. Fax: (617) 769-8763. Quarterly.

Gastroenterology and Hepatology MEDLINE. MEP, 124 Mt. Auburn St., Cambridge, MA 02138. Phone: (800) 342-1338. Fax: (617) 868-7738. Quarterly.

SCISEARCH. Institute for Scientific Information, 3501 Market St., Philadelphia, PA 19104. Phone: (215) 386-0100. Fax: (215) 386-6362.

HANDBOOKS, GUIDES, MANUALS, ATLASES

A Color Atlas of Liver Disease. S. Sherlock, J.A. Summerfield. Mosby-Year Book, 11830 Westline Industrial Drive, St. Louis, MO 63146. Phone: (800) 325-4177. Fax: (314) 432-1380. Second edition 1991.

Handbook of Drug Therapy in Liver and Kidney Disease. Schrier. Little, Brown and Co., 34 Beacon St., Boston, MA 02108. Phone: (617) 227-0730. Fax: (617) 227-0790. 1991.

JOURNALS

Digestion. S. Karger Publishers, Inc., 26 W. Avon Rd., P.O. Box 529, Farmington, CT 06085. Phone: (203) 675-7834. Fax: (203) 675-7302.

Hepatology. Mosby-Year Book, 11830 Westline Industrial Drive, St. Louis, MO 63146. Phone: (800) 325-4177. Fax: (314) 432-1380. Monthly.

Journal of Hepatology. Elsevier Science Publishing Co., Inc., P.O. Box 882, Madison Square Station, New York, NY 10159-2101. Phone: (212) 989-5800. Fax: (212) 633-3990. 6/year.

Seminars in Liver Disease. Thieme Medical Publishers, Inc., 381 Park Ave. S., New York, NY 10016. Phone: (212) 683-5088. Fax: (212) 779-9020. Quarterly.

NEWSLETTERS

Progress. American Liver Foundation, 1425 Pompton Ave., Cedar Grove, NJ 07009. Phone: (800) 223-0179. Quarterly.

ONLINE DATABASES

EMBASE. Elsevier Science Publishing Co., Inc., P.O. Box 882, Madison Square Station, New York, NY 10159-2101. Phone: (212) 989-5800. Fax: (212) 633-3990.

MEDLINE. National Library of Medicine, 8600 Rockville Pike, Bethesda, MD 20894. Phone: (800) 638-8480.

SciSearch. Institute for Scientific Information, 3501 Market St., Philadelphia, PA 19104. Phone: (215) 386-0100. Fax: (215) 386-6362.

RESEARCH CENTERS, INSTITUTES, CLEARINGHOUSES

National Digestive Diseases Information Clearinghouse (NDDIC). P.O. Box NDDIC, Bethesda, MD 20892. Phone: (301) 468-6344.

TEXTBOOKS AND MONOGRAPHS

Autoimmune Liver Diseases. Edward L. Krawitt, Russell H. Wiesner. Raven Press, 1185 Avenue of the Americas, New York, NY 10036. Phone: (212) 930-9500. Fax: (212) 869-3495. 1991.

Biopsy Diagnosis of Liver Disease. Snover. Williams & Wilkins, 428 East Preston St., Baltimore, MD 21202. Phone: (800) 638-0672. Fax: (800) 447-8438. 1992.

Complications of Chronic Liver Disease. Rector. Mosby-Year Book, 11830 Westline Industrial Drive, St. Louis, MO 63146. Phone: (800) 325-4177. Fax: (314) 432-1380. 1992.

Diseases of the Gastrointestinal Tract and Liver. D.J.C. Shearman and others. Churchill Livingstone Inc., 650 Ave. of the Americas, New York, NY 10011. Phone: (212) 819-5400. Fax: (212) 302-6598. Second edition 1989.

Diseases of the Liver. Leon Schiff, Eugenee R. Schiff. J.B. Lippincott Co., 227 E. Washington Square, Philadelphia, PA 19106-3780. Phone: (215) 238-4200. Fax: (215) 238-4227. Sixth edition 1987.

Diseases of the Liver and Biliary System. Sherlock. Blackwell Scientific Publications, Inc., 3 Cambridge Ctr., Cambridge, MA 02142. Phone: (800) 759-6102. Ninth edition 1992.

Essentials of Clinical Hepatology. Charles F. Gholson, Bruce R. Bacon. Mosby-Year Book, 11830 Westline Industrial Drive, St. Louis, MO 63146. Phone: (800) 325-4177. Fax: (314) 432-1380. 1992.

Hepatology: A Textbook of Liver Disease. David Zakim, Thomas D. Boyer. W.B. Saunders Co., The Curtis Center, Independence Square W., Philadelphia, PA 19106-3399. Phone: (215) 238-7800. Second edition 1990.

Liver and Biliary Diseases. Neil Kaplowitz. Williams & Wilkins, 428 East Preston St., Baltimore, MD 21202. Phone: (800) 638-0672. Fax: (800) 447-8438. 1992.

The Liver and Biliary System. Gitnick. Mosby-Year Book, 11830 Westline Industrial Drive, St. Louis, MO 63146. Phone: (800) 325-4177. Fax: (314) 432-1380. 1991.

Liver Diseases. Leavy. Mosby-Year Book, 11830 Westline Industrial Drive, St. Louis, MO 63146. Phone: (800) 325-4177. Fax: (314) 432-1380. 1991.

Liver Diseases and Renal Complications. Paolo Gentilini, Irwin M. Arias, Vincente Arroyo, et. al.. Raven Press, 1185 Avenue of the Americas, New York, NY 10036. Phone: (212) 930-9500. Fax: (212) 869-3495. 1990.

Liver Function. Derek Cramp, Ewart Carson (eds.). Routledge, Chapman & Hall, Inc., 29 W. 35th St., New York, NY 10001-2291. Phone: (212) 244-3336. 1990.

Progress in Liver Diseases. Hans Popper, Fenton Schaffner (eds.). W.B. Saunders Co., The Curtis Center, Independence Square W., Philadelphia, PA 19106-3399. Phone: (215) 238-7800. Irregular.

Textbook of Liver and Biliary Surgery. William C. Meyers, R. Scott Jones. J.B. Lippincott Co., 227 E. Washington Square, Philadelphia, PA 19106-3780. Phone: (215) 238-4200. Fax: (215) 238-4227. 1990.

Viral Hepatitis and Liver Disease. Arie J. Zuckerman (ed.). John Wiley & Sons, Inc., 605 Third Ave., New York, NY 10158-0012. Phone: (212) 850-6000. Fax: (212) 850-6088. 1988.

Wright's Liver and Biliary Disease. G.H. Millward-Sadler, M. Arthur. W.B. Saunders Co., The Curtis Center, Independence Square W., Philadelphia, PA 19106-3399. Phone: (215) 238-7800. Third edition 1991.

LONG TERM CARE

See also: HEALTH INSURANCE; NURSING HOMES

ABSTRACTING, INDEXING, AND CURRENT AWARENESS PUBLICATIONS

Cumulative Index to Nursing and Allied Health Literature. Glendale Adventist Medical Center, P.O. Box 871, Glendale, CA 91209. Phone: (818) 409-8005. Bimonthly.

Hospital Literature Index. American Hospital Association, 840 N. Lake Shore Dr., Chicago, IL 60611. Phone: (800) 242-2626. Fax: (312) 280-6015. Quarterly.

Index Medicus. U.S. National Library of Medicine, 8600 Rockville Pike, Bethesda, MD 20894. Phone: (800) 638-8480. Monthly.

MEDOC: Index to U.S. Government Publications in the Medical and Health Sciences. Spencer S. Eccles Health Sciences Library, University of Utah, Bldg. 589, Salt Lake City, UT 84112. Phone: (801) 581-5268. Quarterly.

ASSOCIATIONS, PROFESSIONAL SOCIETIES, ADVOCACY AND SUPPORT GROUPS

American Association of Retired Persons. 1909 K St. N.W., Washington, DC 20049. Phone: (202) 872-4700.

Foundation for Hospice and Homecare (FHH). 519 C St. NE, Stanton Park, Washington, DC 20002. Phone: (202) 547-6586.

Health Insurance Association of America. 1025 Connecticut Ave. N.W., Washington, DC 20036. Phone: (202) 223-7780.

National Association of Insurance Commissioners. 120 W. 12th St., No. 1100, Kansas City, MO 64105. Phone: (816) 842-3600.

National Foundation for Long Term Health Care (NFLTHC). 1200 15th St. N.W., Washington, DC 20005. Phone: (202) 659-3148.

CD-ROM DATABASES

Nursing and Allied Health (CINAHL) on CD-ROM. CINAHL, 1509 Wilson Terrace, P.O. Box 871, Glendale, CA 91209-0871. Phone: (818) 409-8005.

HANDBOOKS, GUIDES, MANUALS, ATLASES

Care Plan Manual for Long Term Care. Connie S. March. American Hospital Association, 840 N. Lake Shore Dr.,

Chicago, IL 60611. Phone: (800) 242-2626. Fax: (312) 280-6015. 1988.

Guide to the Nursing Home Industry. Health Care Investment Analysts, Inc., 300 E. Lombard St., Baltimore, MD 21202. Phone: (410) 576-9600. Fax: (410) 783-0575. 1992.

JOURNALS

Nursing Homes and Senior Citizen Care. International Publishing Group, 4959 Commerce Pkwy., Cleveland, OH 44128. Phone: (216) 464-1210. Fax: (216) 464-1835. 6/year.

ONLINE DATABASES

AgeLine. American Association of Retired Persons, 601 E. St. NW, Washington, DC 20049. Phone: (202) 434-6231. Bimonthly.

EMBASE. Elsevier Science Publishing Co., Inc., P.O. Box 882, Madison Square Station, New York, NY 10159-2101. Phone: (212) 989-5800. Fax: (212) 633-3990.

MEDLINE. National Library of Medicine, 8600 Rockville Pike, Bethesda, MD 20894. Phone: (800) 638-8480.

Nursing and Allied Health (CINAHL). CINAHL, 1509 Wilson Terrace, P.O. Box 871, Glendale, CA 91209-0871. Phone: (818) 409-8005.

SciSearch. Institute for Scientific Information, 3501 Market St., Philadelphia, PA 19104. Phone: (215) 386-0100. Fax: (215) 386-6362.

POPULAR WORKS AND PATIENT EDUCATION

How to Choose a Nursing Home: A Guide to Quality Caring. Joanne Meshinsky. Avon Books, 1350 Ave. of the Americas, 2nd Flr., New York, NY 10019. Phone: (800) 238-0658. 1991.

RESEARCH CENTERS, INSTITUTES, CLEARINGHOUSES

Center for Aging. University of Alabama at Birmingham. Community Health Service Bldg., Room 118, 933 S. 19th St., Birmingham, AL 35294. Phone: (205) 934-3260. Fax: (205) 934-7239.

Center for Geriatrics, Gerontology, and Long-Term Care. Columbia University. 100 Haven Ave., Tower 3-29F, New York, NY 10032. Phone: (212) 781-0600.

Center on Health and Aging. Atlanta University. 223 James P. Brawley Dr. S.W., Atlanta, GA 30313. Phone: (404) 653-8610.

TEXTBOOKS AND MONOGRAPHS

Being a Long-Term Care Nursing Assistant. Connie A. Will, Judith B. Eighmy. Prentice Hall, 113 Sylvan Ave., Rt. 9W, Prentice Hall Bldg., Englewood Cliffs, NJ 07632. Phone: (201) 767-5937. 1991.

LOU GEHRIG'S DISEASE

See: AMYOTROPHIC LATERAL SCLEROSIS; NEUROMUSCULAR DISORDERS

LUNG CANCER

See also: CANCER

ABSTRACTING, INDEXING, AND CURRENT AWARENESS PUBLICATIONS

Current Contents/Clinical Medicine. Institute for Scientific Information, 3501 Market St., Philadelphia, PA 19104. Phone: (800) 523-1850. Fax: (215) 386-6362. Weekly.

Excerpta Medica. Section 16: Cancer. Elsevier Science Publishing Co., Inc., P.O. Box 882, Madison Square Station, New York, NY 10159-2101. Phone: (212) 989-5800. Fax: (212) 633-3990. 32/year.

ICRDB Cancergram: Lung Cancer--Diagnosis, Treatment. U.S. Government Printing Office, Superintendent of Documents, P.O. Box 371954, Pittsburgh, PA 15250-7954. Phone: (202) 783-3238. Fax: (202) 512-2250. Monthly.

Index Medicus. U.S. National Library of Medicine, 8600 Rockville Pike, Bethesda, MD 20894. Phone: (800) 638-8480. Monthly.

Research Alert: Cancer of the Respiratory System. Institute for Scientific Information, 3501 Market St., Philadelphia, PA 19104. Phone: (800) 523-1850. Fax: (215) 386-6362. Weekly.

Research Alert: Lung Cancer. Institute for Scientific Information, 3501 Market St., Philadelphia, PA 19104. Phone: (800) 523-1850. Fax: (215) 386-6362. Weekly.

Science Citation Index. Institute for Scientific Information, 3501 Market St., Philadelphia, PA 19104. Phone: (800) 523-1850. Fax: (215) 386-6362. Bimonthly.

ANNUALS AND REVIEWS

Current Pulmonology. Mosby-Year Book, 11830 Westline Industrial Drive, St. Louis, MO 63146. Phone: (800) 325-4177. Fax: (314) 432-1380.

In Development New Medicines for Older Americans. 1991 Annual Survey. More Medicines in Testing for Cancer Than for Any Other Disease of Aging. Pharmaceutical Manufacturers Association, 1100 15th St. N.W., Washington, DC 20005. Phone: (202) 835-3400. 1991.

ASSOCIATIONS, PROFESSIONAL SOCIETIES, ADVOCACY AND SUPPORT GROUPS

American Cancer Society (ACS). 1599 Clifton Rd. N.E., Atlanta, GA 30329. Phone: (404) 320-3333.

BIBLIOGRAPHIES

Lung Cancer Acquired by Radon Gas. National Technical Information Service, 5285 Port Royal Rd., Springfield, VA 22161. Phone: (703) 487-4650. Fax: (703) 321-8547. Mar. 1978-Nov. 1989 PB90-853839/CBY.

CD-ROM DATABASES

Cancer-CD. SilverPlatter Information, Inc., River Ridge Office Park, 100 River Ridge Rd., Norwood, MA 02062. Phone: (617) 769-2599. Fax: (617) 769-8763. Quarterly.

SCISEARCH. Institute for Scientific Information, 3501 Market St., Philadelphia, PA 19104. Phone: (215) 386-0100. Fax: (215) 386-6362.

ENCYCLOPEDIAS, DICTIONARIES, WORD BOOKS

Oncology Words. Stedman. Williams & Wilkins, 428 East Preston St., Baltimore, MD 21202. Phone: (800) 638-0672. Fax: (800) 447-8438. 1992.

HANDBOOKS, GUIDES, MANUALS, ATLASES

Atlas of Lung Cancer. Turner. Raven Press, 1185 Ave. of the Americas, New York, NY 10036. Phone: (212) 930-9500. Fax: (212) 869-3495. 1992.

JOURNALS

American Journal of Clinical Oncology. Raven Press, 1185 Ave. of the Americas, New York, NY 10036. Phone: (212) 930-9500. Fax: (212) 869-3495. Bimonthly.

CA - A Cancer Journal for Clinicians. J.B. Lippincott Co., 227 E. Washington Square, Philadelphia, PA 19106-3780. Phone: (215) 238-4200. Fax: (215) 238-4227. Bimonthly.

Cancer Causes and Control. Rapid Communications of Oxford Ltd., The Old Malthouse, Paradise St., Oxford OX1 1LD, England. Phone: 44-865-790447. Fax: 44-865-244012. 6/year.

Chest. American College of Chest Physicians, 911 Busse Hwy., Park Ridge, IL 60068. Phone: (708) 698-2200. Fax: (708) 698-1791. Monthly.

Journal of the National Cancer Institute. Superintendent of Documents, P.O. Box 371954, Pittsburgh, PA 15250-7954. Fax: (202) 512-2233. Semimonthly.

Journal of Surgical Oncology. John Wiley & Sons, Inc., 605 Third Ave., New York, NY 10158-0012. Phone: (212) 850-6000. Fax: (212) 850-6088. Monthly.

Lung Cancer. Elsevier Science Publishing Co., Inc., P.O. Box 882, Madison Square Station, New York, NY 10159-2101. Phone: (212) 989-5800. Fax: (212) 633-3990. 6/year.

ONLINE DATABASES

Cancer Weekly. CDC AIDS Weekly/NCI Cancer Weekly, 206 Rogers St. NE, Suite 104, P.O. Box 5528, Atlanta, GA 30317. Phone: (404) 377-8895. Weekly.

CANCERLIT. U.S. National Cancer Institute, International Cancer Information Center, Building 82, Room 102, Bethesda, MD 20892. Phone: (301) 496-7403. Fax: (301) 480-8105. Monthly.

Clinical Protocols. U.S. National Cancer Institute, International Cancer Information Center, Building 82, Room 102, Bethesda, MD 20892. Phone: (301) 496-7403. Fax: (301) 480-8105.

EMBASE. Elsevier Science Publishing Co., Inc., P.O. Box 882, Madison Square Station, New York, NY 10159-2101. Phone: (212) 989-5800. Fax: (212) 633-3990.

MEDLINE. National Library of Medicine, 8600 Rockville Pike, Bethesda, MD 20894. Phone: (800) 638-8480.

Physician Data Query (PDQ) Cancer Information File. U.S. National Cancer Institute, International Cancer Information Center, Building 82, Room 102, Bethesda, MD 20892. Phone: (301) 496-7403. Fax: (301) 480-8105. Monthly.

Physician Data Query (PDQ) Directory File. U.S. National Cancer Institute, International Cancer Information Center, Building 82, Room 102, Bethesda, MD 20892. Phone: (301) 496-7403. Fax: (301) 480-8105. Monthly.

Physician Data Query (PDQ) Protocol File. U.S. National Cancer Institute, International Cancer Information Center, Building 82, Room 102, Bethesda, MD 20892. Phone: (301) 496-7403. Fax: (301) 480-8105. Monthly.

SciSearch. Institute for Scientific Information, 3501 Market St., Philadelphia, PA 19104. Phone: (215) 386-0100. Fax: (215) 386-6362.

POPULAR WORKS AND PATIENT EDUCATION

Cancervive: The Challenge of Life After Cancer. Susan Nessim, Judith Ellis. Houghton Mifflin Co., 1 Beacon St., Boston, MA 02108. Phone: (800) 225-3362. 1991.

Everyone's Guide to Cancer Therapy: How Cancer is Diagnosed, Treated, and Managed on a Day to Day Basis. Malin Dollinger, Ernest H. Rosenbaum, Greg Cable. Andrews & McMeel, 4900 Main St., Kansas City, MO 64112. Phone: (800) 826-4216. 1991.

Lung Cancer Chronicles. Hohn A. Meyer. Rutgers University Press, 109 Church St., New Brunswick, NJ 08901. Phone: (800) 446-9323. 1990.

RESEARCH CENTERS, INSTITUTES, CLEARINGHOUSES

Cancer Information Service (CIS). Office of Cancer Communications, National Cancer Institute, Bldg. 31, Rm. 10A24, 9000 Rockville Pike, Bethesda, MD 20892. Phone: (800) 4CA-NCER.

TEXTBOOKS AND MONOGRAPHS

Cancer Medicine. James F. Holland, Emil Frei, Robert C. Bast Jr., and others. Williams & Wilkins, 428 East Preston St., Baltimore, MD 21202. Phone: (800) 638-0672. Fax: (800) 447-8438. Third edition 1992.

Cancer: Principles and Practice of Oncology. Vincent T. DeVita. J.B. Lippincott Co., 227 E. Washington Square, Philadelphia, PA 19106-3780. Phone: (215) 238-4200. Fax: (215) 238-4227. 1989 3rd edtion.

Cancer Treatment. Charles M. Haskell. W.B. Saunders Co., The Curtis Center, Independence Square W., Philadelphia, PA 19106-3399. Phone: (215) 238-7800. Third edition 1990.

Chest Medicine: Essentials of Pulmonary and Critical Care Medicine. George. Williams & Wilkins, 428 East Preston St., Baltimore, MD 21202. Phone: (800) 638-0672. Fax: (800) 447-8438. Second edition 1990.

Pathology of the Lung. W.H. Thurlbeck (ed.). Thieme Medical Publishers, Inc., 381 Park Ave. S., New York, NY 10016. Phone: (212) 683-5088. Fax: (212) 779-9020. 1988.

Textbook of Pulmonary Diseases. Gerald L. Baum, Emanuel Wolinsky (eds.). Little, Brown and Company, 34 Beacon St., Boston, MA 02108. Phone: (617) 227-0730. Fourth edition Two volumes 1989.

LUNG DISEASES

See also: RESPIRATORY THERAPY;
RESPIRATORY TRACT INFECTIONS

ABSTRACTING, INDEXING, AND CURRENT AWARENESS PUBLICATIONS

Current Contents/Clinical Medicine. Institute for Scientific Information, 3501 Market St., Philadelphia, PA 19104. Phone: (800) 523-1850. Fax: (215) 386-6362. Weekly.

Excerpta Medica. Section 15: Chest Diseases, Thoracic Surgery and Tuberculosis. Elsevier Science Publishing Co., Inc., P.O. Box 882, Madison Square Station, New York, NY 10159-2101. Phone: (212) 989-5800. Fax: (212) 633-3990. 20/year.

Index Medicus. U.S. National Library of Medicine, 8600 Rockville Pike, Bethesda, MD 20894. Phone: (800) 638-8480. Monthly.

Research Alert: Asthma, Emphysema & Bronchitis; Pulmonary Diseases, Chronic (COPD). Institute for Scientific Information, 3501 Market St., Philadelphia, PA 19104. Phone: (800) 523-1850. Fax: (215) 386-6362. Weekly.

Research Alert: Cancer of the Respiratory System. Institute for Scientific Information, 3501 Market St., Philadelphia, PA 19104. Phone: (800) 523-1850. Fax: (215) 386-6362. Weekly.

Science Citation Index. Institute for Scientific Information, 3501 Market St., Philadelphia, PA 19104. Phone: (800) 523-1850. Fax: (215) 386-6362. Bimonthly.

ANNUALS AND REVIEWS

Chest Surgery Clinics of North America. W.B. Saunders Co., The Curtis Center, Independence Square W., Philadelphia, PA 19106-3399. Phone: (215) 238-7800. Quarterly.

Clinics in Chest Medicine. W.B. Saunders Co., The Curtis Center, Independence Square W., Philadelphia, PA 19106-3399. Phone: (215) 238-7800. Quarterly.

Current Pulmonology. Mosby-Year Book, 11830 Westline Industrial Drive, St. Louis, MO 63146. Phone: (800) 325-4177. Fax: (314) 432-1380.

Progress in Respiration Research. S. Karger Publishers, Inc., 26 West Avon Rd., P.O. Box 529, Farmington, CT 06085. Phone: (203) 675-7834. Fax: (203) 675-7302. Irregular.

Year Book of Pulmonary Diseases. Mosby-Year Book, 11830 Westline Industrial Drive, St. Louis, MO 63146. Phone: (800) 325-4177. Fax: (314) 432-1380. Annual.

ASSOCIATIONS, PROFESSIONAL SOCIETIES, ADVOCACY AND SUPPORT GROUPS

American Lung Association (ALA). 1740 Broadway, New York, NY 10019. Phone: (212) 315-8700. Fax: (212) 265-5642.

Emphysema Anonymous, Inc. (EAI). P.O. Box 3224, Seminole, FL 34642. Phone: (813) 391-9977.

Vermont Pulmonary Specialized Center of Research. College of Medicine, Dept. of PHysiology, Given E-211, Burlington, VT 05405-0068. Phone: (802) 656-4338. Fax: (802) 656-8786.

CD-ROM DATABASES

SCISEARCH. Institute for Scientific Information, 3501 Market St., Philadelphia, PA 19104. Phone: (215) 386-0100. Fax: (215) 386-6362.

HANDBOOKS, GUIDES, MANUALS, ATLASES

Color Atlas of Clinical Applications of Fiberoptic Bronchoscopy. Kitamura. Mosby-Year Book, 11830 Westline Industrial Drive, St. Louis, MO 63146. Phone: (800) 325-4177. Fax: (314) 432-1380. 1991.

A Color Atlas of Respiratory Diseases. D. Geraint, James Peter, R. Studdy. Mosby-Year Book, 11830 Westline Industrial Drive, St. Louis, MO 63146. Phone: (800) 325-4177. Fax: (314) 432-1380. 1993.

Manual of Clinical Problems in Pulmonary Medicine: With Annotated Key References. Richard A. Bordow, Kenneth M. Moser (eds.). Little, Brown and Company, 34 Beacon St., Boston, MA 02108. Phone: (617) 227-0730. Third edition 1991.

Manual of Pulmonary Function Testing. Gregg Rupper. Mosby-Year Book, 11830 Westline Industrial Drive, St. Louis, MO 63146. Phone: (800) 325-4177. Fax: (314) 432-1380. 5th edition, 1991.

Pulmonary Diseases & Disorders: Companion Handbook. Alfred P. Fishman. McGraw-Hill, Inc., 1221 Avenue of the Americas, 28th Floor, New York, NY 10020. Phone: (212) 512-4228. Second edition 1992.

JOURNALS

Chest. American College of Chest Physicians, 911 Busse Hwy., Park Ridge, IL 60068. Phone: (708) 698-2200. Fax: (708) 698-1791. Monthly.

Experimental Lung Research. Taylor & Francis Inc., 1900 Frost Rd., Suite 101, Bristol, PA 19007-1598. Phone: (800) 821-8312. Fax: (215) 785-5515. Bimonthly.

Heart & Lung: The Journal of Critical Care. Mosby-Year Book, 11830 Westline Industrial Drive, St. Louis, MO 63146. Phone: (800) 325-4177. Fax: (314) 432-1380. Bimonthly.

The Journal of Heart and Lung Transplantation. Mosby-Year Book, 11830 Westline Industrial Drive, St. Louis, MO 63146. Phone: (800) 325-4177. Fax: (314) 432-1380. Bimonthly.

Lung. Springer-Verlag New York Inc., 175 Fifth Ave., New York, NY 10010. Phone: (212) 460-1500. Fax: (212) 473-6272.

Respiratory Medicine. Balliere Tindall, 24-28 Oval Rd., London NW1 7DX, England.

Seminars in Respiratory Medicine. Thieme Medical Publishers, Inc., 381 Park Ave. S., New York, NY 10016. Phone: (212) 683-5088. Fax: (212) 779-9020. Quarterly.

NEWSLETTERS

Batting the Breeze. Emphysema Anonymous, Inc., P.O. Box 3224, Seminole, FL 34642. Phone: (813) 391-9977. Bimonthly.

ONLINE DATABASES

EMBASE. Elsevier Science Publishing Co., Inc., P.O. Box 882, Madison Square Station, New York, NY 10159-2101. Phone: (212) 989-5800. Fax: (212) 633-3990.

MEDLINE. National Library of Medicine, 8600 Rockville Pike, Bethesda, MD 20894. Phone: (800) 638-8480.

SciSearch. Institute for Scientific Information, 3501 Market St., Philadelphia, PA 19104. Phone: (215) 386-0100. Fax: (215) 386-6362.

POPULAR WORKS AND PATIENT EDUCATION

The Chronic Bronchitis and Emphysema Handbook. Francois Haas, Sheila Sperber Haas. John Wiley & Sons, Inc., 605 Third Ave., New York, NY 10158-0012. Phone: (212) 850-6000. Fax: (212) 850-6088. 1990.

Living Well with Chronic Asthma, Bronchitis, and Emphysema: A Complete Guide to Coping with Chronic Lung Disease. Myra B. Shayevitz, Berton R. Shayevitz. Consumer Reports Books, 9180 LeSaint Dr., Fairfield, OH 45014. Phone: (513) 860-1178. 1991.

RESEARCH CENTERS, INSTITUTES, CLEARINGHOUSES

National Heart, Lung, and Blood Institute. 4733 Bethesda Ave., Ste. 530, Bethesda, MD 20814. Phone: (301) 951-3260.

National Jewish Center for Immunology and Respiratory Medicine. 1400 Jackson St., Denver, CO 80206. Phone: (303) 388-4461.

Occupational Lung Disease Center. Tulane University. School of Medicine, 1700 Perdido St., New Orleans, LA 70112. Phone: (504) 588-5265. Fax: (504) 588-5035.

TEXTBOOKS AND MONOGRAPHS

Biopsy Techniques in Pulmonary Disorders. Ko Pen Wang. Raven Press, 1185 Avenue of the Americas, New York, NY 10036. Phone: (212) 930-9500. Fax: (212) 869-3495. 1989.

Chest Medicine: Essentials of Pulmonary and Critical Care Medicine. George. Williams & Wilkins, 428 East Preston St., Baltimore, MD 21202. Phone: (800) 638-0672. Fax: (800) 447-8438. Second edition 1990.

Clinical Pulmonary Medicine. Lyle D. Victor (ed.). Little, Brown and Company, 34 Beacon St., Boston, MA 02108. Phone: (617) 227-0730. 1992.

Decision Making in Pulmonary Medicine. Karlinsky. Mosby-Year Book, 11830 Westline Industrial Drive, St. Louis, MO 63146. Phone: (800) 325-4177. Fax: (314) 432-1380. 1991.

Diagnostic Bronchoscopy: A Teaching Manual. Stradling. Churchill Livingstone Inc., 650 Ave. of the Americas, New York, NY 10011. Phone: (212) 819-5400. Fax: (212) 302-6598. Sixth edition 1991.

Eagan's Fundamentals of Respiratory Care. Scanlan. Mosby-Year Book, 11830 Westline Industrial Drive, St. Louis, MO 63146. Phone: (800) 325-4177. Fax: (314) 432-1380. Fifth editin 1990.

Foundations of Respiratory Care. Pierson. Churchill Livingstone Inc., 650 Ave. of the Americas, New York, NY 10011. Phone: (212) 819-5400. Fax: (212) 302-6598. 1992.

Lung Injury. Crystal. Raven Press, 1185 Ave. of the Americas, New York, NY 10036. Phone: (212) 930-9500. Fax: (212) 869-3495. 1992.

The Lung: Scientific Foundations. Ronald G. Crystal, John B. West (eds.). Raven Press, 1185 Avenue of the Americas, New York, NY 10036. Phone: (212) 930-9500. Fax: (212) 869-3495. Two volumes 1991.

Pathology of Asbestos-Related Diseases. Roggli. Little, Brown and Co., 34 Beacon St., Boston, MA 02108. Phone: (617) 227-0730. Fax: (617) 227-0790. 1992.

Pathology of the Lung. W.H. Thurlbeck (ed.). Thieme Medical Publishers, Inc., 381 Park Ave. S., New York, NY 10016. Phone: (212) 683-5088. Fax: (212) 779-9020. 1988.

Pleural Disease. Light. Williams & Wilkins, 428 East Preston St., Baltimore, MD 21202. Phone: (800) 638-0672. Fax: (800) 447-8438. Second edition 1990.

Pulmonary and Critical Care Medicine. Roger C. Bone (ed.). Mosby-Year Book, 11830 Westline Industrial Drive, St. Louis, MO 63146. Phone: (800) 325-4177. Fax: (314) 432-1380. 1992.

Pulmonary Rehabilitation. Hodgkin. J.B. Lippincott Co., 227 E. Washington Square, Philadelphia, PA 19106-3780. Phone: (215) 238-4200. Fax: (215) 238-4227. 1993.

Respiratory Care. Pryor. Churchill Livingstone Inc., 650 Ave. of the Americas, New York, NY 10011. Phone: (212) 819-5400. Fax: (212) 302-6598. 1991.

Respiratory Medicine. R.A.L. Brewis and others. W.B. Saunders Co., The Curtis Center, Independence Square W., Philadelphia, PA 19106-3399. Phone: (215) 238-7800. 1990.

Synopsis of Clinical Pulmonary Disease. Mitchell. Mosby-Year Book, 11830 Westline Industrial Drive, St. Louis, MO 63146. Phone: (800) 325-4177. Fax: (314) 432-1380. Fourth edition 1989.

Textbook of Pulmonary Diseases. Gerald L. Baum, Emanuel Wolinsky (eds.). Little, Brown and Company, 34 Beacon St., Boston, MA 02108. Phone: (617) 227-0730. Fourth edition Two volumes 1989.

Update: Pulmonary Diseases and Disorders. Fishman. McGraw-Hill Inc., 11 West 19th St., New York, NY 10011. Phone: (212) 337-5001. Fax: (212) 337-4092. 1992.

LUPUS ERYTHEMATOSUS

ABSTRACTING, INDEXING, AND CURRENT AWARENESS PUBLICATIONS

Current Contents/Clinical Medicine. Institute for Scientific Information, 3501 Market St., Philadelphia, PA 19104. Phone: (800) 523-1850. Fax: (215) 386-6362. Weekly.

Excerpta Medica. Section 31. Arthritis and Rheumatism. Elsevier Science Publishing Co., Inc., P.O. Box 882, Madison Square Station, New York, NY 10159-2101. Phone: (212) 989-5800. Fax: (212) 633-3990. 8/year.

Index Medicus. U.S. National Library of Medicine, 8600 Rockville Pike, Bethesda, MD 20894. Phone: (800) 638-8480. Monthly.

Research Alert: Systemic Lupus Erythematosus. Institute for Scientific Information, 3501 Market St., Philadelphia, PA 19104. Phone: (800) 523-1850. Fax: (215) 386-6362. Weekly.

Science Citation Index. Institute for Scientific Information, 3501 Market St., Philadelphia, PA 19104. Phone: (800) 523-1850. Fax: (215) 386-6362. Bimonthly.

ASSOCIATIONS, PROFESSIONAL SOCIETIES, ADVOCACY AND SUPPORT GROUPS

The American Lupus Society (TALS). 2914 Del Amo Blvd., Ste. 922, Torrance, CA 90503. Phone: (213) 542-8891.

Lupus Foundation of America (LFA). 1717 Massachusetts Ave. N.W., Ste. 203, Washington, DC 20036. Phone: (202) 328-4550. Fax: (202) 328-9052.

National Lupus Erythematosus Foundation (NLEF). 2635 N. 1st St., Ste. 206, San Jose, CA 95134. Phone: (408) 954-8600.

CD-ROM DATABASES

SCISEARCH. Institute for Scientific Information, 3501 Market St., Philadelphia, PA 19104. Phone: (215) 386-0100. Fax: (215) 386-6362.

JOURNALS

American Journal of Medicine. Reed Publishing USA, 249 W. 17th St., New York, NY 10011. Phone: (212) 645-0067. Fax: (212) 242-6987. Monthly.

Annals of the Rheumatic Diseases. BMJ Publishing Group, BMA House, Tavistock Square, London WC1H 9JR, England. Phone: 071-383 6244/6638. Fax: 071-383 6662. Monthly.

Archives of Dermatology. American Medical Association, 515 N. State St., Chicago, IL 60610. Phone: (312) 464-0183. Fax: (312) 464-5834. Monthly.

Arthritis and Rheumatism. American College of Rheumatology, 17 Executive Park Dr. N.E., Ste. 480, Atlanta, GA 30329. Phone: (404) 633-3777. Fax: (404) 663-1870. Monthly.

British Journal of Rheumatology. Balliere Tindall, 24-28 Oval Rd., London NW1 7DX, England. Bimonthly.

Cutis. Cahners Publishing Co., 249 W. 17th St., New York, NY 10011. Phone: (212) 645-0067. Fax: (212) 242-6987. Monthly.

Journal of the American Academy of Dermatology. Mosby-Year Book, 11830 Westline Industrial Drive, St. Louis, MO 63146. Phone: (800) 325-4177. Fax: (314) 432-1380. Monthly.

Journal of Investigative Dermatology. Elsevier Science Publishing Co., Inc., P.O. Box 882, Madison Square Station, New York, NY 10159-2101. Phone: (212) 989-5800. Fax: (212) 633-3990. Monthly.

Journal of Rheumatology. Journal of Rheumatology Publishing Co., 920 Yonge St., Ste. 115, Toronto, ON, Canada M4W 3C7. Phone: (416) 967-5155. Fax: (416) 967-7556. Monthly.

NEWSLETTERS

Lupus News. Lupus Foundation of America, 111 Pleasant St., No. 27, Watertown, MA 02172. Phone: (617) 924-3034. Quarterly.

Lupus Today. The American Lupus Society, 23751 Madison St., Torrance, CA 90505. Phone: (800) 331-1802. Quarterly.

ONLINE DATABASES

EMBASE. Elsevier Science Publishing Co., Inc., P.O. Box 882, Madison Square Station, New York, NY 10159-2101. Phone: (212) 989-5800. Fax: (212) 633-3990.

MEDLINE. National Library of Medicine, 8600 Rockville Pike, Bethesda, MD 20894. Phone: (800) 638-8480.

SciSearch. Institute for Scientific Information, 3501 Market St., Philadelphia, PA 19104. Phone: (215) 386-0100. Fax: (215) 386-6362.

POPULAR WORKS AND PATIENT EDUCATION

Coping with Lupus: A Guide to Living with Lupus for You and Your Family. Robert H. PHillips. Avery Publishing Group, Inc., 120 Old Broadway, Garden City Park, NY 11040. Phone: (800) 548-5757. 1991.

Lupus: My Serach for a Diagnosis. Eileen Radziunas. Borgo Press, P.O. Box 2845, San Bernardino, CA 92406-2845. Phone: (909) 884-5813. Fax: (909) 888-4942. 1989.

A Woman's Couragous Victory over Lupus. Henrietta Aladjem, Peter H. Schur. Macmillan Publishing Co., 866 Third Ave., New York, NY 10011. Phone: (800) 257-5755. Revised edition 1988.

RESEARCH CENTERS, INSTITUTES, CLEARINGHOUSES

Autoimmune Disease Center. Scripps Clinic and Research Foundation. 10666 N. Torrey Pines Rd., La Jolla, CA 92037. Phone: (619) 554-8686. Fax: (619) 554-6805.

Lupus Study Center. Hahnemann University. 221 N. Broad St., Philadelphia, PA 19107. Phone: (215) 448-7300.

National Arthritis and Musculoskeletal and Skin Diseases Information Clearinghouse (NAMSIC). 9000 Rockville Pike, P.O. Box AMS, Bethesda, MD 20892. Phone: (301) 495-4484. Fax: (301) 587-4352.

TEXTBOOKS AND MONOGRAPHS

Dubois' Lupus Erythematosus. Daniel J. Wallace, Edmund L. Dubois (eds.). Williams & Wilkins, 428 East Preston St., Baltimore, MD 21202. Phone: (800) 638-0672. Fax: (800) 447-8438. Third edition 1987.

LYME DISEASE

See also: ARTHRITIS

ABSTRACTING, INDEXING, AND CURRENT AWARENESS PUBLICATIONS

Current Contents/Clinical Medicine. Institute for Scientific Information, 3501 Market St., Philadelphia, PA 19104. Phone: (800) 523-1850. Fax: (215) 386-6362. Weekly.

Index Medicus. U.S. National Library of Medicine, 8600 Rockville Pike, Bethesda, MD 20894. Phone: (800) 638-8480. Monthly.

Research Alert: Lyme Disease. Institute for Scientific Information, 3501 Market St., Philadelphia, PA 19104. Phone: (800) 523-1850. Fax: (215) 386-6362. Weekly.

Science Citation Index. Institute for Scientific Information, 3501 Market St., Philadelphia, PA 19104. Phone: (800) 523-1850. Fax: (215) 386-6362. Bimonthly.

ASSOCIATIONS, PROFESSIONAL SOCIETIES, ADVOCACY AND SUPPORT GROUPS

Lyme Borreliosis Foundation (LBF). P.O. Box 462, Tolland, CT 06084. Phone: (203) 871-2900. Fax: (203) 870-9789.

BIBLIOGRAPHIES

Lyme Disease. National Technical Information Service, 5285 Port Royal Rd., Springfield, VA 22161. Phone: (703) 487-4650. Fax: (703) 321-8547. Jan. 1978-Apr. 1988 PB88-862685/CBY.

CD-ROM DATABASES

SCISEARCH. Institute for Scientific Information, 3501 Market St., Philadelphia, PA 19104. Phone: (215) 386-0100. Fax: (215) 386-6362

JOURNALS

Arthritis and Rheumatism. American College of Rheumatology, 17 Executive Park Dr. N.E., Ste. 480, Atlanta, GA 30329. Phone: (404) 633-3777. Fax: (404) 663-1870. Monthly.

Journal of Infectious Diseases. University of Chicago Press, P.O. Box 37005, Chicago, IL 60637. Phone: (312) 753-3347. Fax: (312) 753-0811. Monthly.

Journal of Wildlife Diseases. Wildlife Diseases Association, 224 S.E. 16th St., Ames, IA 50010. Phone: (515) 233-1931.

Review of Infectious Diseases. Infectious Diseases Society of America, 5720 S. Woodlawn Ave., Chicago, IL 60637. Phone: (312) 753-3347.

NEWSLETTERS

Bulletin on the Rheumatic Diseases. Arthritis Foundation, 1314 Sprin St., N.W., Atlanta, GA 30309. Phone: (404) 872-7100. Fax: (404) 872-0457. Bimonthly.

ONLINE DATABASES

EMBASE. Elsevier Science Publishing Co., Inc., P.O. Box 882, Madison Square Station, New York, NY 10159-2101. Phone: (212) 989-5800. Fax: (212) 633-3990.

MEDLINE. National Library of Medicine, 8600 Rockville Pike, Bethesda, MD 20894. Phone: (800) 638-8480.

SciSearch. Institute for Scientific Information, 3501 Market St., Philadelphia, PA 19104. Phone: (215) 386-0100. Fax: (215) 386-6362.

POPULAR WORKS AND PATIENT EDUCATION

Lyme Disease. Elaine Landau. Franklin Watts, Inc., 387 Park Ave. S., New York, NY 10016. Phone: (800) 672-6672. 1990.

RESEARCH CENTERS, INSTITUTES, CLEARINGHOUSES

Division of Vector-Borne Infectious Diseases. Centers for Disease Control. U.S. Public Health Service, P.O. Box 2087, Fort Collins, CO 80522-2087. Phone: (303) 221-6400. Fax: (303) 221-6476.

TEXTBOOKS AND MONOGRAPHS

Lyme Disease. L. Reik. Thieme Medical Publishers, Inc., 381 Park Ave. S., New York, NY 10016. Phone: (212) 683-5088. Fax: (212) 779-9020. 1991.

LYMPHATIC DISEASES

See: LEUKEMIA; LYMPHOMAS

LYMPHOMAS

ABSTRACTING, INDEXING, AND CURRENT AWARENESS PUBLICATIONS

Current Contents/Clinical Medicine. Institute for Scientific Information, 3501 Market St., Philadelphia, PA 19104. Phone: (800) 523-1850. Fax: (215) 386-6362. Weekly.

Excerpta Medica. Section 16: Cancer. Elsevier Science Publishing Co., Inc., P.O. Box 882, Madison Square Station, New York, NY 10159-2101. Phone: (212) 989-5800. Fax: (212) 633-3990. 32/year.

Index Medicus. U.S. National Library of Medicine, 8600 Rockville Pike, Bethesda, MD 20894. Phone: (800) 638-8480. Monthly.

Science Citation Index. Institute for Scientific Information, 3501 Market St., Philadelphia, PA 19104. Phone: (800) 523-1850. Fax: (215) 386-6362. Bimonthly.

ASSOCIATIONS, PROFESSIONAL SOCIETIES, ADVOCACY AND SUPPORT GROUPS

American Cancer Society (ACS). 1599 Clifton Rd. N.E., Atlanta, GA 30329. Phone: (404) 320-3333.

CD-ROM DATABASES

Cancer on Disc. CMC ReSearch, Inc., 7150 S.W. Hampton, Suite C-120, Portland, OR 97223. Phone: (800) 262-7668. Fax: (503) 639-1796. Annual.

SCISEARCH. Institute for Scientific Information, 3501 Market St., Philadelphia, PA 19104. Phone: (215) 386-0100. Fax: (215) 386-6362.

JOURNALS

Leukemia & Lymphoma. Harwood Academic Publishers, P.O. Box 768, Cooper Station, New York, NY 10276. Phone: (800) 545-8398. Fax: (212) 654-2549. Monthly.

ONLINE DATABASES

Cancer Weekly. CDC AIDS Weekly/NCI Cancer Weekly, 206 Rogers St. NE, Suite 104, P.O. Box 5528, Atlanta, GA 30317. Phone: (404) 377-8895. Weekly.

CANCERLIT. U.S. National Cancer Institute, International Cancer Information Center, Building 82, Room 102, Bethesda, MD 20892. Phone: (301) 496-7403. Fax: (301) 480-8105. Monthly.

EMBASE. Elsevier Science Publishing Co., Inc., P.O. Box 882, Madison Square Station, New York, NY 10159-2101. Phone: (212) 989-5800. Fax: (212) 633-3990.

MEDLINE. National Library of Medicine, 8600 Rockville Pike, Bethesda, MD 20894. Phone: (800) 638-8480.

Physician Data Query (PDQ) Cancer Information File. U.S. National Cancer Institute, International Cancer Information Center, Building 82, Room 102, Bethesda, MD 20892. Phone: (301) 496-7403. Fax: (301) 480-8105. Monthly.

Physician Data Query (PDQ) Directory File. U.S. National Cancer Institute, International Cancer Information Center, Building 82, Room 102, Bethesda, MD 20892. Phone: (301) 496-7403. Fax: (301) 480-8105. Monthly.

Physician Data Query (PDQ) Protocol File. U.S. National Cancer Institute, International Cancer Information Center, Building 82, Room 102, Bethesda, MD 20892. Phone: (301) 496-7403. Fax: (301) 480-8105. Monthly.

SciSearch. Institute for Scientific Information, 3501 Market St., Philadelphia, PA 19104. Phone: (215) 386-0100. Fax: (215) 386-6362.

POPULAR WORKS AND PATIENT EDUCATION

Everyone's Guide to Cancer Therapy: How Cancer is Diagnosed, Treated, and Managed on a Day to Day Basis. Malin Dollinger, Ernest H. Rosenbaum, Greg Cable. Andrews & McMeel, 4900 Main St., Kansas City, MO 64112. Phone: (800) 826-4216. 1991.

RESEARCH CENTERS, INSTITUTES, CLEARINGHOUSES

Cancer Information Service (CIS). Office of Cancer Communications, National Cancer Institute, Bldg. 31, Rm. 10A24, 9000 Rockville Pike, Bethesda, MD 20892. Phone: (800) 4CA-NCER.

TEXTBOOKS AND MONOGRAPHS

Cancer Medicine. James F. Holland, Emil Frei, Robert C. Bast Jr., and others. Williams & Wilkins, 428 East Preston St., Baltimore, MD 21202. Phone: (800) 638-0672. Fax: (800) 447-8438. Third edition 1992.

Cancer Treatment. Charles M. Haskell. W.B. Saunders Co., The Curtis Center, Independence Square W., Philadelphia, PA 19106-3399. Phone: (215) 238-7800. Third edition 1990.

Hodgkin's Disease: The Consequences of Survival. Mortimer J. Lacher, John Redman. Williams & Wilkins, 428 East Preston St., Baltimore, MD 21202. Phone: (800) 638-0672. Fax: (800) 447-8438. 1990.

Malignant Lymphoma: Biology, Natural History and Treatment. Alan C. Aisenberg. Williams & Wilkins, 428 East Preston St., Baltimore, MD 21202. Phone: (800) 638-0672. Fax: (800) 447-8438. 1991.

Non-Hodgkin's Lymphomas. Ian T. Magrath. Williams & Wilkins, 428 East Preston St., Baltimore, MD 21202. Phone: (800) 638-0672. Fax: (800) 447-8438. 1990.

M

MACULAR DISEASE

See: EYE DISEASES

MALARIA

See also: PARASITIC DISEASES; TROPICAL MEDICINE

ABSTRACTING, INDEXING, AND CURRENT AWARENESS PUBLICATIONS

Current Contents/Clinical Medicine. Institute for Scientific Information, 3501 Market St., Philadelphia, PA 19104. Phone: (800) 523-1850. Fax: (215) 386-6362. Weekly.

Index Medicus. U.S. National Library of Medicine, 8600 Rockville Pike, Bethesda, MD 20894. Phone: (800) 638-8480. Monthly.

Research Alert: Malaria. Institute for Scientific Information, 3501 Market St., Philadelphia, PA 19104. Phone: (800) 523-1850. Fax: (215) 386-6362. Weekly.

Tropical Diseases Bulletin. Bureau of Hygiene and Tropical Diseases, Keppel St., London WC1E 7HT, England. Monthly.

ASSOCIATIONS, PROFESSIONAL SOCIETIES, ADVOCACY AND SUPPORT GROUPS

American Society of Tropical Medicine and Hygiene (ASTMH). 8000 Westpark Dr., Ste. 130, Mc Lean, VA 22102. Phone: (703) 790-1745. Fax: (703) 790-9063.

JOURNALS

American Journal of Tropical Medicine and Hygiene. American Society of Tropical Medicine and Hygiene, LSU School of Medicine, P.O. Box 33932, Shreveport, LA 71130. Phone: (318) 674-5191. Monthly.

Transactions of the Royal Society of Tropical Medicine and Hygiene. Manson House, 26 Portland Pl., London W1N 4EY, England. Bimonthly.

Tropical Doctor. Royal Society of Medicine Services Ltd., 1 Wimpole St., London W1M 8AE, England. Phone: 071-408 2119. Fax: 071-355 3198. Quarterly.

Tropical Medicine and Parasitology. Thieme Medical Publishers, Inc., 381 Park Ave. S., New York, NY 10016. Phone: (212) 683-5088. Fax: (212) 779-9020. Quarterly.

NEWSLETTERS

Travel Medicine Advisor. American Health Consultants, Department ADI-59, P.O. Box 740060, Atlanta, GA 30374. Phone: (800) 559-1032. Fax: (404) 352-1971.

ONLINE DATABASES

EMBASE. Elsevier Science Publishing Co., Inc., P.O. Box 882, Madison Square Station, New York, NY 10159-2101. Phone: (212) 989-5800. Fax: (212) 633-3990.

MEDLINE. National Library of Medicine, 8600 Rockville Pike, Bethesda, MD 20894. Phone: (800) 638-8480.

SciSearch. Institute for Scientific Information, 3501 Market St., Philadelphia, PA 19104. Phone: (215) 386-0100. Fax: (215) 386-6362.

POPULAR WORKS AND PATIENT EDUCATION

The Malaria Capers: More Tales of Parasites and People, Research and Reality. Robert S. Desowitz. W.W. Norton & Co., Inc., 500 Fifth Ave., New York, NY 10110. Phone: (800) 223-2584. 1991.

RESEARCH CENTERS, INSTITUTES, CLEARINGHOUSES

Malaria Branch. Centers for Disease Control, 1600 Clifton Rd. N.E., Atlanta, GA 30333. Phone: (404) 488-4698.

STANDARDS AND STATISTICS SOURCES

Malaria Surrveillance, Annual Summary. Centers for Disease Control, 1600 Clifton Rd. N.E., Atlanta, GA 30333. Phone: (404) 488-4698.

TEXTBOOKS AND MONOGRAPHS

Malaria. Knell. Oxford University Press, 200 Madison Ave., New York, NY 10016. Phone: (212) 679-7300. 1991.

MALNUTRITION

See: NUTRITIONAL DISORDERS

MALOCCLUSION

See: ORTHODONTICS

MALPRACTICE

See also: MEDICAL CONSUMERISM

ABSTRACTING, INDEXING, AND CURRENT AWARENESS PUBLICATIONS

Hospital Literature Index. American Hospital Association, 840 N. Lake Shore Dr., Chicago, IL 60611. Phone: (800) 242-2626. Fax: (312) 280-6015. Quarterly.

Index Medicus. U.S. National Library of Medicine, 8600 Rockville Pike, Bethesda, MD 20894. Phone: (800) 638-8480. Monthly.

ASSOCIATIONS, PROFESSIONAL SOCIETIES, ADVOCACY AND SUPPORT GROUPS

American Bar Association. 750 N. Lakeshore Dr., Chicago, IL 60611.

The Campaign for Women's Health. 666 11th St. N.W., Ste. 700, Washington, DC 20001. Phone: (202) 783-6686.

Public Citizen Health Research Group (PCHRG). 2000 P St. N.W., Ste. 700, Washington, DC 20036. Phone: (202) 872-0320.

BIBLIOGRAPHIES

Malpractice Triangle: Medical, Legal, Insurance Issues. National Technical Information Service, 5285 Port Royal Rd., Springfield, VA 22161. Phone: (703) 487-4650. Fax: (703) 321-8547. Jan. 1970-Dec. 1987 PB88-854187/CBY.

JOURNALS

Journal of Legal Medicine. Shugar Publishing, 32 Mill Rd., Westhampton Beach, NY 11978. Phone: (516) 288-4404. Quarterly.

NEWSLETTERS

Health Facts. Center for Medical Consumers, 237 Thompson St., New York, NY 10012. Phone: (212) 674-7105. Monthly.

Health Letter. Public Citizen Health Research Group, 2000 P St. N.W., Ste. 700, Washington, DC 20036. Phone: (202) 872-0320. Monthly.

People's Medical Society-Newsletter. People's Medical Society, 462 Walnut St., Allentown, PA 18102. Phone: (215) 770-1670. Bimonthly.

ONLINE DATABASES

EMBASE. Elsevier Science Publishing Co., Inc., P.O. Box 882, Madison Square Station, New York, NY 10159-2101. Phone: (212) 989-5800. Fax: (212) 633-3990.

MEDLINE. National Library of Medicine, 8600 Rockville Pike, Bethesda, MD 20894. Phone: (800) 638-8480.

SciSearch. Institute for Scientific Information, 3501 Market St., Philadelphia, PA 19104. Phone: (215) 386-0100. Fax: (215) 386-6362.

POPULAR WORKS AND PATIENT EDUCATION

9000 Questionable Doctors. Sidney Wolfe. Public Citizen Health Resource Group, 2000 P St. N.W., Suite 700, Washington, DC 20036. Phone: (202) 872-0320. 1993.

Medicine on Trial: The Appalling Story of Medical Ineptitude and the Arrogance that Overlooks It. Charles B. Inlander, Lowell S. Levin, Ed Weiner. Random House, Inc., 201 E. 50th St., New York, NY 10022. Phone: (800) 726-0600. 1990.

The Rights of Patients: The Basic ACLU Guide to Patient Rights. George J. Annas. Southern Illinois University Press, P.O. Box 3697, Carbondale, IL 62902-3697. Phone: (618) 453-2281. 1989.

TEXTBOOKS AND MONOGRAPHS

Grand Rounds on Medical Practice. American Medical Association, 515 North State St., Chicago, IL 60610. Phone: (312) 464-0183. Fax: (312) 464-5834. 1990.

The Guide to Medical Professional Liability Insurance. American Medical Association, 515 North State St., Chicago, IL 60610. Phone: (312) 464-0183. Fax: (312) 464-5834. 1991.

Malpractice and Contact Lenses. Harvey M. Rosenwasser. Butterworth-Heinemann, 80 Montvale Ave., Stoneham, MA 02180. Phone: (617) 438-8464. Fax: (617) 279-4851. Updated edition 1991.

Malpractice: Managing Your Defense. R.M. Fish, and others. Medical Economics, Five Paragon Dr., Montvale, NJ 07645-1742. Phone: (800) 232-7379. Fax: (201) 573-4956. 1990.

Preventing Emergency Malpractice. R.M. Fish, M.E. Ehrhardt. Medical Economics, Five Paragon Dr., Montvale, NJ 07645-1742. Phone: (800) 232-7379. Fax: (201) 573-4956. 1989.

MAMMOGRAPHY

See also: BREAST CANCER; DIAGNOSIS; RADIOLOGY

ABSTRACTING, INDEXING, AND CURRENT AWARENESS PUBLICATIONS

Current Contents/Clinical Medicine. Institute for Scientific Information, 3501 Market St., Philadelphia, PA 19104. Phone: (800) 523-1850. Fax: (215) 386-6362. Weekly.

Excerpta Medica. Section 16: Cancer. Elsevier Science Publishing Co., Inc., P.O. Box 882, Madison Square Station, New York, NY 10159-2101. Phone: (212) 989-5800. Fax: (212) 633-3990. 32/year.

Index Medicus. U.S. National Library of Medicine, 8600 Rockville Pike, Bethesda, MD 20894. Phone: (800) 638-8480. Monthly.

Research Alert: Breast Cancer. Institute for Scientific Information, 3501 Market St., Philadelphia, PA 19104. Phone: (800) 523-1850. Fax: (215) 386-6362. Weekly.

Science Citation Index. Institute for Scientific Information, 3501 Market St., Philadelphia, PA 19104. Phone: (800) 523-1850. Fax: (215) 386-6362. Bimonthly.

ANNUALS AND REVIEWS

Current Opinion in Radiology. Current Science Ltd., 20 N. Third St., Philadelphia, PA 19106-2199. Phone: (800) 552-5866. Fax: (215) 574-2270. Bimonthly.

Year Book of Diagnostic Radiology. Mosby-Year Book, 11830 Westline Industrial Drive, St. Louis, MO 63146. Phone: (800) 325-4177. Fax: (314) 432-1380. Annual.

ASSOCIATIONS, PROFESSIONAL SOCIETIES, ADVOCACY AND SUPPORT GROUPS

American Cancer Society (ACS). 1599 Clifton Rd. N.E., Atlanta, GA 30329. Phone: (404) 320-3333.

American College of Radiology (ACR). 1891 Preston White Dr., Reston, VA 22091. Phone: (703) 648-8900.

National Alliance of Breast Cancer Organizations (NABCO). 1180 Ave. of the Americas, 2nd Flr., New York, NY 10036. Phone: (212) 719-0154. Fax: (212) 719-0263.

CD-ROM DATABASES

SCISEARCH. Institute for Scientific Information, 3501 Market St., Philadelphia, PA 19104. Phone: (215) 386-0100. Fax: (215) 386-6362.

DIRECTORIES

Directory of Certified Radiologists. American Board of Medical Specialties, 1 Rotary Center, Suite 805, Evanston, IL 60201. Phone: (708) 491-9091. Biennial.

HANDBOOKS, GUIDES, MANUALS, ATLASES

Atlas of Breast Disease. Volker Barth, Klaus Prechtel. Mosby-Year Book, 11830 Westline Industrial Drive, St. Louis, MO 63146. Phone: (800) 325-4177. Fax: (314) 432-1380. Second edition 1991.

Film Screen Mammography: An Atlas of Instructional Cases. Lawrence W. Bassett, Reza Jahanshahi, Richard H. Gold, et. al.. Raven Press, 1185 Avenue of the Americas, New York, NY 10036. Phone: (212) 930-9500. Fax: (212) 869-3495. 1991.

Manual of Diagnostic Imaging. Straub. Little, Brown and Co., 34 Beacon St., Boston, MA 02108. Phone: (617) 227-0730. Fax: (617) 227-0790. Second edition 1989.

JOURNALS

Journal of Women's Health. Mary Ann Liebert, Inc., 1651 Third Ave., New York, NY 10128. Phone: (212) 289-2300. Fax: (212) 289-4697. Quarterly.

ONLINE DATABASES

EMBASE. Elsevier Science Publishing Co., Inc., P.O. Box 882, Madison Square Station, New York, NY 10159-2101. Phone: (212) 989-5800. Fax: (212) 633-3990.

MEDLINE. National Library of Medicine, 8600 Rockville Pike, Bethesda, MD 20894. Phone: (800) 638-8480.

SciSearch. Institute for Scientific Information, 3501 Market St., Philadelphia, PA 19104. Phone: (215) 386-0100. Fax: (215) 386-6362.

POPULAR WORKS AND PATIENT EDUCATION

Everyone's Guide to Cancer Therapy: How Cancer is Diagnosed, Treated, and Managed on a Day to Day Basis. Malin Dollinger, Ernest H. Rosenbaum, Greg Cable. Andrews & McMeel, 4900 Main St., Kansas City, MO 64112. Phone: (800) 826-4216. 1991.

If It Runs in Your Family: Breast Cancer, Reducing Your Risk. Mary D. Eades. Bantam Books, Inc., 666 Fifth Ave., New York, NY 10103. Phone: (800) 223-6834. 1991.

Women Talk about Breast Surgery: From Diagnosis to Recovery. Amy Gross, Dee Ito. HarperCollins Pubs., Inc., 10 E. 53rd St., New York, NY 10022-5299. Phone: (212) 207-7000. Fax: (800) 242-7737. 1991.

Women's Cancers: How to Prevent Them, How to Treat Them, How to Beat Them. Donna Dawson, Marlene Mersch (eds.). Hunter House, Inc., 2200 Central, Ste. 202, Alameda, CA 94501-4451. Phone: (510) 865-5282. 1992.

RESEARCH CENTERS, INSTITUTES, CLEARINGHOUSES

Cancer Information Service (CIS). Office of Cancer Communications, National Cancer Institute, Bldg. 31, Rm. 10A24, 9000 Rockville Pike, Bethesda, MD 20892. Phone: (800) 4CA-NCER.

Comprehensive Breast Center. Vincent P. Lombardi Cancer Research Center, Georgetown University, Washington, DC 20007. Phone: (202) 687-2117.

STANDARDS AND STATISTICS SOURCES

Early Stage Breast Cancer. Consensus Statement. NIH Consensus Development Conference. June 18-21, 1990. National Institutes of Health, Office of Medical Applications of Research, Federal Bldg., Rm. 618, Bethesda, MD 20892. 1990.

TEXTBOOKS AND MONOGRAPHS

The Female Breast and Its Disorders: Essentials of Diagnosis and Management. George W. Mitchell Jr., Lawrence Bassett. Williams & Wilkins, 428 East Preston St., Baltimore, MD 21202. Phone: (800) 638-0672. Fax: (800) 447-8438. 1990.

Mammographic Interpretation: A Practical Approach. Marc J. Homer. McGraw-Hill, Inc., Health Professions Division, 1221 Avenue of the Americas, 28th Floor, New York, NY 10020. Phone: (212) 512-4228. 1991.

Mammography for Radiologic Technologists. Gini Wentz, Ward C. Parsons. McGraw-Hill Inc., 11 West 19th St., New York, NY 10011. Phone: (212) 337-5001. Fax: (212) 337-4092. 1992.

Textbook of Breast Disease. John H. Isaacs. Mosby-Year Book, 11830 Westline Industrial Drive, St. Louis, MO 63146. Phone: (800) 325-4177. Fax: (314) 432-1380. 1992.

MANIC DISORDER

See: MOOD DISORDERS

MARFAN'S SYNDROME

See: GENETIC DISEASES

MARIJUANA

See also: DRUG ABUSE

ABSTRACTING, INDEXING, AND CURRENT AWARENESS PUBLICATIONS

Excerpta Medica. Section 40: Drug Dependence, Alcohol Abuse and Alcoholism. Elsevier Science Publishing Co., Inc., P.O. Box 882, Madison Square Station, New York, NY 10159-2101. Phone: (212) 989-5800. Fax: (212) 633-3990. 6/year.

Index Medicus. U.S. National Library of Medicine, 8600 Rockville Pike, Bethesda, MD 20894. Phone: (800) 638-8480. Monthly.

Psychological Abstracts. American Psychological Association, 1200 17th St. NW, Washington, DC 20036. Phone: (202) 955-7600. Monthly.

ANNUALS AND REVIEWS

Advances in Alcohol and Substance Abuse. Haworth Press, 10 Alice St., Binghamton, NY 13904-1580. Phone: (803) 429-6784. Fax: (607) 722-1424.

Marijuana. Mark S. Gold. Plenum Publishing Co., 233 Spring St., New York, NY 10013-1578. Phone: (212) 620-8000. Fax: (212) 463-0742. Volume 1 1989.

ASSOCIATIONS, PROFESSIONAL SOCIETIES, ADVOCACY AND SUPPORT GROUPS

Narcotics Association for Children of Alcoholics (NACoA). 31582 Coast Highway, Ste. B, South Laguna, CA 92677-3044. Phone: (714) 499-3889.

National Council on Alcoholism and Drug Dependence, Inc.. 12 W. 21st St., New York, NY 10010. Phone: (212) 206-6770.

BIBLIOGRAPHIES

Drug Abuse, Drug Abuse Prevention, and Drug Testing. National Technical Information Service, 5285 Port Royal Rd., Springfield, VA 22161. Phone: (703) 487-4650. Fax: (703) 321-8547. Jan. 1985-Feb. 1989 PB88-862444/CBY.

Marijuana, Hashish, and Related Compounds. National Technical Information Service, 5285 Port Royal Rd., Springfield, VA 22161. Phone: (703) 487-4650. Fax: (703) 321-8547. June 1970-June 1988 PB88-865456/CBY.

CD-ROM DATABASES

PsycLit. SilverPlatter Information, Inc., River Ridge Office Park, 100 River Ridge Rd., Norwood, MA 02062. Phone: (617) 769-2599. Fax: (617) 769-8763. Quarterly.

ENCYCLOPEDIAS, DICTIONARIES, WORD BOOKS

Encyclopedia of Drug Abuse. Glen Evans, Robert O'Brien, Sidney Cohen, James Fine. Facts on File, Inc., 460 Park Ave. S., New York, NY 10016-7382. Phone: (212) 683-2244. Fax: (212) 683-3633. Third edition 1992.

JOURNALS

American Journal of Drug and Alcohol Abuse. Marcel Dekker, Inc., 270 Madison Ave., New York, NY 10016. Phone: (800) 228-1160.

Journal of Substance Abuse. Ablex Publishing Co., 355 Chestnut St., Norwood, NJ 07648. Phone: (201) 767-8450. Fax: (201) 767-6717. Quarterly.

Journal of Substance Abuse Treatment. Pergamon Press, 660 White Plains Rd., Tarrytown, NY 10591-5153. Phone: (914) 592-7700. Fax: (914) 592-3625. 6/year.

ONLINE DATABASES

Druginfo and Alcohol Use and Abuse. University of Minnesota, College of Pharmacy, Drug Information Services, 3-160 Health Sciences Center, Unit F, 308 Harvard St. Se, Minneapolis, MN 55455. Phone: (612) 624-6492. Quarterly.

EMBASE. Elsevier Science Publishing Co., Inc., P.O. Box 882, Madison Square Station, New York, NY 10159-2101. Phone: (212) 989-5800. Fax: (212) 633-3990.

MEDLINE. National Library of Medicine, 8600 Rockville Pike, Bethesda, MD 20894. Phone: (800) 638-8480.

PsycInfo. SilverPlatter Information, Inc., River Ridge Office Park, 100 River Ridge Rd., Norwood, MA 02062. Phone: (617) 769-2599. Fax: (617) 769-8763. Quarterly.

SciSearch. Institute for Scientific Information, 3501 Market St., Philadelphia, PA 19104. Phone: (215) 386-0100. Fax: (215) 386-6362.

POPULAR WORKS AND PATIENT EDUCATION

The Facts about Drug Use. Barry Stimmel. Consumer Reports Books, 101 Truman Ave., Yonkers, NY 10703. Phone: (914) 378-2000. 1991.

RESEARCH CENTERS, INSTITUTES, CLEARINGHOUSES

LCF Foundation, Inc.. 41 Mall Rd., Burlington, MA 01805. Phone: (617) 273-5100. Fax: (617) 273-8999.

National Clearinghouse for Alcohol and Drug Information (NCADI). P.O. Box 2345, Rockville, MD 20852. Phone: (301) 468-2600.

TEXTBOOKS AND MONOGRAPHS

Marijuana/Cannabinoids: Neurophysiology and Neurobiology. Andrzej Bartke, Laura Murphy. CRC Press, Inc., 2000 Corporate Blvd. N.W., Boca Raton, FL 33431. Phone: (407) 994-0555. Fax: (407) 997-0949. 1992.

MARITAL THERAPY

See also: FAMILY THERAPY; PSYCHOLOGY

ABSTRACTING, INDEXING, AND CURRENT AWARENESS PUBLICATIONS

Psychological Abstracts. American Psychological Association, 1200 17th St. NW, Washington, DC 20036. Phone: (202) 955-7600. Monthly.

ASSOCIATIONS, PROFESSIONAL SOCIETIES, ADVOCACY AND SUPPORT GROUPS

American Association for Marriage and Family Therapy (AAMFT). 1100 17th St. N.W., 10th Flr., Washington, DC 20036. Phone: (202) 452-0109.

Family Therapy Network (FTN). 7705 13th St. N.W., Washington, DC 20012. Phone: (202) 829-2452. Fax: (202) 726-7983.

CD-ROM DATABASES

PsycLit. SilverPlatter Information, Inc., River Ridge Office Park, 100 River Ridge Rd., Norwood, MA 02062. Phone: (617) 769-2599. Fax: (617) 769-8763. Quarterly.

JOURNALS

Family Process. Family Process, 841 Broadway, No. 504, New York, NY 10003. Phone: (212) 565-6517.

Journal of Sex and Marital Therapy. Brunner/Mazel Pubs., 19 Union Sq. W., New York, NY 10003. Phone: (212) 924-3344.

ONLINE DATABASES

PsycInfo. SilverPlatter Information, Inc., River Ridge Office Park, 100 River Ridge Rd., Norwood, MA 02062. Phone: (617) 769-2599. Fax: (617) 769-8763. Quarterly.

POPULAR WORKS AND PATIENT EDUCATION

The Consumer's Guide to Psychotherapy. Louis J. Rosner, Shelley Ross. Simon & Schuster, Inc., 1230 Ave. of the Americas, New York, NY 10020. Phone: (212) 698-7000. 1992.

TEXTBOOKS AND MONOGRAPHS

Principles and Practice of Sex Therapy. Sandra Leiblum, Raymond Rosen (eds.). Guilford Publications, Inc., 72 Spring St., New York, NY 10012. Phone: (800) 365-7006. Fax: (212) 366-6708. 1989.

The Psychology of Marriage: Basic Issues and Applications. Frank Fincham (ed.). Guilford Publications, Inc., 72 Spring St., New York, NY 10012. Phone: (800) 365-7006. Fax: (212) 366-6708. 1990.

Sexual Desire Disorders. Sandra R. Leiblum, Raymond C. Rosen. Guilford Publications, Inc., 72 Spring St., New York, NY 10012. Phone: (800) 365-7006. Fax: (212) 366-6708. 1992.

Transgenerational Family Therapies. Laura Roberts. Guilford Publications, Inc., 72 Spring St., New York, NY 10012. Phone: (800) 365-7006. Fax: (212) 366-6708. 1992.

MARRIAGE COUNSELING

See: MARITAL THERAPY

MASTECTOMY

See: BREAST CANCER

MATERNITY

See: CHILDBIRTH; PREGNANCY

MAXILLOFACIAL SURGERY

See: ORAL SURGERY

MEASLES

See: INFECTIOUS DISEASES

MEDICAID

See: MEDICARE AND MEDICAID

MEDICAL ANTHROPOLOGY

See: FORENSIC MEDICINE

MEDICAL CONSUMERISM

See also: INFORMED CONSENT; MALPRACTICE

ABSTRACTING, INDEXING, AND CURRENT AWARENESS PUBLICATIONS

Consumer Health and Nutrition Index. Alan Rees. Oryx Press, 4041 N. Central, Suite 700, Phoenix, AZ 85012. Phone: (800) 279-6799. Fax: (800) 279-4663. Quarterly.

Medical Abstracts Newsletter. Communi-T Publications, P.O. Box 2170, Teaneck, NJ 07666. Phone: (201) 836-5030. Monthly.

MEDOC: Index to U.S. Government Publications in the Medical and Health Sciences. Spencer S. Eccles Health Sciences Library, University of Utah, Bldg. 589, Salt Lake City, UT 84112. Phone: (801) 581-5268. Quarterly.

ASSOCIATIONS, PROFESSIONAL SOCIETIES, ADVOCACY AND SUPPORT GROUPS

American Association of Retired Persons. 1909 K St. N.W., Washington, DC 20049. Phone: (202) 872-4700.

The Campaign for Women's Health. 666 11th St. N.W., Ste. 700, Washington, DC 20001. Phone: (202) 783-6686.

Institute for Medical Record Economics. 567 Walnut St., Newtonville, MA 02160. Phone: (617) 964-3923.

National Council Against Health Fraud. P.O. Box 1276, Loma Linda, CA 92354. Phone: (714) 824-4690.

People's Medical Society. 462 Walnut St., Allentown, PA 18102. Phone: (215) 770-1670.

Public Citizen Health Research Group (PCHRG). 2000 P St. N.W., Ste. 700, Washington, DC 20036. Phone: (202) 872-0320.

BIBLIOGRAPHIES

Consumer Health Information Source Book. Alan Rees, Catherine Hoffman. Oryx Press, 4041 N. Central, Suite 700, Phoenix, AZ 85012. Phone: (800) 279-6799. Fax: (800) 279-4663. Third edition 1990.

Core Collection in Nursing and the Allied Health Sciences: Books, Journal, Media. Oryx Press, 4041 N. Central, Suite 700, Phoenix, AZ 85012. Phone: (800) 279-ORYX. Fax: (800) 279-4663. 1990.

DIRECTORIES

The Best in Medicine: How and Where to Find the Best Health Care Available. Herbert J. Dietrich, Virginia H. Biddle. Crown Publishing Group, Inc., 201 E. 50th St., New York, NY 10022. Phone: (800) 726-0600. 1990.

National Healthlines Directory. Louanne Marinos. Information Resources Press, 1110 N. Glebe Rd., Ste. 550, Arlington, VA 22201. Phone: (703) 558-8270. Fax: (703) 558-4979. 1992.

NEWSLETTERS

Health Facts. Center for Medical Consumers, 237 Thompson St., New York, NY 10012. Phone: (212) 674-7105. Monthly.

Health Letter. Public Citizen Health Research Group, 2000 P St. N.W., Ste. 700, Washington, DC 20036. Phone: (202) 872-0320. Monthly.

People's Medical Society-Newsletter. People's Medical Society, 462 Walnut St., Allentown, PA 18102. Phone: (215) 770-1670. Bimonthly.

POPULAR WORKS AND PATIENT EDUCATION

150 Ways to Be a Savvy Medical Consumer. Charles B. Inlander. People's Medical Society, 462 Walnut St., Allentown, PA 18102. Phone: (215) 770-1670. 1992.

Best Medicine: Your Essential Guide to Finding Top Doctors, Hospitals and Treatments. Robert Arnot. Addison-Wesley Publishing Co., Rte. 128, Reading, MA 01867. Phone: (800) 447-2226. 1992.

A Doctor's Guide to the Best Medical Care: A Practical, No-Nonsense Evaluation of Your Treatment Options for Over 100 Conditions and Diseases. Michael Oppenheim. Rodale Press, Inc., 33 E. Minor St., Emmaus, PA 18098. Phone: (800) 527-8200. Fax: (215) 967-6263. 1992.

Getting the Most for Your Medical Dollar. Charles B. Inlander, Karla Morales. Random House, Inc., 201 E. 50th St., New York, NY 10022. Phone: (800) 726-0600. 1991.

The Great White Lie: How America's Hospitals Betray Our Trust and Endanger Our Lives. Walt Bogdanich. Simon & Schuster, Inc., 1230 Ave. of the Americas, New York, NY 10020. Phone: (212) 698-7000. 1991.

Health Schemes, Scams, and Frauds. Stephen Barrett. Consumer Reports Books, 101 Truman Ave., Yonkers, NY 10703. Phone: (914) 378-2000. 1990.

The Heart Surgery Trap: Why Most Invasive Procedures Are Unnecessary and How to Avoid Them. Julian Whitaker. Simon & Schuster, Inc., 1230 Ave. of the Americas, New York, NY 10020. Phone: (212) 698-7000. 1992.

Medicine on Trial: The Appalling Story of Medical Ineptitude and the Arrogance that Overlooks It. Charles B. Inlander, Lowell S. Levin, Ed Weiner. Random House, Inc., 201 E. 50th St., New York, NY 10022. Phone: (800) 726-0600. 1990.

Personal Health Reporter. Alan Rees, Charlene Wiley. Gale Research, Inc., 835 Penobscot Bldg., Detroit, MI 48226-4094. Phone: (800) 877-GALE. Fax: (313) 961-6083. 1992.

The Rights of Patients: The Basic ACLU Guide to Patient Rights. George J. Annas. Southern Illinois University Press, P.O. Box 3697, Carbondale, IL 62902-3697. Phone: (618) 453-2281. 1989.

Savvy Patient: How to Be an Active Participant in Your Medical Care. Daniel Stutz. Consumer Reports Books, 101 Truman Ave., Yonkers, NY 10703. Phone: (914) 378-2000. 1990.

So Your Doctor Recommended Surgery. John Lewis. Holt, Rinehart & Winston, 115 W. 18th St., New York, NY 10011. Phone: (800) 488-5233. 1992.

Take This Book to the Gynecologist with You: Consumer's Guide to Women's Health. Gale Malesky. Addison-Wesley Publishing Co., Rte. 128, Reading, MA 01867. Phone: (800) 447-2226. 1991.

Take This Book to the Hospital with You: A Consumer Guide to Surviving Your Hospital Stay. Charles B. Inlander, Ed. Weiner. Random House, Inc., 201 E. 50th St., New York, NY 10022. Phone: (800) 726-0600. 1991.

Take This Book to the Obstetrician with You: Consumer Guide to Pregnancy and Childbirth. Karen Morales. Addison-Wesley Publishing Co., Rte. 128, Reading, MA 01867. Phone: (800) 447-2226. 1991.

Women's Health Alert: What Most Doctors Won't Tell You About. Sidney M. Wolfe. Addison-Wesley Publishing Co., Rte. 128, Reading, MA 01867. Phone: (800) 447-2226. 1990.

Worst Pills, Best Pills. Sidney Wolf and others. 2000 P St. N.W., Ste. 700, Washington, DC 20036. Phone: (202) 872-0320. 1988.

Your Medical Rights: How to Become and Empowered Consumer. Charles B. Inlander. Little, Brown and Co., 34 Beacon St., Boston, MA 02108. Phone: (617) 227-0730. 1990.

RESEARCH CENTERS, INSTITUTES, CLEARINGHOUSES

Center for Medical Consumers and Health Care Information (CMC). 237 Thompson St., New York, NY 10012. Phone: (212) 674-7105. Fax: (212) 674-7100.

MEDICAL DEVICES AND INSTRUMENTATION

See also: PROSTHESES

ABSTRACTING, INDEXING, AND CURRENT AWARENESS PUBLICATIONS

Excerpta Medica. Section 27: Biophysics, Bioengineering and Medical Instrumentation. Elsevier Science Publishing Co., Inc., P.O. Box 882, Madison Square Station, New York, NY 10159-2101. Phone: (212) 989-5800. Fax: (212) 633-3990. 10/year.

Index Medicus. U.S. National Library of Medicine, 8600 Rockville Pike, Bethesda, MD 20894. Phone: (800) 638-8480. Monthly.

ANNUALS AND REVIEWS

Biomedical Sciences Instrumentation. Instrument Society of America, 67 Alexander Dr., P.O. Box 12277, Research Triangle Park, NC 27709. Phone: (919) 549-8411. Fax: (919) 832-0237. Annual.

ASSOCIATIONS, PROFESSIONAL SOCIETIES, ADVOCACY AND SUPPORT GROUPS

Association for the Advancement of Medical Instrumentation (AAMI). 3330 Washington Blvd., Ste. 400, Arlington, VA 22201-4598. Phone: (800) 332-2264. Fax: (703) 276-0793.

BIBLIOGRAPHIES

Blood Pressure Measuring Devices. National Technical Information Service, 5285 Port Royal Rd., Springfield, VA 22161. Phone: (703) 487-4650. Fax: (703) 321-8547. Jan. 1970 to July 1989 PB89-897154/CBY.

Cardiac Monitors: Design and Applications. National Technical Information Service, 5285 Port Royal Rd., Springfield, VA 22161. Phone: (703) 487-4650. Fax: (703) 321-8547. June 1970 to Oct. 1987 PB88-851647/CBY.

Cardiac Pacemakers. National Technical Information Service, 5285 Port Royal Rd., Springfield, VA 22161. Phone: (703) 487-4650. Fax: (703) 321-8547. Jan. 1976 - Oct. 1987. NTIS order no.: PB88-850797/CBY.

Food and Drug Administration (FDA) Medical Devices Regulatory Information. National Technical Information Service, 5285 Port Royal Rd., Springfield, VA 22161. Phone: (703) 487-4650. Fax: (703) 321-8547. June 1975 to Apr. 1989 PB89-851553/CBY.

CD-ROM DATABASES

Health Devices Alerts. DIALOG Information Services, 3460 Hillview Ave., Palo Alto, CA 94304. Phone: (800) 334-2564. Fax: (415) 858-7069. Quarterly.

Healthcare Product Comparison System. DIALOG Information Services, 3460 Hillview Ave., Palo Alto, CA 94304. Phone: (800) 334-2564. Fax: (415) 858-7069. Quarterly.

Medical Devices-On CD-ROM. FD Inc., 600 New Hampshire Ave. NW, Suite 355, Washington, DC 20037. Phone: (800) 332-6623. Fax: (202) 337-0457. Quarterly.

DIRECTORIES

Association for the Advancement of Medical Instrumentation-Membership Directory. Association for the Advancement of Medical Instrumentation, 3330 Washington Blvd., Ste. 400, Arlington, VA 22201-4598. Phone: (703) 525-4890. Fax: (703) 276-0793. Biennial.

Buyers Guide to Medical Equipment Pricing. Medical Economics, Five Paragon Dr., Montvale, NJ 07645-1742. Phone: (800) 222-3045. Fax: (201) 573-4956. Annual.

Health Devices Sourcebook. Vivian H. Coates, Dorothy Woods (eds.). ECRI, 5200 Butler Pike, Plymouth Meeting, PA 19462. Phone: (215) 825-6000. 1990.

Medical Device Register, Domestic Edition. Medical Economics, Five Paragon Dr., Montvale, NJ 07645-1742. Phone: (800) 222-3045. Fax: (201) 573-4956. Annual.

Medical Device Register, International Edition. Medical Economics, Five Paragon Dr., Montvale, NJ 07645-1742. Phone: (800) 222-3045. Fax: (201) 573-4956. Annual.

Product Development Directory. Medical Economics, Five Paragon Dr., Montvale, NJ 07645-1742. Phone: (800) 222-3045. Fax: (201) 573-4956. Annual.

Product SOS. Medical Economics, Five Paragon Dr., Montvale, NJ 07645-1742. Phone: (800) 222-3045. Fax: (201) 573-4956. Annual.

ENCYCLOPEDIAS, DICTIONARIES, WORD BOOKS

Encyclopedia of Medical Devices and Instrumentation. John G. Webster. John Wiley & Sons, Inc., 605 Third Ave., New York, NY 10158-0012. Phone: (212) 850-6000. Fax: (212) 850-6088. 1988.

JOURNALS

Biomedical Instrumentation & Technology. Hanley & Belfus, Inc., 210 S. 13th St., Philadelphia, PA 19107. Phone: (215) 546-7293. Fax: (215) 790-9330. Bimonthly.

Medical Device Technology. Aster Publishing Company, 859 Willamette St., Eugene, OR 97440. Phone: (503) 343-1200.

Medical Devices, Diagnostics and Instrumentation Reports: The Gray Sheet. F-D-C Reports Inc., 5550 Friendship Blvd., Chevy Chase, MD 20815. Phone: (301) 657-9830.

NEWSLETTERS

Devices and Diagnostics Letter. Washington Business Information, Inc., 1117 N. 19th St., Arlington, VA 22209-1978. Phone: (703) 247-3427. Fax: (703) 247-3421. Weekly.

Health Devices Alerts. Emergency Care Research Institute, 5200 Butler Pike, Plymouth Meeting, PA 19462. Phone: (215) 825-6000. Weekly.

ONLINE DATABASES

EMBASE. Elsevier Science Publishing Co., Inc., P.O. Box 882, Madison Square Station, New York, NY 10159-2101. Phone: (212) 989-5800. Fax: (212) 633-3990.

MEDLINE. National Library of Medicine, 8600 Rockville Pike, Bethesda, MD 20894. Phone: (800) 638-8480.

SciSearch. Institute for Scientific Information, 3501 Market St., Philadelphia, PA 19104. Phone: (215) 386-0100. Fax: (215) 386-6362.

RESEARCH CENTERS, INSTITUTES, CLEARINGHOUSES

Biomedical Computer Laboratory. Washington University. 700 S. Euclid, St. Louis, MO 63110. Phone: (314) 362-2135.

Biomedical Computing Laboratory. University of Wisconsin-Madison. Dept. of Electrical and Computer Engineering, 1415 Johnson Dr., Madison, WI 53706. Phone: (608) 263-1581.

Food and Drug Administration. 5600 Fishers Lane, Rockville, MD 20857. Phone: (301) 443-2410.

Knowledge Systems Laboratory. Stanford University. 701 C Welch Rd., Palo Alto, CA 94304. Phone: (415) 723-4878. Fax: (415) 723-5850.

Laboratory of Electronics. Rockefeller University. 1230 York Ave., New York, NY 10021. Phone: (212) 570-8613.

TEXTBOOKS AND MONOGRAPHS

Advanced Medical Instrumentation and Equipment. Susan E. Suthphin. Prentice Hall, 113 Sylvan Ave., Rt. 9W, Prentice Hall Bldg., Englewood Cliffs, NJ 07632. Phone: (201) 767-5937. 1987.

The Medical Device Industry: Technology and Regulation. Estrin. Marcel Dekker, Inc., 270 Madison Ave., New York, NY 10016. Phone: (800) 228-1160. 1990.

New Medical Devices: Invention, Development and Use. National Academy of Engineering. National Academy Press, 2101 Constitution Ave., N.W., Washington, DC 20418. Phone: (800) 642-6242. 1988.

MEDICAL ECONOMICS

See: HEALTH CARE FINANCING

MEDICAL EDUCATION

ABSTRACTING, INDEXING, AND CURRENT AWARENESS PUBLICATIONS

Cumulative Index to Nursing and Allied Health Literature. Glendale Adventist Medical Center, P.O. Box 871, Glendale, CA 91209. Phone: (818) 409-8005. Bimonthly.

Index Medicus. U.S. National Library of Medicine, 8600 Rockville Pike, Bethesda, MD 20894. Phone: (800) 638-8480. Monthly.

ANNUALS AND REVIEWS

Springer Series on Medical Education. Springer Publishing Co., Inc., 536 Broadway, 11th Floor, New York, NY 10012. Phone: (212) 431-4370. Annual.

ASSOCIATIONS, PROFESSIONAL SOCIETIES, ADVOCACY AND SUPPORT GROUPS

Association of Academic Health Centers. 11 Dupont Circle N.W., Washington, DC 20036. Phone: (202) 265-9600.

Association of American Medical Colleges. One Dupont Circle N.W., Suite 200, Washington, DC 20036. Phone: (202) 828-0400.

Council on Medical Education. American Medical Association, 515 N. State St., Chicago, IL 60610. Phone: (312) 464-5000. Fax: (312) 645-4184.

Education and Research Foundation. American Medical Association, 515 N. State St., Chicago, IL 60610. Phone: (312) 464-5000. Fax: (312) 645-4184.

Educational Commission for Foreign Medical Graduates. 3624 Market St., Philadelphia, PA 19104. Phone: (215) 386-5900.

Liaison Committee on Medical Education. Association of American Medical Colleges, One Dupont Circle N.W., Washington, DC 20036. Phone: (202) 828-0670.

National Board of Medical Examiners. 3930 Chestnut St., Philadelphia, PA 19104. Phone: (215) 349-6400.

National League for Nursing (NLN). 350 Hudson St., New York, NY 10014. Phone: (212) 989-9393.

Student National Medical Association. 1012 10th St. N.W., Washington, DC 20001. Phone: (202) 371-1616.

CD-ROM DATABASES

LektureTek. LectureTek, Inc., P.O. Box 34140, Indianapolis, IN 46234-0140. Phone: (800) 243-0248. Fax: (317) 852-5552. Bimonthly.

Nursing and Allied Health (CINAHL) on CD-ROM. CINAHL, 1509 Wilson Terrace, P.O. Box 871, Glendale, CA 91209-0871. Phone: (818) 409-8005.

DIRECTORIES

Association of American Medical Colleges Group on Public Affairs--Membership Directory. Association of American Medical Colleges, One Dupont Circle N.W., Suite 200, Washington, DC 20036. Phone: (202) 828-0400. Annual.

Barron's Guide to Medical and Dental Schools. Barron's Educational Series, Inc., P.O. Box 8040, 250 Wireless Blvd., Hauppauge, NY 11788. Phone: (516) 434-3311. Fax: (516) 434-3723. Biennial.

Curriculum Directory. Association of American Medical Colleges, One Dupont Circle N.W., Suite 200, Washington, DC 20036. Phone: (202) 828-0400. Annual.

Directory of American Medical Education. Association of American Medical Colleges, One Dupont Circle N.W., Suite 200, Washington, DC 20036. Phone: (202) 828-0400. Annual.

Directory of Graduate Medical Programs. American Medical Association, 515 North State St., Chicago, IL 60610. Phone: (312) 464-0183. Fax: (312) 464-5834. Annual.

Directory of Medical Schools Worldwide. U.S. Directory Service, 655 N.W. 128th St., P.O. Box 68-1700, Miami, FL 33168. Phone: (305) 769-1700. Irregular.

Medical School Admission Requirements--United States and Canada. Association of American Medical Colleges, One Dupont Circle N.W., Suite 200, Washington, DC 20036. Phone: (202) 828-0400. Annual.

World Directory of Medical Schools. World Health Organization, Ave. Appia, CH-1211, Geneva 27, Switzerland. Sixth edition 1988.

HANDBOOKS, GUIDES, MANUALS, ATLASES

Handbook of Pharmacy Health Education. Martin. Pharmaceutical Press, Rittenhouse Book Distributors, 511 Feheley Dr., King of Prussia, PA 19406. Phone: (800) 345-6425. Fax: (800) 223-7488. 1991.

JOURNALS

Academic Medicine. Association of American Medical Colleges, 1 Dupont Circle NW, Suite 200, Washington, DC 20036. Phone: (202) 828-0416. Fax: (202) 785-5027. Monthly.

Humane Medicine. Canadian Medical Association, 1867 Alta Vista Drive, Box 8650, Ottawa, ON, Canada K1G 0G8. Phone: (613) 731-9331. Fax: (613) 731-4797. Quarterly.

Journal of Audiovisual Media in Medicine. Butterworth-Heinemann, 80 Montvale Ave., Stoneham, MA 02180. Phone: (617) 438-8464. Fax: (617) 279-4851.

Journal of Pharmacy Teaching. Haworth Press, 10 Alice Street, Binghamton, NY 13904-1580. Phone: (800) 342-9678. Fax: (607) 722-1424. Quarterly.

Media Profiles: The Health Sciences Edition. Olympic Media Information, 100 Vandewater Rd., West Park, NY 12493-0190. Phone: (914) 384-6563. Quarterly.

Medical Education. Blackwell Scientific Publications, Inc., 3 Cambridge Center, Cambridge, MA 02142. Phone: (800) 759-6102.

ONLINE DATABASES

EMBASE. Elsevier Science Publishing Co., Inc., P.O. Box 882, Madison Square Station, New York, NY 10159-2101. Phone: (212) 989-5800. Fax: (212) 633-3990.

MEDLINE. National Library of Medicine, 8600 Rockville Pike, Bethesda, MD 20894. Phone: (800) 638-8480.

Nursing and Allied Health (CINAHL). CINAHL, 1509 Wilson Terrace, P.O. Box 871, Glendale, CA 91209-0871. Phone: (818) 409-8005.

SciSearch. Institute for Scientific Information, 3501 Market St., Philadelphia, PA 19104. Phone: (215) 386-0100. Fax: (215) 386-6362.

RESEARCH CENTERS, INSTITUTES, CLEARINGHOUSES

Center for Research in Medical Education and Health Care. Thomas Jefferson University. Jefferson Medical College, 1025 Walnut St., Rm. 119, Philadelphia, PA 19107. Phone: (215) 955-9807. Fax: (215) 923-6939.

National Resident Matching Program. One American Plaza, No. 807, Evanston, IL 60201. Phone: (312) 328-3440.

MEDICAL ETHICS

See also: DEATH AND DYING

ABSTRACTING, INDEXING, AND CURRENT AWARENESS PUBLICATIONS

Cumulative Index to Nursing and Allied Health Literature. Glendale Adventist Medical Center, P.O. Box 871, Glendale, CA 91209. Phone: (818) 409-8005. Bimonthly.

Excerpta Medica. Section 17: Public Health, Social Medicine and Epidemiology. Elsevier Science Publishing Co., Inc., P.O. Box 882, Madison Square Station, New York, NY 10159-2101. Phone: (212) 989-5800. Fax: (212) 633-3990. 24/year.

Index Medicus. U.S. National Library of Medicine, 8600 Rockville Pike, Bethesda, MD 20894. Phone: (800) 638-8480. Monthly.

Science Citation Index. Institute for Scientific Information, 3501 Market St., Philadelphia, PA 19104. Phone: (800) 523-1850. Fax: (215) 386-6362. Bimonthly.

ANNUALS AND REVIEWS

Bioethics Yearbook. Kluwer Academic Publishers, P.O. Box 358, Accord Station, Hingham, MA 02018-0358. Phone: (617) 871-6600. Fax: (617) 871-6528. Annual.

Biomedical Ethics Reviews. Humana Press, 999 Riverview Dr., Suite 208, Totowa, NJ 07512. Phone: (201) 256-1699. Annual.

Medical Ethics Series. Indiana University Press, 601 N. Morton St., Bloomington, IN 47404-3797. Phone: (812) 855-4203. Irregular.

BIBLIOGRAPHIES

Bibliography of Bioethics. Kennedy Institute of Ethics, National Center for Bioethics Literature, Georgetown University, Washington, DC 20057. Phone: (202) 687-6771. Annual.

CD-ROM DATABASES

Nursing and Allied Health (CINAHL) on CD-ROM. CINAHL, 1509 Wilson Terrace, P.O. Box 871, Glendale, CA 91209-0871. Phone: (818) 409-8005.

SCISEARCH. Institute for Scientific Information, 3501 Market St., Philadelphia, PA 19104. Phone: (215) 386-0100. Fax: (215) 386-6362.

HANDBOOKS, GUIDES, MANUALS, ATLASES

Infertility: A Clinician's Guide to Diagnosis and Treatment. Melvin L. Taymor. Plenum Publishing Co., 233 Spring St., New York, NY 10013-1578. Phone: (212) 620-8000. Fax: (212) 463-0742. 1990.

JOURNALS

Bulletin of Medical Ethics. BMJ Publishing Group, BMA House, Tavistock Square, London WC1H 9JR, England. Phone: 071-383 6244/6638. Fax: 071-383 6662. 10/year.

Cambridge Quarterly of Healthcare Ethics. Cambridge University Press, 40 W. 20th St., New York, NY 10011. Phone: (800) 431-1580. Quarterly.

Hastings Center Report. Hastings Center, 255 Elm Rd., Briarcliff Manor, NY 10510-9974. Phone: (914) 762-8500.

Journal of Genetic Counseling. Human Sciences Press, 233 Spring St., New York, NY 10013-1578. Phone: (800) 221-9369. Fax: (212) 807-1047. Quarterly.

Journal of Medical Ethics. BMJ Publishing Group, BMA House, Tavistock Square, London WC1H 9JR, England. Phone: 071-383 6244/6638. Fax: 071-383 6662. Quarterly.

NEWSLETTERS

Medical Ethics Advisor. American Health Consultants, Department C1290, P.O. Box 740060, Atlanta, GA 30374. Phone: (800) 559-1032. Monthly.

ONLINE DATABASES

EMBASE. Elsevier Science Publishing Co., Inc., P.O. Box 882, Madison Square Station, New York, NY 10159-2101. Phone: (212) 989-5800. Fax: (212) 633-3990.

MEDLINE. National Library of Medicine, 8600 Rockville Pike, Bethesda, MD 20894. Phone: (800) 638-8480.

Nursing and Allied Health (CINAHL). CINAHL, 1509 Wilson Terrace, P.O. Box 871, Glendale, CA 91209-0871. Phone: (818) 409-8005.

SciSearch. Institute for Scientific Information, 3501 Market St., Philadelphia, PA 19104. Phone: (215) 386-0100. Fax: (215) 386-6362.

POPULAR WORKS AND PATIENT EDUCATION

Ethics on Call: A Medical Ethicist Shows How to Take Charge of Life-and-Death Choices. Nancy Dubler, David Nimmons. Random House, Inc., 201 E. 50th St., New York, NY 10022. Phone: (800) 726-0600. 1992.

Euthanasia: The Moral Issues. Robert M. Baird, Stuart E. Rosenbaum (eds.). Prometheus Books, 700 E. Amherst St., Buffalo, NY 14215. Phone: (800) 421-0351. 1989.

What Kind of Life: The Limits of Medical Progress. Daniel Callahan. Simon & Schuster, Inc., 1230 Ave. of the Americas, New York, NY 10020. Phone: (212) 698-7000. 1990.

RESEARCH CENTERS, INSTITUTES, CLEARINGHOUSES

Center for Bioethics. Clinical Research Institute of Montreal, 110 Pine Ave. W., Montreal, PQ, Canada H2W 1R7. Phone: (514) 987-5615. Fax: (514) 987-5695.

Center for Biomedical Ethics. Case Western Reserve University. School of Medicine, Cleveland, OH 44106. Phone: (216) 368-6196.

The Hastings Center. 255 Elm Rd., Briarcliff Manor, NY 10510-9974. Phone: (914) 762-8500. Fax: (914) 762-2124.

Human Life Center. University of Steubenville, Steubenville, OH 43952. Phone: (614) 282-9953.

Institute for Jewish Medical Ethics. 645 14th Ave., San Francisco, CA 94118. Phone: (415) 752-7333. Fax: (415) 752-5851.

Kennedy Institute of Ethics. Georgetown University. Washington, DC 20057. Phone: (202) 687-6774. Fax: (202) 687-6770.

Pope John XXIII Medical Moral Research and Education Center. 186 Forbes Rd., Braintree, MA 02184. Phone: (617) 848-6965. Fax: (617) 849-1309.

STANDARDS AND STATISTICS SOURCES

1992 Code of Medical Ethics: Annotated Current Opinions. American Medical Association, 515 North State St., Chicago, IL 60610. Phone: (312) 464-0183. Fax: (312) 464-5834. 1992.

TEXTBOOKS AND MONOGRAPHS

Annotated Current Opinions of the Council of Ethics & Judicial Affairs. American Medical Association, 515 North State St., Chicago, IL 60610. Phone: (312) 464-0183. Fax: (312) 464-5834. 1990.

Clinical Ethics. Albert R. Jonsen, Mark Siegler, William J. Winslade. McGraw-Hill, Inc., Health Professions Division, 1221 Avenue of the Americas, 28th Floor, New York, NY 10020. Phone: (212) 512-4228. Third edition 1992.

Clinical Medical Ethics: Cases in Practice. Terry M. Perlin. Little, Brown and Company, 34 Beacon St., Boston, MA 02108. Phone: (617) 227-0730. 1992.

Doctors' Decisions: Ethical Conflicts in Medical Practice. G.R. Dunstan, E.A. Shinebourne. Oxford University Press, 200 Madison Ave., New York, NY 10016. Phone: (212) 679-7300. 1989.

Ethical Problems in Dialysis and Transplantation. Carl M. Kjellstrand, John B. Dossetor (eds.). Kluwer Academic Publishers, P.O. Box 358, Accord Station, Hingham, MA 02018-0358. Phone: (617) 871-6600. Fax: (617) 871-6528. 1992.

Ethics in Health Education. Spyros Doxiadis (ed.). John Wiley & Sons, Inc., 605 Third Ave., New York, NY 10158-0012. Phone: (212) 850-6000. Fax: (212) 850-6088. 1990.

Ethics and Law in Health Care and Research. Peter Byrne (ed.). John Wiley & Sons, Inc., 605 Third Ave., New York, NY 10158-0012. Phone: (212) 850-6000. Fax: (212) 850-6088. 1990.

Life Before Birth: The Moral and Legal Status of Embryos and Fetuses. Bonnie Steinbock. Oxford University Press, 200 Madison Ave., New York, NY 10016. Phone: (212) 679-7300. 1992.

Medicine, Medical Ethics and the Value of Life. P. Byrne. John Wiley & Sons, Inc., 605 Third Ave., New York, NY 10158-0012. Phone: (212) 850-6000. Fax: (212) 850-6088. 1989.

Practical Medical Ethics. Grant Gillett, Alastair Campbell, Gareth Jones. Oxford University Press, 200 Madison Ave., New York, NY 10016. Phone: (212) 679-7300. 1992.

Psychiatric Ethics. Sidney Bloch, Paul Chodoff (eds.). Oxford University Press, 200 Madison Ave., New York, NY 10016. Phone: (212) 679-7300. Second edition 1991.

Textbook of Medical Ethics. Erich H. Loewy. Plenum Publishing Co., 233 Spring St., New York, NY 10013-1578. Phone: (212) 620-8000. Fax: (212) 463-0742. 1989.

MEDICAL GENETICS

See: GENETICS

MEDICAL ILLUSTRATION

ABSTRACTING, INDEXING, AND CURRENT AWARENESS PUBLICATIONS

Index Medicus. U.S. National Library of Medicine, 8600 Rockville Pike, Bethesda, MD 20894. Phone: (800) 638-8480. Monthly.

ASSOCIATIONS, PROFESSIONAL SOCIETIES, ADVOCACY AND SUPPORT GROUPS

Association of Medical Illustrators (AMI). 2692 Huguenot Springs Rd., Midlothian, VA 23113. Phone: (804) 794-2908. Fax: (804) 379-8260.

Biological Photographic Association. 115 Stoneridge Dr., Chapel Hill, NC 27514. Phone: (919) 967-8247.

Ophthalmic Photographers Society. c/o Mark Malo, Erie County Medical Center, 462 Grider St., Buffalo, NY 14215. Phone: (716) 898-3940.

DIRECTORIES

Allied Health Education Directory. American Medical Association, 515 North State St., Chicago, IL 60610. Phone: (312) 464-0183. Fax: (312) 464-5834. Annual.

Association of Medical Illustrators--Membership Directory. The Association of Medical Illustrators, 1819 Peachtree St. N.E., Station 560, Atlanta, GA 30309. Phone: (404) 350-7900. Annual.

Biological Photographic Association--Membership Directory. Biological Photographic Association, 115 Stoneridge Dr., Chapel Hill, NC 27514. Phone: (919) 967-8247. Annual.

Medical Illustration Sourcebook. The Association of Medical Illustrators, 1819 Peachtree St. N.E., Station 560, Atlanta, GA 30309. Phone: (404) 350-7900. Biennial.

Ophthalmic Photographers' Society--Directory. Ophthalmic Photographers Society, c/o Mark Malo, Erie County Medical Center, 462 Grider St., Buffalo, NY 14215. Phone: (716) 898-3940. Annual.

JOURNALS

Journal of Audiovisual Media in Medicine. Butterworth-Heinemann, 80 Montvale Ave., Stoneham, MA 02180. Phone: (617) 438-8464. Fax: (617) 279-4851.

ONLINE DATABASES

EMBASE. Elsevier Science Publishing Co., Inc., P.O. Box 882, Madison Square Station, New York, NY 10159-2101. Phone: (212) 989-5800. Fax: (212) 633-3990.

MEDLINE. National Library of Medicine, 8600 Rockville Pike, Bethesda, MD 20894. Phone: (800) 638-8480.

SciSearch. Institute for Scientific Information, 3501 Market St., Philadelphia, PA 19104. Phone: (215) 386-0100. Fax: (215) 386-6362.

RESEARCH CENTERS, INSTITUTES, CLEARINGHOUSES

Center for Medical Illustration. Armed Forces Institute of Pathology, Washington, DC 20306.

MEDICAL LIBRARIES

ABSTRACTING, INDEXING, AND CURRENT AWARENESS PUBLICATIONS

Cumulative Index to Nursing and Allied Health Literature. Glendale Adventist Medical Center, P.O. Box 871, Glendale, CA 91209. Phone: (818) 409-8005. Bimonthly.

Hospital Literature Index. American Hospital Association, 840 N. Lake Shore Dr., Chicago, IL 60611. Phone: (800) 242-2626. Fax: (312) 280-6015. Quarterly.

ASSOCIATIONS, PROFESSIONAL SOCIETIES, ADVOCACY AND SUPPORT GROUPS

Association of Academic Health Sciences Library Directors. c/o Richard Lyders, Houston Academy of Medicine, Texas Medical Center Library, Houston, TX 77030. Phone: (713) 797-1230.

Association of Libraries in the History of the Health Sciences. c/o Mr. Glen Jenkins, Allen Memorial Library, 1100 Euclid Ave., Cleveland, OH 44106. Phone: (216) 368-3649.

Canadian Health Libraries Association. P.O. Box 434, Station K, Toronto, ON, Canada M4P 2G9.

Medical Library Association. 6 N. Michigan Ave., No. 300, Chicago, IL 60602. Phone: (312) 419-9094. Fax: (312) 419-8950.

BIBLIOGRAPHIES

Core Collection of Medical Books and Journals 1992. Howard Hague, Michael Jackson. Medical Information Working Party, Henry Hochland, Haigh and Hochland Ltd., The Precinct Ctr., Oxford Rd., Manchester M13 9QA, England. 1992.

Information Sources in the Medical Sciences. Leslie Morton, Shane Godbolt (eds.). R.R. Bowker Co., 245 W. 17th St., New York, NY 10011. Phone: (800) 521-8110. Fourth edition 1992.

Medical and Health Care Books and Serials in Print. R.R. Bowker Co., 245 W. 17th St., New York, NY 10011. Phone: (800) 521-8110. Fax: (908) 665-6688. Annual.

CD-ROM DATABASES

Nursing and Allied Health (CINAHL) on CD-ROM. CINAHL, 1509 Wilson Terrace, P.O. Box 871, Glendale, CA 91209-0871. Phone: (818) 409-8005.

DIRECTORIES

Medical and Health Information Directory. Karen Backus (ed.). Gale Research, Inc., 835 Penobscot Bldg., Detroit, MI 48226-4094. Phone: (800) 877-4253. Fax: (313) 961-6083. Fifth edition Three volumes 1990.

Medical Library Association-Directory. Medical Library Association, 6 N. Michigan Ave., No. 300, Chicago, IL 60602. Phone: (312) 419-9094. Fax: (312) 419-8950. Annual.

World Directory of Biological and Medical Sciences Libraries. R.R. Bowker Co., 245 W. 17th St., New York, NY 10011. Phone: (800) 521-8110. Fax: (908) 665-6688. 1988.

HANDBOOKS, GUIDES, MANUALS, ATLASES

Handbook of Medical Library Practice. L. Darling, and others. Medical Library Association, 6 N. Michigan Ave., No. 300, Chicago, IL 60602. Phone: (312) 419-9094. Fax: (312) 419-8950. 1988.

Medical Subject Headings: Annotated Alphabetic List. National Library of Medicine, 8600 Rockville Pike, Bethesda, MD 20894. Phone: (800) 638-8480. 1992.

Medical Subject Headings: Tree Structures. National Library of Medicine, 8600 Rockville Pike, Bethesda, MD 20894. Phone: (800) 638-8480. 1992.

JOURNALS

Bulletin of the Medical Library Association. Medical Library Association, Six N. Michigan Ave., Chicago, IL 60602. Phone: (312) 419-9094. Fax: (312) 419-8950. Quarterly.

Health Libraries Review. Blackwell Scientific Publications, Inc., 3 Cambridge Center, Cambridge, MA 02142. Phone: (800) 759-6102.

Medical Reference Series Quarterly. Haworth Press, 10 Alice St., Binghamton, NY 13904-1580. Phone: (803) 429-6784. Fax: (607) 722-1424. Quarterly.

NEWSLETTERS

MLA News. Medical Library Association, 6 N. Michigan Ave., No. 300, Chicago, IL 60602. Phone: (312) 419-9094. Fax: (312) 419-8950.

ONLINE DATABASES

Nursing and Allied Health (CINAHL). CINAHL, 1509 Wilson Terrace, P.O. Box 871, Glendale, CA 91209-0871. Phone: (818) 409-8005.

RESEARCH CENTERS, INSTITUTES, CLEARINGHOUSES

Knowledge Systems Laboratory. Stanford University. 701 C Welch Rd., Palo Alto, CA 94304. Phone: (415) 723-4878. Fax: (415) 723-5850.

U.S. National Library of Medicine. 8600 Rockville Pike, Bethesda, MD 20894. Phone: (800) 638-8480.

TEXTBOOKS AND MONOGRAPHS

End User Searching in the Health Sciences. M. Sandra Wood, Ellen Brassil Horak, Bonnie Snow (eds.). Haworth Press, 10 Alice St., Binghamton, NY 13904-1580. Phone: (803) 429-6784. Fax: (607) 722-1424.

Information Searching in Health Care. Renee May Williams, Lynda M. Baker, Joanne G. Marshall. SLACK Inc., 6900 Grove Rd., Thorofare, NJ 08086-9447. Phone: (800) 257-8290. Fax: (609) 853-5991. 1991.

The Integrated Medical Library. Helis Miido. CRC Press, Inc., 2000 Corporate Blvd. N.W., Boca Raton, FL 33431. Phone: (407) 994-0555. Fax: (407) 997-0949. 1991.

MEDICAL AND NURSING INFORMATICS

ABSTRACTING, INDEXING, AND CURRENT AWARENESS PUBLICATIONS

Index Medicus. U.S. National Library of Medicine, 8600 Rockville Pike, Bethesda, MD 20894. Phone: (800) 638-8480. Monthly.

Research Alert: Computer Applications in Medicine. Institute for Scientific Information, 3501 Market St., Philadelphia, PA 19104. Phone: (800) 523-1850. Fax: (215) 386-6362. Weekly.

ANNUALS AND REVIEWS

15th Annual Symposium on Computer Applications in Medical Care. American Medical Informatics Association. McGraw-Hill, Inc., Health Professions Division, 1221 Avenue of the Americas, 28th Floor, New York, NY 10020. Phone: (212) 512-4228. 1992.

ASSOCIATIONS, PROFESSIONAL SOCIETIES, ADVOCACY AND SUPPORT GROUPS

American Association for Medical Systems and Informatics. 1101 Connecticut Ave., Washington, DC 20036. Phone: (202) 857-1189.

American Medical Informatics Association (AMIA). 1101 Connecticut Ave. N.W., Ste. 700, Washington, DC 20036. Phone: (202) 857-1189.

International Medical Informatics Association. c/o Mr. J. Flint, 10 Trench St., Richmond Hill, ON, Canada L4C 4Z3.

MUMPS Users' Group. 4321 Hartwick Rd., No. 100, College Park, MD 20740. Phone: (301) 779-6555.

Special Interest Group on Biomedical Computing. c/o William E. Hammond, Box 2914, Duke University Medical Center, Durham, NC 27710. Phone: (919) 684-6421.

BIBLIOGRAPHIES

Computer Aided Medical Diagnosis. National Technical Information Service, 5285 Port Royal Rd., Springfield, VA 22161. Phone: (703) 487-4650. Fax: (703) 321-8547. May 1986-Jan. 1989 PB89-855100/CBY.

JOURNALS

Academic Medicine. Association of American Medical Colleges, 1 Dupont Circle NW, Suite 200, Washington, DC 20036. Phone: (202) 828-0416. Fax: (202) 785-5027. Monthly.

British Journal of Anaesthesia. BMJ Publishing Group, BMA House, Tavistock Square, London WC1H 9JR, England. Phone: 071-383 6244/6638. Fax: 071-383 6662. Monthly.

Computer Methods and Programs in Biomedicine. Elsevier Science Publishing Co., Inc., P.O. Box 882, Madison Square Station, New York, NY 10159-2101. Phone: (212) 989-5800. Fax: (212) 633-3990. 12/year.

Computers and Biomedical Research. Academic Press, Inc., 1250 Sixth Ave., San Diego, CA 92101-4311. Phone: (619) 699-6345. Fax: (619) 699-6715. Bimonthly.

International Journal of Bio-Medical Computing. Elsevier Science Publishing Co., Inc., P.O. Box 882, Madison Square Station, New York, NY 10159-2101. Phone: (212) 989-5800. Fax: (212) 633-3990. 8/year.

Journal of Dental Education. American Associatoin of Dental Schools, 1625 Massachusetts Ave. N.W., Washington, DC 20036. Phone: (202) 667-9433. Monthly.

M.D. Computing. Springer-Verlag New York Inc., 175 Fifth Ave., New York, NY 10010. Phone: (212) 460-1500. Fax: (212) 473-6272. 6/year.

Medical Informatics: An International Journal of Computing in Health Care. Taylor & Francis Inc., 1900 Frost Rd., Suite 101,

Bristol, PA 19007-1598. Phone: (800) 821-8312. Fax: (215) 785-5515. Quarterly.

Physicians and Computers. Physicians and Computers, 2333 Waukegan Rd., Bannockburn, IL 60015. Phone: (708) 940-8333.

RESEARCH CENTERS, INSTITUTES, CLEARINGHOUSES

Biomedical Information Communication Center. Oregon Health Sciences University. 3181 S.W. Sam Jackson Park Rd., Portland, OR 97201-3098. Phone: (503) 494-4502. Fax: (503) 494-4551.

U.S. National Library of Medicine. 8600 Rockville Pike, Bethesda, MD 20894. Phone: (800) 638-8480.

TEXTBOOKS AND MONOGRAPHS

Computers in Obstetrics and Gynecology. K.J. Dalton, T. Chard (eds.). Elsevier Science Publishing Co., Inc., P.O. Box 882, Madison Square Station, New York, NY 10159-2101. Phone: (212) 989-5800. Fax: (212) 633-3990. 1990.

Computers and Perinatal Medicine. K. Maeda, M. Hogaki, H. Nakano (eds.). Elsevier Science Publishing Co., Inc., P.O. Box 882, Madison Square Station, New York, NY 10159-2101. Phone: (212) 989-5800. Fax: (212) 633-3990. 1990.

Dental Informatics. Abbey. Springer-Verlag New York Inc., 175 Fifth Ave., New York, NY 10010. Phone: (212) 460-1500. Fax: (212) 473-6272. 1992.

Expert Systems and Decision Support in Medicine. O. Rienhoff, B. Schneider (eds.). Springer-Verlag New York Inc., 175 Fifth Ave., New York, NY 10010. Phone: (212) 460-1500. Fax: (212) 473-6272. 1988.

Health Care Computer Systems for the 1990s: Critical Executive Decisions. Bernie Minard. Health Administration Press, 1021 E. Huron St., Ann Arbor, MI 48104-9990. Phone: (313) 764-1380. Fax: (313) 763-1105. 1991.

History of Medical Informatics. Bruce I. Blum, Karen Duncan. Addison-Wesley Publishing Co., Rte. 128, Reading, MA 01867. Phone: (800) 447-2226. 1990.

Managing Computers in Health Care: A Guide for Professionals. John Abbott Worthley, Philip DiSalvio. Health Administration Press, 1021 E. Huron St., Ann Arbor, MI 48104-9990. Phone: (313) 764-1380. Fax: (313) 763-1105. 1989.

Medical Informatics: Computer Applications in Health Care. Edward H. Shortliffe, Leslie E. Perreault, and others. Addison-Wesley Publishing Co., Rte. 128, Reading, MA 01867. Phone: (800) 447-2226. 1990.

Nursing Informatics. M.J. Ball, K.J. Hannah, U. Gerdin-Jelger, H. Peterson (eds.). Springer-Verlag New York Inc., 175 Fifth Ave., New York, NY 10010. Phone: (212) 460-1500. Fax: (212) 473-6272. 1989.

Nursing Informatics '91: Pre-Conference Proceedings. J.P. Turley, S.K. Newbold (eds.). Springer-Verlag New York Inc., 175 Fifth Ave., New York, NY 10010. Phone: (212) 460-1500. Fax: (212) 473-6272. 1991.

Nursing Informatics '91: Proceedings of the Fourth International Conference on Nursing Use of Computers and Information Science. Melbourne, Australia. J. Hovenga, K.J.

Hannah, K.A. McCormick, J. Ronald (eds.). Springer-Verlag New York Inc., 175 Fifth Ave., New York, NY 10010. Phone: (212) 460-1500. Fax: (212) 473-6272. 1991.

MEDICAL RECORDS

ABSTRACTING, INDEXING, AND CURRENT AWARENESS PUBLICATIONS

Cumulative Index to Nursing and Allied Health Literature. Glendale Adventist Medical Center, P.O. Box 871, Glendale, CA 91209. Phone: (818) 409-8005. Bimonthly.

Hospital Literature Index. American Hospital Association, 840 N. Lake Shore Dr., Chicago, IL 60611. Phone: (800) 242-2626. Fax: (312) 280-6015. Quarterly.

Index Medicus. U.S. National Library of Medicine, 8600 Rockville Pike, Bethesda, MD 20894. Phone: (800) 638-8480. Monthly.

ASSOCIATIONS, PROFESSIONAL SOCIETIES, ADVOCACY AND SUPPORT GROUPS

American Association for Medical Transcription (AAMT). P.O. Box 576187, Modesto, CA 95357. Phone: (209) 551-0883. Fax: (209) 551-9317.

American Medical Record Association (AMRA). 919 N. Michigan Ave., Chicago, IL 60611. Phone: (312) 787-2672.

International Federation of Health Records Organizations (IFHRO). c/o Peggy P. Starks, 1123 Mill Springs, Richardson, TX 75080. Phone: (214) 690-9849.

CD-ROM DATABASES

Nursing and Allied Health (CINAHL) on CD-ROM. CINAHL, 1509 Wilson Terrace, P.O. Box 871, Glendale, CA 91209-0871. Phone: (818) 409-8005.

DIRECTORIES

Accredited Educational Programs in Medical Record Administration. American Medical Record Association, 919 N. Michigan Ave., No. 1400, Chicago, IL 60611. Phone: (312) 787-2672.

ENCYCLOPEDIAS, DICTIONARIES, WORD BOOKS

Glossary of Health Care Terms. American Medical Record Association, 919 N. Michigan Ave., Ste. 1400, Chicago, IL 60611. Phone: (312) 787-2672. Third edition 1986.

HANDBOOKS, GUIDES, MANUALS, ATLASES

CPT Coding Made Easy: A Technical Guide. Gabrelle M. Kotoski. Aspen Publishers, Inc., 200 Orchard Ridge Dr., Gaithersburg, MD 20878. Phone: (800) 638-8437. Second edition 1992.

Current Procedural Terminology (CPT). American Medical Association, 515 N. State St., Chicago, IL 60610. Phone: (312) 464-5000. Fax: (312) 645-4184. 1993.

ICD-10: The International Statistical Classification of Diseases & Related Health Problems. American Psychiatric Press, Inc., 1400 K St. N.W., Washington, DC 20005. Phone: (202) 682-6268. Fax: (202) 789-2648. Three volumes 1992.

Medical Transcription Guide: Do's and Don'ts. Marilyn Takahashi Fordney, Marcy Otis Diehl. W.B. Saunders Co., The Curtis Center, Independence Square W., Philadelphia, PA 19106-3399. Phone: (215) 238-7800. 1990.

Research Manual for the Medical Record Profession. Margret Amatayakul. American Medical Record Association, 919 N. Michigan Ave., Ste. 1400, Chicago, IL 60611. Phone: (312) 787-2672. 1985.

JOURNALS

American Medical Record Association Journal. American Medical Record Association, 919 N. Michigan Ave., Ste. 1400, Chicago, IL 60611. Phone: (312) 787-2672. Monthly.

NEWSLETTERS

CPT Assistant. American Medical Association, 515 N. State St., Chicago, IL 60610. Phone: (312) 464-5000. Fax: (312) 645-4184.

ONLINE DATABASES

EMBASE. Elsevier Science Publishing Co., Inc., P.O. Box 882, Madison Square Station, New York, NY 10159-2101. Phone: (212) 989-5800. Fax: (212) 633-3990.

MEDLINE. National Library of Medicine, 8600 Rockville Pike, Bethesda, MD 20894. Phone: (800) 638-8480.

Nursing and Allied Health (CINAHL). CINAHL, 1509 Wilson Terrace, P.O. Box 871, Glendale, CA 91209-0871. Phone: (818) 409-8005.

SciSearch. Institute for Scientific Information, 3501 Market St., Philadelphia, PA 19104. Phone: (215) 386-0100. Fax: (215) 386-6362.

POPULAR WORKS AND PATIENT EDUCATION

How to Read, Review and Summarize Medical Reecords: A Lay Person's Guide. Sandra Williams. Medi-Research & Review, Inc., P.O. Box 30339, Oklahoma City, OK 73140-3339. Phone: (405) 732-2848. 1987.

TEXTBOOKS AND MONOGRAPHS

The Computer-Based Record: An Essential Technology for Health Care. Richard S. Dick, Elaine B. Steen (eds.). National Academy Press, 2101 Constitution Ave., N.W., Washington, DC 20418. Phone: (800) 642-6242. 1991.

Documenting Care: Communication - The Nursing Process and Documentation Standards. Frances T. Fischbach. F.A. Davis Co., 1915 Arch St., Philadelphia, PA 19103. Phone: (800) 523-4049. Fax: (215) 568-5065. 1991.

Healthcare Records: A Practical Legal Guide. Jonathan P. Tomes. Healthcare Financial Management Association, Two Westbrook Corporate Ctr., Ste. 700, Westchester, IL 60154. Phone: (708) 531-9600. Fax: (708) 531-0032. 1990.

Medical Record Examination Review. Susan Pritchard Bailey. American Medical Record Association, 919 N. Michigan Ave., Ste. 1400, Chicago, IL 60611. Phone: (312) 787-2672. Fifth edition 1989.

Medical Record Management. Edna K. Huffman. Physicians' Record Co., 3000 S. Ridgeland Ave., Berwyn, IL 60402. Phone: (800) 323-9268. Ninth edition 1990.

Medical Records Examination Review. S.P. Bruce. Elsevier Science Publishing Co., Inc., P.O. Box 882, Madison Square Station, New York, NY 10159-2101. Phone: (212) 989-5800. Fax: (212) 633-3990. 1989.

Medical Records Management in a Changing Environment. Susan M. Murphy-Muth. Aspen Publishers, Inc., 200 Orchard Ridge Dr., Gaithersburg, MD 20878. Phone: (800) 638-8437. 1987.

Medical Typing and Transcribing: Techniques and Procedures. Mary Diehl, Marilyn Fordney. W.B. Saunders Co., The Curtis Center, Independence Sqare W., Philadelphia, PA 19106-3399. Phone: (215) 238-7800. 3rd edition, 1991.

Organization of Medical Record Departments in Hospitals. Margaret Skurka. American Hospital Association, 840 N. Lake Shore Dr., Chicago, IL 60611. Phone: (800) 242-2626. Fax: (312) 280-6015. Second edition 1988.

Privacy and Confidentiality of Health Care Information. Jo Anne Czecowski Bruce. American Hospital Association, 840 N. Lake Shore Dr., Chicago, IL 60611. Phone: (800) 242-2626. Fax: (312) 280-6015. Second edition 1988.

Today's Challenge: Content of the Health Record. Barbara Glondys. American Medical Record Association, 919 N. Michigan Ave., Ste. 1400, Chicago, IL 60611. Phone: (312) 787-2672. 1988.

MEDICAL SCHOOLS

See: MEDICAL EDUCATION

MEDICAL STATISTICS

See: BIOSTATISTICS

MEDICAL TECHNOLOGY

See also: LABORATORY MEDICINE

ABSTRACTING, INDEXING, AND CURRENT AWARENESS PUBLICATIONS

Excerpta Medica. Section 16: Cancer. Elsevier Science Publishing Co., Inc., P.O. Box 882, Madison Square Station, New York, NY 10159-2101. Phone: (212) 989-5800. Fax: (212) 633-3990. 32/year.

Index Medicus. U.S. National Library of Medicine, 8600 Rockville Pike, Bethesda, MD 20894. Phone: (800) 638-8480. Monthly.

ANNUALS AND REVIEWS

Advances in Pathology and Laboratory Medicine. Mosby-Year Book, 11830 Westline Industrial Drive, St. Louis, MO 63146. Phone: (800) 325-4177. Fax: (314) 432-1380. Annual.

ASSOCIATIONS, PROFESSIONAL SOCIETIES, ADVOCACY AND SUPPORT GROUPS

American Medical Technologists (AMT). 710 Higgins Rd., Park Ridge, IL 60068. Phone: (708) 823-5169. Fax: (708) 823-0458.

American Society for Medical Technology. 2021 L St. N.W., Suite 400, Washington, DC 20036. Phone: (202) 785-3311.

Canadian Society of Laboratory Technologists. P.O. Box 2830, Hamilton, ON, Canada L8N 3N5. Phone: (416) 528-8642. Fax: (416) 528-4968.

Clinical Laboratory Management Association (CLMA). 195 W. Lancaster Ave., Paoli, PA 19301. Phone: (215) 647-8970. Fax: (215) 889-9731.

HANDBOOKS, GUIDES, MANUALS, ATLASES

Clinical Guide to Laboratory Tests. Norbert W. Tietz (ed.). W.B. Saunders Co., The Curtis Center, Independence Square W., Philadelphia, PA 19106-3399. Phone: (215) 238-7800. Second edition 1990.

Interpretation of Diagnostic Tests. Jacques Wallach. Little, Brown and Company, 34 Beacon St., Boston, MA 02108. Phone: (617) 227-0730. Fifth edition 1992.

Laboratory Test Handbook. David S. Jacobs, Bernard L. Kasten Jr., Wayne R. DeMott. Williams & Wilkins, 428 E. Preston St., Baltimore, MD 21202. Phone: (800) 638-0672. Fax: (800) 447-8438. Second edition 19990.

A Manual of Laboratory and Diagnostic Tests. Frances Fischbach. J.B. Lippincott Co., 227 East Washington Square, Philadelphia, PA 19106-3780. Phone: (215) 238-4200. Fax: (215) 238-4227. 1992.

JOURNALS

The Journal of Laboratory and Clinical Medicine. Mosby-Year Book, 11830 Westline Industrial Drive, St. Louis, MO 63146. Phone: (800) 325-4177. Fax: (314) 432-1380. Monthly.

Journal of Nuclear Medicine Technology. Society of Nuclear Medicine, 136 Madison Ave., New York, NY 10016. Phone: (212) 889-0717.

Laboratory Investigation. Williams & Wilkins, 428 E. Preston St., Baltimore, MD 21202. Phone: (800) 638-0672. Fax: (800) 447-8438. Monthly.

Lasers in Surgery and Medicine. John Wiley & Sons, Inc., 605 Third Ave., New York, NY 10158-0012. Phone: (212) 850-6000. Fax: (212) 850-6088. Bimonthly + Supplement 3.

ONLINE DATABASES

EMBASE. Elsevier Science Publishing Co., Inc., P.O. Box 882, Madison Square Station, New York, NY 10159-2101. Phone: (212) 989-5800. Fax: (212) 633-3990.

MEDLINE. National Library of Medicine, 8600 Rockville Pike, Bethesda, MD 20894. Phone: (800) 638-8480.

SciSearch. Institute for Scientific Information, 3501 Market St., Philadelphia, PA 19104. Phone: (215) 386-0100. Fax: (215) 386-6362.

POPULAR WORKS AND PATIENT EDUCATION

Complete Guide to Medical Tests. Griffith H. Winter. Fisher Books, P.O. Box 38040, Tucson, AZ 85740-8040. Phone: (602) 292-9080. 1988.

Medical Tests and Diagnostic Procedures: A Patient's Guide to Just What the Doctor Ordered. Philip Shtasel. HarperCollins

Publishers., Inc., 10 E. 53rd St., New York, NY 10022-5299. Phone: (212) 207-7000. Fax: (800) 242-7737. 1990.

Patient's Guide to Medical Tests. Cathy Pickney. Facts on File, Inc., 460 Park Ave. S., New York, NY 10016-7382. Phone: (212) 683-2244. Fax: (212) 683-3633. Third edition 1987.

RESEARCH CENTERS, INSTITUTES, CLEARINGHOUSES

Office of Technology Assessment. Agency for Health Care Policy and Research, 5600 Fishers Lane, Rockville, MD 20857. Phone: (301) 443-4100.

TEXTBOOKS AND MONOGRAPHS

Clinical Diagnosis & Management by Laboratory Methods. Hohn Bernard Henry (ed.). W.B. Saunders Co., The Curtis Center, Independence Square W., Philadelphia, PA 19106-3399. Phone: (215) 238-7800. 18th edition 1991.

Clinical Laboratory Medicine. Tilton. Mosby-Year Book, 11830 Westline Industrial Drive, St. Louis, MO 63146. Phone: (800) 325-4177. Fax: (314) 432-1380. 1992.

Widmann's Clinical Interpretation of Laboratory Tests. Ronald A. Sacher, Richard A. McPherson, Joseph M. Caompos. F.A. Davis Co., 1915 Arch St., Philadelphia, PA 19103. Phone: (800) 523-4049. Fax: (215) 568-5065. 10th edition, 1991.

MEDICAL TERMINOLOGY

ASSOCIATIONS, PROFESSIONAL SOCIETIES, ADVOCACY AND SUPPORT GROUPS

American Society for Medical Terminology (ASMT). 2021 L St. N.W., Ste. 400, Washington, DC 20036. Phone: (202) 785-3311. Fax: (202) 466-2254.

CD-ROM DATABASES

Stedman's/25 for WordPerfect. Stedman (ed.). Williams & Wilkins, 428 East Preston St., Baltimore, MD 21202. Phone: (800) 638-0672. Fax: (800) 447-8438. 1991.

ENCYCLOPEDIAS, DICTIONARIES, WORD BOOKS

Black's Medical Dictionary. Gordon Macpherson (ed.). Barnes & Noble Books, 4270 Boston Way, Lanham, MD 20706. Phone: (800) 462-6420. 37th edition 1992.

Black's Veterinary Dictionary. Geoffrey West (ed.). Barnes & Noble Books, 4270 Boston Way, Lanham, MD 20706. Phone: (800) 462-6420. 17th edition 1992.

Churchill's Illustrated Medical Dictionary. Churchill Livingstone Inc., 650 Ave. of the Americas, New York, NY 10011. Phone: (212) 819-5400. Fax: (212) 302-6598. 1989.

Clinical Laboratory Word Book. Barbara De Lorenzo. Springhouse Publishing Co., 1111 Bethlehem Pike, Spring House, PA 19477. Phone: (800) 331-3170. Fax: (215) 646-8716. 1992.

The Davis Book of Medical Abbreviations: A Deciphering Guide. Sarah Lu Mitchell-Hatton. F.A. Davis Co., 1915 Arch St., Philadelphia, PA 19103. Phone: (800) 523-4049. Fax: (215) 568-5065. 1991.

Dental and Otolaryngology Word Book. Helen E. Littrell. Springhouse Publishing Co., 1111 Bethlehem Pike, Spring

House, PA 19477. Phone: (800) 331-3170. Fax: (215) 646-8716. 1992.

Dictionary of Immunology. F. Rosen and others (eds.). Macmillan Publishing Co., 866 Third Ave., New York, NY 10011. Phone: (800) 257-5755. 1988.

Dictionary of Medical Acronyms & Abbreviations. Stanley Jablonski. Mosby-Year Book, 11830 Westline Industrial Drive, St. Louis, MO 63146. Phone: (800) 325-4177. Fax: (314) 432-1380. Second edition 1992.

Dictionary of Medical Eponyms. B.G. Firkin. The Parthenon Publishing Group, Inc., 120 Mill Rd., Park Ridge, NJ 07656. Phone: (201) 391-6796. 1987.

Dictionary of Medical Syndromes. S. Magalini and others. J.B. Lippincott Co., 227 E. Washington Square, Philadelphia, PA 19106-3780. Phone: (215) 238-4200. Fax: (215) 238-4227. Third edition 1990.

The Dictionary of Modern Medicine. J.C. Segen. The Parthenon Publishing Group, Inc., 120 Mill Rd., Park Ridge, NJ 07656. Phone: (201) 391-6796. 1992.

Dictionary of Obstetrics & Gynecology. Walter De Gruyter, Inc., 200 Saw Mill River Rd., Hawthorne, NY 10532. Phone: (914) 747-0110. 1988.

Dictionary of Optometry. Michel Millodot. Butterworth-Heinemann, 80 Montvale Ave., Stoneham, MA 02180. Phone: (617) 438-8464. Fax: (617) 279-4851. Second edition 1990.

Dorland's Illustrated Medical Dictionary. W.B. Saunders Co., The Curtis Center, Independence Square W., Philadelphia, PA 19106-3399. Phone: (215) 238-7800. 27th edition 1988.

Encyclopedia and Dictionary of Medicine, Nursing, and Allied Health. Benjamin F. Miller, Claire B. Keane. W.B. Saunders Co., The Curtis Center, Independence Square W., Philadelphia, PA 19106-3399. Phone: (215) 238-7800. Fifth edition 1992.

Glossary of Anatomy and Physiology. Diane Shaw. Springhouse Publishing Co., 1111 Bethlehem Pike, Spring House, PA 19477. Phone: (800) 331-3170. Fax: (215) 646-8716. 1992.

Glossary of Health Care Terms. American Medical Record Association, 919 N. Michigan Ave., Ste. 1400, Chicago, IL 60611. Phone: (312) 787-2672. Third edition 1986.

Glossary of Medical Terminology. Joy Willey. Springhouse Publishing Co., 1111 Bethlehem Pike, Spring House, PA 19477. Phone: (800) 331-3170. Fax: (215) 646-8716. 1992.

Illustrated Medical Dictionary. W.A.N. Dorland. W.B. Saunders Co., The Curtis Center, Independence Square W., Philadelphia, PA 19106-3399. Phone: (215) 238-7800. 27th edition 1988.

Immunologic and AIDS Word Book. Helen E. Littrell. Springhouse Publishing Co., 1111 Bethlehem Pike, Spring House, PA 19477. Phone: (800) 331-3170. Fax: (215) 646-8716. 1992.

Introduction to Medical Terminology. Norma Stevens, Jerene Adler. Springhouse Publishing Co., 1111 Bethlehem Pike, Spring House, PA 19477. Phone: (800) 331-3170. Fax: (215) 646-8716. 1992.

Jablonski's Dictionary of Syndromes & Eponymic Diseases. Stanley Jablonski. Krieger Publishing Co., P.O. Box 9542,

Melbourne, FL 32902-9542. Phone: (407) 724-9542. Fax: (407) 951-3671. Second edition 1991.

The Language of Medicine. Davi-Ellen Chabner. W.B. Saunders Co., The Curtis Center, Independence Sqare W., Philadelphia, PA 19106-3399. Phone: (215) 238-7800. 4th edition, 1991.

Medical Dictionary of the English and German Languages. D.W. Unseld. CRC Press, Inc., 2000 Corporate Blvd. N.W., Boca Raton, FL 33431. Phone: (407) 994-0555. Fax: (407) 997-0949. 10th edition 1991.

Medical Terminology: Building a Vocabulary. Nancy N. Scanlan. Prentice Hall, 113 Sylvan Ave., Rt. 9W, Prentice Hall Bldg., Englewood Cliffs, NJ 07632. Phone: (201) 767-5937. 1988.

The Medical Word Book: A Spelling and Vocabulary Guide to Medical Transcription. Sheila B. Sloane. W.B. Saunders Co., The Curtis Center, Independence Square W., Philadelphia, PA 19106-3399. Phone: (215) 238-7800. Third edition 1991.

Medical Word Book A-Z. Barbara De Lorenzo. Springhouse Publishing Co., 1111 Bethlehem Pike, Spring House, PA 19477. Phone: (800) 331-3170. Fax: (215) 646-8716. 1992.

Medicine, Literature, and Eponyms: Encyclopedia of Medical Eponyms Derived from Literary Characters. Alvin E. Rodin, Jack D. Key. Krieger Publishing Co., P.O. Box 9542, Melbourne, FL 32902-9542. Phone: (407) 724-9542. Fax: (407) 951-3671. 1989.

Mosby's Medical, Nursing, and Allied Health Dictionary. Kenneth N. Anderson, Lois Anderson, Walter D. Glanze (eds.). Mosby-Year Book, 11830 Westline Industrial Dr., St. Louis, MO 63146. Phone: (800) 325-4177. Fax: (314) 432-1380. Third edition 1990.

Neurologic and Psychiatric Word Book. Helen E. Littrell. Springhouse Publishing Co., 1111 Bethlehem Pike, Spring House, PA 19477. Phone: (800) 331-3170. Fax: (215) 646-8716. 1992.

Obstetric and Gynecologic Word Book. Helen E. Littrell. Springhouse Publishing Co., 1111 Bethlehem Pike, Spring House, PA 19477. Phone: (800) 331-3170. Fax: (215) 646-8716. 1992.

Oncologic Word Book. Barbara De Lorenzo. Springhouse Publishing Co., 1111 Bethlehem Pike, Spring House, PA 19477. Phone: (800) 331-3170. Fax: (215) 646-8716. 1992.

Ophthalmic Word Book. Barbara De Lorenzo. Springhouse Publishing Co., 1111 Bethlehem Pike, Spring House, PA 19477. Phone: (800) 331-3170. Fax: (215) 646-8716. 1992.

Orthopedic Word Book. Thomas J. Cittadine. Springhouse Publishing Co., 1111 Bethlehem Pike, Spring House, PA 19477. Phone: (800) 331-3170. Fax: (215) 646-8716. 1992.

Pharmaceutical Word Book. Barbara De Lorenzo. Springhouse Publishing Co., 1111 Bethlehem Pike, Spring House, PA 19477. Phone: (800) 331-3170. Fax: (215) 646-8716. Second edition 1992.

Pharmaceutical Words. Stedman. Williams & Wilkins, 428 East Preston St., Baltimore, MD 21202. Phone: (800) 638-0672. Fax: (800) 447-8438. 1992.

Pocket Glossary of Ophthalmologic Terminology. Joseph Hoffman. SLACK Inc., 6900 Grove Rd., Thorofare, NJ 08086-9447. Phone: (800) 257-8290. Fax: (609) 853-5991. 1990.

Radiologic Word Book. Barbara De Lorenzo. Springhouse Publishing Co., 1111 Bethlehem Pike, Spring House, PA 19477. Phone: (800) 331-3170. Fax: (215) 646-8716. 1992.

Saunders Ophthalmology Word Book. Joyce Adams. W.B. Saunders Co., The Curtis Center, Independence Sqare W., Philadelphia, PA 19106-3399. Phone: (215) 238-7800. 1991.

Spanish-English English-Spanish Medical Dictionary. Onyria Herrera McElroy, Lola L. Grabb. Little, Brown and Company, 34 Beacon St., Boston, MA 02108. Phone: (617) 227-0730. 1992.

Stedman's Abbreviations, Acronyms and Symbols. Practice Management Information Co., 4727 Wilshire Blvd., Suite 300, Los Angeles, CA 90010. Phone: (213) 658-8501. 1992.

Stedman's Medical Dictionary. Williams & Wilkins, 428 E. Preston St., Baltimore, MD 21202. Phone: (800) 638-0672. Fax: (800) 447-8438. 25th edition 1990.

Surgical Word Book. Sam McMillan. Springhouse Publishing Co., 1111 Bethlehem Pike, Spring House, PA 19477. Phone: (800) 331-3170. Fax: (215) 646-8716. 1992.

Taber's Cyclopedic Medical Dictionary. Clayton L. Thomas (ed.). F.A. Davis Co., 1915 Arch St., Philadelphia, PA 19103. Phone: (800) 523-4049. Fax: (215) 568-5065. Seventeenth edition 1993.

HANDBOOKS, GUIDES, MANUALS, ATLASES

Medical Subject Headings: Annotated Alphabetic List. National Library of Medicine, 8600 Rockville Pike, Bethesda, MD 20894. Phone: (800) 638-8480. 1992.

Medical Subject Headings: Tree Structures. National Library of Medicine, 8600 Rockville Pike, Bethesda, MD 20894. Phone: (800) 638-8480. 1992.

Premuted MESH. National Library of Medicine, 8600 Rockville Pike, Bethesda, MD 20894. Phone: (800) 638-8480. 1992.

POPULAR WORKS AND PATIENT EDUCATION

Consumer's Guide to Medical Lingo. Charles B. Inlander. People's Medical Society, 462 Walnut St., Allentown, PA 18102. Phone: (215) 770-1670. 1992.

TEXTBOOKS AND MONOGRAPHS

Brady's Introduction to Medical Terminology. Carol A. Lillis. Appleton & Lange, 25 Van Zant St., East Norwalk, CT 06855. Phone: (800) 423-1359. Fax: (203) 854-9486. 3rd edition, 1989.

Fundamentals of Immunolgy and Allergy. Richard F. Lockey. W.B. Saunders Co., The Curtis Center, Independence Square W., Philadelphia, PA 19106-3399. Phone: (215) 238-7800. 1987.

Learning Medical Terminology: A Worksheet. Miriam Austin, Harvey Austin. Mosby-Year Book, 11830 Westline Industrial Drive, St. Louis, MO 63146. Phone: (800) 325-4177. Fax: (314) 432-1380. 7th edition, 1991.

Medical Terminology: A Short Course. Davi-Ellen Chabner. W.B. Saunders Co., The Curtis Center, Independence Sqare W., Philadelphia, PA 19106-3399. Phone: (215) 238-7800. 1991.

Today's Challenge: Content of the Health Record. Barbara Glondys. American Medical Record Association, 919 N. Michigan Ave., Ste. 1400, Chicago, IL 60611. Phone: (312) 787-2672. 1988.

MEDICARE AND MEDICAID

See also: HEALTH INSURANCE

ABSTRACTING, INDEXING, AND CURRENT AWARENESS PUBLICATIONS

Hospital Literature Index. American Hospital Association, 840 N. Lake Shore Dr., Chicago, IL 60611. Phone: (800) 242-2626. Fax: (312) 280-6015. Quarterly.

Index Medicus. U.S. National Library of Medicine, 8600 Rockville Pike, Bethesda, MD 20894. Phone: (800) 638-8480. Monthly.

MEDOC: Index to U.S. Government Publications in the Medical and Health Sciences. Spencer S. Eccles Health Sciences Library, University of Utah, Bldg. 589, Salt Lake City, UT 84112. Phone: (801) 581-5268. Quarterly.

ANNUALS AND REVIEWS

Nursing Clinics. W.B. Saunders Co., The Curtis Center, Independence Square W., Philadelphia, PA 19106-3399. Phone: (215) 238-7800. Quarterly.

ASSOCIATIONS, PROFESSIONAL SOCIETIES, ADVOCACY AND SUPPORT GROUPS

American Association of Retired Persons. 1909 K St. N.W., Washington, DC 20049. Phone: (202) 872-4700.

Health Care Financing Administration. Oak Meadows Building, 6325 Security Blvd., Baltimore, MD 21207. Phone: (301) 966-6573.

BIBLIOGRAPHIES

Medicare and Medicaid Manuals, Guides, and Guidelines. National Technical Information Service, 5285 Port Royal Rd., Springfield, VA 22161. Phone: (703) 487-4650. Fax: (703) 321-8547. Jan. 1970-May 1989 PB89-863526/CBY.

CD-ROM DATABASES

American Journal of Public Health. MEP, 124 Mt. Auburn St., Cambridge, MA 02138. Phone: (800) 342-1338. Fax: (617) 868-7738. Annual.

HFCA --On CD-ROM. FD Inc., 600 New Hampshire Ave. NW, Suite 355, Washington, DC 20037. Phone: (800) 332-6623. Fax: (202) 337-0457. Monthly.

Journal of the American Medical Association. Macmillan New Media, 124 Mt. Auburn St., Cambridge, MA 02138. Weekly.

New England Journal of Medicine. CMC ReSearch, Inc., 7150 S.W. Hampton, Suite C-120, Portland, OR 97223. Phone: (800) 262-7668. Fax: (503) 639-1796. 3/year.

The New England Journal of Medicine on CD-ROM. MEP, 124 Mt. Auburn St., Cambridge, MA 02138. Phone: (800) 342-1338. Fax: (617) 868-7738. Semiannual.

ENCYCLOPEDIAS, DICTIONARIES, WORD BOOKS

Facts on File Dictionary of Health Care Management. Joseph C. Rhea, and others. Facts On File, Inc., 460 Park Ave. S., New York, NY 10016-7382. Phone: (800) 322-8755. Fax: (212) 683-3633. 1988.

HANDBOOKS, GUIDES, MANUALS, ATLASES

Medicare DRG Handbook: Comparative Clinical & Financial Standards. Health Care Investment Analysts, Inc., 300 E. Lombard St., Baltimore, MD 21202. Phone: (410) 576-9600. Fax: (410) 783-0575. 1992.

The Medicare Survival Guide: A Physician's Handbook to Understanding and Working with Medicare. Denise Kraus. McGraw-Hill, Inc., Health Professions Division, 1221 Avenue of the Americas, 28th Floor, New York, NY 10020. Phone: (212) 512-4228. 1992.

JOURNALS

AARP Bulletin. American Association of Retired Persons, 1909 K St. N.W., Washington, DC 20049. Phone: (202) 872-4700.

American Journal of Public Health. American Public Health Association, 1015 15th St. NW, Washington, DC 20005. Phone: (202) 789-5666. Monthly.

Archives of Internal Medicine. American Medical Association, 515 North State St., Chicago, IL 60610. Phone: (312) 464-0183. Fax: (312) 464-5834. Monthly.

Geriatrics: Medicine for Midlife and Beyond. Edgell Communications, 7500 Old Oak Blvd., Cleveland, OH 44130. Phone: (216) 826-2839. Fax: (216) 891-2726. Monthly.

Health Care Financing Administration Manuals. U.S. National Technical Information Service, 5285 Port Royal Rd., Springfield, VA 22161. Phone: (703) 487-4650. Fax: (703) 321-8547.

Health Care Financing Review. Health Care Financing Administration, Oak Meadows Building, 6325 Security Blvd., Baltimore, MD 21207. Phone: (301) 966-6573.

Hospitals. American Hospital Publishing, Inc., 211 E. Chicago Ave., Ste. 700, Chicago, IL 60611. Phone: (312) 440-6800. Semimonthly.

Journal of the American Geriatrics Society. Williams & Wilkins, 428 E. Preston St., Baltimore, MD 21202. Phone: (800) 638-0672. Fax: (800) 447-8438. Monthly.

The New England Journal of Medicine. Massachusetts Medical Society, 1440 Main St., Waltham, MA 02154-1649. Phone: (617) 893-3800. Fax: (617) 893-0413. Weekly.

Social Security Bulletin. U.S. Government Printing Office, Superintendent of Documents, P.O. Box 371954, Pittsburgh, PA 15250-7954. Phone: (202) 783-3238. Fax: (202) 512-2250. Monthly.

NEWSLETTERS

Medicare Compliance Alert. United Communications Group, 4550 Montgomery Ave., Ste. 700N, Bethesda, MD 20814-3382. Phone: (301) 961-8700. Bimonthly.

Medicare and Medicaid Law Reporter. LRP Publications, 747 Dresher Rd., Ste. 500, P.O. Box 980, Horsham, PA 19044-0980. Phone: (800) 341-7874. Fax: (215) 784-9639. Weekly.

Parent Care Advisor. American Health Consultants, P.O. Box 71266, Chicago, IL 60691-9987. Phone: (800) 688-2421. Monthly.

ONLINE DATABASES

EMBASE. Elsevier Science Publishing Co., Inc., P.O. Box 882, Madison Square Station, New York, NY 10159-2101. Phone: (212) 989-5800. Fax: (212) 633-3990.

MEDLINE. National Library of Medicine, 8600 Rockville Pike, Bethesda, MD 20894. Phone: (800) 638-8480.

SciSearch. Institute for Scientific Information, 3501 Market St., Philadelphia, PA 19104. Phone: (215) 386-0100. Fax: (215) 386-6362.

POPULAR WORKS AND PATIENT EDUCATION

Avoiding the Medicaid Trap. Armond D. Budish. Avon Books, 1350 Ave. of the Americas, 2nd Flr., New York, NY 10019. Phone: (800) 238-0658. 1991.

A Guide for Senior Citizens: Social Security, Medicare, Legal & Tax Assistance Including an Address and Phone Number Directory. Gordon Press Publishers, P.O. Box 459, Bowling Green Sta., New York, NY 10004. Phone: (718) 624-8419. 1991.

Keys to Understanding Medicare. Jim Gaffney. Barron's Educational Series, Inc., P.O. Box 8040, 250 Wireless Blvd., Hauppauge, NY 11788. Phone: (516) 434-3311. Fax: (516) 434-3723. 1991.

Mastering the Medicare Maze: An Essential Guide to Benefits, Appeals and Medigap Insurance. Betsy Abramson, Jeffrey Spitzer-Resnick, Margie Groom, and others. Center for Public Representation, Inc., 121 S. Pinckney St., Madison, WI 53703-1999. Phone: (608) 251-4008. 1991.

Medicare Made Easy: Everything You Need to Know to Make Medicare Work for You. Charles B. Inlander. Addison-Wesley Publishing Co., Rte. 128, Reading, MA 01867. Phone: (800) 447-2226. Revised edition 1991.

Medicare/Medigap: The Essential Guide for Older Americans and Their Families. Carl Oshiro, Harry Snyder. Consumer Reports Books, 9180 LeSaint Dr., Fairfield, OH 45014. Phone: (513) 860-1178. 1990.

RESEARCH CENTERS, INSTITUTES, CLEARINGHOUSES

Agency for Health Care Policy and Research Publications Clearinghouse. P.O. Box 8547, Silver Spring, MD 20907. Phone: (800) 358-9295.

Social Security Administration. 6401 Security Rd., Baltimore, MD 21235. Phone: (301) 965-2736.

STANDARDS AND STATISTICS SOURCES

HCFA Statistics. Health Care Financing Administration, Oak Meadows Building, 6325 Security Blvd., Baltimore, MD 21207. Phone: (301) 966-6573. Annual.

Health Care Financing Program Statistics: Medicare and Medicaid Data Book. Health Care Financing Administration, Oak Meadows Building, 6325 Security Blvd., Baltimore, MD 21207. Phone: (301) 966-6573. Biennial.

Medicare Hospital Mortality Information. Health Care Financing Administration, Oak Meadows Building, 6325 Security Blvd., Baltimore, MD 21207. Phone: (301) 966-6573. Annual.

The Medicare and Medicaid Data Book. U.S. Health Care Financing Administration, 200 Independence Ave. S.W., Baltimore, MD 21218. Phone: (202) 245-6113. Annual.

Medicare/Medicaid Nursing Home Information. U.S. Government Printing Office, Superintendent of Documents, P.O. Box 371954, Pittsburgh, PA 15250-7954. Phone: (202) 783-3238. Fax: (202) 512-2250. Annual.

TEXTBOOKS AND MONOGRAPHS

Medicare: A Strategy for Quality Assurance. Kathleen Lohr (ed.). National Academy of Sciences Press. 2101 Constitution Ave., Washington, DC 20418. Phone: (800) 624-6242. Two vols., 1990.

Medicare/Medicaid Nursing Home Information. Health Care Financing Administration, Oak Meadows Building, 6325 Security Blvd., Baltimore, MD 21207. Phone: (301) 966-6573. 1990.

Medicare and Medigaps: A Guide to Retirement Health Insurance. Susan Hellman, Leonard H. Hellman. Sage Publications, Inc., 2455 Teller Road, P.O. Box 5084, Newbury Park, CA 91320. Phone: (805) 499-0721. Fax: (805) 499-0871. 1991.

MEDICINAL PLANTS

See: HERBAL MEDICINE

MELANOMA

See: SKIN CANCER

MENIERE'S DISEASE

See: OTOLARYNGOLOGY

MENINGITIS

See: INFECTIOUS DISEASES

MENOPAUSE

ABSTRACTING, INDEXING, AND CURRENT AWARENESS PUBLICATIONS

Current Contents/Clinical Medicine. Institute for Scientific Information, 3501 Market St., Philadelphia, PA 19104. Phone: (800) 523-1850. Fax: (215) 386-6362. Weekly.

Excerpta Medica. Section 10: Obstetrics and Gynecology. Elsevier Science Publishing Co., Inc., P.O. Box 882, Madison Square Station, New York, NY 10159-2101. Phone: (212) 989-5800. Fax: (212) 633-3990. 20/year.

Index Medicus. U.S. National Library of Medicine, 8600 Rockville Pike, Bethesda, MD 20894. Phone: (800) 638-8480. Monthly.

Key Obstetrics and Gynecology: Current Literature in Perspective. Mosby-Year Book, 11830 Westline Industrial Drive, St. Louis, MO 63146. Phone: (800) 325-4177. Fax: (314) 432-1380. Quarterly.

Science Citation Index. Institute for Scientific Information, 3501 Market St., Philadelphia, PA 19104. Phone: (800) 523-1850. Fax: (215) 386-6362. Bimonthly.

ASSOCIATIONS, PROFESSIONAL SOCIETIES, ADVOCACY AND SUPPORT GROUPS

American College of Obstetricians and Gynecologists (ACOG). 409 12th St. S.W., Washington, DC 20024-2188. Phone: (202) 638-5577.

North American Menopause Society (NAMS). University Hospitals of Cleveland, 2074 Abington Rd., Cleveland, OH 44106. Phone: (216) 844-3334. Fax: (216) 844-3348.

CD-ROM DATABASES

Excerpta Medica CD: Obstetrics & Gynecology. SilverPlatter Information, Inc., River Ridge Office Park, 100 River Ridge Rd., Norwood, MA 02062. Phone: (617) 769-2599. Fax: (617) 769-8763. Quarterly.

OBGLine. Aries Systems Corporation, One Dundee Park, Andover, MA 01810. Phone: (508) 475-7200. Fax: (508) 474-8860. Monthly or quarterly.

SCISEARCH. Institute for Scientific Information, 3501 Market St., Philadelphia, PA 19104. Phone: (215) 386-0100. Fax: (215) 386-6362.

HANDBOOKS, GUIDES, MANUALS, ATLASES

Handbook of Gynecology and Obstetrics. Brown. Appleton & Lange, 25 Van Zant St., East Norwalk, CT 06855. Phone: (800) 423-1359. Fax: (203) 854-9486. 1992.

Zuspan and Quilligan's Manual of Obstetrics and Gynecology. Jay D. Iams, Frederick P. Zuspan, Edward J. Quilligan. Mosby-Year Book, 11830 Westline Industrial Drive, St. Louis, MO 63146. Phone: (800) 325-4177. Fax: (314) 432-1380. Second edition 1990.

JOURNALS

American Journal of Obstetrics and Gynecology. Mosby-Year Book, 11830 Westline Industrial Drive, St. Louis, MO 63146. Phone: (800) 325-4177. Fax: (314) 432-1380. Monthly.

British Journal of Obstetrics & Gynaecology. Blackwell Publishers, Three Cambridge Center, Cambridge, MA 02142. Phone: (617) 225-0430. Fax: (617) 494-1437. Monthly.

Journal of Clinical Endocrinology & Metabolism. Williams & Wilkins, 428 E. Preston St., Baltimore, MD 21202. Phone: (800) 638-0672. Fax: (900) 447-8438. Monthly.

Journal of Women's Health. Mary Ann Liebert, Inc., 1651 Third Ave., New York, NY 10128. Phone: (212) 289-2300. Fax: (212) 289-4697. Quarterly.

Maturitas. Elsevier Science Publishing Co., Inc., P.O. Box 882, Madison Square Station, New York, NY 10159-2101. Phone: (212) 989-5800. Fax: (212) 633-3990. 4/year.

Obstetrics and Gynecology. Elsevier Science Publishing Co., Inc., P.O. Box 882, Madison Square Station, New York, NY 10159-2101. Phone: (212) 989-5800. Fax: (212) 633-3990. 15/year.

NEWSLETTERS

A Friend Indeed: For Women in the Prime of Life. A Friend Indeed Publications, Inc., Box 515, Place du Parc Sta., Montreal, PQ, Canada H2W 2P1. Phone: (514) 843-5730. 10/yr..

Menopause News. Menopause News, 2074 Union St., San Francisco, CA 94123. 6/year.

National Women's Health Network-Network News. National Women's Health Network, 1325 G St. N.W., Washington, DC 20005. Phone: (202) 347-1140. Bimonthly.

ONLINE DATABASES

EMBASE. Elsevier Science Publishing Co., Inc., P.O. Box 882, Madison Square Station, New York, NY 10159-2101. Phone: (212) 989-5800. Fax: (212) 633-3990.

MEDLINE. National Library of Medicine, 8600 Rockville Pike, Bethesda, MD 20894. Phone: (800) 638-8480.

SciSearch. Institute for Scientific Information, 3501 Market St., Philadelphia, PA 19104. Phone: (215) 386-0100. Fax: (215) 386-6362.

POPULAR WORKS AND PATIENT EDUCATION

Doctor Discusses Menopause and Estrogens. Edward M. Davis, Dona Meilach. Budlong Press, 5915 Northwest Hwy., Chicago, IL 60631. 1990.

Estrogen: A Complete Guide to Reversing the Effects of Menopause Using Hormone Replacement Therapy. Lila Nachtigall, Joan R. Heilman. HarperCollins Pubs., Inc., 10 E. 53rd St., New York, NY 10022-5299. Phone: (212) 207-7000. Fax: (800) 242-7737. Revised edition 1991.

Hormones, Hot Flashes & Mood Swings: Living Through the Ups & Downs of Menopause. Clark Gillespie. HarperCollins Pubs., Inc., 10 E. 53rd St., New York, NY 10022-5299. Phone: (212) 207-7000. Fax: (800) 242-7737. 1989.

Hysterectomy - Before and After: A Comprehensive Guide to Preventing, Preparing for, and Maximizing Health after Hysterectomy - With Essential Information. Winnifred B. Cutler. HarperCollins Pubs., Inc., 10 E. 53rd St., New York, NY 10022-5299. Phone: (212) 207-7000. Fax: (800) 242-7737. 1990.

Managing Your Menopause. Wulf H. Utian. Prentice Hall, 113 Sylvan Ave., Rt. 9W, Prentice Hall Bldg., Englewood Cliffs, NJ 07632. Phone: (201) 767-5937. 1991.

Menopause: A Guide for Women and the Men Who Love Them. Winnifred B. Cutler. W.W. Norton & Co., Inc., 500 Fifth Ave., New York, NY 10110. Phone: (800) 223-2584. 1991.

Menopause: All Your Questions Answered. Contemporary Books, Inc., 180 N. Michigan Ave., Chicago, IL 60601. Phone: (312) 782-9181. 1987.

The Menopause Self-Help Book. Susan M. Lark. Celestial Arts Publishing Co., P.O. Box 7327, Berkeley, CA 94707. Phone: (800) 841-2665.

Menopause and the Years Ahead. Mary Beard, Lindsay Curtis. Fisher Books, P.O. Box 38040, Tucson, AZ 85740-8040. Phone: (602) 292-9080. Revised edition 1991.

Natural Menopause: The Complete Guide to a Woman's Most Misunderstood Passage. Susan Perry, Katherine O'Harlan. Addison-Wesley Publishing Co., Rte. 128, Reading, MA 01867. Phone: (800) 447-2226. 1992.

The New Our Bodies, Ourselves: The Updated and Expanded Edition. The Boston Women's Health Book Collective. Simon & Schuster, 1230 Ave. of the Americas, New York, NY 10020. Phone: (800) 223-2348. Fax: (800) 284-0735. 1992.

Take This Book to the Gynecologist with You: Consumer's Guide to Women's Health. Gale Malesky. Addison-Wesley Publishing Co., Rte. 128, Reading, MA 01867. Phone: (800) 447-2226. 1991.

RESEARCH CENTERS, INSTITUTES, CLEARINGHOUSES

Center for the Mature Woman. Medical College of Pennsylvania. 3300 Henry Ave., Philadelphia, PA 19129. Phone: (215) 842-7180.

Division of Reproductive Endocrinology. University of Tennessee. 956 Ct. Ave., Room D328, Memphis, TN 38163. Phone: (901) 528-5859.

Queen Elizabeth Hospital Research Institute. 550 University Ave., Toronto, ON, Canada M5G 2A2. Phone: (416) 672-4218.

TEXTBOOKS AND MONOGRAPHS

Menopause: Evaluation, Treatment and Health Concerns. Charles B. Hammond, Florence P. Haseltine, Isaac Schiff. John Wiley & Sons, Inc., 605 Third Ave., New York, NY 10158-0012. Phone: (212) 850-6000. Fax: (212) 850-6088. 1989.

Premenstrual, Postpartum, and Menopausal Mood Disorders. Laurence M. Demers, John L. McGuire, Audrey Phillips, et. al.. Williams & Wilkins, 428 East Preston St., Baltimore, MD 21202. Phone: (800) 638-0672. Fax: (800) 447-8438. 1990.

Transdermal Estrogen Replacement for Menopausal Women. George F. Birdwood (ed.). Hogrefe & Huber Publishers, P.O. Box 51, Lewiston, NY 14092. Phone: (716) 282-1610. 1988.

MENSTRUATION

See also: PREMENSTRUAL SYNDROME

ABSTRACTING, INDEXING, AND CURRENT AWARENESS PUBLICATIONS

Current Contents/Clinical Medicine. Institute for Scientific Information, 3501 Market St., Philadelphia, PA 19104. Phone: (800) 523-1850. Fax: (215) 386-6362. Weekly.

Excerpta Medica. Section 10: Obstetrics and Gynecology. Elsevier Science Publishing Co., Inc., P.O. Box 882, Madison Square Station, New York, NY 10159-2101. Phone: (212) 989-5800. Fax: (212) 633-3990. 20/year.

Science Citation Index. Institute for Scientific Information, 3501 Market St., Philadelphia, PA 19104. Phone: (800) 523-1850. Fax: (215) 386-6362. Bimonthly.

ANNUALS AND REVIEWS

Obstetrics and Gynecology Clinics. W.B. Saunders Co., The Curtis Center, Independence Square W., Philadelphia, PA 19106-3399. Phone: (215) 238-7800. Quarterly.

ASSOCIATIONS, PROFESSIONAL SOCIETIES, ADVOCACY AND SUPPORT GROUPS

American College of Obstetricians and Gynecologists (ACOG). 409 12th St. S.W., Washington, DC 20024-2188. Phone: (202) 638-5577.

Society for Menstrual Cycle Research. c/o Ava Tayman, 600 Maryland Ave. S.W., No. 300E, Washington, DC 20024. Phone: (202) 488-0970.

CD-ROM DATABASES

Excerpta Medica CD: Obstetrics & Gynecology. SilverPlatter Information, Inc., River Ridge Office Park, 100 River Ridge Rd., Norwood, MA 02062. Phone: (617) 769-2599. Fax: (617) 769-8763. Quarterly.

OBGLine. Aries Systems Corporation, One Dundee Park, Andover, MA 01810. Phone: (508) 475-7200. Fax: (508) 474-8860. Monthly or quarterly.

SCISEARCH. Institute for Scientific Information, 3501 Market St., Philadelphia, PA 19104. Phone: (215) 386-0100. Fax: (215) 386-6362.

HANDBOOKS, GUIDES, MANUALS, ATLASES

Manual of Outpatient Gynecology. Carol Havens, Nancy Sullivan, Patty Tilton. Little, Brown and Company, 34 Beacon St., Boston, MA 02108. Phone: (617) 227-0730. Second edition 1991.

Zuspan and Quilligan's Manual of Obstetrics and Gynecology. Jay D. Iams, Frederick P. Zuspan, Edward J. Quilligan. Mosby-Year Book, 11830 Westline Industrial Drive, St. Louis, MO 63146. Phone: (800) 325-4177. Fax: (314) 432-1380. Second edition 1990.

JOURNALS

Journal of Women's Health. Mary Ann Liebert, Inc., 1651 Third Ave., New York, NY 10128. Phone: (212) 289-2300. Fax: (212) 289-4697. Quarterly.

NEWSLETTERS

National Women's Health Network-Network News. National Women's Health Network, 1325 G St. N.W., Washington, DC 20005. Phone: (202) 347-1140. Bimonthly.

ONLINE DATABASES

EMBASE. Elsevier Science Publishing Co., Inc., P.O. Box 882, Madison Square Station, New York, NY 10159-2101. Phone: (212) 989-5800. Fax: (212) 633-3990.

MEDLINE. National Library of Medicine, 8600 Rockville Pike, Bethesda, MD 20894. Phone: (800) 638-8480.

SciSearch. Institute for Scientific Information, 3501 Market St., Philadelphia, PA 19104. Phone: (215) 386-0100. Fax: (215) 386-6362.

POPULAR WORKS AND PATIENT EDUCATION

The A-Z of Women's Health. Derek Llewellyn-Jones. Oxford University Press, Inc., 200 Madison Ave., New York, NY 10016. Phone: (800) 451-7556. Second edition 1991.

The New Our Bodies, Ourselves: The Updated and Expanded Edition. The Boston Women's Health Book Collective. Simon & Schuster, 1230 Ave. of the Americas, New York, NY 10020. Phone: (800) 223-2348. Fax: (800) 284-0735. 1992.

Understanding Your Body: Every Woman's Guide to a Lifetime of Health. Felicia Stewart, Felicia Guest, Gary Stewart, R. Hatcher. Bantam Books, Inc., 666 Fifth Ave., New York, NY 10103. Phone: (800) 223-6834. 1987.

TEXTBOOKS AND MONOGRAPHS

Functional Disorders of the Menstrual Cycle. M.G. Brush, E.M. Goudsmit (eds.). John Wiley & Sons, Inc., 605 Third Ave., New York, NY 10158-0012. Phone: (212) 850-6000. Fax: (212) 850-6088. 1988.

The Menstrual Cycle. Michael Ferin, Raphael Jewelewicz, Michele Warren. Oxford University Press, 200 Madison Ave., New York, NY 10016. Phone: (212) 679-7300. 1992.

Menstrual Cycle and Its Disorders. K.M. Pirke, and others (eds.). Springer-Verlag New York Inc., 175 Fifth Ave., New York, NY 10010. Phone: (212) 460-1500. Fax: (212) 473-6272. 1989.

MENTAL DISORDERS

See: DEPRESSION; MOOD DISORDERS; PERSONALITY DISORDERS; PSYCHIATRIC DISORDERS; SCHIZOPHRENIA

MENTAL HEALTH

ABSTRACTING, INDEXING, AND CURRENT AWARENESS PUBLICATIONS

Adolescent Mental Health Abstracts. Center for Adolescent Health, Washington University, Box 1196, St. Louis, MO 63130. Phone: (314) 889-5824. Quarterly.

Current Contents/Clinical Medicine. Institute for Scientific Information, 3501 Market St., Philadelphia, PA 19104. Phone: (800) 523-1850. Fax: (215) 386-6362. Weekly.

Excerpta Medica. Section 32: Psychiatry. Elsevier Science Publishing Co., Inc., P.O. Box 882, Madison Square Station, New York, NY 10159-2101. Phone: (212) 989-5800. Fax: (212) 633-3990. 20/year.

Index Medicus. U.S. National Library of Medicine, 8600 Rockville Pike, Bethesda, MD 20894. Phone: (800) 638-8480. Monthly.

Psychological Abstracts. American Psychological Association, 1200 17th St. NW, Washington, DC 20036. Phone: (202) 955-7600. Monthly.

Science Citation Index. Institute for Scientific Information, 3501 Market St., Philadelphia, PA 19104. Phone: (800) 523-1850. Fax: (215) 386-6362. Bimonthly.

ASSOCIATIONS, PROFESSIONAL SOCIETIES, ADVOCACY AND SUPPORT GROUPS

American Mental Health Fund. 2735 Hartland Rd., Ste. 302, Falls Church, VA 22043. Phone: (703) 573-2200. Fax: (703) 207-9894.

Canadian Psychiatric Association. 294 Albert St., Suite 204, Ottawa, ON, Canada K1P 6E6. Phone: (613) 234-2815. Fax: (613) 234-9857.

Canadian Psychological Association. Chemin Vincent, Old Chelsea, PQ, Canada J0X 2N0. Phone: (819) 827-3927. Fax: (819) 827-4639.

Mental Illness Foundation. 7 Penn Plaza, New York, NY 10001. Phone: (212) 629-0755.

National Alliance for the Mentally Ill (NAMI). 2101 Wilson Blvd., Ste. 302, Arlington, VA 22201. Phone: (703) 524-7600. Fax: (703) 524-9094.

National Depressive and Manic Depressive Association (NDMDA). 53 W. Jackson Blvd., Ste. 505, Chicago, IL 60604. Phone: (312) 939-2442. Fax: (312) 939-1241.

National Mental Health Association (NMHA). 1021 Prince St., Alexandria, VA 22314-2971. Phone: (703) 684-7722. Fax: (703) 684-5968.

National Mental Health Consumers Association. 311 S. Juniper St., Philadelphia, PA 19107. Phone: (215) 735-2465.

World Federation for Mental Health. 1021 Prince St., Alexandria, VA 22314. Phone: (703) 684-7722.

BIBLIOGRAPHIES

National Alliance for the Mentally Ill-Annotated Reading List. National Alliance for the Mentally Ill, 2101 Wilson Blvd., Ste. 302, Arlington, VA 22201. Phone: (703) 524-7600. Fax: (703) 524-9094. Irregular.

CD-ROM DATABASES

Excerpta Medica CD: Psychiatry. SilverPlatter Information, Inc., River Ridge Office Park, 100 River Ridge Rd., Norwood, MA 02062. Phone: (617) 769-2599. Fax: (617) 769-8763. Quarterly.

PsycLit. SilverPlatter Information, Inc., River Ridge Office Park, 100 River Ridge Rd., Norwood, MA 02062. Phone: (617) 769-2599. Fax: (617) 769-8763. Quarterly.

SCISEARCH. Institute for Scientific Information, 3501 Market St., Philadelphia, PA 19104. Phone: (215) 386-0100. Fax: (215) 386-6362.

Year Books on Disc. CMC ReSearch, Inc., 7150 S.W. Hampton, Suite C-120, Portland, OR 97223. Phone: (800) 262-7668. Fax: (503) 639-1796. Annual includes Year Books of Cardiology, Dermatology, Diagnostic Radiology, Drug Therapy, Emergency Medicine, Family Practice, Medicine, Neurology and Neurosurgery, Obstetrics and Gynecology, Oncology, Pediatrics, and Psychiatry and Applied Mental Health.

DIRECTORIES

Mental Health Directory. National Institute of Mental Health, 5600 Fishers Ln., Rm. 15C-05, Rockville, MD 20857. Phone: (301) 443-4513. Irregular.

HANDBOOKS, GUIDES, MANUALS, ATLASES

Getting Help: A Consumer's Guide to Therapy. Christine Amner. Paragon House Publishers, 90 Fifth Ave., New York, NY 10011. Phone: (800) 727-2466. 1991.

JOURNALS

Bulletin of the Menninger Clinic: A Journal for the Mental Health Professions. The Menninger Clinic, Box 829, Topeka, KS 66601-0829. Phone: (913) 273-7500. Fax: (913) 273-8625. Quarterly.

NEWSLETTERS

Harvard Mental Health Letter. Harvard Medical School Publications Group, 164 Longwood Ave., Boston, MA 02115. Monthly.

ONLINE DATABASES

EMBASE. Elsevier Science Publishing Co., Inc., P.O. Box 882, Madison Square Station, New York, NY 10159-2101. Phone: (212) 989-5800. Fax: (212) 633-3990.

MEDLINE. National Library of Medicine, 8600 Rockville Pike, Bethesda, MD 20894. Phone: (800) 638-8480.

Mental Health Abstracts. IFI/Plenum Data Company, 302 Swann Ave., Alexandria, VA 22301. Phone: (800) 368-3093. Monthly.

PsycInfo. SilverPlatter Information, Inc., River Ridge Office Park, 100 River Ridge Rd., Norwood, MA 02062. Phone: (617) 769-2599. Fax: (617) 769-8763. Quarterly.

SciSearch. Institute for Scientific Information, 3501 Market St., Philadelphia, PA 19104. Phone: (215) 386-0100. Fax: (215) 386-6362.

Suicide Information and Education. Suicide Information Education Center, 1615 10th Ave. S.W., Calgary, AB, Canada. Phone: (403) 245-3900.

POPULAR WORKS AND PATIENT EDUCATION

The Columbia University College of Physicians and Surgeons Complete Home Guide to Mental and Emotional Health. Frederic I. Kass, John M. Oldham, Herbert Pardes, and others. Holt, Rinehart & Winston, 115 W. 18th St., New York, NY 10011. Phone: (800) 488-5233. 1992.

Family Mental Health Encyclopedia. Frank Bruno. John Wiley & Sons, Inc., 605 Third Ave., New York, NY 10158-0012. Phone: (212) 850-6000. Fax: (212) 850-6088. 1991.

Know Your Own Mind: The Comprehensive One-Volume Home Reference Guide to Mental Health. Jane Knowles. HarperCollins Pubs., Inc., 10 E. 53rd St., New York, NY 10022-5299. Phone: (212) 207-7000. 1992.

Psychotherapy Today: A Consumer's Guide to Choosing the Right Therapist. Ronald W. Pies. Skidmore-Roth Publishing, 1001 Wall St., El Paso, TX 79915-1012. Phone: (800) 825-3150. 1991.

RESEARCH CENTERS, INSTITUTES, CLEARINGHOUSES

Clarke Institute of Psychiatry. 250 College St., Toronto, ON, Canada M5T 1R8. Phone: (416) 979-0940. Fax: (416) 979-7871.

Eastern Pennsylvania Psychiatric Institute. Medical College of Pennsylvania. 3200 Henry Ave., Philadelphia, PA 19129. Phone: (215) 842-4000. Fax: (215) 843-7384.

Hogg Foundation for Mental Health. University of Texas. Austin, TX 78713-7998. Phone: (512) 471-5041. Fax: (512) 471-9608.

Institute for Mental Health Research. State University of New York at Stony Brook. Dept. of Psychiatry and Behavioral Science, Stony Brook, NY 11794. Phone: (516) 444-2990. Fax: (516) 444-7534.

Institute for Psychosomatic and Psychiatric Research and Training. Humana Hospital Michael Reese, Lake Shore Dr. at 31st St., Chicago, IL 60616. Phone: (312) 791-3877. Fax: (312) 567-7440.

Menninger Clinic Department of Research. Box 829, Topeka, KS 66601. Phone: (913) 273-7500. Fax: (913) 273-8625.

Missouri Institute of Mental Health. University of Missouri-Columbia. 5247 Fyler Ave., St. Louis, MO 63139-1494. Phone: (314) 644-8787. Fax: (314) 644-8834.

National Institute of Mental Health (NIMH). 5600 Fishers Ln., Room 15C-05, Rockville, MD 20857. Phone: (301) 443-4513.

National Resource Center on Homelessness and Mental Illness. 262 Delaware Ave., Delmar, NY 12054. Phone: (800) 444-7415.

Western Psychiatric Institute and Clinic. University of Pittsburgh. 3811 O'Hara St., Pittsburgh, PA 15213. Phone: (412) 624-2360. Fax: (412) 624-1881.

STANDARDS AND STATISTICS SOURCES

Mental Health National Statistics: Mental Health Service System Reports, Series CN. U.S. Government Printing Office, Superintendent of Documents, P.O. Box 371954, Pittsburgh, PA 15250-7954. Phone: (202) 783-3238. Fax: (202) 512-2250.

Mental Health, U.S.. U.S. Government Printing Office, Superintendent of Documents, P.O. Box 371954, Pittsburgh, PA 15250-7954. Phone: (202) 783-3238. Fax: (202) 512-2250. Biennial.

TEXTBOOKS AND MONOGRAPHS

Mental Health and Illness. R. Kosky, H. Eshkevari, V.J. Carr. Butterworth-Heinemann, 80 Montvale Ave., Stoneham, MA 02180. Phone: (617) 438-8464. Fax: (617) 279-4851. 1991.

Mental Health Policy for Older Americans: Protecting Minds at Risk. Barry Foger, and others. American Psychiatric Press, 1400 K St. N.W., Washington, DC 20005. Phone: (202) 682-6000. Fax: (202) 682-6114. 1990.

MENTAL RETARDATION

See also: BIRTH DEFECTS

ABSTRACTING, INDEXING, AND CURRENT AWARENESS PUBLICATIONS

General Science Index. H.W. Wilson Co., 950 University Ave., Bronx, NY 10452. Phone: (800) 367-6770.

Index Medicus. U.S. National Library of Medicine, 8600 Rockville Pike, Bethesda, MD 20894. Phone: (800) 638-8480. Monthly.

Psychological Abstracts. American Psychological Association, 1200 17th St. NW, Washington, DC 20036. Phone: (202) 955-7600. Monthly.

Research Alert: Mental Retardation. Institute for Scientific Information, 3501 Market St., Philadelphia, PA 19104. Phone: (800) 523-1850. Fax: (215) 386-6362. Weekly.

Science Citation Index. Institute for Scientific Information, 3501 Market St., Philadelphia, PA 19104. Phone: (800) 523-1850. Fax: (215) 386-6362. Bimonthly.

ASSOCIATIONS, PROFESSIONAL SOCIETIES, ADVOCACY AND SUPPORT GROUPS

American Association on Mental Retardation (AAMR). 1719 Kalorama Rd., N.W., Washington, DC 20009. Phone: (202) 387-1958.

Association for Retarded Citizens of the United States. P.O. Box 6109, Arlington, TX 76005. Phone: (817) 640-0204.

Mental Retardation Association of America. 211 E. Third S., Ste. 214, Salt Lake City, UT 84111. Phone: (801) 328-1575.

CD-ROM DATABASES

PsycLit. SilverPlatter Information, Inc., River Ridge Office Park, 100 River Ridge Rd., Norwood, MA 02062. Phone: (617) 769-2599. Fax: (617) 769-8763. Quarterly.

SCISEARCH. Institute for Scientific Information, 3501 Market St., Philadelphia, PA 19104. Phone: (215) 386-0100. Fax: (215) 386-6362.

JOURNALS

American Journal of Human Genetics. University of Chicago Press, P.O. Box 37005, Chicago, IL 60637. Phone: (312) 753-3347. Fax: (312) 753-0811. Monthly.

American Journal on Mental Retardation. American Association on Mental Retardation, 1719 Kalorama Rd NW, Washington, DC 20009-2583. Phone: (202) 387-1968. Fax: (202) 387-2193. Bimonthly.

Archives of Disease in Childhood. BMJ Publishing Group, BMA House, Tavistock Square, London WC1H 9JR, England. Phone: 071-383 6244/6638. Fax: 071-383 6662. Monthly.

British Journal of Psychiatry. Royal Society of Medicine Services Ltd., 1 Wimpole St., London W1M 8AE, England. Phone: 071-408 2119. Fax: 071-355 3198. Monthly.

Journal of Medical Genetics. BMJ Publishing Group, BMA House, Tavistock Square, London WC1H 9JR, England. Phone: 071-383 6244/6638. Fax: 071-383 6662. Monthly.

Mental Retardation. American Association on Mental Retardation, 1719 Kalorama Rd NW, Washington, DC 20009-2583. Phone: (202) 387-1968. Fax: (202) 387-2193. Bimonthly.

NEWSLETTERS

American Association on Mental Retardation-News and Notes. American Association on Mental Retardation, 1719 Kalorama Rd., N.W., Washington, DC 20009. Phone: (202) 387-1968. Bimonthly.

ONLINE DATABASES

EMBASE. Elsevier Science Publishing Co., Inc., P.O. Box 882, Madison Square Station, New York, NY 10159-2101. Phone: (212) 989-5800. Fax: (212) 633-3990.

MEDLINE. National Library of Medicine, 8600 Rockville Pike, Bethesda, MD 20894. Phone: (800) 638-8480.

Mental Health Abstracts. IFI/Plenum Data Company, 302 Swann Ave., Alexandria, VA 22301. Phone: (800) 368-3093. Monthly.

PsycInfo. SilverPlatter Information, Inc., River Ridge Office Park, 100 River Ridge Rd., Norwood, MA 02062. Phone: (617) 769-2599. Fax: (617) 769-8763. Quarterly.

SciSearch. Institute for Scientific Information, 3501 Market St., Philadelphia, PA 19104. Phone: (215) 386-0100. Fax: (215) 386-6362.

POPULAR WORKS AND PATIENT EDUCATION

Children with Mental Retardation: A Parents' Guide. Romayne Smith (ed.). Woodbine House, 5615 Fishers Ln., Rockville, MD 20852. Phone: (800) 843-7323. 1992.

RESEARCH CENTERS, INSTITUTES, CLEARINGHOUSES

Child Development and Mental Retardation Center. University of Washington. WJ-10, Seattle, WA 98195. Phone: (206) 543-3224.

Joseph P. Kennedy Jr. Foundation. 1350 New York Ave., Washington, DC 20005. Phone: (202) 393-1250.

Joseph P. Kennedy Jr. Mental Retardation Research Center. Wyle Children's Hospital, 950 E. 59th St., Chicago, IL 60637. Phone: (312) 702-6428.

Nisonger Center for Mental Retardation and Developmental Disabilities. Ohio State University. 1581 Dodd Dr., Columbus, OH 43210-1296. Phone: (614) 292-8365. Fax: (614) 292-3727.

TEXTBOOKS AND MONOGRAPHS

Mental Retardation: Developing Pharmacotherapies. John J. Ratey (ed.). American Psychiatric Press, Inc., 1400 K St. NW,

Washington, DC 20005. Phone: (202) 682-6268. Fax: (202) 789-2648. 1991.

Mental Retardation and Mental Illness Assessment, Treatment, and Service for the Dually Diagnosed. Robert Fletcher, Frank Menolascino. D.C. Heath & Co., 125 Spring St., Lexington, MA 02173. Phone: (800) 235-3565.

METABOLIC DISORDERS

ABSTRACTING, INDEXING, AND CURRENT AWARENESS PUBLICATIONS

Biological Abstracts. BIOSIS, 2100 Arch St., Philadelphia, PA 19103-1399. Phone: (800) 523-4800. Fax: (215) 587-2016.

Current Contents/Clinical Medicine. Institute for Scientific Information, 3501 Market St., Philadelphia, PA 19104. Phone: (800) 523-1850. Fax: (215) 386-6362. Weekly.

Current Contents/Life Sciences. Institute for Scientific Information, 3501 Market St., Philadelphia, PA 19104. Phone: (215) 386-0100. Fax: (215) 386-6362.

Endocrinology Abstracts. Cambridge Scientific Abstracts, 7200 Wisconsin Ave., Bethesda, MD 20814-4823. Phone: (800) 843-7751. Fax: (301) 961-6720. Monthly.

Excerpta Medica. Section 6: Internal Medicine. Elsevier Science Publishers, P.O. Box 882, Madison Square Station, New York, NY 10159-2101. Phone: (212) 633-3950. Fax: (212) 633-3990. 24/year.

Index Medicus. U.S. National Library of Medicine, 8600 Rockville Pike, Bethesda, MD 20894. Phone: (800) 638-8480. Monthly.

Research Alert: Obesity & Energy Metabolism. Institute for Scientific Information, 3501 Market St., Philadelphia, PA 19104. Phone: (800) 523-1850. Fax: (215) 386-6362. Weekly.

Science Citation Index. Institute for Scientific Information, 3501 Market St., Philadelphia, PA 19104. Phone: (800) 523-1850. Fax: (215) 386-6362. Bimonthly.

ANNUALS AND REVIEWS

Advances in Endocrinology and Metabolism. Mosby-Year Book, 11830 Westline Industrial Drive, St. Louis, MO 63146. Phone: (800) 325-4177. Fax: (314) 432-1380. Annual.

Advances in Metabolic Disorders. Academic Press, Inc., 1250 Sixth Ave., San Diego, CA 92101-4311. Phone: (619) 699-6345. Fax: (619) 699-6715.

Contemporary Metabolism. Plenum Publishing Co., 233 Spring St., New York, NY 10013-1578. Phone: (212) 620-8000. Fax: (212) 463-0742. Irregular.

Endocrinology and Metabolism Clinics. W.B. Saunders Co., The Curtis Center, Independence Square W., Philadelphia, PA 19106-3399. Phone: (215) 238-7800. Quarterly.

ASSOCIATIONS, PROFESSIONAL SOCIETIES, ADVOCACY AND SUPPORT GROUPS

Hemochromatosis Research Foundation. P.O. Box 8569, Albany, NY 12208. Phone: (518) 489-0972.

Metabolic Information Network. P.O. Box 670847, Dallas, TX 75367-0847. Phone: (800) 945-2188.

National Center for the Study of Wilson's Disease (NCSWD). 5447 Palisade Ave., Bronx, NY 10471. Phone: (212) 892-5119. Fax: (212) 863-7572.

National Gaucher Foundation (NGF). 1424 K St. N.W., 4th Flr., Washington, DC 20005. Phone: (202) 393-2777. Fax: (202) 393-5541.

CD-ROM DATABASES

Biological Abstracts on Compact Disc. BIOSIS, 2100 Arch St., Philadelphia, PA 19103-1399. Phone: (800) 523-4800. Fax: (215) 587-2016. Quarterly.

SCISEARCH. Institute for Scientific Information, 3501 Market St., Philadelphia, PA 19104. Phone: (215) 386-0100. Fax: (215) 386-6362.

JOURNALS

Hormone and Metabolic Research. Thieme Medical Publishers, Inc., 381 Park Ave. S., New York, NY 10016. Phone: (212) 683-5088. Fax: (212) 779-9020. Monthly.

Journal of Clinical Endocrinology & Metabolism. Williams & Wilkins, 428 E. Preston St., Baltimore, MD 21202. Phone: (800) 638-0672. Fax: (900) 447-8438. Monthly.

Journal of Inherited Metabolic Disease. Kluwer Academic Publishers, P.O. Box 358, Accord Station, Hingham, MA 02018-0358. Phone: (617) 871-6600. Fax: (617) 871-6528. 6/year.

Metabolism: Clinical and Experimental. W.B. Saunders Co., The Curtis Center, Independence Square W., Philadelphia, PA 19106-3399. Phone: (215) 238-7800.

Trends in Endocrinology and Metabolism. Elsevier Science Publishing Co., Inc., P.O. Box 882, Madison Square Station, New York, NY 10159-2101. Phone: (212) 989-5800. Fax: (212) 633-3990. 10/year.

ONLINE DATABASES

BIOSIS Previews. BIOSIS, 2100 Arch St., Philadelphia, PA 19103-1399. Phone: (800) 523-4800. Fax: (215) 587-2016.

EMBASE. Elsevier Science Publishing Co., Inc., P.O. Box 882, Madison Square Station, New York, NY 10159-2101. Phone: (212) 989-5800. Fax: (212) 633-3990.

MEDLINE. National Library of Medicine, 8600 Rockville Pike, Bethesda, MD 20894. Phone: (800) 638-8480.

SciSearch. Institute for Scientific Information, 3501 Market St., Philadelphia, PA 19104. Phone: (215) 386-0100. Fax: (215) 386-6362.

RESEARCH CENTERS, INSTITUTES, CLEARINGHOUSES

Center for Endocrinology, Metabolism and Nutrition. 10-555 Searle, 303 Chicago Ave., Chicago, IL 60611. Phone: (708) 908-8023. Fax: (312) 908-9032.

TEXTBOOKS AND MONOGRAPHS

Current Therapy in Endocrinology and Metabolism. C. Wayne Bardin (ed.). Mosby-Year Book, 11830 Westline Industrial

Drive, St. Louis, MO 63146. Phone: (800) 325-4177. Fax: (314) 432-1380. Fourth edition 1991.

Endocrinology and Metabolism. Philip Felig, John D. Baxter, Lawrence A. Frohman. McGraw-Hill, Inc., Health Professions Division, 1221 Avenue of the Americas, 28th Floor, New York, NY 10020. Phone: (212) 512-4228. Third edition 1992.

Metabolic Bone Disease and Clinically Related Disorders. Louis V. Avioli, Stephen M. Krane. W.B. Saunders Co., The Curtis Center, Independence Square W., Philadelphia, PA 19106-3399. Phone: (215) 238-7800. Second edition 1990.

Principles and Practice of Endocrinology and Metabolism. Kenneth L. Becker, John P. Bilezikian, William J Bremner. J.B. Lippincott Co., 227 East Washington Square, Philadelphia, PA 19106-3780. Phone: (215) 238-4200. Fax: (215) 238-4227. 1990.

MICROBIOLOGY

ABSTRACTING, INDEXING, AND CURRENT AWARENESS PUBLICATIONS

Biological Abstracts. BIOSIS, 2100 Arch St., Philadelphia, PA 19103-1399. Phone: (800) 523-4800. Fax: (215) 587-2016.

Current Contents/Life Sciences. Institute for Scientific Information, 3501 Market St., Philadelphia, PA 19104. Phone: (215) 386-0100. Fax: (215) 386-6362.

Excerpta Medica. Section 4: Microbiology, Mycology, Parasitology and Virology. Elsevier Science Publishers, P.O. Box 882, Madison Square Station, New York, NY 10159-2101. Phone: (212) 633-3950. Fax: (212) 633-3990. 32/year.

Index Medicus. U.S. National Library of Medicine, 8600 Rockville Pike, Bethesda, MD 20894. Phone: (800) 638-8480. Monthly.

Microbiology Abstracts. Section A: Industrial & Applied Microbiology. Cambridge Scientific Abstracts, 7200 Wisconsin Ave., Bethesda, MD 20814-4823. Phone: (800) 843-7751. Fax: (301) 961-6720. Monthly.

Microbiology Abstracts. Section B: Bacteriology. Cambridge Scientific Abstracts, 7200 Wisconsin Ave., Bethesda, MD 20814-4823. Phone: (800) 843-7751. Fax: (301) 961-6720. Monthly.

Microbiology Abstracts. Section C: Algology, Mycology & Protozoology. Cambridge Scientific Abstracts, 7200 Wisconsin Ave., Bethesda, MD 20814-4823. Phone: (800) 843-7751. Fax: (301) 961-6720. Monthly.

Science Citation Index. Institute for Scientific Information, 3501 Market St., Philadelphia, PA 19104. Phone: (800) 523-1850. Fax: (215) 386-6362. Bimonthly.

ANNUALS AND REVIEWS

Advances in Applied Microbiology. Academic Press, Inc., 1250 Sixth Ave., San Diego, CA 92101-4311. Phone: (619) 699-6345. Fax: (619) 699-6715. Irregular.

Advances in Microbial Physiology. Academic Press, Inc., 1250 Sixth Ave., San Diego, CA 92101-4311. Phone: (619) 699-6345. Fax: (619) 699-6715. Irregular.

Annual Review of Microbiology. Annual Reviews Inc., 4139 El Camino Way, P.O. Box 10139, Palo Alto, CA 94303-0897. Phone: (415) 493-4400. Fax: (415) 855-9815. Annual.

Contributions to Microbiology and Immunology. S. Karger Publishers, Inc., 26 West Avon Rd., P.O. Box 529, Farmington, CT 06085. Phone: (203) 675-7834. Fax: (203) 675-7302. Irregular.

Critical Reviews in Microbiology. CRC Press, Inc., 2000 Corporate Blvd. N.W., Boca Raton, FL 33431. Phone: (407) 994-0555. Fax: (407) 997-0949. Quarterly.

Current Topics in Microbiology and Immunology. Springer-Verlag New York, Inc., 175 Fifth Ave., New York, NY 10010. Phone: (212) 460-1500. Fax: (212) 473-6272. Irregular.

FEMS Microbiology Reviews. Elsevier Science Publishing Co., Inc., P.O. Box 882, Madison Square Station, New York, NY 10159-2101. Phone: (212) 989-5800. Fax: (212) 633-3990. 8/year.

Reviews in Medical Microbiology. Churchill Livingstone Inc., 650 Avenue of the Americas, New York, NY 10011. Phone: (212) 819-5400. Fax: (212) 302-6598. Quarterly.

Year Book of Clinical Microbiology. CRC Press, Inc., 2000 Corporate Blvd. N.W., Boca Raton, FL 33431. Phone: (407) 994-0555. Fax: (407) 997-0949. Annual.

ASSOCIATIONS, PROFESSIONAL SOCIETIES, ADVOCACY AND SUPPORT GROUPS

American Society for Microbiology. 1325 Massachusetts Ave. N.W., Washington, DC 20005. Phone: (202) 737-3600.

Foundation for Microbiology. National MS Society, 205 E. 42nd St., New York, NY 10017. Phone: (212) 986-3240.

CD-ROM DATABASES

Biological Abstracts on Compact Disc. BIOSIS, 2100 Arch St., Philadelphia, PA 19103-1399. Phone: (800) 523-4800. Fax: (215) 587-2016. Quarterly.

Biotechnology Citation Index. Institute for Scientific Information, 3501 Market St., Philadelphia, PA 19104. Phone: (215) 386-0100. Fax: (215) 386-6362. Bimonthly.

Cambridge Microbiology Abstracts Series. Cambridge Scientific Abstracts, 7200 Wisconsin Ave., Bethesda, MD 20814-4823. Phone: (800) 843-7751. Fax: (301) 961-6720.

SCISEARCH. Institute for Scientific Information, 3501 Market St., Philadelphia, PA 19104. Phone: (215) 386-0100. Fax: (215) 386-6362.

ENCYCLOPEDIAS, DICTIONARIES, WORD BOOKS

Encyclopedia of Microbiology. Joshua Lederberg. Academic Press, Inc., 1250 Sixth Ave., San Diego, CA 92101-4311. Phone: (619) 699-6345. Fax: (619) 699-6715. Four volumes 1992.

HANDBOOKS, GUIDES, MANUALS, ATLASES

Color Atlas and Textbook of Diagnostic Microbiology. Koneman. J.B. Lippincott Co., 227 E. Washington Square, Philadelphia, PA 19106-3780. Phone: (215) 238-4200. Fax: (215) 238-4227. Fourth edition 1992.

Manual of Clinical Microbiology. A. Balows and others. American Society for Microbiology, 1325 Massachusetts Ave N.W., Washington, DC 20005. Phone: (202) 737-3600. 5th edition 1991.

JOURNALS

Antonie van Leeuwenhoek: Journal of General and Molecular Biology. Kluwer Academic Publishers, P.O. Box 358, Accord Station, Hingham, MA 02018-0358. Phone: (617) 871-6600. Fax: (617) 871-6528. 12/year.

Applied and Environmental Microbiology. American Society for Microbiology, 1325 Massachusetts Ave. N.W., Washington, DC 20005. Phone: (202) 737-3600.

Applied Microbiology and Biotechnology. Springer-Verlag New York Inc., 175 Fifth Ave., New York, NY 10010. Phone: (212) 460-1500. Fax: (212) 473-6272.

Clinical Microbiology Review. American Society for Microbiology, 1325 Massachusetts Ave. N.W., Washington, DC 20005. Phone: (202) 737-3600.

Clinical Microbiology Reviews. American Society for Microbiology, 1325 Massachusetts Ave. NW, Washington, DC 20005-4171. Phone: (202) 737-3600. Fax: (202) 737-0368. Quarterly.

Diagnostic Microbiology and Infectious Disease. Elsevier Science Publishing Co., Inc., P.O. Box 882, Madison Square Station, New York, NY 10159-2101. Phone: (212) 989-5800. Fax: (212) 633-3990. 8/year.

FEMS Microbiology Ecology. Elsevier Science Publishing Co., Inc., P.O. Box 882, Madison Square Station, New York, NY 10159-2101. Phone: (212) 989-5800. Fax: (212) 633-3990. 8/year.

FEMS Mircobiology Immunology. Elsevier Science Publishing Co., Inc., P.O. Box 882, Madison Square Station, New York, NY 10159-2101. Phone: (212) 989-5800. Fax: (212) 633-3990. 6/year.

Journal of Clinical Microbiology. American Society for Microbiology, 1325 Massachusetts Ave. N.W., Washington, DC 20005. Phone: (202) 737-3600.

Journal of Medical Microbiology. Churchill Livingstone Inc., 650 Avenue of the Americas, New York, NY 10011. Phone: (212) 819-5400. Fax: (212) 302-6598. Monthly.

Microbiological Reviews. American Society for Microbiology, 1325 Massachusetts Ave. N.W., Washington, DC 20005. Phone: (202) 737-3600.

Research in Microbiology. Elsevier Science Publishing Co., Inc., P.O. Box 882, Madison Square Station, New York, NY 10159-2101. Phone: (212) 989-5800. Fax: (212) 633-3990. 9/year.

World Journal of Microbiology and Biotechnology. Rapid Communications of Oxford Ltd., The Old Malthouse, Paradise St., Oxford OX1 1LD, England. Phone: 44-865-790447. Fax: 44-865-244012. 6/year.

NEWSLETTERS

Clinical Microbiology Newsletter. Elsevier Science Publishing Co., Inc., P.O. Box 882, Madison Square Station, New York,

NY 10159-2101. Phone: (212) 989-5800. Fax: (212) 633-3990. 24/year.

ONLINE DATABASES

BIOSIS Previews. BIOSIS, 2100 Arch St., Philadelphia, PA 19103-1399. Phone: (800) 523-4800. Fax: (215) 587-2016.

CSA Life Sciences Collection. Cambridge Scientific Abstracts, 7200 Wisconsin Ave., Bethesda, MD 20814-4823. Phone: (800) 843-7751. Fax: (301) 961-6720.

EMBASE. Elsevier Science Publishing Co., Inc., P.O. Box 882, Madison Square Station, New York, NY 10159-2101. Phone: (212) 989-5800. Fax: (212) 633-3990.

MEDLINE. National Library of Medicine, 8600 Rockville Pike, Bethesda, MD 20894. Phone: (800) 638-8480.

SciSearch. Institute for Scientific Information, 3501 Market St., Philadelphia, PA 19104. Phone: (215) 386-0100. Fax: (215) 386-6362.

RESEARCH CENTERS, INSTITUTES, CLEARINGHOUSES

Boston Biomedical Research Institute. 20 Staniford St., Boston, MA 02114. Phone: (617) 742-2010.

Coriell Institute for Medical Research (Camden). 401 Haddon Ave., Camden, NJ 08103. Phone: (609) 966-7377. Fax: (609) 964-0254.

Microbiology Laboratories. Box 672, Dept. of Microbiology, University of Rochester, 601 Elmwood Ave., Rochester, NY 14642. Phone: (716) 275-3405.

TEXTBOOKS AND MONOGRAPHS

Basic Medical Microbiology. Jawetz. Appleton & Lange, 25 Van Zant St., East Norwalk, CT 06855. Phone: (800) 423-1359. Fax: (203) 854-9486. 19th edition 1991.

Fields Virology. Bernard N. Fields, David M. Knipe (eds.). Raven Press, 1185 Avenue of the Americas, New York, NY 10036. Phone: (212) 930-9500. Fax: (212) 869-3495. Second edition. Two volumes. 1990.

Medical Microbiology. Samuel Baron (ed.). Churchill Livingstone Inc., 650 Avenue of the Americas, New York, NY 10011. Phone: (212) 819-5400. Fax: (212) 302-6598. Third edition 1991.

Medical Microbiology and Immunology. Levinson. Appleton & Lange, 25 Van Zant St., East Norwalk, CT 06855. Phone: (800) 423-1359. Fax: (203) 854-9486. Second edition 1992.

Microbiology. Davis. J.B. Lippincott Co., 227 E. Washington Square, Philadelphia, PA 19106-3780. Phone: (215) 238-4200. Fax: (215) 238-4227. Fourth edition 1991.

Trends in Microbiology. P. Sajdl, M. Kocur (eds.). Rapid Communications of Oxford Ltd., The Old Malthouse, Paradise St., Oxford OX1 1LD, England. Phone: 44-865-790447. Fax: 44-865-244012. 1992.

Zinsser Microbiology. Joklik. Appleton & Lange, 25 Van Zant St., East Norwalk, CT 06855. Phone: (800) 423-1359. Fax: (203) 854-9486. 20th edition 1992.

MICROSURGERY

ABSTRACTING, INDEXING, AND CURRENT AWARENESS PUBLICATIONS

Excerpta Medica. Section 8: Neurology and Neurosurgery. Elsevier Science Publishers, P.O. Box 882, Madison Square Station, New York, NY 10159-2101. Phone: (212) 633-3950. Fax: (212) 633-3990. 32/year.

Index Medicus. U.S. National Library of Medicine, 8600 Rockville Pike, Bethesda, MD 20894. Phone: (800) 638-8480. Monthly.

Science Citation Index. Institute for Scientific Information, 3501 Market St., Philadelphia, PA 19104. Phone: (800) 523-1850. Fax: (215) 386-6362. Bimonthly.

ASSOCIATIONS, PROFESSIONAL SOCIETIES, ADVOCACY AND SUPPORT GROUPS

American Board of Neurological Microsurgery. 2320 Rancho Drive, No. 108, Las Vegas, NV 89102.

CD-ROM DATABASES

SCISEARCH. Institute for Scientific Information, 3501 Market St., Philadelphia, PA 19104. Phone: (215) 386-0100. Fax: (215) 386-6362.

HANDBOOKS, GUIDES, MANUALS, ATLASES

Microsurgery: Transplantation-Replantation. An Atlas-Text. Harry J. Buneke. Williams & Wilkins, 428 East Preston St., Baltimore, MD 21202. Phone: (800) 638-0672. Fax: (800) 447-8438. 1991.

JOURNALS

Journal of Reconstructive Microsurgery. Thieme Medical Publishers, Inc., 381 Park Ave. S., New York, NY 10016. Phone: (212) 683-5088. Fax: (212) 779-9020.

Microsurgery. John Wiley & Sons, Inc., 605 Third Ave., New York, NY 10158-0012. Phone: (212) 850-6000. Fax: (212) 850-6088. Bimonthly.

Neurosurgery. Williams & Wilkins, 428 E. Preston St., Baltimore, MD 21202. Phone: (800) 638-0672. Fax: (800) 447-8438. Monthly.

ONLINE DATABASES

EMBASE. Elsevier Science Publishing Co., Inc., P.O. Box 882, Madison Square Station, New York, NY 10159-2101. Phone: (212) 989-5800. Fax: (212) 633-3990.

MEDLINE. National Library of Medicine, 8600 Rockville Pike, Bethesda, MD 20894. Phone: (800) 638-8480.

SciSearch. Institute for Scientific Information, 3501 Market St., Philadelphia, PA 19104. Phone: (215) 386-0100. Fax: (215) 386-6362.

RESEARCH CENTERS, INSTITUTES, CLEARINGHOUSES

Reconstructive Microsurgery and Transplantation Laboratories. Dept. of Surgery, University of California, Irvine, Irvine, CA 92717. Phone: (714) 856-5880.

TEXTBOOKS AND MONOGRAPHS

Head and Neck Microsurgery. William M. Swartz, Joseph C. Banis. Williams & Wilkins, 428 East Preston St., Baltimore, MD 21202. Phone: (800) 638-0672. Fax: (800) 447-8438. 1992.

Microsurgery. Buncke. Williams & Wilkins, 428 East Preston St., Baltimore, MD 21202. Phone: (800) 638-0672. Fax: (800) 447-8438. 1991.

MIDWIFERY

See also: CHILDBIRTH

ABSTRACTING, INDEXING, AND CURRENT AWARENESS PUBLICATIONS

Cumulative Index to Nursing and Allied Health Literature. Glendale Adventist Medical Center, P.O. Box 871, Glendale, CA 91209. Phone: (818) 409-8005. Bimonthly.

Index Medicus. U.S. National Library of Medicine, 8600 Rockville Pike, Bethesda, MD 20894. Phone: (800) 638-8480. Monthly.

International Nursing Index. American Journal of Nursing Co., 555 W. 57th St., New York, NY 10019. Phone: (212) 582-8820. Quarterly.

Nursing and Midwifery Index. CLN Publications, c/o Bournemouth University, Dorset House Library, Talbot Campus, Fern Barrow, Poole, Dorset BH12 5BB, England. Monthly.

ASSOCIATIONS, PROFESSIONAL SOCIETIES, ADVOCACY AND SUPPORT GROUPS

American College of Nurse-Midwives (ACNM). 1522 K St. N.W., Ste. 1000, Washington, DC 20005. Phone: (202) 289-0171. Fax: (202) 289-4395.

Consortium for Nurse-Midwifery, Inc. (CNMI). 1911 W. 233rd St., Torrance, CA 90501. Phone: (213) 539-9801.

Midwives Alliance of North America (MANA). 30 S. Main, Concord, NH 03301. Phone: (603) 225-9586.

National Association of Parents and Professionals for Safe Alternatives in Childbirth. Route 1, Box 646, Marble Hill, MO 63764. Phone: (314) 238-2010.

CD-ROM DATABASES

Nursing and Allied Health (CINAHL) on CD-ROM. CINAHL, 1509 Wilson Terrace, P.O. Box 871, Glendale, CA 91209-0871. Phone: (818) 409-8005.

DIRECTORIES

Directory of Nurse-Midwifery Practices. American College of Nurse-Midwives, 1522 K St. N.W., Ste. 1000, Washington, DC 20005. Phone: (202) 289-0171. Fax: (202) 289-4395.

ENCYCLOPEDIAS, DICTIONARIES, WORD BOOKS

Bailliere's Midwive's Dictionary. Margaret Adams. W.B. Saunders Co., The Curtis Center, Independence Square W., Philadelphia, PA 19106-3399. Phone: (215) 238-7800. Seventh edition 1991.

JOURNALS

The Birth Gazette. The Birth Gazette, 42 The Farm, Summertown, TN 38483. Phone: (615) 904-2519.

Journal of Nurse-Midwifery. Elsevier Science Publishing Co., Inc., P.O. Box 882, Madison Square Station, New York, NY 10159-2101. Phone: (212) 989-5800. Fax: (212) 633-3990. 6/year.

Midwifery. Churchill Livingstone Inc., 650 Avenue of the Americas, New York, NY 10011. Phone: (212) 819-5400. Fax: (212) 302-6598. Quarterly.

Mothering Magazine. Mothering Magazine, P.O. Box 1690, Santa Fe, NM 87504. Phone: (505) 984-8116.

ONLINE DATABASES

EMBASE. Elsevier Science Publishing Co., Inc., P.O. Box 882, Madison Square Station, New York, NY 10159-2101. Phone: (212) 989-5800. Fax: (212) 633-3990.

MEDLINE. National Library of Medicine, 8600 Rockville Pike, Bethesda, MD 20894. Phone: (800) 638-8480.

Nursing and Allied Health (CINAHL). CINAHL, 1509 Wilson Terrace, P.O. Box 871, Glendale, CA 91209-0871. Phone: (818) 409-8005.

SciSearch. Institute for Scientific Information, 3501 Market St., Philadelphia, PA 19104. Phone: (215) 386-0100. Fax: (215) 386-6362.

POPULAR WORKS AND PATIENT EDUCATION

The Midwife Challenge. Sheila Kitzinger. HarperCollins Pubs., Inc., 10 E. 53rd St., New York, NY 10022-5299. Phone: (212) 207-7000. Fax: (800) 242-7737. 1991.

The New Our Bodies, Ourselves: The Updated and Expanded Edition. The Boston Women's Health Book Collective. Simon & Schuster, 1230 Ave. of the Americas, New York, NY 10020. Phone: (800) 223-2348. Fax: (800) 284-0735. 1992.

RESEARCH CENTERS, INSTITUTES, CLEARINGHOUSES

Seattle Midwifery School. 2524 16th Ave. S., No. 300, Seattle, WA 98144. Phone: (206) 322-8834.

TEXTBOOKS AND MONOGRAPHS

Heart and Hands: A Midwife's Guide to Pregnancy and Birth. Elizabeth Davis. Celestial Arts Publishing Co., P.O. Box 7327, Berkeley, CA 94707. Phone: (800) 841-2665.

Helpers in Childbirth: Midwifery Today. Ann Oakley, Susanne Houd (eds.). Taylor & Francis Inc., 1900 Frost Rd., Suite 101, Bristol, PA 19007-1598. Phone: (800) 821-8312. Fax: (215) 785-5515. 1990.

MIGRAINE

See: HEADACHE

MISCARRIAGE

See: PREGNANCY COMPLICATIONS

MITRAL VALVE DISORDERS

See: HEART DISEASES

MOLECULAR BIOLOGY

ABSTRACTING, INDEXING, AND CURRENT AWARENESS PUBLICATIONS

Current Contents/Life Sciences. Institute for Scientific Information, 3501 Market St., Philadelphia, PA 19104. Phone: (215) 386-0100. Fax: (215) 386-6362.

Index Medicus. U.S. National Library of Medicine, 8600 Rockville Pike, Bethesda, MD 20894. Phone: (800) 638-8480. Monthly.

Science Citation Index. Institute for Scientific Information, 3501 Market St., Philadelphia, PA 19104. Phone: (800) 523-1850. Fax: (215) 386-6362. Bimonthly.

ANNUALS AND REVIEWS

Annual Review of Cell Biology. Annual Reviews Inc., 4139 El Camino Way, P.O. Box 10139, Palo Alto, CA 94303-0897. Phone: (415) 493-4400. Fax: (415) 855-9815. Annual.

Cell Membranes, Methods and Reviews. Plenum Publishing Co., 233 Spring St., New York, NY 10013-1578. Phone: (212) 620-8000. Fax: (212) 463-0742.

Critical Reviews in Biochemistry and Molecular Biology. CRC Press, Inc., 2000 Corporate Blvd. N.W., Boca Raton, FL 33431. Phone: (407) 994-0555. Fax: (407) 997-0949. Bimonthly.

International Review of Cytology. Academic Press, Inc., 1250 Sixth Ave., San Diego, CA 92101-4311. Phone: (619) 699-6345. Fax: (619) 699-6715.

Progress in Molecular and Subcellular Biology. Springer-Verlag New York Inc., 175 Fifth Ave., New York, NY 10010. Phone: (212) 460-1500. Fax: (212) 473-6272.

CD-ROM DATABASES

Biotechnology Citation Index. Institute for Scientific Information, 3501 Market St., Philadelphia, PA 19104. Phone: (215) 386-0100. Fax: (215) 386-6362. Bimonthly.

LASERGENE. DNASTAR, Inc., 1228 S. Park St., Madison, WI 53715. Phone: (658) 258-7420. Fax: (608) 258-7439. Quarterly.

SCISEARCH. Institute for Scientific Information, 3501 Market St., Philadelphia, PA 19104. Phone: (215) 386-0100. Fax: (215) 386-6362.

JOURNALS

Antisense Research and Development. Mary Ann Liebert, Inc., 1651 Third Ave., New York, NY 10128. Phone: (212) 289-2300. Fax: (212) 289-4697. Quarterly.

Cell. Cell Press, 50 Church St., Cambridge, MA 02138.

Cell Growth & Differentiation. American Association for Cancer Research, Public Ledger Bldg., Suite 816, Philadelphia, PA 19106-3483. Phone: (215) 440-9300. Fax: (215) 440-9354. Monthly.

Journal of Molecular Biology. Academic Press, Inc., 1250 Sixth Ave., San Diego, CA 92101-4311. Phone: (619) 699-6345. Fax: (619) 699-6715.

Molecular and Cellular Biology. American Society for Microbiology, 1325 Massachusetts Ave. N.W., Washington, DC 20005. Phone: (202) 737-3600.

ONLINE DATABASES

EMBASE. Elsevier Science Publishing Co., Inc., P.O. Box 882, Madison Square Station, New York, NY 10159-2101. Phone: (212) 989-5800. Fax: (212) 633-3990.

MEDLINE. National Library of Medicine, 8600 Rockville Pike, Bethesda, MD 20894. Phone: (800) 638-8480.

SciSearch. Institute for Scientific Information, 3501 Market St., Philadelphia, PA 19104. Phone: (215) 386-0100. Fax: (215) 386-6362.

RESEARCH CENTERS, INSTITUTES, CLEARINGHOUSES

Institute for Molecular Biology and Biotechnology. McMaster University. Life Sciences Bldg., Room 425, 1280 Main St. W., Hamilton, ON, Canada L8S 4K1. Phone: (416) 525-9140. Fax: (416) 521-2955.

TEXTBOOKS AND MONOGRAPHS

Human Retroviruses. Jerome E. Groopman, Irvin S.Y. Chen, Myron Essex, et al.. John Wiley & Sons, Inc., 605 Third Ave., New York, NY 10158-0012. Phone: (212) 850-6000. Fax: (212) 850-6088. 1990.

Molecular Biology of Autoimmune Disease. Springer-Verlag New York Inc., 175 Fifth Ave., New York, NY 10010. Phone: (212) 460-1500. Fax: (212) 473-6272.

Molecular Biology of Cancer Genes. Mels Sluyber. Routledge, Chapman & Hall, Inc., 29 W. 35th St., New York, NY 10001-2291. Phone: (212) 244-3336. 1990.

Molecular Biology of the Cardiovascular System. Shu Chien. Williams & Wilkins, 428 East Preston St., Baltimore, MD 21202. Phone: (800) 638-0672. Fax: (800) 447-8438. 1990.

MONOCLONAL ANTIBODIES

ABSTRACTING, INDEXING, AND CURRENT AWARENESS PUBLICATIONS

BIOSIS/CAS Selects: Monoclonal Antibodies. BIOSIS, 2100 Arch St., Philadelphia, PA 19103-1399. Phone: (215) 587-4800. Fax: (215) 587-2016. Biweekly.

Biotechnology Research Abstracts. Cambridge Scientific Abstracts, 7200 Wisconsin Ave., Bethesda, MD 20814-4823. Phone: (800) 843-7751. Fax: (301) 961-6720. Bimonthly.

CA Selects: Monoclonal Antibodies. Chemical Abstracts Service, 2540 Olentangy River Road, P.O. Box 3012, Columbus, OH 43210-0012. Phone: (800) 848-6538. Biweekly.

Chemical Abstracts. Chemical Abstracts Service, 2540 Olentangy River Rd., P.O. Box 3012, Columbus, OH 43210-0012. Phone: (800) 848-6538.

Current Biotechnology Abstracts. Royal Society of Chemistry, Burlington House, Piccadilly, London W1V 0BN, England. Monthly.

Current Contents/Clinical Medicine. Institute for Scientific Information, 3501 Market St., Philadelphia, PA 19104. Phone: (800) 523-1850. Fax: (215) 386-6362. Weekly.

Current Contents/Life Sciences. Institute for Scientific Information, 3501 Market St., Philadelphia, PA 19104. Phone: (215) 386-0100. Fax: (215) 386-6362.

Excerpta Medica. Section 26: Immunology, Serology and Transplantation. Elsevier Science Publishing Co., Inc., P.O. Box 882, Madison Square Station, New York, NY 10159-2101. Phone: (212) 989-5800. Fax: (212) 633-3990. 32/year.

Index Medicus. U.S. National Library of Medicine, 8600 Rockville Pike, Bethesda, MD 20894. Phone: (800) 638-8480. Monthly.

Research Alert: Immunology-Antibodies/Immunoglobulins. Institute for Scientific Information, 3501 Market St., Philadelphia, PA 19104. Phone: (800) 523-1850. Fax: (215) 386-6362. Weekly.

Research Alert: Monoclonal Antibodies, Hybridomas. Institute for Scientific Information, 3501 Market St., Philadelphia, PA 19104. Phone: (800) 523-1850. Fax: (215) 386-6362. Weekly.

Science Citation Index. Institute for Scientific Information, 3501 Market St., Philadelphia, PA 19104. Phone: (800) 523-1850. Fax: (215) 386-6362. Bimonthly.

ANNUALS AND REVIEWS

Annual Review of Immunology. Annual Reviews Inc., 4139 El Camino Way, P.O. Box 10139, Palo Alto, CA 94303-0897. Phone: (415) 493-4400. Fax: (415) 855-9815. Annual.

BIBLIOGRAPHIES

Genetic Engineering: Monoclonal Antibodies. National Technical Information Service, 5285 Port Royal Rd., Springfield, VA 22161. Phone: (703) 487-4650. Fax: (703) 321-8547. Jan. 1978-Jan. 1989 PB88-855515/CBY.

Oncology Overview: Application of Monoclonal Antibodies in Clinical Oncology. David Berd (ed.). U.S. Government Printing Office, Superintendent of Documents, P.O. Box 371954, Pittsburgh, PA 15250-7954. Phone: (202) 783-3238. Fax: (202) 512-2250. 1990.

CD-ROM DATABASES

SCISEARCH. Institute for Scientific Information, 3501 Market St., Philadelphia, PA 19104. Phone: (215) 386-0100. Fax: (215) 386-6362.

DIRECTORIES

Monoclonal Antibodies. Theta Corporation, Theta Bldg., Middlefield, CT 06455. Phone: (203) 349-1054. Fax: (203) 349-1227. Irregular.

JOURNALS

Cancer Research. Williams & Wilkins, 428 East Preston St., Baltimore, MD 21202. Phone: (800) 638-0672. Fax: (800) 447-8438. Semimonthly.

International Journal of Cancer. John Wiley & Sons, Inc., 605 Third Ave., New York, NY 10158-0012. Phone: (212) 850-6000. Fax: (212) 850-6088. 18/year.

Journal of General Virology. Society for Gernal Microbiology, Harvest House, 62 London Rd., Reading, Berks. RG1 5AS, England. Phone: 07348-61345. Fax: 07343-14112. Monthly.

Journal of Immunology. Williams & Wilkins, 428 E. Preston St., Baltimore, MD 21202. Phone: (800) 638-0672. Fax: (800) 447-8438. Semimonthly.

Monoclonal Antibodies. Mary Ann Liebert, Inc., 1651 Third Ave., New York, NY 10128. Phone: (212) 289-2300. Fax: (212) 289-4697. Quarterly.

ONLINE DATABASES

Biotechnology Abstracts. Derwent Publications Ltd., Rochdale House, 128 Theobalds Rd., London WC1X BRP, England. Phone: 071-242 5823. Fax: 071-405 3630. Monthly.

CA File (Chemical Abstracts File). Chemical Abstracts Service, 2540 Olentangy River Rd., P.O. Box 3012, Columbus, OH 43210-0012. Phone: (800) 848-6538.

EMBASE. Elsevier Science Publishing Co., Inc., P.O. Box 882, Madison Square Station, New York, NY 10159-2101. Phone: (212) 989-5800. Fax: (212) 633-3990.

MEDLINE. National Library of Medicine, 8600 Rockville Pike, Bethesda, MD 20894. Phone: (800) 638-8480.

SciSearch. Institute for Scientific Information, 3501 Market St., Philadelphia, PA 19104. Phone: (215) 386-0100. Fax: (215) 386-6362.

RESEARCH CENTERS, INSTITUTES, CLEARINGHOUSES

Boston Biomedical Research Institute. 20 Staniford St., Boston, MA 02114. Phone: (617) 742-2010.

Center for Advanced Biotechnology and Medicine. 679 Hoes Lane, Piscataway, NJ 08854-5638. Phone: (201) 463-5311. Fax: (201) 463-5318.

Coriell Institute for Medical Research (Camden). 401 Haddon Ave., Camden, NJ 08103. Phone: (609) 966-7377. Fax: (609) 964-0254.

Department of Immunology. University of Toronto. Medical Sciences Bldg., Toronto, ON, Canada M5S 1A8. Phone: (416) 978-6382. Fax: (416) 978-1938.

Fred Hutchinson Cancer Research Center. 1124 Columbia St., Seattle, WA 98104. Phone: (206) 467-5000. Fax: (206) 467-5268.

Immunobiology Research Group. University of Montreal. 2900 Blvd. Edouard-Montpetit, C.P. 6128, Succursale "A", Montreal, PQ, Canada H3C 3J7. Phone: (514) 343-6273. Fax: (514) 343-5701.

Immunology Research Program. Duke University. Medical Center, Box 3010, Durham, NC 27710. Phone: (919) 684-4119. Fax: (919) 684-8982.

TEXTBOOKS AND MONOGRAPHS

Clinical Applications of Monoclonal Antibodies. R. Hubbard, V. Marks (eds.). Plenum Publishing Co., 233 Spring St., New York, NY 10013-1578. Phone: (212) 620-8000. Fax: (212) 463-0742. 1988.

Making Monoclonals: A Practical Beginner's Guide to the Protection and Characterization of Monoclonal Antibodies Against Bacteria and Viruses. Dianne G. Newell, Brian W. McBride, Stuart A. Clark. Cambridge University Press, 40 W. 20th St., New York, NY 10011. Phone: (800) 431-1580. 1991.

Monoclonal Antibodies: Applications in Clinical Oncology. A. Epenetos. Routledge, Chapman & Hall, Inc., 29 W. 35th St., New York, NY 10001-2291. Phone: (212) 244-3336. 1991.

Monoclonal Antibodies Therapy. H. Waldmann (ed.). S. Karger Publishers, Inc., 26 W. Avon Rd., P.O. Box 529, Farmington, CT 06085. Phone: (203) 675-7834. Fax: (203) 675-7302. 1988.

Monoclonal Antibodies for Therapy, Prevention and in Vivo Diagnosis of Human Disease. H. Van de Donk, W. Hennessen (eds.). S. Karger Publishers, Inc., 26 West Avon Rd., P.O. Box 529, Farmington, CT 06085. Phone: (203) 675-7834. Fax: (203) 675-7302. 1990.

The Present and Future Role of Monoclonal Antibodies in the Management of Cancer: 24th Annual San Francisco Cancer Symposium, San Francisco, CA. J.M. Vaeth, J.L. Meyer (eds.). S. Karger Publishers, Inc., 26 West Avon Rd., P.O. Box 529, Farmington, CT 06085. Phone: (203) 675-7834. Fax: (203) 675-7302. 1990.

Therapeutic Monoclonal Antibodies. J. Larrick, C. Borrebaeck. Macmillan Publishing Co., 866 Third Ave., New York, NY 10011. Phone: (800) 257-5755. 1990.

MONONUCLEOSIS

See: INFECTIOUS DISEASES

MOOD DISORDERS

See also: DEPRESSION; PSYCHIATRIC DISORDERS

ABSTRACTING, INDEXING, AND CURRENT AWARENESS PUBLICATIONS

Current Contents/Clinical Medicine. Institute for Scientific Information, 3501 Market St., Philadelphia, PA 19104. Phone: (800) 523-1850. Fax: (215) 386-6362. Weekly.

Excerpta Medica. Section 32: Psychiatry. Elsevier Science Publishing Co., Inc., P.O. Box 882, Madison Square Station, New York, NY 10159-2101. Phone: (212) 989-5800. Fax: (212) 633-3990. 20/year.

Index Medicus. U.S. National Library of Medicine, 8600 Rockville Pike, Bethesda, MD 20894. Phone: (800) 638-8480. Monthly.

Psychological Abstracts. American Psychological Association, 1200 17th St. NW, Washington, DC 20036. Phone: (202) 955-7600. Monthly.

Science Citation Index. Institute for Scientific Information, 3501 Market St., Philadelphia, PA 19104. Phone: (800) 523-1850. Fax: (215) 386-6362. Bimonthly.

ASSOCIATIONS, PROFESSIONAL SOCIETIES, ADVOCACY AND SUPPORT GROUPS

American Orthopsychiatric Association (ORTHO). 19 W. 44th St., No. 1616, New York, NY 10036. Phone: (212) 354-5770. Fax: (212) 302-9463.

American Psychiatric Association (APA). 1400 K St. N.W., Washington, DC 20005. Phone: (202) 682-6000. Fax: (202) 682-6114.

American Psychological Association (APA). 1200 17th St. N.W., Washington, DC 20036. Phone: (202) 955-7600. Fax: (703) 525-5191.

Canadian Psychiatric Association. 294 Albert St., Suite 204, Ottawa, ON, Canada K1P 6E6. Phone: (613) 234-2815. Fax: (613) 234-9857.

Canadian Psychological Association. Chemin Vincent, Old Chelsea, PQ, Canada J0X 2N0. Phone: (819) 827-3927. Fax: (819) 827-4639.

Foundation for Depression and Manic Depression (FDMD). 7 E. 67th St., New York, NY 10021. Phone: (212) 772-3400.

National Depressive and Manic Depressive Association (NDMDA). 53 W. Jackson Blvd., Ste. 505, Chicago, IL 60604. Phone: (312) 939-2442. Fax: (312) 939-1241.

CD-ROM DATABASES

Excerpta Medica CD: Psychiatry. SilverPlatter Information, Inc., River Ridge Office Park, 100 River Ridge Rd., Norwood, MA 02062. Phone: (617) 769-2599. Fax: (617) 769-8763. Quarterly.

PsycLit. SilverPlatter Information, Inc., River Ridge Office Park, 100 River Ridge Rd., Norwood, MA 02062. Phone: (617) 769-2599. Fax: (617) 769-8763. Quarterly.

SCISEARCH. Institute for Scientific Information, 3501 Market St., Philadelphia, PA 19104. Phone: (215) 386-0100. Fax: (215) 386-6362.

ENCYCLOPEDIAS, DICTIONARIES, WORD BOOKS

The Encyclopedia of Depression. Roberta Roesch, Stanley W. Jackson. Facts on File, Inc., 460 Park Ave. S., New York, NY 10016-7382. Phone: (212) 683-2244. Fax: (212) 683-3633. 1990.

Psychiatry Words. Stedman. Williams & Wilkins, 428 East Preston St., Baltimore, MD 21202. Phone: (800) 638-0672. Fax: (800) 447-8438. 1992.

HANDBOOKS, GUIDES, MANUALS, ATLASES

Getting Help: A Consumer's Guide to Therapy. Christine Amner. Paragon House Publishers, 90 Fifth Ave., New York, NY 10011. Phone: (800) 727-2466. 1991.

JOURNALS

Harvard Review of Psychiatry. Mosby-Year Book, 11830 Westline Industrial Drive, St. Louis, MO 63146. Phone: (800) 325-4177. Fax: (314) 432-1380. Bimonthly.

Journal of Affective Disorders. Elsevier Science Publishing Co., Inc., P.O. Box 882, Madison Square Station, New York, NY 10159-2101. Phone: (212) 989-5800. Fax: (212) 633-3990. 12/year.

NEWSLETTERS

Harvard Mental Health Letter. Harvard Medical School Publications Group, 164 Longwood Ave., Boston, MA 02115. Monthly.

ONLINE DATABASES

EMBASE. Elsevier Science Publishing Co., Inc., P.O. Box 882, Madison Square Station, New York, NY 10159-2101. Phone: (212) 989-5800. Fax: (212) 633-3990.

MEDLINE. National Library of Medicine, 8600 Rockville Pike, Bethesda, MD 20894. Phone: (800) 638-8480.

Mental Health Abstracts. IFI/Plenum Data Company, 302 Swann Ave., Alexandria, VA 22301. Phone: (800) 368-3093. Monthly.

SciSearch. Institute for Scientific Information, 3501 Market St., Philadelphia, PA 19104. Phone: (215) 386-0100. Fax: (215) 386-6362.

POPULAR WORKS AND PATIENT EDUCATION

Feeling Good: The New Mood Therapy. Burns. Avon Books, 1350 Ave. of the Americas, 2nd Flr., New York, NY 10019. Phone: (800) 238-0658. 1992.

Life on a Roller Coaster: Coping with the Ups and Downs of Mood Disorders. Ekkehard Othmer. Berkley Publishing Group, 200 Madison Ave., New York, NY 10016. Phone: (212) 866-5930. 1991.

Overcoming Depression. Demitri Papolos, Janice Papolos. HarperCollins Pubs., Inc., 10 E. 53rd St., New York, NY 10022-5299. Phone: (212) 207-7000. Fax: (800) 242-7737. Revised edition 1992.

TEXTBOOKS AND MONOGRAPHS

Biological Aspects of Affective Disorders. Roger Horton, Cornelius Katona (eds.). Academic Press, Inc., 1250 Sixth Ave., San Diego, CA 92101-4311. Phone: (619) 699-6345. Fax: (619) 699-6715. 1991.

Brain Imaging in Affective Disorders. Peter Hauser (ed.). American Psychiatric Press, Inc., 1400 K St. N.W., Washington, DC 20005. Phone: (202) 682-6268. Fax: (202) 789-2648. 1991.

Comorbitity of Mood and Anxiety Disorders. Jack D. Maser, C. Robert Cloninger (eds.). American Psychiatric Press, Inc., 1400 K St. NW, Washington, DC 20005. Phone: (202) 682-6268. Fax: (202) 789-2648. 1990.

Depression and Mania. Anastasios Georgotas, Robert Cancro (eds.). Elsevier Science Publishing Co., Inc., P.O. Box 882, Madison Square Station, New York, NY 10159-2101. Phone: (212) 989-5800. Fax: (212) 633-3990. 1988.

Depressive Disorders: Facts, Theories, and Treatment Methods. Benjamin B. Wolman, George Striker (eds.). John Wiley & Sons, Inc., 605 Third Ave., New York, NY 10158-0012. Phone: (212) 850-6000. Fax: (212) 850-6088. 1990.

The Genetics of Mood Disorders. Ming T. Tsuang, Stephen V. Faraone. Johns Hopkins University Press, 701 W. 40th St., Suite 275, Baltimore, MD 21211-2190. Phone: (800) 537-5487. Fax: (410) 516-6998. 1990.

Premenstrual, Postpartum, and Menopausal Mood Disorders. Laurence M. Demers, John L. McGuire, Audrey Phillips, et. al.. Williams & Wilkins, 428 East Preston St., Baltimore, MD 21202. Phone: (800) 638-0672. Fax: (800) 447-8438. 1990.

Refractory Depression. Jay D. Amsterdam. Raven Press, 1185 Avenue of the Americas, New York, NY 10036. Phone: (212) 930-9500. Fax: (212) 869-3495. Advances in Neuropsychiatry and Psychopharmacology. Volume 2. 1991.

Seasonal Affective Disorder. C. Thompson, T. Silverstone (eds.). Rapid Communications of Oxford Ltd., The Old Malthouse, Paradise St., Oxford OX1 1LD, England. Phone: 44-865-790447. Fax: 44-865-244012. 1989.

Seasonal Affective Disorders. Chris Thompson, Trevor Silverstone (eds.). Sheridan House, Inc., 145 Palisade St., Dobbs Ferry, NY 10522. Phone: (914) 693-2410. 1989.

MORBIDITY

See: VITAL STATISTICS

MORTALITY

See: VITAL STATISTICS

MOUTH CANCER

See: ORAL CANCER

MOUTH DISEASES

See also: DENTISTRY; ORAL SURGERY; PERIODONTICS

ABSTRACTING, INDEXING, AND CURRENT AWARENESS PUBLICATIONS

Current Contents/Clinical Medicine. Institute for Scientific Information, 3501 Market St., Philadelphia, PA 19104. Phone: (800) 523-1850. Fax: (215) 386-6362. Weekly.

Dental Abstracts. Mosby-Year Book, 11830 Westline Industrial Drive, St. Louis, MO 63146. Phone: (800) 325-4177. Fax: (314) 432-1380. Bimonthly.

Index to Dental Literature. American Dental Association, 211 E. Chicago Ave., Chicago, IL 60611-2678. Phone: (800) 947-4746. Fax: (312) 440-3542. Quarterly.

Index Medicus. U.S. National Library of Medicine, 8600 Rockville Pike, Bethesda, MD 20894. Phone: (800) 638-8480. Monthly.

Science Citation Index. Institute for Scientific Information, 3501 Market St., Philadelphia, PA 19104. Phone: (800) 523-1850. Fax: (215) 386-6362. Bimonthly.

ANNUALS AND REVIEWS

Year Book of Dentistry. Mosby-Year Book, 11830 Westline Industrial Drive, St. Louis, MO 63146. Phone: (800) 325-4177. Fax: (314) 432-1380. Annual.

ASSOCIATIONS, PROFESSIONAL SOCIETIES, ADVOCACY AND SUPPORT GROUPS

American Academy of Oral Pathology. c/o Dean K. White, Dept. of Oral Pathology, College of Dentistry, University of Kentucky, Lexington, KY 40536.

American Academy of Periodontology. 211 E. Chicago Ave., Chicago, IL 60611. Phone: (312) 787-5518.

American Board of Oral Pathology. 1121 W. Michigan St., Indiana University School of Dentistry, Indianapolis, IN 46202. Phone: (317) 274-7668.

American Dental Association (ADA). 211 E. Chicago Ave., Chicago, IL 60611. Phone: (312) 440-2500.

CD-ROM DATABASES

SCISEARCH. Institute for Scientific Information, 3501 Market St., Philadelphia, PA 19104. Phone: (215) 386-0100. Fax: (215) 386-6362.

DIRECTORIES

American Dental Directory. American Dental Association, 211 E. Chicago Ave., Chicago, IL 60611-2678. Phone: (800) 947-4746. Fax: (312) 440-3542. Annual.

HANDBOOKS, GUIDES, MANUALS, ATLASES

Atlas of Disease of the Oral Mucosa. J.J. Pindborg. Mosby-Year Book, 11830 Westline Industrial Drive, St. Louis, MO 63146. Phone: (800) 325-4177. Fax: (314) 432-1380. Fifth edition 1992.

Clinical Atlas of Clinical Oral Pathology. Neville. Williams & Wilkins, 428 E. Preston St., Baltimore, MD 21202. Phone: (800) 638-0672. Fax: (800) 447-8438. 1991.

Colby, Kerr, and Robinson's Color Atlas of Oral Pathology. Hamilton B.G. Robinson, Arthur S. Miller. J.B. Lippincott Co., 227 East Washington Square, Philadelphia, PA 19106-3780. Phone: (215) 238-4200. Fax: (215) 238-4227. Fifth edition 1990.

Color Atlas of Common Oral Diseases. Robert P. Langlais, Craig S. Miller. Williams & Wilkins, 428 E. Preston St., Baltimore, MD 21202. Phone: (800) 638-0672. Fax: (800) 447-8438. 1992.

Color Atlas of Oral Diseases. G. Laskaris. Thieme Medical Publishers, Inc., 381 Park Ave. S., New York, NY 10016. Phone: (212) 683-5088. Fax: (212) 779-9020. 1988.

A Color Atlas of Orofacial Diseases. W.R. Tyldesley. Mosby-Year Book, 11830 Westline Industrial Drive, St. Louis, MO 63146. Phone: (800) 325-4177. Fax: (314) 432-1380. Second edition 1991.

JOURNALS

Journal of the American Dental Association. American Dental Association, 211 E. Chicago Ave., Chicago, IL 60611-2678. Phone: (800) 947-4746. Fax: (312) 440-3542. Monthly.

Journal of Dentistry. Butterworth-Heinemann, 80 Montvale Ave., Stoneham, MA 02180. Phone: (617) 438-8464. Fax: (617) 279-4851. Bimonthly.

Journal of Periodontology. American Academy of Periodontology, 211 E. Chicago Ave., Chicago, IL 60611. Phone: (312) 787-5518.

Oral Surgery, Oral Medicine, Oral Pathology. Mosby-Year Book, 11830 Westline Industrial Drive, St. Louis, MO 63146. Phone: (800) 325-4177. Fax: (314) 432-1380. Monthly.

ONLINE DATABASES

EMBASE. Elsevier Science Publishing Co., Inc., P.O. Box 882, Madison Square Station, New York, NY 10159-2101. Phone: (212) 989-5800. Fax: (212) 633-3990.

MEDLINE. National Library of Medicine, 8600 Rockville Pike, Bethesda, MD 20894. Phone: (800) 638-8480.

SciSearch. Institute for Scientific Information, 3501 Market St., Philadelphia, PA 19104. Phone: (215) 386-0100. Fax: (215) 386-6362.

POPULAR WORKS AND PATIENT EDUCATION

Complete Guide to Dental Health: How to Avoid Being Overcharged and Overtreated. Jay Friedman. Consumer Reports Books, 9180 LeSaint Dr., Fairfield, OH 45014. Phone: (513) 860-1178. 1991.

The Mount Sinai Medical Center Family Guide to Dental Health. Jack Klatell, Andrew Kaplan, Gray Williams Jr.. Macmillan Publishing Co., Inc., 866 Third Ave., New York, NY 10022. Phone: (800) 257-5755. 1992.

RESEARCH CENTERS, INSTITUTES, CLEARINGHOUSES

National Institute of Dental Research. NIH Bldg. 31, Rm. 2C-35, 9000 Rockville Pike, Bethesda, MD 20892. Phone: (301) 496-4261.

TEXTBOOKS AND MONOGRAPHS

Burket's Oral Medicine. Malcolm A. Lynch, Vernon J. Brightman, Martin Greenberg. J.B. Lippincott Co., 227 East Washington Square, Philadelphia, PA 19106-3780. Phone: (215) 238-4200. Fax: (215) 238-4227. Ninth edition 1992.

Clinical Virology in Oral Medicine and Dentistry. Crispian Scully, Lakshman Samaranayake. Cambridge University Press, 40 W. 20th St., New York, NY 10011. Phone: (800) 431-1580. 1992.

Glickman's Clinical Periodontology. Fermin A. Carranza Jr. (ed.). W.B. Saunders Co., The Curtis Center, Independence Square W., Philadelphia, PA 19106-3399. Phone: (215) 238-7800. Seventh edition 1990.

Oral Disease in the Tropics. Prabhu. Oxford University Press, 200 Madison Ave., New York, NY 10016. Phone: (212) 679-7300. 1992.

Oral Pathology. Ash. Williams & Wilkins, 428 East Preston St., Baltimore, MD 21202. Phone: (800) 638-0672. Fax: (800) 447-8438. Sixth edition 1992.

Periodontal Diseases: Basic Phenomena, Clinical Management, and Occlusal and Resorative Interrelationships. Saul Schluger,

Ralph A. Yuodelis, Roy C. Page, et. al.. Williams & Wilkins, 428 E. Preston St., Baltimore, MD 21202. Phone: (800) 638-0672. Fax: (800) 447-8438. Second edition 1990.

MRI (MAGNETIC RESONANCE IMAGING)

See also: DIAGNOSIS; NUCLEAR MEDICINE; TOMOGRAPHY

ABSTRACTING, INDEXING, AND CURRENT AWARENESS PUBLICATIONS

Current Contents/Clinical Medicine. Institute for Scientific Information, 3501 Market St., Philadelphia, PA 19104. Phone: (800) 523-1850. Fax: (215) 386-6362. Weekly.

Excerpta Medica. Section 23: Nuclear Medicine. Elsevier Science Publishers, P.O. Box 882, Madison Square Station, New York, NY 10159-2101. Phone: (212) 633-3950. Fax: (212) 633-3990. 20/year.

Index Medicus. U.S. National Library of Medicine, 8600 Rockville Pike, Bethesda, MD 20894. Phone: (800) 638-8480. Monthly.

Research Alert: Imaging Techniques-CT, MR, PET, SPECT. Institute for Scientific Information, 3501 Market St., Philadelphia, PA 19104. Phone: (800) 523-1850. Fax: (215) 386-6362. Weekly.

Science Citation Index. Institute for Scientific Information, 3501 Market St., Philadelphia, PA 19104. Phone: (800) 523-1850. Fax: (215) 386-6362. Bimonthly.

ANNUALS AND REVIEWS

Advances in Magnetic and Optical Resonance. Academic Press, Inc., 1250 Sixth Ave., San Diego, CA 92101-4311. Phone: (619) 699-6345. Fax: (619) 699-6715. Irregular.

Critical Reviews in Diagnostic Imaging. CRC Press, Inc., 2000 Corporate Blvd. N.W., Boca Raton, FL 33431. Phone: (407) 994-0555. Fax: (407) 997-0949. Bimonthly.

Neuroimaging Clinics of North America. W.B. Saunders Co., The Curtis Center, Independence Square W., Philadelphia, PA 19106-3399. Phone: (215) 238-7800. Quarterly.

Year Book of Diagnostic Radiology. Mosby-Year Book, 11830 Westline Industrial Drive, St. Louis, MO 63146. Phone: (800) 325-4177. Fax: (314) 432-1380. Annual.

Year Book of Nuclear Medicine. Mosby-Year Book, 11830 Westline Industrial Drive, St. Louis, MO 63146. Phone: (800) 325-4177. Fax: (314) 432-1380. Annual.

ASSOCIATIONS, PROFESSIONAL SOCIETIES, ADVOCACY AND SUPPORT GROUPS

American Society of Neuroimaging (ASN). 2221 University Ave. S.E., Ste. 340, Minneapolis, MN 55414. Phone: (612) 378-7240.

Computerized Medical Imaging Society (CMIS). National Biomedical Research Foundation, Georgetown University Medical Ctr., 3900 Reservoir Rd. N.W., Washington, DC 20007. Phone: (202) 687-2121.

Council on Diagnostic Imaging. P.O. Box 1655, Ashtabula, OH 44004. Phone: (216) 993-7213.

Radiological Society of North America (RSNA). 2021 Spring Rd., Ste. 600, Oak Brook, IL 60521. Phone: (708) 571-2670. Fax: (708) 571-7837.

Society for Magnetic Resonance Imaging (SMRI). 213 W. Institute Pl., Ste. 501, Chicago, IL 60610. Phone: (312) 751-2590. Fax: (312) 951-6474.

BIBLIOGRAPHIES

Nuclear Magnetic Resonance: Applications in Medical Diagnosis. National Technical Information Service, 5285 Port Royal Rd., Springfield, VA 22161. Phone: (703) 487-4650. Fax: (703) 321-8547. Jan. 1978-July 1988 PB88-866900/CBY.

Nuclear Magnetic Resonance as a Diagnostic Tool. National Technical Information Service, 5285 Port Royal Rd., Springfield, VA 22161. Phone: (703) 487-4650. Fax: (703) 321-8547. Jan. 1970-July 1988 PB88-866926/CBY.

CD-ROM DATABASES

Electronic MRI Manual. Aries Systems Corporation, One Dundee Park, Andover, MA 01810. Phone: (508) 475-7200. Fax: (508) 474-8860. Irregular.

Excerpta Medica CD: Radiology & Nuclear Medicine. SilverPlatter Information, Inc., River Ridge Office Park, 100 River Ridge Rd., Norwood, MA 02062. Phone: (617) 769-2599. Fax: (617) 769-8763. Quarterly.

SCISEARCH. Institute for Scientific Information, 3501 Market St., Philadelphia, PA 19104. Phone: (215) 386-0100. Fax: (215) 386-6362.

DIRECTORIES

Directory of Certified Nuclear Medicine Specialists. American Board of Medical Specialties, 1 Rotary Center, Suite 805, Evanston, IL 60201. Phone: (708) 491-9091. Biennial.

HANDBOOKS, GUIDES, MANUALS, ATLASES

Manual of Clinical Magnetic Resonance Imaging. Jay P. Heiken, Jeffrey J. Brown (eds.). Raven Press, 1185 Avenue of the Americas, New York, NY 10036. Phone: (212) 930-9500. Fax: (212) 869-3495. Second edition 1991.

Manual of Clinical MRI. Heiken. Raven Press, 1185 Ave. of the Americas, New York, NY 10036. Phone: (212) 930-9500. Fax: (212) 869-3495. Second edition 1991.

Manual of Diagnostic Imaging. Straub. Little, Brown and Co., 34 Beacon St., Boston, MA 02108. Phone: (617) 227-0730. Fax: (617) 227-0790. Second edition 1989.

MRI Atlas of the Brain. William G. Bradley, Graeme Bydder. Raven Press, 1185 Avenue of the Americas, New York, NY 10036. Phone: (212) 930-9500. Fax: (212) 869-3495. 1990.

MRI Atlas of the Spine. Kenneth R. Maravilla, Wendy A. Cohen. Raven Press, 1185 Avenue of the Americas, New York, NY 10036. Phone: (212) 930-9500. Fax: (212) 869-3495. 1991.

MRI Manual. Lufkin. Mosby-Year Book, 11830 Westline Industrial Drive, St. Louis, MO 63146. Phone: (800) 325-4177. Fax: (314) 432-1380. 1990.

Nuclear Medicine. Datz. Mosby-Year Book, 11830 Westline Industrial Drive, St. Louis, MO 63146. Phone: (800) 325-4177. Fax: (314) 432-1380. 1988.

Pocket Atlas of Cardiac and Thoracic MRI. Brown. Raven Press, 1185 Ave. of the Americas, New York, NY 10036. Phone: (212) 930-9500. Fax: (212) 869-3495. 1989.

Pocket Atlas of Spinal MRI. Czervionke. Raven Press, 1185 Ave. of the Americas, New York, NY 10036. Phone: (212) 930-9500. Fax: (212) 869-3495. 1989.

Practical MRI Atlas of Neonatal Brain Development. A. James Barkovich, Charles L. Truwit. Raven Press, 1185 Avenue of the Americas, New York, NY 10036. Phone: (212) 930-9500. Fax: (212) 869-3495. 1990.

Workbook for MRI and CT of the Head and Neck. Anthony Mancuso, and others. Williams & Wilkins, 428 East Preston St., Baltimore, MD 21202. Phone: (800) 638-0672. Fax: (800) 447-8438. 2nd edition, 1988.

JOURNALS

Imaging. Rapid Communications of Oxford Ltd., The Old Malthouse, Paradise St., Oxford OX1 1LD, England. Phone: 44-865-790447. Fax: 44-865-244012. 4/year.

Magnetic Resonance Imaging. Pergamon Press, 660 White Plains Rd., Tarrytown, NY 10591-5153. Phone: (914) 592-7700. Fax: (914) 592-3625.

Magnetic Resonance in Medicine. Academic Press, Inc., 1250 Sixth Ave., San Diego, CA 92101-4311. Phone: (619) 699-6345. Fax: (619) 699-6715.

Magnetic Resonance Quarterly. Raven Press, 1185 Avenue of the Americas, New York, NY 10036. Phone: (212) 930-9500. Fax: (212) 869-3495. Quarterly.

Radiology. Radiological Society of North America, 2021 Spring Rd., Ste. 600, Oak Brook, IL 60521. Phone: (708) 571-2670.

ONLINE DATABASES

EMBASE. Elsevier Science Publishing Co., Inc., P.O. Box 882, Madison Square Station, New York, NY 10159-2101. Phone: (212) 989-5800. Fax: (212) 633-3990.

MEDLINE. National Library of Medicine, 8600 Rockville Pike, Bethesda, MD 20894. Phone: (800) 638-8480.

SciSearch. Institute for Scientific Information, 3501 Market St., Philadelphia, PA 19104. Phone: (215) 386-0100. Fax: (215) 386-6362.

RESEARCH CENTERS, INSTITUTES, CLEARINGHOUSES

Magnetic Resonance Imaging Center. 9450 Grogan's Mill Rd., Baylor College of Medicine, The Woodlands, TX 77380. Phone: (713) 363-4844.

Magnetic Resonance Systems Research Laboratory. Durand Bldg., Stanford University, Stanford, CA 94305. Phone: (415) 725-5638.

Mayo Biomedical Imaging Resource. Mayo Clinic. 200 First St. SW, Rochester, MN 55901. Phone: (507) 284-4937. Fax: (507) 284-1632.

Pittsburgh MRI Institute. 3260 5th Ave., Pittsburgh, PA 15213. Phone: (412) 647-6679.

TEXTBOOKS AND MONOGRAPHS

Clincal Brain Imaging. Mazziotta. F.A. Davis Co., 1915 Arch St., Philadelphia, PA 19103. Phone: (800) 523-4049. Fax: (215) 568-5065. 1992.

Clinical Imaging. Eisenberg. Aspen Publishers, Inc., 200 Orchard Ridge Dr., Gaithersburg, MD 20878. Phone: (800) 638-8437. Second edition 1992.

Clinical Magnetic Resonance Imaging. R.R. Edelman, J.R. Hesselink. W.B. Saunders Co., The Curtis Center, Independence Sqare W., Philadelphia, PA 19106-3399. Phone: (215) 238-7800. 1990.

Cranial MRI. Bisese. McGraw-Hill Inc., 11 West 19th St., New York, NY 10011. Phone: (212) 337-5001. Fax: (212) 337-4092. 1991.

Essentials of Diagnostic Imaging. Guebert. Mosby-Year Book, 11830 Westline Industrial Drive, St. Louis, MO 63146. Phone: (800) 325-4177. Fax: (314) 432-1380. 1992.

Fundamentals of Magnetic Resonance Imaging. Chakeres. Williams & Wilkins, 428 East Preston St., Baltimore, MD 21202. Phone: (800) 638-0672. Fax: (800) 447-8438. 1992.

An Introduction to Magnetic Resonance Medicine. P.A. Rinck (ed.). Thieme Medical Publishers, Inc., 381 Park Ave. S., New York, NY 10016. Phone: (212) 683-5088. Fax: (212) 779-9020. 1990.

Magnetic Resonance Imaging. David Stark, William Bradley Jr.. Mosby-Year Book, 11830 Westline Industrial Drive, St. Louis, MO 63146. Phone: (800) 325-4177. Fax: (314) 432-1380. 2nd edition, 1991.

Magnetic Resonance Imaging: Basic Principles. Stuart Wesley Young. Raven Press, 1185 Avenue of the Americas, New York, NY 10036. Phone: (212) 930-9500. Fax: (212) 869-3495. Second edition 1988.

Magnetic Resonance Imaging of the Brain and Spine. Scott W. Atlas. Raven Press, 1185 Avenue of the Americas, New York, NY 10036. Phone: (212) 930-9500. Fax: (212) 869-3495. 1991.

Magnetic Resonance Imaging and Computed Tomography of the Head and Spine. C. Barrie Grossman. Williams & Wilkins, 428 East Preston St., Baltimore, MD 21202. Phone: (800) 638-0672. Fax: (800) 447-8438. 1990.

MRI Angiography. James E. Potchen, Alexander Gottschalk. Mosby-Year Book, 11830 Westline Industrial Drive, St. Louis, MO 63146. Phone: (800) 325-4177. Fax: (314) 432-1380. 1992.

MRI of the Spine. Modic. Mosby-Year Book, 11830 Westline Industrial Drive, St. Louis, MO 63146. Phone: (800) 325-4177. Fax: (314) 432-1380. Second edition 1992.

Orthopaedic MRI. Pomeranz. J.B. Lippincott Co., 227 East Washington Square, Philadelphia, PA 19106-3780. Phone: (215) 238-4200. Fax: (215) 238-4227. 1991.

Understanding MRI. Jeffrey H. Newhouse, Jonathan I. Wiener. Little, Brown and Company, 34 Beacon St., Boston, MA 02108. Phone: (617) 227-0730. 1991.

MULTIPLE SCLEROSIS

ABSTRACTING, INDEXING, AND CURRENT AWARENESS PUBLICATIONS

Current Contents/Clinical Medicine. Institute for Scientific Information, 3501 Market St., Philadelphia, PA 19104. Phone: (800) 523-1850. Fax: (215) 386-6362. Weekly.

Excerpta Medica. Section 8: Neurology and Neurosurgery. Elsevier Science Publishers, P.O. Box 882, Madison Square Station, New York, NY 10159-2101. Phone: (212) 633-3950. Fax: (212) 633-3990. 32/year.

Index Medicus. U.S. National Library of Medicine, 8600 Rockville Pike, Bethesda, MD 20894. Phone: (800) 638-8480. Monthly.

Research Alert: Multiple Sclerosis. Institute for Scientific Information, 3501 Market St., Philadelphia, PA 19104. Phone: (800) 523-1850. Fax: (215) 386-6362. Weekly.

Science Citation Index. Institute for Scientific Information, 3501 Market St., Philadelphia, PA 19104. Phone: (800) 523-1850. Fax: (215) 386-6362. Bimonthly.

ASSOCIATIONS, PROFESSIONAL SOCIETIES, ADVOCACY AND SUPPORT GROUPS

National Multiple Sclerosis Society (NMSS). 205 E. 42nd St., New York, NY 10017. Phone: (800) 624-8236. Fax: (212) 986-7981.

CD-ROM DATABASES

CSA Neurosciences Abstracts on CD-ROM. Cambridge Scientific Abstracts, 7200 Wisconsin Ave., Bethesda, MD 20814-4823. Phone: (800) 843-7751. Fax: (301) 961-6720.

SCISEARCH. Institute for Scientific Information, 3501 Market St., Philadelphia, PA 19104. Phone: (215) 386-0100. Fax: (215) 386-6362.

JOURNALS

Archives of Neurology. American Medical Association, 515 North State St., Chicago, IL 60610. Phone: (312) 464-0183. Fax: (312) 464-5834. Monthly.

Journal of the Autonomic Nervous System. Elsevier Science Publishing Co., Inc., P.O. Box 882, Madison Square Station, New York, NY 10159-2101. Phone: (212) 989-5800. Fax: (212) 633-3990. 12/year.

MS News. Multiple Sclerosis Society, 25 Effie Rd., London W1R 7LE, England.

Neurology. Edgell Communications, 7500 Old Oak Blvd., Cleveland, OH 44130. Phone: (216) 826-2839. Fax: (216) 891-2726. Monthly.

NEWSLETTERS

Inside MS. National Multiple Sclerosis Society, 205 E. 42nd St., New York, NY 10017. Phone: (212) 986-3240. Quarterly.

ONLINE DATABASES

EMBASE. Elsevier Science Publishing Co., Inc., P.O. Box 882, Madison Square Station, New York, NY 10159-2101. Phone: (212) 989-5800. Fax: (212) 633-3990.

MEDLINE. National Library of Medicine, 8600 Rockville Pike, Bethesda, MD 20894. Phone: (800) 638-8480.

SciSearch. Institute for Scientific Information, 3501 Market St., Philadelphia, PA 19104. Phone: (215) 386-0100. Fax: (215) 386-6362.

POPULAR WORKS AND PATIENT EDUCATION

Multiple Sclerosis. Louis J. Rosner, Shelley Ross. Simon & Schuster, Inc., 1230 Ave. of the Americas, New York, NY 10020. Phone: (212) 698-7000. 1992.

Multiple Sclerosis: A Guide for Patients and Their Families. Labe C. Scheinberg, Nancy J. Holland. Raven Press, 1185 Avenue of the Americas, New York, NY 10036. Phone: (212) 930-9500. Fax: (212) 869-3495. Second edition 1987.

Multiple Sclerosis Fact Book. Richard Lechtenberg. F.A. Davis Co., 1915 Arch St., Philadelphia, PA 19103. Phone: (800) 523-4049. Fax: (215) 568-5065. 1988.

Understanding Multiple Sclerosis. Robert Shuman, Janice Schwartz. Macmillan Publishing Co., 866 Third Ave., New York, NY 10011. Phone: (800) 257-5755. 1988.

RESEARCH CENTERS, INSTITUTES, CLEARINGHOUSES

Amyotrophic Lateral Sclerosis/Multiple Sclerosis Center. University of Maryland, 22 S. Greene St., Baltimore, MD 21201. Phone: (301) 328-5605.

Medical Rehabilitation Research and Training Center for Multiple Sclerosis. Albert Einstein College of Medicine, Yeshiva University, 1300 Morris Park Dr., Bronx, NY 10461. Phone: (212) 430-2682.

Mellen Center for Multiple Sclerosis Treatment and Research. Cleveland Clinic Foundation, 9500 Euclid Ave, Cleveland, OH 44195. Phone: (216) 444-6800.

Multiple Sclerosis Center. Rush University, 1725 W. Hamson St., Chicago, IL 60612. Phone: (312) 942-8011.

TEXTBOOKS AND MONOGRAPHS

McAlpine's Multiple Sclerosis. W.B. Matthews, A. Compston, Christopher N. Martyn. Churchill Livingstone Inc., 650 Avenue of the Americas, New York, NY 10011. Phone: (212) 819-5400. Fax: (212) 302-6598. Second edition 1991.

Multiple Sclerosis: Approaches to Management. Lorraine DeSouza, Jo Campling (eds.). Routledge, Chapman, & Hall, 29 W. 35th St., New York, NY 10001-2291. Phone: (212) 244-3336. 1990.

Recent Advances in Multiple Sclerosis Therapy: Proceedings of the Vth Congress of the European Committee for Treatment and Research in Multiple Sclerosis. R.E. Gonsette, P. Delmotte (eds.). Elsevier Science Publishing Co., Inc., P.O. Box 882, Madison Square Station, New York, NY 10159-2101. Phone: (212) 989-5800. Fax: (212) 633-3990. 1989.

MUMPS

See: INFECTIOUS DISEASES

MUSCULAR DYSTROPHY

See also: NEUROMUSCULAR DISORDERS

ABSTRACTING, INDEXING, AND CURRENT AWARENESS PUBLICATIONS

Current Contents/Clinical Medicine. Institute for Scientific Information, 3501 Market St., Philadelphia, PA 19104. Phone: (800) 523-1850. Fax: (215) 386-6362. Weekly.

Excerpta Medica. Section 8: Neurology and Neurosurgery. Elsevier Science Publishers, P.O. Box 882, Madison Square Station, New York, NY 10159-2101. Phone: (212) 633-3950. Fax: (212) 633-3990. 32/year.

Index Medicus. U.S. National Library of Medicine, 8600 Rockville Pike, Bethesda, MD 20894. Phone: (800) 638-8480. Monthly.

Science Citation Index. Institute for Scientific Information, 3501 Market St., Philadelphia, PA 19104. Phone: (800) 523-1850. Fax: (215) 386-6362. Bimonthly.

ASSOCIATIONS, PROFESSIONAL SOCIETIES, ADVOCACY AND SUPPORT GROUPS

Families of Spinal Muscular Atrophy. P.O. Box 1465, Highland Park, IL 60035. Phone: (312) 432-5551.

Muscular Dystrophy Association (MDA). 810 7th Ave., New York, NY 10019. Phone: (212) 586-0808. Fax: (212) 763-2003.

CD-ROM DATABASES

CSA Neurosciences Abstracts on CD-ROM. Cambridge Scientific Abstracts, 7200 Wisconsin Ave., Bethesda, MD 20814-4823. Phone: (800) 843-7751. Fax: (301) 961-6720.

SCISEARCH. Institute for Scientific Information, 3501 Market St., Philadelphia, PA 19104. Phone: (215) 386-0100. Fax: (215) 386-6362.

JOURNALS

MDA Newsmagazine. Muscular Dystrophy Association, 810 Seventh Ave., New York, NY 10019. Phone: (212) 765-2003.

Muscle and Nerve. John Wiley & Sons, Inc., 605 Third Ave., New York, NY 10158-0012. Phone: (212) 850-6000. Fax: (212) 850-6088.

Search. Muscular Dystrophy Group of Great Britain and Northern Ireland, Nattrass House, 35 Macaulay Rd., Clapham, London SW4 OQP, England. Phone: 071-7208055.

ONLINE DATABASES

EMBASE. Elsevier Science Publishing Co., Inc., P.O. Box 882, Madison Square Station, New York, NY 10159-2101. Phone: (212) 989-5800. Fax: (212) 633-3990.

MEDLINE. National Library of Medicine, 8600 Rockville Pike, Bethesda, MD 20894. Phone: (800) 638-8480.

SciSearch. Institute for Scientific Information, 3501 Market St., Philadelphia, PA 19104. Phone: (215) 386-0100. Fax: (215) 386-6362.

RESEARCH CENTERS, INSTITUTES, CLEARINGHOUSES

Jerry Lewis Neuromuscular Center. 2100 Pierce Ave., Vanderbilt University, Nashville, TN 37212. Phone: (615) 322-2989.

Jerry Lewis Neuromuscular Disease Center. New York University, 400 E. 34th St., New York, NY 10016. Phone: (212) 340-6350.

Jerry Lewis Neuromuscular Disease Research Center. Baylor College of Medicine, One Baylor Plaza, Houston, TX 77030. Phone: (713) 799-5971.

Jerry Lewis Neuromuscular Research Center. Washington University, 600 South Euclid Ave., Box 8111, St. Louis, MO 63110. Phone: (314) 362-6981.

TEXTBOOKS AND MONOGRAPHS

Myology. A. Engel, B.Q. Banker. McGraw Hill, 11 W. 19th St., New York, NY 10011. Phone: (212) 337-5001. Fax: (212) 337-4092. 1986.

MUSCULOSKELETAL DISEASES

See: BONE AND JOINT DISEASES; NEUROMUSCULAR DISORDERS

MYASTHENIA GRAVIS

See also: NEUROMUSCULAR DISORDERS

ABSTRACTING, INDEXING, AND CURRENT AWARENESS PUBLICATIONS

Excerpta Medica. Section 8: Neurology and Neurosurgery. Elsevier Science Publishers, P.O. Box 882, Madison Square Station, New York, NY 10159-2101. Phone: (212) 633-3950. Fax: (212) 633-3990. 32/year.

General Science Index. H.W. Wilson Co., 950 University Ave., Bronx, NY 10452. Phone: (800) 367-6770.

Index Medicus. U.S. National Library of Medicine, 8600 Rockville Pike, Bethesda, MD 20894. Phone: (800) 638-8480. Monthly.

Science Citation Index. Institute for Scientific Information, 3501 Market St., Philadelphia, PA 19104. Phone: (800) 523-1850. Fax: (215) 386-6362. Bimonthly.

ASSOCIATIONS, PROFESSIONAL SOCIETIES, ADVOCACY AND SUPPORT GROUPS

Myasthenia Gravis Foundation (MG). 53 W. Jackson Blvd., Ste. 1352, Chicago, IL 60604. Phone: (312) 427-6252. Fax: (312) 427-9437.

CD-ROM DATABASES

CSA Neurosciences Abstracts on CD-ROM. Cambridge Scientific Abstracts, 7200 Wisconsin Ave., Bethesda, MD 20814-4823. Phone: (800) 843-7751. Fax: (301) 961-6720.

SCISEARCH. Institute for Scientific Information, 3501 Market St., Philadelphia, PA 19104. Phone: (215) 386-0100. Fax: (215) 386-6362.

JOURNALS

Journal of Neuroimmunology. Elsevier Science Publishing Co., Inc., P.O. Box 882, Madison Square Station, New York, NY 10159-2101. Phone: (212) 989-5800. Fax: (212) 633-3990. 18/year.

Neurology. Edgell Communications, 7500 Old Oak Blvd., Cleveland, OH 44130. Phone: (216) 826-2839. Fax: (216) 891-2726. Monthly.

ONLINE DATABASES

EMBASE. Elsevier Science Publishing Co., Inc., P.O. Box 882, Madison Square Station, New York, NY 10159-2101. Phone: (212) 989-5800. Fax: (212) 633-3990.

MEDLINE. National Library of Medicine, 8600 Rockville Pike, Bethesda, MD 20894. Phone: (800) 638-8480.

SciSearch. Institute for Scientific Information, 3501 Market St., Philadelphia, PA 19104. Phone: (215) 386-0100. Fax: (215) 386-6362.

TEXTBOOKS AND MONOGRAPHS

Merritt's Textbook of Neurology. Lewis P. Rowland (ed.). Williams & Wilkins, 428 E. Preston St., Baltimore, MD 21202. Phone: (800) 638-0672. Fax: (800) 447-8438. Eighth edition 1989.

Neurology and General Medicine. Michael J. Aminoff (ed.). Churchill Livingstone Inc., 650 Ave. of the Americas, New York, NY 10011. Phone: (212) 819-5400. Fax: (212) 302-6598. 1989.

MYCOSIS

See: INFECTIOUS DISEASES

MYELITIS

See: SPINAL DISEASES

MYOCARDIAL INFARCTION

See: HEART DISEASES

MYOPIA

See: VISION DISORDERS

N

NAIL DISEASES

See: DERMATOLOGIC DISEASES

NARCOLEPSY

See: SLEEP DISORDERS

NATURAL CHILDBIRTH

See: CHILDBIRTH

NEARSIGHTEDNESS

See: VISION DISORDERS

NEONATOLOGY

See also: INTENSIVE CARE; PERINATOLOGY

ABSTRACTING, INDEXING, AND CURRENT AWARENESS PUBLICATIONS

Current Contents/Clinical Medicine. Institute for Scientific Information, 3501 Market St., Philadelphia, PA 19104. Phone: (800) 523-1850. Fax: (215) 386-6362. Weekly.

Excerpta Medica. Section 7: Pediatrics and Pediatric Surgery. Elsevier Science Publishing Co., Inc., P.O. Box 882, Madison Square Station, New York, NY 10159-2101. Phone: (212) 989-5800. Fax: (212) 633-3990. 24/year.

Index Medicus. U.S. National Library of Medicine, 8600 Rockville Pike, Bethesda, MD 20894. Phone: (800) 638-8480. Monthly.

Science Citation Index. Institute for Scientific Information, 3501 Market St., Philadelphia, PA 19104. Phone: (800) 523-1850. Fax: (215) 386-6362. Bimonthly.

ANNUALS AND REVIEWS

Year Book of Neonatal and Perinatal Medicine. Mosby-Year Book, 11830 Westline Industrial Drive, St. Louis, MO 63146. Phone: (800) 325-4177. Fax: (314) 432-1380. Annual.

ASSOCIATIONS, PROFESSIONAL SOCIETIES, ADVOCACY AND SUPPORT GROUPS

NAACOG: The Organization for Obstetric, Gynecologic and Neonatal Nurses. 409 12th St. S.W., Washington, DC 20024. Phone: (202) 638-0026.

Wee-Life Parents. W10957 Rodney Dr., Lodi, WI 53555. Phone: (608) 592-4648.

CD-ROM DATABASES

SCISEARCH. Institute for Scientific Information, 3501 Market St., Philadelphia, PA 19104. Phone: (215) 386-0100. Fax: (215) 386-6362.

DIRECTORIES

Directory of Medical Specialists. Marquis Who's Who, 3002 Glenview Rd., Wilmette, IL 60091. Phone: (800) 621-9669. Fax: (708) 441-2264. Biennial.

Directory of Physicians in the United States. American Medical Association, 515 North State St., Chicago, IL 60610. Phone: (312) 464-0183. Fax: (312) 464-5834. Biennial.

HANDBOOKS, GUIDES, MANUALS, ATLASES

Handbook of Neonatal Intensive Care. Merenstein. Mosby-Year Book, 11830 Westline Industrial Drive, St. Louis, MO 63146. Phone: (800) 325-4177. Fax: (314) 432-1380. Second edition 1989.

Manual of Neonatal Care. John P. Cloherty, Ann R. Stark. Little, Brown and Co., 34 Beacon St., Boston, MA 02108. Phone: (617) 227-0730. Fax: (617) 227-0790. 3rd edition, 1991.

Neonatal Intensive Care Handbook. Goetzman. Mosby-Year Book, 11830 Westline Industrial Drive, St. Louis, MO 63146. Phone: (800) 325-4177. Fax: (314) 432-1380. Second edition 1991.

Neonatology. Gomella. Appleton & Lange, 25 Van Zant St., East Norwalk, CT 06855. Phone: (800) 423-1359. Fax: (203) 854-9486. Second edition 1992.

Resident's Handbook of Neonatology. Perlman. Mosby-Year Book, 11830 Westline Industrial Drive, St. Louis, MO 63146. Phone: (800) 325-4177. Fax: (314) 432-1380. 1992.

JOURNALS

Biology of the Neonate. S. Karger Publishers, Inc., 26 W. Avon Rd., P.O. Box 529, Farmington, CT 06085. Phone: (203) 675-7834. Fax: (203) 675-7302.

Journal of Pediatrics. Mosby-Year Book, 11830 Westline Industrial Drive, St. Louis, MO 63146. Phone: (800) 325-4177. Fax: (314) 432-1380. Monthly.

Journal of Perinatology. Appleton & Lange, 25 Van Zant St., East Norwalk, CT 06855. Phone: (800) 423-1359. Fax: (203) 854-9486. Quarterly.

Pediatrics. American Academy of Pediatrics, 141 Northwest Point Rd., Elk Grove Village, IL 60009-0927. Phone: (708) 228-5005. Fax: (708) 228-5097. Monthly.

Screening: Journal of the International Society of Neonatal Screening. Elsevier Science Publishing Co., Inc., P.O. Box 882, Madison Square Station, New York, NY 10159-2101. Phone: (212) 989-5800. Fax: (212) 633-3990. 4/year.

ONLINE DATABASES

EMBASE. Elsevier Science Publishing Co., Inc., P.O. Box 882, Madison Square Station, New York, NY 10159-2101. Phone: (212) 989-5800. Fax: (212) 633-3990.

MEDLINE. National Library of Medicine, 8600 Rockville Pike, Bethesda, MD 20894. Phone: (800) 638-8480.

SciSearch. Institute for Scientific Information, 3501 Market St., Philadelphia, PA 19104. Phone: (215) 386-0100. Fax: (215) 386-6362.

POPULAR WORKS AND PATIENT EDUCATION

Your Premature Baby: Everything You Need to Know About the Problems, Treatment and Parenting of Premature Infants. Frank P. Manginello, Theresa Foy DiGeronimo. John Wiley & Sons, Inc., 605 Third Ave., New York, NY 10158-0012. Phone: (212) 850-6000. Fax: (212) 850-6088. 1991.

RESEARCH CENTERS, INSTITUTES, CLEARINGHOUSES

Neonatology Research Laboratory. College of Medicine, University of Nebraska at Omaha, 42nd and Dewey, Omaha, NE 68105. Phone: (402) 559-7340.

Neonatology Research Units. University of Southern California, 1240 Mission Rd., Los Angeles, CA 90033. Phone: (213) 226-3406.

TEXTBOOKS AND MONOGRAPHS

Disorders of the Placenta, Fetus and Neonate: Diagnosis and Clinical Significance. Richard L. Naeye. Mosby-Year Book, 11830 Westline Industrial Drive, St. Louis, MO 63146. Phone: (800) 325-4177. Fax: (314) 432-1380. 1992.

Essentials of Pediatric Intensive Care. Levin. Quality Publications, P.O. Box 1060, Abilene, TX 79604. Phone: (800) 359-7708. 1990.

Fetal and Neonatal Cardiology. Walker A. Long. W.B. Saunders Co., The Curtis Center, Independence Square W., Philadelphia, PA 19106-3399. Phone: (215) 238-7800. 1990.

Fetal, Neonatal, and Infant Cardiac Disease. James H. Moller, William A. Neal (eds.). Appleton & Lange, 25 Van Zant Street, East Norwalk, CT 06855. Phone: (800) 423-1359. Fax: (203) 854-9486. 1990.

Fetal and Neonatal Physiology. Richard A. Polin, William W. Fox. W.B. Saunders Co., The Curtis Center, Independence

Sqare W., Philadelphia, PA 19106-3399. Phone: (215) 238-7800. 1992.

Infectious Diseases of the Fetus and Newborn Infant. Jack Remington, Jerome Klein. W.B. Saunders Co., The Curtis Center, Independence Sqare W., Philadelphia, PA 19106-3399. Phone: (215) 238-7800. Third Edition 1990.

Neonatal Emergencies. Donn. Futura Publishing Co., Inc., P.O. Box 330, Mount Kisco, NY 10549. Phone: (914) 666-7528. 1991.

Neonatal Heart Disease. Freedom. Springer-Verlag New York Inc., 175 Fifth Ave., New York, NY 10010. Phone: (212) 460-1500. Fax: (212) 473-6272. 1992.

Neonatal and Perinatal Medicine: Diseases of the Fetus and Infant. Avory Fanaroff, Richard Martin. Mosby-Year Book, 11830 Westline Industrial Drive, St. Louis, MO 63146. Phone: (800) 325-4177. Fax: (314) 432-1380. 5th edition, 1992.

Neonatal Therapeutics. Yeh. Mosby-Year Book, 11830 Westline Industrial Drive, St. Louis, MO 63146. Phone: (800) 325-4177. Fax: (314) 432-1380. Second edition 1991.

Neonatology. Avery. J.B. Lippincott Co., 227 E. Washington Square, Philadelphia, PA 19106-3780. Phone: (215) 238-4200. Fax: (215) 238-4227. Fourth edition 1993.

Normal Infant Development. Flehmig. Thieme Medical Publishers, Inc., 381 Park Ave. S., New York, NY 10016. Phone: (212) 683-5088. Fax: (212) 779-9020. 1992.

Preterm Birth: Causes, Prevention, and Management. Fritz A. Fuchs, Anna-Ritta Fuchs, Phillip G. Stubblefield. McGraw-Hill, Inc., Health Professions Division, 1221 Avenue of the Americas, 28th Floor, New York, NY 10020. Phone: (212) 512-4228. Second edition 1992.

Textbook of Neonatal Infections. D. Isaacs, Richard Moxon. Butterworth-Heinemann, 80 Montvale Ave., Stoneham, MA 02180. Phone: (617) 438-8464. Fax: (617) 279-4851. 1991.

Textbook of Pediatric Intensive Care. Rogers. Williams & Wilkins, 428 East Preston St., Baltimore, MD 21202. Phone: (800) 638-0672. Fax: (800) 447-8438. Two volumes. Second edition. 1992.

Tumors of the Newborn and Infant. Isaacs. Mosby-Year Book, 11830 Westline Industrial Drive, St. Louis, MO 63146. Phone: (800) 325-4177. Fax: (314) 432-1380. 1991.

NEOPLASMS

See: CANCER

NEPHRITIS

See: KIDNEY DISEASES; TRANSPLANTATION

NERVOUS SYSTEM DISEASES

See: NEUROLOGIC DISORDERS

NEURAL TUBE DEFECTS

See: BIRTH DEFECTS

NEUROANATOMY

See: ANATOMY

NEUROLOGIC DISORDERS

See also: BRAIN DISEASES;
CEREBROVASCULAR DISEASES; DEMENTIA;
NEUROLOGY; NEUROSURGERY

ABSTRACTING, INDEXING, AND CURRENT AWARENESS PUBLICATIONS

Core Journals in Clinical Neurology. Elsevier Science Publishing Co., Inc., P.O. Box 882, Madison Square Station, New York, NY 10159-2101. Phone: (212) 989-5800. Fax: (212) 633-3990. 11/year.

Current Contents/Clinical Medicine. Institute for Scientific Information, 3501 Market St., Philadelphia, PA 19104. Phone: (800) 523-1850. Fax: (215) 386-6362. Weekly.

Current Contents/Life Sciences. Institute for Scientific Information, 3501 Market St., Philadelphia, PA 19104. Phone: (215) 386-0100. Fax: (215) 386-6362.

Digest of Neurology and Psychiatry. Institute of Living, 400 Washington St., Hartford, CT 06106. Phone: (203) 241-6824. Monthly.

Excerpta Medica. Section 8: Neurology and Neurosurgery. Elsevier Science Publishers, P.O. Box 882, Madison Square Station, New York, NY 10159-2101. Phone: (212) 633-3950. Fax: (212) 633-3990. 32/year.

Index Medicus. U.S. National Library of Medicine, 8600 Rockville Pike, Bethesda, MD 20894. Phone: (800) 638-8480. Monthly.

Key Neurology and Neurosurgery: Current Literature in Perspective. Mosby-Year Book, 11830 Westline Industrial Drive, St. Louis, MO 63146. Phone: (800) 325-4177. Fax: (314) 432-1380. Quarterly.

ANNUALS AND REVIEWS

Annual Review of Neuroscience. Annual Reviews Inc., 4139 El Camino Way, P.O. Box 10139, Palo Alto, CA 94303-0897. Phone: (415) 493-4400. Fax: (415) 855-9815. Annual.

Current Neurology. Mosby-Year Book, 11830 Westline Industrial Drive, St. Louis, MO 63146. Phone: (800) 325-4177. Fax: (314) 432-1380. Annual.

Current Opinion in Neurology & Neurosurgery. Current Science Ltd., 20 N. Third St., Philadelphia, PA 19106-2199. Phone: (800) 552-5866. Fax: (215) 574-2270. Bimonthly.

Developments in Neurology. Elsevier Science Publishing Co., Inc., P.O. Box 882, Madison Square Station, New York, NY 10159-2101. Phone: (212) 989-5800. Fax: (212) 633-3990. Irregular.

Neurologic Clinics. W.B. Saunders Co., The Curtis Center, Independence Square W., Philadelphia, PA 19106-3399. Phone: (215) 238-7800. Quarterly.

Neuroscience and Biobehavioral Reviews. Pergamon Press, 660 White Plains Rd., Tarrytown, NY 10591-5153. Phone: (914) 592-7700. Fax: (914) 592-3625. Quarterly.

Progress in Brain Research. Elsevier Science Publishing Co., Inc., P.O. Box 882, Madison Square Station, New York, NY 10159-2101. Phone: (212) 989-5800. Fax: (212) 633-3990. Irregular.

Progress in Neuropathology. Raven Press, 1185 Avenue of the Americas, New York, NY 10036. Phone: (212) 930-9500. Fax: (212) 869-3495. Irregular.

Year Book of Neurology and Neurosurgery. Mosby-Year Book, 11830 Westline Industrial Drive, St. Louis, MO 63146. Phone: (800) 325-4177. Fax: (314) 432-1380. Annual.

Year Book of Neuroradiology. Mosby-Year Book, 11830 Westline Industrial Drive, St. Louis, MO 63146. Phone: (800) 325-4177. Fax: (314) 432-1380. Annual.

ASSOCIATIONS, PROFESSIONAL SOCIETIES, ADVOCACY AND SUPPORT GROUPS

Amyotrophic Lateral Sclerosis Association (ALSA). 21021 Ventura Blvd., Ste. 321, Woodland Hills, CA 91364. Phone: (818) 340-7500. Fax: (818) 340-2060.

Guillain-Barre Syndrome Foundation International (GBSFI). P.O. Box 262, Wynnewood, PA 19096. Phone: (215) 667-0131.

Huntington's Disease Society of America (HDSA). 140 W. 22nd St., 6th Fl., New York, NY 10011-2420. Phone: (212) 242-1968. Fax: (212) 243-2443.

National Ataxia Foundation (NAF). 600 Twelve Oaks Ctr., 15500 Wayzata Blvd., Wayzata, MN 55391. Phone: (612) 473-7666. Fax: (612) 473-9289.

National Neurofibromatosis Foundation (NNFF). 141 5th Ave., Ste. 75, New York, NY 10010. Phone: (212) 460-8980.

National Parkinson Foundation (NPF). 1501 NW 9th Ave., Miami, FL 33136. Phone: (305) 547-6666.

National Tuberous Sclerosis Association. 8000 Corporate Dr., Ste. 120, Landover, MD 20785. Phone: (800) 225-6872.

CD-ROM DATABASES

CSA Neurosciences Abstracts on CD-ROM. Cambridge Scientific Abstracts, 7200 Wisconsin Ave., Bethesda, MD 20814-4823. Phone: (800) 843-7751. Fax: (301) 961-6720.

Excerpta Medica CD: Neurosciences. SilverPlatter Information, Inc., River Ridge Office Park, 100 River Ridge Rd., Norwood, MA 02062. Phone: (617) 769-2599. Fax: (617) 769-8763. Quarterly.

Neuroscience Citation Index. Institute for Scientific Information, 3501 Market St., Philadelphia, PA 19104. Phone: (800) 523-1857. Fax: (215) 386-6362. Bimonthly.

Year Books on Disc. CMC ReSearch, Inc., 7150 S.W. Hampton, Suite C-120, Portland, OR 97223. Phone: (800) 262-7668. Fax: (503) 639-1796. Annual includes Year Books of Cardiology, Dermatology, Diagnostic Radiology, Drug

Therapy, Emergency Medicine, Family Practice, Medicine, Neurology and Neurosurgery, Obstetrics and Gynecology, Oncology, Pediatrics, and Psychiatry and Applied Mental Health.

DIRECTORIES

Directory of Certified Neurologists. American Board of Medical Specialties, 1 Rotary Center, Suite 805, Evanston, IL 60201. Phone: (708) 491-9091. Biennial.

HANDBOOKS, GUIDES, MANUALS, ATLASES

A Color Atlas of Clinical Neurology. Malcolm R. Parsons. Mosby-Year Book, 11830 Westline Industrial Drive, St. Louis, MO 63146. Phone: (800) 325-4177. Fax: (314) 432-1380. Second edition 1992.

Handbook of Neurology. Warlow. Blackwell Scientific Publications, Inc., 3 Cambridge Ctr., Cambridge, MA 02142. Phone: (800) 759-6102. 1991.

Manual of Clinical Problems in Neurology. Mohr. Little, Brown and Co., 34 Beacon St., Boston, MA 02108. Phone: (617) 227-0730. Second edition 1989.

Manual of Neurologic Therapy. Samuels. Little, Brown and Co., 34 Beacon St., Boston, MA 02108. Phone: (617) 227-0730. Fax: (617) 227-0790. Fourth edition 1991.

Manual of Neurology: Diagnosis and Therapy. Martin A. Samuels (ed.). Little, Brown and Company, 34 Beacon St., Boston, MA 02108. Phone: (617) 227-0730. Fourth edition 1991.

JOURNALS

Archives of Neurology. American Medical Association, 515 North State St., Chicago, IL 60610. Phone: (312) 464-0183. Fax: (312) 464-5834. Monthly.

Clinical Neuropharmacology. Raven Press, 1185 Avenue of the Americas, New York, NY 10036. Phone: (212) 930-9500. Fax: (212) 869-3495. Bimonthly.

Dementia. S. Karger Publishers, Inc., 26 West Avon Rd., P.O. Box 529, Farmington, CT 06085. Phone: (203) 675-7834. Fax: (203) 675-7302. Bimonthly.

Journal of Child Neurology. Mosby-Year Book, 11830 Westline Industrial Drive, St. Louis, MO 63146. Phone: (800) 325-4177. Fax: (314) 432-1380. Quarterly.

Journal of Geriatric Psychiatry and Neurology. Mosby-Year Book, 11830 Westline Industrial Drive, St. Louis, MO 63146. Phone: (800) 325-4177. Fax: (314) 432-1380. Quarterly.

Journal of the Neurological Sciences. Elsevier Science Publishing Co., Inc., P.O. Box 882, Madison Square Station, New York, NY 10159-2101. Phone: (212) 989-5800. Fax: (212) 633-3990. 12/year.

Journal of Neurology, Neurosurgery & Psychiatry. BMJ Publishing Group, BMA House, Tavistock Square, London WC1H 9JR, England. Phone: 071-383 6244/6638. Fax: 071-383 6662. Monthly.

Pediatric Neurology. Pediatric Neurology, Box 486, Mayo Bldg., Harvard St. at E. River Rd., Minneapolis, MN 55455. Phone: (612) 625-7466. Fax: (612) 625-7950. Bimonthly.

NEWSLETTERS

American Parkinson Disease Association-Newsletter. American Parkinson Disease Association, 116 John St., Ste. 417, New York, NY 10038. Phone: (212) 732-9550. Quarterly.

Neuroscience Newsletter. Society for Neuroscience, 11 Dupont Circle N.W., Suite 500, Washington, DC 20036. Phone: (202) 462-6688. Bimonthly.

ONLINE DATABASES

EMBASE. Elsevier Science Publishing Co., Inc., P.O. Box 882, Madison Square Station, New York, NY 10159-2101. Phone: (212) 989-5800. Fax: (212) 633-3990.

EPIL. Epilepsy Foundation of America, National Epilepsy Library, 4351 Garden City Dr., Landover, MD 20785. Phone: (800) EFA-4050. Fax: (301) 577-2684.

MEDLINE. National Library of Medicine, 8600 Rockville Pike, Bethesda, MD 20894. Phone: (800) 638-8480.

SciSearch. Institute for Scientific Information, 3501 Market St., Philadelphia, PA 19104. Phone: (215) 386-0100. Fax: (215) 386-6362.

RESEARCH CENTERS, INSTITUTES, CLEARINGHOUSES

Brain Development Research Center. University of North Carolina at Chapel Hill. CB 7250, Chapel Hill, NC 27599-7250. Phone: (919) 966-2405. Fax: (919) 966-1844.

Brain Research Foundation. 208 S. LaSalle St., Chicago, IL 60604. Phone: (312) 782-4311.

Brain Research Institute. UCLA Center for Health Sciences, University of California, Los Angeles, CA 90024. Phone: (213) 825-5061.

Center for Neurological Diseases. University of Miami. 1501 N.W. 9th Ave., P.O. Box 016960, Miami, FL 33136. Phone: (305) 547-6732.

Center for Neuroscience. University of Tennessee. 875 Monroe Ave., Memphis, TN 38163. Phone: (901) 528-5956. Fax: (901) 528-7193.

TEXTBOOKS AND MONOGRAPHS

Carpal Tunnel Syndrome: A Comprehensive Approach to Early Diagnosis and Treatment. Mark P. Koniuch, John J. Palazzo (eds.). SLACK Inc., 6900 Grove Rd., Thorofare, NJ 08086-9447. Phone: (800) 257-8290. Fax: (609) 853-5991. 1992.

Clinical Neurology. Simon. Appleton & Lange, 25 Van Zant St., East Norwalk, CT 06855. Phone: (800) 423-1359. Fax: (203) 854-9486. Second edition 1992.

Guillain-Barre Syndrome. Allan H. Ropper, Eelco F.M. Wijdicks. F.A. Davis Co., 1915 Arch St., Philadelphia, PA 19103. Phone: (800) 523-4049. Fax: (215) 568-5065. Contemporary Neurology. Series No. 34. 1991.

Infections of the Central Nervous System. W. Michael Scheld, Richard J. Whitley, David T. Durack. Raven Press, 1185 Avenue of the Americas, New York, NY 10036. Phone: (212) 930-9500. Fax: (212) 869-3495. 1991.

Merritt's Textbook of Neurology. Lewis P. Rowland (ed.). Williams & Wilkins, 428 E. Preston St., Baltimore, MD 21202.

Phone: (800) 638-0672. Fax: (800) 447-8438. Eighth edition 1989.

Nerve Injuries and Their Repair: A Critical Appraisal. Sir Sydney Sunderland. Churchill Livingstone Inc., 650 Avenue of the Americas, New York, NY 10011. Phone: (212) 819-5400. Fax: (212) 302-6598. 1991.

Neurologic Emergencies: Recognition and Management. Michael Salcman. Raven Press, 1185 Avenue of the Americas, New York, NY 10036. Phone: (212) 930-9500. Fax: (212) 869-3495. Second edition 1990.

Neurology and General Medicine. Michael J. Aminoff (ed.). Churchill Livingstone Inc., 650 Ave. of the Americas, New York, NY 10011. Phone: (212) 819-5400. Fax: (212) 302-6598. 1989.

Tunnel Syndromes. Marko Pecina, Jelena Krmpotic-Nemanci, Drew D Markeiwitz. CRC Press, Inc., 2000 Corporate Blvd. N.W., Boca Raton, FL 33431. Phone: (407) 994-0555. Fax: (407) 997-0949. 1992.

NEUROLOGY

See also: NEUROLOGIC DISORDERS;
NEUROSURGERY

ABSTRACTING, INDEXING, AND CURRENT AWARENESS PUBLICATIONS

Biological Abstracts. BIOSIS, 2100 Arch St., Philadelphia, PA 19103-1399. Phone: (800) 523-4800. Fax: (215) 587-2016.

Core Journals in Clinical Neurology. Elsevier Science Publishing Co., Inc., P.O. Box 882, Madison Square Station, New York, NY 10159-2101. Phone: (212) 989-5800. Fax: (212) 633-3990. 11/year.

Current Contents/Life Sciences. Institute for Scientific Information, 3501 Market St., Philadelphia, PA 19104. Phone: (215) 386-0100. Fax: (215) 386-6362.

Digest of Neurology and Psychiatry. Institute of Living, 400 Washington St., Hartford, CT 06106. Phone: (203) 241-6824. Monthly.

Excerpta Medica. Section 8: Neurology and Neurosurgery. Elsevier Science Publishers, P.O. Box 882, Madison Square Station, New York, NY 10159-2101. Phone: (212) 633-3950. Fax: (212) 633-3990. 32/year.

Index Medicus. U.S. National Library of Medicine, 8600 Rockville Pike, Bethesda, MD 20894. Phone: (800) 638-8480. Monthly.

Key Neurology and Neurosurgery: Current Literature in Perspective. Mosby-Year Book, 11830 Westline Industrial Drive, St. Louis, MO 63146. Phone: (800) 325-4177. Fax: (314) 432-1380. Quarterly.

Science Citation Index. Institute for Scientific Information, 3501 Market St., Philadelphia, PA 19104. Phone: (800) 523-1850. Fax: (215) 386-6362. Bimonthly.

ANNUALS AND REVIEWS

Advances in Neurology. Raven Press, 1185 Avenue of the Americas, New York, NY 10036. Phone: (212) 930-9500. Fax: (212) 869-3495. Irregular.

Annual Review of Neuroscience. Annual Reviews Inc., 4139 El Camino Way, P.O. Box 10139, Palo Alto, CA 94303-0897. Phone: (415) 493-4400. Fax: (415) 855-9815. Annual.

Current Neurology. Mosby-Year Book, 11830 Westline Industrial Drive, St. Louis, MO 63146. Phone: (800) 325-4177. Fax: (314) 432-1380. Annual.

Current Opinion in Neurology & Neurosurgery. Current Science Ltd., 20 N. Third St., Philadelphia, PA 19106-2199. Phone: (800) 552-5866. Fax: (215) 574-2270. Bimonthly.

Developments in Neurology. Elsevier Science Publishing Co., Inc., P.O. Box 882, Madison Square Station, New York, NY 10159-2101. Phone: (212) 989-5800. Fax: (212) 633-3990. Irregular.

Neurologic Clinics. W.B. Saunders Co., The Curtis Center, Independence Square W., Philadelphia, PA 19106-3399. Phone: (215) 238-7800. Quarterly.

Neuroscience and Biobehavioral Reviews. Pergamon Press, 660 White Plains Rd., Tarrytown, NY 10591-5153. Phone: (914) 592-7700. Fax: (914) 592-3625. Quarterly.

Year Book of Neurology and Neurosurgery. Mosby-Year Book, 11830 Westline Industrial Drive, St. Louis, MO 63146. Phone: (800) 325-4177. Fax: (314) 432-1380. Annual.

ASSOCIATIONS, PROFESSIONAL SOCIETIES, ADVOCACY AND SUPPORT GROUPS

American Academy of Neurology (AAN). 2221 University Ave. S.E., Ste. 335, Minneapolis, MN 55414. Phone: (612) 623-8115.

American Board of Psychiatry and Neurology (ABPN). 500 Lake Cook Rd., Ste. 335, Deerfield, IL 60015. Phone: (708) 945-7900.

American Neurological Association (ANA). 2221 University St. S.E., Ste. 350, Minneapolis, MN 55414. Phone: (612) 378-3290.

CD-ROM DATABASES

Biological Abstracts on Compact Disc. BIOSIS, 2100 Arch St., Philadelphia, PA 19103-1399. Phone: (800) 523-4800. Fax: (215) 587-2016. Quarterly.

CSA Neurosciences Abstracts on CD-ROM. Cambridge Scientific Abstracts, 7200 Wisconsin Ave., Bethesda, MD 20814-4823. Phone: (800) 843-7751. Fax: (301) 961-6720.

Excerpta Medica CD: Neurosciences. SilverPlatter Information, Inc., River Ridge Office Park, 100 River Ridge Rd., Norwood, MA 02062. Phone: (617) 769-2599. Fax: (617) 769-8763. Quarterly.

SCISEARCH. Institute for Scientific Information, 3501 Market St., Philadelphia, PA 19104. Phone: (215) 386-0100. Fax: (215) 386-6362.

Year Books on Disc. CMC ReSearch, Inc., 7150 S.W. Hampton, Suite C-120, Portland, OR 97223. Phone: (800) 262-7668. Fax: (503) 639-1796. Annual includes Year Books of Cardiology, Dermatology, Diagnostic Radiology, Drug Therapy, Emergency Medicine, Family Practice, Medicine, Neurology and Neurosurgery, Obstetrics and Gynecology, Oncology, Pediatrics, and Psychiatry and Applied Mental Health.

DIRECTORIES

Directory of Certified Neurological Surgeons. American Board of Medical Specialties, 1 Rotary Center, Suite 805, Evanston, IL 60201. Phone: (708) 491-9091. Biennial.

Directory of Certified Neurologists. American Board of Medical Specialties, 1 Rotary Center, Suite 805, Evanston, IL 60201. Phone: (708) 491-9091. Biennial.

Directory of Medical Specialists. Marquis Who's Who, 3002 Glenview Rd., Wilmette, IL 60091. Phone: (800) 621-9669. Fax: (708) 441-2264. Biennial.

Directory of Physicians in the United States. American Medical Association, 515 North State St., Chicago, IL 60610. Phone: (312) 464-0183. Fax: (312) 464-5834. Biennial.

ENCYCLOPEDIAS, DICTIONARIES, WORD BOOKS

Neurologic and Psychiatric Word Book. Helen E. Littrell. Springhouse Publishing Co., 1111 Bethlehem Pike, Spring House, PA 19477. Phone: (800) 331-3170. Fax: (215) 646-8716. 1992.

HANDBOOKS, GUIDES, MANUALS, ATLASES

Clinical Neurology. C. David Marsden, Timothy J. Fowler (eds.). Raven Press, 1185 Avenue of the Americas, New York, NY 10036. Phone: (212) 930-9500. Fax: (212) 869-3495. 1989.

Handbook of Neurology. Warlow. Blackwell Scientific Publications, Inc., 3 Cambridge Ctr., Cambridge, MA 02142. Phone: (800) 759-6102. 1991.

Handbook of Symptom Oriented Neurology. W. Olson, and others. Mosby-Year Book, 11830 Westline Industrial Drive, St. Louis, MO 63146. Phone: (800) 325-4177. Fax: (314) 432-1380. 1989.

Manual of Clinical Problems in Neurology. Mohr. Little, Brown and Co., 34 Beacon St., Boston, MA 02108. Phone: (617) 227-0730. Second edition 1989.

Manual of Neurologic Therapy. Samuels. Little, Brown and Co., 34 Beacon St., Boston, MA 02108. Phone: (617) 227-0730. Fax: (617) 227-0790. Fourth edition 1991.

Manual of Neurology: Diagnosis and Therapy. Martin A. Samuels (ed.). Little, Brown and Company, 34 Beacon St., Boston, MA 02108. Phone: (617) 227-0730. Fourth edition 1991.

Principles of Neurology: Companion Handbook. Raymond D. Adams, Maurice Victor. McGraw-Hill, Inc., Health Professions Division, 1221 Avenue of the Americas, 28th Floor, New York, NY 10020. Phone: (212) 512-4228. Fourth edition 1991.

JOURNALS

Annals of Neurology. Little, Brown and Co., 34 Beacon St., Boston, MA 02108. Phone: (617) 227-0730. Fax: (617) 227-0790. Monthly.

Archives of Neurology. American Medical Association, 515 North State St., Chicago, IL 60610. Phone: (312) 464-0183. Fax: (312) 464-5834. Monthly.

Brain Research. Elsevier Science Publishing Co., Inc., P.O. Box 882, Madison Square Station, New York, NY 10159-2101. Phone: (212) 989-5800. Fax: (212) 633-3990. 101/year.

Clinical Neuropharmacology. Raven Press, 1185 Avenue of the Americas, New York, NY 10036. Phone: (212) 930-9500. Fax: (212) 869-3495. Bimonthly.

Journal of the Autonomic Nervous System. Elsevier Science Publishing Co., Inc., P.O. Box 882, Madison Square Station, New York, NY 10159-2101. Phone: (212) 989-5800. Fax: (212) 633-3990. 12/year.

Journal of Comparative Neurology. John Wiley & Sons, Inc., 605 Third Ave., New York, NY 10158-0012. Phone: (212) 850-6000. Fax: (212) 850-6088. 48/year.

Journal of Neuroimmunology. Elsevier Science Publishing Co., Inc., P.O. Box 882, Madison Square Station, New York, NY 10159-2101. Phone: (212) 989-5800. Fax: (212) 633-3990. 18/year.

Journal of the Neurological Sciences. Elsevier Science Publishing Co., Inc., P.O. Box 882, Madison Square Station, New York, NY 10159-2101. Phone: (212) 989-5800. Fax: (212) 633-3990. 12/year.

Journal of Neurology. Springer-Verlag New York Inc., 175 Fifth Ave., New York, NY 10010. Phone: (212) 460-1500. Fax: (212) 473-6272.

Journal of Neurology, Neurosurgery & Psychiatry. BMJ Publishing Group, BMA House, Tavistock Square, London WC1H 9JR, England. Phone: 071-383 6244/6638. Fax: 071-383 6662. Monthly.

Journal of Neuropsychiatry and Clinical Neurosciences. American Psychiatric Press, 1400 K St. N.W., Washington, DC 20005. Phone: (202) 682-6000. Fax: (202) 682-6114. Quarterly.

Neurology. Edgell Communications, 7500 Old Oak Blvd., Cleveland, OH 44130. Phone: (216) 826-2839. Fax: (216) 891-2726. Monthly.

Neuroscience. Pergamon Press, 660 White Plains Rd., Tarrytown, NY 10591-5153. Phone: (914) 592-7700. Fax: (914) 592-3625.

Seminars in Neurology. Thieme Medical Publishers, Inc., 381 Park Ave. S., New York, NY 10016. Phone: (212) 683-5088. Fax: (212) 779-9020. Quarterly.

NEWSLETTERS

Neurology Alert. American Health Consultants, Department C1290, P.O. Box 740060, Atlanta, GA 30374. Phone: (800) 559-1032. Fax: (404) 352-1971. Monthly.

ONLINE DATABASES

BIOSIS Previews. BIOSIS, 2100 Arch St., Philadelphia, PA 19103-1399. Phone: (800) 523-4800. Fax: (215) 587-2016.

CSA Life Sciences Collection. Cambridge Scientific Abstracts, 7200 Wisconsin Ave., Bethesda, MD 20814-4823. Phone: (800) 843-7751. Fax: (301) 961-6720.

EMBASE. Elsevier Science Publishing Co., Inc., P.O. Box 882, Madison Square Station, New York, NY 10159-2101. Phone: (212) 989-5800. Fax: (212) 633-3990.

MEDLINE. National Library of Medicine, 8600 Rockville Pike, Bethesda, MD 20894. Phone: (800) 638-8480.

SciSearch. Institute for Scientific Information, 3501 Market St., Philadelphia, PA 19104. Phone: (215) 386-0100. Fax: (215) 386-6362.

RESEARCH CENTERS, INSTITUTES, CLEARINGHOUSES

Brain Development Research Center. University of North Carolina at Chapel Hill. CB 7250, Chapel Hill, NC 27599-7250. Phone: (919) 966-2405. Fax: (919) 966-1844.

Brain Information Service (BIS). University of California Brain Information Service, Ctr. for Health Sciences, Rm. 43-367, Los Angeles, CA 90024. Phone: (213) 825-3417.

Brain Research Foundation. 208 S. LaSalle St., Chicago, IL 60604. Phone: (312) 782-4311.

Center for Neuroscience. University of Tennessee. 875 Monroe Ave., Memphis, TN 38163. Phone: (901) 528-5956. Fax: (901) 528-7193.

TEXTBOOKS AND MONOGRAPHS

The Autonomic Nervous System: An Introduction to Basic and Clinical Concepts. Otto Appenzeller. Elsevier Science Publishing Co., Inc., P.O. Box 882, Madison Square Station, New York, NY 10159-2101. Phone: (212) 989-5800. Fax: (212) 633-3990. Fourth edition 1990.

Basic Neurology. John Gilroy. McGraw-Hill, Inc., Health Professions Division, 1221 Avenue of the Americas, 28th Floor, New York, NY 10020. Phone: (212) 512-4228. Second edition 1990.

Clinical Neuroanatomy for Medical Students. Richard S. Snell. Little, Brown and Company, 34 Beacon St., Boston, MA 02108. Phone: (617) 227-0730. Third edition 1992.

Clinical Neurology. Michael Swash, John Oxbury (eds.). Churchill Livingstone Inc., 650 Avenue of the Americas, New York, NY 10011. Phone: (212) 819-5400. Fax: (212) 302-6598. Two volumes 1991.

Comprehensive Neurology. Roger N. Rosenberg. Raven Press, 1185 Avenue of the Americas, New York, NY 10036. Phone: (212) 930-9500. Fax: (212) 869-3495. 1991.

Emergent & Urgent Neurology. William J. Welner. J.B. Lippincott Co., 227 East Washington Square, Philadelphia, PA 19106-3780. Phone: (215) 238-4200. Fax: (215) 238-4227. 1992.

The Epilepsies: Diagnosis and Management. Ernst Niedermeyer. Williams & Wilkins, 428 E. Preston St., Baltimore, MD 21202. Phone: (800) 638-0672. Fax: (800) 447-8438. 1990.

The Management of Pain. John J. Bonica, John D. Loeser, C. Richard Chapman, et. al.. Williams & Wilkins, 428 East Preston St., Baltimore, MD 21202. Phone: (800) 638-0672. Fax: (800) 447-8438. Second edition. Two volumes. 1990.

Merritt's Textbook of Neurology. Lewis P. Rowland (ed.). Williams & Wilkins, 428 E. Preston St., Baltimore, MD 21202. Phone: (800) 638-0672. Fax: (800) 447-8438. Eighth edition 1989.

Neurology in Clinical Practice. Walter G. Bradley, Robert B. Daroff, Gerald M. Fenichel (eds.). Butterworth-Heinemann, 80 Montvale Ave., Stoneham, MA 02180. Phone: (617) 438-8464. Fax: (617) 279-4851. 1991.

Neurology and General Medicine. Michael J. Aminoff (ed.). Churchill Livingstone Inc., 650 Ave. of the Americas, New York, NY 10011. Phone: (212) 819-5400. Fax: (212) 302-6598. 1989.

Neurology for the Non-Neurologist. William J. Weiner, Christopher Goetz. J.B. Lippincott Co., 227 East Washington Square, Philadelphia, PA 19106-3780. Phone: (215) 238-4200. Fax: (215) 238-4227. 1989.

Principles of Neurology. Raymond D. Adams, Maurice Victor. McGraw-Hill, Inc., Health Professions Division, 1221 Avenue of the Americas, 28th Floor, New York, NY 10020. Phone: (212) 512-4228. Fourth edition 1989.

Synopsis of Neurology. Richard Lechtenberg. Williams & Wilkins, 428 E. Preston St., Baltimore, MD 21202. Phone: (800) 638-0672. Fax: (800) 447-8438. 1991.

Textbook of Child Neurology. John H. Menkes. Williams & Wilkins, 428 E. Preston St., Baltimore, MD 21202. Phone: (800) 638-0672. Fax: (800) 447-8438. 1990.

NEUROMUSCULAR DISORDERS

See also: AMYOTROPHIC LATERAL SCLEROSIS; MUSCULAR DYSTROPHY; MYASTHENIA GRAVIS; PARKINSON'S DISEASE

ABSTRACTING, INDEXING, AND CURRENT AWARENESS PUBLICATIONS

Current Contents/Clinical Medicine. Institute for Scientific Information, 3501 Market St., Philadelphia, PA 19104. Phone: (800) 523-1850. Fax: (215) 386-6362. Weekly.

Current Contents/Life Sciences. Institute for Scientific Information, 3501 Market St., Philadelphia, PA 19104. Phone: (215) 386-0100. Fax: (215) 386-6362.

Excerpta Medica. Section 8: Neurology and Neurosurgery. Elsevier Science Publishers, P.O. Box 882, Madison Square Station, New York, NY 10159-2101. Phone: (212) 633-3950. Fax: (212) 633-3990. 32/year.

Index Medicus. U.S. National Library of Medicine, 8600 Rockville Pike, Bethesda, MD 20894. Phone: (800) 638-8480. Monthly.

Science Citation Index. Institute for Scientific Information, 3501 Market St., Philadelphia, PA 19104. Phone: (800) 523-1850. Fax: (215) 386-6362. Bimonthly.

ANNUALS AND REVIEWS

In Development New Medicines for Arthritis. Pharmaceutical Manufacturers Association, 1100 15th St. N.W., Washington, DC 20005. Phone: (202) 835-3400. Annual.

ASSOCIATIONS, PROFESSIONAL SOCIETIES, ADVOCACY AND SUPPORT GROUPS

ALS and Neuromuscular Research Foundation (ALSNRF). Pacific Presbyterian Medical Ctr., 2351 Clay St., No. 416, San Francisco, CA 94115. Phone: (415) 923-3604.

Amyotrophic Lateral Sclerosis Association (ALSA). 21021 Ventura Blvd., Ste. 321, Woodland Hills, CA 91364. Phone: (818) 340-7500. Fax: (818) 340-2060.

Charcot-Marie-Tooth Association (CMTA). Crozer Mills Enterprise Ctr., 600 Upland Ave., Philadelphia, PA 19105. Phone: (215) 499-7486.

Families of Spinal Muscular Atrophy. P.O. Box 1465, Highland Park, IL 60035. Phone: (312) 432-5551.

Friedreich's Ataxia Group in America (FAGA). P.O. Box 11116, Oakland, CA 94611-0116. Phone: (415) 655-0833.

Muscular Dystrophy Association (MDA). 810 7th Ave., New York, NY 10019. Phone: (212) 586-0808. Fax: (212) 765-2003.

Myasthenia Gravis Foundation (MG). 53 W. Jackson Blvd., Ste. 1352, Chicago, IL 60604. Phone: (312) 427-6252. Fax: (312) 427-9437.

CD-ROM DATABASES

Excerpta Medica CD: Neurosciences. SilverPlatter Information, Inc., River Ridge Office Park, 100 River Ridge Rd., Norwood, MA 02062. Phone: (617) 769-2599. Fax: (617) 769-8763. Quarterly.

SCISEARCH. Institute for Scientific Information, 3501 Market St., Philadelphia, PA 19104. Phone: (215) 386-0100. Fax: (215) 386-6362.

JOURNALS

Journal of the Autonomic Nervous System. Elsevier Science Publishing Co., Inc., P.O. Box 882, Madison Square Station, New York, NY 10159-2101. Phone: (212) 989-5800. Fax: (212) 633-3990. 12/year.

Journal of Neurology. Springer-Verlag New York Inc., 175 Fifth Ave., New York, NY 10010. Phone: (212) 460-1500. Fax: (212) 473-6272.

Neurology. Edgell Communications, 7500 Old Oak Blvd., Cleveland, OH 44130. Phone: (216) 826-2839. Fax: (216) 891-2726. Monthly.

ONLINE DATABASES

Combined Health Information Database (CHID). U.S. National Institutes of Health, P.O. Box NDIC, Bethesda, MD 20892. Phone: (301) 496-2162. Fax: (301) 770-5164. Quarterly.

EMBASE. Elsevier Science Publishing Co., Inc., P.O. Box 882, Madison Square Station, New York, NY 10159-2101. Phone: (212) 989-5800. Fax: (212) 633-3990.

MEDLINE. National Library of Medicine, 8600 Rockville Pike, Bethesda, MD 20894. Phone: (800) 638-8480.

SciSearch. Institute for Scientific Information, 3501 Market St., Philadelphia, PA 19104. Phone: (215) 386-0100. Fax: (215) 386-6362.

POPULAR WORKS AND PATIENT EDUCATION

Chronic Muscle Pain Syndrome. Paul Davidson. Random House, Inc., 201 E. 50th St., New York, NY 10022. Phone: (800) 726-0600. 1989.

RESEARCH CENTERS, INSTITUTES, CLEARINGHOUSES

Dystonia Medical Research Foundation. 8383 Wilshire Blvd., Beverly Hills, CA 90211. Phone: (213) 852-1630.

Jerry Lewis Neuromuscular Disease Center. New York University, 400 E. 34th St., New York, NY 10016. Phone: (212) 340-6350.

Jerry Lewis Neuromuscular Disease Research Center. Baylor College of Medicine, One Baylor Plaza, Houston, TX 77030. Phone: (713) 799-5971.

Jerry Lewis Neuromuscular Research Center. Washington University, 600 South Euclid Ave., Box 8111, St. Louis, MO 63110. Phone: (314) 362-6981.

National Arthritis and Musculoskeletal and Skin Diseases Information Clearinghouse (NAMSIC). 9000 Rockville Pike, P.O. Box AMS, Bethesda, MD 20892. Phone: (301) 495-4484. Fax: (301) 587-4352.

National Institute of Neurological Disorders and Stroke. 9000 Rockville Pike, Bethesda, MD 20892. Phone: (301) 496-5679.

NIDRR Research and Training Center. School of Medicine, University of California, Davis, Davis, CA 95616. Phone: (916) 752-2903.

TEXTBOOKS AND MONOGRAPHS

Tardive Dyskinesia: A Task Force Report of the American Psychiatric Association. John M. Kane. American Psychiatric Press, Inc., 1400 K St. NW, Washington, DC 20005. Phone: (202) 682-6268. Fax: (202) 789-2648. 1992.

NEUROSES

See: ANXIETY; DEPRESSION; MENTAL HEALTH; MOOD DISORDERS; PSYCHIATRIC DISORDERS; PSYCHOANALYSIS

NEUROSURGERY

See also: NEUROLOGIC DISORDERS

ABSTRACTING, INDEXING, AND CURRENT AWARENESS PUBLICATIONS

Core Journals in Clinical Neurology. Elsevier Science Publishing Co., Inc., P.O. Box 882, Madison Square Station, New York, NY 10159-2101. Phone: (212) 989-5800. Fax: (212) 633-3990. 11/year.

Current Contents/Clinical Medicine. Institute for Scientific Information, 3501 Market St., Philadelphia, PA 19104. Phone: (800) 523-1850. Fax: (215) 386-6362. Weekly.

Excerpta Medica. Section 8: Neurology and Neurosurgery. Elsevier Science Publishers, P.O. Box 882, Madison Square Station, New York, NY 10159-2101. Phone: (212) 633-3950. Fax: (212) 633-3990. 32/year.

Index Medicus. U.S. National Library of Medicine, 8600 Rockville Pike, Bethesda, MD 20894. Phone: (800) 638-8480. Monthly.

Key Neurology and Neurosurgery: Current Literature in Perspective. Mosby-Year Book, 11830 Westline Industrial Drive, St. Louis, MO 63146. Phone: (800) 325-4177. Fax: (314) 432-1380. Quarterly.

Science Citation Index. Institute for Scientific Information, 3501 Market St., Philadelphia, PA 19104. Phone: (800) 523-1850. Fax: (215) 386-6362. Bimonthly.

ANNUALS AND REVIEWS

Current Opinion in Neurology & Neurosurgery. Current Science Ltd., 20 N. Third St., Philadelphia, PA 19106-2199. Phone: (800) 552-5866. Fax: (215) 574-2270. Bimonthly.

Neurosurgery Clinics. W.B. Saunders Co., The Curtis Center, Independence Square W., Philadelphia, PA 19106-3399. Phone: (215) 238-7800. Quarterly.

Progress in Neurological Surgery. S. Karger Publishers, Inc., 26 West Avon Rd., P.O. Box 529, Farmington, CT 06085. Phone: (203) 675-7834. Fax: (203) 675-7302. Irregular.

Year Book of Neurology and Neurosurgery. Mosby-Year Book, 11830 Westline Industrial Drive, St. Louis, MO 63146. Phone: (800) 325-4177. Fax: (314) 432-1380. Annual.

ASSOCIATIONS, PROFESSIONAL SOCIETIES, ADVOCACY AND SUPPORT GROUPS

American Academy of Neurological and Orthopaedic Surgeons (FAANaOS). 2320 Rancho Dr., Ste. 108, Las Vegas, NV 89102. Phone: (702) 385-6886.

American Association of Neurological Surgeons (AANS). 22 S. Washington St., Ste. 100, Park Ridge, IL 60068. Phone: (708) 692-9500. Fax: (708) 692-2589.

American Board of Neurological and Orthopaedic Medicine and Surgery. 2320 Rancho Dr., Ste. 108, Las Vegas, NV 89102-4592. Phone: (702) 385-6886.

American Board of Neurological Surgery (ABNS). 6550 Fannin St., No. 2139, Houston, TX 77030-2722. Phone: (713) 790-6015.

Society of Neurological Surgeons. c/o James I. Ausman, Dept. of Neurosurgery, Henry Ford Hospital, 2799 W. Grand Blvd., Detroit, MI 48202. Phone: (313) 876-1340.

CD-ROM DATABASES

Excerpta Medica CD: Neurosciences. SilverPlatter Information, Inc., River Ridge Office Park, 100 River Ridge Rd., Norwood, MA 02062. Phone: (617) 769-2599. Fax: (617) 769-8763. Quarterly.

Neuroscience Citation Index. Institute for Scientific Information, 3501 Market St., Philadelphia, PA 19104. Phone: (800) 523-1857. Fax: (215) 386-6362. Bimonthly.

SCISEARCH. Institute for Scientific Information, 3501 Market St., Philadelphia, PA 19104. Phone: (215) 386-0100. Fax: (215) 386-6362.

Year Books on Disc. CMC ReSearch, Inc., 7150 S.W. Hampton, Suite C-120, Portland, OR 97223. Phone: (800) 262-

7668. Fax: (503) 639-1796. Annual includes Year Books of Cardiology, Dermatology, Diagnostic Radiology, Drug Therapy, Emergency Medicine, Family Practice, Medicine, Neurology and Neurosurgery, Obstetrics and Gynecology, Oncology, Pediatrics, and Psychiatry and Applied Mental Health.

DIRECTORIES

Directory of Certified Neurological Surgeons. American Board of Medical Specialties, 1 Rotary Center, Suite 805, Evanston, IL 60201. Phone: (708) 491-9091. Biennial.

HANDBOOKS, GUIDES, MANUALS, ATLASES

Atlas of Operative Neurosurgical Technique. Volume I: Cranial Operations. Donlin M. Long. Williams & Wilkins, 428 East Preston St., Baltimore, MD 21202. Phone: (800) 638-0672. Fax: (800) 447-8438. 1988.

Atlas of Spinal Surgery. Donlin M. Long. Williams & Wilkins, 428 E. Preston St., Baltimore, MD 21202. Phone: (800) 638-0672. Fax: (800) 447-8438. 1992.

Neurosurgical Operative Atlas. Setti S. Rengachary, Robert H. Wilkins (eds.). Williams & Wilkins, 428 East Preston St., Baltimore, MD 21202. Phone: (800) 638-0672. Fax: (800) 447-8438. Biennial.

JOURNALS

Journal of Child Neurology. Mosby-Year Book, 11830 Westline Industrial Drive, St. Louis, MO 63146. Phone: (800) 325-4177. Fax: (314) 432-1380. Quarterly.

Journal of Neurology, Neurosurgery & Psychiatry. BMJ Publishing Group, BMA House, Tavistock Square, London WC1H 9JR, England. Phone: 071-383 6244/6638. Fax: 071-383 6662. Monthly.

Journal of Neurosurgery. American Association of Neurological Surgeons, 22 S. Washington St., Park Ridge, IL 60068. Phone: (708) 692-9500.

Neurochiurgia. Thieme Medical Publishers, Inc., 381 Park Ave. S., New York, NY 10016. Phone: (212) 683-5088. Fax: (212) 779-9020. Bimonthly.

Neurosurgery. Williams & Wilkins, 428 E. Preston St., Baltimore, MD 21202. Phone: (800) 638-0672. Fax: (800) 447-8438. Monthly.

Neurosurgery Quarterly. Raven Press, 1185 Avenue of the Americas, New York, NY 10036. Phone: (212) 930-9500. Fax: (212) 869-3495. Quarterly.

Surgical Neurology. Elsevier Science Publishing Co., Inc., P.O. Box 882, Madison Square Station, New York, NY 10159-2101. Phone: (212) 989-5800. Fax: (212) 633-3990. Monthly.

NEWSLETTERS

Contemporary Neurosurgery: A Biweekly Review of Clinical Practice. Williams & Wilkins, 428 E. Preston St., Baltimore, MD 21202. Phone: (800) 638-0672. Fax: (800) 447-8438. Biweekly.

ONLINE DATABASES

EMBASE. Elsevier Science Publishing Co., Inc., P.O. Box 882, Madison Square Station, New York, NY 10159-2101. Phone: (212) 989-5800. Fax: (212) 633-3990.

MEDLINE. National Library of Medicine, 8600 Rockville Pike, Bethesda, MD 20894. Phone: (800) 638-8480.

SciSearch. Institute for Scientific Information, 3501 Market St., Philadelphia, PA 19104. Phone: (215) 386-0100. Fax: (215) 386-6362.

TEXTBOOKS AND MONOGRAPHS

Clinical Neurology: Proceedings of the Congress of Neurological Surgeons, Altlanta, GA, 1989. Peter McL. Black. Williams & Wilkins, 428 East Preston St., Baltimore, MD 21202. Phone: (800) 638-0672. Fax: (800) 447-8438. Volume 37, 1990.

Essentials of Neurosurgery: A Guide to Clinical Practice. Marshall B. Allen, Ross H. Miller. McGraw-Hill, Inc., Health Professions Division, 1221 Avenue of the Americas, 28th Floor, New York, NY 10020. Phone: (212) 512-4228. 1992.

Lumbar Spine Surgery: Indications, Techniques, Failures, and Alternatives. Joseph C. Cauthen (ed.). Williams & Wilkins, 428 E. Preston St., Baltimore, MD 21202. Phone: (800) 638-0672. Fax: (800) 447-8438. Second edition 1988.

Neurology and Neurosurgery Illustrated. K.W. Lindsay and others. Churchill Livingstone Inc., 650 Ave. of the Americas, New York, NY 10011. Phone: (212) 819-5400. Fax: (212) 302-6598. Second edition 1991.

Neurosurgery: The Scientific Basis of Clinical Practice. Crockard. Blackwell Scientific Publications, Inc., 3 Cambridge Ctr., Cambridge, MA 02142. Phone: (800) 759-6102. Second edition 1992.

Patient Care in Neurosurgery. Oyesiku. Little, Brown and Co., 34 Beacon St., Boston, MA 02108. Phone: (617) 227-0730. Fax: (617) 227-0790. Third edition 1990.

Plastic Techniques in Neurosurgery. J.T. Goodrich, K.D. Post, R. Argamaso. Thieme Medical Publishers, Inc., 381 Park Ave. S., New York, NY 10016. Phone: (212) 683-5088. Fax: (212) 779-9020. 1991.

Principles of Neurosurgery. Robert G. Grossman (ed.). Raven Press, 1185 Avenue of the Americas, New York, NY 10036. Phone: (212) 930-9500. Fax: (212) 869-3495. 1991.

Reoperative Neurosurgery. Little. Williams & Wilkins, 428 East Preston St., Baltimore, MD 21202. Phone: (800) 638-0672. Fax: (800) 447-8438. 1992.

Techniques in Neurosurgery. Charles B. Wilson. Williams & Wilkins, 428 E. Preston St., Baltimore, MD 21202. Phone: (800) 638-0672. Fax: (800) 447-8438. 1991.

Ultrasound in Neurosurgery. Jonathan M. Rubin, William F. Chandler, and others. Raven Press, 1185 Avenue of the Americas, New York, NY 10036. Phone: (212) 930-9500. Fax: (212) 869-3495. 1990.

NITRATES

See: FOOD ADDITIVES

NMR

See: MRI (MAGNETIC RESONANCE IMAGING)

NON-PRESCRIPTION DRUGS

See also: DRUGS

ABSTRACTING, INDEXING, AND CURRENT AWARENESS PUBLICATIONS

General Science Index. H.W. Wilson Co., 950 University Ave., Bronx, NY 10452. Phone: (800) 367-6770.

International Pharmaceutical Abstracts. American Society of Hospital Pharmacists, 4630 Montgomery Ave., Bethesda, MD 20814. Phone: (301) 657-3000. Fax: (301) 657-1641. Semimonthly.

ASSOCIATIONS, PROFESSIONAL SOCIETIES, ADVOCACY AND SUPPORT GROUPS

Nonprescription Drug Manufacturers Association. 1150 Connecticut Ave. N.W., Washington, DC 20036. Phone: (202) 429-9260.

The Proprietary Association. 1150 Connecticut Ave. N.W., Washington, DC 20030. Phone: (202) 429-9260.

CD-ROM DATABASES

1993 PDR Library on CD-ROM. Medical Economics, Five Paragon Dr., Montvale, NJ 07645-1742. Phone: (800) 232-7379. Fax: (201) 573-4956. 1993.

International Pharmaceutical Abstracts. SilverPlatter Information, Inc., River Ridge Office Park, 100 River Ridge Rd., Norwood, MA 02062. Phone: (617) 769-2599. Fax: (617) 769-8763. Quarterly.

PDR on CD-ROM. Medical Economics, Five Paragon Dr., Montvale, NJ 07645-1742. Phone: (800) 222-3045. Fax: (201) 573-4956. 3/year.

HANDBOOKS, GUIDES, MANUALS, ATLASES

USP-DI Volume III: Approved Drug Products and Legal Requirements. U.S. Pharmacopeial Convention, Inc., 12601 Twinbrook Parkway, Rockville, MD 20852. Phone: (800) 227-8772. Annual.

ONLINE DATABASES

International Pharmaceutical Abstracts. American Society of Hospital Pharmacists, 4630 Montgomery Ave., Bethesda, MD 20814. Phone: (301) 657-3000. Fax: (301) 657-1641. Monthly.

POPULAR WORKS AND PATIENT EDUCATION

About Your Medicines. United States Pharmacopeial Convention, Inc., 12601 Twinbrook Parkway, Rockville, MD 20852. Phone: (800) 227-8772. Fax: (301) 816-8148. Sixth edition 1992.

Advice for the Patient. United States Pharmacopeial Convention, Inc., 12601 Twinbrook Parkway, Rockville, MD 20852. Phone: (800) 227-8772. Fax: (301) 816-8148. 1989.

Complete Guide to Prescription & Non-Prescription Drugs. H. Winter Griffith. Putnam Publishing Group, 200 Madison Ave., New York, NY 10016. Phone: (800) 631-8571. Revised edition 1992.

Graedons' Best Medicine: From Herbal Remedies to High-Tech Rx Breakthroughs. Joe Graedon, Teresa Graedon. Bantam Books, Inc., 666 Fifth Ave., New York, NY 10103. Phone: (800) 223-6834. 1991.

Guide to Prescription and Over-the-Counter Drugs: Brand Name Drugs, Generic Drugs, Vitamins, Minerals, Food Additives. American Medical Association Staff. Random House, Inc., 201 E. 50th St., New York, NY 10022. Phone: (800) 726-0600. 1988.

Zimmerman's Complete Guide to Nonprescription Drugs. David Zimmerman. Visible Ink Press, 835 Penobscot Bldg., Detroit, MI 48226.

RESEARCH CENTERS, INSTITUTES, CLEARINGHOUSES

Food and Drug Administration. 5600 Fishers Lane, Rockville, MD 20857. Phone: (301) 443-2410.

NON-STEROIDAL ANTI-INFLAMMATORY AGENTS

See: DRUGS

NOSE DISEASES

See: OTOLARYNGOLOGY

NUCLEAR MEDICINE

See also: DIAGNOSIS; MRI (MAGNETIC RESONANCE IMAGING); TOMOGRAPHY

ABSTRACTING, INDEXING, AND CURRENT AWARENESS PUBLICATIONS

Current Contents/Clinical Medicine. Institute for Scientific Information, 3501 Market St., Philadelphia, PA 19104. Phone: (800) 523-1850. Fax: (215) 386-6362. Weekly.

Current Contents/Life Sciences. Institute for Scientific Information, 3501 Market St., Philadelphia, PA 19104. Phone: (215) 386-0100. Fax: (215) 386-6362.

Excerpta Medica. Section 23: Nuclear Medicine. Elsevier Science Publishers, P.O. Box 882, Madison Square Station, New York, NY 10159-2101. Phone: (212) 633-3950. Fax: (212) 633-3990. 20/year.

Index Medicus. U.S. National Library of Medicine, 8600 Rockville Pike, Bethesda, MD 20894. Phone: (800) 638-8480. Monthly.

Research Alert: Nuclear Medicine. Institute for Scientific Information, 3501 Market St., Philadelphia, PA 19104. Phone: (800) 523-1850. Fax: (215) 386-6362. Weekly.

Science Citation Index. Institute for Scientific Information, 3501 Market St., Philadelphia, PA 19104. Phone: (800) 523-1850. Fax: (215) 386-6362. Bimonthly.

ANNUALS AND REVIEWS

Neuroimaging Clinics of North America. W.B. Saunders Co., The Curtis Center, Independence Square W., Philadelphia, PA 19106-3399. Phone: (215) 238-7800. Quarterly.

Nuclear Medicine Annual. Raven Press, 1185 Avenue of the Americas, New York, NY 10036. Phone: (212) 930-9500. Fax: (212) 869-3495. Annual.

Recent Advances in Nuclear Medicine. W.B. Saunders Co., The Curtis Center, Independence Sqare W., Philadelphia, PA 19106-3399. Phone: (215) 238-7800.

Year Book of Nuclear Medicine. Mosby-Year Book, 11830 Westline Industrial Drive, St. Louis, MO 63146. Phone: (800) 325-4177. Fax: (314) 432-1380. Annual.

ASSOCIATIONS, PROFESSIONAL SOCIETIES, ADVOCACY AND SUPPORT GROUPS

American Board of Nuclear Medicine (ABMN). 900 Veteran Ave., Los Angeles, CA 90024-1786. Phone: (213) 825-6787. Fax: (213) 825-9433.

American College of Nuclear Medicine (ACNM). P.O. Box 5887, Columbus, GA 31906. Phone: (404) 322-8049.

American College of Nuclear Physicians (ACNP). 1101 Connecticut Ave. N.W., Ste. 700, Washington, DC 20036. Phone: (202) 857-1135. Fax: (202) 223-4579.

Society of Nuclear Medicine (SNM). 136 Madison Ave., 8th Flr., New York, NY 10016-6760. Phone: (212) 889-0717. Fax: (212) 545-0221.

BIBLIOGRAPHIES

Nuclear Magnetic Resonance: Applications in Medical Diagnosis. National Technical Information Service, 5285 Port Royal Rd., Springfield, VA 22161. Phone: (703) 487-4650. Fax: (703) 321-8547. Jan. 1978-July 1988 PB88-866900/CBY.

Nuclear Magnetic Resonance as a Diagnostic Tool. National Technical Information Service, 5285 Port Royal Rd., Springfield, VA 22161. Phone: (703) 487-4650. Fax: (703) 321-8547. Jan. 1970-July 1988 PB88-866926/CBY.

CD-ROM DATABASES

Excerpta Medica CD: Radiology & Nuclear Medicine. SilverPlatter Information, Inc., River Ridge Office Park, 100 River Ridge Rd., Norwood, MA 02062. Phone: (617) 769-2599. Fax: (617) 769-8763. Quarterly.

RadLine. Aries Systems Corporation, One Dundee Park, Andover, MA 01810. Phone: (508) 475-7200. Fax: (508) 474-8860. Quarterly.

SCISEARCH. Institute for Scientific Information, 3501 Market St., Philadelphia, PA 19104. Phone: (215) 386-0100. Fax: (215) 386-6362.

DIRECTORIES

Directory of Certified Nuclear Medicine Specialists. American Board of Medical Specialties, 1 Rotary Center, Suite 805, Evanston, IL 60201. Phone: (708) 491-9091. Biennial.

ENCYCLOPEDIAS, DICTIONARIES, WORD BOOKS

Dictionary and Handbook of Nuclear Medicine and Clinical Imaging. Mario P. Iturralde. CRC Press, Inc., 2000 Corporate Blvd. N.W., Boca Raton, FL 33431. Phone: (407) 994-0555. Fax: (407) 997-0949. 1990.

HANDBOOKS, GUIDES, MANUALS, ATLASES

Manual of Diagnostic Imaging. Straub. Little, Brown and Co., 34 Beacon St., Boston, MA 02108. Phone: (617) 227-0730. Fax: (617) 227-0790. Second edition 1989.

Nuclear Medicine. Datz. Mosby-Year Book, 11830 Westline Industrial Drive, St. Louis, MO 63146. Phone: (800) 325-4177. Fax: (314) 432-1380. 1988.

JOURNALS

Clinical Nuclear Medicine. J.B. Lippincott Co., 227 E. Washington Square, Philadelphia, PA 19106-3780. Phone: (215) 238-4200. Fax: (215) 238-4227.

European Journal of Nuclear Medicine. Springer-Verlag New York Inc., 175 Fifth Ave., New York, NY 10010. Phone: (212) 460-1500. Fax: (212) 473-6272.

Journal of Nuclear Medicine. Society of Nuclear Medicine, 136 Madison Ave., New York, NY 10016. Phone: (212) 889-0717.

Journal of Nuclear Medicine Technology. Society of Nuclear Medicine, 136 Madison Ave., New York, NY 10016. Phone: (212) 889-0717.

Seminars in Nuclear Medicine. W.B. Saunders Co., The Curtis Center, Independence Sqare W., Philadelphia, PA 19106-3399. Phone: (215) 238-7800.

ONLINE DATABASES

EMBASE. Elsevier Science Publishing Co., Inc., P.O. Box 882, Madison Square Station, New York, NY 10159-2101. Phone: (212) 989-5800. Fax: (212) 633-3990.

MEDLINE. National Library of Medicine, 8600 Rockville Pike, Bethesda, MD 20894. Phone: (800) 638-8480.

SciSearch. Institute for Scientific Information, 3501 Market St., Philadelphia, PA 19104. Phone: (215) 386-0100. Fax: (215) 386-6362.

RESEARCH CENTERS, INSTITUTES, CLEARINGHOUSES

Diagnostic Imaging Science Center. University of Washington. Dept. of Radiology, SB-05, Seattle, WA 98195. Phone: (206) 543-0873. Fax: (206) 543-3495.

Nuclear Medicine Division. University Hospital, University of Michigan, Ann Arbor, MI 48109. Phone: (313) 936-5388.

TEXTBOOKS AND MONOGRAPHS

Cardiac Nuclear Medicine. Myron C. Gerson. McGraw-Hill, Inc., Health Professions Division, 1221 Avenue of the Americas, 28th Floor, New York, NY 10020. Phone: (212) 512-4228. Second edition 1991.

Clinical Nuclear Medicine. M.N. Maisey. Routledge, Chapman & Hall, Inc., 29 W. 35th St., New York, NY 10001-2291. Phone: (212) 244-3336. Second edition 1990.

Clinical Practice of Nuclear Medicine. Taylor. Churchill Livingstone Inc., 650 Ave. of the Americas, New York, NY 10011. Phone: (212) 819-5400. Fax: (212) 302-6598. 1991.

Introductory Physics of Nuclear Medicine. Ramesh Chandra. Williams & Wilkins, 428 East Preston St., Baltimore, MD 21202. Phone: (800) 638-0672. Fax: (800) 447-8438. Fourth edition 1992.

Nuclear Medicine: Quantitative Analysis in Imaging and Function. H.A.E. Schmidt, J. Chambron (eds.). John Wiley & Sons, Inc., 605 Third Ave., New York, NY 10158-0012. Phone: (212) 850-6000. Fax: (212) 850-6088. 1990.

Principles and Practice of Nuclear Medicine. Paul J. Early, D. Bruce Sodee. Mosby-Year Book, 11830 Westline Industrial Drive, St. Louis, MO 63146. Phone: (800) 325-4177. Fax: (314) 432-1380. Second edition 1992.

NURSE ANESTHETISTS

See: ANESTHESIOLOGY; NURSING

NURSE PRACTITIONERS

See: NURSING; NURSING EDUCATION

NURSING

ABSTRACTING, INDEXING, AND CURRENT AWARENESS PUBLICATIONS

AACN Nursing Scan in Critical Care. NURSECOM, Inc., 1211 Locust St., Philadelphia, PA 19107. Phone: (215) 545-7222. Bimonthly.

Cumulative Index to Nursing and Allied Health Literature. Glendale Adventist Medical Center, P.O. Box 871, Glendale, CA 91209. Phone: (818) 409-8005. Bimonthly.

ENA's Nursing Scan in Emergency Care. NURSECOM, Inc., 1211 Locust St., Philadelphia, PA 19107. Phone: (215) 545-7222. Bimonthly.

Index Medicus. U.S. National Library of Medicine, 8600 Rockville Pike, Bethesda, MD 20894. Phone: (800) 638-8480. Monthly.

International Nursing Index. American Journal of Nursing Co., 555 W. 57th St., New York, NY 10019. Phone: (212) 582-8820. Quarterly.

Nursing Abstracts. Nursing Abstracts Co., Inc., P.O. Box 295, Forest Hills, NY 11375. Bimonthly.

Nursing Scan in Research: Application for Clinical Practice. NURSECOM, Inc., 1211 Locust St., Philadelphia, PA 19107. Phone: (215) 545-7222. Bimonthly.

ONS Nursing Scan in Oncology. NURSECOM, Inc., 1211 Locust St., Philadelphia, PA 19107. Phone: (215) 545-7222. Bimonthly.

ANNUALS AND REVIEWS

Annual Review of Nursing Research. Springer Publishing Co., Inc., 536 Broadway, 11th Floor, New York, NY 10012. Phone: (212) 431-4370. Annual.

Critical Care Nursing Clinics of North America. W.B. Saunders Co., The Curtis Center, Independence Square W., Philadelphia, PA 19106-3399. Phone: (215) 238-7800. Quarterly.

Mosby's Comprehensive Review of Nursing. Mosby-Year Book, 11830 Westline Industrial Drive, St. Louis, MO 63146. Phone: (800) 325-4177. Fax: (314) 432-1380. Irregular.

Nursing Clinics. W.B. Saunders Co., The Curtis Center, Independence Square W., Philadelphia, PA 19106-3399. Phone: (215) 238-7800. Quarterly.

Perpectives in Nursing. National League for Nursing, 350 Hudson St., New York, NY 10014. Phone: (212) 989-9393. Biennial.

ASSOCIATIONS, PROFESSIONAL SOCIETIES, ADVOCACY AND SUPPORT GROUPS

American Academy of Nursing (AAN). 2420 Pershing Rd., Kansas City, MO 64108. Phone: (816) 474-5720. Fax: (816) 471-4903.

American Association of Critical-Care Nurses (AACN). 1 Civic Plaza, Newport Beach, CA 92660. Phone: (714) 644-9310. Fax: (714) 640-4903.

American Nurses' Association (ANA). 2420 Pershing Rd., Kansas City, MO 64108. Phone: (816) 474-5720. Fax: (816) 471-4903.

Canadian Nurses Association. 50 The Driveway, Ottawa, ON, Canada K2P 1E2. Phone: (613) 237-2133. Fax: (613) 237-3520.

NAACOG: The Organization for Obstetric, Gynecologic and Neonatal Nurses. 409 12th St. S.W., Washington, DC 20024. Phone: (202) 638-0026.

National League for Nursing (NLN). 350 Hudson St., New York, NY 10014. Phone: (212) 989-9393.

BIBLIOGRAPHIES

Core Collection in Nursing and the Allied Health Sciences: Books, Journal, Media. Oryx Press, 4041 N. Central, Suite 700, Phoenix, AZ 85012. Phone: (800) 279-ORYX. Fax: (800) 279-4663. 1990.

CD-ROM DATABASES

CD Plus/CINAHL. CD Plus, 333 7th Ave., 6th Floor, New York, NY 10001. Phone: (212) 563-3006. Monthly.

Nursing and Allied Health (CINAHL-CD) on Compact Cambridge. Cambridge Scientific Abstracts, 7200 Wisconsin Ave., Bethesda, MD 20814-4823. Phone: (800) 843-7751. Fax: (301) 961-6720. Monthly.

Nursing and Allied Health (CINAHL) on CD-ROM. CINAHL, 1509 Wilson Terrace, P.O. Box 871, Glendale, CA 91209-0871. Phone: (818) 409-8005.

Nursing and Allied Health (CINAHL-CD) on SilverPlatter. SilverPlatter Information, Inc., River Ridge Office Park, 100 River Ridge Rd., Norwood, MA 02062. Phone: (617) 769-2599. Fax: (617) 769-8763. Bimonthly.

Nursing INDISC. Knowledge Access International, 2685 Marine Way, Suite 1305, Mountain View, CA 94043. Phone: (800) 252-9273. Fax: (415) 964-2027. Quarterly.

DIRECTORIES

Directory of Nursing Homes 1991-1992. Oryx Press, 4041 N. Central, Suite 700, Phoenix, AZ 85012. Phone: (800) 279-ORYX. Fax: (800) 279-4663. 1991.

ENCYCLOPEDIAS, DICTIONARIES, WORD BOOKS

Mosby's Medical, Nursing, and Allied Health Dictionary. Kenneth N. Anderson, Lois Anderson, Walter D. Glanze (eds.). Mosby-Year Book, 11830 Westline Industrial Dr., St. Louis, MO 63146. Phone: (800) 325-4177. Fax: (314) 432-1380. Third edition 1990.

Nurse's Book of Advice. Springhouse Publishing Co., 1111 Bethlehem Pike, Spring House, PA 19477. Phone: (800) 331-3170. Fax: (215) 646-8716. 1992.

The Nurse's Dictionary. Christine Brooker (ed.). Faber & Faber, Inc., 50 Cross St., Winchester, MA 01890. Phone: (617) 721-1427. 30th edition 1989.

HANDBOOKS, GUIDES, MANUALS, ATLASES

Health Assessment: An Illustrated Pocket Guide. June Thompson, Arden Bowers. Mosby-Year Book, 11830 Westline Industrial Drive, St. Louis, MO 63146. Phone: (800) 325-4177. Fax: (314) 432-1380. 3rd edition, 1992.

Illustrated Manual of Nursing Practice. Springhouse Publishing Co., 1111 Bethlehem Pike, Spring House, PA 19477. Phone: (800) 331-3170. Fax: (215) 646-8716. 1991.

Lippincott Manual of Nursing Practice. J.B. Lippincott Co., 227 E. Washington Square, Philadelphia, PA 19106-3780. Phone: (215) 238-4200. Fax: (215) 238-4227. Fifth edition 1991.

Manual of Nursing Diagnosis. Marjory Gordon. Mosby-Year Book, 11830 Westline Industrial Drive, St. Louis, MO 63146. Phone: (800) 325-4177. Fax: (314) 432-1380. Irregular.

Nurse's Quick Reference. Springhouse Publishing Co., 1111 Bethlehem Pike, Spring House, PA 19477. Phone: (800) 331-3170. Fax: (215) 646-8716. 1990.

JOURNALS

American Journal of Nursing. American Journal of Nursing Co., 555 W. 57th St., New York, NY 10019. Phone: (212) 582-8820. Monthly.

Geriatric Nursing. Mosby-Year Book, 11830 Westline Industrial Drive, St. Louis, MO 63146. Phone: (800) 325-4177. Fax: (314) 432-1380. Bimonthly.

Heart & Lung: The Journal of Critical Care. Mosby-Year Book, 11830 Westline Industrial Drive, St. Louis, MO 63146. Phone: (800) 325-4177. Fax: (314) 432-1380. Bimonthly.

Intensive Care Nursing. Churchill Livingstone Inc., 650 Avenue of the Americas, New York, NY 10011. Phone: (212) 819-5400. Fax: (212) 302-6598. Quarterly.

Issues in Comprehensive Pediatric Nursing. Taylor & Francis Inc., 1900 Frost Rd., Suite 101, Bristol, PA 19007-1598. Phone: (800) 821-8312. Fax: (215) 785-5515. Quarterly.

Issues in Mental Health Nursing. Taylor & Francis Inc., 1900 Frost Rd., Suite 101, Bristol, PA 19007-1598. Phone: (800) 821-8312. Fax: (215) 785-5515. Quarterly.

Journal of Emergency Nursing. Mosby-Year Book, 11830 Westline Industrial Drive, St. Louis, MO 63146. Phone: (800) 325-4177. Fax: (314) 432-1380. Bimonthly.

Journal of ET Nursing. Mosby-Year Book, 11830 Westline Industrial Drive, St. Louis, MO 63146. Phone: (800) 325-4177. Fax: (314) 432-1380. Bimonthly.

Journal of Gerontological Nursing. SLACK Inc., 6900 Grove Rd., Thorofare, NJ 08086-9447. Phone: (800) 257-8290. Fax: (609) 853-5991. Monthly.

Journal of Pediatric Health Care. Mosby-Year Book, 11830 Westline Industrial Drive, St. Louis, MO 63146. Phone: (800) 325-4177. Fax: (314) 432-1380. Bimonthly.

Journal of Vascular Nursing. Mosby-Year Book, 11830 Westline Industrial Drive, St. Louis, MO 63146. Phone: (800) 325-4177. Fax: (314) 432-1380. Quarterly.

The Nurse Practitioner: The American Journal of Primary Health Care. Vernon Publications, Inc., 3000 Northup Way, Suite 200, Box 96043, Bellevue, WA 98009. Phone: (206) 827-9900. Monthly.

Nursing Administration Quarterly. Aspen Publishers, Inc., 200 Orchard Ridge Dr., Gaithersburg, MD 20878. Phone: (800) 638-8437. Quarterly.

Nursing Diagnosis. J.B. Lippincott Co., 227 E. Washington Square, Philadelphia, PA 19106-3780. Phone: (215) 238-4200. Fax: (215) 238-4227. Quarterly.

Nursing Management. Nursing Management, 103 N. 2nd St., West Dundee, IL 60118. Phone: (708) 426-6100. Fax: (708) 426-6416. Monthly.

Nursing Outlook. Mosby-Year Book, 11830 Westline Industrial Drive, St. Louis, MO 63146. Phone: (800) 325-4177. Fax: (314) 432-1380. Bimonthly.

Nursing Research. American Journal of Nursing Co., 555 W. 57th St., New York, NY 10019-2961. Phone: (212) 582-8820. Bimonthly.

Nursing Science Quarterly. Chestnut House Publications, P.O. Box 22492, Pittsburgh, PA 15222-0492. Quarterly.

Professional Nurse. Mosby-Year Book, 11830 Westline Industrial Drive, St. Louis, MO 63146. Phone: (800) 325-4177. Fax: (314) 432-1380. Monthly.

RN. Medical Economics, Five Paragon Dr., Montvale, NJ 07645-1742. Phone: (800) 222-3045. Fax: (201) 573-4956. Monthly.

Urologic Nursing. Mosby-Year Book, 11830 Westline Industrial Drive, St. Louis, MO 63146. Phone: (800) 325-4177. Fax: (314) 432-1380. Quarterly.

NEWSLETTERS

The American Nurse. American Nurses' Association, 2420 Pershing Rd., Kansas City, MO 64108. Phone: (816) 474-5720. 10/year.

ONLINE DATABASES

EMBASE. Elsevier Science Publishing Co., Inc., P.O. Box 882, Madison Square Station, New York, NY 10159-2101. Phone: (212) 989-5800. Fax: (212) 633-3990.

MEDLINE. National Library of Medicine, 8600 Rockville Pike, Bethesda, MD 20894. Phone: (800) 638-8480.

Nursing and Allied Health (CINAHL). CINAHL, 1509 Wilson Terrace, P.O. Box 871, Glendale, CA 91209-0871. Phone: (818) 409-8005.

Nursing93. Springhouse Publishing Co., 1111 Bethlehem Pike, Spring House, PA 19477. Phone: (800) 331-3170. Fax: (215) 646-8716. Monthly.

SciSearch. Institute for Scientific Information, 3501 Market St., Philadelphia, PA 19104. Phone: (215) 386-0100. Fax: (215) 386-6362.

RESEARCH CENTERS, INSTITUTES, CLEARINGHOUSES

Center for Nursing and Health Services Research. University of Maryland, 655 W. Lombard St., Baltimore, MD 21201. Phone: (301) 328-7848.

Center for Nursing Research. Ohio State University, 1585 Neil Ave., Columbus, OH 43210. Phone: (614) 292-5371.

Center for Nursing Research and Evaluation. University of Wisconsin-Milwaukee, P.O. Box 413, 1909 E. Hartford Ave., Milwaukee, WI 53201. Phone: (414) 963-5647.

TEXTBOOKS AND MONOGRAPHS

Clinical Pharmacology and Nursing. Charold L. Baer, Bradley R. Williams. Springhouse Publishing Co., 1111 Bethlehem Pike, Spring House, PA 19477. Phone: (800) 331-3170. Fax: (215) 646-8716. Second edition 1992.

Fundamentals of Nursing: Concepts, Process and Practice. Barbara Kozier, Glenora Erb, Rita Olivieri. Addison-Wesley Nursing, 390 Bridge Parkway, Redwood City, CA 94065. Phone: (800) 950-5544. Fourth edition 1991.

Medical-Surgical Nursing: Concepts and Clinical Practice. Wilma J. Phipps, and others. Mosby-Year Book, 11830 Westline Industrial Drive, St. Louis, MO 63146. Phone: (800) 325-4177. Fax: (314) 432-1380. 1991.

The Nursing Experience: Trends, Challenges, and Transitions. Lucie Young Kelly. McGraw-Hill Inc., 11 West 19th St., New York, NY 10011. Phone: (212) 337-5001. Fax: (212) 337-4092. Second edition 1992.

Nursing Interventions: Essential Nursing Treatments. Glonci M. Bulechek, Joanne McCloskey. W.B. Saunders Co., The Curtis Center, Independence Sqare W., Philadelphia, PA 19106-3399. Phone: (215) 238-7800. 2nd edition, 1992.

Nursing Procedures. Springhouse Publishing Co., 1111 Bethlehem Pike, Spring House, PA 19477. Phone: (800) 331-3170. Fax: (215) 646-8716. 1992.

NURSING EDUCATION

ABSTRACTING, INDEXING, AND CURRENT AWARENESS PUBLICATIONS

Cumulative Index to Nursing and Allied Health Literature. Glendale Adventist Medical Center, P.O. Box 871, Glendale, CA 91209. Phone: (818) 409-8005. Bimonthly.

Index Medicus. U.S. National Library of Medicine, 8600 Rockville Pike, Bethesda, MD 20894. Phone: (800) 638-8480. Monthly.

International Nursing Index. American Journal of Nursing Co., 555 W. 57th St., New York, NY 10019. Phone: (212) 582-8820. Quarterly.

Nursing Abstracts. Nursing Abstracts Co., Inc., P.O. Box 295, Forest Hills, NY 11375. Bimonthly.

ANNUALS AND REVIEWS

Springer Series on the Teaching of Nursing. Springer Publishing Co., Inc., 536 Broadway, 11th Floor, New York, NY 10012. Phone: (212) 431-4370. Irregular.

ASSOCIATIONS, PROFESSIONAL SOCIETIES, ADVOCACY AND SUPPORT GROUPS

American Association of Colleges of Nursing. One Dupont Circle N.W., Washington, DC 20036. Phone: (202) 463-6930.

American Nurses' Association (ANA). 2420 Pershing Rd., Kansas City, MO 64108. Phone: (816) 474-5720. Fax: (816) 471-4903.

National League for Nursing (NLN). 350 Hudson St., New York, NY 10014. Phone: (212) 989-9393.

BIBLIOGRAPHIES

AJN Multimedia Catalog 1991-1992. American Journal of Nursing Co., 555 W. 57th St., New York, NY 10019. Phone: (212) 582-8820. 1991.

CD-ROM DATABASES

Nursing and Allied Health (CINAHL) on CD-ROM. CINAHL, 1509 Wilson Terrace, P.O. Box 871, Glendale, CA 91209-0871. Phone: (818) 409-8005.

DIRECTORIES

Education for Nursing: The Diploma Way. National League for Nursing, 350 Hudson St., New York, NY 10014. Phone: (800) 669-1656. Annual.

Graduate Education in Nursing. National League for Nursing, 350 Hudson St., New York, NY 10014. Phone: (800) 669-1656. Annual.

JOURNALS

Journal of Continuing Education in Nursing. SLACK Inc., 6900 Grove Rd., Thorofare, NJ 08086-9447. Phone: (800) 257-8290. Fax: (609) 853-5991.

Journal of Nursing Education. SLACK Inc., 6900 Grove Rd., Thorofare, NJ 08086-9447. Phone: (800) 257-8290. Fax: (609) 853-5991. Monthly.

Journal of Nursing Staff Development. J.B. Lippincott Co., 227 E. Washington Square, Philadelphia, PA 19106-3780. Phone: (215) 238-4200. Fax: (215) 238-4227.

Journal of Professional Nursing. W.B. Saunders Co., The Curtis Center, Independence Sqare W., Philadelphia, PA 19106-3399. Phone: (215) 238-7800.

Nurse Education Today. Churchill Livingstone Inc., 650 Ave. of the Americas, New York, NY 10011. Phone: (212) 819-5400. Fax: (212) 302-6598.

Nurse Educator. J.B. Lippincott Co., 227 E. Washington Square, Philadelphia, PA 19106-3780. Phone: (215) 238-4200. Fax: (215) 238-4227.

The Nurse Practitioner: The American Journal of Primary Health Care. Vernon Publications, Inc., 3000 Northup Way, Suite 200, Box 96043, Bellevue, WA 98009. Phone: (206) 827-9900. Monthly.

Nursing Outlook. Mosby-Year Book, 11830 Westline Industrial Drive, St. Louis, MO 63146. Phone: (800) 325-4177. Fax: (314) 432-1380. Bimonthly.

ONLINE DATABASES

Nursing and Allied Health (CINAHL). CINAHL, 1509 Wilson Terrace, P.O. Box 871, Glendale, CA 91209-0871. Phone: (818) 409-8005.

TEXTBOOKS AND MONOGRAPHS

Curriculum Building in Nursing. Em. O. Bevis. National League for Nursing, 350 Hudson St., New York, NY 10014. Phone: (800) 669-1656. 3rd edition, 1989.

Innovative Teaching Strategies in Nursing. Barbara Fuszard. Aspen Publishers, Inc., 200 Orchard Ridge Dr., Gaithersburg, MD 20878. Phone: (800) 638-8437. 1989.

A Nuts-and-Bolts Approach to Teaching Nursing. Victoria Scholcraft. Springer Publishing Co., Inc., 536 Broadway, 11th Floor, New York, NY 10012. Phone: (212) 431-4370. 1989.

Review of Research in Nursing Education. National League for Nursing, 350 Hudson St., New York, NY 10014. Phone: (800) 669-1656.

Teaching Nursing. Sandra D'Young. Addison-Wesley Publishing Co., Rte. 128, Reading, MA 01867. Phone: (800) 447-2226. 1990.

Toward a Caring Curriculum: A New Pedagogy for Nursing. Em. O. Bevis, Jean Watson. National League for Nursing, 350 Hudson St., New York, NY 10014. Phone: (800) 669-1656. 1989.

NURSING HOMES

See also: HEALTH CARE ADMINISTRATION;
LONG TERM CARE

ABSTRACTING, INDEXING, AND CURRENT AWARENESS PUBLICATIONS

Cumulative Index to Nursing and Allied Health Literature. Glendale Adventist Medical Center, P.O. Box 871, Glendale, CA 91209. Phone: (818) 409-8005. Bimonthly.

Hospital Literature Index. American Hospital Association, 840 N. Lake Shore Dr., Chicago, IL 60611. Phone: (800) 242-2626. Fax: (312) 280-6015. Quarterly.

MEDOC: Index to U.S. Government Publications in the Medical and Health Sciences. Spencer S. Eccles Health Sciences Library, University of Utah, Bldg. 589, Salt Lake City, UT 84112. Phone: (801) 581-5268. Quarterly.

ASSOCIATIONS, PROFESSIONAL SOCIETIES, ADVOCACY AND SUPPORT GROUPS

American Association of Retired Persons. 1909 K St. N.W., Washington, DC 20049. Phone: (202) 872-4700.

American College of Health Care Administrators (ACHCA). 325 S. Patrick St., Alexandria, VA 22314. Phone: (703) 549-5822. Fax: (703) 739-7901.

American Health Care Association (AHCA). 1201 L St. N.W., Washington, DC 20005. Phone: (202) 842-4444. Fax: (202) 842-3860.

Nursing Home Advisory and Research Council. P.O. Box 18820, Cleveland Heights, OH 44118. Phone: (216) 321-0403.

CD-ROM DATABASES

HFCA --On CD-ROM. FD Inc., 600 New Hampshire Ave. NW, Suite 355, Washington, DC 20037. Phone: (800) 332-6623. Fax: (202) 337-0457. Monthly.

Nursing and Allied Health (CINAHL) on CD-ROM. CINAHL, 1509 Wilson Terrace, P.O. Box 871, Glendale, CA 91209-0871. Phone: (818) 409-8005.

DIRECTORIES

Directory of Members. American Association of Homes for the Aging, 1129 20th St. N.W., No. 400, Washington, DC 20036. Phone: (202) 296-5960.

Directory of Nursing Homes 1991-1992. Oryx Press, 4041 N. Central, Suite 700, Phoenix, AZ 85012. Phone: (800) 279-ORYX. Fax: (800) 279-4663. 1991.

Directory of U.S. Nursing Homes and Nursing Home Chains. Medical Economics, Five Paragon Dr., Montvale, NJ 07645-1742. Phone: (800) 222-3045. Fax: (201) 573-4956. Annual.

Nursing Home Chain Directory. SMG Marketing Group, 1242 N. LaSalle Dr., Chicago, IL 60610. Phone: (312) 642-3026.

ENCYCLOPEDIAS, DICTIONARIES, WORD BOOKS

Health Care Terms. Vergil N. Slee, Debora A. Slee. Tringa Press, P.O. Box 8181, St. Paul, MN 55108. Second edition 1991.

HANDBOOKS, GUIDES, MANUALS, ATLASES

Care Plan Manual for Long Term Care. Connie S. March. American Hospital Association, 840 N. Lake Shore Dr., Chicago, IL 60611. Phone: (800) 242-2626. Fax: (312) 280-6015. 1988.

Guide to the Nursing Home Industry. Health Care Investment Analysts, Inc., 300 E. Lombard St., Baltimore, MD 21202. Phone: (410) 576-9600. Fax: (410) 783-0575. 1992.

JOURNALS

Nursing Homes and Senior Citizen Care. International Publishing Group, 4959 Commerce Pkwy., Cleveland, OH 44128. Phone: (216) 464-1210. Fax: (216) 464-1835. 6/year.

ONLINE DATABASES

Health Planning and Administration. U.S. National Library of Medicine, MEDLARS Management Section, 8600 Rockville Pike, Bethesda, MD 20894. Phone: (800) 638-8480. Monthly.

Nursing and Allied Health (CINAHL). CINAHL, 1509 Wilson Terrace, P.O. Box 871, Glendale, CA 91209-0871. Phone: (818) 409-8005.

POPULAR WORKS AND PATIENT EDUCATION

Choosing a Nursing Home. Seth Goldsmith. Prentice Hall, 113 Sylvan Ave., Rt. 9W, Prentice Hall Bldg., Englewood Cliffs, NJ 07632. Phone: (201) 767-5937. 1990.

How to Choose a Nursing Home: A Guide to Quality Caring. Joanne Meshinsky. Avon Books, 1350 Ave. of the Americas, 2nd Flr., New York, NY 10019. Phone: (800) 238-0658. 1991.

Nursing Home: The Complete Guide. Brumby Forrest. Facts on File, Inc., 460 Park Ave. S., New York, NY 10016-7382. Phone: (212) 683-2244. Fax: (212) 683-3633. 1990.

Nursing Homes: The Complete Guide for Families. Mary Brumby Forrest, Christopher Forrest, Richard Forrest. Facts on File, Inc., 460 Park Ave. S., New York, NY 10016-7382. Phone: (212) 683-2244. Fax: (212) 683-3633. 1990.

RESEARCH CENTERS, INSTITUTES, CLEARINGHOUSES

Agency for Health Care Policy and Research Publications Clearinghouse. P.O. Box 8547, Silver Spring, MD 20907. Phone: (800) 358-9295.

STANDARDS AND STATISTICS SOURCES

Discharges from Nursing Homes: 1985 National Nursing Home Survey. National Center for Health Statistics, 6525 Belcrest Rd., Rm. 1064, Hyattsville, MD 20782. Phone: (301) 436-8500. PHS 90-1764 1990.

Medicare/Medicaid Nursing Home Information. U.S. Government Printing Office, Superintendent of Documents, P.O. Box 371954, Pittsburgh, PA 15250-7954. Phone: (202) 783-3238. Fax: (202) 512-2250. Annual.

Mental Illness in Nursing Homes: United States, 1985. National Center for Health Statistics, 6525 Belcrest Rd., Rm. 1064, Hyattsville, MD 20782. Phone: (301) 436-8500. PHS 91-1766 1991.

TEXTBOOKS AND MONOGRAPHS

Medical Care in the Nursing Home. Joseph G. Ouslander, Dan Osterwell, John Morley. McGraw-Hill, Inc., Health Professions Division, 1221 Avenue of the Americas, 28th Floor, New York, NY 10020. Phone: (212) 512-4228. 1991.

Medicare/Medicaid Nursing Home Information. Health Care Financing Administration, Oak Meadows Building, 6325 Security Blvd., Baltimore, MD 21207. Phone: (301) 966-6573. 1990.

NURSING INFORMATICS

See: MEDICAL AND NURSING
INFORMATICS

NURSING SCHOOLS

See: NURSING EDUCATION

NUTRITION

See also: VITAMINS AND MINERALS

ABSTRACTING, INDEXING, AND CURRENT AWARENESS PUBLICATIONS

Biological Abstracts. BIOSIS, 2100 Arch St., Philadelphia, PA 19103-1399. Phone: (800) 523-4800. Fax: (215) 587-2016.

BIOSIS/CAS Selects: Cancer & Nutrition. BIOSIS, 2100 Arch St., Philadelphia, PA 19103-1399. Phone: (215) 587-4800. Fax: (215) 587-2016. Biweekly.

BIOSIS/CAS Selects: Nutrition & Immunology. BIOSIS, 2100 Arch St., Philadelphia, PA 19103-1399. Phone: (215) 587-4800. Fax: (215) 587-2016. Biweekly.

CA Selects: Nutritional Aspects of Cancer. Chemical Abstracts Service, 2540 Olentangy River Road, P.O. Box 3012, Columbus, OH 43210-0012. Phone: (800) 848-6538. Biweekly.

CAB Abstracts. C.A.B. International, 845 N. Park Ave., Tucson, AZ 85719. Phone: (800) 528-4841.

Consumer Health and Nutrition Index. Alan Rees. Oryx Press, 4041 N. Central, Suite 700, Phoenix, AZ 85012. Phone: (800) 279-6799. Fax: (800) 279-4663. Quarterly.

Index Medicus. U.S. National Library of Medicine, 8600 Rockville Pike, Bethesda, MD 20894. Phone: (800) 638-8480. Monthly.

MEDOC: Index to U.S. Government Publications in the Medical and Health Sciences. Spencer S. Eccles Health Sciences Library, University of Utah, Bldg. 589, Salt Lake City, UT 84112. Phone: (801) 581-5268. Quarterly.

Nutrition Abstracts and Reviews. Series A: Human and Experimental. C.A.B. International, 845 N. Park Ave., Tucson, AZ 85719. Phone: (800) 528-4841. Monthly.

Research Alert: Nutrition-Human. Institute for Scientific Information, 3501 Market St., Philadelphia, PA 19104. Phone: (800) 523-1850. Fax: (215) 386-6362. Weekly.

Science Citation Index. Institute for Scientific Information, 3501 Market St., Philadelphia, PA 19104. Phone: (800) 523-1850. Fax: (215) 386-6362. Bimonthly.

ANNUALS AND REVIEWS

Advances in Food and Nutrition Research. Academic Press, Inc., 1250 Sixth Ave., San Diego, CA 92101-4311. Phone: (619) 699-6345. Fax: (619) 699-6715. Irregular.

Annual Review of Nutrition. Annual Reviews Inc., 4139 El Camino Way, P.O. Box 10139, Palo Alto, CA 94303-0897. Phone: (415) 493-4400. Fax: (415) 855-9815. Annual.

Critical Reviews in Food Science and Nutrition. CRC Press, Inc., 2000 Corporate Blvd. N.W., Boca Raton, FL 33431. Phone: (407) 994-0555. Fax: (407) 997-0949. 8/year.

Nutrition Research Reviews. Cambridge University Press, 40 W. 20th St., New York, NY 10011. Phone: (800) 431-1580. Annual.

ASSOCIATIONS, PROFESSIONAL SOCIETIES, ADVOCACY AND SUPPORT GROUPS

American College of Nutrition. 9650 Rockville Pike, Bethesda, MD 20814. Phone: (301) 530-7110.

American Dietetic Association (ADA). 216 W. Jackson Blvd., Ste. 800, Chicago, IL 60606. Phone: (312) 899-0040. Fax: (312) 899-1979.

American Institute of Nutrition (AIN). 9650 Rockville Pike, Bethesda, MD 20814. Phone: (301) 530-7050.

American Society for Clinical Nutrition (ASCN). 9650 Rockville Pike, Bethesda, MD 20814. Phone: (301) 530-7110.

American Society for Parenteral and Enteral Nutrition (ASPEN). 8630 Fenton St., No. 412, Silver Spring, MD 20910-3803. Phone: (301) 587-6315.

Nutrition Education Association. P.O. Box 20301, 3647 Glen Haven, Houston, TX 77225. Phone: (713) 665-2946.

Society for Nutrition Education (SNE). 1700 Broadway, Ste. 300, Oakland, CA 94612. Phone: (415) 444-7133.

The Vegetarian Resource Group. P.O. Box 1463, Baltimore, MD 21203.

BIBLIOGRAPHIES

Adult/Patient Nutrition Education Materials. Food and Nutrition Center, National Agricultural Library, 10301 Baltimore Blvd., Beltsville, MD 20705. Jan. 1982 to Sept. 1990.

Dietary Fiber: Content in Foods. National Technical Information Service, 5285 Port Royal Rd., Springfield, VA 22161. Phone: (703) 487-4650. Fax: (703) 321-8547. Jan. 1972-Nov. 1989.

Food and Nutrition Microcomputer Software List. Food and Nutrition Center, National Agricultural Library, 10301 Baltimore Blvd., Beltsville, MD 20705. June 1991.

Infant Nutrition. Food and Nutrition Center, National Agricultural Library, 10301 Baltimore Blvd., Beltsville, MD 20705. January 1987 to March 1991.

Literature Search on: Eating Healthy When Eating Out. National Heart, Lung, and Blood Institute Education-Programs Information Center, 4733 Bethesda Ave., Ste. 530, Bethesda, MD 20814. Phone: (301) 951-3260. Monthly.

Nutri-Topics. Food and Nutrition Center, National Agricultural Library, 10301 Baltimore Blvd., Beltsville, MD 20705.

Nutri-Topics: Adolescent Pregnancy and Nutrition. Food and Nutrition Center, National Agricultural Library, 10301 Baltimore Blvd., Beltsville, MD 20705.

Nutri-Topics: Children's Literature on Food and Nutrition. Food and Nutrition Center, National Agricultural Library, 10301 Baltimore Blvd., Beltsville, MD 20705.

Nutri-Topics: Nutrition and Cardiovascular Disease. Food and Nutrition Center, National Agricultural Library, 10301 Baltimore Blvd., Beltsville, MD 20705.

Nutri-Topics: Nutrition and Diabetes. Food and Nutrition Center, National Agricultural Library, 10301 Baltimore Blvd., Beltsville, MD 20705.

Nutri-Topics: Nutrition and the Elderly. Food and Nutrition Center, National Agricultural Library, 10301 Baltimore Blvd., Beltsville, MD 20705.

Nutri-Topics: Nutrition and the Handicapped. Food and Nutrition Center, National Agricultural Library, 10301 Baltimore Blvd., Beltsville, MD 20705.

Nutri-Topics: Nutrition for Infants and Toddlers. Food and Nutrition Center, National Agricultural Library, 10301 Baltimore Blvd., Beltsville, MD 20705.

Nutri-Topics: Sensible Nutrition. Food and Nutrition Center, National Agricultural Library, 10301 Baltimore Blvd., Beltsville, MD 20705.

Nutri-Topics: Sports Nutrition. Food and Nutrition Center, National Agricultural Library, 10301 Baltimore Blvd., Beltsville, MD 20705.

Nutri-Topics: Vegetarian Nutrition. Food and Nutrition Center, National Agricultural Library, 10301 Baltimore Blvd., Beltsville, MD 20705.

Nutri-Topics: Weight Control. Food and Nutrition Center, National Agricultural Library, 10301 Baltimore Blvd., Beltsville, MD 20705.

Nutrition and AIDS. Food and Nutrition Center, National Agricultural Library, 10301 Baltimore Blvd., Beltsville, MD 20705. May 1991.

Nutrition Education Resource Guide: An Annotated Bibliography of Educational Materials for the WIC and SCF Programs Supplement 1. Food and Nutrition Center, National Agricultural Library, 10301 Baltimore Blvd., Beltsville, MD 20705.

Quick Bibliography Series. Nutrition and the Elderly. National Agricultural Library, Public Services Division, Rm. 111, Beltsville, MD 20705. Jan. 1987-May 1990.

Sources of Free or Low-Cost Food and Nutrition Materials. Food and Nutrition Center, National Agricultural Library, 10301 Baltimore Blvd., Beltsville, MD 20705. Fall 1991.

CD-ROM DATABASES

Biological Abstracts on Compact Disc. BIOSIS, 2100 Arch St., Philadelphia, PA 19103-1399. Phone: (800) 523-4800. Fax: (215) 587-2016. Quarterly.

CABCD (CAB Abstracts on CD-ROM). C.A.B. International, 845 N. Park Ave., Tucson, AZ 85719. Phone: (800) 528-4841.

Human Nutrition on CD-ROM. C.A.B. International, 845 N. Park Ave., Tucson, AZ 85719. Phone: (800) 528-4841. Quarterly.

SCISEARCH. Institute for Scientific Information, 3501 Market St., Philadelphia, PA 19104. Phone: (215) 386-0100. Fax: (215) 386-6362.

DIRECTORIES

Directory of Dietetic Programs. American Dietetic Association, 216 W. Jackson Blvd., Ste. 800, Chicago, IL 60606. Phone: (312) 899-0040. Fax: (312) 899-1979. Annual.

Directory of Food and Nutrition Information for Professionals and Consumers. Robyn C. Frank, Holly Berry Irving. Oryx Press, 4041 N. Central, Suite 700, Phoenix, AZ 85012. Phone: (800) 279-ORYX. Fax: (800) 279-4663. 1992.

Directory of Registered Dietitians. American Dietetic Association, 216 W. Jackson Blvd., Chicago, IL 60606. Phone: (800) 621-6469.

ENCYCLOPEDIAS, DICTIONARIES, WORD BOOKS

Recommended Dietary Allowances. National Research Council. National Academy Press, 2101 Constitution Ave., N.W., Washington, DC 20418. Phone: (800) 642-6242. Tenth edition 1989.

HANDBOOKS, GUIDES, MANUALS, ATLASES

Bowes and Church's Food Values of Portions Commonly Used. Jean A.T. Pennington. J.B. Lippincott Co., 227 E. Washington Square, Philadelphia, PA 19106-3780. Phone: (215) 238-4200. Fax: (215) 238-4227. 16th edition, 1993.

Dietician's Patient Education Manual. Aspen Publishers, Inc., 200 Orchard Ridge Dr., Gaithersburg, MD 20878. Phone: (800) 638-8437. 1991.

Handbook of Clinical Nutrition. Roland Weinsier, and others (eds.). Mosby-Year Book, 11830 Westline Industrial Drive, St. Louis, MO 63146. Phone: (800) 325-4177. Fax: (314) 432-1380. 1989.

Handbook of Surgical Nutrition. Van Way. J.B. Lippincott Co., 227 E. Washington Square, Philadelphia, PA 19106-3780. Phone: (215) 238-4200. Fax: (215) 238-4227. 1992.

Manual of Nutritional Therapy. Alpers. Little, Brown and Co., 34 Beacon St., Boston, MA 02108. Phone: (617) 227-0730. Fax: (617) 227-0790. Second edition 1988.

JOURNALS

American Journal of Clinical Nutrition. Waverly Press, 428 E. Preston St., Baltimore, MD 21202. Phone: (800) 638-0672. Fax: (800) 447-8438. Monthly.

British Journal of Nutrition. Cambridge University Press, 40 W. 20th St., New York, NY 10011. Phone: (800) 431-1580. Bimonthly.

Clinical Nutrition. Churchill Livingstone Inc., 650 Avenue of the Americas, New York, NY 10011. Phone: (212) 819-5400. Fax: (212) 302-6598. 6/year.

Journal of the American College of Nutrition. John Wiley & Sons, Inc., 605 Third Ave., New York, NY 10158-0012. Phone: (212) 850-6000. Fax: (212) 850-6088. Bimonthly.

Journal of the American Dietetic Association. American Dietetic Association, 216 W. Jackson Blvd., Suite 800, Chicago, IL 60606-6995. Phone: (312) 899-0040. 12/year.

Journal of Nutrition. American Institute of Nutrition, 9650 Rockville Pike, Bethesda, MD 20814. Phone: (301) 530-7027.

Journal of Nutrition Education. Williams & Wilkins, 428 E. Preston St., Baltimore, MD 21202. Phone: (800) 638-0672. Fax: (800) 447-8438. Bimonthly.

Journal of Nutrition for the Elderly. Annette B. Natow, Jo-Ann Heslin (eds.). Haworth Press, 10 Alice Street, Binghamton, NY

13904-1580. Phone: (800) 3HA-WORTH. Fax: (607) 722-1424. Quarterly.

Nutrition Today. Williams & Wilkins, 428 E. Preston St., Baltimore, MD 21202. Phone: (800) 638-0672. Fax: (800) 447-8438. Bimonthly.

Proceedings of the Nutrition Society. Cambridge University Press, 40 W. 20th St., New York, NY 10011. Phone: (800) 431-1580. 3/year.

Vegetarian Journal. The Vegetarian Resource Group, P.O. Box 1463, Baltimore, MD 21203. Bimonthly.

NEWSLETTERS

AICR Newsletter. American Institute for Cancer Research (AICR), 1759 R St. N.W., Washington, DC 20009-2552. Phone: (202) 328-7744. Fax: (800) 843-8114. Quarterly.

Dairy Council Digest. National Dairy Council, 6300 N. River Rd., Rosemont, IL 60018. Bimonthly.

Environmental Nutrition. Environmental Nutrition, Inc., 52 Riverside Dr., New York, NY 10024. Phone: (212) 362-0424. Monthly.

Nutrition Action Healthletter. Center for Science in the Public Interest, 1501 16th St. N.W., Washington, DC 20036. Phone: (202) 332-9110. Fax: (202) 265-4954. 10/year.

Nutrition Forum. George F. Stickley Co., P.O. Box 1747, Allentown, PA 18105. Phone: (215) 437-1795. Bimonthly.

Nutrition & the M.D.. PM, Inc., P.O. Box 2468, Van Nuys, CA 91404-2160. Phone: (800) 365-2468. Monthly.

Nutrition News. National Dairy Council, 6300 N. River Rd., Rosemont, IL 60018. Phone: (312) 696-1020. Quarterly.

Tufts University Diet & Nutrition Letter. Tufts University, 203 Harrison Ave., Boston, MA 02111. Phone: (800) 274-7581. Monthly.

ONLINE DATABASES

BIOSIS Previews. BIOSIS, 2100 Arch St., Philadelphia, PA 19103-1399. Phone: (800) 523-4800. Fax: (215) 587-2016.

EMBASE. Elsevier Science Publishing Co., Inc., P.O. Box 882, Madison Square Station, New York, NY 10159-2101. Phone: (212) 989-5800. Fax: (212) 633-3990.

MEDLINE. National Library of Medicine, 8600 Rockville Pike, Bethesda, MD 20894. Phone: (800) 638-8480.

SciSearch. Institute for Scientific Information, 3501 Market St., Philadelphia, PA 19104. Phone: (215) 386-0100. Fax: (215) 386-6362.

POPULAR WORKS AND PATIENT EDUCATION

The 8-Week Cholesterol Cure: How to Lower Your Blood Cholesterol by Up to 40 Percent Without Drugs or Deprivation. Robert E. Kowalski. HarperCollins Publishers., Inc., 10 E. 53rd St., New York, NY 10022-5299. Phone: (212) 207-7000. Fax: (800) 242-7737. Revised edition 1990.

American Heart Association Cookbook. Ballantine Books, 201 E. 50th St., New York, NY 10022. Phone: (800) 733-3000.

Cholesterol & Children: A Parent's Guide to Giving Children a Future Free of Heart Disease. Robert E. Kowalski. HarperCollins Publishers, Inc., 10 E. 53rd St., New York, NY 10022-5299. Phone: (800) 242-7737. 1989.

The Duke University Medical Center Book of Diet and Fitness. Michael Hamilton. Fawcett Book Group, 201 E. 50th St., New York, NY 10022. Phone: (800) 733-3000. 1991.

Food Pharmacy Guide to Good Eating. Jean Carper. Bantam Books, Inc., 666 Fifth Ave., New York, NY 10103. Phone: (800) 223-6834. 1992.

How Many Calories? How Much Fat? Guide to Calculating the Nutritional Content of the Foods You Eat. Rosemary Baskin. Consumer Reports Books, 9180 LeSaint Dr., Fairfield, OH 45014. Phone: (513) 860-1178. 1992.

Mount Sinai School of Medicine Complete Book of Nutrition. Victor Herbert. St. Martin's Press, 175 Fifth Ave., New York, NY 10010. Phone: (212) 674-5151. 1990.

Nutrition for the Chemotherapy Patient. Janet Ramstack. Bull Publishing Co., 110 Gilbert Ave., Menlo Park, CA 94025. Phone: (800) 676-2855. 1990.

The Pregnancy Nutrition Counter. Annette B. Natow Jo-Ann Hoslin. Pocket Books, Inc., 1230 Ave. of the Americas, New York, NY 10020. Phone: (800) 223-2348. Fax: (800) 284-0735. 1992.

Prevention Magazine's Complete Nutrition Reference Handbook: Over 1,000 Foods and Meals Analyzed and Rated for Health Effect. Mark Bricklin. Rodale Press, Inc., 33 E. Minor St., Emmaus, PA 18098. Phone: (800) 527-8200. Fax: (215) 967-6263. 1992.

The Tufts University Guide to Total Nutrition. Stanley Gershoff, Catherine Whitney. HarperCollins Publishers., Inc., 10 E. 53rd St., New York, NY 10022-5299. Phone: (212) 207-7000. Fax: (800) 242-7737. 1990.

RESEARCH CENTERS, INSTITUTES, CLEARINGHOUSES

Children's Nutrition Research Center. Baylor College of Medicine, 1100 Bates St., Houston, TX 77030. Phone: (713) 799-6006.

Clinical Nutrition Research Unit. University of Alabama at Birmingham. Dept. of Nutrition Sciences, P.O. Box 501, UAB Station, Birmingham, AL 35294. Phone: (205) 934-5218.

Clinical Nutrition Research Unit. University of Chicago. 5841 S. Maryland Ave., Box 223, Chicago, IL 60637. Phone: (312) 702-6741.

Food and Nutrition Information Center (FNIC). Department of Agriculture, National Agricultural Library, Rm. 304, 10301 Baltimore Blvd., Beltsville, MD 20705. Phone: (301) 344-3719.

Human Nutrition Information Service (HNIS). Department of Agriculture, 6505 Belcrest Rd., West Hyattsville, MD 20782. Phone: (301) 436-7725.

McGill Nutrition and Food Science Centre. McGill University. Royal Victoria Hospital, 687 Pine Ave. W., Montreal, PQ, Canada H3A 1A1. Phone: (514) 842-1231. Fax: (514) 982-0893.

National Dairy Board Institute for Nutrition and Cardiovascular Research. Oregon Health Sciences University.

Division of Nephrology and Hypertension, 3181 SW Sam Jackson Park Rd., L463, Portland, OR 97201. Phone: (503) 494-8490.

USDA Children's Nutrition Research Center. Baylor College of Medicine, 1100 Bates St., Houston, TX 77030. Phone: (713) 798-7000.

USDA Grand Forks Human Nutrition Research Center. 2420 Second Ave. N, P.O. Box 7166, University Station, Grand Forks, ND 58202. Phone: (701) 795-8353. Fax: (701) 795-8395.

USDA Human Nutrition Research Center on Aging.. Tufts University, 711 Washington St., Boston, MA 02111. Phone: (617) 556-3330. Fax: (617) 556-3295.

TEXTBOOKS AND MONOGRAPHS

Basic Nutrition and Diet Therapy. Sue Rodwell Williams. Mosby-Year Book, 11830 Westline Industrial Drive, St. Louis, MO 63146. Phone: (800) 325-4177. Fax: (314) 432-1380. Ninth edition 1992.

Cancer and Nutrition. Alfin-Slater. Plenum Publishing Co., 233 Spring St., New York, NY 10013-1578. Phone: (212) 620-8000. Fax: (212) 463-0742. 1991.

Developmental Nutrition. Norman Kretchmer. CRC Press, Inc., 2000 Corporate Blvd. N.W., Boca Raton, FL 33431. Phone: (407) 994-0555. Fax: (407) 997-0949. 1992.

Diet and Health: Implications for Reducing Chronic Disease Risk. National Research Council. National Academy Press, 2101 Constitution Ave., NW, Washington, DC 20418. Phone: (800) 642-6242. 1989.

Essentials of Clinical Nutrition. Roland L. Weinsier, Sarah L. Morgan. Mosby-Year Book, 11830 Westline Industrial Drive, St. Louis, MO 63146. Phone: (800) 325-4177. Fax: (314) 432-1380. 1992.

Essentials of Nutrition and Diet Therapy. S.R. Williams. Mosby-Year Book, 11830 Westline Industrial Drive, St. Louis, MO 63146. Phone: (800) 325-4177. Fax: (314) 432-1380. Fifth edition 1990.

Geriatric Nutrition. Chernoff. Aspen Publishers, Inc., 200 Orchard Ridge Dr., Gaithersburg, MD 20878. Phone: (800) 638-8437. 1991.

Improving America's Diet and Health: From Recommendations to Action. Paul R. Thomas (ed.). National Academy Press, 2101 Constitution Ave., NW, Washington, DC 20418. Phone: (800) 642-6242. 1991.

Introductory Nutrition and Diet Therapy. Marian Maltese Eschelman. J.B. Lippincott Co., 227 E. Washington Square, Philadelphia, PA 19106-3780. Phone: (215) 238-4200. Fax: (215) 238-4227. Second edition 1991.

Nutritional Care of the Terminally Ill. Charlotte R. Gallagher-Allred. Aspen Publishers, Inc., 200 Orchard Ridge Dr., Gaithersburg, MD 20878. Phone: (800) 638-8437. 1989.

Textbook of Pediatric Nutrition. McLaren. Churchill Livingstone Inc., 650 Ave. of the Americas, New York, NY 10011. Phone: (212) 819-5400. Fax: (212) 302-6598. Third edition 1991.

NUTRITIONAL DISORDERS

See also: OBESITY; VITAMINS AND MINERALS

ABSTRACTING, INDEXING, AND CURRENT AWARENESS PUBLICATIONS

Current Contents/Clinical Medicine. Institute for Scientific Information, 3501 Market St., Philadelphia, PA 19104. Phone: (800) 523-1850. Fax: (215) 386-6362. Weekly.

Current Contents/Life Sciences. Institute for Scientific Information, 3501 Market St., Philadelphia, PA 19104. Phone: (215) 386-0100. Fax: (215) 386-6362.

Index Medicus. U.S. National Library of Medicine, 8600 Rockville Pike, Bethesda, MD 20894. Phone: (800) 638-8480. Monthly.

Science Citation Index. Institute for Scientific Information, 3501 Market St., Philadelphia, PA 19104. Phone: (800) 523-1850. Fax: (215) 386-6362. Bimonthly.

ASSOCIATIONS, PROFESSIONAL SOCIETIES, ADVOCACY AND SUPPORT GROUPS

American Society for Clinical Nutrition (ASCN). 9650 Rockville Pike, Bethesda, MD 20814. Phone: (301) 530-7110.

American Society for Parenteral and Enteral Nutrition (ASPEN). 8630 Fenton St., No. 412, Silver Spring, MD 20910-3803. Phone: (301) 587-6315.

BIBLIOGRAPHIES

Nutri-Topics: Diet and Cancer. Food and Nutrition Center, National Agricultural Library, 10301 Baltimore Blvd., Beltsville, MD 20705.

Nutri-Topics: Nutrition and Alcohol. Food and Nutrition Center, National Agricultural Library, 10301 Baltimore Blvd., Beltsville, MD 20705.

Nutri-Topics: Nutrition and Cardiovascular Disease. Food and Nutrition Center, National Agricultural Library, 10301 Baltimore Blvd., Beltsville, MD 20705.

CD-ROM DATABASES

SCISEARCH. Institute for Scientific Information, 3501 Market St., Philadelphia, PA 19104. Phone: (215) 386-0100. Fax: (215) 386-6362.

HANDBOOKS, GUIDES, MANUALS, ATLASES

A Color Atlas of Nutritional Disorders. D.S. McLaren. Mosby-Year Book, 11830 Westline Industrial Drive, St. Louis, MO 63146. Phone: (800) 325-4177. Fax: (314) 432-1380. 1988.

Color Atlas of Obesity. Roland Jung. Mosby-Year Book, 11830 Westline Industrial Drive, St. Louis, MO 63146. Phone: (800) 325-4177. Fax: (314) 432-1380. 1991.

Manual of Nutritional Therapy. Alpers. Little, Brown and Co., 34 Beacon St., Boston, MA 02108. Phone: (617) 227-0730. Fax: (617) 227-0790. Second edition 1988.

Mayo Clinic Diet Manual. Cecilia M. Pemberton. Mosby-Year Book, 11830 Westline Industrial Drive, St. Louis, MO 63146. Phone: (800) 325-4177. Fax: (314) 432-1380. 1988.

JOURNALS

Nutrition and Clinical Practice. Williams & Wilkins, 428 East Preston St., Baltimore, MD 21202. Phone: (800) 638-0672. Fax: (800) 447-8438.

Nutrition Today. Williams & Wilkins, 428 E. Preston St., Baltimore, MD 21202. Phone: (800) 638-0672. Fax: (800) 447-8438. Bimonthly.

Proceedings of the Nutrition Society. Cambridge University Press, 40 W. 20th St., New York, NY 10011. Phone: (800) 431-1580. 3/year.

NEWSLETTERS

Nutrition & the M.D.. PM, Inc., P.O. Box 2468, Van Nuys, CA 91404-2160. Phone: (800) 365-2468. Monthly.

ONLINE DATABASES

EMBASE. Elsevier Science Publishing Co., Inc., P.O. Box 882, Madison Square Station, New York, NY 10159-2101. Phone: (212) 989-5800. Fax: (212) 633-3990.

MEDLINE. National Library of Medicine, 8600 Rockville Pike, Bethesda, MD 20894. Phone: (800) 638-8480.

SciSearch. Institute for Scientific Information, 3501 Market St., Philadelphia, PA 19104. Phone: (215) 386-0100. Fax: (215) 386-6362.

POPULAR WORKS AND PATIENT EDUCATION

The IBD Nutrition Book. Jan K. Greenwood. John Wiley & Sons, Inc., 605 Third Ave., New York, NY 10158-0012. Phone: (212) 850-6000. Fax: (212) 850-6088. 1992.

RESEARCH CENTERS, INSTITUTES, CLEARINGHOUSES

Cleveland Clinic Foundation Research Institute. 9500 Euclid Ave., Cleveland, OH 44195-5210. Phone: (216) 444-3900. Fax: (216) 444-3279.

TEXTBOOKS AND MONOGRAPHS

Cardiovascular Disease: Prevention and Treatment. Penny M. Kris-Etherton (ed.). American Dietetic Association, 216 W. Jackson Blvd., Suite 800, Chicago, IL 60606-6995. Phone: (312) 899-0040. 1990.

Clinical Nutrition for the House Officer. Albert. Williams & Wilkins, 428 East Preston St., Baltimore, MD 21202. Phone: (800) 638-0672. Fax: (800) 447-8438. 1992.

Introductory Nutrition and Diet Therapy. Marian Maltese Eschelman. J.B. Lippincott Co., 227 E. Washington Square, Philadelphia, PA 19106-3780. Phone: (215) 238-4200. Fax: (215) 238-4227. Second edition 1991.

Krause's Food, Nutrition and Diet Therapy. L. Kathleen Mahan, Marian Arlen. W.B. Saunders Co., The Curtis Center, Independence Sqare W., Philadelphia, PA 19106-3399. Phone: (215) 238-7800. 8th edition, 1992.

Nutrition and Diagnosis-Related Care. Sylvia Escott Stump. Williams & Wilkins, 428 East Preston St., Baltimore, MD 21202. Phone: (800) 638-0672. Fax: (800) 447-8438. Third edition 1992.

Obesity. Bjorntarp. J.B. Lippincott Co., 227 E. Washington Square, Philadelphia, PA 19106-3780. Phone: (215) 238-4200. Fax: (215) 238-4227. 1992.

Obesity and Related Diseases. J.S. Garrow. Churchill Livingstone Inc., 650 Ave. of the Americas, New York, NY 10011. Phone: (212) 819-5400. Fax: (212) 302-6598. Second edition 1988.

Primary Hyperlipoproteinemias. George Steiner, Eleazar Shafrir. McGraw-Hill, Inc., Health Professions Division, 1221 Avenue of the Americas, 28th Floor, New York, NY 10020. Phone: (212) 512-4228. 1991.

Working Group Report on Management of Patients with Hypertension and High Blood Cholesterol. National Heart, Lung, and Blood Institute, 4733 Bethesda Ave., Ste. 530, Bethesda, MD 20814. Phone: (301) 951-3260. NIH Pub. No. 90-2361 1990.

O

OBESITY

See also: NUTRITIONAL DISORDERS;
WEIGHT CONTROL DIETS

ABSTRACTING, INDEXING, AND CURRENT AWARENESS PUBLICATIONS

Current Contents/Clinical Medicine. Institute for Scientific Information, 3501 Market St., Philadelphia, PA 19104. Phone: (800) 523-1850. Fax: (215) 386-6362. Weekly.

Index Medicus. U.S. National Library of Medicine, 8600 Rockville Pike, Bethesda, MD 20894. Phone: (800) 638-8480. Monthly.

Research Alert: Obesity & Energy Metabolism. Institute for Scientific Information, 3501 Market St., Philadelphia, PA 19104. Phone: (800) 523-1850. Fax: (215) 386-6362. Weekly.

ASSOCIATIONS, PROFESSIONAL SOCIETIES, ADVOCACY AND SUPPORT GROUPS

American Dietetic Association (ADA). 216 W. Jackson Blvd., Ste. 800, Chicago, IL 60606. Phone: (312) 899-0040. Fax: (312) 899-1979.

American Society of Bariatric Physicians. 5600 S. Quebec, Englewood, CO 80111. Phone: (303) 779-4833.

The Obesity Foundation (TOF). 5600 S. Quebec, Ste. 160-D, Englewood, CO 80111. Phone: (303) 779-4833.

Overeaters Anonymous. 1246 S. LaCienega Blvd., Rm. 203, Los Angeles, CA 90035. Phone: (213) 618-8835.

BIBLIOGRAPHIES

Childhood Obesity and Cardiovascular Disease. Food and Nutrition Center, National Agricultural Library, 10301 Baltimore Blvd., Beltsville, MD 20705. January 1985 - May 1990.

DIRECTORIES

American Society of Bariatric Physicians-Directory. American Society of Bariatric Physicians, 5600 S. Quebec, Ste. 160-D, Englewood, CO 80111. Phone: (303) 779-4833. Fax: (303) 779-4834. Annual.

HANDBOOKS, GUIDES, MANUALS, ATLASES

Color Atlas of Obesity. Roland Jung. Mosby-Year Book, 11830 Westline Industrial Drive, St. Louis, MO 63146. Phone: (800) 325-4177. Fax: (314) 432-1380. 1991.

JOURNALS

American Journal of Clinical Nutrition. Waverly Press, 428 E. Preston St., Baltimore, MD 21202. Phone: (800) 638-0672. Fax: (800) 447-8438. Monthly.

Appetite. Academic Press, Inc., 1250 Sixth Ave., San Diego, CA 92101-4311. Phone: (619) 699-6345. Fax: (619) 699-6715.

International Journal of Obesity. Macmillan Publishing Co., 866 Third Ave., New York, NY 10011. Phone: (800) 257-5755.

Journal of the American Dietetic Association. American Dietetic Association, 216 W. Jackson Blvd., Suite 800, Chicago, IL 60606-6995. Phone: (312) 899-0040. 12/year.

Journal of Clinical Endocrinology & Metabolism. Williams & Wilkins, 428 E. Preston St., Baltimore, MD 21202. Phone: (800) 638-0672. Fax: (900) 447-8438. Monthly.

Journal of Nutrition. American Institute of Nutrition, 9650 Rockville Pike, Bethesda, MD 20814. Phone: (301) 530-7027.

Metabolism: Clinical and Experimental. W.B. Saunders Co., The Curtis Center, Independence Sqare W., Philadelphia, PA 19106-3399. Phone: (215) 238-7800.

Obesity & Health: Current Research and Related Issues. Healthy Living Institute, Route 2, Box 905, Hettinger, ND 58639. Phone: (701) 567-2845. Bimonthly.

Obesity Surgery. Rapid Communications of Oxford Ltd., The Old Malthouse, Paradise St., Oxford OX1 1LD, England. Phone: 44-865-790447. Fax: 44-865-244012. 4/year.

ONLINE DATABASES

EMBASE. Elsevier Science Publishing Co., Inc., P.O. Box 882, Madison Square Station, New York, NY 10159-2101. Phone: (212) 989-5800. Fax: (212) 633-3990.

MEDLINE. National Library of Medicine, 8600 Rockville Pike, Bethesda, MD 20894. Phone: (800) 638-8480.

SciSearch. Institute for Scientific Information, 3501 Market St., Philadelphia, PA 19104. Phone: (215) 386-0100. Fax: (215) 386-6362.

POPULAR WORKS AND PATIENT EDUCATION

Fat Oppression and Psychotherapy: A Feminist Perspective. Laura S. Brown, Esther D. Rothblum (eds.). Haworth Press, 10 Alice Street, Binghamton, NY 13904-1580. Phone: (800) 3HA-WORTH. Fax: (607) 722-1424. 1990.

How Many Calories? How Much Fat? Guide to Calculating the Nutritional Content of the Foods You Eat. Rosemary Baskin.

Consumer Reports Books, 9180 LeSaint Dr., Fairfield, OH 45014. Phone: (513) 860-1178. 1992.

Keep Coming Back: The Spiritual Journey of Recovery in Overeaters Anonymous. Elisabeth L.. HarperCollins Pubs., Inc., 10 E. 53rd St., New York, NY 10022-5299. Phone: (212) 207-7000. Fax: (800) 242-7737. 1989.

Now That You've Lost It: How to Maintain Your Best Weight. Joyce D. Hash. Bull Publishing Co., 110 Gilbert Ave., Menlo Park, CA 94025. Phone: (800) 676-2855. 1992.

Overcoming Overeating. Jane R. Hirschman, Carol H. Munter. Addison-Wesley Publishing Co., Rte. 128, Reading, MA 01867. Phone: (800) 447-2226. 1988.

A Parent's Guide to Eating Disorders and Obesity. Martha M. Jablow. Bantam Doubleday Dell, 666 Fifth Ave., New York, NY 10103. Phone: (800) 223-6834. 1992.

RESEARCH CENTERS, INSTITUTES, CLEARINGHOUSES

Children's Nutrition Research Center. Baylor College of Medicine, 1100 Bates St., Houston, TX 77030. Phone: (713) 799-6006.

Department of Psychiatry, University of Pittsburgh. Western Psychiatric Institute & Clinic, 3811 O'Hara St., Pittsburgh, PA 15231. Phone: (412) 624-2448.

Division of Endocrinology, Metabolism and Nutrition. College of Medicine, University of Vermont, Burlington, VT 05405. Phone: (802) 656-2530.

Division of Gastroenterology and Nutrition. Dept. of Pediatrics, New England Medical Center Hospitals, P.O. Box 213, Boston, MA 02111. Phone: (617) 956-0132.

Obesity Research Center. St. Luke's-Roosevelt Hospital, 411 W. 114th St., Ste. 3D, New York, NY 10025. Phone: (212) 523-3570.

Obesity Research Group. Dept. of Psychiatry, University of Pennsylvania, 133 S. 36th St., Philadelphia, PA 19104. Phone: (215) 989-7314.

STANDARDS AND STATISTICS SOURCES

Gastrointestinal Surgery for Severe Obesity. Consensus Statement. NIH Consensus Development Conference. March 25-27, 1991. National Institutes of Health, Office of Medical Applications of Research, Federal Bldg., Rm. 618, Bethesda, MD 20892. 1990.

TEXTBOOKS AND MONOGRAPHS

Obesity. Bjorntarp. J.B. Lippincott Co., 227 E. Washington Square, Philadelphia, PA 19106-3780. Phone: (215) 238-4200. Fax: (215) 238-4227. 1992.

Obesity and Related Diseases. J.S. Garrow. Churchill Livingstone Inc., 650 Ave. of the Americas, New York, NY 10011. Phone: (212) 819-5400. Fax: (212) 302-6598. Second edition 1988.

Obesity: Towards a Molecular Approach (UCLA Symposia on Molecular and Cellular Biology). George A. Bray, Daniel Ricquier, Bruce M. Spiegelman (eds.). John Wiley & Sons, Inc., 605 Third Ave., New York, NY 10158-0012. Phone: (212) 850-6000. Fax: (212) 850-6088. 1990.

OBSESSIVE COMPULSIVE DISORDER

See: PSYCHIATRIC DISORDERS

OBSTETRICS AND GYNECOLOGY

See also: CHILDBIRTH; GYNECOLOGIC DISORDERS; HYSTERECTOMY; PREGNANCY; PREGNANCY COMPLICATIONS

ABSTRACTING, INDEXING, AND CURRENT AWARENESS PUBLICATIONS

ACOG Current Journal Review. Elsevier Science Publishing Co., Inc., P.O. Box 882, Madison Square Station, New York, NY 10159-2101. Phone: (212) 989-5800. Fax: (212) 633-3990. Bimonthly.

Core Journals in Obstetrics and Gynecology. Elsevier Science Publishing Co., Inc., P.O. Box 882, Madison Square Station, New York, NY 10159-2101. Phone: (212) 989-5800. Fax: (212) 633-3990. 11/year.

Current Contents/Clinical Medicine. Institute for Scientific Information, 3501 Market St., Philadelphia, PA 19104. Phone: (800) 523-1850. Fax: (215) 386-6362. Weekly.

Excerpta Medica. Section 10: Obstetrics and Gynecology. Elsevier Science Publishing Co., Inc., P.O. Box 882, Madison Square Station, New York, NY 10159-2101. Phone: (212) 989-5800. Fax: (212) 633-3990. 20/year.

Index Medicus. U.S. National Library of Medicine, 8600 Rockville Pike, Bethesda, MD 20894. Phone: (800) 638-8480. Monthly.

Key Obstetrics and Gynecology: Current Literature in Perspective. Mosby-Year Book, 11830 Westline Industrial Drive, St. Louis, MO 63146. Phone: (800) 325-4177. Fax: (314) 432-1380. Quarterly.

Science Citation Index. Institute for Scientific Information, 3501 Market St., Philadelphia, PA 19104. Phone: (800) 523-1850. Fax: (215) 386-6362. Bimonthly.

ANNUALS AND REVIEWS

Contemporary Management in Obstetrics and Gynecology. Churchill Livingstone Inc., 650 Avenue of the Americas, New York, NY 10011. Phone: (212) 819-5400. Fax: (212) 302-6598. Quarterly.

Contemporary Reviews in Obstetrics and Gynaecology. Butterworth-Heinemann, 80 Montvale Ave., Stoneham, MA 02180. Phone: (617) 438-8464. Fax: (617) 279-4851. Quarterly.

Contributions to Gynecology and Obstetrics. S. Karger Publishers, Inc., 26 West Avon Rd., P.O. Box 529, Farmington, CT 06085. Phone: (203) 675-7834. Fax: (203) 675-7302. Irregular.

Current Obstetric Medicine. Mosby-Year Book, 11830 Westline Industrial Drive, St. Louis, MO 63146. Phone: (800) 325-4177. Fax: (314) 432-1380. Biennial.

Current Obstetrics and Gynaecology. Churchill Livingstone Inc., 650 Avenue of the Americas, New York, NY 10011. Phone: (212) 819-5400. Fax: (212) 302-6598. Quarterly.

Current Opinion in Obstetrics & Gynecology. Current Science Group, 20 N. Third St., Philadelphia, PA 19106-2199. Phone: (800) 552-5866. Fax: (215) 574-2270. Bimonthly.

Current Problems in Obstetrics, Gynecology and Fertility. Mosby-Year Book, 11830 Westline Industrial Drive, St. Louis, MO 63146. Phone: (800) 325-4177. Fax: (314) 432-1380. Monthly.

Obstetrical and Gynecological Survey. Williams & Wilkins, 428 E. Preston St., Baltimore, MD 21202. Phone: (800) 638-0672. Fax: (800) 447-8438. Monthly.

Obstetrics & Gynecology: Annual Review. Alemany Press, Inc., Sylvan Ave., Rte. 9W, PHR Building, PHR Dept., Englewood Cliffs, NJ 07632. Phone: (800) 227-2375. Irregular.

Obstetrics and Gynecology Clinics. W.B. Saunders Co., The Curtis Center, Independence Square W., Philadelphia, PA 19106-3399. Phone: (215) 238-7800. Quarterly.

Obstetrics and Gynecology Review. McGraw-Hill Inc., 11 West 19th St., New York, NY 10011. Phone: (212) 337-5001. Fax: (212) 337-4092. Annual.

Recent Advances in Obstetrics and Gynecology. Churchill Livingstone, 650 Avenue of the Americas, New York, NY 10011. Phone: (212) 819-5400. Fax: (212) 302-6598. Irregular.

Year Book of Obstetrics and Gynecology. Mosby-Year Book, 11830 Westline Industrial Drive, St. Louis, MO 63146. Phone: (800) 325-4177. Fax: (314) 432-1380. Annual.

ASSOCIATIONS, PROFESSIONAL SOCIETIES, ADVOCACY AND SUPPORT GROUPS

American Association of Gynecological Laparoscopists (AAGL). 13021 E. Florence Ave., Santa Fe Springs, CA 90670. Phone: (213) 946-8774.

American Board of Obstetrics and Gynecology (ABOG). 4225 Roosevelt Way N.E., Suite 305, Seattle, WA 98105. Phone: (206) 547-4884.

American College of Nurse-Midwives (ACNM). 1522 K St. N.W., Ste. 1000, Washington, DC 20005. Phone: (202) 289-0171. Fax: (202) 289-4395.

American College of Obstetricians and Gynecologists (ACOG). 409 12th St. S.W., Washington, DC 20024-2188. Phone: (202) 638-5577.

American Gynecological and Obstetrical Society (AGOS). 601 Elmwood Ave., P.O. Box 668, Rochester, NY 14642. Phone: (716) 275-5201.

The Campaign for Women's Health. 666 11th St. N.W., Ste. 700, Washington, DC 20001. Phone: (202) 783-6686.

NAACOG: The Organization for Obstetric, Gynecologic and Neonatal Nurses. 409 12th St. S.W., Washington, DC 20024. Phone: (202) 638-0026.

CD-ROM DATABASES

Clinical Problems in Obstetrics: Critical Care Obstetrics. Catanzarite. Williams & Wilkins, 428 East Preston St.,

Baltimore, MD 21202. Phone: (800) 638-0672. Fax: (800) 447-8438. 1989.

Clinical Problems in Obstetrics: Hypertension and Preeclampsia. Catanzarite. Williams & Wilkins, 428 East Preston St., Baltimore, MD 21202. Phone: (800) 638-0672. Fax: (800) 447-8438. 1989.

Critical Care Obstetrics: Clinical Cases. Valerion A. Catanzarite. Williams & Wilkins, 428 East Preston St., Baltimore, MD 21202. Phone: (800) 638-0672. Fax: (800) 447-8438. 1989.

Critical Care Obstetrics: Obstetric Infections. Valerion A. Catanzarite. Williams & Wilkins, 428 East Preston St., Baltimore, MD 21202. Phone: (800) 638-0672. Fax: (800) 447-8438. 1989.

Excerpta Medica CD: Obstetrics & Gynecology. SilverPlatter Information, Inc., River Ridge Office Park, 100 River Ridge Rd., Norwood, MA 02062. Phone: (617) 769-2599. Fax: (617) 769-8763. Quarterly.

OBGLine. Aries Systems Corporation, One Dundee Park, Andover, MA 01810. Phone: (508) 475-7200. Fax: (508) 474-8860. Monthly or quarterly.

Obstetrics and Gynecology. CMC ReSearch, Inc., 7150 S.W. Hampton, Suite C-120, Portland, OR 97223. Phone: (800) 262-7668. Fax: (503) 639-1796. Annual.

Obstetrics and Gynecology MEDLINE. MEP, 124 Mt. Auburn St., Cambridge, MA 02138. Phone: (800) 342-1338. Fax: (617) 868-7738. Quarterly.

SCISEARCH. Institute for Scientific Information, 3501 Market St., Philadelphia, PA 19104. Phone: (215) 386-0100. Fax: (215) 386-6362.

Year Books on Disc. CMC ReSearch, Inc., 7150 S.W. Hampton, Suite C-120, Portland, OR 97223. Phone: (800) 262-7668. Fax: (503) 639-1796. Annual includes Year Books of Cardiology, Dermatology, Diagnostic Radiology, Drug Therapy, Emergency Medicine, Family Practice, Medicine, Neurology and Neurosurgery, Obstetrics and Gynecology, Oncology, Pediatrics, and Psychiatry and Applied Mental Health.

DIRECTORIES

Directory of Certified Obstetricians and Gynecologists. American Board of Medical Specialties, 1 Rotary Center, Suite 805, Evanston, IL 60201. Phone: (708) 491-9091. Biennial.

Directory of Medical Specialists. Marquis Who's Who, 3002 Glenview Rd., Wilmette, IL 60091. Phone: (800) 621-9669. Fax: (708) 441-2264. Biennial.

Directory of Physicians in the United States. American Medical Association, 515 North State St., Chicago, IL 60610. Phone: (312) 464-0183. Fax: (312) 464-5834. Biennial.

ENCYCLOPEDIAS, DICTIONARIES, WORD BOOKS

Bailliere's Midwive's Dictionary. Margaret Adams. W.B. Saunders Co., The Curtis Center, Independence Square W., Philadelphia, PA 19106-3399. Phone: (215) 238-7800. Seventh edition 1991.

Dictionary of Obstetrics & Gynecology. Walter De Gruyter, Inc., 200 Saw Mill River Rd., Hawthorne, NY 10532. Phone: (914) 747-0110. 1988.

The Illustrated Dictionary of Pregnancy & Childbirth. Carl Jones. Meadowbrook Press, 18318 Minnetonka Blvd., Deephaven, MN 55391. Phone: (800) 338-2232. 1990.

Obstetric & Gynecologic Terminology. Helen E. Littrell. Slack, Inc., 6900 Grove Rd., Thorofare, NJ 08086-9447. Phone: (800) 257-8290. 1990.

Obstetric and Gynecologic Word Book. Helen E. Littrell. Springhouse Publishing Co., 1111 Bethlehem Pike, Spring House, PA 19477. Phone: (800) 331-3170. Fax: (215) 646-8716. 1992.

Obstetric and Gynecological Words. Stedman. Williams & Wilkins, 428 East Preston St., Baltimore, MD 21202. Phone: (800) 638-0672. Fax: (800) 447-8438. 1992.

Surgery on File: Obstetrics and Gynecology. The Diagram Group. Facts on File, Inc., 460 Park Ave. S., New York, NY 10016-7382. Phone: (212) 683-2244. 1988.

HANDBOOKS, GUIDES, MANUALS, ATLASES

Acute Obstetrics: A Practical Guide. Marth C.S. Heppard, Thomas J. Garite. Mosby-Year Book, 11830 Westline Industrial Drive, St. Louis, MO 63146. Phone: (800) 325-4177. Fax: (314) 432-1380. 1991.

An Atlas of Ultrasonography in Obstetrics and Gynecology. A. Kurjak (ed.). The Parthenon Publishing Group, Inc., 120 Mill Rd., Park Ridge, NJ 07656. Phone: (201) 391-6796. 1992.

Color Atlas of Childbirth and Obstetric Techniques. F.A. Al-Azzawi. Mosby-Year Book, 11830 Westline Industrial Drive, St. Louis, MO 63146. Phone: (800) 325-4177. Fax: (314) 432-1380. 1991.

Handbook of Gynecology and Obstetrics. Brown. Appleton & Lange, 25 Van Zant St., East Norwalk, CT 06855. Phone: (800) 423-1359. Fax: (203) 854-9486. 1992.

Handbook of Obstetrics and Gynecology. Ralph C. Benson, Martin Pernoll. McGraw-Hill, Inc., Health Professions Division, 1221 Avenue of the Americas, 28th Floor, New York, NY 10020. Phone: (212) 512-4228. Ninth edition 1992.

Manual of Obstetrics: Diagnosis and Therapy. Kenneth R. Niswander, Arthur T. Evans (eds.). Little, Brown and Company, 34 Beacon St., Boston, MA 02108. Phone: (617) 227-0730. Fourth edition 1991.

Manual of Outpatient Gynecology. Carol Havens, Nancy Sullivan, Patty Tilton. Little, Brown and Company, 34 Beacon St., Boston, MA 02108. Phone: (617) 227-0730. Second edition 1991.

OB-GYN Secrets: Questions You Will Be Asked...On Rounds, In the Clinic, In the OR, On Oral Exams. Helen M. Frederickson, Louise Wilkins-Haug. Mosby-Year Book, 11830 Westline Industrial Drive, St. Louis, MO 63146. Phone: (800) 325-4177. Fax: (314) 432-1380. 1991.

The Obstetric Anesthesia Handbook. Sanjay Datta. Mosby-Year Book, 11830 Westline Industrial Drive, St. Louis, MO 63146. Phone: (800) 325-4177. Fax: (314) 432-1380. 1991.

Obstetrical and Perinatal Infections. David Charles. Mosby-Year Book, 11830 Westline Industrial Drive, St. Louis, MO 63146. Phone: (800) 325-4177. Fax: (314) 432-1380. 1992.

Obstetrics on Call: A Clinical Manual. David C. Shaver, Sharon Phelan. McGraw-Hill, Inc., 1221 Avenue of the Americas, 28th Floor, New York, NY 10020. Phone: (212) 512-4228. 1992.

Obstetrics and Gynecology On Call. Ira Horowitz, Leonard Gomella. Appleton & Lange, 25 Van Zant St., East Norwalk, CT 06855. Phone: (800) 423-1359. Fax: (203) 854-9486. 1991.

A Pocket Book of Obstetrics & Gynecology. N.O. Sjoberg, B. Astedt (eds.). The Parthenon Publishing Group, Inc., 120 Mill Rd., Park Ridge, NJ 07656. Phone: (201) 391-6796. 1989.

A Pocket Obstetrics & Gynaecology. Stanley G. Clayton, John R. Newton (eds.). Churchill Livingstone, 650 Avenue of the Americas, New York, NY 10011. Phone: (212) 819-5400. Fax: (212) 302-6598. 11th edition 1988.

Quick Reference to Ob/Gyn Procedures. Barber and others. J.B. Lippincott Co., 227 E. Washington Square, Philadelphia, PA 19106-3780. Phone: (215) 238-4200. Fax: (215) 238-4227. Third edition 1990.

Zuspan and Quilligan's Manual of Obstetrics and Gynecology. Jay D. Iams, Frederick P. Zuspan, Edward J. Quilligan. Mosby-Year Book, 11830 Westline Industrial Drive, St. Louis, MO 63146. Phone: (800) 325-4177. Fax: (314) 432-1380. Second edition 1990.

JOURNALS

American Journal of Obstetrics and Gynecology. Mosby-Year Book, 11830 Westline Industrial Drive, St. Louis, MO 63146. Phone: (800) 325-4177. Fax: (314) 432-1380. Monthly.

British Journal of Obstetrics & Gynaecology. Blackwell Publishers, Three Cambridge Center, Cambridge, MA 02142. Phone: (617) 225-0430. Fax: (617) 494-1437. Monthly.

Clinical Obstetrics and Gynecology. J.B. Lippincott Co., 227 East Washington Square, Philadelphia, PA 19106-3780. Phone: (215) 238-4200. Fax: (215) 238-4227. Quarterly.

Clinical Practice of Gynecology. Elsevier Science Publishing Co., Inc., P.O. Box 882, Madison Square Station, New York, NY 10159-2101. Phone: (212) 989-5800. Fax: (212) 633-3990.

Contemporary OB/GYN. Medical Economics, Five Paragon Dr., Montvale, NJ 07645-1742. Phone: (800) 222-3045. Fax: (201) 573-4956. Monthly.

European Journal of Obstetrics & Gynecology and Reproductive Biology. Elsevier Science Publishing Co., Inc., P.O. Box 882, Madison Square Station, New York, NY 10159-2101. Phone: (212) 989-5800. Fax: (212) 633-3990. 15/year.

Fertility and Sterility. American Fertility Society, 2140 11th Ave., Suite 200, Birmingham, AL 35205-2800. Phone: (205) 933-8494. Fax: (205) 930-9904. Monthly.

Gynecologic Oncology. Academic Press, Inc., 1250 Sixth Ave., San Diego, CA 92101-4311. Phone: (619) 699-6345. Fax: (619) 699-6715. Monthly.

International Journal of Gynecology and Obstetrics. Elsevier Science Publishing Co., Inc., P.O. Box 882, Madison Square Station, New York, NY 10159-2101. Phone: (212) 989-5800. Fax: (212) 633-3990. 12/year.

Journal of Reproduction and Fertility. Journals of Reproduction and Fertility Ltd., 22 Newmarket Rd., Cambridge CB5 8DT, England. Phone: 0223-351809. Fax: 0223-359754. Bimonthly.

Journal of Women's Health. Mary Ann Liebert, Inc., 1651 Third Ave., New York, NY 10128. Phone: (212) 289-2300. Fax: (212) 289-4697. Quarterly.

Obstetrics and Gynecology. Elsevier Science Publishing Co., Inc., P.O. Box 882, Madison Square Station, New York, NY 10159-2101. Phone: (212) 989-5800. Fax: (212) 633-3990. 15/year.

NEWSLETTERS

ACOG Newsletter. American College of Obstetricians and Gynecologists, 409 12th St. S.W., Washington, DC 20024-2188. Phone: (202) 638-5577. Monthly.

National Women's Health Network-Network News. National Women's Health Network, 1325 G St. N.W., Washington, DC 20005. Phone: (202) 347-1140. Bimonthly.

OB/GYN Clinical Alert. American Health Consultants, Department C1290, P.O. Box 740060, Atlanta, GA 30374. Phone: (800) 559-1032. Fax: (404) 352-1971. Monthly.

ONLINE DATABASES

EMBASE. Elsevier Science Publishing Co., Inc., P.O. Box 882, Madison Square Station, New York, NY 10159-2101. Phone: (212) 989-5800. Fax: (212) 633-3990.

MEDIS. Mead Data Central, P.O. Box 1830, Dayton, OH 45401. Phone: (800) 227-4908.

MEDLINE. National Library of Medicine, 8600 Rockville Pike, Bethesda, MD 20894. Phone: (800) 638-8480.

Obstetrical and Gynecological Survey. Williams & Wilkins, 428 E. Preston St., Baltimore, MD 21202. Phone: (800) 638-0672. Fax: (800) 447-8438.

SciSearch. Institute for Scientific Information, 3501 Market St., Philadelphia, PA 19104. Phone: (215) 386-0100. Fax: (215) 386-6362.

Standards for Obstetric-Gynecologic Services. American College of Obstetricians & Gynecologists, 409 12th St. S.W., Washington, DC 20024. Phone: (202) 638-5577. BRS Colleague. Sixth edition. 1985.

POPULAR WORKS AND PATIENT EDUCATION

The A-Z of Women's Health. Derek Llewellyn-Jones. Oxford University Press, Inc., 200 Madison Ave., New York, NY 10016. Phone: (800) 451-7556. Second edition 1991.

The Complete Guide to Women's Health. Bruce Shepard, Carroll Shepard. Viking Penguin, 375 Hudson St., New York, NY 10014-3657. Phone: (800) 331-4624. Second revised edition 1990.

Dr. Susan Love's Breast Book. Susan M. Love. Addison-Wesley Nursing, 390 Bridge Parkway, Redwood City, CA 94065. Phone: (800) 950-5544. 1990.

Every Woman's Medical Handbook. Marie Stoppard. Ballantine Books, Inc., 201 E. 50th St., New York, NY 10022. Phone: (800) 733-3000. 1991.

The Illustrated Book of Pregnancy and Childbirth. Margaret Martin. Facts on File, Inc., 460 Park Ave. S., New York, NY 10016-7382. Phone: (212) 683-2244. Fax: (212) 683-3633. 1991.

The New Our Bodies, Ourselves: The Updated and Expanded Edition. The Boston Women's Health Book Collective. Simon & Schuster, 1230 Ave. of the Americas, New York, NY 10020. Phone: (800) 223-2348. Fax: (800) 284-0735. 1992.

Take This Book to the Gynecologist with You: Consumer's Guide to Women's Health. Gale Malesky. Addison-Wesley Publishing Co., Rte. 128, Reading, MA 01867. Phone: (800) 447-2226. 1991.

Take This Book to the Obstetrician with You: Consumer Guide to Pregnancy and Childbirth. Karen Morales. Addison-Wesley Publishing Co., Rte. 128, Reading, MA 01867. Phone: (800) 447-2226. 1991.

Understanding Your Body: Every Woman's Guide to a Lifetime of Health. Felicia Stewart, Felicia Guest, Gary Stewart, R. Hatcher. Bantam Books, Inc., 666 Fifth Ave., New York, NY 10103. Phone: (800) 223-6834. 1987.

Women Talk about Gynecological Surgery: How to Go Through It in the Calmest, Smartest Way, from Diagnosis to Recovery. Amy Gross, Dee Ito. Crown Publishers, Inc., 201 E. 50th St., New York, NY 10022. Phone: (212) 572-2600. 1991.

RESEARCH CENTERS, INSTITUTES, CLEARINGHOUSES

ACOG Resource Center. American College of Obstetricians and Gynecologists, 600 Maryland Ave. S.W., Ste. 300 E., Washington, DC 20024-2588. Phone: (202) 863-2518.

TEXTBOOKS AND MONOGRAPHS

Appleton & Lange's Review of Obstetrics and Gynecology. Louis A. Vontver, Thomas M. Julian. Appleton & Lange, 25 Van Zant St., East Norwalk, CT 06855. Phone: (800) 423-1359. Fax: (203) 854-9486. Fourth edition 1989.

Clinical Gynecological Endocrinology and Infertility. Leon Speroff, Robert H. Glass, Nathan G. Kase. Williams & Wilkins, 428 East Preston St., Baltimore, MD 21202. Phone: (800) 638-0672. Fax: (800) 447-8438. Fourth edition 1988.

Computers in Obstetrics and Gynecology. K.J. Dalton, T. Chard (eds.). Elsevier Science Publishing Co., Inc., P.O. Box 882, Madison Square Station, New York, NY 10159-2101. Phone: (212) 989-5800. Fax: (212) 633-3990. 1990.

Current Obstetric and Gynecologic Diagnosis and Treatment. Martin L. Pernoll. Appleton & Lange, 25 Van Zant St., East Norwalk, CT 06855. Phone: (800) 423-1359. Fax: (203) 854-9486. Seventh Edition 1991.

Current Therapy in Obstetrics and Gynecology. Edward J. Quilligan, Frederick P. Zuspan. W.B. Saunders Co., The Curtis Center, Independence Square W., Philadelphia, PA 19106-3399. Phone: (215) 238-7800. Third edition 1990.

Danforth's Obstetrics and Gynecology. James R. Scott, Philip J. DiSaia, Charles B. Hammond, et. al.. J.B. Lippincott Co., 227 East Washington Square, Philadelphia, PA 19106-3780. Phone: (215) 238-4200. Fax: (215) 238-4227. Sixth edition 1990.

Douglas-Stromme's Operative Obstetrics. Frederick P. Zuspan, Edward J. Quilligan. Appleton & Lange, 25 Van Zant St., East

Norwalk, CT 06855. Phone: (800) 423-1359. Fax: (203) 854-9486. Fifth edition 1988.

Genetics in Obstetrics and Gynecology. Joe Leigh Simpson, Mitchell S. Golbus. W.B. Saunders Co., The Curtis Center, Independence Sqare W., Philadelphia, PA 19106-3399. Phone: (215) 238-7800. 2nd edition, 1992.

Green's Gynecology: Essentials of Clinical Practice. Daniel L. Clarke-Pearson, M. Yusoff Dawood. Little, Brown and Co., 34 Beacon St., Boston, MA 02108. Phone: (617) 227-0730. Fourth edition 1990.

Gynecologic Oncology. Malcolm Coppleson, John M. Monaghan, C. Paul Morrow, et. al.. Churchill Livingstone Inc., 650 Avenue of the Americas, New York, NY 10011. Phone: (212) 819-5400. Fax: (212) 302-6598. Second edition. Two volumes. 1991.

Gynecology: Principles and Practice. Zev Rosenwaks, Fred Benjamin, Martin L. Stone, et. al.. McGraw-Hill, Inc., Health Professions Division, 1221 Avenue of the Americas, 28th Floor, New York, NY 10020. Phone: (212) 512-4228. Second edition 1992.

Illustrated Textbook of Obstetrics. Chamberlain. Raven Press, 1185 Ave. of the Americas, New York, NY 10036. Phone: (212) 930-9500. Fax: (212) 869-3495. Second edition 1992.

Kistner's Gynecology: Principles and Practice. Kenneth J. Ryan, and others (eds.). Mosby-Year Book, 11830 Westline Industrial Drive, St. Louis, MO 63146. Phone: (800) 325-4177. Fax: (314) 432-1380. Fifth edition 1990.

Maternal-Fetal Medicine: Principles and Practice. Robert K. Creasy, Robert Resnik. W.B. Saunders Co., The Curtis Center, Independence Square W., Philadelphia, PA 19106-3399. Phone: (215) 238-7800. Second edition 1989.

Medical Disorders During Pregnancy. William M. Barron, Marshall D. Lindheimer (eds.). Mosby-Year Book, 11830 Westline Industrial Drive, St. Louis, MO 63146. Phone: (800) 325-4177. Fax: (314) 432-1380. 1991.

Novak's Textbook of Gynecolgy. Howard W. Wentz III, Anne Colston, Burnett, Lonnie Jones. Williams & Wilkins, 428 East Preston St., Baltimore, MD 21202. Phone: (800) 638-0672. Fax: (800) 447-8438. Eleventh edition 1988.

Obstetrics and Gynecology. Mimi C. Berman (ed.). J.B. Lippincott Co., 227 East Washington Square, Philadelphia, PA 19106-3780. Phone: (215) 238-4200. Fax: (215) 238-4227. 1991.

Obstetrics: Normal and Problem Pregnancies. Steven G. Gabbe, Jennifer R. Niebyl, Joe Leigh Simpson (eds.). Churchill Livingstone Inc., 650 Avenue of the Americas, New York, NY 10011. Phone: (212) 819-5400. Fax: (212) 302-6598. Second edition 1991.

Office Gynecology. Morton A. Stenchever. Mosby-Year Book, 11830 Westline Industrial Drive, St. Louis, MO 63146. Phone: (800) 325-4177. Fax: (314) 432-1380. 1991.

Operative Obstetrics. Leslie Iffy, Joseph Appuzio, Anthony M. Vintzileos. McGraw-Hill Inc., 11 West 19th St., New York, NY 10011. Phone: (212) 337-5001. Fax: (212) 337-4092. Second edition 1992.

Practical Guide to High-Risk Pregnancy and Delivery. Fernando Arias. Mosby-Year Book, 11830 Westline Industrial

Drive, St. Louis, MO 63146. Phone: (800) 325-4177. Fax: (314) 432-1380. Second edition 1992.

Principles and Practice of Clinical Gynecology. Nathan G. Kase, Allan B. Weingold, David M. Gershenson, et. al.. Churchill Livingstone, 650 Avenue of the Americas, New York, NY 10011. Phone: (212) 819-5400. Fax: (212) 302-6598. Second edition 1990.

Principles and Practice of Ultrasonography in Obstetrics and Gynecology. Arthur C. Fleishcer, Roberto Romero, Frank Manning, et. al.. Appleton & Lange, 25 Van Zant St., East Norwalk, CT 06855. Phone: (800) 423-1359. Fax: (203) 854-9486. Fourth edition 1990.

Scientific Foundations of Obstetrics and Gynecology. Elliot E. Philipp, Marcus E. Setchell. Butterworth-Heinemann, 80 Montvale Ave., Stoneham, MA 02180. Phone: (617) 438-8464. Fax: (617) 279-4851. Fourth edition 1991.

The Unborn Patient: Prenatal Diagnosis and Treatment. Michael R. Harrison, Mitchell S. Golbus, Roy A. Filly. W.B. Saunders Co., The Curtis Center, Independence Square W., Philadelphia, PA 19106-3399. Phone: (215) 238-7800. Second edition 1991.

Williams Obstetrics. F. Gary Cunningham, Paul C. MacDonald, Norman F. Gant, et. al.. Appleton & Lange, 25 Van Zant St., East Norwalk, CT 06855. Phone: (800) 423-1359. Fax: (203) 854-9486. 18th edition 1989.

OCCUPATIONAL HEALTH AND SAFETY

See also: INDUSTRIAL TOXICOLOGY; TOXICOLOGY

ABSTRACTING, INDEXING, AND CURRENT AWARENESS PUBLICATIONS

BIOSIS/CAS Selects: Occupational Exposure. BIOSIS, 2100 Arch St., Philadelphia, PA 19103-1399. Phone: (215) 587-4800. Fax: (215) 587-2016. Biweekly.

CA Selects: Chemical Hazards, Health, & Safety. Chemical Abstracts Service, 2540 Olentangy River Road, P.O. Box 3012, Columbus, OH 43210-0012. Phone: (800) 848-6538. Biweekly.

CA Selects: Occupational Exposure & Hazards. Chemical Abstracts Service, 2540 Olentangy River Road, P.O. Box 3012, Columbus, OH 43210-0012. Phone: (800) 848-6538. Biweekly.

Chemical Abstracts. Chemical Abstracts Service, 2540 Olentangy River Rd., P.O. Box 3012, Columbus, OH 43210-0012. Phone: (800) 848-6538.

Excerpta Medica. Section 35: Occupational Health and Industrial Medicine. Elsevier Science Publishing Co., Inc., P.O. Box 882, Madison Square Station, New York, NY 10159-2101. Phone: (212) 989-5800. Fax: (212) 633-3990. 16/year.

Health and Science Safety Abstracts. Cambridge Scientific Abstracts, 7200 Wisconsin Ave., Bethesda, MD 20814-4823. Phone: (800) 843-7751. Fax: (301) 961-6720. 10/year.

Index Medicus. U.S. National Library of Medicine, 8600 Rockville Pike, Bethesda, MD 20894. Phone: (800) 638-8480. Monthly.

MEDOC: Index to U.S. Government Publications in the Medical and Health Sciences. Spencer S. Eccles Health Sciences Library, University of Utah, Bldg. 589, Salt Lake City, UT 84112. Phone: (801) 581-5268. Quarterly.

Research Alert: Industrial & Occupational Medicine. Institute for Scientific Information, 3501 Market St., Philadelphia, PA 19104. Phone: (800) 523-1850. Fax: (215) 386-6362. Weekly.

Safety and Health at Work. International Occupational Safety and Health Information Centre, International Labour Office, CH-1211, Geneva 22, Switzerland. 6/year.

Science Citation Index. Institute for Scientific Information, 3501 Market St., Philadelphia, PA 19104. Phone: (800) 523-1850. Fax: (215) 386-6362. Bimonthly.

Selected Abstracts on Occupational Diseases. Great Britain Dept. of Health and Social Security, Alexander Fleming House, Elephant and Castle, London SE1 6BY, England. Quarterly.

ANNUALS AND REVIEWS

Annual Review of Public Health. Annual Reviews Inc., 4139 El Camino Way, P.O. Box 10139, Palo Alto, CA 94303-0897. Phone: (415) 493-4400. Fax: (415) 855-9815. Annual.

Physical Medicine and Rehabilitation Clinics of North America. W.B. Saunders Co., The Curtis Center, Independence Square W., Philadelphia, PA 19106-3399. Phone: (215) 238-7800. Quarterly.

Year Book of Occupational and Environmental Medicine. Mosby-Year Book, 11830 Westline Industrial Drive, St. Louis, MO 63146. Phone: (800) 325-4177. Fax: (314) 432-1380. Annual.

ASSOCIATIONS, PROFESSIONAL SOCIETIES, ADVOCACY AND SUPPORT GROUPS

American Academy of Occupational Medicine. 55 W. Seegers Rd., Arlington Heights, IL 60005. Phone: (312) 228-6850.

American College of Occupational Medicine (ACOM). 55 W. Seegers Rd., Arlington Heights, IL 60005. Phone: (708) 228-6850. Fax: (708) 228-1856.

American Occupational Medical Association. 55 W. Seegers Rd., Arlington Heights, IL 60005. Phone: (312) 228-6850.

Society for Occupational and Environmental Health. 2021 K St. N.W., Suite 305, Washington, DC 20006.

BIBLIOGRAPHIES

Lead Exposure: Public and Occupational Health Hazards. National Technical Information Service, 5285 Port Royal Rd., Springfield, VA 22161. Phone: (703) 487-4650. Fax: (703) 321-8547. Jan. 1978 to Apr. 1989. PB89-860928/CBY.

Occupational Health: Stress. National Technical Information Service, 5285 Port Royal Rd., Springfield, VA 22161. Phone: (703) 487-4650. Fax: (703) 321-8547. Jan. 1985-May 1989 PB89-862304/CBY.

CD-ROM DATABASES

CCINFOdisc. Canadian Centre for Occupational Health and Safety (CCOHS), 250 Main St. E., Hamilton, ON, Canada L8N 1H6. Phone: (416) 572-2981. Fax: (416) 572-2206.

MSDS Reference File. Occupational Health Services, Inc., 450 7th Ave., Suite 2407, New York, NY 10123. Phone: (212) 967-1100. Quarterly.

OSH-ROM. SilverPlatter Information, Inc., River Ridge Office Park, 100 River Ridge Rd., Norwood, MA 02062. Phone: (617) 769-2599. Fax: (617) 769-8763. Quarterly.

PolTox. Cambridge Scientific Abstracts, 7200 Wisconsin Ave., Bethesda, MD 20814-4823. Phone: (800) 843-7751. Fax: (301) 961-6720. Quarterly.

SCISEARCH. Institute for Scientific Information, 3501 Market St., Philadelphia, PA 19104. Phone: (215) 386-0100. Fax: (215) 386-6362.

TOXLINE. SilverPlatter Information, Inc., River Ridge Office Park, 100 River Ridge Rd., Norwood, MA 02062. Phone: (617) 769-2599. Fax: (617) 769-8763. Quarterly.

TOXLINE Plus. SilverPlatter Information, Inc., River Ridge Office Park, 100 River Ridge Rd., Norwood, MA 02062. Phone: (617) 769-2599. Fax: (617) 769-8763. Quarterly.

DIRECTORIES

American College of Occupational Medicine-Membership Directory. American College of Occupational Medicine, 55 W. Seegers Rd., Arlington Heights, IL 60005. Phone: (708) 228-6850. Annual.

Directory of Medical Specialists. Marquis Who's Who, 3002 Glenview Rd., Wilmette, IL 60091. Phone: (800) 621-9669. Fax: (708) 441-2264. Biennial.

Directory of Physicians in the United States. American Medical Association, 515 North State St., Chicago, IL 60610. Phone: (312) 464-0183. Fax: (312) 464-5834. Biennial.

ENCYCLOPEDIAS, DICTIONARIES, WORD BOOKS

Lead: Occupational Health Hazards. National Technical Information Service, 5285 Port Royal Rd., Springfield, VA 22161. Phone: (703) 487-4650. Fax: (703) 321-8547. Jan. 1970 to Apr. 1989. PB89-860191/CBY.

HANDBOOKS, GUIDES, MANUALS, ATLASES

Handbook of Occupational Medicine. McCunney. Little, Brown and Co., 34 Beacon St., Boston, MA 02108. Phone: (617) 227-0730. Fax: (617) 227-0790. 1988.

Preventing Occupational Disease and Injury. James L. Weeks, Barry S. Levy, Gregory R. Wagner (eds.). American Public Health Association, 1015 15th St. N.W., Washington, DC 20005. Phone: (202) 789-5600. Fax: (202) 789-5661. 1991.

JOURNALS

AAOHN Journal. SLACK Inc., 6900 Grove Rd., Thorofare, NJ 08086-9447. Phone: (800) 257-8290. Fax: (609) 853-5991. Monthly American Association of Occupational Health Nurses.

American Journal of Industrial Medicine. John Wiley & Sons, Inc., 605 Third Ave., New York, NY 10158-0012. Phone: (212) 850-6000. Fax: (212) 850-6088. Monthly.

American Journal of Infection Control. Mosby-Year Book, 11830 Westline Industrial Drive, St. Louis, MO 63146. Phone: (800) 325-4177. Fax: (314) 432-1380. Bimonthly.

British Journal of Industrial Medicine. BMJ Publishing Group, BMA House, Tavistock Square, London WC1H 9JR, England. Phone: 071-383-6244. Fax: 071-383-6662.

Journal of Occupational Medicine. Williams & Wilkins, 428 E. Preston St., Baltimore, MD 21202. Phone: (800) 638-0672. Fax: (900) 447-8438. Monthly.

Journal of Occupational Rehabilitation. Plenum Publishing Co., 233 Spring St., New York, NY 10013-1578. Phone: (212) 620-8000. Fax: (212) 463-0742. Quarterly.

Occupational Medicine. Butterworth-Heinemann, 80 Montvale Ave., Stoneham, MA 02180. Phone: (617) 438-8464. Fax: (617) 279-4851. Quarterly.

NEWSLETTERS

Occupational Health Management. American Health Consultants, P.O. Box 740060, Atlanta, GA 30374. Phone: (800) 688-2421. Fax: (404) 352-1971. Monthly.

Occupational Health and Safety Letter. Business Publishers Inc., 951 Pershing Dr., Silver Spring, MD 20910. Phone: (301) 587-6300.

Occupational Safety and Health Reporter. The Bureau of National Affairs Inc., 1231 25th St. N.W., Washington, DC 20037. Phone: (800) 452-7773.

ONLINE DATABASES

CA File (Chemical Abstracts File). Chemical Abstracts Service, 2540 Olentangy River Rd., P.O. Box 3012, Columbus, OH 43210-0012. Phone: (800) 848-6538.

Hazardline. Occupational Health Services Inc., 450 7th Ave., No. 2407, New York, NY 10123. Phone: (212) 967-1100.

TOXLINE. U.S. National Library of Medicine, Toxicology Information Program, 8600 Rockville Pike, Bethesda, MD 20894. Phone: (800) 638-8480. Monthly.

RESEARCH CENTERS, INSTITUTES, CLEARINGHOUSES

Canadian Centre for Occupational Health and Safety. 250 Main St. E., Hamilton, ON, Canada L8N 1H6. Phone: (416) 572-2981. Fax: (416) 572-2206.

Division of Occupational and Environmental Medicine. University of California, Davis, Davis, CA 95616. Phone: (916) 752-4256.

Institute of Occupational Health and Safety. West Virginia University. WVU School of Medicine, Morgantown, WV 26506. Phone: (304) 293-3693.

Milbank Memorial Fund. One E. 75th St., New York, NY 10021. Phone: (212) 570-4805.

Occupational Health and Safety Institute. Dept. of Industrial Engineering, Texas A & M University, College Station, TX 77843. Phone: (409) 845-5531.

Technical Information Branch. Clearinghouse for Occupational Safety and Health Information. 4676 Columbia Pkwy., Cincinnati, OH 45226. Phone: (800) 35N-IOSH.

TEXTBOOKS AND MONOGRAPHS

Cancer Prevention Strategies in the Workplace. Charles E. Becker, Molly Joel Coye (eds.). Taylor & Francis Inc., 1900 Frost Rd., Suite 101, Bristol, PA 19007-1598. Phone: (800) 821-8312. Fax: (215) 785-5515. 1986.

Concerning the Carers: Occupational Health for Health Care Workers. J.A. Lunn, H.A. Waldron. Butterworth-Heinemann, 80 Montvale Ave., Stoneham, MA 02180. Phone: (617) 438-8464. Fax: (617) 279-4851. 1991.

Environmental and Occupational Medicine. William N. Rom (ed.). Little, Brown and Company, 34 Beacon St., Boston, MA 02108. Phone: (617) 227-0730. Second edition 1992.

Occupational Health Practice. H.A. Waldron. Butterworth-Heinemann, 80 Montvale Ave., Stoneham, MA 02180. Phone: (617) 438-8464. Fax: (617) 279-4851. Third edition 1989.

Occupational Health Services: A Guide to Program Planning and Management. William L. Newkirk, Lynn D. Jones (eds.). American Hospital Association, 840 N. Lake Shore Dr., Chicago, IL 60611. Phone: (800) 242-2626. Fax: (312) 280-6015. 1989.

Occupational Low Back Pain. Pope. Mosby-Year Book, 11830 Westline Industrial Drive, St. Louis, MO 63146. Phone: (800) 325-4177. Fax: (314) 432-1380. 1991.

Occupational Medicine. Zenz. Mosby-Year Book, 11830 Westline Industrial Drive, St. Louis, MO 63146. Phone: (800) 325-4177. Fax: (314) 432-1380. Second edition 1988.

OCCUPATIONAL THERAPY

See also: ALLIED HEALTH EDUCATION; REHABILITATION

ABSTRACTING, INDEXING, AND CURRENT AWARENESS PUBLICATIONS

Cumulative Index to Nursing and Allied Health Literature. Glendale Adventist Medical Center, P.O. Box 871, Glendale, CA 91209. Phone: (818) 409-8005. Bimonthly.

Excerpta Medica. Section 19: Rehabilitation and Physical Medicine. Elsevier Science Publishing Co., Inc., P.O. Box 882, Madison Square Station, New York, NY 10159-2101. Phone: (212) 989-5800. Fax: (212) 633-3990. 8/year.

Index Medicus. U.S. National Library of Medicine, 8600 Rockville Pike, Bethesda, MD 20894. Phone: (800) 638-8480. Monthly.

International Nursing Index. American Journal of Nursing Co., 555 W. 57th St., New York, NY 10019. Phone: (212) 582-8820. Quarterly.

Occupational Therapy Index. Medical Information Service, British Library, Boston Spa, Wetherby, W. Yorkshire LS23 7BQ, England. Phone: 0937-546039. Fax: 0937-546236. Monthly.

ASSOCIATIONS, PROFESSIONAL SOCIETIES, ADVOCACY AND SUPPORT GROUPS

American Occupational Therapy Association (AOTA). 1383 Piccard Dr., Ste. 301, Rockville, MD 20850-4375. Phone: (301) 948-9626. Fax: (301) 948-5512.

American Occupational Therapy Certification Board (AOTCB). 1383 Piccard Dr., Ste. 105, Rockville, MD 20850. Phone: (301) 990-7979.

CD-ROM DATABASES

Nursing and Allied Health (CINAHL) on CD-ROM. CINAHL, 1509 Wilson Terrace, P.O. Box 871, Glendale, CA 91209-0871. Phone: (818) 409-8005.

DIRECTORIES

Occupational Therapists Register. Occupational Therapists Board, 184 Kennington Park Rd., London SE11, England.

Occupational Therapy Education Programs. American Occupational Therapy Association, 1383 Picard Dr., P.O. Box 1725, Rockville, MD 20850. Phone: (301) 948-9626.

ENCYCLOPEDIAS, DICTIONARIES, WORD BOOKS

Mosby's Medical, Nursing, and Allied Health Dictionary. Kenneth N. Anderson, Lois Anderson, Walter D. Glanze (eds.). Mosby-Year Book, 11830 Westline Industrial Dr., St. Louis, MO 63146. Phone: (800) 325-4177. Fax: (314) 432-1380. Third edition 1990.

HANDBOOKS, GUIDES, MANUALS, ATLASES

Preventing Occupational Disease and Injury. James I. Weeks, Barry S. Levy, Gregory R. Wagner (eds.). American Public Health Association, 1015 15th St. N.W., Washington, DC 20005. Phone: (202) 789-5600. Fax: (202) 789-5661. 1991.

JOURNALS

American Journal of Occupational Therapy. American Occupational Therapy Association, 1383 Piccard Dr., P.O. Box 1725, Rockville, MD 20849-1725. Phone: (301) 948-9626. Fax: (301) 948-5512. Monthly.

Assistive Technology. Resna Press, 1101 Connecticut Ave. NW, Suite 700, Washington, DC 20036. Phone: (202) 857-1199. Quarterly.

British Journal of Occupational Therapy. College of Occupational Therapists Ltd., 20 Rede Place, Bayswater, London W2 4TU, England. Monthly.

International Journal of Rehabilitation Research. Heidelberger Verlagsantalt in Druckerei GmbH, Edition Schindele, Hans-Bunte-Str. 18, D-6900 Heidelberg, Germany.

Journal of Occupational Rehabilitation. Plenum Publishing Co., 233 Spring St., New York, NY 10013-1578. Phone: (212) 620-8000. Fax: (212) 463-0742. Quarterly.

Journal of Vocational Rehabilitation. Butterworth-Heinemann, 80 Montvale Ave., Stoneham, MA 02180. Phone: (617) 438-8464. Fax: (617) 279-4851. Quarterly.

The Occupational Therapy Journal of Research. SLACK Inc., 6900 Grove Rd., Thorofare, NJ 08086-9447. Phone: (800) 257-8290. Fax: (609) 853-5991. Monthly.

Physical Therapy. American Physical Therapy Association, 1111 N. Fairfax St., Alexandria, VA 22314-1488. Phone: (703) 684-2782. Fax: (703) 684-7343. Monthly.

ONLINE DATABASES

ABLEDATA. Newington Children's Hospital, Adaptive Equipment Center, 181 E. Cedar St., Newington, CT 06111. Phone: (800) 344-5405. Monthly.

EMBASE. Elsevier Science Publishing Co., Inc., P.O. Box 882, Madison Square Station, New York, NY 10159-2101. Phone: (212) 989-5800. Fax: (212) 633-3990.

MEDLINE. National Library of Medicine, 8600 Rockville Pike, Bethesda, MD 20894. Phone: (800) 638-8480.

Nursing and Allied Health (CINAHL). CINAHL, 1509 Wilson Terrace, P.O. Box 871, Glendale, CA 91209-0871. Phone: (818) 409-8005.

SciSearch. Institute for Scientific Information, 3501 Market St., Philadelphia, PA 19104. Phone: (215) 386-0100. Fax: (215) 386-6362.

TEXTBOOKS AND MONOGRAPHS

Clinical Decision Making in Occupational Therapy. Nancy N. Kari, Jean A. Kalscheur. SLACK Inc., 6900 Grove Rd., Thorofare, NJ 08086-9447. Phone: (800) 257-8290. Fax: (609) 853-5991. 1992.

Concepts of Occupational Therapy. Kathlyn L. Reed, Sharon Nelson Sanderson. Williams & Wilkins, 428 East Preston St., Baltimore, MD 21202. Phone: (800) 638-0672. Fax: (800) 447-8438. Third edition 1992.

Conceptual Models of Occupational Therapy. Gary Kielhofner. F.A. Davis Co., 1915 Arch St., Philadelphia, PA 19103. Phone: (800) 523-4049. Fax: (215) 568-5065. 1992.

Occupational Therapy and Activities Health: Toward Health Through Activities. Simme Cynkin, Anne Mazur Robinson. Little, Brown and Company, 34 Beacon St., Boston, MA 02108. Phone: (617) 227-0730. 1989.

Occupational Therapy Consultation: Theory, Principles, and Practice. Evelyn Jaffe, Cynthia Fuchs Epstein. Mosby-Year Book, 11830 Westline Industrial Drive, St. Louis, MO 63146. Phone: (800) 325-4177. Fax: (314) 432-1380. 1992.

Occupational Therapy: Overcoming Human Performance Deficits. Charles Christiansen (ed.). SLACK Inc., 6900 Grove Rd., Thorofare, NJ 08086-9447. Phone: (800) 257-8290. Fax: (609) 853-5991. 1991.

Occupational Therapy for Physical Dysfunction. Catherine Anne Trombly (ed.). Williams & Wilkins, 428 East Preston St., Baltimore, MD 21202. Phone: (800) 638-0672. Fax: (800) 447-8438. Third edition 1989.

Occupational Therapy: Practice Skills for Physical Dysfunction. Lorraine Williams Pedretti, Barbara Zoltan. Mosby-Year Book, 11830 Westline Industrial Drive, St. Louis, MO 63146. Phone: (800) 325-4177. Fax: (314) 432-1380. Third edition 1990.

Occupational Therapy: Principles and Practice. Alice Punwar. Williams & Wilkins, 428 East Preston St., Baltimore, MD 21202. Phone: (800) 638-0672. Fax: (800) 447-8438. 1988.

Occupational Therapy: Work Related Programs and Assessments. Karen Jacobs. Little, Brown and Company, 34 Beacon St., Boston, MA 02108. Phone: (617) 227-0730. Second edition 1991.

Willard and Spackman's Occupational Therapy. Helen L. Hopkins, Helen P. Smith. J.B. Lippincott Co., 227 E. Washington Square, Philadelphia, PA 19106-3780. Phone: (215) 238-4200. Fax: (215) 238-4227. 1993.

ONCOLOGY

See also: CANCER

ABSTRACTING, INDEXING, AND CURRENT AWARENESS PUBLICATIONS

Current Contents/Clinical Medicine. Institute for Scientific Information, 3501 Market St., Philadelphia, PA 19104. Phone: (800) 523-1850. Fax: (215) 386-6362. Weekly.

Current Contents/Life Sciences. Institute for Scientific Information, 3501 Market St., Philadelphia, PA 19104. Phone: (215) 386-0100. Fax: (215) 386-6362.

Excerpta Medica. Section 16: Cancer. Elsevier Science Publishing Co., Inc., P.O. Box 882, Madison Square Station, New York, NY 10159-2101. Phone: (212) 989-5800. Fax: (212) 633-3990. 32/year.

ICRDB Cancergram: CNS Malignancies--Diagnosis, Treatment. U.S. Government Printing Office, Superintendent of Documents, P.O. Box 371954, Pittsburgh, PA 15250-7954. Phone: (202) 783-3238. Fax: (202) 512-2250. Monthly.

ICRDB Cancergram: Endocrine Tumors--Diagnosis, Treatment, Pathophysiology. U.S. Government Printing Office, Superintendent of Documents, P.O. Box 371954, Pittsburgh, PA 15250-7954. Phone: (202) 783-3238. Fax: (202) 512-2250. Monthly.

ICRDB Cancergram: Lymphomas--Diagnosis, Treatment. U.S. Government Printing Office, Superintendent of Documents, P.O. Box 371954, Pittsburgh, PA 15250-7954. Phone: (202) 783-3238. Fax: (202) 512-2250. Monthly.

ICRDB Cancergram: Pediatric Oncology. U.S. Government Printing Office, Superintendent of Documents, P.O. Box 371954, Pittsburgh, PA 15250-7954. Phone: (202) 783-3238. Fax: (202) 512-2250. Monthly.

ICRDB Cancergram: Rehabilitation and Supportive Care. U.S. Government Printing Office, Superintendent of Documents, P.O. Box 371954, Pittsburgh, PA 15250-7954. Phone: (202) 783-3238. Fax: (202) 512-2250. Monthly.

ICRDB Cancergram: Upper Gastrointestinal Tumors-- Diagnosis, Treatment. U.S. Government Printing Office, Superintendent of Documents, P.O. Box 371954, Pittsburgh, PA 15250-7954. Phone: (202) 783-3238. Fax: (202) 512-2250. Monthly.

Index Medicus. U.S. National Library of Medicine, 8600 Rockville Pike, Bethesda, MD 20894. Phone: (800) 638-8480. Monthly.

ONS Nursing Scan in Oncology. NURSECOM, Inc., 1211 Locust St., Philadelphia, PA 19107. Phone: (215) 545-7222. Bimonthly.

Research Alert: Cancer Immunology & Immunotherapy. Institute for Scientific Information, 3501 Market St., Philadelphia, PA 19104. Phone: (800) 523-1850. Fax: (215) 386-6362. Weekly.

Research Alert: Oncogenes & Viral Carcinogenesis. Institute for Scientific Information, 3501 Market St., Philadelphia, PA 19104. Phone: (800) 523-1850. Fax: (215) 386-6362. Weekly.

Science Citation Index. Institute for Scientific Information, 3501 Market St., Philadelphia, PA 19104. Phone: (800) 523-1850. Fax: (215) 386-6362. Bimonthly.

ANNUALS AND REVIEWS

Advances in Cancer Research. Academic Press, Inc., 1250 Sixth Ave., San Diego, CA 92101-4311. Phone: (619) 699-6345. Fax: (619) 699-6715. Irregular.

Cambridge Medical Reviews: Haematological Oncology. A.C. Newland, Alan Burnett, Armand Keating, Ja Armitage. Cambridge University Press, 40 W. 20th St., New York, NY 10011. Phone: (800) 431-1580. Volume 1 1992.

Contemporary Hematology/Oncology. Plenum Publishing Co., 233 Spring St., New York, NY 10013-1578. Phone: (212) 620-8000. Fax: (212) 463-0742. Irregular.

Critical Reviews in Oncogenesis. CRC Press, Inc., 2000 Corporate Blvd. N.W., Boca Raton, FL 33431. Phone: (407) 994-0555. Fax: (407) 997-0949. 6/year.

Critical Reviews in Oncology/Hematology. Elsevier Science Publishing Co., Inc., P.O. Box 882, Madison Square Station, New York, NY 10159-2101. Phone: (212) 989-5800. Fax: (212) 633-3990. Quarterly.

Current Opinion in Oncology. Current Science Ltd., 20 N. Third St., Philadelphia, PA 19106-2199. Phone: (800) 552-5866. Fax: (215) 574-2270. Bimonthly.

Developments in Oncology. Kluwer Academic Publishers, P.O. Box 358, Accord Station, Hingham, MA 02018-0358. Phone: (617) 871-6600. Fax: (617) 871-6528. Irregular.

Frontiers of Radiation Therapy and Oncology. S. Karger Publishers, Inc., 26 West Avon Rd., P.O. Box 529, Farmington, CT 06085. Phone: (203) 675-7834. Fax: (203) 675-7302. Irregular.

Hematology/Oncology Clinics. W.B. Saunders Co., The Curtis Center, Independence Square W., Philadelphia, PA 19106-3399. Phone: (215) 238-7800. Bimonthly.

Important Advances in Oncology. Vincent T. Devita, Samuel Hellman, Steven A. Rosenberg, et. al.. J.B. Lippincott Co., 227 East Washington Square, Philadelphia, PA 19106-3780. Phone: (215) 238-4200. Fax: (215) 238-4227. Annual.

In Development New Medicines for Older Americans. 1991 Annual Survey. More Medicines in Testing for Cancer Than for Any Other Disease of Aging. Pharmaceutical Manufacturers Association, 1100 15th St. N.W., Washington, DC 20005. Phone: (202) 835-3400. 1991.

Seminars in Oncology. W.B. Saunders Co., The Curtis Center, Independence Square W., Philadelphia, PA 19106-3399. Phone: (215) 238-7800. Bimonthly.

Surgical Oncology Clinics of North America. W.B. Saunders Co., The Curtis Center, Independence Square W., Philadelphia, PA 19106-3399. Phone: (215) 238-7800. Quarterly.

Year Book of Oncology. Mosby-Year Book, 11830 Westline Industrial Drive, St. Louis, MO 63146. Phone: (800) 325-4177. Fax: (314) 432-1380. Annual.

ASSOCIATIONS, PROFESSIONAL SOCIETIES, ADVOCACY AND SUPPORT GROUPS

American Cancer Society (ACS). 1599 Clifton Rd. N.E., Atlanta, GA 30329. Phone: (404) 320-3333.

American Society of Clinical Oncology. 435 N. Michigan Ave., No. 1717, Chicago, IL 60611. Phone: (312) 644-0828.

Society of Surgical Oncology. 13 Elm St., P.O. Box 1565, Manchester by the Sea, MD 01944. Phone: (508) 526-8330.

BIBLIOGRAPHIES

Oncology Overview: Application of Monoclonal Antibodies in Clinical Oncology. David Berd (ed.). U.S. Government Printing Office, Superintendent of Documents, P.O. Box 371954, Pittsburgh, PA 15250-7954. Phone: (202) 783-3238. Fax: (202) 512-2250. 1990.

CD-ROM DATABASES

Cancer-CD. SilverPlatter Information, Inc., River Ridge Office Park, 100 River Ridge Rd., Norwood, MA 02062. Phone: (617) 769-2599. Fax: (617) 769-8763. Quarterly.

Cancer on Disc. CMC ReSearch, Inc., 7150 S.W. Hampton, Suite C-120, Portland, OR 97223. Phone: (800) 262-7668. Fax: (503) 639-1796. Annual.

Cancerlit. Aries Systems Corporation, One Dundee Park, Andover, MA 01810. Phone: (508) 475-7200. Fax: (508) 474-8860. Quarterly.

Cancerlit CD-ROM. Cambridge Scientific Abstracts, 7200 Wisconsin Ave., Bethesda, MD 20814-4823. Phone: (800) 843-7751. Fax: (301) 961-6720. Quarterly.

CD Plus/CancerLit. CD Plus, 333 7th Ave., 6th Floor, New York, NY 10001. Phone: (212) 563-3006. Monthly.

Morbidity Mortality Weekly Report. MEP, 124 Mt. Auburn St., Cambridge, MA 02138. Phone: (800) 342-1338. Fax: (617) 868-7738. Annual.

OncoDisc. J.B. Lippincott Co., 227 East Washington Square, Philadelphia, PA 19106-3780. Phone: (215) 238-4200. Fax: (215) 238-4227. Bimonthly.

Physician's Data Query (PDQ). Cambridge Scientific Abstracts, 7200 Wisconsin Ave., Bethesda, MD 20814-4823. Phone: (800) 843-7751. Fax: (301) 961-6720. Quarterly.

SCISEARCH. Institute for Scientific Information, 3501 Market St., Philadelphia, PA 19104. Phone: (215) 386-0100. Fax: (215) 386-6362.

Year Books on Disc. CMC ReSearch, Inc., 7150 S.W. Hampton, Suite C-120, Portland, OR 97223. Phone: (800) 262-7668. Fax: (503) 639-1796. Annual includes Year Books of Cardiology, Dermatology, Diagnostic Radiology, Drug Therapy, Emergency Medicine, Family Practice, Medicine, Neurology and Neurosurgery, Obstetrics and Gynecology, Oncology, Pediatrics, and Psychiatry and Applied Mental Health.

DIRECTORIES

Directory of Medical Specialists. Marquis Who's Who, 3002 Glenview Rd., Wilmette, IL 60091. Phone: (800) 621-9669. Fax: (708) 441-2264. Biennial.

Directory of Physicians in the United States. American Medical Association, 515 North State St., Chicago, IL 60610. Phone: (312) 464-0183. Fax: (312) 464-5834. Biennial.

ENCYCLOPEDIAS, DICTIONARIES, WORD BOOKS

The Cancer Dictionary. Roberta Altman, Michael J. Sarg. Facts on File, Inc., 460 Park Ave. S., New York, NY 10016-7382. Phone: (212) 683-2244. Fax: (212) 683-3633. 1992.

Oncologic Word Book. Barbara De Lorenzo. Springhouse Publishing Co., 1111 Bethlehem Pike, Spring House, PA 19477. Phone: (800) 331-3170. Fax: (215) 646-8716. 1992.

Oncology Words. Stedman. Williams & Wilkins, 428 East Preston St., Baltimore, MD 21202. Phone: (800) 638-0672. Fax: (800) 447-8438. 1992.

A Word Book in Oncology and Hematology: With Special Reference to AIDS. Sheila B. Sloane. Mosby-Year Book, 11830 Westline Industrial Drive, St. Louis, MO 63146. Phone: (800) 325-4177. Fax: (314) 432-1380. 1992.

HANDBOOKS, GUIDES, MANUALS, ATLASES

Atlas of Diagnostic Oncology. Skarin. Raven Press, 1185 Ave. of the Americas, New York, NY 10036. Phone: (212) 930-9500. Fax: (212) 869-3495. 1991.

Atlas of Surgical Oncology. John M. Daly, Blake Cady. Mosby-Year Book, 11830 Westline Industrial Drive, St. Louis, MO 63146. Phone: (800) 325-4177. Fax: (314) 432-1380. 1992.

Manual of Clinical Oncology. D.K. Hossfeld, C.D. Sherman, R.R. Love, F.X. Bosch (eds.). Springer-Verlag New York Inc., 175 Fifth Ave., New York, NY 10010. Phone: (212) 460-1500. Fax: (212) 473-6272. Fifth edition 1990.

Manual of Oncologic Therapeutics 1991-1992. Robert E. Wittes. J.B. Lippincott Co., 227 East Washington Square, Philadelphia, PA 19106-3780. Phone: (215) 238-4200. Fax: (215) 238-4227. 1991.

Manual of Quantitative Pathology in Cancer Diagnosis and Prognosis. J.P. Baak. Springer-Verlag New York, Inc., 175 Fifth Ave., New York, NY 10010. Phone: (212) 460-1500. Fax: (212) 473-6272. Second edition 1991.

Manual for Staging of Cancer. Oliver H. Beahrs. J.B. Lippincott Co., 227 E. Washington Square, Philadelphia, PA 19106-3780. Phone: (215) 238-4200. Fax: (215) 238-4227. Third edition 1988.

TNM Classification of Malignant Tumors. Springer-Verlag New York Inc., 175 Fifth Ave., New York, NY 10010. Phone: (212) 460-1500. Fax: (212) 473-6272. 4th ed., rev..

JOURNALS

American Journal of Clinical Oncology. Raven Press, 1185 Ave. of the Americas, New York, NY 10036. Phone: (212) 930-9500. Fax: (212) 869-3495. Bimonthly.

Annals of Oncology. Kluwer Academic Publishers, P.O. Box 358, Accord Station, Hingham, MA 02018-0358. Phone: (617) 871-6600. Fax: (617) 871-6528. 10/year.

Cancer Causes and Control. Rapid Communications of Oxford Ltd., The Old Malthouse, Paradise St., Oxford OX1 1LD, England. Phone: 44-865-790447. Fax: 44-865-244012. 6/year.

Cancer Research. Williams & Wilkins, 428 East Preston St., Baltimore, MD 21202. Phone: (800) 638-0672. Fax: (800) 447-8438. Semimonthly.

Cancer Therapy Update. Kluwer Academic Publishers, P.O. Box 358, Accord Station, Hingham, MA 02018-0358. Phone: (617) 871-6600. Fax: (617) 871-6528. 6/year.

Contemporary Oncology. Medical Economics, Five Paragon Dr., Montvale, NJ 07645-1742. Phone: (800) 222-3045. Fax: (201) 573-4956. 10/year.

European Journal of Cancer. Pergamon Press, 660 White Plains Rd., Tarrytown, NY 10591-5153. Phone: (914) 592-7700. Fax: (914) 592-3625. 14/year.

Frontiers of Radiation Therapy and Oncology. S. Karger Publishers, Inc., 26 W. Avon Rd., P.O. Box 529, Farmington, CT 06085. Phone: (203) 675-7834. Fax: (203) 675-7302.

International Journal of Hyperthermia. Taylor & Francis Inc., 1900 Frost Rd., Suite 101, Bristol, PA 19007-1598. Phone: (800) 821-8312. Fax: (215) 785-5515. Bimonthly.

International Journal of Radiation Oncology-Biology-Physics. Pergamon Press, 660 White Plains Rd., Tarrytown, NY 10591-5153. Phone: (914) 592-7700. Fax: (914) 592-3625. 15/year.

Journal of Clinical Oncology. W.B. Saunders Co., The Curtis Center, Independence Square W., Philadelphia, PA 19106-3399. Phone: (215) 238-7800. Monthly.

Journal of the National Cancer Institute. Superintendent of Documents, P.O. Box 371954, Pittsburgh, PA 15250-7954. Fax: (202) 512-2233. Semimonthly.

Journal of Surgical Oncology. John Wiley & Sons, Inc., 605 Third Ave., New York, NY 10158-0012. Phone: (212) 850-6000. Fax: (212) 850-6088. Monthly.

Morbidity and Mortality Weekly Report. Massachusetts Medical Society, 1440 Main St., Waltham, MA 02154-1649. Phone: (617) 893-3800. Fax: (617) 893-0413. Weekly.

National Cancer Institute. Journal. U.S. National Cancer Institute, 9030 Old Georgetown Rd., Bldg. 82, Room 103, Bethesda, MD 20892. Phone: (301) 496-7186. Monthly.

Oncology Research: An International Journal. Pergamon Press, Inc., 395 Saw Mill River Rd., Elmsford, NY 10523. Phone: (914) 592-7700. Fax: (914) 592-3625. 12/year.

Radiotherapy and Oncology. Elsevier Science Publishing Co., Inc., P.O. Box 882, Madison Square Station, New York, NY 10159-2101. Phone: (212) 989-5800. Fax: (212) 633-3990. 12/year.

NEWSLETTERS

Clinical Oncology Alert. American Health Consultants, Department C1290, P.O. Box 740060, Atlanta, GA 30374. Phone: (800) 559-1032. Fax: (404) 352-1971. Monthly.

NCI Cancer Weekly. Charles W. Henderson, P.O. Box 5528, Atlanta, GA 30307-0527. Phone: (404) 377-8895. Weekly.

Oncology Times. J.B. Lippincott Co., 227 East Washington Square, Philadelphia, PA 19106-3780. Phone: (215) 238-4200. Fax: (215) 238-4227. Monthly.

ONLINE DATABASES

Cancer Weekly. CDC AIDS Weekly/NCI Cancer Weekly, 206 Rogers St. NE, Suite 104, P.O. Box 5528, Atlanta, GA 30317. Phone: (404) 377-8895. Weekly.

CANCERLIT. U.S. National Cancer Institute, International Cancer Information Center, Building 82, Room 102, Bethesda, MD 20892. Phone: (301) 496-7403. Fax: (301) 480-8105. Monthly.

CANCERNET (International Database on Oncology). CANCERNET/Centre National de la Recherche Scientifique, 15 quai Anatole France, F-75700 Paris, France. Phone: 01-46771616.

Cancerquest Online. CDC AIDS Weekly/NCI Cancer Weekly, 206 Rogers St. NE, Suite 104, P.O. Box 5528, Atlanta, GA 30317. Phone: (404) 377-8895. Weekly.

Clinical Protocols. U.S. National Cancer Institute, International Cancer Information Center, Building 82, Room 102, Bethesda, MD 20892. Phone: (301) 496-7403. Fax: (301) 480-8105.

EMBASE. Elsevier Science Publishing Co., Inc., P.O. Box 882, Madison Square Station, New York, NY 10159-2101. Phone: (212) 989-5800. Fax: (212) 633-3990.

MEDLINE. National Library of Medicine, 8600 Rockville Pike, Bethesda, MD 20894. Phone: (800) 638-8480.

Physician Data Query (PDQ) Cancer Information File. U.S. National Cancer Institute, International Cancer Information Center, Building 82, Room 102, Bethesda, MD 20892. Phone: (301) 496-7403. Fax: (301) 480-8105. Monthly.

Physician Data Query (PDQ) Directory File. U.S. National Cancer Institute, International Cancer Information Center, Building 82, Room 102, Bethesda, MD 20892. Phone: (301) 496-7403. Fax: (301) 480-8105. Monthly.

Physician Data Query (PDQ) Protocol File. U.S. National Cancer Institute, International Cancer Information Center, Building 82, Room 102, Bethesda, MD 20892. Phone: (301) 496-7403. Fax: (301) 480-8105. Monthly.

SciSearch. Institute for Scientific Information, 3501 Market St., Philadelphia, PA 19104. Phone: (215) 386-0100. Fax: (215) 386-6362.

POPULAR WORKS AND PATIENT EDUCATION

Everyone's Guide to Cancer Therapy: How Cancer is Diagnosed, Treated, and Managed on a Day to Day Basis. Malin Dollinger, Ernest H. Rosenbaum, Greg Cable. Andrews & McMeel, 4900 Main St., Kansas City, MO 64112. Phone: (800) 826-4216. 1991.

Options: The Alternative Cancer Therapy Book. Richard Walters. Avery Publishing Group, Inc., 120 Old Broadway, Garden City Park, NY 11040. Phone: (800) 548-5757. 1992.

RESEARCH CENTERS, INSTITUTES, CLEARINGHOUSES

Cancer Center. University of Iowa. 20 Medical Laboratories, Iowa City, IA 52242. Phone: (319) 335-7905.

Cancer Information Service (CIS). Office of Cancer Communications, National Cancer Institute, Bldg. 31, Rm.

10A24, 9000 Rockville Pike, Bethesda, MD 20892. Phone: (800) 4CA-NCER.

Cancer Research Institute. New England Deaconess Hospital, 185 Pilgrim, Boston, MA 02215. Phone: (617) 732-8016.

Comprehensive Cancer Center. Columbia University. 701 W. 168th St., New York, NY 10032. Phone: (212) 305-6921. Fax: (212) 305-6889.

Comprehensive Cancer Center. University of Alabama at Birmingham. University Station, Birmingham, AL 35294. Phone: (205) 934-5077. Fax: (205) 934-1608.

Dana Farber Cancer Institute. 44 Binney St., Boston, MA 02115. Phone: (617) 732-3000.

Fred Hutchinson Cancer Research Center. 1124 Columbia St., Seattle, WA 98104. Phone: (206) 467-5000. Fax: (206) 467-5268.

Memorial Sloan-Kettering Cancer Center. 1275 York Ave., New York, NY 10021. Phone: (212) 355-0060.

National Cancer Institute of Canada. 10 Alcorn Ave., Ste. 200, Toronto, ON, Canada M4V 3B1.

Oncology Center. Johns Hopkins University. 600 N. Wolfe St., Baltimore, MD 21205. Phone: (301) 955-8800. Fax: (301) 955-1904.

Vincent T. Lombardi Cancer Research Center. Georgetown University. 3800 Reservoir Rd. NW, Podium Level, Washington, DC 20007. Phone: (202) 687-2110. Fax: (202) 687-6402.

STANDARDS AND STATISTICS SOURCES

Atlas of U.S. Cancer Mortality Among Nonwhites: 1950-1980. L.W. Pickle, T.J. Manson, and others. U.S. Government Printing Office, Superintendent of Documents, P.O. Box 371954, Pittsburgh, PA 15250-7954. Phone: (202) 783-3238. Fax: (202) 512-2250. NIH90-1582, 1990.

Cancer Facts and Figures. American Cancer Society, 1599 Clifton Rd., N.E., Atlanta, GA 30329-4251. Phone: (404) 320-3333. Annual.

Cancer Statistics. American Cancer Society, 1599 Clifton Rd., N.E., Atlanta, GA 30329-4251. Phone: (800) 227-2345. Annual.

National Cancer Institute Annual Report. U.S. Government Printing Office, Superintendent of Documents, P.O. Box 371954, Pittsburgh, PA 15250-7954. Phone: (202) 783-3238. Fax: (202) 512-2250. 1989.

TEXTBOOKS AND MONOGRAPHS

Adjuncts to Cancer Surgery. Steven G. Economou, Thomas R. Witt, Daniel J. Deziel, et. al.. Williams & Wilkins, 428 East Preston St., Baltimore, MD 21202. Phone: (800) 638-0672. Fax: (800) 447-8438. 1991.

The Basic Science of Oncology. Ian F. Tannock, Richard P. Hill. McGraw-Hill, Inc., Health Professions Division, 1221 Avenue of the Americas, 28th Floor, New York, NY 10020. Phone: (212) 512-4228. Second edition 1992.

Cancer Medicine. James F. Holland, Emil Frei, Robert C. Bast Jr., and others. Williams & Wilkins, 428 East Preston St.,

Baltimore, MD 21202. Phone: (800) 638-0672. Fax: (800) 447-8438. Third edition 1992.

Cancer: Principles and Practice of Oncology. Vincent T. DeVita. J.B. Lippincott Co., 227 E. Washington Square, Philadelphia, PA 19106-3780. Phone: (215) 238-4200. Fax: (215) 238-4227. 1989 3rd edtion.

Cancer Treatment. Charles M. Haskell. W.B. Saunders Co., The Curtis Center, Independence Square W., Philadelphia, PA 19106-3399. Phone: (215) 238-7800. Third edition 1990.

Cancer Treatment by Hyperthermia, Radiation and Drugs. Tadayoshi Matsuda (ed.). Taylor & Francis Inc., 1900 Frost Rd., Suite 101, Bristol, PA 19007-1598. Phone: (800) 821-8312. Fax: (215) 785-5515. 1991.

Comprehensive Textbook of Oncology. A.R. Moossa, Stephen C. Schimpff, Martin C. Robson. Williams & Wilkins, 428 East Preston St., Baltimore, MD 21202. Phone: (800) 638-0672. Fax: (800) 447-8438. Second edition. Two volumes. 1991.

Current Therapy in Oncology. John L. Niederhuber and others. Mosby-Year Book, 11830 Westline Industrial Drive, St. Louis, MO 63146. Phone: (800) 325-4177. Fax: (314) 432-1380. 1992.

Gynecologic Oncology. Malcolm Coppleson, John M. Monaghan, C. Paul Morrow, et. al.. Churchill Livingstone Inc., 650 Avenue of the Americas, New York, NY 10011. Phone: (212) 819-5400. Fax: (212) 302-6598. Second edition. Two volumes. 1991.

Medical Oncology: Basic Principles and Clinical Management of Cancer. Paul Calabresi, Philip S. Schein. McGraw-Hill, Inc., Health Professions Division, 1221 Avenue of the Americas, 28th Floor, New York, NY 10020. Phone: (212) 512-4228. Second edition 1992.

Molecular Foundations of Oncology. Samuel Broder (ed.). Williams & Wilkins, 428 East Preston St., Baltimore, MD 21202. Phone: (800) 638-0672. Fax: (800) 447-8438. 1991.

Oncogenes. Cooper. Jones & Bartlett Publishers, Inc., 20 Park Plaza, Boston, MA 02116. Phone: (800) 832-0034. 1990.

Tumors of the Newborn and Infant. Isaacs. Mosby-Year Book, 11830 Westline Industrial Drive, St. Louis, MO 63146. Phone: (800) 325-4177. Fax: (314) 432-1380. 1991.

Urological Oncology. Alderson Smith. John Wiley & Sons, Inc., 605 Third Ave., New York, NY 10158-0012. Phone: (212) 850-6000. Fax: (212) 850-6088. 1991.

OPHTHALMOLOGY

See also: EYE DISEASES; EYE SURGERY; OPTOMETRY; VISION DISORDERS

ABSTRACTING, INDEXING, AND CURRENT AWARENESS PUBLICATIONS

Core Journals in Ophthalmology. Elsevier Science Publishing Co., Inc., P.O. Box 882, Madison Square Station, New York, NY 10159-2101. Phone: (212) 989-5800. Fax: (212) 633-3990. 11/year.

Current Contents/Clinical Medicine. Institute for Scientific Information, 3501 Market St., Philadelphia, PA 19104. Phone: (800) 523-1850. Fax: (215) 386-6362. Weekly.

Excerpta Medica. Section 12: Ophthalmology. Elsevier Science Publishing Co., Inc., P.O. Box 882, Madison Square Station, New York, NY 10159-2101. Phone: (212) 989-5800. Fax: (212) 633-3990. 16/year.

Index Medicus. U.S. National Library of Medicine, 8600 Rockville Pike, Bethesda, MD 20894. Phone: (800) 638-8480. Monthly.

Key Ophthalmology: Current Literature in Perspective. Mosby-Year Book, 11830 Westline Industrial Drive, St. Louis, MO 63146. Phone: (800) 325-4177. Fax: (314) 432-1380. Quarterly.

Ophthalmic Literature. Institute of Ophthalmology, Judd St., London WC1H 9QS, England. 7/year.

Research Alert: Ophthalmology. Institute for Scientific Information, 3501 Market St., Philadelphia, PA 19104. Phone: (800) 523-1850. Fax: (215) 386-6362. Weekly.

Science Citation Index. Institute for Scientific Information, 3501 Market St., Philadelphia, PA 19104. Phone: (800) 523-1850. Fax: (215) 386-6362. Bimonthly.

ANNUALS AND REVIEWS

Current Opinion in Ophthalmology. Current Science Ltd., 20 N. Third St., Philadelphia, PA 19106-2199. Phone: (800) 552-5866. Fax: (215) 574-2270. Bimonthly.

Ophthalmology Clinics. W.B. Saunders Co., The Curtis Center, Independence Square W., Philadelphia, PA 19106-3399. Phone: (215) 238-7800. Quarterly.

Year Book of Ophthalmology. Mosby-Year Book, 11830 Westline Industrial Drive, St. Louis, MO 63146. Phone: (800) 325-4177. Fax: (314) 432-1380. Annual.

ASSOCIATIONS, PROFESSIONAL SOCIETIES, ADVOCACY AND SUPPORT GROUPS

American Academy of Ophthalmology (AAO). 655 Beach St., San Francisco, CA 94109. Phone: (415) 561-8500. Fax: (415) 561-8533.

American Association for Pediatric Ophthalmology. 655 Beach St., P.O. Box 3832, San Francisco, CA 94119. Phone: (415) 561-8505.

American Board of Ophthalmology (ABO). 111 Presidential Blvd., Ste. 241, Bala-Cynwyd, PA 19004. Phone: (215) 664-1175.

American Ophthalmological Society. 200 First St. N.W., Rochester, MN 55905. Phone: (507) 284-3726.

American Society of Contemporary Ophthalmology (ASCO). 233 E. Erie St., St. 710, Chicago, IL 60611. Phone: (312) 951-1400.

Canadian Ophthalmological Society. 1525 Carling Ave., No. 610, Ottawa, ON, Canada K1Z 8R9. Phone: (613) 729-6779. Fax: (613) 729-7209.

CD-ROM DATABASES

SCISEARCH. Institute for Scientific Information, 3501 Market St., Philadelphia, PA 19104. Phone: (215) 386-0100. Fax: (215) 386-6362.

DIRECTORIES

ABMS Directory of Certified Ophthalmologists. American Board of Medical Specialties, One Rotary Center, No. 805, Evanston, IL 60201. Phone: (312) 491-9091.

Directory of Certified Ophthalmologists. American Board of Medical Specialties, 1 Rotary Center, Suite 805, Evanston, IL 60201. Phone: (708) 491-9091. Biennial.

Directory of Medical Specialists. Marquis Who's Who, 3002 Glenview Rd., Wilmette, IL 60091. Phone: (800) 621-9669. Fax: (708) 441-2264. Biennial.

ENCYCLOPEDIAS, DICTIONARIES, WORD BOOKS

Ophthalmic Terminology. Stein. Mosby-Year Book, 11830 Westline Industrial Drive, St. Louis, MO 63146. Phone: (800) 325-4177. Fax: (314) 432-1380. Third edition 1992.

Ophthalmic Word Book. Barbara De Lorenzo. Springhouse Publishing Co., 1111 Bethlehem Pike, Spring House, PA 19477. Phone: (800) 331-3170. Fax: (215) 646-8716. 1992.

Ophthalmology Words. Stedman. Williams & Wilkins, 428 East Preston St., Baltimore, MD 21202. Phone: (800) 638-0672. Fax: (800) 447-8438. 1992.

Pocket Glossary of Ophthalmologic Terminology. Joseph Hoffman. SLACK Inc., 6900 Grove Rd., Thorofare, NJ 08086-9447. Phone: (800) 257-8290. Fax: (609) 853-5991. 1990.

Stedman's Ophthalmology Word Book. Williams & Wilkins, 428 East Preston St., Baltimore, MD 21202. Phone: (800) 638-0672. Fax: (800) 447-8438. 1991.

HANDBOOKS, GUIDES, MANUALS, ATLASES

Atlas of Ophthalmic Surgery. Norman S. Jaffe (ed.). J.B. Lippincott Co., 227 E. Washington Square, Philadelphia, PA 19106-3780. Phone: (215) 238-4200. Fax: (215) 238-4227. 1990.

Handbook of Ophthalmology. Gardner. Appleton & Lange, 25 Van Zant St., East Norwalk, CT 06855. Phone: (800) 423-1359. Fax: (203) 854-9486. 1987.

Manual of Clinical Problems in Opththalmology. Gittinger. Little, Brown and Co., 34 Beacon St., Boston, MA 02108. Phone: (617) 227-0730. 1988.

Ophthalmic Surgery: Cataracts. Richard P. Kratz, and others. J.B. Lippincott Co., 227 E. Washington Square, Philadelphia, PA 19106-3780. Phone: (215) 238-4200. Fax: (215) 238-4227. 1991.

Physician's Desk Reference for Ophthalmology. Medical Economics, Five Paragon Dr., Montvale, NJ 07645-1742. Phone: (800) 222-3045. Fax: (201) 573-4956. Annual.

JOURNALS

American Journal of Ophthalmology. Ophthalmic Publishing Co., 435 N. Michigan Ave., Chicago, IL 60611. Phone: (312) 787-3853.

Annals of Otology, Rhinology & Laryngology. Annals Publishing Co., 4507 Laclede Ave., St. Louis, MO 63108. Phone: (314) 367-4987. Fax: (314) 367-4988. Monthly.

Archives of Ophthalmology. American Medical Association, 515 North State St., Chicago, IL 60610. Phone: (312) 464-0183. Fax: (312) 464-5834. Monthly.

British Journal of Ophthalmology. BMJ Publishing Group, BMA House, Tavistock Square, London WC1H 9JR, England. Phone: 071-383 6244/6638. Fax: 071-383 6662. Monthly.

International Ophthalmology. Kluwer Academic Publishers, P.O. Box 358, Accord Station, Hingham, MA 02018-0358. Phone: (617) 871-6600. Fax: (617) 871-6528. 6/year.

Journal of Pediatric Ophthalmology and Strabismus. SLACK Inc., 6900 Grove Rd., Thorofare, NJ 08086-9447. Phone: (800) 257-8290. Fax: (609) 853-5991.

Ophthalmic Research. S. Karger Publishers, Inc., 26 W. Avon Rd., P.O. Box 529, Farmington, CT 06085. Phone: (203) 675-7834. Fax: (203) 675-7302.

Ophthalmic Surgery. SLACK Inc., 6900 Grove Rd., Thorofare, NJ 08086-9447. Phone: (800) 257-8290. Fax: (609) 853-5991. Monthly.

Ophthalmology. J.B. Lippincott Co., 227 E. Washington Square, Philadelphia, PA 19106-3780. Phone: (215) 238-4200. Fax: (215) 238-4227.

Ophthalmology Report. Mosby-Year Book, 11830 Westline Industrial Drive, St. Louis, MO 63146. Phone: (800) 325-4177. Fax: (314) 432-1380.

Survey of Ophthalmology. Survey of Ophthalmology, Inc., Suite 4, 7 Kent St., Brookline, MA 02146. Phone: (617) 566-2138. Fax: (617) 566-4019. Bimonthly.

NEWSLETTERS

Ophthalmology Alert. American Health Consultants, Department C1290, P.O. Box 740060, Atlanta, GA 30374. Phone: (800) 559-1032. Monthly.

ONLINE DATABASES

EMBASE. Elsevier Science Publishing Co., Inc., P.O. Box 882, Madison Square Station, New York, NY 10159-2101. Phone: (212) 989-5800. Fax: (212) 633-3990.

MEDIS. Mead Data Central, P.O. Box 1830, Dayton, OH 45401. Phone: (800) 227-4908.

MEDLINE. National Library of Medicine, 8600 Rockville Pike, Bethesda, MD 20894. Phone: (800) 638-8480.

SciSearch. Institute for Scientific Information, 3501 Market St., Philadelphia, PA 19104. Phone: (215) 386-0100. Fax: (215) 386-6362.

RESEARCH CENTERS, INSTITUTES, CLEARINGHOUSES

Laboratory for Ophthalmic Research. Emory University, Atlanta, GA 30322. Phone: (404) 321-0111.

Wilmer Ophthalmological Institute. Johns Hopkins University. 601 N. Broadway, Baltimore, MD 21205. Phone: (301) 955-6846. Fax: (301) 955-0675.

TEXTBOOKS AND MONOGRAPHS

Decision Making in Ophthalmology. Richard van Heuven, Johan T. Zwaan. Mosby-Year Book, 11830 Westline Industrial

Drive, St. Louis, MO 63146. Phone: (800) 325-4177. Fax: (314) 432-1380. 1992.

The Eye in Systemic Disease. Jack J. Kanski, D. Thomas. Butterworth-Heinemann, 80 Montvale Ave., Stoneham, MA 02180. Phone: (617) 438-8464. Fax: (617) 279-4851. Second edition 1990.

General Ophthalmology. Vaughn. Appleton & Lange, 25 Van Zant St., East Norwalk, CT 06855. Phone: (800) 423-1359. Fax: (203) 854-9486. 13th edition 1992.

Ocular Pathology: Clinical Applications and Self-Assessment. David J. Apple, Maurice F. Rabb. Mosby-Year Book, 11830 Westline Industrial Drive, St. Louis, MO 63146. Phone: (800) 325-4177. Fax: (314) 432-1380. 1991.

Ophthalmic Surgery: Principles and Concepts. George Spaeth (ed.). W.B. Saunders Co., The Curtis Center, Independence Sqare W., Philadelphia, PA 19106-3399. Phone: (215) 238-7800. 1990.

Ophthalmology: A Diagnostic Text. William H. Coles. Williams & Wilkins, 428 East Preston St., Baltimore, MD 21202. Phone: (800) 638-0672. Fax: (800) 447-8438. 1989.

Ophthalmology: Principles and Concepts. Frank Newell. Mosby-Year Book, 11830 Westline Industrial Drive, St. Louis, MO 63146. Phone: (800) 325-4177. Fax: (314) 432-1380. 7th edition, 1992.

OPTOMETRY

See also: OPHTHALMOLOGY; VISION
DISORDERS

ABSTRACTING, INDEXING, AND CURRENT AWARENESS PUBLICATIONS

Index Medicus. U.S. National Library of Medicine, 8600 Rockville Pike, Bethesda, MD 20894. Phone: (800) 638-8480. Monthly.

Optometry: Current Literature in Perspective. Mosby-Year Book, 11830 Westline Industrial Drive, St. Louis, MO 63146. Phone: (800) 325-4177. Fax: (314) 432-1380. Quarterly.

ASSOCIATIONS, PROFESSIONAL SOCIETIES, ADVOCACY AND SUPPORT GROUPS

American Academy of Optometry (AAO). 5530 Wisconsin Ave. N.W., Ste. 1149, Washington, DC 20015. Phone: (301) 652-0905. Fax: (301) 656-0989.

American Optometric Association (AOA). 243 N. Lindbergh Blvd., St. Louis, MO 63141. Phone: (314) 991-4100. Fax: (314) 991-4101.

Association of Schools and Colleges of Optometry. 6110 Executive Blvd., No. 514, Rockville, MD 20852. Phone: (301) 231-5944.

Canadian Association of Optometrists. 1785 Alta Vista Dr., Suite 301, Ottawa, ON, Canada K1G 3Y6. Phone: (613) 738-4412. Fax: (613) 738-7161.

National Association of Optometrists and Opticians. 18903 S. Miles Rd., Cleveland, OH 44128. Phone: (216) 475-8925.

National Board of Examiners in Optometry. 5530 Wisconsin Ave. N.W., Ste. 805, Washington, DC 20015. Phone: (301) 652-5192. Fax: (301) 907-0013.

DIRECTORIES

Blue Book of Optometrists. Butterworth-Heinemann, 80 Montvale Ave., Stoneham, MA 02180. Phone: (617) 438-8464. Fax: (617) 279-4851. Biennial.

ENCYCLOPEDIAS, DICTIONARIES, WORD BOOKS

Dictionary of Optometry. Michel Millodot. Butterworth-Heinemann, 80 Montvale Ave., Stoneham, MA 02180. Phone: (617) 438-8464. Fax: (617) 279-4851. Second edition 1990.

Ophthalmic Terminology. Stein. Mosby-Year Book, 11830 Westline Industrial Drive, St. Louis, MO 63146. Phone: (800) 325-4177. Fax: (314) 432-1380. Third edition 1992.

Ophthalmology Words. Stedman. Williams & Wilkins, 428 East Preston St., Baltimore, MD 21202. Phone: (800) 638-0672. Fax: (800) 447-8438. 1992.

HANDBOOKS, GUIDES, MANUALS, ATLASES

The Optometry Handbook. R.D. Llewellyn. Butterworth-Heinemann, 80 Montvale Ave., Stoneham, MA 02180. Phone: (617) 438-8464. Fax: (617) 279-4851. 1991.

JOURNALS

American Optometric Association Journal. American Optometric Association, 243 N. Lindbergh Blvd., St. Louis, MO 63141. Phone: (314) 991-4100.

The Journal of the British Contact Lens Association. Mosby-Year Book, 11830 Westline Industrial Drive, St. Louis, MO 63146. Phone: (800) 325-4177. Fax: (314) 432-1380. Quarterly.

Optometry Clinics. Appleton & Lange, 25 Van Zant St., East Norwalk, CT 06855. Phone: (800) 423-1359. Fax: (203) 854-9486. Quarterly.

Optometry and Vision Science. Williams & Wilkins, 428 E. Preston St., Baltimore, MD 21202. Phone: (800) 638-0672. Fax: (800) 447-8438. Monthly.

ONLINE DATABASES

EMBASE. Elsevier Science Publishing Co., Inc., P.O. Box 882, Madison Square Station, New York, NY 10159-2101. Phone: (212) 989-5800. Fax: (212) 633-3990.

MEDLINE. National Library of Medicine, 8600 Rockville Pike, Bethesda, MD 20894. Phone: (800) 638-8480.

SciSearch. Institute for Scientific Information, 3501 Market St., Philadelphia, PA 19104. Phone: (215) 386-0100. Fax: (215) 386-6362.

RESEARCH CENTERS, INSTITUTES, CLEARINGHOUSES

Eye Institute. Pennsylvania College of Optometry. 13th & Spencer Sts., Philadelphia, PA 19141. Phone: (215) 276-6000. Fax: (215) 276-6082.

STANDARDS AND STATISTICS SOURCES

Annual Survey of Optometric Educational Institutions. Association of Schools and Colleges of Optometry, 6110

Executive Blvd., No. 514, Rockville, MD 20852. Phone: (301) 231-5944. Annual.

TEXTBOOKS AND MONOGRAPHS

Optometry. Keith Edwards, Richard Llewellyn. Butterworth-Heinemann, 80 Montvale Ave., Stoneham, MA 02180. Phone: (617) 438-8464. Fax: (617) 279-4851. 1988.

Pediatric Optometry. Jerome Rosner, Joy Rosner. Butterworth-Heinemann, 80 Montvale Ave., Stoneham, MA 02180. Phone: (617) 438-8464. Fax: (617) 279-4851. 2nd edition, 1989.

ORAL CANCER

See also: CANCER

ABSTRACTING, INDEXING, AND CURRENT AWARENESS PUBLICATIONS

Current Contents/Clinical Medicine. Institute for Scientific Information, 3501 Market St., Philadelphia, PA 19104. Phone: (800) 523-1850. Fax: (215) 386-6362. Weekly.

Excerpta Medica. Section 16: Cancer. Elsevier Science Publishing Co., Inc., P.O. Box 882, Madison Square Station, New York, NY 10159-2101. Phone: (212) 989-5800. Fax: (212) 633-3990. 32/year.

Index Medicus. U.S. National Library of Medicine, 8600 Rockville Pike, Bethesda, MD 20894. Phone: (800) 638-8480. Monthly.

Science Citation Index. Institute for Scientific Information, 3501 Market St., Philadelphia, PA 19104. Phone: (800) 523-1850. Fax: (215) 386-6362. Bimonthly.

ANNUALS AND REVIEWS

In Development New Medicines for Older Americans. 1991 Annual Survey. More Medicines in Testing for Cancer Than for Any Other Disease of Aging. Pharmaceutical Manufacturers Association, 1100 15th St. N.W., Washington, DC 20005. Phone: (202) 835-3400. 1991.

ASSOCIATIONS, PROFESSIONAL SOCIETIES, ADVOCACY AND SUPPORT GROUPS

American Cancer Society (ACS). 1599 Clifton Rd. N.E., Atlanta, GA 30329. Phone: (404) 320-3333.

CD-ROM DATABASES

Cancer on Disc. CMC ReSearch, Inc., 7150 S.W. Hampton, Suite C-120, Portland, OR 97223. Phone: (800) 262-7668. Fax: (503) 639-1796. Annual.

Physician's Data Query (PDQ). Cambridge Scientific Abstracts, 7200 Wisconsin Ave., Bethesda, MD 20814-4823. Phone: (800) 843-7751. Fax: (301) 961-6720. Quarterly.

SCISEARCH. Institute for Scientific Information, 3501 Market St., Philadelphia, PA 19104. Phone: (215) 386-0100. Fax: (215) 386-6362.

ENCYCLOPEDIAS, DICTIONARIES, WORD BOOKS

Oncology Words. Stedman. Williams & Wilkins, 428 East Preston St., Baltimore, MD 21202. Phone: (800) 638-0672. Fax: (800) 447-8438. 1992.

HANDBOOKS, GUIDES, MANUALS, ATLASES

Atlas of Disease of the Oral Mucosa. J.J. Pindborg. Mosby-Year Book, 11830 Westline Industrial Drive, St. Louis, MO 63146. Phone: (800) 325-4177. Fax: (314) 432-1380. Fifth edition 1992.

A Color Atlas of Orofacial Diseases. W.R. Tyldesley. Mosby-Year Book, 11830 Westline Industrial Drive, St. Louis, MO 63146. Phone: (800) 325-4177. Fax: (314) 432-1380. Second edition 1991.

JOURNALS

Cancer Causes and Control. Rapid Communications of Oxford Ltd., The Old Malthouse, Paradise St., Oxford OX1 1LD, England. Phone: 44-865-790447. Fax: 44-865-244012. 6/year.

Journal of the National Cancer Institute. Superintendent of Documents, P.O. Box 371954, Pittsburgh, PA 15250-7954. Fax: (202) 512-2233. Semimonthly.

Journal of Oral and Maxillofacial Surgery. W.B. Saunders Co., The Curtis Center, Independence Square W., Philadelphia, PA 19106-3399. Phone: (215) 238-7800. Monthly.

Journal of Oral Pathology and Medicine. Munksgaard International Publishers Ltd., P.O. Box 2148, DK-1016 Copenhagen K, Denmark. Phone: 33-127030. Fax: 33-129387.

Journal of Surgical Oncology. John Wiley & Sons, Inc., 605 Third Ave., New York, NY 10158-0012. Phone: (212) 850-6000. Fax: (212) 850-6088. Monthly.

Oral Surgery, Oral Medicine, Oral Pathology. Mosby-Year Book, 11830 Westline Industrial Drive, St. Louis, MO 63146. Phone: (800) 325-4177. Fax: (314) 432-1380. Monthly.

ONLINE DATABASES

Cancer Weekly. CDC AIDS Weekly/NCI Cancer Weekly, 206 Rogers St. NE, Suite 104, P.O. Box 5528, Atlanta, GA 30317. Phone: (404) 377-8895. Weekly.

CANCERLIT. U.S. National Cancer Institute, International Cancer Information Center, Building 82, Room 102, Bethesda, MD 20892. Phone: (301) 496-7403. Fax: (301) 480-8105. Monthly.

Clinical Protocols. U.S. National Cancer Institute, International Cancer Information Center, Building 82, Room 102, Bethesda, MD 20892. Phone: (301) 496-7403. Fax: (301) 480-8105.

EMBASE. Elsevier Science Publishing Co., Inc., P.O. Box 882, Madison Square Station, New York, NY 10159-2101. Phone: (212) 989-5800. Fax: (212) 633-3990.

MEDLINE. National Library of Medicine, 8600 Rockville Pike, Bethesda, MD 20894. Phone: (800) 638-8480.

Physician Data Query (PDQ) Cancer Information File. U.S. National Cancer Institute, International Cancer Information Center, Building 82, Room 102, Bethesda, MD 20892. Phone: (301) 496-7403. Fax: (301) 480-8105. Monthly.

Physician Data Query (PDQ) Directory File. U.S. National Cancer Institute, International Cancer Information Center, Building 82, Room 102, Bethesda, MD 20892. Phone: (301) 496-7403. Fax: (301) 480-8105. Monthly.

Physician Data Query (PDQ) Protocol File. U.S. National Cancer Institute, International Cancer Information Center, Building 82, Room 102, Bethesda, MD 20892. Phone: (301) 496-7403. Fax: (301) 480-8105. Monthly.

SciSearch. Institute for Scientific Information, 3501 Market St., Philadelphia, PA 19104. Phone: (215) 386-0100. Fax: (215) 386-6362.

POPULAR WORKS AND PATIENT EDUCATION

Cancervive: The Challenge of Life After Cancer. Susan Nessim, Judith Ellis. Houghton Mifflin Co., 1 Beacon St., Boston, MA 02108. Phone: (800) 225-3362. 1991.

RESEARCH CENTERS, INSTITUTES, CLEARINGHOUSES

Cancer Information Service (CIS). Office of Cancer Communications, National Cancer Institute, Bldg. 31, Rm. 10A24, 9000 Rockville Pike, Bethesda, MD 20892. Phone: (800) 4CA-NCER.

TEXTBOOKS AND MONOGRAPHS

Cancer Medicine. James F. Holland, Emil Frei, Robert C. Bast Jr., and others. Williams & Wilkins, 428 East Preston St., Baltimore, MD 21202. Phone: (800) 638-0672. Fax: (800) 447-8438. Third edition 1992.

Cancer: Principles and Practice of Oncology. Vincent T. DeVita. J.B. Lippincott Co., 227 E. Washington Square, Philadelphia, PA 19106-3780. Phone: (215) 238-4200. Fax: (215) 238-4227. 1989 3rd edtion.

Cancer Treatment. Charles M. Haskell. W.B. Saunders Co., The Curtis Center, Independence Square W., Philadelphia, PA 19106-3399. Phone: (215) 238-7800. Third edition 1990.

Head and Neck Oncology for the General Surgeon. Paul E. Preece, and others. Mosby-Year Book, 11830 Westline Industrial Drive, St. Louis, MO 63146. Phone: (800) 325-4177. Fax: (314) 432-1380. 1991.

Oral Cancer: Epidemiology, Etiology and Pathology. Colin Smith, Jens J. Pindborg, William H. Binnie (eds.). Taylor & Francis Inc., 1900 Frost Rd., Suite 101, Bristol, PA 19007-1598. Phone: (800) 821-8312. Fax: (215) 785-5515. 1990.

Risk Markers for Oral Diseases. Volume 2: Oral Cancer. N.W. Johnson (ed.). Cambridge University Press, 40 W. 20th St., New York, NY 10011. Phone: (800) 431-1580. 1991.

ORAL SURGERY

See also: DENTISTRY; ENDODONTICS;
MOUTH DISEASES; PERIODONTICS

ABSTRACTING, INDEXING, AND CURRENT AWARENESS PUBLICATIONS

Current Contents/Clinical Medicine. Institute for Scientific Information, 3501 Market St., Philadelphia, PA 19104. Phone: (800) 523-1850. Fax: (215) 386-6362. Weekly.

Index to Dental Literature. American Dental Association, 211 E. Chicago Ave., Chicago, IL 60611-2678. Phone: (800) 947-4746. Fax: (312) 440-3542. Quarterly.

Index Medicus. U.S. National Library of Medicine, 8600 Rockville Pike, Bethesda, MD 20894. Phone: (800) 638-8480. Monthly.

Science Citation Index. Institute for Scientific Information, 3501 Market St., Philadelphia, PA 19104. Phone: (800) 523-1850. Fax: (215) 386-6362. Bimonthly.

ANNUALS AND REVIEWS

Oral and Maxillofacial Surgery Clinics. W.B. Saunders Co., The Curtis Center, Independence Square W., Philadelphia, PA 19106-3399. Phone: (215) 238-7800. Quarterly.

ASSOCIATIONS, PROFESSIONAL SOCIETIES, ADVOCACY AND SUPPORT GROUPS

Academy for Implants and Transplants. P.O. Box 223, Springfield, VA 22150. Phone: (703) 457-0001.

American Academy of Implant Dentistry. 6900 Grove St., Thorofare, NJ 08086. Phone: (609) 848-7027.

American Academy of Oral Medicine. 222 S. Bemistone Ave., St. Louis, MO 63105. Phone: (314) 721-3753.

American Association of Oral and Maxillofacial Surgeons (AAOMS). 9700 W. Bryn Mawr, Rosemont, IL 60018. Phone: (800) 822-6637. Fax: (708) 678-6286.

American Board of Oral and Maxillofacial Surgery (ABOMS). 625 N. Michigan Ave., Ste. 1820, Chicago, IL 60611. Phone: (312) 642-0070.

CD-ROM DATABASES

SCISEARCH. Institute for Scientific Information, 3501 Market St., Philadelphia, PA 19104. Phone: (215) 386-0100. Fax: (215) 386-6362.

HANDBOOKS, GUIDES, MANUALS, ATLASES

Atlas of Oral and Maxillofacial Surgery. David A. Keith. W.B. Saunders Co., The Curtis Center, Independence Square W., Philadelphia, PA 19106-3399. Phone: (215) 238-7800. 1992.

Massachusetts General Hospital Manual of Oral and Maxillofacial Surgery. R. Bruce Donoff. Mosby-Year Book, 11830 Westline Industrial Drive, St. Louis, MO 63146. Phone: (800) 325-4177. Fax: (314) 432-1380. Second edition 1992.

JOURNALS

British Journal of Oral and Maxillofacial Surgery. Churchill Livingstone Inc., 650 Avenue of the Americas, New York, NY 10011. Phone: (212) 819-5400. Fax: (212) 302-6598. 6/year.

Implant Dentistry. Williams & Wilkins, 428 E. Preston St., Baltimore, MD 21202. Phone: (800) 638-0672. Fax: (800) 447-8438. Quarterly.

Journal of Oral and Maxillofacial Surgery. W.B. Saunders Co., The Curtis Center, Independence Square W., Philadelphia, PA 19106-3399. Phone: (215) 238-7800. Monthly.

Oral Surgery, Oral Medicine, Oral Pathology. Mosby-Year Book, 11830 Westline Industrial Drive, St. Louis, MO 63146. Phone: (800) 325-4177. Fax: (314) 432-1380. Monthly.

NEWSLETTERS

Dental Implantology Update. American Health Consultants, Department C1290, P.O. Box 740060, Atlanta, GA 30374. Phone: (800) 559-1032. Monthly.

Implant Update. Academy for Implants and Transplants, P.O. Box 223, Springfield, VA 22150. Phone: (703) 451-0001. Quarterly.

ONLINE DATABASES

EMBASE. Elsevier Science Publishing Co., Inc., P.O. Box 882, Madison Square Station, New York, NY 10159-2101. Phone: (212) 989-5800. Fax: (212) 633-3990.

MEDLINE. National Library of Medicine, 8600 Rockville Pike, Bethesda, MD 20894. Phone: (800) 638-8480.

SciSearch. Institute for Scientific Information, 3501 Market St., Philadelphia, PA 19104. Phone: (215) 386-0100. Fax: (215) 386-6362.

RESEARCH CENTERS, INSTITUTES, CLEARINGHOUSES

National Institute of Dental Research. NIH Bldg. 31, Rm. 2C-35, 9000 Rockville Pike, Bethesda, MD 20892. Phone: (301) 496-4261.

TEXTBOOKS AND MONOGRAPHS

Contemporary Implant Dentistry. Carl E. Misch. Mosby-Year Book, 11830 Westline Industrial Drive, St. Louis, MO 63146. Phone: (800) 325-4177. Fax: (314) 432-1380. 1992.

Contemporary Oral and Maxillofacial Surgery. Larry J. Peterson. Mosby-Year Book, 11830 Westline Industrial Drive, St. Louis, MO 63146. Phone: (800) 325-4177. Fax: (314) 432-1380. 1992.

Dental Implants: Principles and Practice. Charles A. Babbush. W.B. Saunders Co., The Curtis Center, Independence Square W., Philadelphia, PA 19106-3399. Phone: (215) 238-7800. 1992.

Modern Practice in Orthognathic and Reconstructive Surgery. William H. Bell. W.B. Saunders Co., The Curtis Center, Independence Square W., Philadelphia, PA 19106-3399. Phone: (215) 238-7800. Three volumes 1992.

Oral Implantology. A. Schroeder, F. Sutter, G. Krekeler. Thieme Medical Publishers, Inc., 381 Park Ave. S., New York, NY 10016. Phone: (212) 683-5088. Fax: (212) 779-9020. 1991.

Oral Surgery. Gordon W. Pedersen. W.B. Saunders Co., The Curtis Center, Independence Square W., Philadelphia, PA 19106-3399. Phone: (215) 238-7800. 1988.

Principles of Oral and Maxillofacial Surgery. Larry J. Peterson, A. Thomas Indresano, Robert Marciani. J.B. Lippincott Co., 227 East Washington Square, Philadelphia, PA 19106-3780. Phone: (215) 238-4200. Fax: (215) 238-4227. Three volumes 1992.

Surgical Management of Impacted Teeth. Charles C. Alling III, John F. Helfrick, Rocklin Alling. W.B. Saunders Co., The Curtis Center, Independence Square W., Philadelphia, PA 19106-3399. Phone: (215) 238-7800. 1992.

ORGAN TRANSPLANTS

See: TRANSPLANTATION

ORPHAN DRUGS

See also: DRUGS

ABSTRACTING, INDEXING, AND CURRENT AWARENESS PUBLICATIONS

Current Contents/Life Sciences. Institute for Scientific Information, 3501 Market St., Philadelphia, PA 19104. Phone: (215) 386-0100. Fax: (215) 386-6362.

Excerpta Medica. Section 30: Clinical and Experimental Pharmacology. Elsevier Science Publishing Co., Inc., P.O. Box 882, Madison Square Station, New York, NY 10159-2101. Phone: (212) 989-5800. Fax: (212) 633-3990. 32/year.

Index Medicus. U.S. National Library of Medicine, 8600 Rockville Pike, Bethesda, MD 20894. Phone: (800) 638-8480. Monthly.

International Pharmaceutical Abstracts. American Society of Hospital Pharmacists, 4630 Montgomery Ave., Bethesda, MD 20814. Phone: (301) 657-3000. Fax: (301) 657-1641. Semimonthly.

ANNUALS AND REVIEWS

In Development Orphan Drugs. Pharmaceutical Manufacturers Association, 1100 15th St. N.W., Washington, DC 20005. Phone: (202) 835-3400. Annual.

ASSOCIATIONS, PROFESSIONAL SOCIETIES, ADVOCACY AND SUPPORT GROUPS

National Organization for Rare Disorders. P.O. Box 8927, New Fairfield, CT 06812. Phone: (800) 999-6673.

Office of Orphan Products Development. Food and Drug Administration, 5600 Fishers Lane, Rm. HF 35, Rockville, MD 20857. Phone: (301) 443-4903.

Pharmaceutical Manufacturers Association Commission on Drugs for Rare Diseases. 1100 15th St. N.W., Washington, DC 20005. Phone: (202) 835-3550.

CD-ROM DATABASES

Excerpta Medica CD: Drugs & Pharmacology. SilverPlatter Information, Inc., River Ridge Office Park, 100 River Ridge Rd., Norwood, MA 02062. Phone: (617) 769-2599. Fax: (617) 769-8763. Quarterly.

Journal of the American Medical Association. Macmillan New Media, 124 Mt. Auburn St., Cambridge, MA 02138. Weekly.

New England Journal of Medicine. CMC ReSearch, Inc., 7150 S.W. Hampton, Suite C-120, Portland, OR 97223. Phone: (800) 262-7668. Fax: (503) 639-1796. 3/year.

The New England Journal of Medicine on CD-ROM. MEP, 124 Mt. Auburn St., Cambridge, MA 02138. Phone: (800) 342-1338. Fax: (617) 868-7738. Semiannual.

JOURNALS

American Journal of Hospital Pharmacy. American Society of Hospital Pharmacists, c/o Jean Rogers, Dir. Mkt. Services, 4630 Montgomery Ave., Bethesda, MD 20814. Phone: (301) 657-3000. Monthly.

The New England Journal of Medicine. Massachusetts Medical Society, 1440 Main St., Waltham, MA 02154-1649. Phone: (617) 893-3800. Fax: (617) 893-0413. Weekly.

NEWSLETTERS

Orphan Disease Update. National Organization for Rare Disorders (NORD), P.O. Box 8923, New Fairfield, CT 06812. Phone: (203) 746-6518. 3/year.

ONLINE DATABASES

EMBASE. Elsevier Science Publishing Co., Inc., P.O. Box 882, Madison Square Station, New York, NY 10159-2101. Phone: (212) 989-5800. Fax: (212) 633-3990.

MEDLINE. National Library of Medicine, 8600 Rockville Pike, Bethesda, MD 20894. Phone: (800) 638-8480.

Orphan Drug Database. National Organization for Rare Disorders, P.O. Box 8927, New Fairfield, CT 06812. Phone: (800) 999-6673.

SciSearch. Institute for Scientific Information, 3501 Market St., Philadelphia, PA 19104. Phone: (215) 386-0100. Fax: (215) 386-6362.

RESEARCH CENTERS, INSTITUTES, CLEARINGHOUSES

National Information Center for Orphan Drugs and Rare Diseases. P.O. Box 1133, Washington, DC 20013-1133. Phone: (800) 456-3505.

Office of Consumer Affairs. Food and Drug Administration. 5600 Fishers Ln., HFE-50, Rockville, MD 20857. Phone: (301) 443-3170.

TEXTBOOKS AND MONOGRAPHS

Orphan Diseases and Orphan Drugs. I. Herbert Scheinberg, J.M. Walshe (eds.). St. Martin's Press, 175 Fifth Ave., New York, NY 10010. Phone: (212) 674-5151. 1989.

ORTHODONTICS

See also: DENTISTRY

ABSTRACTING, INDEXING, AND CURRENT AWARENESS PUBLICATIONS

Dental Abstracts. Mosby-Year Book, 11830 Westline Industrial Drive, St. Louis, MO 63146. Phone: (800) 325-4177. Fax: (314) 432-1380. Bimonthly.

Index to Dental Literature. American Dental Association, 211 E. Chicago Ave., Chicago, IL 60611-2678. Phone: (800) 947-4746. Fax: (312) 440-3542. Quarterly.

Index Medicus. U.S. National Library of Medicine, 8600 Rockville Pike, Bethesda, MD 20894. Phone: (800) 638-8480. Monthly.

ANNUALS AND REVIEWS

Year Book of Dentistry. Mosby-Year Book, 11830 Westline Industrial Drive, St. Louis, MO 63146. Phone: (800) 325-4177. Fax: (314) 432-1380. Annual.

ASSOCIATIONS, PROFESSIONAL SOCIETIES, ADVOCACY AND SUPPORT GROUPS

American Association of Orthodontists (AAO). 460 N. Lindbergh Blvd., St. Louis, MO 63141-7883. Phone: (314) 993-1700. Fax: (314) 997-1745.

American Board of Orthodontics (ABO). 225 S. Meramec Ave., St. Louis, MO 63105. Phone: (314) 727-5039.

American Orthodontic Society. 9550 Forest Lane, No. 215, Dallas, TX 75243. Phone: (214) 343-0805.

American Society for the Study of Orthodontics. 50-12 204th St., Oakland Gardens, NY 11364. Phone: (212) 224-8898.

Angle Orthodontists Research and Education Foundation. 100 W. Lawrence St., Appleton, WI 54911.

DIRECTORIES

American Board of Orthodontics-Directory of Diplomates. American Board of Orthodontics, 225 S. Meremec Ave., St. Louis, MO 63105. Phone: (314) 727-5039.

HANDBOOKS, GUIDES, MANUALS, ATLASES

Atlas of Adult Orthodontics: Functional and Esthetic Enhancement. Manuel H. Marka, Herman Corn. Williams & Wilkins, 428 E. Preston St., Baltimore, MD 21202. Phone: (800) 638-0672. Fax: (800) 447-8438. 1989.

Handbook of Orthodontics. Robert Moyers. Mosby-Year Book, 11830 Westline Industrial Drive, St. Louis, MO 63146. Phone: (800) 325-4177. Fax: (314) 432-1380. 4th edition, 1988.

JOURNALS

American Journal of Orthodontics and Dentofacial Orthopedics. Mosby-Year Book, 11830 Westline Industrial Drive, St. Louis, MO 63146. Phone: (800) 325-4177. Fax: (314) 432-1380. Monthly.

Angle Orthodontist. Angle Orthodontists Research and Education Foundation, 100 W. Lawrence St., Appleton, WI 54911.

Journal of Clinical Orthodontics. 1828 Pearl St., Boulder, CO 80302. Phone: (303) 443-1720.

Oral Surgery, Oral Medicine, Oral Pathology. Mosby-Year Book, 11830 Westline Industrial Drive, St. Louis, MO 63146. Phone: (800) 325-4177. Fax: (314) 432-1380. Monthly.

NEWSLETTERS

American Orthodontic Society-Newsletter. American Orthodontic Society, 9550 Forest Ln., Ste. 215, Dallas, TX 75243. Phone: (800) 448-1601. Quarterly.

ONLINE DATABASES

EMBASE. Elsevier Science Publishing Co., Inc., P.O. Box 882, Madison Square Station, New York, NY 10159-2101. Phone: (212) 989-5800. Fax: (212) 633-3990.

MEDLINE. National Library of Medicine, 8600 Rockville Pike, Bethesda, MD 20894. Phone: (800) 638-8480.

SciSearch. Institute for Scientific Information, 3501 Market St., Philadelphia, PA 19104. Phone: (215) 386-0100. Fax: (215) 386-6362.

POPULAR WORKS AND PATIENT EDUCATION

The Mount Sinai Medical Center Family Guide to Dental Health. Jack Klatell, Andrew Kaplan, Gray Williams Jr.. Macmillan Publishing Co., Inc., 866 Third Ave., New York, NY 10022. Phone: (800) 257-5755. 1992.

RESEARCH CENTERS, INSTITUTES, CLEARINGHOUSES

National Institute of Dental Research. NIH Bldg. 31, Rm. 2C-35, 9000 Rockville Pike, Bethesda, MD 20892. Phone: (301) 496-4261.

TEXTBOOKS AND MONOGRAPHS

Contemporary Orthodontics. William R. Proffit. Mosby-Year Book, 11830 Westline Industrial Drive, St. Louis, MO 63146. Phone: (800) 325-4177. Fax: (314) 432-1380. Second edition 1992.

Retention and Stability in Orthodontics. Ravindra Nanda, Charles J. Burstone. W.B. Saunders Co., The Curtis Center, Independence Square W., Philadelphia, PA 19106-3399. Phone: (215) 238-7800. 1992.

ORTHOPEDIC SURGERY

See: ORTHOPEDICS

ORTHOPEDICS

See also: FRACTURES; HAND SURGERY; KNEE SURGERY; PROSTHESES; SPORTS MEDICINE; SURGERY

ABSTRACTING, INDEXING, AND CURRENT AWARENESS PUBLICATIONS

Current Contents/Clinical Medicine. Institute for Scientific Information, 3501 Market St., Philadelphia, PA 19104. Phone: (800) 523-1850. Fax: (215) 386-6362. Weekly.

Excerpta Medica. Section 33: Orthopedic Surgery. Elsevier Science Publishing Co., Inc., P.O. Box 882, Madison Square Station, New York, NY 10159-2101. Phone: (212) 989-5800. Fax: (212) 633-3990. 10/year.

Index Medicus. U.S. National Library of Medicine, 8600 Rockville Pike, Bethesda, MD 20894. Phone: (800) 638-8480. Monthly.

Science Citation Index. Institute for Scientific Information, 3501 Market St., Philadelphia, PA 19104. Phone: (800) 523-1850. Fax: (215) 386-6362. Bimonthly.

ANNUALS AND REVIEWS

Advances in Orthopaedic Surgery. Data Trace Medical Publishers, Inc., P.O. Box 1239, Brooklandville, MD 21022. Phone: (410) 494-4994. Fax: (410) 494-0515. Bimonthly.

Current Opinion in Orthopaedics. Current Science Ltd., 20 N. Third St., Philadelphia, PA 19106-2199. Phone: (800) 552-5866. Fax: (215) 574-2270. Bimonthly.

Current Orthopaedics. Churchill Livingstone Inc., 650 Avenue of the Americas, New York, NY 10011. Phone: (212) 819-5400. Fax: (212) 302-6598. Quarterly.

Orthopaedic Physical Therapy Clinics of North America. W.B. Saunders Co., The Curtis Center, Independence Square W., Philadelphia, PA 19106-3399. Phone: (215) 238-7800. Quarterly.

Orthopedic Clinics. W.B. Saunders Co., The Curtis Center, Independence Square W., Philadelphia, PA 19106-3399. Phone: (215) 238-7800. Quarterly.

Year Book of Hand Surgery. Mosby-Year Book, 11830 Westline Industrial Drive, St. Louis, MO 63146. Phone: (800) 325-4177. Fax: (314) 432-1380. Annual.

Year Book of Orthopedics. Mosby-Year Book, 11830 Westline Industrial Drive, St. Louis, MO 63146. Phone: (800) 325-4177. Fax: (314) 432-1380. Annual.

Year Book of Sports Medicine. Mosby-Year Book, 11830 Westline Industrial Drive, St. Louis, MO 63146. Phone: (800) 325-4177. Fax: (314) 432-1380. Annual.

ASSOCIATIONS, PROFESSIONAL SOCIETIES, ADVOCACY AND SUPPORT GROUPS

American Academy of Orthopedic Surgeons (AAOS). 222 S. Prospect Ave., Park Ridge, IL 60068-4058. Phone: (708) 823-7186. Fax: (708) 823-8125.

American Board of Orthopedic Surgery (ABOS). 737 N. Michigan Ave., Ste. 1150, Chicago, IL 60611. Phone: (312) 664-9444.

American Orthopaedic Society for Sports Medicine (AOSSM). 2250 E. Devon Ave., Ste. 115, Des Plaines, IL 60018. Phone: (708) 836-7000. Fax: (708) 803-8653.

Conservative Orthopedics International Association (COIA). 1811 Monroe, Dearborn, MI 48124. Phone: (313) 563-0360.

CD-ROM DATABASES

Ortholine. Aries Systems Corporation, One Dundee Park, Andover, MA 01810. Phone: (508) 475-7200. Fax: (508) 474-8860. Monthly or quarterly.

SCISEARCH. Institute for Scientific Information, 3501 Market St., Philadelphia, PA 19104. Phone: (215) 386-0100. Fax: (215) 386-6362.

DIRECTORIES

Directory of Certified Orthopaedic Surgeons. American Board of Medical Specialties, 1 Rotary Center, Suite 805, Evanston, IL 60201. Phone: (708) 491-9091. Biennial.

Directory of Medical Specialists. Marquis Who's Who, 3002 Glenview Rd., Wilmette, IL 60091. Phone: (800) 621-9669. Fax: (708) 441-2264. Biennial.

Directory of Physicians in the United States. American Medical Association, 515 North State St., Chicago, IL 60610. Phone: (312) 464-0183. Fax: (312) 464-5834. Biennial.

ENCYCLOPEDIAS, DICTIONARIES, WORD BOOKS

CRC Handbook of Orthopaedic Terminology. Ray F. Kilcoyne, Edward L. Farrar. CRC Press, Inc., 2000 Corporate Blvd. N.W., Boca Raton, FL 33431. Phone: (407) 994-0555. Fax: (407) 997-0949. 1990.

Handbook of Orthopedic Terminology. Kilcoyne. CRC Press, Inc., 2000 Corporate Blvd. N.W., Boca Raton, FL 33431. Phone: (407) 994-0555. Fax: (407) 997-0949. 1991.

Orthopedic Word Book. Thomas J. Cittadine. Springhouse Publishing Co., 1111 Bethlehem Pike, Spring House, PA 19477. Phone: (800) 331-3170. Fax: (215) 646-8716. 1992.

Orthopedic Words. Stedman. Williams & Wilkins, 428 East Preston St., Baltimore, MD 21202. Phone: (800) 638-0672. Fax: (800) 447-8438. 1992.

Surgery on File: Orthopedics and Trauma Surgery. The Diagram Group. Facts on File, Inc., 460 Park Ave. S., New York, NY 10016-7382. Phone: (212) 683-2244. 1988.

HANDBOOKS, GUIDES, MANUALS, ATLASES

Atlas of Orthopaedic Surgical Approaches. C.L. Colton, A.J. Hall (eds.). Butterworth-Heinemann, 80 Montvale Ave., Stoneham, MA 02180. Phone: (617) 438-8464. Fax: (617) 279-4851. 1991.

Manual of Emergency Orthopedics. William M. Green, Robert W. Derlet, Timothy Dray. Williams & Wilkins, 428 East Preston St., Baltimore, MD 21202. Phone: (800) 638-0672. Fax: (800) 447-8438. 1992.

Manual of Rheumatology and Outpatient Orthopedic Disorders: Diagnosis and Therapy. Stephen Paget, John F. Beary, Charles L. Christian, et. al.. Little, Brown and Company, 34 Beacon St., Boston, MA 02108. Phone: (617) 227-0730. Third edition 1992.

Synopsis of Orthopedics. H.S. An (ed.). Thieme Medical Publishers, Inc., 381 Park Ave. S., New York, NY 10016. Phone: (212) 683-5088. Fax: (212) 779-9020. 1991.

JOURNALS

Clinical Orthopedics and Related Research. J.B. Lippincott Co., 227 E. Washington Square, Philadelphia, PA 19106-3780. Phone: (215) 238-4200. Fax: (215) 238-4227.

Foot & Ankle. Williams & Wilkins, 428 E. Preston St., Baltimore, MD 21202. Phone: (800) 638-0672. Fax: (800) 447-8438. 9/year.

Journal of Bone and Joint Surgery: American Volume. Journal of Bone and Joint Surgery, Inc., 10 Shattuck St., Boston, MA 02115. Phone: (617) 734-2835. 10/year.

Journal of Orthopaedic Research. Raven Press, 1185 Avenue of the Americas, New York, NY 10036. Phone: (212) 930-9500. Fax: (212) 869-3495. Bimonthly.

Journal of Orthopaedic and Sports Physical Therapy. Williams & Wilkins, 428 E. Preston St., Baltimore, MD 21202. Phone: (800) 638-0672. Fax: (800) 447-8438. Monthly.

Journal of Shoulder and Elbow Surgery. Mosby-Year Book, 11830 Westline Industrial Drive, St. Louis, MO 63146. Phone: (800) 325-4177. Fax: (314) 432-1380. Bimonthly.

Orthopedics. SLACK Inc., 6900 Grove Rd., Thorofare, NJ 08086-9447. Phone: (800) 257-8290. Fax: (609) 853-5991. Monthly.

Seminars in Orthopedics. W.B. Saunders Co., The Curtis Center, Independence Sqare W., Philadelphia, PA 19106-3399. Phone: (215) 238-7800.

ONLINE DATABASES

EMBASE. Elsevier Science Publishing Co., Inc., P.O. Box 882, Madison Square Station, New York, NY 10159-2101. Phone: (212) 989-5800. Fax: (212) 633-3990.

MEDIS. Mead Data Central, P.O. Box 1830, Dayton, OH 45401. Phone: (800) 227-4908.

MEDLINE. National Library of Medicine, 8600 Rockville Pike, Bethesda, MD 20894. Phone: (800) 638-8480.

SciSearch. Institute for Scientific Information, 3501 Market St., Philadelphia, PA 19104. Phone: (215) 386-0100. Fax: (215) 386-6362.

RESEARCH CENTERS, INSTITUTES, CLEARINGHOUSES

Orthopaedic Biomechanics Laboratory. Shriners Hospital for Crippled Children, 1701 19th Ave., San Francisco, CA 94112. Phone: (415) 665-1100.

Orthopaedic Research Laboratories. 600 N. Wolfe St., Johns Hopkins Hospital, Baltimore, MD 21205. Phone: (301) 955-7976.

TEXTBOOKS AND MONOGRAPHS

Current Orthopaedic Practice. Philip Yeoman, Daniel M. Spangler (eds.). Butterworth-Heinemann, 80 Montvale Ave., Stoneham, MA 02180. Phone: (617) 438-8464. Fax: (617) 279-4851. 1991.

Current Surgical Diagnosis and Treatment. L.W. Way. Appleton & Lange, 25 Van Zant St., East Norwalk, CT 06855. Phone: (800) 423-1359. Fax: (203) 854-9486. Ninth edition 1990.

Flynn's Hand Surgery. Jupiter. Williams & Wilkins, 428 East Preston St., Baltimore, MD 21202. Phone: (800) 638-0672. Fax: (800) 447-8438. Fourth edition 1992.

The Hand Book. Ariyan. McGraw-Hill Inc., 11 West 19th St., New York, NY 10011. Phone: (212) 337-5001. Fax: (212) 337-4092. 1989.

Hip Arthroplasty. Harlan C. Amstutz (ed.). Churchill Livingstone Inc., 650 Avenue of the Americas, New York, NY 10011. Phone: (212) 819-5400. Fax: (212) 302-6598. 1991.

Joint Replacement. Coombs. Mosby-Year Book, 11830 Westline Industrial Drive, St. Louis, MO 63146. Phone: (800) 325-4177. Fax: (314) 432-1380. 1990.

Joint Replacement Arthroplasty. Bernard F. Morrey (ed.). Churchill Livingstone Inc., 650 Avenue of the Americas, New York, NY 10011. Phone: (212) 819-5400. Fax: (212) 302-6598. 1991.

Operative Hand Surgery. Green. Churchill Livingstone Inc., 650 Ave. of the Americas, New York, NY 10011. Phone: (212) 819-5400. Fax: (212) 302-6598. Second edition. Three volumes. 1988.

Orthopaedic Infections. Robert D. D'Ambrosia, Robert L. Marier (eds.). SLACK Inc., 6900 Grove Rd., Thorofare, NJ 08086-9447. Phone: (800) 257-8290. Fax: (609) 853-5991. 1989.

Orthopaedic MRI. Pomeranz. J.B. Lippincott Co., 227 East Washington Square, Philadelphia, PA 19106-3780. Phone: (215) 238-4200. Fax: (215) 238-4227. 1991.

Orthopaedic Rehabilitation. Vernon L. Nickel, Michael J. Botte (eds.). Churchill Livingstone Inc., 650 Avenue of the Americas, New York, NY 10011. Phone: (212) 819-5400. Fax: (212) 302-6598. Second edition 1991.

Orthopaedics. George Bentley, Robert B. Greer III (eds.). Butterworth-Heinemann, 80 Montvale Ave., Stoneham, MA 02180. Phone: (617) 438-8464. Fax: (617) 279-4851. Fourth edition 1991.

Practical Orthopedics. Lonnie R. Mercier, Fred J. Pettid, Dean F. Tamisea, et. al.. Mosby-Year Book, 11830 Westline Industrial Drive, St. Louis, MO 63146. Phone: (800) 325-4177. Fax: (314) 432-1380. Third edition 1991.

Primary and Revision Total Hip Replacement. Ross K. Leighton, James P. Waddell (eds.). SLACK Inc., 6900 Grove Rd., Thorofare, NJ 08086-9447. Phone: (800) 257-8290. Fax: (609) 853-5991. 1992.

Rehabilitation of the Hand. Hunter. Mosby-Year Book, 11830 Westline Industrial Drive, St. Louis, MO 63146. Phone: (800) 325-4177. Fax: (314) 432-1380. Third edition 1990.

OSTEOARTHRITIS

See: ARTHRITIS

OSTEOPATHY

ABSTRACTING, INDEXING, AND CURRENT AWARENESS PUBLICATIONS

Index Medicus. U.S. National Library of Medicine, 8600 Rockville Pike, Bethesda, MD 20894. Phone: (800) 638-8480. Monthly.

ASSOCIATIONS, PROFESSIONAL SOCIETIES, ADVOCACY AND SUPPORT GROUPS

American Academy of Osteopathic Surgeons (ACOS). 123 N. Henry St., Alexandria, VA 22314. Phone: (703) 684-0416.

American Academy of Osteopathy (AAO). P.O. Box 750, 1127 Mt. Vernon Rd., Newark, OH 43055. Phone: (614) 366-7911.

American Association of Colleges of Osteopathic Medicine. 6110 Executive Blvd., No. 405, Rockville, MD 20852. Phone: (201) 468-0990.

American College of General Practitioners in Osteopathic Medicine and Surgery (ACGPOMS). 330 E. Algonquin, Arlington Heights, IL 60005. Phone: (708) 228-6090.

American Osteopathic Association (AOA). 142 E. Ontario St., Chicago, IL 60611. Phone: (800) 621-1773. Fax: (312) 280-5893.

DIRECTORIES

Yearbook and Directory of Osteopathic Phyicians. American Osteopathic Association, 142 E. Ontario St., Chicago, IL 60611. Phone: (312) 280-5800. Annual.

JOURNALS

Journal of the American Osteopathic Association. American Osteopathic Association, 142 Ontario St., Chicago, IL 60611. Phone: (312) 280-5800.

Journal of Osteopathic Education. Gerneral Council of Registered Osteopaths, 56 London St., Reading, Berks. RG1 4SQ, England.

Journal of Osteopathic Sports Medicine. American Osteopathic Academy of Sports Medicine, P.O. Box 623, Middleton, WI 53562-0623.

NEWSLETTERS

American Academy of Osteopathy-Quarterly Newsletter. American Academy of Osteopathy, 12 W. Locust St., P.O.Box 750, Newark, OH 43055. Phone: (614) 349-8701. Quarterly.

ONLINE DATABASES

EMBASE. Elsevier Science Publishing Co., Inc., P.O. Box 882, Madison Square Station, New York, NY 10159-2101. Phone: (212) 989-5800. Fax: (212) 633-3990.

MEDLINE. National Library of Medicine, 8600 Rockville Pike, Bethesda, MD 20894. Phone· (800) 638-8480.

OLIO. American Osteopathic Association, 142 E. Ontario St., Chicago, IL 60611-2864. Phone: (800) 621-1773. Monthly.

SciSearch. Institute for Scientific Information, 3501 Market St., Philadelphia, PA 19104. Phone: (215) 386-0100. Fax: (215) 386-6362.

OSTEOPOROSIS

See also: BONE AND JOINT DISEASES

ABSTRACTING, INDEXING, AND CURRENT AWARENESS PUBLICATIONS

CA Selects: Osteoporosis & Related Bone Loss. Chemical Abstracts Service, 2540 Olentangy River Road, P.O. Box 3012, Columbus, OH 43210-0012. Phone: (800) 848-6538. Biweekly.

Chemical Abstracts. Chemical Abstracts Service, 2540 Olentangy River Rd., P.O. Box 3012, Columbus, OH 43210-0012. Phone: (800) 848-6538.

Current Contents/Clinical Medicine. Institute for Scientific Information, 3501 Market St., Philadelphia, PA 19104. Phone: (800) 523-1850. Fax: (215) 386-6362. Weekly.

Index Medicus. U.S. National Library of Medicine, 8600 Rockville Pike, Bethesda, MD 20894. Phone: (800) 638-8480. Monthly.

Science Citation Index. Institute for Scientific Information, 3501 Market St., Philadelphia, PA 19104. Phone: (800) 523-1850. Fax: (215) 386-6362. Bimonthly.

ANNUALS AND REVIEWS

In Development New Medicines for Arthritis. Pharmaceutical Manufacturers Association, 1100 15th St. N.W., Washington, DC 20005. Phone: (202) 835-3400. Annual.

ASSOCIATIONS, PROFESSIONAL SOCIETIES, ADVOCACY AND SUPPORT GROUPS

National Osteoporosis Foundation. 1625 Eye St. N.W., Ste. 1011, Washington, DC 20006. Phone: (202) 223-2226.

BIBLIOGRAPHIES

Osteoporosis: Causes and Treatment. National Technical Information Service, 5285 Port Royal Rd., Springfield, VA 22161. Phone: (703) 487-4650. Fax: (703) 321-8547. Jan. 1970-May 1988 PB88-863899/CBY.

Osteoporosis: Prevention and Product Marketing. National Technical Information Service, 5285 Port Royal Rd., Springfield, VA 22161. Phone: (703) 487-4650. Fax: (703) 321-8547. Jan. 1985-Feb. 1989 PB89-857239/CBY.

CD-ROM DATABASES

SCISEARCH. Institute for Scientific Information, 3501 Market St., Philadelphia, PA 19104. Phone: (215) 386-0100. Fax: (215) 386-6362.

HANDBOOKS, GUIDES, MANUALS, ATLASES

An Atlas of Osteoporosis. J.C. Stevenson, M.S. Marsh. The Parthenon Publishing Group, Inc., 120 Mill Rd., Park Ridge, NJ 07656. Phone: (201) 391-6796. 1992.

JOURNALS

American Journal of Clinical Nutrition. Waverly Press, 428 E. Preston St., Baltimore, MD 21202. Phone: (800) 638-0672. Fax: (800) 447-8438. Monthly.

Journal of Bone and Joint Surgery: American Volume. Journal of Bone and Joint Surgery, Inc., 10 Shattuck St., Boston, MA 02115. Phone: (617) 734-2835. 10/year.

Journal of Clinical Endocrinology & Metabolism. Williams & Wilkins, 428 E. Preston St., Baltimore, MD 21202. Phone: (800) 638-0672. Fax: (900) 447-8438. Monthly.

ONLINE DATABASES

CA File (Chemical Abstracts File). Chemical Abstracts Service, 2540 Olentangy River Rd., P.O. Box 3012, Columbus, OH 43210-0012. Phone: (800) 848-6538.

EMBASE. Elsevier Science Publishing Co., Inc., P.O. Box 882, Madison Square Station, New York, NY 10159-2101. Phone: (212) 989-5800. Fax: (212) 633-3990.

MEDLINE. National Library of Medicine, 8600 Rockville Pike, Bethesda, MD 20894. Phone: (800) 638-8480.

SciSearch. Institute for Scientific Information, 3501 Market St., Philadelphia, PA 19104. Phone: (215) 386-0100. Fax: (215) 386-6362.

POPULAR WORKS AND PATIENT EDUCATION

Keys to Understanding Osteoporosis. Jan Rozek. Barron's Educational Series, Inc., P.O. Box 8040, 250 Wireless Blvd.,

Hauppauge, NY 11788. Phone: (516) 434-3311. Fax: (516) 434-3723. 1992.

Osteoporosis: The Silent Thief. Williams Peck, Louis Avioli. HarperCollins Publishers, Inc., 10 E. 53rd St., New York, NY 10022-5299. Phone: (212) 207-7000. Fax: (800) 242-7737. 1988.

RESEARCH CENTERS, INSTITUTES, CLEARINGHOUSES

National Institute of Arthritis and Musculoskeletal and Skin Diseases. NIH Bldg. 31, 9000 Rockville Pike, Bethesda, MD 20892. Phone: (301) 496-4353.

Osteoporosis Center. University of Connecticut. 208 Farm Hollow, Ste. C, 309 Farmington Ave., Farmington, CT 06030. Phone: (203) 679-3855. Fax: (203) 679-1258.

TEXTBOOKS AND MONOGRAPHS

Osteoporosis: Etiology, Diagnosis, and Management. B.L. Riggs, L.J. Melton. Raven Press, 1185 Ave. of the Americas, New York, NY 10036. Phone: (212) 930-9500. Fax: (212) 869-3495. 1988.

Osteoporosis, Pathogenesis and Management. R.M. Francis. Kluwer Academic Publishers, P.O. Box 358, Accord Station, Hingham, MA 02018-0358. Phone: (617) 871-6600. Fax: (617) 871-6528. 1990.

Osteoporosis: Prevention, Management, Treatment. Harris H. McIlwain, Debra Fulghum Bruce, Joe Silverfield. John Wiley & Sons, Inc., 605 Third Ave., New York, NY 10158-0012. Phone: (212) 850-6000. Fax: (212) 850-6088. 1988.

OSTOMY

See: COLORECTAL SURGERY; STOMA

OTOLARYNGOLOGY

ABSTRACTING, INDEXING, AND CURRENT AWARENESS PUBLICATIONS

Current Contents/Clinical Medicine. Institute for Scientific Information, 3501 Market St., Philadelphia, PA 19104. Phone: (800) 523-1850. Fax: (215) 386-6362. Weekly.

Excerpta Medica. Section 11: Otorhinolaryngology. Elsevier Science Publishing Co., Inc., P.O. Box 882, Madison Square Station, New York, NY 10159-2101. Phone: (212) 989-5800. Fax: (212) 633-3990. 16/year.

Index Medicus. U.S. National Library of Medicine, 8600 Rockville Pike, Bethesda, MD 20894. Phone: (800) 638-8480. Monthly.

ANNUALS AND REVIEWS

Advances in Otolaryngology. Mosby-Year Book, 11830 Westline Industrial Drive, St. Louis, MO 63146. Phone: (800) 325-4177. Fax: (314) 432-1380. Annual.

Otolaryngologic Clinics. W.B. Saunders Co., The Curtis Center, Independence Square W., Philadelphia, PA 19106-3399. Phone: (215) 238-7800. Bimonthly.

Year Book of Otolaryngology-Head and Neck Surgery. Mosby-Year Book, 11830 Westline Industrial Drive, St. Louis, MO 63146. Phone: (800) 325-4177. Fax: (314) 432-1380. Annual.

ASSOCIATIONS, PROFESSIONAL SOCIETIES, ADVOCACY AND SUPPORT GROUPS

American Academy of Otolaryngology - Head and Neck Surgery (AAO-HNS). 1 Prince St., Alexandria, VA 22314. Phone: (703) 836-4444. Fax: (703) 683-5100.

American Board of Otolaryngology (ABO). 5615 Kirby Dr., Ste. 936, Houston, TX 77005. Phone: (713) 528-6200.

CD-ROM DATABASES

Pediatric Cough. Hoffer. Williams & Wilkins, 428 East Preston St., Baltimore, MD 21202. Phone: (800) 638-0672. Fax: (800) 447-8438. 1990.

DIRECTORIES

Directory of Certified Otolaryngologists. American Board of Medical Specialties, 1 Rotary Center, Suite 805, Evanston, IL 60201. Phone: (708) 491-9091. Biennial.

Directory of Medical Specialists. Marquis Who's Who, 3002 Glenview Rd., Wilmette, IL 60091. Phone: (800) 621-9669. Fax: (708) 441-2264. Biennial.

Directory of Physicians in the United States. American Medical Association, 515 North State St., Chicago, IL 60610. Phone: (312) 464-0183. Fax: (312) 464-5834. Biennial.

ENCYCLOPEDIAS, DICTIONARIES, WORD BOOKS

Dental and Otolaryngology Word Book. Helen E. Littrell. Springhouse Publishing Co., 1111 Bethlehem Pike, Spring House, PA 19477. Phone: (800) 331-3170. Fax: (215) 646-8716. 1992.

HANDBOOKS, GUIDES, MANUALS, ATLASES

Clinical Manual of Otolaryngology. Davidson. McGraw-Hill Inc., 11 West 19th St., New York, NY 10011. Phone: (212) 337-5001. Fax: (212) 337-4092. Second edition 1992.

A Color Atlas of Ear, Nose and Throat Diagnosis. T.R. Bull (ed.). Mosby-Year Book, 11830 Westline Industrial Drive, St. Louis, MO 63146. Phone: (800) 325-4177. Fax: (314) 432-1380. 2nd edition.

Manual of Otolaryngology: Diagnosis and Treatment. Strome Marshall, Marving Fried, James Kelly (eds.). Little, Brown and Company, 34 Beacon St., Boston, MA 02108. Phone: (617) 227-0730. Second edition 1992.

Otolaryngology On Call. Terence M. Davidson. McGraw-Hill, Inc., 1221 Avenue of the Americas, 28th Floor, New York, NY 10020. Phone: (212) 512-4228. Second edition 1992.

JOURNALS

American Journal of Otolaryngology. W.B. Saunders Co., The Curtis Center, Independence Sqare W., Philadelphia, PA 19106-3399. Phone: (215) 238-7800.

American Journal of Otology. Mosby-Year Book, 11830 Westline Industrial Drive, St. Louis, MO 63146. Phone: (800) 325-4177. Fax: (314) 432-1380.

Annals of Otology, Rhinology & Laryngology. Annals Publishing Co., 4507 Laclede Ave., St. Louis, MO 63108. Phone: (314) 367-4987. Fax: (314) 367-4988. Monthly.

Archives of Otolaryngology-Head & Neck Surgery. American Medical Association, 515 North State St., Chicago, IL 60610. Phone: (312) 464-0183. Fax: (312) 464-5834. Monthly.

Clinical Otolaryngology. Blackwell Scientific Publications, Inc., 3 Cambridge Ctr., Cambridge, MA 02142. Phone: (800) 759-6102. Bimonthly.

Ear, Nose and Throat Journal. Little, Brown and Co., 34 Beacon St., Boston, MA 02108. Phone: (617) 227-0730. Fax: (617) 227-0790.

International Journal of Pediatric Otorhinolaryngology. Elsevier Science Publishing Co., Inc., P.O. Box 882, Madison Square Station, New York, NY 10159-2101. Phone: (212) 989-5800. Fax: (212) 633-3990. 6/year.

Journal of Laryngology and Otology. Headley Bros. Ltd., Invicta Press, Ashford, Kent TN24 8HH, England. Monthly.

Laryngoscope. Trialogical Foundation Inc., 9216 Clayton Rd., St. Louis, MO 63124. Phone: (314) 997-5070.

ONLINE DATABASES

EMBASE. Elsevier Science Publishing Co., Inc., P.O. Box 882, Madison Square Station, New York, NY 10159-2101. Phone: (212) 989-5800. Fax: (212) 633-3990.

MEDIS. Mead Data Central, P.O. Box 1830, Dayton, OH 45401. Phone: (800) 227-4908.

MEDLINE. National Library of Medicine, 8600 Rockville Pike, Bethesda, MD 20894. Phone: (800) 638-8480.

SciSearch. Institute for Scientific Information, 3501 Market St., Philadelphia, PA 19104. Phone: (215) 386-0100. Fax: (215) 386-6362.

TEXTBOOKS AND MONOGRAPHS

Clinical Geriatric Otorhinolaryngology. Kashima. Mosby-Year Book, 11830 Westline Industrial Drive, St. Louis, MO 63146. Phone: (800) 325-4177. Fax: (314) 432-1380. Second edition 1992.

Clinical Otoscopy: An Introduction to Ear Diseases. Michael Hawke, Malcolm Keene, Peter W. Alberti. Churchill Livingstone Inc., 650 Avenue of the Americas, New York, NY 10011. Phone: (212) 819-5400. Fax: (212) 302-6598. Second edition 1990.

Core Otolaryngology. Koufman. J.B. Lippincott Co., 227 E. Washington Square, Philadelphia, PA 19106-3780. Phone: (215) 238-4200. Fax: (215) 238-4227. 1990.

Diseases of the Nose, Throat, Ear, head, and Neck. Ballenger. Williams & Wilkins, 428 East Preston St., Baltimore, MD 21202. Phone: (800) 638-0672. Fax: (800) 447-8438. 14th edition 1991.

Diseases of the Vocal Tract. Gould. Mosby-Year Book, 11830 Westline Industrial Drive, St. Louis, MO 63146. Phone: (800) 325-4177. Fax: (314) 432-1380. 1992.

Ear, Nose and Throat Diseases. Becker. Thieme Medical Publishers, Inc., 381 Park Ave. S., New York, NY 10016.

Phone: (212) 683-5088. Fax: (212) 779-9020. Fourth edition 1991.

Essentials of Otolaryngology. Frank E. Lucente, Steven M. Sobol. Raven Press, 1185 Avenue of the Americas, New York, NY 10036. Phone: (212) 930-9500. Fax: (212) 869-3495. Second edition 1988.

A New Short Textbook of Otolaryngology. M.S. McCormick, W.J. Primrose. Sheridan House, Inc., 145 Palisade St., Dobbs Ferry, NY 10522. Phone: (914) 693-2410. Third edition 1992.

Otolaryngology. Cummings. Mosby-Year Book, 11830 Westline Industrial Drive, St. Louis, MO 63146. Phone: (800) 325-4177. Fax: (314) 432-1380. Four volumes. Second edition. 1992.

Otolaryngology-Head and Neck Surgery. Charles W. Cummings, John M. Frederickson, Lee H. Harker. Mosby-Year Book, 11830 Westline Industrial Drive, St. Louis, MO 63146. Phone: (800) 325-4177. Fax: (314) 432-1380. Second edition 1992.

Practical Endoscopic Sinus Surgery. Vijay K. Anand, William R. Panje. McGraw-Hill, Inc., Health Professions Division, 1221 Avenue of the Americas, 28th Floor, New York, NY 10020. Phone: (212) 512-4228. 1992.

Synopsis of Otolaryngology. Roger Gray, Maurice R. Hawthorne. Butterworth-Heinemann, 80 Montvale Ave., Stoneham, MA 02180. Phone: (617) 438-8464. Fax: (617) 279-4851. Fifth edition 1991.

Textbook of Otolaryngology. Deweese. Mosby-Year Book, 11830 Westline Industrial Drive, St. Louis, MO 63146. Phone: (800) 325-4177. Fax: (314) 432-1380. Seventh edition 1988.

OTOLARYNGOLOGY - HEAD AND NECK SURGERY

ABSTRACTING, INDEXING, AND CURRENT AWARENESS PUBLICATIONS

Excerpta Medica. Section 11: Otorhinolaryngology. Elsevier Science Publishing Co., Inc., P.O. Box 882, Madison Square Station, New York, NY 10159-2101. Phone: (212) 989-5800. Fax: (212) 633-3990. 16/year.

ANNUALS AND REVIEWS

Advances in Otolaryngology. Mosby-Year Book, 11830 Westline Industrial Drive, St. Louis, MO 63146. Phone: (800) 325-4177. Fax: (314) 432-1380. Annual.

Otolaryngologic Clinics. W.B. Saunders Co., The Curtis Center, Independence Square W., Philadelphia, PA 19106-3399. Phone: (215) 238-7800. Bimonthly.

ASSOCIATIONS, PROFESSIONAL SOCIETIES, ADVOCACY AND SUPPORT GROUPS

American Academy of Otolaryngology - Head and Neck Surgery (AAO-HNS). 1 Prince St., Alexandria, VA 22314. Phone: (703) 836-4444. Fax: (703) 683-5100.

American Board of Otolaryngology (ABO). 5615 Kirby Dr., Ste. 936, Houston, TX 77005. Phone: (713) 528-6200.

DIRECTORIES

Directory of Certified Otolaryngologists. American Board of Medical Specialties, 1 Rotary Center, Suite 805, Evanston, IL 60201. Phone: (708) 491-9091. Biennial.

ENCYCLOPEDIAS, DICTIONARIES, WORD BOOKS

Surgery on File: Eye, Ear, Nose and Throat Surgery. The Diagram Group. Facts on File, Inc., 460 Park Ave. S., New York, NY 10016-7382. Phone: (212) 683-2244. 1988.

HANDBOOKS, GUIDES, MANUALS, ATLASES

Atlas of Head and Neck Surgery. Johns. Mosby-Year Book, 11830 Westline Industrial Drive, St. Louis, MO 63146. Phone: (800) 325-4177. Fax: (314) 432-1380. Volume I 1990.

JOURNALS

Annals of Otology, Rhinology & Laryngology. Annals Publishing Co., 4507 Laclede Ave., St. Louis, MO 63108. Phone: (314) 367-4987. Fax: (314) 367-4988. Monthly.

Archives of Otolaryngology-Head & Neck Surgery. American Medical Association, 515 North State St., Chicago, IL 60610. Phone: (312) 464-0183. Fax: (312) 464-5834. Monthly.

Journal of Laryngology and Otology. Headley Bros. Ltd., Invicta Press, Ashford, Kent TN24 8HH, England. Monthly.

POPULAR WORKS AND PATIENT EDUCATION

Looking Forward: A Guidebook for the Laryngectomee. R.L. Keith. Thieme Medical Publishers, Inc., 381 Park Ave. S., New York, NY 10016. Phone: (212) 683-5088. Fax: (212) 779-9020. Second edition 1991.

TEXTBOOKS AND MONOGRAPHS

Complications in Head and Neck Surgery. Dana Eisele. Mosby-Year Book, 11830 Westline Industrial Drive, St. Louis, MO 63146. Phone: (800) 325-4177. Fax: (314) 432-1380. 2nd edition, 1992.

Essential Otolaryngology of the Head and Neck. Lee. Elsevier Science Publishing Co., Inc., P.O. Box 882, Madison Square Station, New York, NY 10159-2101. Phone: (212) 989-5800. Fax: (212) 633-3990. Fifth edition 1991.

Head and Neck Microsurgery. William M. Swartz, Joseph C. Banis. Williams & Wilkins, 428 East Preston St., Baltimore, MD 21202. Phone: (800) 638-0672. Fax: (800) 447-8438. 1992.

Otolaryngology-Head and Neck Surgery. Charles W. Cummings, John M. Frederickson, Lee H. Harker. Mosby-Year Book, 11830 Westline Industrial Drive, St. Louis, MO 63146. Phone: (800) 325-4177. Fax: (314) 432-1380. Second edition 1992.

Reconstruction of the Lip. K.H. Calhoun, C.M. Stiernberg (eds.). Thieme Medical Publishers, Inc., 381 Park Ave. S., New York, NY 10016. Phone: (212) 683-5088. Fax: (212) 779-9020. 1991.

OTORHINOLARYNGOLOGIC DISEASES

See: OTOLARYNGOLOGY

OVARIAN CANCER

See also: CANCER

ABSTRACTING, INDEXING, AND CURRENT AWARENESS PUBLICATIONS

Core Journals in Obstetrics and Gynecology. Elsevier Science Publishing Co., Inc., P.O. Box 882, Madison Square Station, New York, NY 10159-2101. Phone: (212) 989-5800. Fax: (212) 633-3990. 11/year.

Current Contents/Clinical Medicine. Institute for Scientific Information, 3501 Market St., Philadelphia, PA 19104. Phone: (800) 523-1850. Fax: (215) 386-6362. Weekly.

Excerpta Medica. Section 10: Obstetrics and Gynecology. Elsevier Science Publishing Co., Inc., P.O. Box 882, Madison Square Station, New York, NY 10159-2101. Phone: (212) 989-5800. Fax: (212) 633-3990. 20/year.

Excerpta Medica. Section 16: Cancer. Elsevier Science Publishing Co., Inc., P.O. Box 882, Madison Square Station, New York, NY 10159-2101. Phone: (212) 989-5800. Fax: (212) 633-3990. 32/year.

ICRDB Cancergram: Gynecologic Tumors--Diagnosis, Treatment. U.S. Government Printing Office, Superintendent of Documents, P.O. Box 371954, Pittsburgh, PA 15250-7954. Phone: (202) 783-3238. Fax: (202) 512-2250. Monthly.

Index Medicus. U.S. National Library of Medicine, 8600 Rockville Pike, Bethesda, MD 20894. Phone: (800) 638-8480. Monthly.

Research Alert: Cancer-Female Reproductive Tract. Institute for Scientific Information, 3501 Market St., Philadelphia, PA 19104. Phone: (800) 523-1850. Fax: (215) 386-6362. Weekly.

Science Citation Index. Institute for Scientific Information, 3501 Market St., Philadelphia, PA 19104. Phone: (800) 523-1850. Fax: (215) 386-6362. Bimonthly.

ANNUALS AND REVIEWS

Advances in Cancer Research. Academic Press, Inc., 1250 Sixth Ave., San Diego, CA 92101-4311. Phone: (619) 699-6345. Fax: (619) 699-6715. Irregular.

Critical Reviews in Oncogenesis. CRC Press, Inc., 2000 Corporate Blvd. N.W., Boca Raton, FL 33431. Phone: (407) 994-0555. Fax: (407) 997-0949. 6/year.

Critical Reviews in Oncology/Hematology. Elsevier Science Publishing Co., Inc., P.O. Box 882, Madison Square Station, New York, NY 10159-2101. Phone: (212) 989-5800. Fax: (212) 633-3990. Quarterly.

Current Opinion in Oncology. Current Science Ltd., 20 N. Third St., Philadelphia, PA 19106-2199. Phone: (800) 552-5866. Fax: (215) 574-2270. Bimonthly.

Current Problems in Cancer. Mosby-Year Book, 11830 Westline Industrial Drive, St. Louis, MO 63146. Phone: (800) 325-4177. Fax: (314) 432-1380. Bimonthly.

In Development New Medicines for Older Americans. 1991 Annual Survey. More Medicines in Testing for Cancer Than for Any Other Disease of Aging. Pharmaceutical Manufacturers Association, 1100 15th St. N.W., Washington, DC 20005. Phone: (202) 835-3400. 1991.

Progress in Cancer Research and Therapy. Raven Press, 1185 Avenue of the Americas, New York, NY 10036. Phone: (212) 930-9500. Fax: (212) 869-3495. Irregular.

Seminars in Oncology. W.B. Saunders Co., The Curtis Center, Independence Square W., Philadelphia, PA 19106-3399. Phone: (215) 238-7800. Bimonthly.

Seminars in Surgical Oncology. John Wiley & Sons, Inc., 605 Third Ave., New York, NY 10158-0012. Phone: (212) 850-6000. Fax: (212) 850-6088. Quarterly.

Year Book of Oncology. Mosby-Year Book, 11830 Westline Industrial Drive, St. Louis, MO 63146. Phone: (800) 325-4177. Fax: (314) 432-1380. Annual.

ASSOCIATIONS, PROFESSIONAL SOCIETIES, ADVOCACY AND SUPPORT GROUPS

American Cancer Society (ACS). 1599 Clifton Rd. N.E., Atlanta, GA 30329. Phone: (404) 320-3333.

Society of Gynecologic Oncologists. 111 Wacker Dr., Chicago, IL 60601. Phone: (312) 644-6610.

CD-ROM DATABASES

Cancer-CD. SilverPlatter Information, Inc., River Ridge Office Park, 100 River Ridge Rd., Norwood, MA 02062. Phone: (617) 769-2599. Fax: (617) 769-8763. Quarterly.

Cancer on Disc. CMC ReSearch, Inc., 7150 S.W. Hampton, Suite C-120, Portland, OR 97223. Phone: (800) 262-7668. Fax: (503) 639-1796. Annual.

Cancerlit. Aries Systems Corporation, One Dundee Park, Andover, MA 01810. Phone: (508) 475-7200. Fax: (508) 474-8860. Quarterly.

Cancerlit CD-ROM. Cambridge Scientific Abstracts, 7200 Wisconsin Ave., Bethesda, MD 20814-4823. Phone: (800) 843-7751. Fax: (301) 961-6720. Quarterly.

Excerpta Medica CD: Obstetrics & Gynecology. SilverPlatter Information, Inc., River Ridge Office Park, 100 River Ridge Rd., Norwood, MA 02062. Phone: (617) 769-2599. Fax: (617) 769-8763. Quarterly.

OncoDisc. J.B. Lippincott Co., 227 East Washington Square, Philadelphia, PA 19106-3780. Phone: (215) 238-4200. Fax: (215) 238-4227. Bimonthly.

SCISEARCH. Institute for Scientific Information, 3501 Market St., Philadelphia, PA 19104. Phone: (215) 386-0100. Fax: (215) 386-6362.

Year Books on Disc. CMC ReSearch, Inc., 7150 S.W. Hampton, Suite C-120, Portland, OR 97223. Phone: (800) 262-7668. Fax: (503) 639-1796. Annual includes Year Books of Cardiology, Dermatology, Diagnostic Radiology, Drug Therapy, Emergency Medicine, Family Practice, Medicine,

Neurology and Neurosurgery, Obstetrics and Gynecology, Oncology, Pediatrics, and Psychiatry and Applied Mental Health.

ENCYCLOPEDIAS, DICTIONARIES, WORD BOOKS

Oncology Words. Stedman. Williams & Wilkins, 428 East Preston St., Baltimore, MD 21202. Phone: (800) 638-0672. Fax: (800) 447-8438. 1992.

HANDBOOKS, GUIDES, MANUALS, ATLASES

Manual of Gynecologic Oncology. J.H. Shepherd, J.M. Monaghan (eds.). Churchill Livingstone Inc., 650 Ave. of the Americas, New York, NY 10011. Phone: (212) 819-5400. Fax: (212) 302-6598. 1989.

Manual of Gynecologic Oncology and Gynecology. M. Steven Piver. Little, Brown and Company, 34 Beacon St., Boston, MA 02108. Phone: (617) 227-0730. 1989.

JOURNALS

American Journal of Clinical Oncology. Raven Press, 1185 Ave. of the Americas, New York, NY 10036. Phone: (212) 930-9500. Fax: (212) 869-3495. Bimonthly.

American Journal of Obstetrics and Gynecology. Mosby-Year Book, 11830 Westline Industrial Drive, St. Louis, MO 63146. Phone: (800) 325-4177. Fax: (314) 432-1380. Monthly.

British Journal of Obstetrics & Gynaecology. Blackwell Publishers, Three Cambridge Center, Cambridge, MA 02142. Phone: (617) 225-0430. Fax: (617) 494-1437. Monthly.

Cancer. J.B. Lippincott Co., 227 East Washington Square, Philadelphia, PA 19106-3780. Phone: (215) 238-4200. Fax: (215) 238-4227. Semimonthly.

Cancer Causes and Control. Rapid Communications of Oxford Ltd., The Old Malthouse, Paradise St., Oxford OX1 1LD, England. Phone: 44-865-790447. Fax: 44-865-244012. 6/year.

Gynecologic Oncology. Academic Press, Inc., 1250 Sixth Ave., San Diego, CA 92101-4311. Phone: (619) 699-6345. Fax: (619) 699-6715. Monthly.

Journal of Clinical Oncology. W.B. Saunders Co., The Curtis Center, Independence Square W., Philadelphia, PA 19106-3399. Phone: (215) 238-7800. Monthly.

Journal of the National Cancer Institute. Superintendent of Documents, P.O. Box 371954, Pittsburgh, PA 15250-7954. Fax: (202) 512-2233. Semimonthly.

Journal of Women's Health. Mary Ann Liebert, Inc., 1651 Third Ave., New York, NY 10128. Phone: (212) 289-2300. Fax: (212) 289-4697. Quarterly.

Obstetrics and Gynecology. Elsevier Science Publishing Co., Inc., P.O. Box 882, Madison Square Station, New York, NY 10159-2101. Phone: (212) 989-5800. Fax: (212) 633-3990. 15/year.

ONLINE DATABASES

Cancer Weekly. CDC AIDS Weekly/NCI Cancer Weekly, 206 Rogers St. NE, Suite 104, P.O. Box 5528, Atlanta, GA 30317. Phone: (404) 377-8895. Weekly.

CANCERLIT. U.S. National Cancer Institute, International Cancer Information Center, Building 82, Room 102, Bethesda, MD 20892. Phone: (301) 496-7403. Fax: (301) 480-8105. Monthly.

CANCERNET (International Database on Oncology). CANCERNET/Centre National de la Recherche Scientifique, 15 quai Anatole France, F-75700 Paris, France. Phone: 01-46771616.

Clinical Protocols. U.S. National Cancer Institute, International Cancer Information Center, Building 82, Room 102, Bethesda, MD 20892. Phone: (301) 496-7403. Fax: (301) 480-8105.

EMBASE. Elsevier Science Publishing Co., Inc., P.O. Box 882, Madison Square Station, New York, NY 10159-2101. Phone: (212) 989-5800. Fax: (212) 633-3990.

MEDLINE. National Library of Medicine, 8600 Rockville Pike, Bethesda, MD 20894. Phone: (800) 638-8480.

Physician Data Query (PDQ) Cancer Information File. U.S. National Cancer Institute, International Cancer Information Center, Building 82, Room 102, Bethesda, MD 20892. Phone: (301) 496-7403. Fax: (301) 480-8105. Monthly.

Physician Data Query (PDQ) Protocol File. U.S. National Cancer Institute, International Cancer Information Center, Building 82, Room 102, Bethesda, MD 20892. Phone: (301) 496-7403. Fax: (301) 480-8105. Monthly.

SciSearch. Institute for Scientific Information, 3501 Market St., Philadelphia, PA 19104. Phone: (215) 386-0100. Fax: (215) 386-6362.

POPULAR WORKS AND PATIENT EDUCATION

Cancervive: The Challenge of Life After Cancer. Susan Nessim, Judith Ellis. Houghton Mifflin Co., 1 Beacon St., Boston, MA 02108. Phone: (800) 225-3362. 1991.

Every Woman's Medical Handbook. Marie Stoppard. Ballantine Books, Inc., 201 E. 50th St., New York, NY 10022. Phone: (800) 733-3000. 1991.

If It Runs In Your Family: Ovarian and Uterine Cancer. Sherilynn J. Hummel. Bantam Books, Inc., 666 Fifth Ave., New York, NY 10103. Phone: (800) 223-6834. 1992.

Women Talk about Gynecological Surgery: From Diagnosis to Recovery. Amy Gross, Dee Ito. HarperCollins Pubs., Inc., 10 E. 53rd St., New York, NY 10022-5299. Phone: (212) 207-7000. Fax: (800) 242-7737. 1992.

Women's Cancers: How to Prevent Them, How to Treat Them, How to Beat Them. Donna Dawson, Marlene Mersch (eds.). Hunter House, Inc., 2200 Central, Ste. 202, Alameda, CA 94501-4451. Phone: (510) 865-5282. 1992.

RESEARCH CENTERS, INSTITUTES, CLEARINGHOUSES

Cancer Information Service (CIS). Office of Cancer Communications, National Cancer Institute, Bldg. 31, Rm. 10A24, 9000 Rockville Pike, Bethesda, MD 20892. Phone: (800) 4CA-NCER.

Gynecologic Oncology Group. 1234 Market St., No. 1945, Philadelphia, PA 19107.

Ohio State University Comprehensive Cancer Center. 410 W. 12th Ave., Columbus, OH 43210. Phone: (614) 293-8729.

TEXTBOOKS AND MONOGRAPHS

Cancer: Principles and Practice of Oncology. Vincent T. DeVita. J.B. Lippincott Co., 227 E. Washington Square, Philadelphia, PA 19106-3780. Phone: (215) 238-4200. Fax: (215) 238-4227. 1989 3rd edtion.

Chemotherapy of Gynecologic Cancer. Gunter Deppe (ed.). John Wiley & Sons, Inc., 605 Third Ave., New York, NY 10158-0012. Phone: (212) 850-6000. Fax: (212) 850-6088. Second edition 1989.

Clinical Gynecologic Oncology. Philip J. DiSaia, William T. Creasman. Mosby-Year Book, 11830 Westline Industrial Drive, St. Louis, MO 63146. Phone: (800) 325-4177. Fax: (314) 432-1380. Fourth edition 1992.

Gynecologic Oncology. Robert C. Knapp, Ross Berkowitz. McGraw-Hill Inc., 11 West 19th St., New York, NY 10011. Phone: (212) 337-5001. Fax: (212) 337-4092. Second edition 1992.

Gynecological Cancer. P. Bellfort, and others (eds.). The Parthenon Publishing Group, Inc., 120 Mill Rd., Park Ridge, NJ 07656. Phone: (201) 391-6796. 1989 Advances in Gynecology & Obstetrics Series.

Multimodal Treatment of Ovarian Cancer. Pier Franco Conte, Nicola Ragni, Riccardo Rosso, et. al.. Raven Press, 1185 Avenue of the Americas, New York, NY 10036. Phone: (212) 930-9500. Fax: (212) 869-3495. European Organization for Research and Treatment of Cancer [EORTC] Monograph Series, Vol. 20 1989.

Ovarian Cancer. Stephen C. Rubin, Gregory P. Sutton. McGraw-Hill, Inc., Health Professions Division, 1221 Avenue of the Americas, 28th Floor, New York, NY 10020. Phone: (212) 512-4228. 1992.

Ovarian Pathology. F. Nogales. Springer-Verlag New York Inc., 175 Fifth Ave., New York, NY 10010. Phone: (212) 460-1500. Fax: (212) 473-6272. 1989 Current Topics in Pathology Series, Volume 78.

Principles and Practice of Gynecologic Oncology. William J. Hoskins, and others. J.B. Lippincott Co., 227 E. Washington Square, Philadelphia, PA 19106-3780. Phone: (215) 238-4200. Fax: (215) 238-4227. 1992.

TeLinde's Operative Gynecology. John D. Thompson, John A. Rock. J.B. Lippincott Co., 227 East Washington Square, Philadelphia, PA 19106-3780. Phone: (215) 238-4200. Fax: (215) 238-4227. Seventh edition 1991.

OVER-THE-COUNTER DRUGS

See: NON-PRESCRIPTION DRUGS

P

PACEMAKERS

See: HEART DISEASES; MEDICAL DEVICES AND INSTRUMENTATION

PAGET'S DISEASE

See: BONE AND JOINT DISEASES

PAIN

See also: HEADACHE

ABSTRACTING, INDEXING, AND CURRENT AWARENESS PUBLICATIONS

Current Contents/Clinical Medicine. Institute for Scientific Information, 3501 Market St., Philadelphia, PA 19104. Phone: (800) 523-1850. Fax: (215) 386-6362. Weekly.

Index Medicus. U.S. National Library of Medicine, 8600 Rockville Pike, Bethesda, MD 20894. Phone: (800) 638-8480. Monthly.

ANNUALS AND REVIEWS

Advances in Pain Research and Therapy. Raven Press, 1185 Ave. of the Americas, New York, NY 10036. Phone: (212) 930-9500. Fax: (212) 869-3495. Irregular.

Current Management of Pain. Kluwer Academic Publishers, P.O. Box 358, Accord Station, Hingham, MA 02018-0358. Phone: (617) 871-6600. Fax: (617) 871-6528. Irregular.

ASSOCIATIONS, PROFESSIONAL SOCIETIES, ADVOCACY AND SUPPORT GROUPS

American Chronic Pain Association (ACPA). 257 Old Haymaker Rd., Monroeville, PA 15146. Phone: (412) 856-9672.

American Pain Society (APS). 5700 Old Orchard Rd., 1st Flr., Skokie, IL 60077-1024. Phone: (708) 966-5595. Fax: (708) 966-9418.

International Association for the Study of Pain (IASP). 909 NE 43rd St., Ste. 306, Seattle, WA 98105. Phone: (206) 547-6409. Fax: (206) 547-1703.

National Committee on the Treatment of Intractable Pain (NCTIP). P.O. Box 9553, Friendship Sta., Washington, DC 20016. Phone: (202) 965-7617.

National Headache Foundation. 5252 N. Western Ave., Chicago, IL 60625. Phone: (312) 878-7715. Fax: (312) 878-2782.

DIRECTORIES

Directory of Pain Treatment Centers in the U.S. and Canada. Oryx Press, 4041 N. Central, Suite 700, Phoenix, AZ 85012. Phone: (800) 279-ORYX. Fax: (800) 279-4663. 1989.

International Association for the Study of Pain-Directory of Members. International Association for the Study of Pain, 909 NE 43rd St., St. 306, Seattle, WA 98105. Phone: (206) 547-6409. Fax: (206) 547-1703.

HANDBOOKS, GUIDES, MANUALS, ATLASES

Handbook of Chronic Pain Management. C. David Tollison, C. Glenn Trent, John R. Satterthwaite. Williams & Wilkins, 428 E. Preston St., Baltimore, MD 21202. Phone: (800) 638-0672. Fax: (800) 447-8438. 1988.

Manual of Pain Management. Carol A. Warfield (ed.). J.B. Lippincott Co., 227 East Washington Square, Philadelphia, PA 19106-3780. Phone: (215) 238-4200. Fax: (215) 238-4227. 1991.

The Pain Clinic Manual. Stephen E. Abram, J. David Haddox, Robert E. Kettler (eds.). J.B. Lippincott Co., 227 East Washington Square, Philadelphia, PA 19106-3780. Phone: (215) 238-4200. Fax: (215) 238-4227. 1990.

JOURNALS

Clinical Journal of Pain. Raven Press, 1185 Avenue of the Americas, New York, NY 10036. Phone: (212) 930-9500. Fax: (212) 869-3495. Quarterly.

Journal of Pain and Symptom Management. Elsevier Science Publishing Co., Inc., P.O. Box 882, Madison Square Station, New York, NY 10159-2101. Phone: (212) 989-5800. Fax: (212) 633-3990. 8/year.

Journal of Pharmaceutical Care in Pain & Symptom Control. Haworth Press, 10 Alice Street, Binghamton, NY 13904-1580. Phone: (800) 3HA-WORTH. Fax: (607) 722-1424. Quarterly.

Pain. Elsevier Science Publishing Co., Inc., P.O. Box 882, Madison Square Station, New York, NY 10159-2101. Phone: (212) 989-5800. Fax: (212) 633-3990. 12/year.

Pain Digest: An International Journal. Springer Publishing Co., Inc., 536 Broadway, 11th Floor, New York, NY 10012. Phone: (212) 431-4370. Quarterly.

Pain and Headache. S. Karger Publishers, Inc., 26 West Avon Rd., P.O. Box 529, Farmington, CT 06085. Phone: (203) 675-7834. Fax: (203) 675-7302. Irregular.

Topics in Pain Management: Current Concepts and Treatment Strategies. Williams & Wilkins, 428 E. Preston St., Baltimore, MD 21202. Phone: (800) 638-0672. Fax: (800) 447-8438. Monthly.

ONLINE DATABASES

EMBASE. Elsevier Science Publishing Co., Inc., P.O. Box 882, Madison Square Station, New York, NY 10159-2101. Phone: (212) 989-5800. Fax: (212) 633-3990.

MEDLINE. National Library of Medicine, 8600 Rockville Pike, Bethesda, MD 20894. Phone: (800) 638-8480.

SciSearch. Institute for Scientific Information, 3501 Market St., Philadelphia, PA 19104. Phone: (215) 386-0100. Fax: (215) 386-6362.

POPULAR WORKS AND PATIENT EDUCATION

The Challenge of Pain. Ronald Melzack, Patrick Wall. Viking Penguin, 375 Hudson St., New York, NY 10014-3657. Phone: (800) 331-4624. 1989.

Chronic Muscle Pain Syndrome. Paul Davidson. Random House, Inc., 201 E. 50th St., New York, NY 10022. Phone: (800) 726-0600. 1989.

Defeating Pain: The War Against a Silent Epidemic. Patrick D. Wall, Mervyn Jones. Plenum Publishing Co., 233 Spring St., New York, NY 10013-1578. Phone: (212) 620-8000. Fax: (212) 463-0742. 1991.

The Fight Against Pain. Charles B. Stacy, Andrew S. Kaplan, Gray Williams. Consumer Reports Books, 9180 LeSaint Dr., Fairfield, OH 45014. Phone: (513) 860-1178. 1992.

The Prevention Pain-Relief System: A Total Program for Relieving Any Pain in Your Body. Editors of Prevention Magazine. Rodale Press, Inc., 33 E. Minor St., Emmaus, PA 18098. Phone: (800) 527-8200. Fax: (215) 967-6263. 1992.

You Can Relieve Pain: How Guided Imagery Can Help You Reduce Pain or Eliminate It Altogether. Ken Dachman, John Lyons. HarperCollins Pubs., Inc., 10 E. 53rd St., New York, NY 10022-5299. Phone: (212) 207-7000. Fax: (800) 242-7737. 1991.

RESEARCH CENTERS, INSTITUTES, CLEARINGHOUSES

Division of Pain Management. Department of Anesthesia, Massachusetts General Hospital, Boston, MA 02114.

Pain Center. University of Alabama at Birmingham. UAB Medical Center, 1813 6th Ave., Birmingham, AL 35233. Phone: (205) 934-6174.

Pain Management Program. Dept. of Anesthesiology and Critical Care Medicine, University of Pennsylvaniea, 3400 Spruce St., Philadelphia, PA 19102.

TEXTBOOKS AND MONOGRAPHS

Acute Pain Management in Adults: Operative Procedures. Quick Reference Guide for Clinicians. Agency for Health Care Policy and Research, 18-12 Parklawn Bldg., Rockville, MD 20857. Phone: (301) 443-4100. AHCPR Pub. No. 92-0019.

Acute Pain Management in Infants, Children, and Adolescents: Operative and Medical Procedures. Quick Reference Guide for Clinicians. Agency for Health Care Policy and Research, 18-12 Parklawn Bldg., Rockville, MD 20857. Phone: (301) 443-4100. AHCPR Pub. No. 92-0020.

Acute Pain: Mechanisms and Management. Raymond S. Sinatra, Allen H. Hord, Brian Ginsberg, et. al.. Mosby-Year Book, 11830 Westline Industrial Drive, St. Louis, MO 63146. Phone: (800) 325-4177. Fax: (314) 432-1380. 1992.

Decision Making in Pain Management. Somayaji Ramamurthy, James N. Rogers. Mosby-Year Book, 11830 Westline Industrial Drive, St. Louis, MO 63146. Phone: (800) 325-4177. Fax: (314) 432-1380. 1992.

Differential Diagnosis of Acute Pain. Stanley L. Wiener. McGraw-Hill, Inc., Health Professions Division, 1221 Avenue of the Americas, 28th Floor, New York, NY 10020. Phone: (212) 512-4228. 1992.

Low Back Pain: An Historical and Contemporary Overview of the Occupational, Medical and Psychosocial Issues of Chronic Back Pain. Peter Mandell, Marvin H. Lipton, Joseph Burnstein, and others. SLACK Inc., 6900 Grove Rd., Thorofare, NJ 08086-9447. Phone: (800) 257-8290. Fax: (609) 853-5991. 1989.

The Management of Pain. John J. Bonica, John D. Loeser, C. Richard Chapman, et. al.. Williams & Wilkins, 428 East Preston St., Baltimore, MD 21202. Phone: (800) 638-0672. Fax: (800) 447-8438. Second edition. Two volumes. 1990.

Pain Management. Judith Watt-Wattson (ed.). Mosby-Year Book, 11830 Westline Industrial Drive, St. Louis, MO 63146. Phone: (800) 325-4177. Fax: (314) 432-1380. 1992.

Pain: Mechanisms and Management. Howard L. Fields. McGraw-Hill Inc., 11 West 19th St., New York, NY 10011. Phone: (212) 337-5001. Fax: (212) 337-4092. Second edition 1992.

Patient-Controlled Analgesia. F.M. Ferrante, and others (eds.). Blackwell Scientific Publications, Inc., 3 Cambridge Center, Cambridge, MA 02142. Phone: (800) 759-6102. 1990.

Textbook of Pain. Patrick D. Wall, Ronald Metzack (eds.). Churchill Livingstone Inc., 650 Avenue of the Americas, New York, NY 10011. Phone: (212) 819-5400. Fax: (212) 302-6598. Second edition 1989.

PANCREATIC CANCER

See also: CANCER

ABSTRACTING, INDEXING, AND CURRENT AWARENESS PUBLICATIONS

Current Contents/Clinical Medicine. Institute for Scientific Information, 3501 Market St., Philadelphia, PA 19104. Phone: (800) 523-1850. Fax: (215) 386-6362. Weekly.

Excerpta Medica. Section 16: Cancer. Elsevier Science Publishing Co., Inc., P.O. Box 882, Madison Square Station, New York, NY 10159-2101. Phone: (212) 989-5800. Fax: (212) 633-3990. 32/year.

Excerpta Medica. Section 48: Gastroenterology. Elsevier Science Publishing Co., Inc., P.O. Box 882, Madison Square

Station, New York, NY 10159-2101. Phone: (212) 989-5800. Fax: (212) 633-3990. 20/year.

Index Medicus. U.S. National Library of Medicine, 8600 Rockville Pike, Bethesda, MD 20894. Phone: (800) 638-8480. Monthly.

Science Citation Index. Institute for Scientific Information, 3501 Market St., Philadelphia, PA 19104. Phone: (800) 523-1850. Fax: (215) 386-6362. Bimonthly.

ANNUALS AND REVIEWS

In Development New Medicines for Older Americans. 1991 Annual Survey. More Medicines in Testing for Cancer Than for Any Other Disease of Aging. Pharmaceutical Manufacturers Association, 1100 15th St. N.W., Washington, DC 20005. Phone: (202) 835-3400. 1991.

ASSOCIATIONS, PROFESSIONAL SOCIETIES, ADVOCACY AND SUPPORT GROUPS

American Cancer Society (ACS). 1599 Clifton Rd. N.E., Atlanta, GA 30329. Phone: (404) 320-3333.

American College of Gastroenterology (ACG). 4222 King St., Alexandria, VA 22302. Phone: (703) 549-4440.

American Gastroenterological Association (AGA). 6900 Grove Rd., Thorofare, NJ 08086. Phone: (609) 848-9218. Fax: (609) 853-5991.

National Foundation for Cancer Research (NFCR). 7315 Wisconsin Ave., Ste. 332W, Bethesda, MD 20814. Phone: (800) 321-2875. Fax: (301) 654-5824.

CD-ROM DATABASES

Cancer-CD. SilverPlatter Information, Inc., River Ridge Office Park, 100 River Ridge Rd., Norwood, MA 02062. Phone: (617) 769-2599. Fax: (617) 769-8763. Quarterly.

Cancerlit CD-ROM. Cambridge Scientific Abstracts, 7200 Wisconsin Ave., Bethesda, MD 20814-4823. Phone: (800) 843-7751. Fax: (301) 961-6720. Quarterly.

Excerpta Medica CD: Gastroenterology. SilverPlatter Information, Inc., River Ridge Office Park, 100 River Ridge Rd., Norwood, MA 02062. Phone: (617) 769-2599. Fax: (617) 769-8763. Quarterly.

SCISEARCH. Institute for Scientific Information, 3501 Market St., Philadelphia, PA 19104. Phone: (215) 386-0100. Fax: (215) 386-6362.

ENCYCLOPEDIAS, DICTIONARIES, WORD BOOKS

Oncology Words. Stedman. Williams & Wilkins, 428 East Preston St., Baltimore, MD 21202. Phone: (800) 638-0672. Fax: (800) 447-8438. 1992.

HANDBOOKS, GUIDES, MANUALS, ATLASES

Atlas of Operative Surgery: Gallbladder, Bile Ducts, Pancreas. K. Kremer, W. Lierse, W. Platzer, and others. Thieme Medical Publishers, Inc., 381 Park Ave. S., New York, NY 10016. Phone: (212) 683-5088. Fax: (212) 779-9020. 1991.

JOURNALS

American Journal of Gastroenterology. Williams & Wilkins, 428 E. Preston St., Baltimore, MD 21202. Phone: (800) 638-0672. Fax: (800) 447-8438. Monthly.

CA - A Cancer Journal for Clinicians. J.B. Lippincott Co., 227 E. Washington Square, Philadelphia, PA 19106-3780. Phone: (215) 238-4200. Fax: (215) 238-4227. Bimonthly.

Cancer Causes and Control. Rapid Communications of Oxford Ltd., The Old Malthouse, Paradise St., Oxford OX1 1LD, England. Phone: 44-865-790447. Fax: 44-865-244012. 6/year.

Journal of the National Cancer Institute. Superintendent of Documents, P.O. Box 371954, Pittsburgh, PA 15250-7954. Fax: (202) 512-2233. Semimonthly.

ONLINE DATABASES

CANCERLIT. U.S. National Cancer Institute, International Cancer Information Center, Building 82, Room 102, Bethesda, MD 20892. Phone: (301) 496-7403. Fax: (301) 480-8105. Monthly.

Clinical Protocols. U.S. National Cancer Institute, International Cancer Information Center, Building 82, Room 102, Bethesda, MD 20892. Phone: (301) 496-7403. Fax: (301) 480-8105.

EMBASE. Elsevier Science Publishing Co., Inc., P.O. Box 882, Madison Square Station, New York, NY 10159-2101. Phone: (212) 989-5800. Fax: (212) 633-3990.

MEDLINE. National Library of Medicine, 8600 Rockville Pike, Bethesda, MD 20894. Phone: (800) 638-8480.

Physician Data Query (PDQ) Cancer Information File. U.S. National Cancer Institute, International Cancer Information Center, Building 82, Room 102, Bethesda, MD 20892. Phone: (301) 496-7403. Fax: (301) 480-8105. Monthly.

Physician Data Query (PDQ) Directory File. U.S. National Cancer Institute, International Cancer Information Center, Building 82, Room 102, Bethesda, MD 20892. Phone: (301) 496-7403. Fax: (301) 480-8105. Monthly.

SciSearch. Institute for Scientific Information, 3501 Market St., Philadelphia, PA 19104. Phone: (215) 386-0100. Fax: (215) 386-6362.

POPULAR WORKS AND PATIENT EDUCATION

Cancervive: The Challenge of Life After Cancer. Susan Nessim, Judith Ellis. Houghton Mifflin Co., 1 Beacon St., Boston, MA 02108. Phone: (800) 225-3362. 1991.

Everyone's Guide to Cancer Therapy: How Cancer is Diagnosed, Treated, and Managed on a Day to Day Basis. Malin Dollinger, Ernest H. Rosenbaum, Greg Cable. Andrews & McMeel, 4900 Main St., Kansas City, MO 64112. Phone: (800) 826-4216. 1991.

Gut Reactions: Understanding Symptoms of the Digestive Tract. W.G. Thompson. Plenum Publishing Co., 233 Spring St., New York, NY 10013-1578. Phone: (323) 620-8000. Fax: (212) 463-0742. 1989.

RESEARCH CENTERS, INSTITUTES, CLEARINGHOUSES

Cancer Information Service (CIS). Office of Cancer Communications, National Cancer Institute, Bldg. 31, Rm. 10A24, 9000 Rockville Pike, Bethesda, MD 20892. Phone: (800) 4CA-NCER.

National Digestive Diseases Information Clearinghouse (NDDIC). P.O. Box NDDIC, Bethesda, MD 20892. Phone: (301) 468-6344.

TEXTBOOKS AND MONOGRAPHS

Cancer: Principles and Practice of Oncology. Vincent T. DeVita. J.B. Lippincott Co., 227 E. Washington Square, Philadelphia, PA 19106-3780. Phone: (215) 238-4200. Fax: (215) 238-4227. 1989 3rd edtion.

Disorders of the Pancreas: Current Issues in Diagnosis and Management. Gerard P. Burns, Simmy Bank. McGraw-Hill, Inc., Health Professions Division, 1221 Avenue of the Americas, 28th Floor, New York, NY 10020. Phone: (212) 512-4228. 1992.

Gastrointestinal Disease: Pathophysiology, Diagnosis, Management. Marvin H. Sleisenger, John. S. Fordtran. W.B. Saunders Co., The Curtis Center, Independence Square W., Philadelphia, PA 19106-3399. Phone: (215) 238-7800. Fourth edition. Two volumes. 1989.

PANCREATIC DISORDERS

See: GASTROINTESTINAL DISORDERS;
PANCREATIC CANCER

PANIC DISORDER

ABSTRACTING, INDEXING, AND CURRENT AWARENESS PUBLICATIONS

Current Contents/Clinical Medicine. Institute for Scientific Information, 3501 Market St., Philadelphia, PA 19104. Phone: (800) 523-1850. Fax: (215) 386-6362. Weekly.

ASSOCIATIONS, PROFESSIONAL SOCIETIES, ADVOCACY AND SUPPORT GROUPS

American Psychiatric Association (APA). 1400 K St. N.W., Washington, DC 20005. Phone: (202) 682-6000. Fax: (202) 682-6114.

American Psychological Association (APA). 1200 17th St. N.W., Washington, DC 20036. Phone: (202) 955-7600. Fax: (703) 525-5191.

Anxiety Disorders Association of America. 6000 Executive Blvd., Ste. 200, Rockville, MD 20852.

CD-ROM DATABASES

PsycLit. SilverPlatter Information, Inc., River Ridge Office Park, 100 River Ridge Rd., Norwood, MA 02062. Phone: (617) 769-2599. Fax: (617) 769-8763. Quarterly.

HANDBOOKS, GUIDES, MANUALS, ATLASES

Diagnosis and Treatment of Anxiety Disorders: A Physician's Handbook. Thomas J. McGlynn, Harry L. Metcalf (eds.).

American Psychiatric Press, Inc., 1400 K St. NW, Washington, DC 20005. Phone: (202) 682-6268. Fax: (202) 789-2648. 1989.

JOURNALS

American Journal of Psychiatry. American Psychiatric Press, Inc., 1400 K St. NW, Washington, DC 20005. Phone: (202) 682-6268. Fax: (202) 789-2648. Monthly.

Archives of General Psychiatry. American Medical Association, 515 North State St., Chicago, IL 60610. Phone: (312) 464-0183. Fax: (312) 464-5834. Monthly.

Psychiatric Annals. SLACK Inc., 6900 Grove Rd., Thorofare, NJ 08086-9447. Phone: (800) 257-8290. Fax: (609) 853-5991.

ONLINE DATABASES

PsycInfo. SilverPlatter Information, Inc., River Ridge Office Park, 100 River Ridge Rd., Norwood, MA 02062. Phone: (617) 769-2599. Fax: (617) 769-8763. Quarterly.

POPULAR WORKS AND PATIENT EDUCATION

Anxiety Disorders and Phobias. Aaron T. Beck, Gary Emery, Ruth L. Greenberg. HarperCollins Publishers, Inc., 10 E. 53rd St., New York, NY 10022-5299. Phone: (800) 242-7737. 1990.

Living with Stress and Anxiety. Bob Whitmore. St. Martin's Press, 175 Fifth Ave., New York, NY 10010. Phone: (212) 674-5151. 1992.

Panic Disorder in the Medical Setting. Wayne J. Katon. American Psychiatric Press, Inc., 1400 K St. N.W., Washington, DC 20005. Phone: (202) 682-6268. Fax: (202) 789-2648. 1990.

Panic Disorder: The Great Pretender. H.M. Zal. Plenum Publishing Co., 233 Spring St., New York, NY 10013-1578. Phone: (212) 620-8000. Fax: (212) 463-0742. 1990.

RESEARCH CENTERS, INSTITUTES, CLEARINGHOUSES

Panic Campaign. Room 15C-05, 5600 Fishers Lane, National Institute of Mental Health, Rockville, MD 20857.

STANDARDS AND STATISTICS SOURCES

Panic. Consensus Statement. NIH Consensus Development Conference. September 25-27, 1991. National Institutes of Health, Office of Medical Applications of Research, Federal Bldg., Rm. 618, Bethesda, MD 20892. 1991.

TEXTBOOKS AND MONOGRAPHS

Anxiety and Its Disorders. D.H. Barlow. Guilford Publications, Inc., 72 Spring St., New York, NY 10012. Phone: (800) 365-7006. Fax: (212) 966-6708. 1988.

Clinical Aspects of Panic Disorder. James C. Ballenger (ed.). John Wiley & Sons, Inc., 605 Third Ave., New York, NY 10158-0012. Phone: (212) 850-6000. Fax: (212) 850-6088. 1990.

The Clinical Management of Anxiety Disorders. William Coryell, George Winokur (eds.). Oxford University Press, 200 Madison Ave., New York, NY 10016. Phone: (212) 679-7300. 1991.

Comorbitity of Mood and Anxiety Disorders. Jack D. Maser, C. Robert Cloninger (eds.). American Psychiatric Press, Inc., 1400 K St. NW, Washington, DC 20005. Phone: (202) 682-6268. Fax: (202) 789-2648. 1990.

PAP SMEAR

See: DIAGNOSIS; GYNECOLOGIC DISORDERS

PAPILLOMA

See: CANCER

PARALYSIS

See also: SPINAL CORD INJURIES

ABSTRACTING, INDEXING, AND CURRENT AWARENESS PUBLICATIONS

Index Medicus. U.S. National Library of Medicine, 8600 Rockville Pike, Bethesda, MD 20894. Phone: (800) 638-8480. Monthly.

ASSOCIATIONS, PROFESSIONAL SOCIETIES, ADVOCACY AND SUPPORT GROUPS

American Paralysis Association (APA). P.O. Box 187, Short HillS, NJ 07078. Phone: (201) 379-2690.

American Paraplegia Society (APS). 75-20 Astoria Blvd., Jackson Heights, NY 11370. Phone: (718) 803-3782.

American Spinal Injury Association (ASIA). 250 E. Superior, Rm. 619, Chicago, IL 60611. Phone: (312) 908-3425.

National Spinal Cord Injury Association (NSCIA). 600 W. Cummings Park, Ste. 2000, Woburn, MA 01801. Phone: (800) 962-9629. Fax: (617) 935-8369.

Paralyzed Veterans of America (PVA). 801 18th St. N.W., Washington, DC 20006. Phone: (202) 872-1300.

Spinal Cord Society (SCS). Wendell Rd., Fergus Falls, MN 56537. Phone: (218) 739-5252. Fax: (218) 739-5262.

JOURNALS

Paraplegia. Churchill Livingstone Inc., 650 Ave. of the Americas, New York, NY 10011. Phone: (212) 819-5400. Fax: (212) 302-6598. 9/year.

Spine. J.B. Lippincott Co., 227 E. Washington Square, Philadelphia, PA 19106-3780. Phone: (215) 238-4200. Fax: (215) 238-4227. 11/year.

NEWSLETTERS

Paraplegia News. Paralyzed Veterans of America, 801 18th St. N.W., Washington, DC 20006. Monthly.

ONLINE DATABASES

EMBASE. Elsevier Science Publishing Co., Inc., P.O. Box 882, Madison Square Station, New York, NY 10159-2101. Phone: (212) 989-5800. Fax: (212) 633-3990.

MEDLINE. National Library of Medicine, 8600 Rockville Pike, Bethesda, MD 20894. Phone: (800) 638-8480.

SciSearch. Institute for Scientific Information, 3501 Market St., Philadelphia, PA 19104. Phone: (215) 386-0100. Fax: (215) 386-6362.

POPULAR WORKS AND PATIENT EDUCATION

Spinal Cord Injury: A Guide for Patient and Family. Lynn Phillips, Mark N. Ozer, Peter Axelson, and others. Raven Press, 1185 Avenue of the Americas, New York, NY 10036. Phone: (212) 930-9500. Fax: (212) 869-3495. 1987.

TEXTBOOKS AND MONOGRAPHS

The Management of Quadriplegia. Gale Whiteneck, and others. Demos Publications, 156 Fifth Ave., Suite 1018, New York, NY 10010. Phone: (212) 255-8768. 1989.

PARAMEDICS

See: EMERGENCY MEDICAL TECHNICIANS

PARANOIA

See: PSYCHIATRIC DISORDERS

PARAPHILIAS

See: SEXUAL DISORDERS

PARASITIC DISEASES

See also: INFECTIOUS DISEASES; MALARIA; TROPICAL MEDICINE

ABSTRACTING, INDEXING, AND CURRENT AWARENESS PUBLICATIONS

CAB Abstracts. C.A.B. International, 845 N. Park Ave., Tucson, AZ 85719. Phone: (800) 528-4841.

Current Contents/Clinical Medicine. Institute for Scientific Information, 3501 Market St., Philadelphia, PA 19104. Phone: (800) 523-1850. Fax: (215) 386-6362. Weekly.

Current Contents/Life Sciences. Institute for Scientific Information, 3501 Market St., Philadelphia, PA 19104. Phone: (215) 386-0100. Fax: (215) 386-6362.

Excerpta Medica. Section 4: Microbiology, Mycology, Parasitology and Virology. Elsevier Science Publishers, P.O. Box 882, Madison Square Station, New York, NY 10159-2101. Phone: (212) 633-3950. Fax: (212) 633-3990. 32/year.

Helminthological Abstracts. C.A.B. International, 845 N. Park Ave., Tucson, AZ 85719. Phone: (800) 528-4841. Monthly.

Index Medicus. U.S. National Library of Medicine, 8600 Rockville Pike, Bethesda, MD 20894. Phone: (800) 638-8480. Monthly.

Microbiology Abstracts. Section C: Algology, Mycology & Protozoology. Cambridge Scientific Abstracts, 7200 Wisconsin Ave., Bethesda, MD 20814-4823. Phone: (800) 843-7751. Fax: (301) 961-6720. Monthly.

Tropical Diseases Bulletin. Bureau of Hygiene and Tropical Diseases, Keppel St., London WC1E 7HT, England. Monthly.

ANNUALS AND REVIEWS

Advances in Parasitology. Academic Press, Inc., 1250 Sixth Ave., San Diego, CA 92101-4311. Phone: (619) 699-6345. Fax: (619) 699-6715. Irregular.

Contributions to Microbiology and Immunology. S. Karger Publishers, Inc., 26 West Avon Rd., P.O. Box 529, Farmington, CT 06085. Phone: (203) 675-7834. Fax: (203) 675-7302. Irregular.

ASSOCIATIONS, PROFESSIONAL SOCIETIES, ADVOCACY AND SUPPORT GROUPS

National Pediculosis Association. P.O. Box 149, Newton, MA 02161. Phone: (800) 464-NPA.

CD-ROM DATABASES

CABCD (CAB Abstracts on CD-ROM). C.A.B. International, 845 N. Park Ave., Tucson, AZ 85719. Phone: (800) 528-4841.

HANDBOOKS, GUIDES, MANUALS, ATLASES

A Color Atlas of Tropical Medicine and Parasitology. W. Peters, H.M. Giles. Mosby-Year Book, 11830 Westline Industrial Drive, St. Louis, MO 63146. Phone: (800) 325-4177. Fax: (314) 432-1380. Third edition 1989.

A Guide to Human Helminths. D.W.T. Crompton, I. Coombs. Taylor & Francis Inc., 1900 Frost Rd., Suite 101, Bristol, PA 19007-1598. Phone: (800) 821-8312. Fax: (215) 785-5515. 1991.

JOURNALS

Annals of Tropical Medicine and Parasitology. Academic Press, Inc., 1250 Sixth Ave., San Diego, CA 92101-4311. Phone: (619) 699-6345. Fax: (619) 699-6715. Bimonthly.

Journal of Tropical Medicine and Hygiene. Blackwell Scientific Publications, Inc., 3 Cambridge Ctr., Cambridge, MA 02142. Phone: (800) 759-6102. Bimonthly.

Molecular and Biochemical Parasitology. Elsevier Science Publishing Co., Inc., P.O. Box 882, Madison Square Station, New York, NY 10159-2101. Phone: (212) 989-5800. Fax: (212) 633-3990. 14/year.

Parasitology Today. Elsevier Science Publishing Co., Inc., P.O. Box 882, Madison Square Station, New York, NY 10159-2101. Phone: (212) 989-5800. Fax: (212) 633-3990. 12+1/year.

Tropical Medicine and Parasitology. Thieme Medical Publishers, Inc., 381 Park Ave. S., New York, NY 10016. Phone: (212) 683-5088. Fax: (212) 779-9020. Quarterly.

NEWSLETTERS

Travel Medicine Advisor. American Health Consultants, Department ADI-59, P.O. Box 740060, Atlanta, GA 30374. Phone: (800) 559-1032. Fax: (404) 352-1971.

ONLINE DATABASES

EMBASE. Elsevier Science Publishing Co., Inc., P.O. Box 882, Madison Square Station, New York, NY 10159-2101. Phone: (212) 989-5800. Fax: (212) 633-3990.

MEDLINE. National Library of Medicine, 8600 Rockville Pike, Bethesda, MD 20894. Phone: (800) 638-8480.

SciSearch. Institute for Scientific Information, 3501 Market St., Philadelphia, PA 19104. Phone: (215) 386-0100. Fax: (215) 386-6362.

POPULAR WORKS AND PATIENT EDUCATION

The Malaria Capers: More Tales of Parasites and People, Research and Reality. Robert S. Desowitz. W.W. Norton & Co., Inc., 500 Fifth Ave., New York, NY 10110. Phone: (800) 223-2584. 1991.

RESEARCH CENTERS, INSTITUTES, CLEARINGHOUSES

Laboratory for Biochemical Parasitology. Division of Infectious Diseases, University of Colorado, Box 168, 4200 E. 9th St., Denver, CO 80262. Phone: (303) 270-7233.

Laboratory of Experimental Chemotherapy for Parasitology. Rockefeller University, 1230 York Ave., New York, NY 10021. Phone: (212) 570-8232.

TEXTBOOKS AND MONOGRAPHS

Hookworm Disease: Current Status and New Directions. G.A. Schad, K.S. Warren (eds.). Taylor & Francis Inc., 1900 Frost Rd., Suite 101, Bristol, PA 19007-1598. Phone: (800) 821-8312. Fax: (215) 785-5515. 1990.

Medical Parasitology: A Self-Instructional Text. Ruth Leventhal, Russell F. Cheadle. F.A. Davis Co., 1915 Arch St., Philadelphia, PA 19103. Phone: (800) 523-4049. Fax: (215) 568-5065. Third edition 1989.

Parasitic Disease. Katz. Springer-Verlag New York Inc., 175 Fifth Ave., New York, NY 10010. Phone: (212) 460-1500. Fax: (212) 473-6272. Second edition 1989.

Schistosomes: Development, Reproduction and Host Relations. Paul F. Basch. Oxford University Press, 200 Madison Ave., New York, NY 10016. Phone: (212) 679-7300. 1991.

Tropical Medicine: A Clinical Text. K.M. Cahill, W. O'Brien. Butterworth-Heinemann, 80 Montvale Ave., Stoneham, MA 02180. Phone: (617) 438-8464. Fax: (617) 279-4851. 1990.

Tropical Medicine and Parasitology. Robert Goldsmith, Donald Heyneman. Appleton & Lange, 25 Van Zant St., East Norwalk, CT 06855. Phone: (800) 423-1359. Fax: (203) 854-9486. 1989.

PARASITOLOGY

See: PARASITIC DISEASES

PARKINSON'S DISEASE

See also: NEUROLOGIC DISORDERS

ABSTRACTING, INDEXING, AND CURRENT AWARENESS PUBLICATIONS

Current Contents/Clinical Medicine. Institute for Scientific Information, 3501 Market St., Philadelphia, PA 19104. Phone: (800) 523-1850. Fax: (215) 386-6362. Weekly.

Excerpta Medica. Section 8: Neurology and Neurosurgery. Elsevier Science Publishers, P.O. Box 882, Madison Square Station, New York, NY 10159-2101. Phone: (212) 633-3950. Fax: (212) 633-3990. 32/year.

Index Medicus. U.S. National Library of Medicine, 8600 Rockville Pike, Bethesda, MD 20894. Phone: (800) 638-8480. Monthly.

Science Citation Index. Institute for Scientific Information, 3501 Market St., Philadelphia, PA 19104. Phone: (800) 523-1850. Fax: (215) 386-6362. Bimonthly.

ANNUALS AND REVIEWS

Current Neurology. Mosby-Year Book, 11830 Westline Industrial Drive, St. Louis, MO 63146. Phone: (800) 325-4177. Fax: (314) 432-1380. Annual.

Neurologic Clinics. W.B. Saunders Co., The Curtis Center, Independence Square W., Philadelphia, PA 19106-3399. Phone: (215) 238-7800. Quarterly.

ASSOCIATIONS, PROFESSIONAL SOCIETIES, ADVOCACY AND SUPPORT GROUPS

American Parkinson Disease Association (APDA). 60 Bay St., Ste. 401, Staten Island, NY 10301. Phone: (212) 981-8001. Fax: (718) 981-4399.

National Parkinson Foundation (NPF). 1501 NW 9th Ave., Miami, FL 33136. Phone: (305) 547-6666.

Parkinson's Disease Foundation (PDF). William Black Medical Research Bldg., Columbia Presbyterian Medical Ctr., 650 W. 168th St., New York, NY 10032. Phone: (212) 923-4700. Fax: (212) 923-4778.

United Parkinson Foundation (UPF). 360 W. Superior St., Chicago, IL 60610. Phone: (312) 664-2344.

BIBLIOGRAPHIES

Parkinson's Disease. National Technical Information Service, 5285 Port Royal Rd., Springfield, VA 22161. Phone: (703) 487-4650. Fax: (703) 321-8547. Jan. 1978-July 1989 PB90-85458/CBY.

CD-ROM DATABASES

Excerpta Medica CD: Neurosciences. SilverPlatter Information, Inc., River Ridge Office Park, 100 River Ridge Rd., Norwood, MA 02062. Phone: (617) 769-2599. Fax: (617) 769-8763. Quarterly.

SCISEARCH. Institute for Scientific Information, 3501 Market St., Philadelphia, PA 19104. Phone: (215) 386-0100. Fax: (215) 386-6362.

HANDBOOKS, GUIDES, MANUALS, ATLASES

Drugs for the Treatment of Parkinson's Disease. D.B. Caine (ed.). Springer-Verlag New York Inc., 175 Fifth Ave., New York, NY 10010. Phone: (212) 460-1500. Fax: (212) 473-6272. 1989.

Manual of Neurology: Diagnosis and Therapy. Martin A. Samuels (ed.). Little, Brown and Company, 34 Beacon St., Boston, MA 02108. Phone: (617) 227-0730. Fourth edition 1991.

Parkinson's Handbook. Dwight C. McGoon. W.W. Norton & Co., Inc., 500 Fifth Ave., New York, NY 10110. Phone: (800) 223-2584. 1990.

JOURNALS

Annals of Neurology. Little, Brown and Co., 34 Beacon St., Boston, MA 02108. Phone: (617) 227-0730. Fax: (617) 227-0790. Monthly.

Archives of Neurology. American Medical Association, 515 North State St., Chicago, IL 60610. Phone: (312) 464-0183. Fax: (312) 464-5834. Monthly.

Journal of Neurology, Neurosurgery & Psychiatry. BMJ Publishing Group, BMA House, Tavistock Square, London WC1H 9JR, England. Phone: 071-383 6244/6638. Fax: 071-383 6662. Monthly.

NEWSLETTERS

American Parkinson Disease Association-Newsletter. American Parkinson Disease Association, 116 John St., Ste. 417, New York, NY 10038. Phone: (212) 732-9550. Quarterly.

Parkinson Report. National Parkinson Foundation, 1501 N.W. 9th Ave., Bob Hope Rd., Miami, FL 33136. Phone: (800) 327-4545. Quarterly.

Parkinson's Disease Foundation-Newsletter. Parkinson's Disease Foundation, 650 W. 168th St., New York, NY 10032. Phone: (800) 457-6676. Fax: (212) 923-4778. Quarterly.

ONLINE DATABASES

EMBASE. Elsevier Science Publishing Co., Inc., P.O. Box 882, Madison Square Station, New York, NY 10159-2101. Phone: (212) 989-5800. Fax: (212) 633-3990.

MEDLINE. National Library of Medicine, 8600 Rockville Pike, Bethesda, MD 20894. Phone: (800) 638-8480.

SciSearch. Institute for Scientific Information, 3501 Market St., Philadelphia, PA 19104. Phone: (215) 386-0100. Fax: (215) 386-6362.

POPULAR WORKS AND PATIENT EDUCATION

Caring for the Parkinson Patient: A Care-Giver Guide. Raye L. Dippel, J. Thomas Hutton (eds.). Prometheus Books, 700 E. Amherst St., Buffalo, NY 14215. Phone: (800) 421-0351. 1989.

Living with Parkinson's: A Guide for the Patient and Caregiver. David Carroll. HarperCollins Pubs., Inc., 10 E. 53rd St., New York, NY 10022-5299. Phone: (212) 207-7000. Fax: (800) 242-7737. 1992.

Living Well with Parkinson's. Glenna Wotton Atwood, Lila Green Hunnewell. John Wiley & Sons, Inc., 605 Third Ave.,

New York, NY 10158-0012. Phone: (212) 850-6000. Fax: (212) 850-6088. 1991.

Parkinson's Disease: A Guide for Patient and Family. Roger C. Duvoisin. Raven Press, 1185 Ave. of the Americas, New York, NY 10036. Phone: (212) 930-9500. Fax: (212) 869-3495. Third edition 1991.

Parkinson's Disease: The Facts. G. Stern. Oxford University Press, 200 Madison Ave., New York, NY 10016. Phone: (212) 679-7300. 1990.

RESEARCH CENTERS, INSTITUTES, CLEARINGHOUSES

Clinical Center for Research in Parkinson's and Allied Disorders. City University of New York, Mt. Sinai School of Medicine, 1 Gustave Levy Place, New York, NY 10029. Phone: (212) 650-7301.

William T. Gossett Parkinson's Disease Center. Henry Ford Hospital, Dept. of Neurology, 2799 W. Grand Blvd., Detroit, MI 48202. Phone: (313) 876-2858.

TEXTBOOKS AND MONOGRAPHS

Alzheimer's and Parkinson's Diseases: Recent Advances in Research and Clinical Management. H.J. Altman, B.N. Altman (eds.). Plenum Publishing Co., 233 Spring St., New York, NY 10013-1578. Phone: (212) 620-800. Fax: (212) 463-0742. 1990.

Long Term Clinical Care of Parkinson's Disease. T. Nakanishi. S. Karger Publishers, Inc., 26 W. Avon Rd., P.O. Box 529, Farmington, CT 06085. Phone: (203) 675-7834. Fax: (203) 675-7302. 1990.

Merritt's Textbook of Neurology. Lewis P. Rowland (ed.). Williams & Wilkins, 428 E. Preston St., Baltimore, MD 21202. Phone: (800) 638-0672. Fax: (800) 447-8438. Eighth edition 1989.

Parkinson's Disease: Anatomy, Pathology, and Therapy. Max B. Streifler, Amos D. Korczyn, Eldad Melamed, et. al.. Raven Press, 1185 Avenue of the Americas, New York, NY 10036. Phone: (212) 930-9500. Fax: (212) 869-3495. Advances in Neurology. Volume 53. 1990.

Progress in Parkinson Research. F. Hefti, W.J. Weiner (eds.). Plenum Publishing Co., 233 Spring St., New York, NY 10013-1578. Phone: (212) 620-800. Fax: (212) 463-0742. 1989.

The Scientific Basis for the Treatment of Parkinson's Disease. C.W. Olanow, A.N. Lieberman (eds.). The Parthenon Publishing Group, Inc., 120 Mill Rd., Park Ridge, NJ 07656. Phone: (201) 391-6796. 1992.

PATHOLOGY

ABSTRACTING, INDEXING, AND CURRENT AWARENESS PUBLICATIONS

Current Contents/Life Sciences. Institute for Scientific Information, 3501 Market St., Philadelphia, PA 19104. Phone: (215) 386-0100. Fax: (215) 386-6362.

Excerpta Medica. Section 5: General Pathology and Pathological Anatomy. Elsevier Science Publishers, P.O. Box 882, Madison Square Station, New York, NY 10159-2101. Phone: (212) 633-3950. Fax: (212) 633-3990. 24/year.

Index Medicus. U.S. National Library of Medicine, 8600 Rockville Pike, Bethesda, MD 20894. Phone: (800) 638-8480. Monthly.

Research Alert: Pathology-Experimental. Institute for Scientific Information, 3501 Market St., Philadelphia, PA 19104. Phone: (800) 523-1850. Fax: (215) 386-6362. Weekly.

Science Citation Index. Institute for Scientific Information, 3501 Market St., Philadelphia, PA 19104. Phone: (800) 523-1850. Fax: (215) 386-6362. Bimonthly.

ANNUALS AND REVIEWS

Advances in Pathology and Laboratory Medicine. Mosby-Year Book, 11830 Westline Industrial Drive, St. Louis, MO 63146. Phone: (800) 325-4177. Fax: (314) 432-1380. Annual.

Current Topics in Pathology. Springer-Verlag New York Inc., 175 Fifth Ave., New York, NY 10010. Phone: (212) 460-1500. Fax: (212) 473-6272.

International Review of Experimental Pathology. Academic Press, Inc., 1250 Sixth Ave., San Diego, CA 92101-4311. Phone: (619) 699-6345. Fax: (619) 699-6715.

Pathology Annual. Appleton & Lange, 25 Van Zant St., East Norwalk, CT 06855. Phone: (800) 423-1359. Fax: (203) 854-9486. Annual.

Year Book of Pathology and Clinical Pathology. Mosby-Year Book, 11830 Westline Industrial Drive, St. Louis, MO 63146. Phone: (800) 325-4177. Fax: (314) 432-1380. Annual.

ASSOCIATIONS, PROFESSIONAL SOCIETIES, ADVOCACY AND SUPPORT GROUPS

American Academy of Oral Pathology. c/o Dean K. White, Dept. of Oral Pathology, College of Dentistry, University of Kentucky, Lexington, KY 40536.

American Association of Pathologists (AAP). 9650 Rockville Pike, Bethesda, MD 20814. Phone: (301) 530-7130.

American Board of Oral Pathology. 1121 W. Michigan St., Indiana University School of Dentistry, Indianapolis, IN 46202. Phone: (317) 274-7668.

American Board of Pathology (ABP). Lincoln Ctr., 5401 W. Kennedy Blvd., P.O. Box 25915, Tampa, FL 33622. Phone: (813) 286-2444.

American Society of Clinical Pathologists. 2100 W. Harrison, Chicago, IL 60612. Phone: (312) 768-1330.

College of American Pathologists (CAP). 325 Waukegan Rd., Northfield, IL 60093-2750. Phone: (708) 446-8800. Fax: (708) 446-8807.

CD-ROM DATABASES

Excerpta Medica CD: Pathology. SilverPlatter Information, Inc., River Ridge Office Park, 100 River Ridge Rd., Norwood, MA 02062. Phone: (617) 769-2599. Fax: (617) 769-8763. Quarterly.

PathLine. Aries Systems Corporation, One Dundee Park, Andover, MA 01810. Phone: (508) 475-7200. Fax: (508) 474-8860. Quarterly.

SCISEARCH. Institute for Scientific Information, 3501 Market St., Philadelphia, PA 19104. Phone: (215) 386-0100. Fax: (215) 386-6362.

DIRECTORIES

Directory of Certified Pathologists. American Board of Medical Specialties, 1 Rotary Center, Suite 805, Evanston, IL 60201. Phone: (708) 491-9091. Biennial.

ENCYCLOPEDIAS, DICTIONARIES, WORD BOOKS

Pathology Words. Stedman. Williams & Wilkins, 428 East Preston St., Baltimore, MD 21202. Phone: (800) 638-0672. Fax: (800) 447-8438. 1992.

HANDBOOKS, GUIDES, MANUALS, ATLASES

A Color Atlas of General Pathology. Austin Gresham. Mosby-Year Book, 11830 Westline Industrial Drive, St. Louis, MO 63146. Phone: (800) 325-4177. Fax: (314) 432-1380. 1992.

Color Atlas of Trauma Pathology. Fischer. Mosby-Year Book, 11830 Westline Industrial Drive, St. Louis, MO 63146. Phone: (800) 325-4177. Fax: (314) 432-1380. 1991.

Royal College of Surgeon's Atlas of Surgical Pathology. Turk. Raven Press, 1185 Ave. of the Americas, New York, NY 10036. Phone: (212) 930-9500. Fax: (212) 869-3495. 1992.

JOURNALS

American Journal of Clinical Pathology. J.B. Lippincott Co., 227 E. Washington Square, Philadelphia, PA 19106-3780. Phone: (215) 238-4200. Fax: (215) 238-4227. Monthly.

American Journal of Pathology. J.B. Lippincott Co., 227 E. Washington Square, Philadelphia, PA 19106-3780. Phone: (215) 238-4200. Fax: (215) 238-4227. Monthly.

American Journal of Surgical Pathology. Raven Press, 1185 Avenue of the Americas, New York, NY 10036. Phone: (212) 930-9500. Fax: (212) 869-3495. Monthly.

Archives of Pathology & Laboratory Medicine. American Medical Association, 515 North State St., Chicago, IL 60610. Phone: (312) 464-0183. Fax: (312) 464-5834. Monthly.

Human Pathology. W.B. Saunders Co., The Curtis Center, Independence Sqare W., Philadelphia, PA 19106-3399. Phone: (215) 238-7800.

International Journal of Gynecological Pathology. Raven Press, 1185 Ave. of the Americas, New York, NY 10036. Phone: (212) 930-9500. Fax: (212) 869-3495.

Journal of Clinical Pathology. BMJ Publishing Group, BMA House, Tavistock Square, London WC1H 9JR, England. Phone: 071-383 6244/6638. Fax: 071-383 6662. Monthly.

Journal of Pathology. John Wiley & Sons, Inc., 605 Third Ave., New York, NY 10158-0012. Phone: (212) 850-6000. Fax: (212) 850-6088. Monthly.

Laboratory Investigation. Williams & Wilkins, 428 E. Preston St., Baltimore, MD 21202. Phone: (800) 638-0672. Fax: (800) 447-8438. Monthly.

Modern Pathology. Williams & Wilkins, 428 E. Preston St., Baltimore, MD 21202. Phone: (800) 638-0672. Fax: (800) 447-8438. Bimonthly.

Seminars in Diagnostic Pathology. W.B. Saunders Co., The Curtis Center, Independence Sqare W., Philadelphia, PA 19106-3399. Phone: (215) 238-7800.

ONLINE DATABASES

EMBASE. Elsevier Science Publishing Co., Inc., P.O. Box 882, Madison Square Station, New York, NY 10159-2101. Phone: (212) 989-5800. Fax: (212) 633-3990.

MEDLINE. National Library of Medicine, 8600 Rockville Pike, Bethesda, MD 20894. Phone: (800) 638-8480.

SciSearch. Institute for Scientific Information, 3501 Market St., Philadelphia, PA 19104. Phone: (215) 386-0100. Fax: (215) 386-6362.

RESEARCH CENTERS, INSTITUTES, CLEARINGHOUSES

Institute of Pathology. School of Medicine, Case Western Reserve University, Cleveland, OH 44106. Phone: (216) 368-5172.

Mallory Institute of Pathology Foundation. 784 Massachusetts Ave., Boston, MA 02118. Phone: (617) 536-3842.

TEXTBOOKS AND MONOGRAPHS

Ackerman's Surgical Pathology. Juan Rosai. Mosby-Year Book, 11830 Westline Industrial Drive, St. Louis, MO 63146. Phone: (800) 325-4177. Fax: (314) 432-1380. 7th edition, 1989.

Anderson's Pathology. John M. Kibsanc. Mosby-Year Book, 11830 Westline Industrial Drive, St. Louis, MO 63146. Phone: (800) 325-4177. Fax: (314) 432-1380.

Boyd's Textbook of Pathology. A.C. Ritchic. Williams & Wilkins, 428 East Preston St., Baltimore, MD 21202. Phone: (800) 638-0672. Fax: (800) 447-8438. 9th edition 1990.

Concise Pathology. Chandrasoma. Appleton & Lange, 25 Van Zant St., East Norwalk, CT 06855. Phone: (800) 423-1359. Fax: (203) 854-9486. 1991.

Forensic Pathology. Knight. Oxford University Press, 200 Madison Ave., New York, NY 10016. Phone: (212) 679-7300. 1991.

Introduction to General Pathology. W.G. Spector, T.D. Spector. Churchill Livingstone Inc., 650 Ave. of the Americas, New York, NY 10011. Phone: (212) 819-5400. Fax: (212) 302-6598. Third edition 1989.

Pathologic Basis of Disease: A Self-Assessment and Review. Carolyn Compton. W.B. Saunders Co., The Curtis Center, Independence Square W., Philadelphia, PA 19106-3399. Phone: (215) 238-7800. Third edition 1989.

Pathology. W.A.D. Anderson J.M. Kissane. Mosby-Year Book, 11830 Westline Industrial Drive, St. Louis, MO 63146. Phone: (800) 325-4177. Fax: (314) 432-1380. Two volumes. Ninth edition. 1989.

Pathology of Asbestos-Related Diseases. Roggli. Little, Brown and Co., 34 Beacon St., Boston, MA 02108. Phone: (617) 227-0730. Fax: (617) 227-0790. 1992.

Pathology for Gynaecologists. Fox. Williams & Wilkins, 428 East Preston St., Baltimore, MD 21202. Phone: (800) 638-0672. Fax: (800) 447-8438. Second edition 1991.

Pathology Illustrated. A.D.T. Govan and others. Churchill Livingstone Inc., 650 Ave. of the Americas, New York, NY 10011. Phone: (212) 819-5400. Fax: (212) 302-6598. Third edition 1991.

Pathology of Infectious Diseases. Von Lichtenberg. Raven Press, 1185 Ave. of the Americas, New York, NY 10036. Phone: (212) 930-9500. Fax: (212) 869-3495. 1991.

Pathology of Reproductive Failure. Kraus. Williams & Wilkins, 428 East Preston St., Baltimore, MD 21202. Phone: (800) 638-0672. Fax: (800) 447-8438. 1991.

PATIENT EDUCATION

See also: CONSUMER HEALTH
INFORMATION

ABSTRACTING, INDEXING, AND CURRENT AWARENESS PUBLICATIONS

Consumer Health and Nutrition Index. Alan Rees. Oryx Press, 4041 N. Central, Suite 700, Phoenix, AZ 85012. Phone: (800) 279-6799. Fax: (800) 279-4663. Quarterly.

Cumulative Index to Nursing and Allied Health Literature. Glendale Adventist Medical Center, P.O. Box 871, Glendale, CA 91209. Phone: (818) 409-8005. Bimonthly.

Hospital Literature Index. American Hospital Association, 840 N. Lake Shore Dr., Chicago, IL 60611. Phone: (800) 242-2626. Fax: (312) 280-6015. Quarterly.

Index Medicus. U.S. National Library of Medicine, 8600 Rockville Pike, Bethesda, MD 20894. Phone: (800) 638-8480. Monthly.

International Nursing Index. American Journal of Nursing Co., 555 W. 57th St., New York, NY 10019. Phone: (212) 582-8820. Quarterly.

Medical Abstracts Newsletter. Communi-T Publications, P.O. Box 2170, Teaneck, NJ 07666. Phone: (201) 836-5030. Monthly.

MEDOC: Index to U.S. Government Publications in the Medical and Health Sciences. Spencer S. Eccles Health Sciences Library, University of Utah, Bldg. 589, Salt Lake City, UT 84112. Phone: (801) 581-5268. Quarterly.

ASSOCIATIONS, PROFESSIONAL SOCIETIES, ADVOCACY AND SUPPORT GROUPS

American Council on Pharmaceutical Education. 311 W. Superior St., No. 512, Chicago, IL 60610. Phone: (312) 664-3575.

Association for the Advancement of Health Education (AAHE). 1900 Association Dr., Reston, VA 22091. Phone: (703) 476-3437.

Health Education Foundation. 600 New Hampshire Ave. N.W., Washington, DC 20037. Phone: (202) 338-3501.

Health Sciences Communications Association. 6105 Lindell Blvd., St. Louis, MO 63112. Phone: (314) 725-4722.

National Center for Health Education (NCHE). 30 E. 29th St., 3rd Flr., New York, NY 10016. Phone: (212) 689-1886. Fax: (212) 689-1728.

National Council on Patient Information and Education (NCPIE). 666 11th St. N.W., Ste. 810, Washington, DC 20001. Phone: (202) 347-6711.

BIBLIOGRAPHIES

Adult/Patient Nutrition Education Materials. Food and Nutrition Center, National Agricultural Library, 10301 Baltimore Blvd., Beltsville, MD 20705. Jan. 1982 to Sept. 1990.

Consumer Health Information Source Book. Alan Rees, Catherine Hoffman. Oryx Press, 4041 N. Central, Suite 700, Phoenix, AZ 85012. Phone: (800) 279-6799. Fax: (800) 279-4663. Third edition 1990.

Keyguide to Information Sources in Pharmacy. Mansell Publishing, Casselle PLC, Villiers House, 41-47 Strand, London WC2N 5JE, England. Phone: 71-8394900.

Patient Education Sourcebook: Volume II. Christine Frank (ed.). Health Sciences Communications Association, 6105 Lindell Blvd., St. Louis, MO 63112. Phone: (314) 725-4722. 1990.

CD-ROM DATABASES

Family Doctor. CMC ReSearch, Inc., 7150 S.W. Hampton, Suite C-120, Portland, OR 97223. Phone: (800) 262-7668. Fax: (503) 639-1796. Irregular.

Personal Medical Library CD-ROM. EBSCO Publishing, P.O. Box 325, Topsfield, MA 01983. Phone: (800) 221-1826. Fax: (508) 887-3923.

DIRECTORIES

Accredited Professional Programs of Colleges and Schools of Pharmacy. American Council on Pharmaceutical Education, 311 W. Superior St., No. 512, Chicago, IL 60610. Phone: (312) 664-3575.

American Association of Colleges of Pharmacy Roster of Teaching Personnel in Colleges and Schools of Pharmacy. American Association of Colleges of Pharmacy, 1426 Prince St., Alexandria, VA 22314. Phone: (703) 739-2330.

National Healthlines Directory. Louanne Marinos. Information Resources Press, 1110 N. Glebe Rd., Ste. 550, Arlington, VA 22201. Phone: (703) 558-8270. Fax: (703) 558-4979. 1992.

Pharmacy School Admission Requirements. American Association of Colleges of Pharmacy, 1426 Prince St., Alexandria, VA 22314. Phone: (703) 739-2330.

ENCYCLOPEDIAS, DICTIONARIES, WORD BOOKS

Surgery on File: Eye, Ear, Nose and Throat Surgery. The Diagram Group. Facts on File, Inc., 460 Park Ave. S., New York, NY 10016-7382. Phone: (212) 683-2244. 1988.

Surgery on File: General Surgery. The Diagram Group. Facts on File, Inc., 460 Park Ave. S., New York, NY 10016-7382. Phone: (212) 683-2244. 1988.

Surgery on File: Obstetrics and Gynecology. The Diagram Group. Facts on File, Inc., 460 Park Ave. S., New York, NY 10016-7382. Phone: (212) 683-2244. 1988.

Surgery on File: Orthopedics and Trauma Surgery. The Diagram Group. Facts on File, Inc., 460 Park Ave. S., New York, NY 10016-7382. Phone: (212) 683-2244. 1988.

Surgery on File: Pediatrics. The Diagram Group. Facts on File, Inc., 460 Park Ave. S., New York, NY 10016-7382. Phone: (212) 683-2244. 1988.

HANDBOOKS, GUIDES, MANUALS, ATLASES

Dietician's Patient Education Manual. Aspen Publishers, Inc., 200 Orchard Ridge Dr., Gaithersburg, MD 20878. Phone: (800) 638-8437. 1991.

Handbook of Patient Education. Ann Haggard. Aspen Publishers, Inc., 200 Orchard Ridge Dr., Gaithersburg, MD 20878. Phone: (800) 638-8437. 1989.

JOURNALS

Patient Education and Counseling. Elsevier Science Publishing Co., Inc., P.O. Box 882, Madison Square Station, New York, NY 10159-2101. Phone: (212) 989-5800. Fax: (212) 633-3990. Bimonthly.

ONLINE DATABASES

Combined Health Information Database (CHID). U.S. National Institutes of Health, P.O. Box NDIC, Bethesda, MD 20892. Phone: (301) 496-2162. Fax: (301) 770-5164. Quarterly.

EMBASE. Elsevier Science Publishing Co., Inc., P.O. Box 882, Madison Square Station, New York, NY 10159-2101. Phone: (212) 989-5800. Fax: (212) 633-3990.

Health Periodicals Database. Information Access Company, 362 Lakeside Dr., Foster City, CA 94404. Phone: (800) 227-8431. Weekly.

MEDLINE. National Library of Medicine, 8600 Rockville Pike, Bethesda, MD 20894. Phone: (800) 638-8480.

SciSearch. Institute for Scientific Information, 3501 Market St., Philadelphia, PA 19104. Phone: (215) 386-0100. Fax: (215) 386-6362.

POPULAR WORKS AND PATIENT EDUCATION

Patient Drug Facts. Bernie R. Olin III (ed.). J.B. Lippincott Co., 227 E. Washington Square, Philadelphia, PA 19106-3780. Phone: (215) 238-4200. Fax: (215) 238-4227. Quarterly.

Personal Health Reporter. Alan Rees, Charlene Wiley. Gale Research, Inc., 835 Penobscot Bldg., Detroit, MI 48226-4094. Phone: (800) 877-GALE. Fax: (313) 961-6083. 1992.

TEXTBOOKS AND MONOGRAPHS

Client Teaching Guides for Home Health Care. Donna Meyers. Aspen Publishers, Inc., 200 Orchard Ridge Dr., Gaithersburg, MD 20878. Phone: (800) 638-8437. 1989.

Communicating with Cancer Patients and Their Families. Andrew Bliztwer and others (eds.). Charles Press Publishers, P.O. Box 15715, Philadelphia, PA 19123. Phone: (215) 735-3665. 1990.

Consumer Health Information: Managing Hospital Based Centers. Salvinija Kemaghan, Barbara Gilott. American Hospital Association, 840 N. Lake Shore Dr., Chicago, IL 60611. Phone: (312) 280-6000. Fax: (312) 280-5979. 1991.

Effective Patient Education: A Guide to Increased Compliance. Donna R. Falvo. Aspen Publishers, Inc., 200 Orchard Ridge Dr., Gaithersburg, MD 20878. Phone: (800) 638-8437. 1985.

Ethics in Health Education. Spyros Doxiadis (ed.). John Wiley & Sons, Inc., 605 Third Ave., New York, NY 10158-0012. Phone: (212) 850-6000. Fax: (212) 850-6088. 1990.

Instructions for Patients. H. Winter Griffith. W.B. Saunders Co., The Curtis Center, Independence Square W., Philadelphia, PA 19106-3399. Phone: (215) 238-7800. 1989.

Management and Education of the Diabetic Patient. Robert J. Metz, James W. Benson. W.B. Saunders Co., The Curtis Center, Independence Square W., Philadelphia, PA 19106-3399. Phone: (215) 238-7800. 1988.

Managing Consumer Health Information Services. Alan Rees. Oryx Press, 4041 N. Central, Suite 700, Phoenix, AZ 85012. Phone: (800) 279-ORYX. Fax: (800) 279-4663. 1991.

Managing Hospital-Based Patient Education. Barbara E. Giloth, (ed.). American Hospital Publishing, Inc., P.O. Box 92683, Chicago, IL 60675-2683. Phone: (800) 242-2626. Fax: (312) 280-6015.

Preconceptual Health Promotion: A Practical Guide. Robert C. Cefalo, Merry K. Moos. Aspen Publishers, Inc., 200 Orchard Ridge Dr., Gaithersburg, MD 20878. Phone: (800) 638-8437. 1988.

The Process of Patient Education. Redman. Mosby-Year Book, 11830 Westline Industrial Drive, St. Louis, MO 63146. Phone: (800) 325-4177. Fax: (314) 432-1380. 1988.

Teaching Patients with Acute Conditions. Matt Cahill (ed.). Springhouse Publishing Co., 1111 Bethlehem Pike, Spring House, PA 19477. Phone: (800) 331-3170. Fax: (215) 646-8716. 1992.

Teaching Patients with Chronic Conditions. Matt Cahill (ed.). Springhouse Publishing Co., 1111 Bethlehem Pike, Spring House, PA 19477. Phone: (800) 331-3170. Fax: (215) 646-8716. 1992.

PEDIATRICS

ABSTRACTING, INDEXING, AND CURRENT AWARENESS PUBLICATIONS

Combined Cumulative Index to Pediatrics. Numarc Book Corporation, 60 Alcona Ave., Buffalo, NY 14226. Phone: (716) 834-1390. Annual.

Core Journals in Pediatrics. Elsevier Science Publishing Co., Inc., P.O. Box 882, Madison Square Station, New York, NY 10159-2101. Phone: (212) 989-5800. Fax: (212) 633-3990. 11/year.

Current Contents/Clinical Medicine. Institute for Scientific Information, 3501 Market St., Philadelphia, PA 19104. Phone: (800) 523-1850. Fax: (215) 386-6362. Weekly.

Excerpta Medica. Section 7: Pediatrics and Pediatric Surgery. Elsevier Science Publishing Co., Inc., P.O. Box 882, Madison Square Station, New York, NY 10159-2101. Phone: (212) 989-5800. Fax: (212) 633-3990. 24/year.

Index Medicus. U.S. National Library of Medicine, 8600 Rockville Pike, Bethesda, MD 20894. Phone: (800) 638-8480. Monthly.

Science Citation Index. Institute for Scientific Information, 3501 Market St., Philadelphia, PA 19104. Phone: (800) 523-1850. Fax: (215) 386-6362. Bimonthly.

ANNUALS AND REVIEWS

Advances in Pediatrics. Mosby-Year Book, 11830 Westline Industrial Drive, St. Louis, MO 63146. Phone: (800) 325-4177. Fax: (314) 432-1380. Annual.

Current Opinion in Pediatrics. Current Science Ltd., 20 N. Third St., Philadelphia, PA 19106-2199. Phone: (800) 552-5866. Fax: (215) 574-2270. Bimonthly.

Current Paediatrics. Churchill Livingstone Inc., 650 Avenue of the Americas, New York, NY 10011. Phone: (212) 819-5400. Fax: (212) 302-6598. Quarterly.

Current Pediatric Diagnosis and Treatment. Appleton & Lange, 25 Van Zant St., East Norwalk, CT 06855. Phone: (800) 423-1359. Fax: (203) 854-9486. Biennial.

Current Problems in Pediatrics. Mosby-Year Book, 11830 Westline Industrial Drive, St. Louis, MO 63146. Phone: (800) 325-4177. Fax: (314) 432-1380. 10/year.

Pediatric Annals. SLACK Inc., 6900 Grove Rd., Thorofare, NJ 08086-9447. Phone: (800) 257-8290. Fax: (609) 853-5991. Monthly.

Pediatric Clinics. W.B. Saunders Co., The Curtis Center, Independence Square W., Philadelphia, PA 19106-3399. Phone: (215) 238-7800. Bimonthly.

Year Book of Pediatrics. Mosby-Year Book, 11830 Westline Industrial Drive, St. Louis, MO 63146. Phone: (800) 325-4177. Fax: (314) 432-1380. Annual.

ASSOCIATIONS, PROFESSIONAL SOCIETIES, ADVOCACY AND SUPPORT GROUPS

American Academy of Pediatrics (AAP). 141 Northwest Point Blvd., P.O. Box 927, Elk Grove Village, IL 60009-0927. Phone: (708) 228-5005. Fax: (708) 228-5097.

American Board of Pediatrics (ABP). 111 Silver Cedar Ct., Chapel Hill, NC 27514. Phone: (919) 929-0461.

American Pediatric Society. c/o Audrey Brown M.D., Dept. of Pediatrics, SUNY Health Science Center, Brooklyn, NY 11207. Phone: (718) 270-1692.

Association for the Care of Children's Health (ACCH). 7910 Woodmont Ave., Ste. 300, Bethesda, MD 20814. Phone: (301) 654-6549. Fax: (301) 986-4553.

BIBLIOGRAPHIES

Childhood Obesity and Cardiovascular Disease. Food and Nutrition Center, National Agricultural Library, 10301 Baltimore Blvd., Beltsville, MD 20705. January 1985 - May 1990.

Infant Nutrition. Food and Nutrition Center, National Agricultural Library, 10301 Baltimore Blvd., Beltsville, MD 20705. January 1987 to March 1991.

Nutri-Topics: Nutrition for Infants and Toddlers. Food and Nutrition Center, National Agricultural Library, 10301 Baltimore Blvd., Beltsville, MD 20705.

CD-ROM DATABASES

Pediatric Cough. Hoffer. Williams & Wilkins, 428 East Preston St., Baltimore, MD 21202. Phone: (800) 638-0672. Fax: (800) 447-8438. 1990.

Pediatric Infectious Disease Journal. CMC ReSearch, Inc., 7150 S.W. Hampton, Suite C-120, Portland, OR 97223. Phone: (800) 262-7668. Fax: (503) 639-1796. Annual.

Pediatric Library. CMC ReSearch, Inc., 7150 S.W. Hampton, Suite C-120, Portland, OR 97223. Phone: (800) 262-7668. Fax: (503) 639-1796. Annual.

Pediatrics on Disc. CMC ReSearch, Inc., 7150 S.W. Hampton, Suite C-120, Portland, OR 97223. Phone: (800) 262-7668. Fax: (503) 639-1796. Annual.

Pediatrics MEDLINE. MEP, 124 Mt. Auburn St., Cambridge, MA 02138. Phone: (800) 342-1338. Fax: (617) 868-7738. Quarterly.

Pediatrics in Review/Red Book. CMC ReSearch, Inc., 7150 S.W. Hampton, Suite C-120, Portland, OR 97223. Phone: (800) 262-7668. Fax: (503) 639-1796. Annual.

SCISEARCH. Institute for Scientific Information, 3501 Market St., Philadelphia, PA 19104. Phone: (215) 386-0100. Fax: (215) 386-6362.

Year Books on Disc. CMC ReSearch, Inc., 7150 S.W. Hampton, Suite C-120, Portland, OR 97223. Phone: (800) 262-7668. Fax: (503) 639-1796. Annual includes Year Books of Cardiology, Dermatology, Diagnostic Radiology, Drug Therapy, Emergency Medicine, Family Practice, Medicine, Neurology and Neurosurgery, Obstetrics and Gynecology, Oncology, Pediatrics, and Psychiatry and Applied Mental Health.

DIRECTORIES

Directory of Certified Pediatricians. American Board of Medical Specialties, 1 Rotary Center, Suite 805, Evanston, IL 60201. Phone: (708) 491-9091. Biennial.

Directory of Medical Specialists. Marquis Who's Who, 3002 Glenview Rd., Wilmette, IL 60091. Phone: (800) 621-9669. Fax: (708) 441-2264. Biennial.

Directory of Physicians in the United States. American Medical Association, 515 North State St., Chicago, IL 60610. Phone: (312) 464-0183. Fax: (312) 464-5834. Biennial.

ENCYCLOPEDIAS, DICTIONARIES, WORD BOOKS

Surgery on File: Pediatrics. The Diagram Group. Facts on File, Inc., 460 Park Ave. S., New York, NY 10016-7382. Phone: (212) 683-2244. 1988.

HANDBOOKS, GUIDES, MANUALS, ATLASES

A Color Atlas of Pediatric Infectious Diseases. C.A. Hart. Mosby-Year Book, 11830 Westline Industrial Drive, St. Louis, MO 63146. Phone: (800) 325-4177. Fax: (314) 432-1380. 1992.

Handbook of Pediatric Emergencies. Baldwin. Little, Brown and Co., 34 Beacon St., Boston, MA 02108. Phone: (617) 227-0730. Fax: (617) 227-0790. 1989.

Handbook of Pediatric Infectious Disease and Antimicrobial Therapy. Stanford T. Shulman, Julie Kim, William

MacKendrick. Mosby-Year Book, 11830 Westline Industrial Drive, St. Louis, MO 63146. Phone: (800) 325-4177. Fax: (314) 432-1380. 1992.

Handbook of Pediatric Intensive Care. Mark C. Rogers (ed.). Williams & Wilkins, 428 East Preston St., Baltimore, MD 21202. Phone: (800) 638-0672. Fax: (800) 447-8438. 1989.

Handbook of Pediatrics. Merenstein. Appleton & Lange, 25 Van Zant St., East Norwalk, CT 06855. Phone: (800) 423-1359. Fax: (203) 854-9486. 16th edition 1991.

The Harriet Lane Handbook: A Manual for Pediatric House Officers. Mary G. Greene (ed.). Mosby-Year Book, 11830 Westline Industrial Drive, St. Louis, MO 63146. Phone: (800) 325-4177. Fax: (314) 432-1380. 1991.

Manual of Clinical Problems in Pediatrics. Roberts. Little, Brown and Co., 34 Beacon St., Boston, MA 02108. Phone: (617) 227-0730. Fax: (617) 227-0790. Third edition 1990.

Manual of Pediatric Physical Diagnosis. Barness. Mosby-Year Book, 11830 Westline Industrial Drive, St. Louis, MO 63146. Phone: (800) 325-4177. Fax: (314) 432-1380. Sixth edition 1991.

Manual of Pediatric Therapeutics. Graef. Little, Brown and Co., 34 Beacon St., Boston, MA 02108. Phone: (617) 227-0730. Fourth edition 1988.

Pediatric Cardiology Handbook. Park. Mosby-Year Book, 11830 Westline Industrial Drive, St. Louis, MO 63146. Phone: (800) 325-4177. Fax: (314) 432-1380. 1991.

Pediatric Drug Handbook. Benitz. Mosby-Year Book, 11830 Westline Industrial Drive, St. Louis, MO 63146. Phone: (800) 325-4177. Fax: (314) 432-1380. Second edition 1988.

Pediatric Pocket Companion. Michael D. Harari. Butterworth-Heinemann, 80 Montvale Ave., Stoneham, MA 02180. Phone: (617) 438-8464. Fax: (617) 279-4851. 1990.

Silver, Kempe, Bruyn and Fulginiti's Handbook of Pediatrics. Merenstein. Appleton & Lange, 25 Van Zant St., East Norwalk, CT 06855. Phone: (800) 423-1359. Fax: (203) 854-9486. 16th edition 1991.

JOURNALS

American Journal of Diseases of Children. American Medical Association, 515 North State St., Chicago, IL 60610. Phone: (312) 464-0183. Fax: (312) 464-5834. Monthly.

Archives of Disease in Childhood. BMJ Publishing Group, BMA House, Tavistock Square, London WC1H 9JR, England. Phone: 071-383 6244/6638. Fax: 071-383 6662. Monthly.

Clinical Pediatrics. J.B. Lippincott Co., 227 E. Washington Square, Philadelphia, PA 19106-3780. Phone: (215) 238-4200. Fax: (215) 238-4227.

Contemporary Pediatrics. Medical Economics, Five Paragon Dr., Montvale, NJ 07645-1742. Phone: (800) 222-3045. Fax: (201) 573-4956. Monthly.

International Journal of Pediatric Otorhinolaryngology. Elsevier Science Publishing Co., Inc., P.O. Box 882, Madison

Square Station, New York, NY 10159-2101. Phone: (212) 989-5800. Fax: (212) 633-3990. 6/year.

Journal of Child Neurology. Mosby-Year Book, 11830 Westline Industrial Drive, St. Louis, MO 63146. Phone: (800) 325-4177. Fax: (314) 432-1380. Quarterly.

Journal of Pediatric Gastroenterology and Nutrition. Raven Press, 1185 Ave. of the Americas, New York, NY 10036. Phone: (212) 930-9500. Fax: (212) 869-3495.

Journal of Pediatric Health Care. Mosby-Year Book, 11830 Westline Industrial Drive, St. Louis, MO 63146. Phone: (800) 325-4177. Fax: (314) 432-1380. Bimonthly.

Journal of Pediatrics. Mosby-Year Book, 11830 Westline Industrial Drive, St. Louis, MO 63146. Phone: (800) 325-4177. Fax: (314) 432-1380. Monthly.

The Pediatric Infectious Disease Journal. Williams & Wilkins, 428 E. Preston St., Baltimore, MD 21202. Phone: (800) 638-0672. Fax: (800) 447-8438. Monthly.

Pediatric Neurology. Pediatric Neurology, Box 486, Mayo Bldg., Harvard St. at E. River Rd., Minneapolis, MN 55455. Phone: (612) 625-7466. Fax: (612) 625-7950. Bimonthly.

Pediatric Research: An International Journal of Clinical, Laboratory, and Developmental Investigation. Williams & Wilkins, 428 E. Preston St., Baltimore, MD 21202. Phone: (800) 638-0672. Fax: (800) 447-8438. Monthly.

Pediatrics. American Academy of Pediatrics, 141 Northwest Point Rd., Elk Grove Village, IL 60009-0927. Phone: (708) 228-5005. Fax: (708) 228-5097. Monthly.

NEWSLETTERS

Child Health Alert. Child Health Alert, Inc., P.O. Box 338, Newton Highlands, MA 02161. Monthly.

Parents' Pediatric Report. IGM Enterprises, Inc., Box 155, 77 Ives St., Providence, RI 02906. Monthly.

ONLINE DATABASES

EMBASE. Elsevier Science Publishing Co., Inc., P.O. Box 882, Madison Square Station, New York, NY 10159-2101. Phone: (212) 989-5800. Fax: (212) 633-3990.

MEDIS. Mead Data Central, P.O. Box 1830, Dayton, OH 45401. Phone: (800) 227-4908.

MEDLINE. National Library of Medicine, 8600 Rockville Pike, Bethesda, MD 20894. Phone: (800) 638-8480.

SciSearch. Institute for Scientific Information, 3501 Market St., Philadelphia, PA 19104. Phone: (215) 386-0100. Fax: (215) 386-6362.

POPULAR WORKS AND PATIENT EDUCATION

The Baby Book: The Most Comprehensive Guide to Infant Care. William Sears, Martha Sears. Little, Brown and Co., 34 Beacon St., Boston, MA 02108. Phone: (617) 227-0730. Fax: (617) 227-0790. 1992.

The Baby & Child Emergency First-Aid Handbook. Mitchell Einzig (ed.). Simon & Schuster, 1230 Ave. of the Americas, New York, NY 10020. Phone: (800) 223-2348. Fax: (800) 284-0735. 1992.

Childhood Symptoms: Every Parent's Guide to Childhood Illnesses. Edward R. Brace, John P. Pacanaowski. HarperCollins Pubs., Inc., 10 E. 53rd St., New York, NY 10022-5299. Phone: (212) 207-7000. Revised edition 1992.

The Columbia University College of Physicians and Surgeons Complete Guide to Early Child Care. Genell Subak-Sharpe (ed.). Random House, Inc., 201 E. 50th St., New York, NY 10022. Phone: (800) 726-0600. 1990.

Complete Guide to Choosing Child Care. Judy Berezin. Random House, Inc., 201 E. 50th St., New York, NY 10022. Phone: (800) 726-0600. 1983.

The Complete Mothercare Manual. Rosalind Y. Ting, Herbert Brant, Kenneth S. Holt. Simon & Schuster, 1230 Ave. of the Americas, New York, NY 10020. Phone: (800) 223-2348. Fax: (800) 284-0735. Revised edition, 1992.

Curing Infant Colic: The 7-Minute Program for Soothing the Fussy Way. Bruce Taubman. Bantam Books, Inc., 666 Fifth Ave., New York, NY 10103. Phone: (800) 223-6834. 1990.

Dr. Mom's Parenting Guide: Commonsense Guidance for the Life of Your Child. Marianne E. Neifert. Viking Penguin, 375 Hudson St., New York, NY 10014-3657. Phone: (800) 331-4624. 1991.

Dr. Spock's Baby and Child Care. Benjamin Spock, Michael Rothenberg. Pocket Books, Inc., 1230 Ave. of the Americas, New York, NY 10020. Phone: (212) 698-7000. 1992.

The Good Housekeeping Illustrated Book of Pregnancy and Baby Care. William Morrow & Company, Inc., 1350 Ave. of the Americas, New York, NY 10019. Phone: (800) 237-0657. 1990.

Infants and Mothers: Differences in Development. T. Berry Brazelton. Bantam Doubleday Dell, 666 Fifth Ave., New York, NY 10103. Phone: (800) 223-6834. 1983.

Taking Care of Your Child: A Parents' Guide to Medical Care. Robert H. Pantell, James F. Fries, Donald M. Vickery. Addison-Wesley Nursing, 390 Bridge Parkway, Redwood City, CA 94065. Phone: (800) 950-5544. Third edition 1990.

What to Expect the First Year. Arlene Eisenberg, Heidi E. Murkoff, Sandee E. Hathaway. Workman Publishing Co., Inc., 708 Broadway, New York, NY 10003. Phone: (800) 722-7202. 1988.

Your Baby & Child. Penelope Leach. Random House, Inc., 201 E. 50th St., New York, NY 10022. Phone: (800) 726-0600. Revised edition 1989.

Your Child's Recovery: A Parent's Guide for the Child with a Life-Threatening Illness. Barbara A. Dailey. Facts on File, Inc., 460 Park Ave. S., New York, NY 10016-7382. Phone: (212) 683-2244. Fax: (212) 683-3633. 1991.

Your Child's Symptoms: A Parent's Guide to Understanding Pediatric Medicine. Bruce Taubman. Simon & Schuster, 1230 Ave. of the Americas, New York, NY 10020. Phone: (800) 223-2348. Fax: (800) 284-0735. 1992.

RESEARCH CENTERS, INSTITUTES, CLEARINGHOUSES

Children's Hospital Oakland Research Institute. 747 52nd St., Oakland, CA 94609. Phone: (415) 428-3502. Fax: (415) 428-3608.

Children's Hospital Research Foundation (Cincinnati). Elland & Bethesda Aves., Cincinnati, OH 45229. Phone: (513) 559-4411. Fax: (513) 559-7194.

Cystic Fibrosis and Pediatric Pulmonary Center. Case Western Reserve University. 2101 Adelbert Rd., Cleveland, OH 44106. Phone: (216) 844-3267. Fax: (216) 844-5916.

Department of Research. American Academy of Pediatrics. 141 Northwest Point Blvd., P.O. Box 927, Elk Grove Village, IL 60009-0927. Phone: (708) 228-5005. Fax: (708) 228-5097.

National Clearinghouse on Family Support and Children's Mental Health. Portland State University, P.O. Box 751, Portland, OR 97202-0751. Phone: (800) 628-1696.

St. Jude Children's Research Hospital. 332 N. Laureldale, P.O. Box 318, Memphis, TN 38101. Phone: (901) 522-0300. Fax: (901) 525-2720.

STANDARDS AND STATISTICS SOURCES

Incidence and Impact of Selected Infectious Diseases in Childhood. National Center for Health Statistics, 6525 Belcrest Rd., Rm. 1064, Hyattsville, MD 20782. Phone: (301) 436-8500. PHS 91-1508 1991.

TEXTBOOKS AND MONOGRAPHS

Ambulatory Pediatric Care. Dershewitz. J.B. Lippincott Co., 227 E. Washington Square, Philadelphia, PA 19106-3780. Phone: (215) 238-4200. Fax: (215) 238-4227. Second edition 1992.

Behavioral Pediatrics. Graydanaus. Springer-Verlag New York Inc., 175 Fifth Ave., New York, NY 10010. Phone: (212) 460-1500. Fax: (212) 473-6272. 1992.

Clinical Pediatric Endocrinology. Hung. Mosby-Year Book, 11830 Westline Industrial Drive, St. Louis, MO 63146. Phone: (800) 325-4177. Fax: (314) 432-1380. 1992.

Essentials of Pediatric Intensive Care. Levin. Quality Publications, P.O. Box 1060, Abilene, TX 79604. Phone: (800) 359-7708. 1990.

Infectious Diseases of Children. Saul Krugman, Samuel L. Katz, Anne A. Gershon, et. al.. Mosby-Year Book, 11830 Westline Industrial Drive, St. Louis, MO 63146. Phone: (800) 325-4177. Fax: (314) 432-1380. Ninth edition 1992.

Nelson Textbook of Pediatrics. Richard E. Behrman, Victor C. Vaughan. W.B. Saunders Co., The Curtis Center, Independence Sqare W., Philadelphia, PA 19106-3399. Phone: (215) 238-7800. 14th edition, 1992.

Pediatric Critical Care. Fuhrman. Mosby-Year Book, 11830 Westline Industrial Drive, St. Louis, MO 63146. Phone: (800) 325-4177. Fax: (314) 432-1380. 1992.

Pediatric Emergency Medicine. Barkin. Mosby-Year Book, 11830 Westline Industrial Drive, St. Louis, MO 63146. Phone: (800) 325-4177. Fax: (314) 432-1380. 1992.

Pediatric Epilepsy. Dodson. Demos Publications, Inc., 156 Fifth Ave., Ste. 1018, New York, NY 10010. Phone: (212) 255-8768. 1992.

Pediatric Medicine. Avery. Williams & Wilkins, 428 East Preston St., Baltimore, MD 21202. Phone: (800) 638-0672. Fax: (800) 447-8438. 1989.

Pediatric Trauma. Martin R. Eichelberger. Mosby-Year Book, 11830 Westline Industrial Drive, St. Louis, MO 63146. Phone: (800) 325-4177. Fax: (314) 432-1380. 1992.

Practical Approach to Pediatric Endocrinology. Bacon. Mosby-Year Book, 11830 Westline Industrial Drive, St. Louis, MO 63146. Phone: (800) 325-4177. Fax: (314) 432-1380. Third edition 1990.

Primary Pediatric Care. Hoekelman. Mosby-Year Book, 11830 Westline Industrial Drive, St. Louis, MO 63146. Phone: (800) 325-4177. Fax: (314) 432-1380. Second edition 1992.

Rudolph's Pediatrics. Abraham M. Rudolph, Julien Hoffman. Appleton & Lange, 25 Van Zant St., East Norwalk, CT 06855. Phone: (800) 423-1359. Fax: (203) 854-9486. 19th edition 1991.

The Science and Practice of Pediatric Cardiology. Arthur Garson Jr., J. Timothy Bricker, Dan G. McNamara. Williams & Wilkins, 428 East Preston St., Baltimore, MD 21202. Phone: (800) 638-0672. Fax: (800) 447-8438. Three volumes 1990.

Textbook of Pediatric Emergency Medicine. Gary Fleisher, Stephen Ludwig (eds.). Williams & Wilkins, 428 East Preston St., Baltimore, MD 21202. Phone: (800) 638-0672. Fax: (800) 447-8438. Second edition 1988.

Textbook of Pediatric Infectious Diseases. Ralph D. Feigin, James D. Cherry. W.B. Saunders Co., The Curtis Center, Independence Square W., Philadelphia, PA 19106-3399. Phone: (215) 238-7800. Second edition. Two volumes. 1987.

Textbook of Pediatric Nutrition. McLaren. Churchill Livingstone Inc., 650 Ave. of the Americas, New York, NY 10011. Phone: (212) 819-5400. Fax: (212) 302-6598. Third edition 1991.

PEDICULOSIS

See: PARASITIC DISEASES

PEDOPHILIA

See: CHILD ABUSE; SEXUAL DISORDERS

PEER REVIEW

See: QUALITY ASSURANCE

PENICILLINS

See: ANTIBIOTICS

PENILE CANCER

See: CANCER

PEPTIC ULCERS

See: ULCERS

PERICARDITIS

See: HEART DISEASES

PERINATOLOGY

See also: FETAL DEVELOPMENT; NEONATOLOGY; PREGNANCY COMPLICATIONS

ABSTRACTING, INDEXING, AND CURRENT AWARENESS PUBLICATIONS

Current Contents/Clinical Medicine. Institute for Scientific Information, 3501 Market St., Philadelphia, PA 19104. Phone: (800) 523-1850. Fax: (215) 386-6362. Weekly.

Excerpta Medica. Section 7: Pediatrics and Pediatric Surgery. Elsevier Science Publishing Co., Inc., P.O. Box 882, Madison Square Station, New York, NY 10159-2101. Phone: (212) 989-5800. Fax: (212) 633-3990. 24/year.

Index Medicus. U.S. National Library of Medicine, 8600 Rockville Pike, Bethesda, MD 20894. Phone: (800) 638-8480. Monthly.

Research Alert: Fetal Medicine. Institute for Scientific Information, 3501 Market St., Philadelphia, PA 19104. Phone: (800) 523-1850. Fax: (215) 386-6362. Weekly.

Science Citation Index. Institute for Scientific Information, 3501 Market St., Philadelphia, PA 19104. Phone: (800) 523-1850. Fax: (215) 386-6362. Bimonthly.

ANNUALS AND REVIEWS

Reviews in Perinatal Medicine. Emile M. Scarpelli, Ermelando V. Cosmi (eds.). John Wiley & Sons, Inc., 605 Third Ave., New York, NY 10158-0012. Phone: (212) 850-6000. Fax: (212) 850-6088. 1989.

Year Book of Neonatal and Perinatal Medicine. Mosby-Year Book, 11830 Westline Industrial Drive, St. Louis, MO 63146. Phone: (800) 325-4177. Fax: (314) 432-1380. Annual.

ASSOCIATIONS, PROFESSIONAL SOCIETIES, ADVOCACY AND SUPPORT GROUPS

National Perinatal Association (NPA). 101 1/2 S. Union St., Alexandria, VA 22314. Phone: (703) 549-5523.

Society of Obstetric Anesthesia and Perinatology. c/o Chief of Anesthesia, 2722 Colby, Ste. 507, Everett, WA 98201. Phone: (206) 259-6616.

CD-ROM DATABASES

SCISEARCH. Institute for Scientific Information, 3501 Market St., Philadelphia, PA 19104. Phone: (215) 386-0100. Fax: (215) 386-6362.

DIRECTORIES

Directory of Medical Specialists. Marquis Who's Who, 3002 Glenview Rd., Wilmette, IL 60091. Phone: (800) 621-9669. Fax: (708) 441-2264. Biennial.

Directory of Physicians in the United States. American Medical Association, 515 North State St., Chicago, IL 60610. Phone: (312) 464-0183. Fax: (312) 464-5834. Biennial.

HANDBOOKS, GUIDES, MANUALS, ATLASES

Guidelines for Perinatal Care. American Academy of Pediatrics, 141 Northwest Point Blvd., P.O. Box 927, Elk Grove Village, IL 60009-0927. Phone: (800) 433-9016. Fax: (708) 228-1281. Third edition 1992.

Handbook of Perinatal Infections. John L. Sever, John W. Larsen Jr., John H. Grossman III. Little, Brown and Company, 34 Beacon St., Boston, MA 02108. Phone: (617) 227-0730. Second edition 1988.

Obstetrical and Perinatal Infections. David Charles. Mosby-Year Book, 11830 Westline Industrial Drive, St. Louis, MO 63146. Phone: (800) 325-4177. Fax: (314) 432-1380. 1992.

JOURNALS

American Journal of Perinatology. Thieme Medical Publishers, Inc., 381 Park Ave. S., New York, NY 10016. Phone: (212) 683-5088. Fax: (212) 779-9020. Bimonthly.

Biology of the Neonate. S. Karger Publishers, Inc., 26 W. Avon Rd., P.O. Box 529, Farmington, CT 06085. Phone: (203) 675-7834. Fax: (203) 675-7302.

Clinics in Perinatology. W.B. Saunders Co., The Curtis Center, Independence Square W., Philadelphia, PA 19106-3399. Phone: (215) 238-7800. Quarterly.

Journal of Perinatal Medicine. Walter de Gruyter and Co., Genthiner Str. 17, W-1000 Berlin 30, Germany. Phone: 030 26005-251.

Journal of Perinatology. Appleton & Lange, 25 Van Zant St., East Norwalk, CT 06855. Phone: (800) 423-1359. Fax: (203) 854-9486. Quarterly.

Seminars in Perinatology. W.B. Saunders Co., The Curtis Center, Independence Sqare W., Philadelphia, PA 19106-3399. Phone: (215) 238-7800.

NEWSLETTERS

Perinatal Press, Inc.-Newsletter. Perinatal Press, Inc., Perinatal Center, Sutter Memorial Hospital, 5275 F St., Sacramento, CA 95819. Phone: (916) 733-1750. 6/year.

ONLINE DATABASES

EMBASE. Elsevier Science Publishing Co., Inc., P.O. Box 882, Madison Square Station, New York, NY 10159-2101. Phone: (212) 989-5800. Fax: (212) 633-3990.

MEDLINE. National Library of Medicine, 8600 Rockville Pike, Bethesda, MD 20894. Phone: (800) 638-8480.

SciSearch. Institute for Scientific Information, 3501 Market St., Philadelphia, PA 19104. Phone: (215) 386-0100. Fax: (215) 386-6362.

POPULAR WORKS AND PATIENT EDUCATION

Intensive Caring: New Hope for High-Risk Pregnancy. Dianne Hales. Random House, Inc., 201 E. 50th St., New York, NY 10022. Phone: (800) 726-0600. 1990.

When Pregnancy Isn't Perfect: A Layperson's Guide to Complications in Pregnancy. Laurie Rich. Viking Penguin, 375 Hudson St., New York, NY 10014-3657. Phone: (800) 331-4624. 1991.

RESEARCH CENTERS, INSTITUTES, CLEARINGHOUSES

Prenatal Clinical Research Center. Case Western Reserve University. 3395 Scranton Rd., Cleveland, OH 44109. Phone: (216) 459-4246.

TEXTBOOKS AND MONOGRAPHS

Abnormal Fetal Growth. Divon. Elsevier Science Publishing Co., Inc., P.O. Box 882, Madison Square Station, New York, NY 10159-2101. Phone: (212) 989-5800. Fax: (212) 633-3990. 1991.

Computers and Perinatal Medicine. K. Maeda, M. Hogaki, H. Nakano (eds.). Elsevier Science Publishing Co., Inc., P.O. Box 882, Madison Square Station, New York, NY 10159-2101. Phone: (212) 989-5800. Fax: (212) 633-3990. 1990.

Fetal Heart Rate Monitoring. Freeman. Williams & Wilkins, 428 East Preston St., Baltimore, MD 21202. Phone: (800) 638-0672. Fax: (800) 447-8438. Second edition 1991.

Fetal and Neonatal Cardiology. Walker A. Long. W.B. Saunders Co., The Curtis Center, Independence Square W., Philadelphia, PA 19106-3399. Phone: (215) 238-7800. 1990.

Fetal and Neonatal Physiology. Richard A. Polin, William W. Fox. W.B. Saunders Co., The Curtis Center, Independence Sqare W., Philadelphia, PA 19106-3399. Phone: (215) 238-7800. 1992.

Infectious Diseases of the Fetus and Newborn Infant. Jack Remington, Jerome Klein. W.B. Saunders Co., The Curtis Center, Independence Sqare W., Philadelphia, PA 19106-3399. Phone: (215) 238-7800. Third Edition 1990.

Introduction to Fetal Medicine. M.J. Whittle, R.J. Morrow. Butterworth-Heinemann, 80 Montvale Ave., Stoneham, MA 02180. Phone: (617) 438-8464. Fax: (617) 279-4851. 1991.

Maternal, Fetal, and Neonatal Physiology: A Clinical Perspective. Susan Tucker Blackburn, Donna Lee Loper. W.B. Saunders Co., The Curtis Center, Independence Sqare W., Philadelphia, PA 19106-3399. Phone: (215) 238-7800. 1992.

Medicine of the Fetus and Mother. Reece. J.B. Lippincott Co., 227 E. Washington Square, Philadelphia, PA 19106-3780. Phone: (215) 238-4200. Fax: (215) 238-4227. 1992.

Neonatal and Perinatal Medicine: Diseases of the Fetus and Infant. Avory Fanaroff, Richard Martin. Mosby-Year Book, 11830 Westline Industrial Drive, St. Louis, MO 63146. Phone: (800) 325-4177. Fax: (314) 432-1380. 5th edition, 1992.

Practical Guide to High-Risk Pregnancy and Delivery. Fernando Arias. Mosby-Year Book, 11830 Westline Industrial Drive, St. Louis, MO 63146. Phone: (800) 325-4177. Fax: (314) 432-1380. Second edition 1992.

The Unborn Patient: Prenatal Diagnosis and Treatment. Michael R. Harrison, Mitchell S. Golbus, Roy A. Filly. W.B. Saunders Co., The Curtis Center, Independence Square W., Philadelphia, PA 19106-3399. Phone: (215) 238-7800. Second edition 1991.

PERIODONTAL DISEASES

See: PERIODONTICS

PERIODONTICS

See also: DENTISTRY; MOUTH DISEASES;
ORAL SURGERY

ABSTRACTING, INDEXING, AND CURRENT AWARENESS PUBLICATIONS

Dental Abstracts. Mosby-Year Book, 11830 Westline Industrial Drive, St. Louis, MO 63146. Phone: (800) 325-4177. Fax: (314) 432-1380. Bimonthly.

Index to Dental Literature. American Dental Association, 211 E. Chicago Ave., Chicago, IL 60611-2678. Phone: (800) 947-4746. Fax: (312) 440-3542. Quarterly.

Index Medicus. U.S. National Library of Medicine, 8600 Rockville Pike, Bethesda, MD 20894. Phone: (800) 638-8480. Monthly.

ANNUALS AND REVIEWS

Year Book of Dentistry. Mosby-Year Book, 11830 Westline Industrial Drive, St. Louis, MO 63146. Phone: (800) 325-4177. Fax: (314) 432-1380. Annual.

ASSOCIATIONS, PROFESSIONAL SOCIETIES, ADVOCACY AND SUPPORT GROUPS

American Academy of Periodontology (AAP). 211 E. Chicago Ave., Ste. 1400, Chicago, IL 60611. Phone: (312) 787-5518.

American Board of Periodontology (ABP). Baltimore College of Dental Surgery, University of Maryland, 666 W. Baltimore St., Baltimore, MD 21201. Phone: (301) 328-2432.

American Dental Association (ADA). 211 E. Chicago Ave., Chicago, IL 60611. Phone: (312) 440-2500.

HANDBOOKS, GUIDES, MANUALS, ATLASES

Color Atlas of Periodontology. Ian Waite, J. Dermot Strahan. Mosby-Year Book, 11830 Westline Industrial Drive, St. Louis, MO 63146. Phone: (800) 325-4177. Fax: (314) 432-1380. Second edition 1990.

Periodontology. K.H. Rateitschak, E.M. Rateitschak, H.F. Wolf, et. al.. Thieme Medical Publishers, Inc., 381 Park Ave. S., New York, NY 10016. Phone: (212) 683-5088. Fax: (212) 779-9020. Color Atlas of Dental Medicine. Volume 1. 1989.

JOURNALS

Journal of Clinical Periodontology. Munksgaard International Publishers Ltd., P.O. Box 2148, DK-1016 Copenhagen K, Denmark. Phone: 33-127030. Fax: 33-129387. 10/year.

Journal of Periodontology. American Academy of Periodontology, 211 E. Chicago Ave., Chicago, IL 60611. Phone: (312) 787-5518.

NEWSLETTERS

Soft Tissue Care for GPs. American Health Consultants, Department C1290, P.O. Box 740060, Atlanta, GA 30374. Phone: (800) 559-1032. Monthly.

ONLINE DATABASES

EMBASE. Elsevier Science Publishing Co., Inc., P.O. Box 882, Madison Square Station, New York, NY 10159-2101. Phone: (212) 989-5800. Fax: (212) 633-3990.

MEDLINE. National Library of Medicine, 8600 Rockville Pike, Bethesda, MD 20894. Phone: (800) 638-8480.

SciSearch. Institute for Scientific Information, 3501 Market St., Philadelphia, PA 19104. Phone: (215) 386-0100. Fax: (215) 386-6362.

RESEARCH CENTERS, INSTITUTES, CLEARINGHOUSES

Clinical Research Center for Periodontal Diseases. 520 N. 12th St., Virginia Commonwealth University, Richmond, VA 23298. Phone: (804) 786-9185.

National Institute of Dental Research. NIH Bldg. 31, Rm. 2C-35, 9000 Rockville Pike, Bethesda, MD 20892. Phone: (301) 496-4261.

Periodontal Disease Clinical Research Center. Foster Hall, SUNY Buffalo, Buffalo, NY 14214. Phone: (716) 831-2854.

TEXTBOOKS AND MONOGRAPHS

Advances in Periodontics. Thomas G. Wilson Jr., and others (eds.) Quintessence Publishing Co., Inc., 870 Oak Creek Dr., Lombard, IL 60148-6405. Phone: (800) 621-0387. 1992.

Contemporary Periodontics. Robert J. Genco, Henry M. Goldman, D. Walter Cohen. Mosby-Year Book, 11830 Westline Industrial Drive, St. Louis, MO 63146. Phone: (800) 325-4177. Fax: (314) 432-1380. 1990.

Essentials of Periodontics. Philip M. Hoag, Elizabeth A. Pawlak. Mosby-Year Book, 11830 Westline Industrial Drive, St. Louis, MO 63146. Phone: (800) 325-4177. Fax: (314) 432-1380. 4th edition, 1990.

Glickman's Clinical Periodontology. Fermin A. Carranza Jr. (ed.). W.B. Saunders Co., The Curtis Center, Independence Square W., Philadelphia, PA 19106-3399. Phone: (215) 238-7800. Seventh edition 1990.

Periodontal Diseases: Basic Phenomena, Clinical Management, and Occlusal and Resorative Interrelationships. Saul Schluger, Ralph A. Yuodelis, Roy C. Page, et. al.. Williams & Wilkins, 428 E. Preston St., Baltimore, MD 21202. Phone: (800) 638-0672. Fax: (800) 447-8438. Second edition 1990.

Periodontal Therapy. Claude N. Nabers, William H. Stalker. Mosby-Year Book, 11830 Westline Industrial Drive, St. Louis, MO 63146. Phone: (800) 325-4177. Fax: (314) 432-1380. 1990.

Risk Markers for Oral Diseases. Volume 3: Periodontal Diseases. N.W. Johnson (ed.). Cambridge University Press, 40 W. 20th St., New York, NY 10011. Phone: (800) 431-1580. 1991.

PERITONEAL DIALYSIS

See: KIDNEY DIALYSIS

PERSONALITY DISORDERS

See also: PSYCHIATRIC DISORDERS

ABSTRACTING, INDEXING, AND CURRENT AWARENESS PUBLICATIONS

Excerpta Medica. Section 32: Psychiatry. Elsevier Science Publishing Co., Inc., P.O. Box 882, Madison Square Station, New York, NY 10159-2101. Phone: (212) 989-5800. Fax: (212) 633-3990. 20/year.

Index Medicus. U.S. National Library of Medicine, 8600 Rockville Pike, Bethesda, MD 20894. Phone: (800) 638-8480. Monthly.

Psychological Abstracts. American Psychological Association, 1200 17th St. NW, Washington, DC 20036. Phone: (202) 955-7600. Monthly.

ASSOCIATIONS, PROFESSIONAL SOCIETIES, ADVOCACY AND SUPPORT GROUPS

American Orthopsychiatric Association (ORTHO). 19 W. 44th St., No. 1616, New York, NY 10036. Phone: (212) 354-5770. Fax: (212) 302-9463.

American Psychiatric Association (APA). 1400 K St. N.W., Washington, DC 20005. Phone: (202) 682-6000. Fax: (202) 682-6114.

Canadian Psychiatric Association. 294 Albert St., Suite 204, Ottawa, ON, Canada K1P 6E6. Phone: (613) 234-2815. Fax: (613) 234-9857.

Canadian Psychological Association. Chemin Vincent, Old Chelsea, PQ, Canada J0X 2N0. Phone: (819) 827-3927. Fax: (819) 827-4639.

CD-ROM DATABASES

Excerpta Medica CD: Psychiatry. SilverPlatter Information, Inc., River Ridge Office Park, 100 River Ridge Rd., Norwood, MA 02062. Phone: (617) 769-2599. Fax: (617) 769-8763. Quarterly.

PsycLit. SilverPlatter Information, Inc., River Ridge Office Park, 100 River Ridge Rd., Norwood, MA 02062. Phone: (617) 769-2599. Fax: (617) 769-8763. Quarterly.

HANDBOOKS, GUIDES, MANUALS, ATLASES

Getting Help: A Consumer's Guide to Therapy. Christine Amner. Paragon House Publishers, 90 Fifth Ave., New York, NY 10011. Phone: (800) 727-2466. 1991.

JOURNALS

American Journal of Psychiatry. American Psychiatric Press, Inc., 1400 K St. NW, Washington, DC 20005. Phone: (202) 682-6268. Fax: (202) 789-2648. Monthly.

Harvard Review of Psychiatry. Mosby-Year Book, 11830 Westline Industrial Drive, St. Louis, MO 63146. Phone: (800) 325-4177. Fax: (314) 432-1380. Bimonthly.

Journal of Clinical Psychology. Clinical Psychology Publishing Co., 4 Corant Sq., Brandon, VT 05733. Phone: (802) 247-6871.

Journal of Personality Disorders. Guilford Publications, Inc., 72 Spring St., New York, NY 10012. Phone: (800) 365-7006. Fax: (212) 366-6708.

NEWSLETTERS

Harvard Mental Health Letter. Harvard Medical School Publications Group, 164 Longwood Ave., Boston, MA 02115. Monthly.

ONLINE DATABASES

EMBASE. Elsevier Science Publishing Co., Inc., P.O. Box 882, Madison Square Station, New York, NY 10159-2101. Phone: (212) 989-5800. Fax: (212) 633-3990.

MEDLINE. National Library of Medicine, 8600 Rockville Pike, Bethesda, MD 20894. Phone: (800) 638-8480.

Mental Health Abstracts. IFI/Plenum Data Company, 302 Swann Ave., Alexandria, VA 22301. Phone: (800) 368-3093. Monthly.

PsycInfo. SilverPlatter Information, Inc., River Ridge Office Park, 100 River Ridge Rd., Norwood, MA 02062. Phone: (617) 769-2599. Fax: (617) 769-8763. Quarterly.

SciSearch. Institute for Scientific Information, 3501 Market St., Philadelphia, PA 19104. Phone: (215) 386-0100. Fax: (215) 386-6362.

POPULAR WORKS AND PATIENT EDUCATION

The Columbia University College of Physicians and Surgeons Complete Home Guide to Mental and Emotional Health. Frederic I. Kass, John M. Oldham, Herbert Pardes, and others. Holt, Rinehart & Winston, 115 W. 18th St., New York, NY 10011. Phone: (800) 488-5233. 1992.

The Consumer's Guide to Psychotherapy. Louis J. Rosner, Shelley Ross. Simon & Schuster, Inc., 1230 Ave. of the Americas, New York, NY 10020. Phone: (212) 698-7000. 1992.

Imbroglio: Rising to the Challenges of Borderline Personality Disorder. Janice M. Carwell. W.W. Norton & Co., Inc., 500 Fifth Ave., New York, NY 10110. Phone: (800) 223-2584. 1992.

TEXTBOOKS AND MONOGRAPHS

Borderline Personality Disorders. Gunderson. American Psychiatric Press, Inc., 1400 K St. N.W., Washington, DC 20005. Phone: (202) 682-6268. Fax: (202) 789-2648. 1984.

The Challenge of the Borderline Patient: Competency in Diagnosis & Treatment. Jerome Kroll. W.W. Norton & Co., Inc., 500 Fifth Ave., New York, NY 10110. Phone: (800) 223-2584. 1988.

Personality Disorders: Diagnosis, Management and Course. Peter J. Tyrer. Butterworth-Heinemann, 80 Montvale Ave., Stoneham, MA 02180. Phone: (617) 438-8464. Fax: (617) 279-4851. 1988.

PERTUSSIS

See: INFECTIOUS DISEASES

PESTICIDES AND HERBICIDES

See also: ENVIRONMENTAL POLLUTANTS

ABSTRACTING, INDEXING, AND CURRENT AWARENESS PUBLICATIONS

CA Selects: Chemical Hazards, Health, & Safety. Chemical Abstracts Service, 2540 Olentangy River Road, P.O. Box 3012, Columbus, OH 43210-0012. Phone: (800) 848-6538. Biweekly.

Excerpta Medica. Section 52: Toxicology. Elsevier Science Publishing Co., Inc., P.O. Box 882, Madison Square Station, New York, NY 10159-2101. Phone: (212) 989-5800. Fax: (212) 633-3990. 20/year.

Index Medicus. U.S. National Library of Medicine, 8600 Rockville Pike, Bethesda, MD 20894. Phone: (800) 638-8480. Monthly.

MEDOC: Index to U.S. Government Publications in the Medical and Health Sciences. Spencer S. Eccles Health Sciences Library, University of Utah, Bldg. 589, Salt Lake City, UT 84112. Phone: (801) 581-5268. Quarterly.

Pestdoc Abstracts Journal. Derwent Publications, Rochdale House, 128 Theobalds Rd., London WC1X 8RP, England.

Pollution Abstracts. Cambridge Scientific Abstracts, 7200 Wisconsin Ave., Bethesda, MD 20814-4823. Phone: (800) 843-7751. Fax: (301) 961-6720. Bimonthly.

Toxicology Abstracts. Cambridge Scientific Abstracts, 7200 Wisconsin Ave., Bethesda, MD 20814-4823. Phone: (800) 843-7751. Fax: (301) 961-6720. Monthly.

BIBLIOGRAPHIES

Pesticide Poisoning and Food Standards for Pesticides. National Technical Information Service, 5285 Port Royal Rd., Springfield, VA 22161. Phone: (703) 487-4650. Fax: (703) 321-8547. Jan. 1978-May 1989.

Pesticide Residues in Foods. Food and Nutrition Center, National Agricultural Library, 10301 Baltimore Blvd., Beltsville, MD 20705. August 1990.

Toxicity of Pesticides. National Technical Information Service, 5285 Port Royal Rd., Springfield, VA 22161. Phone: (703) 487-4650. Fax: (703) 321-8547. Feb. 1987-Oct. 1989 PB90-851072/CBY.

CD-ROM DATABASES

PolTox. Cambridge Scientific Abstracts, 7200 Wisconsin Ave., Bethesda, MD 20814-4823. Phone: (800) 843-7751. Fax: (301) 961-6720. Quarterly.

TOXLINE. SilverPlatter Information, Inc., River Ridge Office Park, 100 River Ridge Rd., Norwood, MA 02062. Phone: (617) 769-2599. Fax: (617) 769-8763. Quarterly.

JOURNALS

Ecotoxicology and Environmental Safety. Academic Press, Inc., 1250 Sixth Ave., San Diego, CA 92101-4311. Phone: (619) 699-6345. Fax: (619) 699-6715.

Journal of Toxicology and Environmental Health. Taylor & Francis Inc., 1900 Frost Rd., Suite 101, Bristol, PA 19007-1598. Phone: (800) 821-8312. Fax: (215) 785-5515. Monthly.

ONLINE DATABASES

EMBASE. Elsevier Science Publishing Co., Inc., P.O. Box 882, Madison Square Station, New York, NY 10159-2101. Phone: (212) 989-5800. Fax: (212) 633-3990.

MEDLINE. National Library of Medicine, 8600 Rockville Pike, Bethesda, MD 20894. Phone: (800) 638-8480.

Pest Control Literature Documentation (PESTDOC). Derwent Publications, Rochdale House, 128 Theobalds Rd., London WC1X 8RP, England.

Pesticide and Toxic Chemical News. Food Chemical News Inc., 1101 Pennsylvania Ave. S.E., Washington, DC 20003. Phone: (202) 544-1980.

Pestline. Occupational Health Services Inc., 450 7th Ave., No. 2407, New York, NY 10123. Phone: (212) 967-1100.

Pollution Abstracts. Cambridge Scientific Abstracts, 7200 Wisconsin Ave., Bethesda, MD 20814-4823. Phone: (800) 843-7751. Fax: (301) 961-6720.

SciSearch. Institute for Scientific Information, 3501 Market St., Philadelphia, PA 19104. Phone: (215) 386-0100. Fax: (215) 386-6362.

TOXLINE. U.S. National Library of Medicine, Toxicology Information Program, 8600 Rockville Pike, Bethesda, MD 20894. Phone: (800) 638-8480. Monthly.

RESEARCH CENTERS, INSTITUTES, CLEARINGHOUSES

Environmental Protection Agency. 401 M St. N.W., Washington, DC 20460. Phone: (202) 382-4700.

TEXTBOOKS AND MONOGRAPHS

Extra Pharmacopeia. J. Reynolds, W. Martindale. Pharmaceutical Press, Rittenhouse Book Distributors, 511 Feheley Dr., King of Prussia, PA 19406. Phone: (800) 345-6425. 29th edition 1989.

Human Toxicology of Pesticides. Fina Petrova Kaloyanova, M.A. El Batawi. CRC Press, Inc., 2000 Corporate Blvd. N.W., Boca Raton, FL 33431. Phone: (407) 994-0555. Fax: (407) 997-0949. 1992.

PHARMACEUTICAL INDUSTRY

See also: DRUGS

ABSTRACTING, INDEXING, AND CURRENT AWARENESS PUBLICATIONS

Chemical Patents Index. Derwent Publications, Rochdale House, 128 Theobalds Rd., London WC1X 8RP, England. Phone: 071-242 5823.

International Pharmaceutical Abstracts. American Society of Hospital Pharmacists, 4630 Montgomery Ave., Bethesda, MD 20814. Phone: (301) 657-3000. Fax: (301) 657-1641. Semimonthly.

ANNUALS AND REVIEWS

In Development Biotechnology Medicines. Pharmaceutical Manufacturers Association, 1100 15th St. N.W., Washington, DC 20005. Phone: (202) 835-3400. Annual.

In Development New Medicines for Arthritis. Pharmaceutical Manufacturers Association, 1100 15th St. N.W., Washington, DC 20005. Phone: (202) 835-3400. Annual.

In Development New Medicines for Children. Pharmaceutical Manufacturers Association, 1100 15th St. N.W., Washington, DC 20005. Phone: (202) 835-3400. Quarterly.

In Development New Medicines for Older Americans. Pharmaceutical Manufacturers Association, 1100 15th St. N.W., Washington, DC 20005. Phone: (202) 835-3400. Annual.

In Development New Medicines for Older Americans. 1991 Annual Survey. 93 Cardiovascular, Cerebrovascular Medicines in Testing for Top Causes of Death. Pharmaceutical Manufacturers Association, 1100 15th St. N.W., Washington, DC 20005. Phone: (202) 835-3400. 1991.

In Development New Medicines for Older Americans. 1991 Annual Survey. 116 Medicines Target 19 Debilitating Diseases. Pharmaceutical Manufacturers Association, 1100 15th St. N.W., Washington, DC 20005. Phone: (202) 835-3400. 1991.

In Development New Medicines for Older Americans. 1991 Annual Survey. 329 Medicines in Testing for 45 Diseases of Aging. Pharmaceutical Manufacturers Association, 1100 15th St. N.W., Washington, DC 20005. Phone: (202) 835-3400. 1991.

In Development New Medicines for Older Americans. 1991 Annual Survey. More Medicines in Testing for Cancer Than for Any Other Disease of Aging. Pharmaceutical Manufacturers Association, 1100 15th St. N.W., Washington, DC 20005. Phone: (202) 835-3400. 1991.

In Development New Medicines for Women. Pharmaceutical Manufacturers Association, 1100 15th St. N.W., Washington, DC 20005. Phone: (202) 835-3400. Annual.

In Development Orphan Drugs. Pharmaceutical Manufacturers Association, 1100 15th St. N.W., Washington, DC 20005. Phone: (202) 835-3400. Annual.

ASSOCIATIONS, PROFESSIONAL SOCIETIES, ADVOCACY AND SUPPORT GROUPS

Generic Pharmaceutical Industry Association. 200 Madison Ave., No. 2404, New York, NY 10016. Phone: (212) 683-1881.

National Association of Pharmaceutical Manufacturers. 747 Third Ave., New York, NY 10017. Phone: (212) 838-3720.

National Pharmaceutical Council. 1894 Preston White Dr., Reston, VA 22091. Phone: (703) 620-6390.

Nonprescription Drug Manufacturers Association. 1150 Connecticut Ave. N.W., Washington, DC 20036. Phone: (202) 429-9260.

Pharmaceutical Manufacturers Association. 1100 15th St. N.W., Washington, DC 20005. Phone: (202) 835-3400.

BIBLIOGRAPHIES

New Drug Approvals in 1991. Pharmaceutical Manufacturers Association, 1100 15th St. N.W., Washington, DC 20005. Phone: (202) 835-3400. 1992.

CD-ROM DATABASES

International Pharmaceutical Abstracts. SilverPlatter Information, Inc., River Ridge Office Park, 100 River Ridge Rd., Norwood, MA 02062. Phone: (617) 769-2599. Fax: (617) 769-8763. Quarterly.

ENCYCLOPEDIAS, DICTIONARIES, WORD BOOKS

Pharmaceutical Word Book. Barbara De Lorenzo. Springhouse Publishing Co., 1111 Bethlehem Pike, Spring House, PA 19477. Phone: (800) 331-3170. Fax: (215) 646-8716. Second edition 1992.

JOURNALS

American Pharmacy. American Pharmaceutical Manufacturers Association, 2215 Constitution Ave. N.W., Washington, DC 20037. Phone: (202) 628-4410.

Drug Topics. Medical Economics, Five Paragon Dr., Montvale, NJ 07645-1742. Phone: (800) 232-7379. Fax: (201) 573-4956.

Drug Topics Red Book. Medical Economics, Five Paragon Dr., Montvale, NJ 07645-1742. Phone: (800) 232-7379. Fax: (201) 573-4956.

Drugs in Prospect. Paul de Haen International, 2750 S. Shoshone St., Englewood, CO 80110. Phone: (800) 438-0296.

Drugs in Research. Paul de Haen International, 2750 S. Shoshone St., Englewood, CO 80110. Phone: (800) 438-0296.

Drugs in Use. Paul de Haen International, 2750 S. Shoshone St., Englewood, CO 80110. Phone: (800) 438-0296.

NEWSLETTERS

Pharmaceutical Representative. Medical Economics, Five Paragon Dr., Montvale, NJ 07645-1742. Phone: (800) 222-3045. Fax: (201) 573-4956. Monthly.

ONLINE DATABASES

International Pharmaceutical Abstracts. American Society of Hospital Pharmacists, 4630 Montgomery Ave., Bethesda, MD 20814. Phone: (301) 657-3000. Fax: (301) 657-1641. Monthly.

Pharmaceutical News Index. UMI/Data Courier, 620 Third St., Louisville, KY 40202. Phone: (800) 626-2475.

POPULAR WORKS AND PATIENT EDUCATION

39 Development AIDS Medicines: Drugs and Vaccines. Pharmaceutical Manufacturers Association, 1100 15th St. N.W., Washington, DC 20005. Phone: (202) 835-3400. Annual.

RESEARCH CENTERS, INSTITUTES, CLEARINGHOUSES

Office of Consumer Affairs. Food and Drug Administration. 5600 Fishers Ln., HFE-50, Rockville, MD 20857. Phone: (301) 443-3170.

PHARMACOLOGY

See also: DRUG HYPERSENSITIVITY; DRUG INTERACTIONS; DRUG TOXICITY; DRUGS

ABSTRACTING, INDEXING, AND CURRENT AWARENESS PUBLICATIONS

Current Contents/Life Sciences. Institute for Scientific Information, 3501 Market St., Philadelphia, PA 19104. Phone: (215) 386-0100. Fax: (215) 386-6362.

Excerpta Medica. Section 30: Clinical and Experimental Pharmacology. Elsevier Science Publishing Co., Inc., P.O. Box 882, Madison Square Station, New York, NY 10159-2101. Phone: (212) 989-5800. Fax: (212) 633-3990. 32/year.

Index Medicus. U.S. National Library of Medicine, 8600 Rockville Pike, Bethesda, MD 20894. Phone: (800) 638-8480. Monthly.

International Pharmaceutical Abstracts. American Society of Hospital Pharmacists, 4630 Montgomery Ave., Bethesda, MD 20814. Phone: (301) 657-3000. Fax: (301) 657-1641. Semimonthly.

PharmIndex. Skyline Publishers, Inc., P.O. Box 1029, University Station, Portland, OR 97207. Phone: (503) 228-6568. Monthly.

Science Citation Index. Institute for Scientific Information, 3501 Market St., Philadelphia, PA 19104. Phone: (800) 523-1850. Fax: (215) 386-6362. Bimonthly.

ANNUALS AND REVIEWS

Advanced Drug Delivery Reviews. Elsevier Science Publishing Co., Inc., P.O. Box 882, Madison Square Station, New York, NY 10159-2101. Phone: (212) 989-5800. Fax: (212) 633-3990. 6/year.

Advances in Drug Research. Academic Press, Inc., 1250 Sixth Ave., San Diego, CA 92101-4311. Phone: (619) 699-6345. Fax: (619) 699-6715. Irregular.

Advances in Pharmaceutical Sciences. Academic Press, Inc., 1250 Sixth Ave., San Diego, CA 92101-4311. Phone: (619) 699-6345. Fax: (619) 699-6715.

Advances in Pharmacology. Academic Press, Inc., 1250 Sixth Ave., San Diego, CA 92101-4311. Phone: (619) 699-6345. Fax: (619) 699-6715. Irregular.

Annual Review of Pharmacology and Toxicology. Annual Reviews Inc., 4139 El Camino Way, P.O. Box 10139, Palo Alto, CA 94303-0897. Phone: (415) 493-4400. Fax: (415) 855-9815. Annual.

Drug Facts and Comparisons. J.B. Lippincott Co., 227 E. Washington Square, Philadelphia, PA 19106-3780. Phone: (215) 238-4200. Fax: (215) 238-4227. Annual.

Pharmacological Reviews. Williams & Wilkins, 428 E. Preston St., Baltimore, MD 21202. Phone: (800) 638-0672. Fax: (800) 447-8438. Quarterly.

Year Book of Pharmacology. CRC Press, Inc., 2000 Corporate Blvd. N.W., Boca Raton, FL 33431. Phone: (407) 994-0555. Fax: (407) 997-0949. Annual.

CD-ROM DATABASES

1993 PDR Library on CD-ROM. Medical Economics, Five Paragon Dr., Montvale, NJ 07645-1742. Phone: (800) 232-7379. Fax: (201) 573-4956. 1993.

Excerpta Medica CD: Drugs & Pharmacology. SilverPlatter Information, Inc., River Ridge Office Park, 100 River Ridge Rd., Norwood, MA 02062. Phone: (617) 769-2599. Fax: (617) 769-8763. Quarterly.

Human Drug Kinetics. Saunders. Oxford University Press, 200 Madison Ave., New York, NY 10016. Phone: (212) 679-7300. 1989.

International Pharmaceutical Abstracts. SilverPlatter Information, Inc., River Ridge Office Park, 100 River Ridge Rd., Norwood, MA 02062. Phone: (617) 769-2599. Fax: (617) 769-8763. Quarterly.

PDR on CD-ROM. Medical Economics, Five Paragon Dr., Montvale, NJ 07645-1742. Phone: (800) 222-3045. Fax: (201) 573-4956. 3/year.

SCISEARCH. Institute for Scientific Information, 3501 Market St., Philadelphia, PA 19104. Phone: (215) 386-0100. Fax: (215) 386-6362.

SEDBASE (Side Effects of Drugs). SilverPlatter Information, Inc., River Ridge Office Park, 100 River Ridge Rd., Norwood, MA 02062. Phone: (617) 769-2599. Fax: (617) 769-8763. Semiannual.

Year Books on Disc. CMC ReSearch, Inc., 7150 S.W. Hampton, Suite C-120, Portland, OR 97223. Phone: (800) 262-7668. Fax: (503) 639-1796. Annual includes Year Books of Cardiology, Dermatology, Diagnostic Radiology, Drug Therapy, Emergency Medicine, Family Practice, Medicine, Neurology and Neurosurgery, Obstetrics and Gynecology, Oncology, Pediatrics, and Psychiatry and Applied Mental Health.

DIRECTORIES

AFHS Drug Information. American Society of Hospital Pharmacists, 4630 Montgomery Ave., Bethesda, MD 20814. Phone: (301) 657-3000. Fax: (301) 652-8278. Annual, updated irregularly.

ENCYCLOPEDIAS, DICTIONARIES, WORD BOOKS

Merck Index: An Encyclopedia of Chemicals and Drugs. Merck & Co., Inc., P.O. Box 2000, Rahway, NJ 07065. Phone: (201) 855-4558. Irregular.

Pharmaceutical Words. Stedman. Williams & Wilkins, 428 East Preston St., Baltimore, MD 21202. Phone: (800) 638-0672. Fax: (800) 447-8438. 1992.

HANDBOOKS, GUIDES, MANUALS, ATLASES

Drug-Test Interactions Handbook. Jack G. Salway. Raven Press, 1185 Avenue of the Americas, New York, NY 10036. Phone: (212) 930-9500. Fax: (212) 869-3495. 1990.

The Handbook of Immunopharmacology. Academic Press, Inc., 1250 Sixth Ave., San Diego, CA 92101-4311. Phone: (619) 699-6345. Fax: (619) 699-6715. Irregular.

Handbook of Pharmacologic Therapeutics. Bogner. Little, Brown and Co., 34 Beacon St., Boston, MA 02108. Phone: (617) 227-0730. Fax: (617) 227-0790. 1988.

Introduction to Drug Therapy. Springhouse Publishing Co., 1111 Bethlehem Pike, Spring House, PA 19477. Phone: (800) 331-3170. Fax: (215) 646-8716. 1992.

Manual of Emergency Medical Therapeutics. Gideon Bosker, Jeffrey S. Jones. Mosby-Year Book, 11830 Westline Industrial Drive, St. Louis, MO 63146. Phone: (800) 325-4177. Fax: (314) 432-1380. 1992.

Pediatric Drug Handbook. Benitz. Mosby-Year Book, 11830 Westline Industrial Drive, St. Louis, MO 63146. Phone: (800) 325-4177. Fax: (314) 432-1380. Second edition 1988.

JOURNALS

Behavioural Pharmacology. Rapid Communications of Oxford Ltd., The Old Malthouse, Paradise St., Oxford OX1 1LD, England. Phone: 44-865-790447. Fax: 44-865-244012. 6/year.

Clinical Neuropharmacology. Raven Press, 1185 Avenue of the Americas, New York, NY 10036. Phone: (212) 930-9500. Fax: (212) 869-3495. Bimonthly.

European Journal of Pharmacology/Environmental Toxicology and Pharmacology Section. Elsevier Science Publishing Co., Inc., P.O. Box 882, Madison Square Station, New York, NY 10159-2101. Phone: (212) 989-5800. Fax: (212) 633-3990. 6/year.

Immunopharmacology. Elsevier Science Publishing Co., Inc., P.O. Box 882, Madison Square Station, New York, NY 10159-2101. Phone: (212) 989-5800. Fax: (212) 633-3990. 6/year.

International Journal of Pharmaceutics. Elsevier Science Publishing Co., Inc., P.O. Box 882, Madison Square Station, New York, NY 10159-2101. Phone: (212) 989-5800. Fax: (212) 633-3990. 33/year.

Journal of Clinical Pharmacology. J.B. Lippincott Co., 227 E. Washington Square, Philadelphia, PA 19106-3780. Phone: (215) 238-4200. Fax: (215) 238-4227.

Journal of Pharmaceutical Sciences. American Pharmaceutical Association, 2215 Constitution Ave. NW, Washington, DC 200037. Phone: (800) 237-2742. Fax: (202) 783-2351. Monthly.

The Journal of Pharmacology and Experimental Therapeutics. Williams & Wilkins, 428 E. Preston St., Baltimore, MD 21202. Phone: (800) 638-0672. Fax: (800) 447-8438. Monthly.

Journal of Pharmacy and Pharmacology. Pharmaceutical Society of Great Britain, 1 Lambeth High St., London SE1 7JN, England.

Molecular Pharmacology. Williams & Wilkins, 428 E. Preston St., Baltimore, MD 21202. Phone: (800) 638-0672. Fax: (800) 447-8438. Monthly.

Pharmaceutical Physician. British Association of Pharmaceutical Physicians, 1 Wimpole St., London W1M 8AE, England. Phone: (44) 71 491 8610. Fax: (44) 71 499 2405. Bimonthly.

Pharmacology and Therapeutics. Pergamon Press, 660 White Plains Rd., Tarrytown, NY 10591-5153. Phone: (914) 592-7700. Fax: (914) 592-3625.

NEWSLETTERS

FDA Drug Bulletin. Food and Drug Administration. Department of Health and Human Services, 5600 Fishers Ln., Rockville, MD 20857. Phone: (301) 443-3220. 3-4/year.

ONLINE DATABASES

EMBASE. Elsevier Science Publishing Co., Inc., P.O. Box 882, Madison Square Station, New York, NY 10159-2101. Phone: (212) 989-5800. Fax: (212) 633-3990.

International Pharmaceutical Abstracts. American Society of Hospital Pharmacists, 4630 Montgomery Ave., Bethesda, MD 20814. Phone: (301) 657-3000. Fax: (301) 657-1641. Monthly.

MEDLINE. National Library of Medicine, 8600 Rockville Pike, Bethesda, MD 20894. Phone: (800) 638-8480.

Pharmline. Regional Drug Information Service, The London Hospital, Whitechapel Rd., London E1 1BB, England. Phone: 071-377 7489. Weekly.

SciSearch. Institute for Scientific Information, 3501 Market St., Philadelphia, PA 19104. Phone: (215) 386-0100. Fax: (215) 386-6362.

POPULAR WORKS AND PATIENT EDUCATION

Pharmacology from A to Z. John Carpenter. St. Martin's Press, 175 Fifth Ave., New York, NY 10010. Phone: (212) 674-5151. 1989.

RESEARCH CENTERS, INSTITUTES, CLEARINGHOUSES

Center for Biomedical Research. University of Kansas. Smissman Research Laboratories, 2099 Constant Ave., Lawrence, KS 66046. Phone: (913) 864-5140.

Department of Pharmacology and Therapeutics. McGill University. 3655 Rue Drummond, Montreal, PQ, Canada H3G 1Y6. Phone: (514) 398-3621. Fax: (514) 398-6690.

Interdisciplinary Program in Cell and Molecular Pharmacology and Experimental Therapeutics. Medical University of South Carolina. 171 Ashley Ave., Charleston, SC 29425. Phone: (803) 792-2471.

Office of Consumer Affairs. Food and Drug Administration. 5600 Fishers Ln., HFE-50, Rockville, MD 20857. Phone: (301) 443-3170.

Pharmacology Research Laboratory. Indiana University. School of Medicine, 635 Barnhill Dr., Indianapolis, IN 46223. Phone: (317) 274-7844. Fax: (317) 274-7714.

Upjohn Center for Clinical Pharmacology. University of Michigan. Medical Center, Ann Arbor, MI 48109. Phone: (313) 764-9121.

TEXTBOOKS AND MONOGRAPHS

Basic and Clinical Pharmacology. Katzung. Appleton & Lange, 25 Van Zant St., East Norwalk, CT 06855. Phone: (800) 423-1359. Fax: (203) 854-9486. Fifth edition 1992.

Clinical Pharmacology and Nursing. Charold L. Baer, Bradley R. Williams. Springhouse Publishing Co., 1111 Bethlehem Pike, Spring House, PA 19477. Phone: (800) 331-3170. Fax: (215) 646-8716. Second edition 1992.

Clinical Pharmacology of Psychotherapeutic Drugs. Leo E. Hollister, John Csernansky. Churchill Livingstone Inc., 650 Avenue of the Americas, New York, NY 10011. Phone: (212) 819-5400. Fax: (212) 302-6598. Third edition 1990.

Essentials of Medical Pharmacology. Kalant. Mosby-Year Book, 11830 Westline Industrial Drive, St. Louis, MO 63146. Phone: (800) 325-4177. Fax: (314) 432-1380. 1991.

Extra Pharmacopeia. J. Reynolds, W. Martindale. Pharmaceutical Press, Rittenhouse Book Distributors, 511 Feheley Dr., King of Prussia, PA 19406. Phone: (800) 345-6425. 29th edition 1989.

Goodman and Gilman's The Pharmacological Basis of Therapeutics. Alfred Goodman Gilman, Theodore W. Rall, Alan S. Nies, et. al.. McGraw-Hill, Inc., 1221 Avenue of the Americas, 28th Floor, New York, NY 10020. Phone: (212) 512-4228. Eighth edition 1990.

Lippincott's Illustrated Reviews: Pharmacology. Richard A. Harvey, Pamela C. Champe. J.B. Lippincott Co., 227 E. Washington Square, Philadelphia, PA 19106-3780. Phone: (215) 238-4200. Fax: (215) 238-4227. 1992.

Melmon and Morrelli's Clinical Pharmacology: Basic Principles of Therapeutics. Kenneth L. Melmon, Howard F. Morrelli, Brian B. Hoffman. McGraw-Hill, Inc., 11 West 19th St., New York, NY 10011. Phone: (212) 337-5001. Fax: (212) 337-4092. Third edition 1992.

Pharmacological Basis of Therapeutics. L. Goodman, A. Gilman. McGraw-Hill Inc., 11 West 19th St., New York, NY 10011. Phone: (212) 337-5001. Fax: (212) 337-4092. 8th edition 1990

Pharmacology. Harvey. J.B. Lippincott Co., 227 E. Washington Square, Philadelphia, PA 19106-3780. Phone: (215) 238-4200. Fax: (215) 238-4227. 1992.

Therapeutic Drugs. Sir Colin Dollery (ed.). Churchill Livingstone Inc., 650 Avenue of the Americas, New York, NY 10011. Phone: (212) 819-5400. Fax: (212) 302-6598. Two volumes 1991.

Wilson and Gisvold's Textbook of Organic Medicinal and Pharmaceutical Chemistry. Delgado. J.B. Lippincott Co., 227 E. Washington Square, Philadelphia, PA 19106-3780. Phone: (215) 238-4200. Fax: (215) 238-4227. Ninth edition 1991.

PHARMACY

See also: DRUGS

ABSTRACTING, INDEXING, AND CURRENT AWARENESS PUBLICATIONS

International Pharmaceutical Abstracts. American Society of Hospital Pharmacists, 4630 Montgomery Ave., Bethesda, MD 20814. Phone: (301) 657-3000. Fax: (301) 657-1641. Semimonthly.

PharmIndex. Skyline Publishers, Inc., P.O. Box 1029, University Station, Portland, OR 97207. Phone: (503) 228-6568. Monthly.

ASSOCIATIONS, PROFESSIONAL SOCIETIES, ADVOCACY AND SUPPORT GROUPS

Academy of Pharmacy Practice and Management (APPM). American Pharmaceutical Association, 2215 Constitution Ave. N.W., Washington, DC 20037. Phone: (202) 628-4410. Fax: (202) 783-2351.

American Association of Colleges of Pharmacy (AACP). 1426 Prince St., Alexandria, VA 22314. Phone: (703) 739-2330.

American Association of Homeopathic Pharmacists. P.O. Box 2273, Falls Church, VA 22042. Phone: (703) 532-3237.

American Pharmaceutical Association (APhA). 2215 Constitution Ave. N.W., Washington, DC 20037. Phone: (202) 628-4410. Fax: (202) 783-2351.

American Society of Hospital Pharmacists (ASHP). 4630 Montgomery Ave., Bethesda, MD 20814. Phone: (301) 657-3000. Fax: (301) 652-8278.

Canadian Society of Hospital Pharmacists. 123 Edward St., Suite 603, Toronto, ON, Canada M5G 1E2.

United States Pharmacopeial Convention (USP). 12601 Twinbrook Pkwy., Rockville, MD 20852. Phone: (800) 227-8772. Fax: (301) 816-8375.

CD-ROM DATABASES

1993 PDR Library on CD-ROM. Medical Economics, Five Paragon Dr., Montvale, NJ 07645-1742. Phone: (800) 232-7379. Fax: (201) 573-4956. 1993.

Drug Data Report on CD-ROM. Prous Science Publishers, Apdo. de Correos 540, E-08080 Barcelona, Spain. Phone: 03 4592220. Fax: 03 2581535. Quarterly.

Drug Information Source on CD-ROM. Cambridge Scientific Abstracts, 7200 Wisconsin Ave., Bethesda, MD 20814-4823. Phone: (800) 843-7751. Fax: (301) 961-6720. Quarterly.

Excerpta Medica CD: Drugs & Pharmacology. SilverPlatter Information, Inc., River Ridge Office Park, 100 River Ridge Rd., Norwood, MA 02062. Phone: (617) 769-2599. Fax: (617) 769-8763. Quarterly.

International Pharmaceutical Abstracts. SilverPlatter Information, Inc., River Ridge Office Park, 100 River Ridge Rd., Norwood, MA 02062. Phone: (617) 769-2599. Fax: (617) 769-8763. Quarterly.

Physician's Desk Reference. Medical Economics, Five Paragon Dr., Montvale, NJ 07645-1742. Phone: (800) 222-3045. Fax: (201) 573-4956. 3/year.

SEDBASE (Side Effects of Drugs). SilverPlatter Information, Inc., River Ridge Office Park, 100 River Ridge Rd., Norwood, MA 02062. Phone: (617) 769-2599. Fax: (617) 769-8763. Semiannual.

DIRECTORIES

American Druggist Blue Book. Hearst Corporation, 60 E. 42nd St., New York, NY 10165. Phone: (212) 297-9680. Fax: (415) 588-6867. Annual.

Red Book. Medical Economics, Five Paragon Dr., Montvale, NJ 07645-1742. Phone: (800) 222-3045. Fax: (201) 573-4956. Annual.

ENCYCLOPEDIAS, DICTIONARIES, WORD BOOKS

Pharmaceutical Word Book. Barbara De Lorenzo. Springhouse Publishing Co., 1111 Bethlehem Pike, Spring House, PA 19477. Phone: (800) 331-3170. Fax: (215) 646-8716. Second edition 1992.

Pharmaceutical Words. Stedman. Williams & Wilkins, 428 East Preston St., Baltimore, MD 21202. Phone: (800) 638-0672. Fax: (800) 447-8438. 1992.

USAN and the USP Dictionary of Drug Names. United States Pharmacopeial Convention, Inc., 12601 Twinbrook Parkway, Rockville, MD 20852. Phone: (800) 227-8772. Fax: (301) 816-8148. Annual.

HANDBOOKS, GUIDES, MANUALS, ATLASES

Physician's Desk Reference. Medical Economics, Five Paragon Dr., Montvale, NJ 07645-1742. Phone: (800) 222-3045. Fax: (201) 573-4956. Annual.

JOURNALS

American Journal of Hospital Pharmacy. American Society of Hospital Pharmacists, c/o Jean Rogers, Dir. Mkt. Services, 4630 Montgomery Ave., Bethesda, MD 20814. Phone: (301) 657-3000. Monthly.

Clinical Pharmacy. American Society of Hospital Pharmacists, 4630 Montgomery Ave., Bethesda, MD 20814. Phone: (301) 657-3000. Fax: (301) 652-8278. Monthly.

Drug Topics. Medical Economics, Five Paragon Dr., Montvale, NJ 07645-1742. Phone: (800) 232-7379. Fax: (201) 573-4956.

Drug Topics Red Book. Medical Economics, Five Paragon Dr., Montvale, NJ 07645-1742. Phone: (800) 232-7379. Fax: (201) 573-4956.

Hospital Pharmacy. J.B. Lippincott Co., 227 E. Washington Square, Philadelphia, PA 19106-3780. Phone: (215) 238-4200. Fax: (215) 238-4227. Monthly.

International Journal of Pharmaceutics. Elsevier Science Publishing Co., Inc., P.O. Box 882, Madison Square Station, New York, NY 10159-2101. Phone: (212) 989-5800. Fax: (212) 633-3990. 33/year.

Journal of Clinical Pharmacy and Therapies. Blackwell Scientific Publications, Inc., 3 Cambridge Center, Cambridge, MA 02142. Phone: (800) 759-6102.

Journal of Pharmaceutical Sciences. American Pharmaceutical Association, 2215 Constitution Ave. NW, Washington, DC 200037. Phone: (800) 237-2742. Fax: (202) 783-2351. Monthly.

Journal of Pharmacy and Pharmacology. Pharmaceutical Society of Great Britain, 1 Lambeth High St., London SE1 7JN, England.

Perspectives in Clinical Pharmacy. Elsevier Science Publishing Co., Inc., P.O. Box 882, Madison Square Station, New York, NY 10159-2101. Phone: (212) 989-5800. Fax: (212) 633-3990. Monthly.

NEWSLETTERS

Drug Utilization Review. American Health Consultants, Department C1290, P.O. Box 740060, Atlanta, GA 30374. Phone: (800) 559-1032. Fax: (404) 352-1971. Monthly.

Pharmacy Today. American Pharmaceutical Association, 2215 Constitution Ave. N.W., Washington, DC 20037. Phone: (202) 628-4410. Biweekly.

ONLINE DATABASES

International Pharmaceutical Abstracts. American Society of Hospital Pharmacists, 4630 Montgomery Ave., Bethesda, MD 20814. Phone: (301) 657-3000. Fax: (301) 657-1641. Monthly.

Pharmline. Regional Drug Information Service, The London Hospital, Whitechapel Rd., London E1 1BB, England. Phone: 071-377 7489. Weekly.

Physician's Desk Reference. Medical Economics, Five Paragon Dr., Montvale, NJ 07645-1742. Phone: (800) 222-3045. Fax: (201) 573-4956. Monthly.

RESEARCH CENTERS, INSTITUTES, CLEARINGHOUSES

Center for the Study of Drug Development. Tufts University, 136 Harrison Ave., Boston, MA 02111. Phone: (617) 956-0070. Fax: (617) 350-8425.

Office of Consumer Affairs. Food and Drug Administration. 5600 Fishers Ln., HFE-50, Rockville, MD 20857. Phone: (301) 443-3170.

Pharmacy Foundation of North Carolina, Inc.. UNC School of Pharmacy, 101 Beard Hall, CB 7360, Chapel Hill, NC 27599. Phone: (919) 966-1121. Fax: (919) 966-6919.

Research Institute of Pharmaceutical Sciences. University of Mississippi. School of Pharmacy, University, MS 38677. Phone: (601) 232-7132. Fax: (601) 232-5118.

TEXTBOOKS AND MONOGRAPHS

Pharmacy Practice: Social and Behavioral Aspects. Albert I. Wertheimer, Mickey Smity. Williams & Wilkins, 428 East Preston St., Baltimore, MD 21202. Phone: (800) 638-0672. Fax: (800) 447-8438. 3rd edition, 1989.

Wilson and Gisvold's Textbook of Organic Medicinal and Pharmaceutical Chemistry. Delgado. J.B. Lippincott Co., 227 E. Washington Square, Philadelphia, PA 19106-3780. Phone: (215) 238-4200. Fax: (215) 238-4227. Ninth edition 1991.

PHENCYCLIDINE

See: DRUG ABUSE

PHENYLKETONURIA

See: METABOLIC DISORDERS

PHLEBITIS

See: VASCULAR DISEASES

PHOBIAS

See: ANXIETY; MENTAL HEALTH; MOOD DISORDERS; PSYCHOANALYSIS

PHOTOSENSITIVITY

See: ALLERGIES

PHYSICAL FITNESS

See: EXERCISE

PHYSICAL MEDICINE

See: REHABILITATION

PHYSICAL THERAPY

See also: ALLIED HEALTH EDUCATION; REHABILITATION

ABSTRACTING, INDEXING, AND CURRENT AWARENESS PUBLICATIONS

Cumulative Index to Nursing and Allied Health Literature. Glendale Adventist Medical Center, P.O. Box 871, Glendale, CA 91209. Phone: (818) 409-8005. Bimonthly.

Excerpta Medica. Section 19: Rehabilitation and Physical Medicine. Elsevier Science Publishing Co., Inc., P.O. Box 882, Madison Square Station, New York, NY 10159-2101. Phone: (212) 989-5800. Fax: (212) 633-3990. 8/year.

Index Medicus. U.S. National Library of Medicine, 8600 Rockville Pike, Bethesda, MD 20894. Phone: (800) 638-8480. Monthly.

International Nursing Index. American Journal of Nursing Co., 555 W. 57th St., New York, NY 10019. Phone: (212) 582-8820. Quarterly.

Physiotherapy Index. Medical Information Service, British Library, Boston Spa, Wetherby, W. Yorkshire LS23 7BQ, England. Phone: 0937-546039. Fax: 0937-546236. Monthly.

ANNUALS AND REVIEWS

Orthopaedic Physical Therapy Clinics of North America. W.B. Saunders Co., The Curtis Center, Independence Square W., Philadelphia, PA 19106-3399. Phone: (215) 238-7800. Quarterly.

ASSOCIATIONS, PROFESSIONAL SOCIETIES, ADVOCACY AND SUPPORT GROUPS

American Academy of Physical Medicine and Rehabilitation (AAPMR). 122 S. Michigan Ave., Ste. 1300, Chicago, IL 60603. Phone: (312) 922-9366. Fax: (312) 922-6754.

American Board of Physical Medicine and Rehabilitation (ABPMR). Norwest Ctr., 21 First St. S.W., Ste. 674, Rochester, MN 55902. Phone: (507) 282-1776.

American Physical Therapy Association (APTA). 111 N. Fairfax St., Alexandria, VA 22314. Phone: (703) 684-2782.

Orthopaedic Section. American Physical Therapy Association. 505 King St., Ste. 103, La Crosse, WI 54601. Phone: (608) 784-0910. Fax: (608) 784-3350.

U.S. Physical Therapy Association (USPTA). 1803 Avon Ln., Arlington Heights, IL 60004.

CD-ROM DATABASES

Nursing and Allied Health (CINAHL) on CD-ROM. CINAHL, 1509 Wilson Terrace, P.O. Box 871, Glendale, CA 91209-0871. Phone: (818) 409-8005.

ENCYCLOPEDIAS, DICTIONARIES, WORD BOOKS

Mosby's Medical, Nursing, and Allied Health Dictionary. Kenneth N. Anderson, Lois Anderson, Walter D. Glanze (eds.). Mosby-Year Book, 11830 Westline Industrial Dr., St. Louis, MO 63146. Phone: (800) 325-4177. Fax: (314) 432-1380. Third edition 1990.

HANDBOOKS, GUIDES, MANUALS, ATLASES

The Home Rehabilitation Program Guide. Paul A. Roggow, Debra K. Berg, Michael D. Lewis. SLACK Inc., 6900 Grove Rd., Thorofare, NJ 08086-9447. Phone: (800) 257-8290. Fax: (609) 853-5991. 1990.

Manual of Physical Therapy. Otto D. Dayton, and others. Churchill Livingstone Inc., 650 Ave. of the Americas, New York, NY 10011. Phone: (212) 819-5400. Fax: (212) 302-6598. 1989.

JOURNALS

American Journal of Physical Medicine & Rehabilitation. Williams & Wilkins, 428 E. Preston St., Baltimore, MD 21202. Phone: (800) 638-0672. Fax: (800) 447-8438. Bimonthly.

Archives of Physical Medicine and Rehabilitation. American Congress of Rehabilitation Medicine, 78 E. Adams, Chicago, IL 60603. Phone: (312) 922-9371. Fax: (312) 922-6754. Monthly.

Assistive Technology. Resna Press, 1101 Connecticut Ave. NW, Suite 700, Washington, DC 20036. Phone: (202) 857-1199. Quarterly.

Clinics in Physical Therapy. Churchill Livingstone Inc., 650 Ave. of the Americas, New York, NY 10011. Phone: (212) 819-5400. Fax: (212) 302-6598.

Journal of Orthopaedic and Sports Physical Therapy. Williams & Wilkins, 428 E. Preston St., Baltimore, MD 21202. Phone: (800) 638-0672. Fax: (800) 447-8438. Monthly.

Journal of Physical Therapy Education. American Physical Therapy Association, 111 N. Fairfax St., Alexandria, VA 22314. Phone: (703) 684-2782.

Pediatric Physical Therapy. Williams & Wilkins, 428 E. Preston St., Baltimore, MD 21202. Phone: (800) 638-0672. Fax: (800) 447-8438. Quarterly.

Physical Therapy. American Physical Therapy Association, 1111 N. Fairfax St., Alexandria, VA 22314-1488. Phone: (703) 684-2782. Fax: (703) 684-7343. Monthly.

Physical Therapy Today. Williams & Wilkins, 428 E. Preston St., Baltimore, MD 21202. Phone: (800) 638-0672. Fax: (800) 447-8438. Quarterly.

Physiotherapy Theroy and Practice. Lawrence Erlbaum Associates, Ltd., 27 Palmeira Masions, Church Rd., Hove, E. Sussex BN3 2FA, England. Phone: 02732-07411. Fax: 02732-5612. 4/year.

ONLINE DATABASES

EMBASE. Elsevier Science Publishing Co., Inc., P.O. Box 882, Madison Square Station, New York, NY 10159-2101. Phone: (212) 989-5800. Fax: (212) 633-3990.

MEDLINE. National Library of Medicine, 8600 Rockville Pike, Bethesda, MD 20894. Phone: (800) 638-8480.

Nursing and Allied Health (CINAHL). CINAHL, 1509 Wilson Terrace, P.O. Box 871, Glendale, CA 91209-0871. Phone: (818) 409-8005.

SciSearch. Institute for Scientific Information, 3501 Market St., Philadelphia, PA 19104. Phone: (215) 386-0100. Fax: (215) 386-6362.

RESEARCH CENTERS, INSTITUTES, CLEARINGHOUSES

Medical Rehabilitation Research and Training Center. New York University, 400 E. 34th St., New York, NY 10016. Phone: (212) 340-6105.

Rehabilitation Institute. 261 Mack Blvd., Detroit, MI 48201. Phone: (313) 494-9731.

TEXTBOOKS AND MONOGRAPHS

Clinical Assessment Procedures in Physical Therapy. M. Lynn Palmer, Marcia E. Epler. J.B. Lippincott Co., 227 E. Washington Square, Philadelphia, PA 19106-3780. Phone: (215) 238-4200. Fax: (215) 238-4227. 1990.

Health Care Management in Physical Therapy. Mark A. Brimer. Charles C. Thomas, Publisher, 2600 S. First St., Springfield, IL 62794-9265. Phone: (800) 250-8980. 1990.

Knee Ligament Rehabilitation. Robert P. Engle (ed.). Churchill Livingstone Inc., 650 Avenue of the Americas, New York, NY 10011. Phone: (212) 819-5400. Fax: (212) 302-6598. 1991.

Management Principles for Physical Therapists. Larry J. Nosse, Deborah G. Friberg. Williams & Wilkins, 428 East Preston St., Baltimore, MD 21202. Phone: (800) 638-0672. Fax: (800) 447-8438. 1992.

Orthopaedic and Sports Physical Therapy. James A. Gould, George J. Davies. Mosby-Year Book, 11830 Westline Industrial Drive, St. Louis, MO 63146. Phone: (800) 325-4177. Fax: (314) 432-1380. Second edition 1990.

Physical Therapy. R.M. Scully, M.R. Barnes. J.B. Lippincott Co., 227 E. Washington Square, Philadelphia, PA 19106-3780. Phone: (215) 238-4200. Fax: (215) 238-4227. 1989.

Practice Issues in Physical Therapy: Current Patterns and Future Directions. Jane S. Mathews (ed.). SLACK Inc., 6900 Grove Rd., Thorofare, NJ 08086-9447. Phone: (800) 257-8290. Fax: (609) 853-5991. 1989.

Tidy's Physiotherapy. A. Thompson and others. Butterworth-Heinemann, 80 Montvale Ave., Stoneham, MA 02180. Phone: (617) 438-8464. Fax: (617) 279-4851. 12th edition 1991.

PHYSICIAN IMPAIRMENT

See: MALPRACTICE

PHYSICIANS

ASSOCIATIONS, PROFESSIONAL SOCIETIES, ADVOCACY AND SUPPORT GROUPS

American Board of Medical Specialties. One Rotary Center, No. 805, Evanston, IL 60201. Phone: (312) 491-9091.

American Medical Association (AMA). 515 N. State St., Chicago, IL 60610. Phone: (312) 464-5000. Fax: (312) 645-4184.

National Medical Association (NMA). 1012 10th St. N.W., Washington, DC 20001. Phone: (202) 347-1895.

BIBLIOGRAPHIES

Physicians: Geographical Distribution. National Technical Information Service, 5285 Port Royal Rd., Springfield, VA 22161. Phone: (703) 487-4650. Fax: (703) 321-8547. Jan. 1970-June 1989 PB89-864334/CBY.

CD-ROM DATABASES

Directory of Physicians in the United States. American Medical Association, 515 North State St., Chicago, IL 60610. Phone: (312) 464-0183. Fax: (312) 464-5834. Annual.

DIRECTORIES

Canadian Medical Directory. Southern Business Communications, Inc., 1450 Don Mills Rd., Don Mills, ON, Canada M3B 2X7. Phone: (416) 445-6641. Fax: (416) 442-2077. Annual.

Directory of Certified Emergency Physicians. American Board of Medical Specialties, 1 Rotary Center, Suite 805, Evanston, IL 60201. Phone: (708) 491-9091. Biennial.

Directory of Medical Specialists. Marquis Who's Who, 3002 Glenview Rd., Wilmette, IL 60091. Phone: (800) 621-9669. Fax: (708) 441-2264. Biennial.

Directory of Physicians in the United States. American Medical Association, 515 North State St., Chicago, IL 60610. Phone: (312) 464-0183. Fax: (312) 464-5834. Biennial.

The National Directory of Medical Practice Opportunities. Jackson and Coker, 115 Perimeter Center Place, Suite 380, Atlanta, GA 30346. Phone: (800) 544-1987. Bimonthly.

Official ABMS Directory of Board Certified Medical Specialists. American Board of Medical Specialties, P.O. Box 1280, Evanston, IL 60204-9913. Phone: (708) 491-9091. Fax: (708) 328-3596. Biennial.

ENCYCLOPEDIAS, DICTIONARIES, WORD BOOKS

Biographical Dictionary of Medicine. Jessica Bendiner Elmer. Facts on File, Inc., 460 Park Ave. S., New York, NY 10016-7382. Phone: (212) 683-2244. Fax: (212) 683-3633. 1990.

JOURNALS

Academic Medicine. Association of American Medical Colleges, 1 Dupont Circle NW, Suite 200, Washington, DC 20036. Phone: (202) 828-0416. Fax: (202) 785-5027. Monthly.

POPULAR WORKS AND PATIENT EDUCATION

Best Medicine: Your Essential Guide to Finding Top Doctors, Hospitals and Treatments. Robert Arnot. Addison-Wesley Publishing Co., Rte. 128, Reading, MA 01867. Phone: (800) 447-2226. 1992.

STANDARDS AND STATISTICS SOURCES

Physician Characteristics and Distribution in the U.S. 1993. American Medical Association, 515 North State St., Chicago, IL 60610. Phone: (312) 464-0183. Fax: (312) 464-5834. 1992.

Physician Marketplace Statistics. American Medical Association, 515 N. State St., Chicago, IL 60610. Phone: (312) 464-5000. Fax: (312) 645-4184. Annual.

Socioeconomic Characteristics of Medical Practice. American Medical Association, 515 N. State St., Chicago, IL 60610. Phone: (312) 464-5000. Fax: (312) 645-4184. Annual.

U.S. Medical Licensure Statisticcs and Current Licensure Requirements. American Medical Association, 515 N. State St., Chicago, IL 60610. Phone: (312) 464-5000. Fax: (312) 645-4184. Annual.

TEXTBOOKS AND MONOGRAPHS

Doctors' Marriages: A Look at the Problems and Their Solutions. Michael F. Myers. Plenum Publishing Co., 233 Spring St., New York, NY 10013-1578. Phone: (212) 620-8000. Fax· (212) 463-0742. 1988.

Leaving the Bedside: The Search for a Nonclinical Medical Career. American Medical Association, 515 N. State St., Chicago, IL 60610. Phone: (312) 464-5000. Fax: (312) 645-4184. 1992.

When Doctors Get Sick. Harvey Mandell, Howard Spiro (eds.). Plenum Publishing Co., 233 Spring St., New York, NY 10013-1578. Phone: (212) 620-8000. Fax: (212) 463-0742. 1987.

PHYSICIANS' ASSISTANTS

See also: ALLIED HEALTH EDUCATION

ABSTRACTING, INDEXING, AND CURRENT AWARENESS PUBLICATIONS

Cumulative Index to Nursing and Allied Health Literature. Glendale Adventist Medical Center, P.O. Box 871, Glendale, CA 91209. Phone: (818) 409-8005. Bimonthly.

Index Medicus. U.S. National Library of Medicine, 8600 Rockville Pike, Bethesda, MD 20894. Phone: (800) 638-8480. Monthly.

ASSOCIATIONS, PROFESSIONAL SOCIETIES, ADVOCACY AND SUPPORT GROUPS

American Academy of Physician Assistants (AAPA). 950 N. Washington St., Alexandria, VA 22314. Phone: (703) 836-2272. Fax: (703) 684-1924.

National Commission on Certification of Physician Assistants (NCCPA). 2845 Henderson Mill Rd. N.E., Atlanta, GA 30341. Phone: (404) 493-9100.

BIBLIOGRAPHIES

Core Collection in Nursing and the Allied Health Sciences: Books, Journal, Media. Oryx Press, 4041 N. Central, Suite 700, Phoenix, AZ 85012. Phone: (800) 279-ORYX. Fax: (800) 279-4663. 1990.

CD-ROM DATABASES

Nursing and Allied Health (CINAHL) on CD-ROM. CINAHL, 1509 Wilson Terrace, P.O. Box 871, Glendale, CA 91209-0871. Phone: (818) 409-8005.

DIRECTORIES

Allied Health Education Directory. American Medical Association, 515 North State St., Chicago, IL 60610. Phone: (312) 464-0183. Fax: (312) 464-5834. Annual.

ENCYCLOPEDIAS, DICTIONARIES, WORD BOOKS

Mosby's Medical, Nursing, and Allied Health Dictionary. Kenneth N. Anderson, Lois Anderson, Walter D. Glanze (eds.). Mosby-Year Book, 11830 Westline Industrial Dr., St. Louis, MO 63146. Phone: (800) 325-4177. Fax: (314) 432-1380. Third edition 1990.

JOURNALS

Journal of the American Academy of Physician Assistants. Mosby-Year Book, 11830 Westline Industrial Drive, St. Louis, MO 63146. Phone: (800) 325-4177. Fax: (314) 432-1380. 10/year.

ONLINE DATABASES

EMBASE. Elsevier Science Publishing Co., Inc., P.O. Box 882, Madison Square Station, New York, NY 10159-2101. Phone: (212) 989-5800. Fax: (212) 633-3990.

MEDLINE. National Library of Medicine, 8600 Rockville Pike, Bethesda, MD 20894. Phone: (800) 638-8480.

Nursing and Allied Health (CINAHL). CINAHL, 1509 Wilson Terrace, P.O. Box 871, Glendale, CA 91209-0871. Phone: (818) 409-8005.

SciSearch. Institute for Scientific Information, 3501 Market St., Philadelphia, PA 19104. Phone: (215) 386-0100. Fax: (215) 386-6362.

TEXTBOOKS AND MONOGRAPHS

Appleton and Lange's Review for the Medical Assistant. Tom Parks. Appleton & Lange, 25 Van Zant St., East Norwalk, CT 06855. Phone: (800) 423-1359. Fax: (203) 854-9486. 3rd edition, 1990.

The Physician Assistant in a Changing Health Care Environment. Gretchen Engle Schafft, James F. Cawley. Aspen Publishers, Inc., 200 Orchard Ridge Dr., Gaithersburg, MD 20878. Phone: (800) 638-8437. 1987.

Physician Assistants: Present and Future Models of Utilization. Sarah F. Zarbock, Kenneth Harbert (eds.). Greenwood Publishing Group, Inc., 88 Post Rd. W., P.O. Box 5007, Westport, CT 06881. Phone: (203) 226-3571. 1986.

Physician's Assistant Examination Review. Richard R. Rahr, Bruce R. Niebuhr (eds.). Elsevier Science Publishing Co., Inc., P.O. Box 882, Madison Square Station, New York, NY 10159-2101. Phone: (212) 989-5800. Fax: (212) 633-3990. Second edition 1991.

Twenty-Eight Allied Health Careers. American Medical Association, 515 North State St., Chicago, IL 60610. Phone: (312) 464-0183. Fax: (312) 464-5834. 1991.

PHYSIOLOGY

ABSTRACTING, INDEXING, AND CURRENT AWARENESS PUBLICATIONS

Current Contents/Life Sciences. Institute for Scientific Information, 3501 Market St., Philadelphia, PA 19104. Phone: (215) 386-0100. Fax: (215) 386-6362.

Excerpta Medica. Section 2: Physiology. Elsevier Science Publishing Co., Inc., P.O. Box 882, Madison Square Station, New York, NY 10159-2101. Phone: (212) 989-5800. Fax: (212) 633-3990. 30/year.

Index Medicus. U.S. National Library of Medicine, 8600 Rockville Pike, Bethesda, MD 20894. Phone: (800) 638-8480. Monthly.

Science Citation Index. Institute for Scientific Information, 3501 Market St., Philadelphia, PA 19104. Phone: (800) 523-1850. Fax: (215) 386-6362. Bimonthly.

ANNUALS AND REVIEWS

Annual Review of Physiology. Annual Reviews Inc., 4139 El Camino Way, P.O. Box 10139, Palo Alto, CA 94303-0897. Phone: (415) 493-4400. Fax: (415) 855-9815. Annual.

ASSOCIATIONS, PROFESSIONAL SOCIETIES, ADVOCACY AND SUPPORT GROUPS

American Physiological Society. 9650 Rockville Pike, Bethesda, MD 20814. Phone: (301) 530-7071.

CD-ROM DATABASES

SCISEARCH. Institute for Scientific Information, 3501 Market St., Philadelphia, PA 19104. Phone: (215) 386-0100. Fax: (215) 386-6362.

ENCYCLOPEDIAS, DICTIONARIES, WORD BOOKS

Anatomy and Physiology Words. Stedman. Williams & Wilkins, 428 East Preston St., Baltimore, MD 21202. Phone: (800) 638-0672. Fax: (800) 447-8438. 1992.

Glossary of Anatomy and Physiology. Diane Shaw. Springhouse Publishing Co., 1111 Bethlehem Pike, Spring House, PA 19477. Phone: (800) 331-3170. Fax: (215) 646-8716. 1992.

HANDBOOKS, GUIDES, MANUALS, ATLASES

Color Atlas of Physiology. A. Despopoulos, S. Silbernagl. Thieme Medical Publishers, Inc., 381 Park Ave. S., New York, NY 10016. Phone: (212) 683-5088. Fax: (212) 779-9020. Fourth edition 1991.

JOURNALS

American Journal of Physiology. American Physiological Society, 9650 Rockville Pike, Bethesda, MD 20814. Phone: (301) 530-7160. Fax: (301) 571-1814. Monthly.

Canadian Journal of Physiology and Pharmacology. National Research Council of Canada, Ottawa, ON, Canada K1A 0R6. Phone: (613) 993-9084. Fax: (613) 852-7656.

Clinical Physiology. Blackwell Scientific Publications, Inc., 3 Cambridge Center, Cambridge, MA 02142. Phone: (800) 759-6102.

European Journal of Applied Physiology. Springer-Verlag New York Inc., 175 Fifth Ave., New York, NY 10010. Phone: (212) 460-1500. Fax: (212) 473-6272. 6/year.

Journal of Applied Physiology. American Physiological Society, 9650 Rockville Pike, Bethesda, MD 20814. Phone: (301) 530-7160. Fax: (301) 571-1814. Monthly.

Journal of Cellular Physiology. John Wiley & Sons, Inc., 605 Third Ave., New York, NY 10158-0012. Phone: (212) 850-6000. Fax: (212) 850-6088.

Journal of General Physiology. Rockefeller University Press, 222 E. 70th St., New York, NY 10021. Phone: (212) 570-8572.

Journal of Physiology. Cambridge University Press, 40 W. 20th St., New York, NY 10011. Phone: (800) 431-1580. Monthly.

Physiological Reviews. American Physiological Society, 9650 Rockville Pike, Bethesda, MD 20814. Phone: (301) 530-7160. Fax: (301) 571-1814. Quarterly.

NEWSLETTERS

The Physiologist. American Physiological Society, 9650 Rockville Pike, Bethesda, MD 20814. Phone: (301) 530-7160. Fax: (301) 571-1814. Bimonthly.

ONLINE DATABASES

EMBASE. Elsevier Science Publishing Co., Inc., P.O. Box 882, Madison Square Station, New York, NY 10159-2101. Phone: (212) 989-5800. Fax: (212) 633-3990.

MEDLINE. National Library of Medicine, 8600 Rockville Pike, Bethesda, MD 20894. Phone: (800) 638-8480.

SciSearch. Institute for Scientific Information, 3501 Market St., Philadelphia, PA 19104. Phone: (215) 386-0100. Fax: (215) 386-6362.

RESEARCH CENTERS, INSTITUTES, CLEARINGHOUSES

Comparative Physiology Lab. Southern Illinois University at Carbondale. 243 Life Science II, Carbondale, IL 62901. Phone: (618) 453-1518.

Institute of Applied Physiology and Medicine. 701 16th Ave., Seattle, WA 98122. Phone: (206) 553-7330. Fax: (206) 553-1717.

TEXTBOOKS AND MONOGRAPHS

Best and Taylor's Physiological Basis of Medical Practice. John B. West (ed.). Williams & Wilkins, 428 East Preston St., Baltimore, MD 21202. Phone: (800) 638-0672. Fax: (800) 447-8438. 1991.

Essential Medical Physiology. Leonard R. Johnson. Raven Press, 1185 Avenue of the Americas, New York, NY 10036. Phone: (212) 930-9500. Fax: (212) 869-3495. 1991.

Essentials of Human Physiology. Ackermann. Mosby-Year Book, 11830 Westline Industrial Drive, St. Louis, MO 63146. Phone: (800) 325-4177. Fax: (314) 432-1380. 1992.

Human Physiology. A.J. Vander and others. McGraw-Hill Inc., 11 West 19th St., New York, NY 10011. Phone: (212) 337-5001. Fax: (212) 337-4092. 5th edition 1989.

Illustrated Physiology. B.R. MacKenna, R. Callander. Churchill Livingstone Inc., 650 Avenue of the Americas, New York, NY 10011. Phone: (212) 819-5400. Fax: (212) 302-6598. Fifth edition 1991.

Physiology. Hsu. Little, Brown and Co., 34 Beacon St., Boston, MA 02108. Phone: (617) 227-0730. Fax: (617) 227-0790. 1987.

Physiology: Essentials of Basic Science. Nicholas Sperelakis, Robert O. Banks. Little, Brown and Company, 34 Beacon St., Boston, MA 02108. Phone: (617) 227-0730. 1992.

Principles of Physiology. Berne. Mosby-Year Book, 11830 Westline Industrial Drive, St. Louis, MO 63146. Phone: (800) 325-4177. Fax: (314) 432-1380. 1990.

Review of Medical Physiology. W.F. Ganong. Appleton & Lange, 25 Van Zant St., East Norwalk, CT 06855. Phone: (800) 423-1359. Fax: (203) 854-9486. 15th edition 1991.

Textbook of Medical Physiology. A.C. Guyton. W.B. Saunders Co., The Curtis Center, Independence Square W., Philadelphia, PA 19106-3399. Phone: (215) 238-7800. 8th edition 1990.

Textbook of Physiology. Berne. Mosby-Year Book, 11830 Westline Industrial Drive, St. Louis, MO 63146. Phone: (800) 325-4177. Fax: (314) 432-1380. Third edition 1992.

PINWORMS

See: PARASITIC DISEASES

PITUITARY CANCER

See: BRAIN CANCER

PITUITARY DISEASE

See: ENDOCRINE DISORDERS

PLANTS, MEDICINAL

See: HERBAL MEDICINE

PLAQUE, DENTAL

See: DENTISTRY

PLASTIC AND COSMETIC SURGERY

See also: HAND SURGERY; SURGERY

ABSTRACTING, INDEXING, AND CURRENT AWARENESS PUBLICATIONS

Current Contents/Clinical Medicine. Institute for Scientific Information, 3501 Market St., Philadelphia, PA 19104. Phone: (800) 523-1850. Fax: (215) 386-6362. Weekly.

Excerpta Medica. Section 34: Plastic Surgery. Elsevier Science Publishing Co., Inc., P.O. Box 882, Madison Square Station, New York, NY 10159-2101. Phone: (212) 989-5800. Fax: (212) 633-3990.

Index Medicus. U.S. National Library of Medicine, 8600 Rockville Pike, Bethesda, MD 20894. Phone: (800) 638-8480. Monthly.

Research Alert: Surgery-Plastic & Reconstructive. Institute for Scientific Information, 3501 Market St., Philadelphia, PA 19104. Phone: (800) 523-1850. Fax: (215) 386-6362. Weekly.

ANNUALS AND REVIEWS

Advances in Plastic and Reconstructive Surgery. Mosby-Year Book, 11830 Westline Industrial Drive, St. Louis, MO 63146. Phone: (800) 325-4177. Fax: (314) 432-1380. Annual.

Clinics in Plastic Surgery. W.B. Saunders Co., The Curtis Center, Independence Square W., Philadelphia, PA 19106-3399. Phone: (215) 238-7800. Quarterly.

Year Book of Plastic and Reconstructive Surgery. Mosby-Year Book, 11830 Westline Industrial Drive, St. Louis, MO 63146. Phone: (800) 325-4177. Fax: (314) 432-1380. Annual.

ASSOCIATIONS, PROFESSIONAL SOCIETIES, ADVOCACY AND SUPPORT GROUPS

American Academy of Cosmetic Surgery (AACS). 159 E. Live Oak Ave., Ste. 204, Arcadia, CA 91006. Phone: (818) 447-1579. Fax: (818) 447-1579.

American Academy of Facial Plastic and Reconstructive Surgery (AAFPRS). 1110 Vermont Ave. N.W., Ste. 220, Washington, DC 20005. Phone: (202) 842-4500. Fax: (202) 371-1514.

American Association for Accreditation of Ambulatory Plastic Surgery Facilities. 505 E. Hawley St., Mundelein, IL 60060. Phone: (312) 949-6058.

American Board of Plastic Surgery (ABPS). 7 Penn Ctr., Ste. 400, 1635 Market St., Philadelphia, PA 19103. Phone: (215) 587-9322.

American Society of Lipo-Suction Surgery (ASLSS). 159 E. Live Oak Ave., No. 204, Arcadia, CA 91006. Phone: (818) 447-1579. Fax: (818) 447-7880.

American Society of Plastic and Reconstructive Surgeons (ASPRS). 444 E. Algonquin Rd., Arlington Heights, IL 60005. Phone: (708) 228-9900. Fax: (708) 228-9131.

BIBLIOGRAPHIES

Current Bibliography of Plastic and Reconstructive Surgery. Plastic Surgery Education Foundation, c/o American Society of Plastic and Reconstructive Surgeons, 444 E. Algonquin Rd., Arlington Heights, IL 60005. Phone: (708) 228-9900. Bimonthly.

DIRECTORIES

Directory of Certified Plastic Surgeons. American Board of Medical Specialties, 1 Rotary Center, Suite 805, Evanston, IL 60201. Phone: (708) 491-9091. Biennial.

HANDBOOKS, GUIDES, MANUALS, ATLASES

Aesthetic Facial Surgery: A Clinical and Surgical Atlas. H. George Brennan. Raven Press, 1185 Ave. of the Americas, New York, NY 10036. Phone: (212) 930-9500. Fax: (212) 869-3495. 1991.

Atlas of Cutaneous Laser Surgery. David B. Apfelberg. Raven Press, 1185 Avenue of the Americas, New York, NY 10036. Phone: (212) 930-9500. Fax: (212) 869-3495. 1991.

Atlas of Suction Assisted Lipectomy. Frederick M. Grazer. Churchill Livingstone Inc., 650 Avenue of the Americas, New York, NY 10011. Phone: (212) 819-5400. Fax: (212) 302-6598. 1991.

Color Atlas of Mammoplasty. P. McKissock. Thieme Medical Publishers, Inc., 381 Park Ave. S., New York, NY 10016. Phone: (212) 683-5088. Fax: (212) 779-9020. 1991.

Handbook of Plastic Surgery. McKinney. Churchill Livingstone Inc., 650 Ave. of the Americas, New York, NY 10011. Phone: (212) 819-5400. Fax: (212) 302-6598. Second edition 1992.

JOURNALS

Annals of Plastic Surgery. Little, Brown and Co., 34 Beacon St., Boston, MA 02108. Phone: (617) 227-0730. Fax: (617) 227-0790.

British Journal of Plastic Surgery. Churchill Livingstone Inc., 650 Avenue of the Americas, New York, NY 10011. Phone: (212) 819-5400. Fax: (212) 302-6598. 6/year.

Facial Plastic Surgery. Thieme Medical Publishers, Inc., 381 Park Ave. S., New York, NY 10016. Phone: (212) 683-5088. Fax: (212) 779-9020. Quarterly.

Journal of Burn Care and Rehabilitation. Mosby-Year Book, 11830 Westline Industrial Drive, St. Louis, MO 63146. Phone: (800) 325-4177. Fax: (314) 432-1380. Bimonthly.

Journal of Dermatologic Surgery and Oncology. Journal of Dermatologic Surgery, Inc., 245 Fifth Ave., New York, NY 10016. Phone: (212) 721-5175. Monthly.

The Journal of Hand Surgery (American Volume). Mosby-Year Book, 11830 Westline Industrial Drive, St. Louis, MO 63146. Phone: (800) 325-4177. Fax: (314) 432-1380. Bimonthly.

Journal of Oral and Maxillofacial Surgery. W.B. Saunders Co., The Curtis Center, Independence Square W., Philadelphia, PA 19106-3399. Phone: (215) 238-7800. Monthly.

Plastic and Reconstructive Surgery. Williams & Wilkins, 428 E. Preston St., Baltimore, MD 21202. Phone: (800) 638-0672. Fax: (800) 447-8438. Monthly.

ONLINE DATABASES

EMBASE. Elsevier Science Publishing Co., Inc., P.O. Box 882, Madison Square Station, New York, NY 10159-2101. Phone: (212) 989-5800. Fax: (212) 633-3990.

MEDLINE. National Library of Medicine, 8600 Rockville Pike, Bethesda, MD 20894. Phone: (800) 638-8480.

SciSearch. Institute for Scientific Information, 3501 Market St., Philadelphia, PA 19104. Phone: (215) 386-0100. Fax: (215) 386-6362.

POPULAR WORKS AND PATIENT EDUCATION

The American Society of Plastic and Reconstructive Surgeon's Guide to Cosmetic Surgery. Josleen Wilson. Simon & Schuster, Inc., 1230 Ave. of the Americas, New York, NY 10020. Phone: (212) 698-7000. 1992.

TEXTBOOKS AND MONOGRAPHS

Aesthetic Facial Surgery. Charles J. Krause. J.B. Lippincott Co., 227 E. Washington Square, Philadelphia, PA 19106-3780. Phone: (215) 238-4200. Fax: (215) 238-4227. 1991.

Aesthetic Plastic Surgery: Rhinoplasty. Rollin K. Daniel (ed.). Little, Brown and Company, 34 Beacon St., Boston, MA 02108. Phone: (617) 227-0730. 1992.

Cosmetic Surgery of the Skin. Coleman. Mosby-Year Book, 11830 Westline Industrial Drive, St. Louis, MO 63146. Phone: (800) 325-4177. Fax: (314) 432-1380. 1991.

Current Surgical Diagnosis and Treatment. L.W. Way. Appleton & Lange, 25 Van Zant St., East Norwalk, CT 06855. Phone: (800) 423-1359. Fax: (203) 854-9486. Ninth edition 1990.

Decision Making in Plastic Surgery. Jeffrey L. Marsh. Mosby-Year Book, 11830 Westline Industrial Drive, St. Louis, MO 63146. Phone: (800) 325-4177. Fax: (314) 432-1380. 1992.

Emergency Plastic Surgery. Richard J. Greco. Little, Brown and Company, 34 Beacon St., Boston, MA 02108. Phone: (617) 227-0730. 1991.

Facial Plastic and Reconstructive Surgery. Papel. Mosby-Year Book, 11830 Westline Industrial Drive, St. Louis, MO 63146. Phone: (800) 325-4177. Fax: (314) 432-1380. 1992.

Fundamental Techniques of Plastic Surgery. McGregor. Churchill Livingstone Inc., 650 Ave. of the Americas, New York, NY 10011. Phone: (212) 819-5400. Fax: (212) 302-6598. Eighth edition 1989.

Grabb and Smith's Plastic Surgery. Smith. Little, Brown and Company, 34 Beacon St., Boston, MA 02108. Phone: (617) 227-0730. Fourth edition 1991.

Maxillofacial and Reconstructive Surgery. Georgiade. Williams & Wilkins, 428 East Preston St., Baltimore, MD 21202. Phone: (800) 638-0672. Fax: (800) 447-8438. Second edition 1991.

Plastic and Reconstructive Surgery of the Breast. Noone. Mosby-Year Book, 11830 Westline Industrial Drive, St. Louis, MO 63146. Phone: (800) 325-4177. Fax: (314) 432-1380. 1991.

Plastic and Reconstructive Surgery of the Head and Neck. Stucker. Mosby-Year Book, 11830 Westline Industrial Drive, St. Louis, MO 63146. Phone: (800) 325-4177. Fax: (314) 432-1380. 1991.

Plastic Surgery. Joseph McCarthy (ed.). W.B. Saunders Co., The Curtis Center, Independence Sqare W., Philadelphia, PA 19106-3399. Phone: (215) 238-7800. 8 volumes, 1990.

Rhinoplasty: State of the Art. Ronal P. Gruber, George C. Peck. Mosby-Year Book, 11830 Westline Industrial Drive, St. Louis, MO 63146. Phone: (800) 325-4177. Fax: (314) 432-1380. 1992.

Surgical Techniques in Cleft Lip and Cleft Palate. Bardach. Mosby-Year Book, 11830 Westline Industrial Drive, St. Louis, MO 63146. Phone: (800) 325-4177. Fax: (314) 432-1380. Second edition 1991.

PLEURISY

See: LUNG DISEASES

PNEUMONIA

See: LUNG DISEASES

PODIATRY

See also: FOOT DISORDERS

ABSTRACTING, INDEXING, AND CURRENT AWARENESS PUBLICATIONS

Gait Study Center. Pennsylvania College of Podiatric Medicine, 8th and Race Sts., Philadelphia, PA 19107. Phone: (215) 629-0300.

Index Medicus. U.S. National Library of Medicine, 8600 Rockville Pike, Bethesda, MD 20894. Phone: (800) 638-8480. Monthly.

ANNUALS AND REVIEWS

American College of Foot Specialists Annual Yearbook. American College of Foot Specialists, 1801 Vauxhall Rd., Union, NJ 07083.

Clinics in Podiatric Medicine and Surgery. W.B. Saunders Co., The Curtis Center, Independence Square W., Philadelphia, PA 19106-3399. Phone: (215) 238-7800. Quarterly.

Year Book of Podiatric Medicine and Surgery. Mosby-Year Book, 11830 Westline Industrial Drive, St. Louis, MO 63146. Phone: (800) 325-4177. Fax: (314) 432-1380. Annual.

ASSOCIATIONS, PROFESSIONAL SOCIETIES, ADVOCACY AND SUPPORT GROUPS

American Association of Colleges of Podiatric Medicine. 6110 Executive Blvd., No. 204, Rockville, MD 20852. Phone: (301) 984-9350.

American Board of Podiatric Surgery (ABPS). 1601 Dolores St., San Francisco, CA 94110-4906. Phone: (415) 826-3200. Fax: (415) 826-4640.

American College of Foot Surgeons. 1601 Dolores St., San Francisco, CA 94110. Phone: (415) 820-3200.

American Podiatric Medical Association (APMA). 9312 Old Georgetown Rd., Bethesda, MD 20814. Phone: (301) 571-9200. Fax: (301) 530-2752.

National Podiatric Medical Association. c/o Raymond E. Lee, 1638 E. 87th St., Chicago, IL 60617. Phone: (312) 374-1616.

DIRECTORIES

American Academy of Foot Surgery Membership Directory. American Ambulatory Foot Surgery Membership Directory, Box 2730, Tuscaloosa, AL 35403. Phone: (205) 758-3678.

HANDBOOKS, GUIDES, MANUALS, ATLASES

A Color Atlas of the Foot in Clinical Diagnosis. Mosby-Year Book, 11830 Westline Industrial Drive, St. Louis, MO 63146. Phone: (800) 325-4177. Fax: (314) 432-1380. 1992.

Manual of Ankle and Foot Arthroscopy. Richard O. Lundeen. Churchill Livingstone Inc., 650 Avenue of the Americas, New York, NY 10011. Phone: (212) 819-5400. Fax: (212) 302-6598. 1991.

Manual of Digital Surgery of the Foot. Michael S. Downey, D. Scot Malay. Churchill Livingstone Inc., 650 Avenue of the Americas, New York, NY 10011. Phone: (212) 819-5400. Fax: (212) 302-6598. 1991.

JOURNALS

American Podiatric Medical Association Journal. American Podiatric Medical Association, 8312 Old Georgetown Rd., Bethesda, MD 20814. Phone: (301) 571-9200.

NEWSLETTERS

American Academy of Podiatry Administration Newsletter. American Academy of Podiatry Administration Newsletter, c/o John Cicero DPM, Ten Meadow Lane, Bloomfield, NJ 07003.

APMA News. American Podiatric Medical Association, 9312 Old Georgetown Rd., Bethesda, MD 20814-1621. Phone: (301) 571-9200. Monthly.

The Podiatrist's Patient Newsletter. Doctor's Press, Inc., Pitney Rd., P.O. Box 11177, Lancaster, PA 17605. Phone: (800) 233-0196. Quarterly.

ONLINE DATABASES

EMBASE. Elsevier Science Publishing Co., Inc., P.O. Box 882, Madison Square Station, New York, NY 10159-2101. Phone: (212) 989-5800. Fax: (212) 633-3990.

MEDLINE. National Library of Medicine, 8600 Rockville Pike, Bethesda, MD 20894. Phone: (800) 638-8480.

SciSearch. Institute for Scientific Information, 3501 Market St., Philadelphia, PA 19104. Phone: (215) 386-0100. Fax: (215) 386-6362.

POPULAR WORKS AND PATIENT EDUCATION

The Complete Foot Book: First Aid for Your Feet. Donald S. Pritt, Morton Walker. Avery Publishing Group, Inc., 120 Old

Broadway, Garden City Park, NY 11040. Phone: (800) 548-5757. 1991.

The Doctor's Sore Foot Book. Daniel M. McGann, L.R. Robinson. William Morrow & Company, Inc., 1350 Ave. of the Americas, New York, NY 10019. Phone: (800) 237-0657. 1991.

The Foot Book: Relief for Overused, Abused and Ailing Feet. Glenn Copeland. John Wiley & Sons, Inc., 605 Third Ave., New York, NY 10158-0012. Phone: (212) 850-6000. Fax: (212) 850-6088. 1992.

TEXTBOOKS AND MONOGRAPHS

Current Therapy in Foot and Ankle Surgery. Mark Myerson. Mosby-Year Book, 11830 Westline Industrial Drive, St. Louis, MO 63146. Phone: (800) 325-4177. Fax: (314) 432-1380. 1993.

Disorders of the Foot and Ankle: Medical and Surgical Management. Melvin Jahss. W.B. Saunders Co., The Curtis Center, Independence Sqare W., Philadelphia, PA 19106-3399. Phone: (215) 238-7800. 1991.

Surgery of the Foot and Ankle. Roger A. Mann, Michael Coughlin. Mosby-Year Book, 11830 Westline Industrial Drive, St. Louis, MO 63146. Phone: (800) 325-4177. Fax: (314) 432-1380. 6th edition, 1992.

POISON CONTROL CENTERS

See: POISONING

POISON IVY

See: ALLERGIES; DERMATOLOGIC DISEASES

POISONING

See also: DRUG TOXICITY; FOOD POISONING; LEAD POISONING

ABSTRACTING, INDEXING, AND CURRENT AWARENESS PUBLICATIONS

Excerpta Medica. Section 52: Toxicology. Elsevier Science Publishing Co., Inc., P.O. Box 882, Madison Square Station, New York, NY 10159-2101. Phone: (212) 989-5800. Fax: (212) 633-3990. 20/year.

Index Medicus. U.S. National Library of Medicine, 8600 Rockville Pike, Bethesda, MD 20894. Phone: (800) 638-8480. Monthly.

International Pharmaceutical Abstracts. American Society of Hospital Pharmacists, 4630 Montgomery Ave., Bethesda, MD 20814. Phone: (301) 657-3000. Fax: (301) 657-1641. Semimonthly.

Research Alert: Detection and Identification of Narcotic Drugs & Poisons. Institute for Scientific Information, 3501 Market St., Philadelphia, PA 19104. Phone: (800) 523-1850. Fax: (215) 386-6362. Weekly.

Toxicology Abstracts. Cambridge Scientific Abstracts, 7200 Wisconsin Ave., Bethesda, MD 20814-4823. Phone: (800) 843-7751. Fax: (301) 961-6720. Monthly.

ASSOCIATIONS, PROFESSIONAL SOCIETIES, ADVOCACY AND SUPPORT GROUPS

American Association of Poison Control Centers. c/o Dr. Ted Tong, Arizona Poison & Drug Information Center, 1501 N. Campbell, Tucson, AZ 85725. Phone: (602) 626-1587.

CD-ROM DATABASES

Morbidity Mortality Weekly Report. MEP, 124 Mt. Auburn St., Cambridge, MA 02138. Phone: (800) 342-1338. Fax: (617) 868-7738. Annual.

TOXLINE. SilverPlatter Information, Inc., River Ridge Office Park, 100 River Ridge Rd., Norwood, MA 02062. Phone: (617) 769-2599. Fax: (617) 769-8763. Quarterly.

DIRECTORIES

Emergency Medicine Magazine List of Poison Control Centers. Cahners Publishing Company, 249 W. 17th St., New York, NY 10011. Phone: (212) 645-0067.

ENCYCLOPEDIAS, DICTIONARIES, WORD BOOKS

Illustrated Dictionary of Poisons. Bob Lewis. CRC Press, Inc., 2000 Corporate Blvd. N.W., Boca Raton, FL 33431. Phone: (407) 994-0555. Fax: (407) 997-0949. 1992.

HANDBOOKS, GUIDES, MANUALS, ATLASES

Handbook of Poisoning. R.H. Dreisbach, W.O. Robertson. Appleton & Lange, 25 Van Zant St., East Norwalk, CT 06855. Phone: (800) 423-1359. Fax: (203) 854-9486. Thirteenth edition 1989.

JOURNALS

Morbidity and Mortality Weekly Report. Massachusetts Medical Society, 1440 Main St., Waltham, MA 02154-1649. Phone: (617) 893-3800. Fax: (617) 893-0413. Weekly.

Toxicology. Elsevier Science Publishing Co., Inc., P.O. Box 882, Madison Square Station, New York, NY 10159-2101. Phone: (212) 989-5800. Fax: (212) 633-3990. 6/year.

ONLINE DATABASES

EMBASE. Elsevier Science Publishing Co., Inc., P.O. Box 882, Madison Square Station, New York, NY 10159-2101. Phone: (212) 989-5800. Fax: (212) 633-3990.

MEDLINE. National Library of Medicine, 8600 Rockville Pike, Bethesda, MD 20894. Phone: (800) 638-8480.

SciSearch. Institute for Scientific Information, 3501 Market St., Philadelphia, PA 19104. Phone: (215) 386-0100. Fax: (215) 386-6362.

TOXLINE. U.S. National Library of Medicine, Toxicology Information Program, 8600 Rockville Pike, Bethesda, MD 20894. Phone: (800) 638-8480. Monthly.

TEXTBOOKS AND MONOGRAPHS

Casarett and Doull's Toxicology: The Basic Science of Poisons. Mary O. Amdur, John Doull, Curtis D. Klaassen. McGraw-Hill, Inc., 1221 Avenue of the Americas, 28th Floor, New York, NY 10020. Phone: (212) 512-4228. Fourth edition 1991.

Clinical Management of Poisoning and Drug Overdose. L.M. Haddad, J.F. Winchester. W.B. Saunders Co., The Curtis Center, Independence Square W., Philadelphia, PA 19106-3399. Phone: (215) 238-7800. Second edition 1990.

Goldfrank's Toxicologic Emergencies. Lewis R. Goldfrank, Neal E. Fomenbaum, Neal A. Lewin, and others. Appleton & Lange, 25 Van Zant St., East Norwalk, CT 06855. Phone: (800) 423-1359. Fax: (203) 854-9486. Fourth edition 1990.

Medical Toxicology: Diagnosis and Treatment of Human Poisoning. Ellerhorn. Elsevier Science Publishing Co., Inc., P.O. Box 882, Madison Square Station, New York, NY 10159-2101. Phone: (212) 989-5800. Fax: (212) 633-3990. 1988.

Poisoning and Drug Overdose. Kent R. Olson. Appleton & Lange, 25 Van Zant St., East Norwalk, CT 06855. Phone: (800) 423-1359. Fax: (203) 854-9486. Biennial 1990.

Poisonous and Medicinal Plants. William H. Blackwell, Thomas J. Cobbe. Prentice Hall, Prentice Hall Bldg., 113 Sylvan Ave., Rt. 9W, Englewood Cliffs, NJ 07632. Phone: (201) 767-5937. 1990.

Toxicologic Emergencies. Goldfrank. Appleton & Lange, 25 Van Zant St., East Norwalk, CT 06855. Phone: (800) 423-1359. Fax: (203) 854-9486. Fourth edition 1990.

POLIOMYELITIS

See: INFECTIOUS DISEASES

POST-TRAUMATIC STRESS DISORDER

See also: STRESS

ABSTRACTING, INDEXING, AND CURRENT AWARENESS PUBLICATIONS

Excerpta Medica. Section 32: Psychiatry. Elsevier Science Publishing Co., Inc., P.O. Box 882, Madison Square Station, New York, NY 10159-2101. Phone: (212) 989-5800. Fax: (212) 633-3990. 20/year.

Index Medicus. U.S. National Library of Medicine, 8600 Rockville Pike, Bethesda, MD 20894. Phone: (800) 638-8480. Monthly.

Psychological Abstracts. American Psychological Association, 1200 17th St. NW, Washington, DC 20036. Phone: (202) 955-7600. Monthly.

ASSOCIATIONS, PROFESSIONAL SOCIETIES, ADVOCACY AND SUPPORT GROUPS

American Psychiatric Association (APA). 1400 K St. N.W., Washington, DC 20005. Phone: (202) 682-6000. Fax: (202) 682-6114.

American Psychological Association (APA). 1200 17th St. N.W., Washington, DC 20036. Phone: (202) 955-7600. Fax: (703) 525-5191.

BIBLIOGRAPHIES

Post-Traumatic Stress Disorder, Rape Trauma, Delayed Stress and Related Conditions: A Bibliography. McFarland & Co.,

Inc., Box 611, Jefferson, NC 28640. Phone: (919) 246-4460. 1986.

CD-ROM DATABASES

Excerpta Medica CD: Psychiatry. SilverPlatter Information, Inc., River Ridge Office Park, 100 River Ridge Rd., Norwood, MA 02062. Phone: (617) 769-2599. Fax: (617) 769-8763. Quarterly.

PsycLit. SilverPlatter Information, Inc., River Ridge Office Park, 100 River Ridge Rd., Norwood, MA 02062. Phone: (617) 769-2599. Fax: (617) 769-8763. Quarterly.

JOURNALS

American Journal of Psychiatry. American Psychiatric Press, Inc., 1400 K St. NW, Washington, DC 20005. Phone: (202) 682-6268. Fax: (202) 789-2648. Monthly.

ONLINE DATABASES

EMBASE. Elsevier Science Publishing Co., Inc., P.O. Box 882, Madison Square Station, New York, NY 10159-2101. Phone: (212) 989-5800. Fax: (212) 633-3990.

MEDLINE. National Library of Medicine, 8600 Rockville Pike, Bethesda, MD 20894. Phone: (800) 638-8480.

PsycInfo. SilverPlatter Information, Inc., River Ridge Office Park, 100 River Ridge Rd., Norwood, MA 02062. Phone: (617) 769-2599. Fax: (617) 769-8763. Quarterly.

SciSearch. Institute for Scientific Information, 3501 Market St., Philadelphia, PA 19104. Phone: (215) 386-0100. Fax: (215) 386-6362.

RESEARCH CENTERS, INSTITUTES, CLEARINGHOUSES

Center for Study of Trauma. University of California, San Francisco. Dept. of Psychiatry, 401 Parnassus, San Francisco, CA 94143-0984. Phone: (415) 476-7344. Fax: (415) 388-4913.

TEXTBOOKS AND MONOGRAPHS

Posttraumatic Stress Disorder: Etiology, Phenomenology, and Treatment. Marion E. Wolf, Aron D. Nosnaim (eds.). American Psychiatric Press, Inc., 1400 K St. NW, Washington, DC 20005. Phone: (202) 682-6268. Fax: (202) 789-2648. 1990.

PRACTICE MANAGEMENT

ABSTRACTING, INDEXING, AND CURRENT AWARENESS PUBLICATIONS

Index to Dental Literature. American Dental Association, 211 E. Chicago Ave., Chicago, IL 60611-2678. Phone: (800) 947-4746. Fax: (312) 440-3542. Quarterly.

Index Medicus. U.S. National Library of Medicine, 8600 Rockville Pike, Bethesda, MD 20894. Phone: (800) 638-8480. Monthly.

ASSOCIATIONS, PROFESSIONAL SOCIETIES, ADVOCACY AND SUPPORT GROUPS

American Academy of Dental Group Practice. 18316 Hermitage Way, Minnetonka, MN 55345. Phone: (612) 474-9285.

American Academy of Dental Practice Administration. c/o Linda Doll, 6134 Cheena Dr., Houston, TX 77096. Phone: (713) 771-2477.

American Dental Association (ADA). 211 E. Chicago Ave., Chicago, IL 60611. Phone: (312) 440-2500.

American Group Practice Association (AGPA). 1422 Duke St., Alexandria, VA 22314. Phone: (703) 838-0033. Fax: (703) 548-1890.

American Medical Association (AMA). 515 N. State St., Chicago, IL 60610. Phone: (312) 464-5000. Fax: (312) 645-4184.

Society of Medical-Dental Management Consultants. 7318 Raytown Rd., Raytown, MO 64133. Phone: (816) 353-8488.

DIRECTORIES

Directory of Medical Office Computer Systems. Vinson J. Hudson. McGraw-Hill, Inc., Health Professions Division, 1221 Avenue of the Americas, 28th Floor, New York, NY 10020. Phone: (212) 512-4228. 1990.

Directory of Practice Parameters. American Medical Association, 515 North State St., Chicago, IL 60610. Phone: (312) 464-0183. Fax: (312) 464-5834. Annual.

HANDBOOKS, GUIDES, MANUALS, ATLASES

Medical Practice Management Manual: A Practical Guide for a Productive Practice. Diane Publishing Co., 600 Upland Ave., Upland, PA 19015. Phone: (215) 499-7415. 1991.

The New Practice Handbook. Maryann Ricardo. McGraw-Hill, Inc., Health Professions Division, 1221 Avenue of the Americas, 28th Floor, New York, NY 10020. Phone: (212) 512-4228. 1991.

The Personnel Management Handbook. Maryann Ricardo. McGraw-Hill, Inc., Health Professions Division, 1221 Avenue of the Americas, 28th Floor, New York, NY 10020. Phone: (212) 512-4228. 1991.

Practice Parameters: A Physician's Guide to their Legal Implications. American Medical Association, 515 N. State St., Chicago, IL 60610. Phone: (312) 464-5000. Fax: (312) 645-4184. 1990.

Relative Values for Physicians, 1991/1992. Relative Value Studies. McGraw-Hill, Inc., Health Professions Division, 1221 Avenue of the Americas, 28th Floor, New York, NY 10020. Phone: (212) 512-4228. 1992 Updated quarterly.

JOURNALS

Journal of Medical Practice Management. Williams & Wilkins, 428 E. Preston St., Baltimore, MD 21202. Phone: (800) 638-0672. Fax: (800) 447-8438. Quarterly.

Medical Economics. Medical Economics, Five Paragon Dr., Montvale, NJ 07645-1742. Phone: (800) 222-3045. Fax: (201) 573-4956. Semimonthly.

NEWSLETTERS

Health Care Marketing and Management. American Health Consultants, Department C1290, P.O. Box 740060, Atlanta, GA 30374. Phone: (800) 559-1032. Monthly.

Practice Parameters Update. American Medical Association, 515 N. State St., Chicago, IL 60610. Phone: (312) 464-5000. Fax: (312) 645-4184.

ONLINE DATABASES

EMBASE. Elsevier Science Publishing Co., Inc., P.O. Box 882, Madison Square Station, New York, NY 10159-2101. Phone: (212) 989-5800. Fax: (212) 633-3990.

MEDLINE. National Library of Medicine, 8600 Rockville Pike, Bethesda, MD 20894. Phone: (800) 638-8480.

SciSearch. Institute for Scientific Information, 3501 Market St., Philadelphia, PA 19104. Phone: (215) 386-0100. Fax: (215) 386-6362.

STANDARDS AND STATISTICS SOURCES

Socioeconomic Characteristics of Medical Practice. American Medical Association, 515 N. State St., Chicago, IL 60610. Phone: (312) 464-5000. Fax: (312) 645-4184. Annual.

TEXTBOOKS AND MONOGRAPHS

The Business Side of Medical Practice. American Medical Association, 515 North State St., Chicago, IL 60610. Phone: (312) 464-0183. Fax: (312) 464-5834. 1988.

Enhancing the Value of Your Medical Practice. American Medical Association, 515 North State St., Chicago, IL 60610. Phone: (312) 464-0183. Fax: (312) 464-5834. 1990.

Management of Pediatric Practice. American Academy of Pediatrics, 141 Northwest Point Blvd., P.O. Box 927, Elk Grove Village, IL 60009-0927. Phone: (800) 433-9016. Fax: (708) 228-1281. Second edition 1991.

Managing Medical Office Personnel. Karen Moawad, Lynne R. Costain. Practice Management Information Co., 4727 Wilshire Blvd., Ste. 300, Los Angeles, CA 90010. Phone: (213) 658-8501. 1991.

Office Computer Systems for Health Professionals: A Cost-Benefit Approach to Assessing Alternative Technologies. James W. Allen. McGraw-Hill, Inc., Health Professions Division, 1221 Avenue of the Americas, 28th Floor, New York, NY 10020. Phone: (212) 512-4228. 1990.

Office Gynecology. Morton A. Stenchever. Mosby-Year Book, 11830 Westline Industrial Drive, St. Louis, MO 63146. Phone: (800) 325-4177. Fax: (314) 432-1380. 1991.

Practice Management for the Dental Team. Betty Ladley Finkbeiner, Jerry Crowe Patt. Mosby-Year Book, 11830 Westline Industrial Drive, St. Louis, MO 63146. Phone: (800) 325-4177. Fax: (314) 432-1380. Third edition 1991.

Private Practice: A Guide to Getting Started. Jack D. McCue, Robert D. Ficalora. Little, Brown and Company, 34 Beacon St., Boston, MA 02108. Phone: (617) 227-0730. 1991.

The Successful Dental Practice: An Introduction. American Dental Association, 211 E. Chicago Ave., Chicago, IL 60611-2678. Phone: (800) 947-4746. Fax: (312) 440-3542. 1991.

Veterinary Practice Management. McCurnin. J.B. Lippincott Co., 227 E. Washington Square, Philadelphia, PA 19106-3780. Phone: (215) 238-4200. Fax: (215) 238-4227. 1989.

PREGNANCY

See also: CHILDBIRTH; OBSTETRICS AND
GYNECOLOGY; PREGNANCY
COMPLICATIONS

ABSTRACTING, INDEXING, AND CURRENT AWARENESS PUBLICATIONS

Core Journals in Obstetrics and Gynecology. Elsevier Science Publishing Co., Inc., P.O. Box 882, Madison Square Station, New York, NY 10159-2101. Phone: (212) 989-5800. Fax: (212) 633-3990. 11/year.

Current Contents/Clinical Medicine. Institute for Scientific Information, 3501 Market St., Philadelphia, PA 19104. Phone: (800) 523-1850. Fax: (215) 386-6362. Weekly.

Excerpta Medica. Section 10: Obstetrics and Gynecology. Elsevier Science Publishing Co., Inc., P.O. Box 882, Madison Square Station, New York, NY 10159-2101. Phone: (212) 989-5800. Fax: (212) 633-3990. 20/year.

Index Medicus. U.S. National Library of Medicine, 8600 Rockville Pike, Bethesda, MD 20894. Phone: (800) 638-8480. Monthly.

Science Citation Index. Institute for Scientific Information, 3501 Market St., Philadelphia, PA 19104. Phone: (800) 523-1850. Fax: (215) 386-6362. Bimonthly.

ANNUALS AND REVIEWS

Contributions to Gynecology and Obstetrics. S. Karger Publishers, Inc., 26 West Avon Rd., P.O. Box 529, Farmington, CT 06085. Phone: (203) 675-7834. Fax: (203) 675-7302. Irregular.

Obstetrics and Gynecology Clinics. W.B. Saunders Co., The Curtis Center, Independence Square W., Philadelphia, PA 19106-3399. Phone: (215) 238-7800. Quarterly.

Year Book of Obstetrics and Gynecology. Mosby-Year Book, 11830 Westline Industrial Drive, St. Louis, MO 63146. Phone: (800) 325-4177. Fax: (314) 432-1380. Annual.

ASSOCIATIONS, PROFESSIONAL SOCIETIES, ADVOCACY AND SUPPORT GROUPS

American College of Nurse-Midwives (ACNM). 1522 K St. N.W., Ste. 1000, Washington, DC 20005. Phone: (202) 289-0171. Fax: (202) 289-4395.

American College of Obstetricians and Gynecologists (ACOG). 409 12th St. S.W., Washington, DC 20024-2188. Phone: (202) 638-5577.

International Childbirth Education Association (ICEA). P.O. Box 20048, Minneapolis, MN 55420-0048. Phone: (612) 854-8660.

BIBLIOGRAPHIES

Nutri-Topics: Adolescent Pregnancy and Nutrition. Food and Nutrition Center, National Agricultural Library, 10301 Baltimore Blvd., Beltsville, MD 20705.

Pregnancy Products: Contraceptives, Pregnancy and Ovulation Kits. National Technical Information Service, 5285 Port Royal Rd., Springfield, VA 22161. Phone: (703) 487-4650. Fax: (703) 321-8547. Jan. 1985-Feb. 1989 PB89-857353/CBY.

CD-ROM DATABASES

Clinical Problems in Obstetrics: Critical Care Obstetrics. Catanzarite. Williams & Wilkins, 428 East Preston St., Baltimore, MD 21202. Phone: (800) 638-0672. Fax: (800) 447-8438. 1989.

Excerpta Medica CD: Obstetrics & Gynecology. SilverPlatter Information, Inc., River Ridge Office Park, 100 River Ridge Rd., Norwood, MA 02062. Phone: (617) 769-2599. Fax: (617) 769-8763. Quarterly.

Maternal Fetal Medicine: Fetal Monitor Interpretation. Valerion A. Catanzarite. Williams & Wilkins, 428 East Preston St., Baltimore, MD 21202. Phone: (800) 638-0672. Fax: (800) 447-8438. 1990.

Obstetrics and Gynecology MEDLINE. MEP, 124 Mt. Auburn St., Cambridge, MA 02138. Phone: (800) 342-1338. Fax: (617) 868-7738. Quarterly.

SCISEARCH. Institute for Scientific Information, 3501 Market St., Philadelphia, PA 19104. Phone: (215) 386-0100. Fax: (215) 386-6362.

ENCYCLOPEDIAS, DICTIONARIES, WORD BOOKS

The Illustrated Dictionary of Pregnancy & Childbirth. Carl Jones. Meadowbrook Press, 18318 Minnetonka Blvd., Deephaven, MN 55391. Phone: (800) 338-2232. 1990.

Obstetric and Gynecologic Word Book. Helen E. Littrell. Springhouse Publishing Co., 1111 Bethlehem Pike, Spring House, PA 19477. Phone: (800) 331-3170. Fax: (215) 646-8716. 1992.

Obstetric and Gynecological Words. Stedman. Williams & Wilkins, 428 East Preston St., Baltimore, MD 21202. Phone: (800) 638-0672. Fax: (800) 447-8438. 1992.

HANDBOOKS, GUIDES, MANUALS, ATLASES

A Guide to Effective Care in Pregnancy and Childbirth. Murray Enkin. Oxford University Press, 200 Madison Ave., New York, NY 10016. Phone: (212) 679-7300. 1990.

Handbook of Gynecology and Obstetrics. Brown. Appleton & Lange, 25 Van Zant St., East Norwalk, CT 06855. Phone: (800) 423-1359. Fax: (203) 854-9486. 1992.

Handbook of Medical Problems During Pregnancy. Richard S. Abrams. Appleton & Lange, 25 Van Zant St., East Norwalk, CT 06855. Phone: (800) 423-1359. Fax: (203) 854-9486. 1989.

Nurse's Clinical Guide to Maternity Care. Aileen MacLaren. Springhouse Publishing Co., 1111 Bethlehem Pike, Spring House, PA 19477. Phone: (800) 331-3170. Fax: (215) 646-8716. 1992.

JOURNALS

American Journal of Obstetrics and Gynecology. Mosby-Year Book, 11830 Westline Industrial Drive, St. Louis, MO 63146. Phone: (800) 325-4177. Fax: (314) 432-1380. Monthly.

British Journal of Obstetrics & Gynaecology. Blackwell Publishers, Three Cambridge Center, Cambridge, MA 02142. Phone: (617) 225-0430. Fax: (617) 494-1437. Monthly.

Journal of Women's Health. Mary Ann Liebert, Inc., 1651 Third Ave., New York, NY 10128. Phone: (212) 289-2300. Fax: (212) 289-4697. Quarterly.

Obstetrics and Gynecology. Elsevier Science Publishing Co., Inc., P.O. Box 882, Madison Square Station, New York, NY 10159-2101. Phone: (212) 989-5800. Fax: (212) 633-3990. 15/ year.

Prenatal Diagnosis. John Wiley & Sons, Inc., 605 Third Ave., New York, NY 10158-0012. Phone: (212) 850-6000. Fax: (212) 850-6088. Monthly.

NEWSLETTERS

ACOG Newsletter. American College of Obstetricians and Gynecologists, 409 12th St. S.W., Washington, DC 20024-2188. Phone: (202) 638-5577. Monthly.

National Women's Health Network-Network News. National Women's Health Network, 1325 G St. N.W., Washington, DC 20005. Phone: (202) 347-1140. Bimonthly.

OB/GYN Clinical Alert. American Health Consultants, Department C1290, P.O. Box 740060, Atlanta, GA 30374. Phone: (800) 559-1032. Fax: (404) 352-1971. Monthly.

ONLINE DATABASES

EMBASE. Elsevier Science Publishing Co., Inc., P.O. Box 882, Madison Square Station, New York, NY 10159-2101. Phone: (212) 989-5800. Fax: (212) 633-3990.

MEDLINE. National Library of Medicine, 8600 Rockville Pike, Bethesda, MD 20894. Phone: (800) 638-8480.

SciSearch. Institute for Scientific Information, 3501 Market St., Philadelphia, PA 19104. Phone: (215) 386-0100. Fax: (215) 386-6362.

POPULAR WORKS AND PATIENT EDUCATION

Birth-Tech: Tests and Technology in Pregnancy and Birth. Anne Charlish, Linda Hughey Holt. Facts on File, Inc., 460 Park Ave. S., New York, NY 10016-7382. Phone: (212) 683-2244. Fax: (212) 683-3633. 1990.

The Complete Mothercare Manual. Rosalind Y. Ting, Herbert Brant, Kenneth S. Holt. Simon & Schuster, 1230 Ave. of the Americas, New York, NY 10020. Phone: (800) 223-2348. Fax: (800) 284-0735. Revised edition, 1992.

Conquering Infertility: A Guide for Couples. Stephen L. Corson. Prentice Hall, 113 Sylvan Ave., Rt. 9W, Prentice Hall Bldg., Englewood Cliffs, NJ 07632. Phone: (201) 767-5937. Revised edition 1991.

Every Woman's Medical Handbook. Marie Stoppard. Ballantine Books, Inc., 201 E. 50th St., New York, NY 10022. Phone: (800) 733-3000. 1991.

Getting Pregnant: A Guide for the Infertile Couple. D. Llewellyn-Jones. Bantam Doubleday Dell, 666 Fifth Ave., New York, NY 10103. Phone: (800) 223-6834. 1991.

Getting Pregnant: What Couples Need to Know Right Now. Niels H. Lauersen, Colette Bouchez. Fawcett Book Group, 201 E. 50th St., New York, NY 10022. Phone: (800) 726-0600. 1992.

A Good Birth, A Safe Birth. Diana Korte, Roberta Scaer. Harvard Common Press, 535 Albany St., Boston, MA 02118. Phone: (617) 423-5803. 3rd edition, 1992.

The Good Housekeeping Illustrated Book of Pregnancy and Baby Care. William Morrow & Company, Inc., 1350 Ave. of the Americas, New York, NY 10019. Phone: (800) 237-0657. 1990.

How to Get Pregnant with the New Technology. Sherman J. Silber. Warner Books, Inc., 666 Fifth Ave., 9th Flr., New York, NY 10103. Phone: (212) 484-2900. 1991.

The Illustrated Book of Pregnancy and Childbirth. Margaret Martin. Facts on File, Inc., 460 Park Ave. S., New York, NY 10016-7382. Phone: (212) 683-2244. Fax: (212) 683-3633. 1991.

Intensive Caring: New Hope for High-Risk Pregnancy. Dianne Hales. Random House, Inc., 201 E. 50th St., New York, NY 10022. Phone: (800) 726-0600. 1990.

A New Life: Pregnancy, Birth and Your Child's First Year - A Comprehensive Guide. John T. Queenan, Carrie N. Queenan (eds.). Little, Brown and Co., 34 Beacon St., Boston, MA 02108. Phone: (617) 227-0730. Second edition 1992.

Open Season: A Survival Guide for Natural Childbirth in the 1990s. Nancy W. Cohen. Greenwood Publishing Group, Inc., 88 Post Rd. W., P.O. Box 5007, Westport, CT 06881. Phone: (203) 226-3571. 1991.

The Pregnancy Nutrition Counter. Annette B. Natow, Jo-Ann Hoslin. Pocket Books, Inc., 1230 Ave. of the Americas, New York, NY 10020. Phone: (800) 223-2348. Fax: (800) 284-0735. 1992.

Understanding Pregnancy and Childbirth. Sheldon H. Cherry. Macmillan Publishing Co., 866 Third Ave., New York, NY 10011. Phone: (800) 257-5755. 1992.

Will It Hurt the Baby?: The Safe Use of Medications During Pregnancy and Breastfeeding. Richard S. Abrams. Addison-Wesley Nursing, 390 Bridge Parkway, Redwood City, CA 94065. Phone: (800) 950-5544. 1990.

Your Pregnancy Month by Month: A Comprehensive Guide and Personal Diary from Conception to Birth. Clark Gillespie. HarperCollins Pubs., Inc., 10 E. 53rd St., New York, NY 10022-5299. Phone: (212) 207-7000. Fax: (800) 242-7737. Fourth edition 1992.

RESEARCH CENTERS, INSTITUTES, CLEARINGHOUSES

ACOG Resource Center. American College of Obstetricians and Gynecologists, 600 Maryland Ave. S.W., Ste. 300 E., Washington, DC 20024-2588. Phone: (202) 863-2518.

National Maternal and Child Health Clearinghouse (NMCHC). 38th and R Sts. N.W., Washington, DC 20057. Phone: (202) 625-8410.

TEXTBOOKS AND MONOGRAPHS

Complications of Pregnancy. Cherry. Williams & Wilkins, 428 East Preston St., Baltimore, MD 21202. Phone: (800) 638-0672. Fax: (800) 447-8438. Fourth edition 1991.

Medical Disorders During Pregnancy. William M. Barron, Marshall D. Lindheimer (eds.). Mosby-Year Book, 11830

Westline Industrial Drive, St. Louis, MO 63146. Phone: (800) 325-4177. Fax: (314) 432-1380. 1991.

Obstetrics: Normal and Problem Pregnancies. Steven G. Gabbe, Jennifer R. Niebyl, Joe Leigh Simpson (eds.). Churchill Livingstone Inc., 650 Avenue of the Americas, New York, NY 10011. Phone: (212) 819-5400. Fax: (212) 302-6598. Second edition 1991.

Practical Guide to High-Risk Pregnancy and Delivery. Fernando Arias. Mosby-Year Book, 11830 Westline Industrial Drive, St. Louis, MO 63146. Phone: (800) 325-4177. Fax: (314) 432-1380. Second edition 1992.

PREGNANCY COMPLICATIONS

See also: OBSTETRICS AND GYNECOLOGY; PERINATOLOGY; PREGNANCY

ABSTRACTING, INDEXING, AND CURRENT AWARENESS PUBLICATIONS

Current Contents/Clinical Medicine. Institute for Scientific Information, 3501 Market St., Philadelphia, PA 19104. Phone: (800) 523-1850. Fax: (215) 386-6362. Weekly.

Excerpta Medica. Section 10: Obstetrics and Gynecology. Elsevier Science Publishing Co., Inc., P.O. Box 882, Madison Square Station, New York, NY 10159-2101. Phone: (212) 989-5800. Fax: (212) 633-3990. 20/year.

Index Medicus. U.S. National Library of Medicine, 8600 Rockville Pike, Bethesda, MD 20894. Phone: (800) 638-8480. Monthly.

ANNUALS AND REVIEWS

Year Book of Obstetrics and Gynecology. Mosby-Year Book, 11830 Westline Industrial Drive, St. Louis, MO 63146. Phone: (800) 325-4177. Fax: (314) 432-1380. Annual.

ASSOCIATIONS, PROFESSIONAL SOCIETIES, ADVOCACY AND SUPPORT GROUPS

American College of Obstetricians and Gynecologists (ACOG). 409 12th St. S.W., Washington, DC 20024-2188. Phone: (202) 638-5577.

American Society for Prophylaxis in Obstetrics (ASPO/LAMAZE). 1840 Wilson Blvd., Ste. 204, Arlington, VA 22201. Phone: (800) 368-4404. Fax: (703) 524-8743.

C/SEC Inc.. Cesarean/Support Education and Concern, 22 Forest Rd., Framingham, MA 01701. Phone: (508) 877-8266.

Intensive Caring Unlimited. 910 Bent Lane, Philadelphia, PA 19118. Phone: (609) 848-1945.

CD-ROM DATABASES

Clinical Problems in Obstetrics: Critical Care Obstetrics. Catanzarite. Williams & Wilkins, 428 East Preston St., Baltimore, MD 21202. Phone: (800) 638-0672. Fax: (800) 447-8438. 1989.

Clinical Problems in Obstetrics: Hypertension and Preeclampsia. Catanzarite. Williams & Wilkins, 428 East Preston St., Baltimore, MD 21202. Phone: (800) 638-0672. Fax: (800) 447-8438. 1989.

Critical Care Obstetrics: Clinical Cases. Valerion A. Catanzarite. Williams & Wilkins, 428 East Preston St., Baltimore, MD 21202. Phone: (800) 638-0672. Fax: (800) 447-8438. 1989.

Critical Care Obstetrics: Obstetric Infections. Valerion A. Catanzarite. Williams & Wilkins, 428 East Preston St., Baltimore, MD 21202. Phone: (800) 638-0672. Fax: (800) 447-8438. 1989.

Obstetrics and Gynecology MEDLINE. MEP, 124 Mt. Auburn St., Cambridge, MA 02138. Phone: (800) 342-1338. Fax: (617) 868-7738. Quarterly.

ENCYCLOPEDIAS, DICTIONARIES, WORD BOOKS

Obstetric and Gynecologic Word Book. Helen E. Littrell. Springhouse Publishing Co., 1111 Bethlehem Pike, Spring House, PA 19477. Phone: (800) 331-3170. Fax: (215) 646-8716. 1992.

Obstetric and Gynecological Words. Stedman. Williams & Wilkins, 428 East Preston St., Baltimore, MD 21202. Phone: (800) 638-0672. Fax: (800) 447-8438. 1992.

HANDBOOKS, GUIDES, MANUALS, ATLASES

Handbook of Gynecology and Obstetrics. Brown. Appleton & Lange, 25 Van Zant St., East Norwalk, CT 06855. Phone: (800) 423-1359. Fax: (203) 854-9486. 1992.

Obstetrical and Perinatal Infections. David Charles. Mosby Year Book, 11830 Westline Industrial Drive, St. Louis, MO 63146. Phone: (800) 325-4177. Fax: (314) 432-1380. 1992.

JOURNALS

American Journal of Perinatology. Thieme Medical Publishers, Inc., 381 Park Ave. S., New York, NY 10016. Phone: (212) 683-5088. Fax: (212) 779-9020. Bimonthly.

Birth. Blackwell Scientific Publications, Inc., 3 Cambridge Center, Cambridge, MA 02142. Phone: (800) 759-6102.

British Journal of Obstetrics & Gynaecology. Blackwell Publishers, Three Cambridge Center, Cambridge, MA 02142. Phone: (617) 225-0430. Fax: (617) 494-1437. Monthly.

Journal of Perinatology. Appleton & Lange, 25 Van Zant St., East Norwalk, CT 06855. Phone: (800) 423-1359. Fax: (203) 854-9486. Quarterly.

Obstetrics and Gynecology. Elsevier Science Publishing Co., Inc., P.O. Box 882, Madison Square Station, New York, NY 10159-2101. Phone: (212) 989-5800. Fax: (212) 633-3990. 15/year.

NEWSLETTERS

National Women's Health Network-Network News. National Women's Health Network, 1325 G St. N.W., Washington, DC 20005. Phone: (202) 347-1140. Bimonthly.

ONLINE DATABASES

EMBASE. Elsevier Science Publishing Co., Inc., P.O. Box 882, Madison Square Station, New York, NY 10159-2101. Phone: (212) 989-5800. Fax: (212) 633-3990.

MEDLINE. National Library of Medicine, 8600 Rockville Pike, Bethesda, MD 20894. Phone: (800) 638-8480.

SciSearch. Institute for Scientific Information, 3501 Market St., Philadelphia, PA 19104. Phone: (215) 386-0100. Fax: (215) 386-6362.

POPULAR WORKS AND PATIENT EDUCATION

Preventing Miscarriage: The Good News. Jonathan Scher, Carol Dix. HarperCollins Pubs., Inc., 10 E. 53rd St., New York, NY 10022-5299. Phone: (212) 207-7000. Fax: (800) 242-7737. 1990.

When Pregnancy Isn't Perfect: A Layperson's Guide to Complications in Pregnancy. Laurie Rich. Viking Penguin, 375 Hudson St., New York, NY 10014-3657. Phone: (800) 331-4624. 1991.

Will It Hurt the Baby?: The Safe Use of Medications During Pregnancy and Breastfeeding. Richard S. Abrams. Addison-Wesley Nursing, 390 Bridge Parkway, Redwood City, CA 94065. Phone: (800) 950-5544. 1990.

TEXTBOOKS AND MONOGRAPHS

Complications of Pregnancy. Cherry. Williams & Wilkins, 428 East Preston St., Baltimore, MD 21202. Phone: (800) 638-0672. Fax: (800) 447-8438. Fourth edition 1991.

Diagnosis and Treatment of Extrauterine Pregnancies. Nicholas Kadar. Raven Press, 1185 Avenue of the Americas, New York, NY 10036. Phone: (212) 930-9500. Fax: (212) 869-3495. 1990.

Ectopic Pregnancy: Pathophysiology and Clinical Management. C.M. Fredericks, J.D. Paulson, G. Holtz. Taylor & Francis Inc., 1900 Frost Rd., Suite 101, Bristol, PA 19007-1598. Phone: (800) 821-8312. Fax: (215) 785-5515. 1989.

High Risk Pregnancy. A.A. Calder, W. Dunlop. Butterworth-Heinemann, 80 Montvale Ave., Stoneham, MA 02180. Phone: (617) 438-8464. Fax: (617) 279-4851. 1991.

Medical Disorders During Pregnancy. William M. Barron, Marshall D. Lindheimer (eds.). Mosby-Year Book, 11830 Westline Industrial Drive, St. Louis, MO 63146. Phone: (800) 325-4177. Fax: (314) 432-1380. 1991.

Obstetrics: Normal and Problem Pregnancies. Steven G. Gabbe, Jennifer R. Niebyl, Joe Leigh Simpson (eds.). Churchill Livingstone Inc., 650 Avenue of the Americas, New York, NY 10011. Phone: (212) 819-5400. Fax: (212) 302-6598. Second edition 1991.

Practical Guide to High-Risk Pregnancy and Delivery. Fernando Arias. Mosby-Year Book, 11830 Westline Industrial Drive, St. Louis, MO 63146. Phone: (800) 325-4177. Fax: (314) 432-1380. Second edition 1992.

Pregnancy and Risk: The Basis of Rational Management. D.K. James, G.M. Stirrat (eds.). John Wiley & Sons, Inc., 605 Third Ave., New York, NY 10158-0012. Phone: (212) 850-6000. Fax: (212) 850-6088. 1989.

Preterm Birth: Causes, Prevention, and Management. Fritz A. Fuchs, Anna-Ritta Fuchs, Phillip G. Stubblefield. McGraw-Hill, Inc., Health Professions Division, 1221 Avenue of the Americas, 28th Floor, New York, NY 10020. Phone: (212) 512-4228. Second edition 1992.

The Unborn Patient: Prenatal Diagnosis and Treatment. Michael R. Harrison, Mitchell S. Golbus, Roy A. Filly. W.B.

Saunders Co., The Curtis Center, Independence Square W., Philadelphia, PA 19106-3399. Phone: (215) 238-7800. Second edition 1991.

PREMATURE INFANTS

See: NEONATOLOGY

PREMENSTRUAL SYNDROME

See also: MENSTRUATION

ABSTRACTING, INDEXING, AND CURRENT AWARENESS PUBLICATIONS

Current Contents/Clinical Medicine. Institute for Scientific Information, 3501 Market St., Philadelphia, PA 19104. Phone: (800) 523-1850. Fax: (215) 386-6362. Weekly.

Excerpta Medica. Section 10: Obstetrics and Gynecology. Elsevier Science Publishing Co., Inc., P.O. Box 882, Madison Square Station, New York, NY 10159-2101. Phone: (212) 989-5800. Fax: (212) 633-3990. 20/year.

Index Medicus. U.S. National Library of Medicine, 8600 Rockville Pike, Bethesda, MD 20894. Phone: (800) 638-8480. Monthly.

Psychological Abstracts. American Psychological Association, 1200 17th St. NW, Washington, DC 20036. Phone: (202) 955-7600. Monthly.

ASSOCIATIONS, PROFESSIONAL SOCIETIES, ADVOCACY AND SUPPORT GROUPS

American College of Obstetricians and Gynecologists (ACOG). 409 12th St. S.W., Washington, DC 20024-2188. Phone: (202) 638-5577.

PMS Access. P.O. Box 9326, Madison, WI 53715. Phone: (800) 222-4767. 800-833-4767 in Wisconsin.

HANDBOOKS, GUIDES, MANUALS, ATLASES

Premenstrual Syndrome: A Clinician's Guide. Sally Severino, Margaret L. Maline. Guilford Publications, Inc., 72 Spring St., New York, NY 10012. Phone: (800) 365-7006. Fax: (212) 366-6708. 1989.

JOURNALS

American Journal of Obstetrics and Gynecology. Mosby-Year Book, 11830 Westline Industrial Drive, St. Louis, MO 63146. Phone: (800) 325-4177. Fax: (314) 432-1380. Monthly.

American Journal of Psychiatry. American Psychiatric Press, Inc., 1400 K St. NW, Washington, DC 20005. Phone: (202) 682-6268. Fax: (202) 789-2648. Monthly.

Obstetrics and Gynecology. Elsevier Science Publishing Co., Inc., P.O. Box 882, Madison Square Station, New York, NY 10159-2101. Phone: (212) 989-5800. Fax: (212) 633-3990. 15/year.

Psychosomatic Medicine. Williams & Wilkins, 428 E. Preston St., Baltimore, MD 21202. Phone: (800) 638-0672. Fax: (800) 447-8438. Bimonthly.

NEWSLETTERS

National Women's Health Network-Network News. National Women's Health Network, 1325 G St. N.W., Washington, DC 20005. Phone: (202) 347-1140. Bimonthly.

ONLINE DATABASES

EMBASE. Elsevier Science Publishing Co., Inc., P.O. Box 882, Madison Square Station, New York, NY 10159-2101. Phone: (212) 989-5800. Fax: (212) 633-3990.

MEDLINE. National Library of Medicine, 8600 Rockville Pike, Bethesda, MD 20894. Phone: (800) 638-8480.

PsycInfo. SilverPlatter Information, Inc., River Ridge Office Park, 100 River Ridge Rd., Norwood, MA 02062. Phone: (617) 769-2599. Fax: (617) 769-8763. Quarterly.

SciSearch. Institute for Scientific Information, 3501 Market St., Philadelphia, PA 19104. Phone: (215) 386-0100. Fax: (215) 386-6362.

POPULAR WORKS AND PATIENT EDUCATION

Complete PMS Medical Treatment Plan. Joseph Martorano. M. Evans and Co., Inc., 216 E. 49th St., New York, NY 10017. Phone: (212) 688-2810. 1992.

Once a Month: The Original Premenstrual Syndrome Handbook. Katharina Dalton. Hunter House, Inc., 2200 Central, Ste. 202, Alameda, CA 94501-4451. Phone: (510) 865-5282. Fourth edition 1990.

PMS: Premenstrual Syndrome: A Guide for Young Women. Gilda Berger. Borgo Press, P.O. Box 2845, San Bernardino, CA 92406-2845. Phone: (909) 884-5813. Fax: (909) 888-4942. Third edition 1991.

Premenstrual Syndrome: A Guide for Young Women. Gilda Berger. Borgo Press, P.O. Box 2845, San Bernardino, CA 92406-2845. Phone: (909) 884-5813. Fax: (909) 888-4942. 3rd edition, 1991.

Premenstrual Syndrome Self-Help Book. Susan M. Lark. Celestial Arts Publishing Co., P.O. Box 7327, Berkeley, CA 94707. Phone: (800) 841-2665.

Women's Health Alert: What Most Doctors Won't Tell You About. Sidney M. Wolfe. Addison-Wesley Publishing Co., Rte. 128, Reading, MA 01867. Phone: (800) 447-2226. 1990.

TEXTBOOKS AND MONOGRAPHS

Premenstrual, Postpartum, and Menopausal Mood Disorders. Laurence M. Demers, John L. McGuire, Audrey Phillips, et. al.. Williams & Wilkins, 428 East Preston St., Baltimore, MD 21202. Phone: (800) 638-0672. Fax: (800) 447-8438. 1990.

The Premenstrual Syndrome. William Keye. W.B. Saunders Co., The Curtis Center, Independence Sqare W., Philadelphia, PA 19106-3399. Phone: (215) 238-7800. 1988.

The Premenstrual Syndromes: New Findings and Controversies. Leslie Gise. Churchill Livingstone Inc., 650 Ave. of the Americas, New York, NY 10011. Phone: (212) 819-5400. Fax: (212) 302-6598. 1988.

PRENATAL CARE

See: PREGNANCY

PRENATAL TESTING

ABSTRACTING, INDEXING, AND CURRENT AWARENESS PUBLICATIONS

Current Contents/Clinical Medicine. Institute for Scientific Information, 3501 Market St., Philadelphia, PA 19104. Phone: (800) 523-1850. Fax: (215) 386-6362. Weekly.

Current Contents/Life Sciences. Institute for Scientific Information, 3501 Market St., Philadelphia, PA 19104. Phone: (215) 386-0100. Fax: (215) 386-6362.

Excerpta Medica. Section 10: Obstetrics and Gynecology. Elsevier Science Publishing Co., Inc., P.O. Box 882, Madison Square Station, New York, NY 10159-2101. Phone: (212) 989-5800. Fax: (212) 633-3990. 20/year.

Index Medicus. U.S. National Library of Medicine, 8600 Rockville Pike, Bethesda, MD 20894. Phone: (800) 638-8480. Monthly.

Science Citation Index. Institute for Scientific Information, 3501 Market St., Philadelphia, PA 19104. Phone: (800) 523-1850. Fax: (215) 386-6362. Bimonthly.

ANNUALS AND REVIEWS

Year Book of Neonatal and Perinatal Medicine. Mosby-Year Book, 11830 Westline Industrial Drive, St. Louis, MO 63146. Phone: (800) 325-4177. Fax: (314) 432-1380. Annual.

ASSOCIATIONS, PROFESSIONAL SOCIETIES, ADVOCACY AND SUPPORT GROUPS

March of Dimes Birth Defects Foundation (MDBDF). 1275 Mamaroneck Ave., White Plains, NY 10605. Phone: (914) 428-7100. Fax: (914) 428-8203.

BIBLIOGRAPHIES

Prenatal Diagnosis: Chorionic Villus Biopsy. National Technical Information Service, 5285 Port Royal Rd., Springfield, VA 22161. Phone: (703) 487-4650. Fax: (703) 321-8547. Jan. 1978-July 1988 PB88-866421/CBY.

CD-ROM DATABASES

Advanced Fetal Monitoring. Catanzarite. Williams & Wilkins, 428 East Preston St., Baltimore, MD 21202. Phone: (800) 638-0672. Fax: (800) 447-8438. 1990.

Critical Concepts of Fetal Monitoring. Blood. Williams & Wilkins, 428 East Preston St., Baltimore, MD 21202. Phone: (800) 638-0672. Fax: (800) 447-8438. 1990.

Maternal Fetal Medicine: Fetal Monitor Interpretation. Valerion A. Catanzarite. Williams & Wilkins, 428 East Preston St., Baltimore, MD 21202. Phone: (800) 638-0672. Fax: (800) 447-8438. 1990.

SCISEARCH. Institute for Scientific Information, 3501 Market St., Philadelphia, PA 19104. Phone: (215) 386-0100. Fax: (215) 386-6362.

HANDBOOKS, GUIDES, MANUALS, ATLASES

Manual of Fetal Assessment. M.J. Whittle, J.P. Neilson. Butterworth-Heinemann, 80 Montvale Ave., Stoneham, MA 02180. Phone: (617) 438-8464. Fax: (617) 279-4851. 1991.

A Practical Guide to Chorion Villus Sampling. David T.Y. Liu. Oxford University Press, 200 Madison Ave., New York, NY 10016. Phone: (212) 679-7300. 1991.

JOURNALS

American Journal of Medical Genetics. John Wiley & Sons, Inc., 605 Third Ave., New York, NY 10158-0012. Phone: (212) 850-6000. Fax: (212) 850-6088. 16/year.

American Journal of Obstetrics and Gynecology. Mosby-Year Book, 11830 Westline Industrial Drive, St. Louis, MO 63146. Phone: (800) 325-4177. Fax: (314) 432-1380. Monthly.

Journal of Clinical Ultrasound. John Wiley & Sons, Inc., 605 Third Ave., New York, NY 10158-0012. Phone: (212) 850-6000. Fax: (212) 850-6088. 9/year.

Journal of Genetic Counseling. Human Sciences Press, 233 Spring St., New York, NY 10013-1578. Phone: (800) 221-9369. Fax: (212) 807-1047. Quarterly.

Journal of Ultrasound in Medicine. American Institute of Ultrasound in Medicine, 11200 Rockville Pike, Suite 205, Rockville, MD 20852-3139. Phone: (800) 638-5352. Fax: (301) 881-7303. Monthly.

Obstetrics and Gynecology. Elsevier Science Publishing Co., Inc., P.O. Box 882, Madison Square Station, New York, NY 10159-2101. Phone: (212) 989-5800. Fax: (212) 633-3990. 15/year.

Prenatal Diagnosis. John Wiley & Sons, Inc., 605 Third Ave., New York, NY 10158-0012. Phone: (212) 850-6000. Fax: (212) 850-6088.

ONLINE DATABASES

EMBASE. Elsevier Science Publishing Co., Inc., P.O. Box 882, Madison Square Station, New York, NY 10159-2101. Phone: (212) 989-5800. Fax: (212) 633-3990.

MEDLINE. National Library of Medicine, 8600 Rockville Pike, Bethesda, MD 20894. Phone: (800) 638-8480.

SciSearch. Institute for Scientific Information, 3501 Market St., Philadelphia, PA 19104. Phone: (215) 386-0100. Fax: (215) 386-6362.

POPULAR WORKS AND PATIENT EDUCATION

The Tentative Pregnancy: Prenatal Diagnosis and the Future of Motherhood. Barbara Katz Rothman. Penguin USA, 375 Hudson St., New York, NY 10014-3657. Phone: (800) 331-4624. 1989.

Which Tests for my Unborn Baby: A Guide to Prenatal Diagnosis. Lachlan De Crespigny, Rhonda Dredge. Oxford University Press, 200 Madison Ave., New York, NY 10016. Phone: (212) 679-7300. 1992.

RESEARCH CENTERS, INSTITUTES, CLEARINGHOUSES

Prenatal Clinical Research Center. Case Western Reserve University. 3395 Scranton Rd., Cleveland, OH 44109. Phone: (216) 459-4246.

Prenatal Diagnostic Center. Baylor College of Medicine, One Baylor Plaza, Houston, TX 77030. Phone: (713) 797-0322.

TEXTBOOKS AND MONOGRAPHS

Disorders of the Placenta, Fetus and Neonate: Diagnosis and Clinical Significance. Richard L. Naeye. Mosby-Year Book, 11830 Westline Industrial Drive, St. Louis, MO 63146. Phone: (800) 325-4177. Fax: (314) 432-1380. 1992.

Fetal Echocardiography. Rudy E. Sabbagha, Samuel Gidding, Janette Strasburger. Appleton & Lange, 25 Van Zant St., East Norwalk, CT 06855. Phone: (800) 423-1359. Fax: (203) 854-9486. 1991.

More Exercises in Fetal Monitoring. Barry S. Schifrin. Mosby-Year Book, 11830 Westline Industrial Drive, St. Louis, MO 63146. Phone: (800) 325-4177. Fax: (314) 432-1380. 1992.

Pre-Natal Diagnosis and Prognosis. R.J. Lifford (ed.). Butterworth-Heinemann, 80 Montvale Ave., Stoneham, MA 02180. Phone: (617) 438-8464. Fax: (617) 279-4851. 1990.

Prenatal Diagnosis in Obstetric Practice. M.J. Whittle, J.M. Conner. Blackwell Scientific Publications, Inc., 3 Cambridge Center, Cambridge, MA 02142. Phone: (800) 759-6102. 1989.

The Unborn Patient: Prenatal Diagnosis and Treatment. Michael R. Harrison, Mitchell S. Golbus, Roy A. Filly. W.B. Saunders Co., The Curtis Center, Independence Square W., Philadelphia, PA 19106-3399. Phone: (215) 238-7800. Second edition 1991.

PRESBYOPIA

See: VISION DISORDERS

PRESENILE DEMENTIA

See: DEMENTIA

PREVENTIVE MEDICINE

ABSTRACTING, INDEXING, AND CURRENT AWARENESS PUBLICATIONS

Excerpta Medica. Section 17: Public Health, Social Medicine and Epidemiology. Elsevier Science Publishing Co., Inc., P.O. Box 882, Madison Square Station, New York, NY 10159-2101. Phone: (212) 989-5800. Fax: (212) 633-3990. 24/year.

Index Medicus. U.S. National Library of Medicine, 8600 Rockville Pike, Bethesda, MD 20894. Phone: (800) 638-8480. Monthly.

Science Citation Index. Institute for Scientific Information, 3501 Market St., Philadelphia, PA 19104. Phone: (800) 523-1850. Fax: (215) 386-6362. Bimonthly.

ASSOCIATIONS, PROFESSIONAL SOCIETIES, ADVOCACY AND SUPPORT GROUPS

American Association for World Health. 1129 20th St. N.W., Ste. 400, Washington, DC 20036. Phone: (202) 466-5883.

American Board of Preventive Medicine (ABPM). Dept. of Community Health, P.O. Box 927, Wright State University School of medicine, Dayton, OH 45401. Phone: (513) 278-6915.

American College of Preventive Medicine (ACPM). 1015 15th St. N.W., Ste. 403, Washington, DC 20005. Phone: (202) 789-0003. Fax: (202) 289-8274.

American Health Foundation (AHF). 320 E. 43rd St., New York, NY 10017. Phone: (212) 953-1900. Fax: (212) 687-2339.

Association of Teachers of Preventive Medicine. 1030 15th St. N.W., No. 410, Washington, DC 20005. Phone: (202) 682-1698.

World Health Organization. Ave. Appia, CH-1211 Geneva 27, Switzerland.

BIBLIOGRAPHIES

Preventive Medicine: Health Education. National Technical Information Service, 5285 Port Royal Rd., Springfield, VA 22161. Phone: (703) 487-4650. Fax: (703) 321-8547. Jan. 1970-May 1988.

CD-ROM DATABASES

SCISEARCH. Institute for Scientific Information, 3501 Market St., Philadelphia, PA 19104. Phone: (215) 386-0100. Fax: (215) 386-6362.

DIRECTORIES

Directory of Certified Preventive Medicine Physicians. American Board of Medical Specialties, 1 Rotary Center, Suite 805, Evanston, IL 60201. Phone: (708) 491-9091. Biennial.

ENCYCLOPEDIAS, DICTIONARIES, WORD BOOKS

Encyclopedia of Health. Chelsea House Publishers, 95 Madison Ave., New York, NY 10016. Phone: (800) 848-2665. Irregular.

HANDBOOKS, GUIDES, MANUALS, ATLASES

The New Handbook of Health and Preventive Medicine. Kurt Butler, Lynn Rayner. Prometheus Books, 700E. Amherst St., Buffalo, NY 14215. Phone: (800) 421-0351. 1990.

JOURNALS

American Journal of Preventive Medicine. Oxford University Press, 200 Madison Ave., New York, NY 10016. Phone: (212) 679-7300.

Preventive Medicine. Academic Press, Inc., 1250 Sixth Ave., San Diego, CA 92101-4311. Phone: (619) 699-6345. Fax: (619) 699-6715.

Preventive Veterinary Medicine. Elsevier Science Publishing Co., Inc., P.O. Box 882, Madison Square Station, New York, NY 10159-2101. Phone: (212) 989-5800. Fax: (212) 633-3990. Monthly.

ONLINE DATABASES

EMBASE. Elsevier Science Publishing Co., Inc., P.O. Box 882, Madison Square Station, New York, NY 10159-2101. Phone: (212) 989-5800. Fax: (212) 633-3990.

MEDLINE. National Library of Medicine, 8600 Rockville Pike, Bethesda, MD 20894. Phone: (800) 638-8480.

SciSearch. Institute for Scientific Information, 3501 Market St., Philadelphia, PA 19104. Phone: (215) 386-0100. Fax: (215) 386-6362.

POPULAR WORKS AND PATIENT EDUCATION

Peace, Love and Healing: Bodymind Communication and the Path to Self-Healing: An Exploration. Bernie S. Siegel. HarperCollins Pubs., Inc., 10 E. 53rd St., New York, NY 10022-5299. Phone: (212) 207-7000. 1990.

The People's Medical Society Health Body Book: Test Yourself for Maximum Health. Charles B. Inlander, Jim Punkre. Viking Penguin, 375 Hudson St., New York, NY 10014-3657. Phone: (800) 331-4624. 1991.

RESEARCH CENTERS, INSTITUTES, CLEARINGHOUSES

Center for Health Promotion and Education. Centers for Disease Control, 1600 Clifton Rd. N.E., Atlanta, GA 30333. Phone: (404) 488-4698.

Center for Health Promotion Research and Development. P.O. Box 20186, University of Texas, Houston, TX 77225. Phone: (713) 792-8540.

Preventive Medicine Research Institute. 2302 Divisadera St., San Francisco, CA 94115. Phone: (415) 346-1557.

Stanford Center for Research in Disease Prevention. Stanford University School of Medicine, 1000 Welch Rd., Palo Alto, CA 94304. Phone: (415) 723-1000.

TEXTBOOKS AND MONOGRAPHS

Healthy People 2000: National Health Promotion and Disease Prevention Objectives. U.S. Dept. of Health and Human Services. U.S. Government Printing Office, Superintendent of Documents, P.O. Box 371954, Pittsburgh, PA 15250-7954. Phone: (202) 783-3238. Fax: (202) 512-2250. 1991.

Maxcy-Rosenau-Last Public Health and Preventive Medicine. J.M. Last (ed.). Appleton & Lange, 25 Van Zant St., East Norwalk, CT 06855. Phone: (800) 423-1359. Fax: (203) 854-9486. 13th edition, 1992.

Prevention in Clinical Practice. Daniel M. Becker, Laurence B. Gardner (eds.). Plenum Publishing Co., 233 Spring St., New York, NY 10013-1578. Phone: (212) 620-8000. Fax: (212) 463-0742. 1988.

PROCTOLOGY

See: COLORECTAL SURGERY; GASTROENTEROLOGY

PROCTOSCOPY

See: ENDOSCOPY

PROFESSIONAL STANDARDS REVIEW ORGANIZATION

See: QUALITY ASSURANCE

PROGERIA

See: ENDOCRINE DISORDERS

PROGESTINS

See: ESTROGEN REPLACEMENT THERAPY; HORMONES

PROSTATE CANCER

ABSTRACTING, INDEXING, AND CURRENT AWARENESS PUBLICATIONS

Current Contents/Clinical Medicine. Institute for Scientific Information, 3501 Market St., Philadelphia, PA 19104. Phone: (800) 523-1850. Fax: (215) 386-6362. Weekly.

Excerpta Medica. Section 16: Cancer. Elsevier Science Publishing Co., Inc., P.O. Box 882, Madison Square Station, New York, NY 10159-2101. Phone: (212) 989-5800. Fax: (212) 633-3990. 32/year.

Excerpta Medica. Section 28: Urology and Nephrology. Elsevier Science Publishing Co., Inc., P.O. Box 882, Madison Square Station, New York, NY 10159-2101. Phone: (212) 989-5800. Fax: (212) 633-3990. 20/year.

ICRDB Cancergram: Genitourinary Cancer--Diagnosis, Treatment. U.S. Government Printing Office, Superintendent of Documents, P.O. Box 371954, Pittsburgh, PA 15250-7954. Phone: (202) 783-3238. Fax: (202) 512-2250. Monthly.

Index Medicus. U.S. National Library of Medicine, 8600 Rockville Pike, Bethesda, MD 20894. Phone: (800) 638-8480. Monthly.

Science Citation Index. Institute for Scientific Information, 3501 Market St., Philadelphia, PA 19104. Phone: (800) 523-1850. Fax: (215) 386-6362. Bimonthly.

ANNUALS AND REVIEWS

EORTC Genitourinary Gourp Monograph 7: Prostate Cancer and Testicular Cancer. W.G. Jones, Donald W.W. Newling (eds.). John Wiley & Sons, Inc., 605 Third Ave., New York, NY 10158-0012. Phone: (212) 850-6000. Fax: (212) 850-6088. 1990.

Urologic Clinics. W.B. Saunders Co., The Curtis Center, Independence Square W., Philadelphia, PA 19106-3399. Phone: (215) 238-7800. Quarterly.

ASSOCIATIONS, PROFESSIONAL SOCIETIES, ADVOCACY AND SUPPORT GROUPS

American Cancer Society (ACS). 1599 Clifton Rd. N.E., Atlanta, GA 30329. Phone: (404) 320-3333.

Prostate Health Council. c/o American Foundation for Urologic Disease, 1120 N. Charles St., No. 401, Baltimore, MD 21201. Phone: (800) 242-2383.

BIBLIOGRAPHIES

Oncology Overview: Current Management of Prostatic Cancer: Diagnosis and Therapy. Peter T. Scardino (ed.). U.S. Government Printing Office, Superintendent of Documents, P.O. Box 371954, Pittsburgh, PA 15250-7954. Phone: (202) 783-3238. Fax: (202) 512-2250. 1990.

Prostate Cancer: Treatment Other Than Surgery. National Technical Information Service, 5285 Port Royal Rd., Springfield, VA 22161. Phone: (703) 487-4650. Fax: (703) 321-8547. Jan. 1978-Nov. 1988 PB89-851430/CBY.

CD-ROM DATABASES

Cancerlit. Aries Systems Corporation, One Dundee Park, Andover, MA 01810. Phone: (508) 475-7200. Fax: (508) 474-8860. Quarterly.

OncoDisc. J.B. Lippincott Co., 227 East Washington Square, Philadelphia, PA 19106-3780. Phone: (215) 238-4200. Fax: (215) 238-4227. Bimonthly.

SCISEARCH. Institute for Scientific Information, 3501 Market St., Philadelphia, PA 19104. Phone: (215) 386-0100. Fax: (215) 386-6362.

HANDBOOKS, GUIDES, MANUALS, ATLASES

Manual of Urologic Surgery. Jackson F. Fowler. Little, Brown and Co., 34 Beacon St., Boston, MA 02108. Phone: (617) 227-0730. Fax: (617) 227-0790. 1990.

JOURNALS

CA - A Cancer Journal for Clinicians. J.B. Lippincott Co., 227 E. Washington Square, Philadelphia, PA 19106-3780. Phone: (215) 238-4200. Fax: (215) 238-4227. Bimonthly.

Journal of the National Cancer Institute. Superintendent of Documents, P.O. Box 371954, Pittsburgh, PA 15250-7954. Fax: (202) 512-2233. Semimonthly.

Journal of Surgical Oncology. John Wiley & Sons, Inc., 605 Third Ave., New York, NY 10158-0012. Phone: (212) 850-6000. Fax: (212) 850-6088. Monthly.

Journal of Urology. Williams & Wilkins, 428 E. Preston St., Baltimore, MD 21202. Phone: (800) 638-0672. Fax: (800) 447-8438. Monthly.

Urology. Cahners Publishing Company, 249 W. 17th St., New York, NY 10011. Phone: (212) 645-0067.

ONLINE DATABASES

CANCERLIT. U.S. National Cancer Institute, International Cancer Information Center, Building 82, Room 102, Bethesda, MD 20892. Phone: (301) 496-7403. Fax: (301) 480-8105. Monthly.

Clinical Protocols. U.S. National Cancer Institute, International Cancer Information Center, Building 82, Room 102, Bethesda, MD 20892. Phone: (301) 496-7403. Fax: (301) 480-8105.

EMBASE. Elsevier Science Publishing Co., Inc., P.O. Box 882, Madison Square Station, New York, NY 10159-2101. Phone: (212) 989-5800. Fax: (212) 633-3990.

MEDLINE. National Library of Medicine, 8600 Rockville Pike, Bethesda, MD 20894. Phone: (800) 638-8480.

Physician Data Query (PDQ) Cancer Information File. U.S. National Cancer Institute, International Cancer Information Center, Building 82, Room 102, Bethesda, MD 20892. Phone: (301) 496-7403. Fax: (301) 480-8105. Monthly.

Physician Data Query (PDQ) Directory File. U.S. National Cancer Institute, International Cancer Information Center, Building 82, Room 102, Bethesda, MD 20892. Phone: (301) 496-7403. Fax: (301) 480-8105. Monthly.

Physician Data Query (PDQ) Protocol File. U.S. National Cancer Institute, International Cancer Information Center, Building 82, Room 102, Bethesda, MD 20892. Phone: (301) 496-7403. Fax: (301) 480-8105. Monthly.

SciSearch. Institute for Scientific Information, 3501 Market St., Philadelphia, PA 19104. Phone: (215) 386-0100. Fax: (215) 386-6362.

POPULAR WORKS AND PATIENT EDUCATION

Cancervive: The Challenge of Life After Cancer. Susan Nessim, Judith Ellis. Houghton Mifflin Co., 1 Deacon St., Boston, MA 02108. Phone: (800) 225-3362. 1991.

The Prostate Book: Sound Advice on Symptoms and Treatment. Stephen Rous. W.W. Norton & Co., Inc., 500 Fifth Ave., New York, NY 10110. Phone: (800) 223-2584. Updated edition 1992.

RESEARCH CENTERS, INSTITUTES, CLEARINGHOUSES

Gastrointestinal Research Group. University of Calgary. Health Sciences Centre, 3330 Hospital Dr. N.W., Calgary, AB, Canada T2N 1N4. Phone: (403) 220-4539. Fax: (403) 270-3353.

TEXTBOOKS AND MONOGRAPHS

Current Genitourinary Cancer Surgery. Dana Crawford, Sakvi Dai (eds.). Williams & Wilkins, 428 East Preston St., Baltimore, MD 21202. Phone: (800) 638-0672. Fax: (800) 447-8438. 1990.

Diagnosis and Management of Genitourinary Cancer. Donald Skinner, Gary Lieskovsky. W.B. Saunders Co., The Curtis Center, Independence Sqare W., Philadelphia, PA 19106-3399. Phone: (215) 238-7800. 1988.

Operative Urology. Fray F. Marshall (ed.). W.B. Saunders Co., The Curtis Center, Independence Sqare W., Philadelphia, PA 19106-3399. Phone: (215) 238-7800. 1991.

Pathology of the Prostate. David G. Bostwck (ed.). Churchill Livingstone Inc., 650 Ave. of the Americas, New York, NY 10011. Phone: (212) 819-5400. Fax: (212) 302-6598. 1990.

Prostate Biopsy Interpretation. Jonathan I. Epstein. Raven Press, 1185 Avenue of the Americas, New York, NY 10036. Phone: (212) 930-9500. Fax: (212) 869-3495. 1989.

Toxic Shock Syndrome. Merlin S. Bergdoll, P. Joan Chesne. CRC Press, Inc., 2000 Corporate Blvd. N.W., Boca Raton, FL 33431. Phone: (407) 994-0555. Fax: (407) 997-0949. 1990.

Treatment Perspectives in Urologic Oncology. Richard D. Williams, Peter R. Carroll. Pergamon Press, 660 White Plains Rd., Tarrytown, NY 10591-5153. Phone: (914) 592-7700. Fax: (914) 592-3625. 1990.

Treatment of Prostatic Cancer-Facts and Controversies. Fritz H. Schroeder. John Wiley & Sons, Inc., 605 Third Ave., New York, NY 10158-0012. Phone: (212) 850-6000. Fax: (212) 850-6088. 1990.

Urological Oncology. Alderson Smith. John Wiley & Sons, Inc., 605 Third Ave., New York, NY 10158-0012. Phone: (212) 850-6000. Fax: (212) 850-6088. 1991.

PROSTATE DISORDERS

ABSTRACTING, INDEXING, AND CURRENT AWARENESS PUBLICATIONS

Current Contents/Clinical Medicine. Institute for Scientific Information, 3501 Market St., Philadelphia, PA 19104. Phone: (800) 523-1850. Fax: (215) 386-6362. Weekly.

Excerpta Medica. Section 28: Urology and Nephrology. Elsevier Science Publishing Co., Inc., P.O. Box 882, Madison Square Station, New York, NY 10159-2101. Phone: (212) 989-5800. Fax: (212) 633-3990. 20/year.

Index Medicus. U.S. National Library of Medicine, 8600 Rockville Pike, Bethesda, MD 20894. Phone: (800) 638-8480. Monthly.

Research Alert: Prostate Disease & Dysfunction. Institute for Scientific Information, 3501 Market St., Philadelphia, PA 19104. Phone: (800) 523-1850. Fax: (215) 386-6362. Weekly.

Science Citation Index. Institute for Scientific Information, 3501 Market St., Philadelphia, PA 19104. Phone: (800) 523-1850. Fax: (215) 386-6362. Bimonthly.

ANNUALS AND REVIEWS

Year Book of Urology. Mosby-Year Book, 11830 Westline Industrial Drive, St. Louis, MO 63146. Phone: (800) 325-4177. Fax: (314) 432-1380. Annual.

ASSOCIATIONS, PROFESSIONAL SOCIETIES, ADVOCACY AND SUPPORT GROUPS

American Board of Urology (ABU). 31700 Telegraph Rd., Ste. 150, Birmingham, MI 48010. Phone: (312) 646-9720.

American Urological Association (AUA). 1120 N. Charles St., Baltimore, MD 21201. Phone: (301) 727-1100. Fax: (301) 625-2390.

Prostate Health Council. c/o American Foundation for Urologic Disease, 1120 N. Charles St., No. 401, Baltimore, MD 21201. Phone: (800) 242-2383.

CD-ROM DATABASES

SCISEARCH. Institute for Scientific Information, 3501 Market St., Philadelphia, PA 19104. Phone: (215) 386-0100. Fax: (215) 386-6362.

DIRECTORIES

Directory of Certified Urologists. American Board of Medical Specialties, 1 Rotary Center, Suite 805, Evanston, IL 60201. Phone: (708) 491-9091. Biennial.

JOURNALS

British Journal of Urology. Churchill Livingstone Inc., 650 Avenue of the Americas, New York, NY 10011. Phone: (212) 819-5400. Fax: (212) 302-6598. Monthly.

Journal of Urology. Williams & Wilkins, 428 E. Preston St., Baltimore, MD 21202. Phone: (800) 638-0672. Fax: (800) 447-8438. Monthly.

The Prostate. John Wiley & Sons, Inc., 605 Third Ave., New York, NY 10158-0012. Phone: (212) 850-6000. Fax: (212) 850-6088. 8/year.

Urological Research. Springer-Verlag New York Inc., 175 Fifth Ave., New York, NY 10010. Phone: (212) 460-1500. Fax: (212) 473-6272.

ONLINE DATABASES

EMBASE. Elsevier Science Publishing Co., Inc., P.O. Box 882, Madison Square Station, New York, NY 10159-2101. Phone: (212) 989-5800. Fax: (212) 633-3990.

MEDLINE. National Library of Medicine, 8600 Rockville Pike, Bethesda, MD 20894. Phone: (800) 638-8480.

SciSearch. Institute for Scientific Information, 3501 Market St., Philadelphia, PA 19104. Phone: (215) 386-0100. Fax: (215) 386-6362.

POPULAR WORKS AND PATIENT EDUCATION

The Prostate Book: Sound Advice on Symptoms and Treatment. Stephen Rous. W.W. Norton & Co., Inc., 500 Fifth Ave., New York, NY 10110. Phone: (800) 223-2584. Updated edition 1992.

Prostate Problems and Their Treatment: Information and Advice for Sufferers. Jeremy Hamand. HarperCollins Pubs., Inc., 10 E. 53rd St., New York, NY 10022-5299. Phone: (212) 207-7000. Fax: (800) 242-7737. 1991.

RESEARCH CENTERS, INSTITUTES, CLEARINGHOUSES

National Kidney and Urologic Diseases Information Clearinghouse (NKUDIC). P.O. Box NKUDIC, 9000 Rockville Pike, Bethesda, MD 20892. Phone: (301) 468-6345.

TEXTBOOKS AND MONOGRAPHS

New Therapies for Benign Prostatic Hypertrophy (BPH)-Proceedings from the DATTA Forum. American Medical Association, 515 North State St., Chicago, IL 60610. Phone: (312) 464-0183. Fax: (312) 464-5834. 1992.

Practical Transurethral Resection. J.P. Blandy, Richard G. Notley. Butterworth-Heinemann, 80 Montvale Ave.,

Stoneham, MA 02180. Phone: (617) 438-8464. Fax: (617) 279-4851. 1991.

Prostate. John M. Fitzpatrick, Robert T. Kane (eds.). Churchill Livingstone Inc., 650 Ave. of the Americas, New York, NY 10011. Phone: (212) 819-5400. Fax: (212) 302-6598. 1989.

Prostate Biopsy Interpretation. Jonathan I. Epstein. Raven Press, 1185 Avenue of the Americas, New York, NY 10036. Phone: (212) 930-9500. Fax: (212) 869-3495. 1989.

Ultrasound of the Prostate. Bruno Fornage. John Wiley & Sons, Inc., 605 Third Ave., New York, NY 10158-0012. Phone: (212) 850-6000. Fax: (212) 850-6088. 1988.

Urologic Surgery. Glenn. J.B. Lippincott Co., 227 E. Washington Square, Philadelphia, PA 19106-3780. Phone: (215) 238-4200. Fax: (215) 238-4227. Fourth edition 1991.

PROSTATE ENLARGEMENT

See: PROSTATE DISORDERS

PROSTATE SURGERY

See: PROSTATE CANCER; PROSTATE DISORDERS

PROSTHESES

See also: BIOMEDICAL ENGINEERING; MEDICAL DEVICES AND INSTRUMENTATION; ORTHOPEDICS

ABSTRACTING, INDEXING, AND CURRENT AWARENESS PUBLICATIONS

Bioengineering and Biotechnology Abstracts. Engineering Information Inc., 345 E. 47th St., New York, NY 10017-2387. Phone: (800) 221-1044. Fax: (212) 832-1857.

Excerpta Medica. Section 19: Rehabilitation and Physical Medicine. Elsevier Science Publishing Co., Inc., P.O. Box 882, Madison Square Station, New York, NY 10159-2101. Phone: (212) 989-5800. Fax: (212) 633-3990. 8/year.

Excerpta Medica. Section 27: Biophysics, Bioengineering and Medical Instrumentation. Elsevier Science Publishing Co., Inc., P.O. Box 882, Madison Square Station, New York, NY 10159-2101. Phone: (212) 989-5800. Fax: (212) 633-3990. 10/year.

Index Medicus. U.S. National Library of Medicine, 8600 Rockville Pike, Bethesda, MD 20894. Phone: (800) 638-8480. Monthly.

ANNUALS AND REVIEWS

Year Book of Rehabilitation. Mosby-Year Book, 11830 Westline Industrial Drive, St. Louis, MO 63146. Phone: (800) 325-4177. Fax: (314) 432-1380. Annual.

ASSOCIATIONS, PROFESSIONAL SOCIETIES, ADVOCACY AND SUPPORT GROUPS

American Orthotic and Prosthetic Association. 717 Pendleton St., Alexandria, VA 22314.

CD-ROM DATABASES

Healthcare Product Comparison System. DIALOG Information Services, 3460 Hillview Ave., Palo Alto, CA 94304. Phone: (800) 334-2564. Fax: (415) 858-7069. Quarterly.

DIRECTORIES

Artificial Breasts Directory. American Business Directories, Inc., 5711 S. 86th Circle, Omaha, NE 68127. Phone: (402) 593-4600. Fax: (402) 331-1505. Annual.

Artificial Limbs Directory. American Business Directories, Inc., 5711 S. 86th Circle, Omaha, NE 68127. Phone: (402) 593-4600. Fax: (402) 331-1505. Annual.

Directory of Certified Orthopaedic Surgeons. American Board of Medical Specialties, 1 Rotary Center, Suite 805, Evanston, IL 60201. Phone: (708) 491-9091. Biennial.

Health Devices Sourcebook. Vivian H. Coates, Dorothy Woods (eds.). ECRI, 5200 Butler Pike, Plymouth Meeting, PA 19462. Phone: (215) 825-6000. 1990.

HANDBOOKS, GUIDES, MANUALS, ATLASES

A Colour Atlas of Contact Lenses. Montague Ruben. Appleton & Lange, 25 Van Zant St., East Norwalk, CT 06855. Phone: (800) 423-1359. Fax: (203) 854-9486. 2nd edition 1988.

JOURNALS

Artificial Organs. Raven Press, 1185 Avenue of the Americas, New York, NY 10036. Phone: (212) 930-9500. Fax: (212) 869-3495. Bimonthly.

Assistive Technology. Resna Press, 1101 Connecticut Ave. NW, Suite 700, Washington, DC 20036. Phone: (202) 857-1199. Quarterly.

Journal of Biomechanics. Pergamon Press, 660 White Plains Rd., Tarrytown, NY 10591-5153. Phone: (914) 592-7700. Fax: (914) 592-3625. Monthly.

Prosthetics and Orthotics International. International Society for Prosthetics and Orthotics, Borgervaenget 5, DK-2100 Copenhagen OE, Denmark.

ONLINE DATABASES

ABLEDATA. Newington Children's Hospital, Adaptive Equipment Center, 181 E. Cedar St., Newington, CT 06111. Phone: (800) 344-5405. Monthly.

EMBASE. Elsevier Science Publishing Co., Inc., P.O. Box 882, Madison Square Station, New York, NY 10159-2101. Phone: (212) 989-5800. Fax: (212) 633-3990.

MEDLINE. National Library of Medicine, 8600 Rockville Pike, Bethesda, MD 20894. Phone: (800) 638-8480.

SciSearch. Institute for Scientific Information, 3501 Market St., Philadelphia, PA 19104. Phone: (215) 386-0100. Fax: (215) 386-6362.

TEXTBOOKS AND MONOGRAPHS

Orthopaedic Rehabilitation. Vernon L. Nickel, Michael J. Botte (eds.). Churchill Livingstone Inc., 650 Avenue of the Americas, New York, NY 10011. Phone: (212) 819-5400. Fax: (212) 302-6598. Second edition 1991.

PROSTHODONTICS

See also: DENTISTRY

ABSTRACTING, INDEXING, AND CURRENT AWARENESS PUBLICATIONS

Dental Abstracts. Mosby-Year Book, 11830 Westline Industrial Drive, St. Louis, MO 63146. Phone: (800) 325-4177. Fax: (314) 432-1380. Bimonthly.

Index to Dental Literature. American Dental Association, 211 E. Chicago Ave., Chicago, IL 60611-2678. Phone: (800) 947-4746. Fax: (312) 440-3542. Quarterly.

Index Medicus. U.S. National Library of Medicine, 8600 Rockville Pike, Bethesda, MD 20894. Phone: (800) 638-8480. Monthly.

ANNUALS AND REVIEWS

Year Book of Dentistry. Mosby-Year Book, 11830 Westline Industrial Drive, St. Louis, MO 63146. Phone: (800) 325-4177. Fax: (314) 432-1380. Annual.

ASSOCIATIONS, PROFESSIONAL SOCIETIES, ADVOCACY AND SUPPORT GROUPS

American Academy of Crown and Bridge Prosthodontics (AACBP). 3302 Gaston Ave., Rm. 330, Dallas, TX 75246. Phone: (214) 828-8370.

American Academy of Implant Prosthodontics. 5555 Peachtree-Dunwoody Rd. N.E., No. 140, Atlanta, GA 30342. Phone: (404) 847-9200.

American Association of Oral and Maxillofacial Surgeons (AAOMS). 9700 W. Bryn Mawr, Rosemont, IL 60018. Phone: (800) 822-6637. Fax: (708) 678-6286.

American Board of Prosthodontics (ABP). P.O. Box 8437, Atlanta, GA 30306. Phone: (404) 876-2625.

American College of Prosthodontists (ACP). 1777 N.E. Loop 410, Ste. 904, San Antonio, TX 78217. Phone: (512) 829-7236.

American Dental Association (ADA). 211 E. Chicago Ave., Chicago, IL 60611. Phone: (312) 440-2500.

DIRECTORIES

American Dental Directory. American Dental Association, 211 E. Chicago Ave., Chicago, IL 60611-2678. Phone: (800) 947-4746. Fax: (312) 440-3542. Annual.

JOURNALS

Implant Dentistry. Williams & Wilkins, 428 E. Preston St., Baltimore, MD 21202. Phone: (800) 638-0672. Fax: (800) 447-8438. Quarterly.

International Journal of Oral Implantology. International Journal of Oral Implantology, Box 912, Upper Montclair, NJ 07043. Phone: (201) 783-6300.

International Journal of Oral and Maxillofacial Implants. Quintessence Publishing Co., 870 Oak Creek Dr., Lombard, IL 60148. Phone: (708) 620-4443. Quarterly.

International Journal of Prosthodontics. Quintessence Publising Co., 870 Oak Creek Dr., Lombard, IL 60148. Phone: (708) 620-4443.

Journal of Oral and Maxillofacial Surgery. W.B. Saunders Co., The Curtis Center, Independence Square W., Philadelphia, PA 19106-3399. Phone: (215) 238-7800. Monthly.

Journal of Prosthetic Dentistry. Mosby-Year Book, 11830 Westline Industrial Drive, St. Louis, MO 63146. Phone: (800) 325-4177. Fax: (314) 432-1380. Monthly.

NEWSLETTERS

Dental Implantology Update. American Health Consultants, Department C1290, P.O. Box 740060, Atlanta, GA 30374. Phone: (800) 559-1032. Monthly.

ONLINE DATABASES

EMBASE. Elsevier Science Publishing Co., Inc., P.O. Box 882, Madison Square Station, New York, NY 10159-2101. Phone: (212) 989-5800. Fax: (212) 633-3990.

MEDLINE. National Library of Medicine, 8600 Rockville Pike, Bethesda, MD 20894. Phone: (800) 638-8480.

SciSearch. Institute for Scientific Information, 3501 Market St., Philadelphia, PA 19104. Phone: (215) 386-0100. Fax: (215) 386-6362.

TEXTBOOKS AND MONOGRAPHS

Boucher's Prosthodontic Treatment for Edentulous Patients. George A. Zarb, Charles L. Bolender, Judson C. Hickey, et. al.. Mosby-Year Book, 11830 Westline Industrial Drive, St. Louis, MO 63146. Phone: (800) 325-4177. Fax: (314) 432-1380. Tenth edition 1990.

Clinical and Laboratory Procedures for Implant Prosthodontics. Edward J. Frederickson, Patrick J. Stevens, Maurice Gress. Mosby-Year Book, 11830 Westline Industrial Drive, St. Louis, MO 63146. Phone: (800) 325-4177. Fax: (314) 432-1380. 1992.

Dental Implants: Principles and Practice. Charles A. Babbush. W.B. Saunders Co., The Curtis Center, Independence Square W., Philadelphia, PA 19106-3399. Phone: (215) 238-7800. 1992.

Endosteal Dental Implants. Ralph V. McKinney. Mosby-Year Book, 11830 Westline Industrial Drive, St. Louis, MO 63146. Phone: (800) 325-4177. Fax: (314) 432-1380. 1991.

Implant Prosthodontics: Surgical and Prosthetic Techiques for Dental Implants. M.J. Fagan, and others. Mosby-Year Book, 11830 Westline Industrial Drive, St. Louis, MO 63146. Phone: (800) 325-4177. Fax: (314) 432-1380. 1990.

Removable Partial Prosthodontics. Joseph E. Grasso, Ernest L. Miller. Mosby-Year Book, 11830 Westline Industrial Drive, St. Louis, MO 63146. Phone: (800) 325-4177. Fax: (314) 432-1380. Third edition 1991.

PSORIASIS

See: DERMATOLOGIC DISEASES

PSRO (PROFESSIONAL STANDARDS REVIEW ORGANIZATION)

See: QUALITY ASSURANCE

PSYCHIATRIC DISORDERS

See also: DEPRESSION; MOOD DISORDERS; PERSONALITY DISORDERS; SCHIZOPHRENIA

ABSTRACTING, INDEXING, AND CURRENT AWARENESS PUBLICATIONS

Current Contents/Clinical Medicine. Institute for Scientific Information, 3501 Market St., Philadelphia, PA 19104. Phone: (800) 523-1850. Fax: (215) 386-6362. Weekly.

Digest of Neurology and Psychiatry. Institute of Living, 400 Washington St., Hartford, CT 06106. Phone: (203) 241-6824. Monthly.

Excerpta Medica. Section 32: Psychiatry. Elsevier Science Publishing Co., Inc., P.O. Box 882, Madison Square Station, New York, NY 10159-2101. Phone: (212) 989-5800. Fax: (212) 633-3990. 20/year.

Index Medicus. U.S. National Library of Medicine, 8600 Rockville Pike, Bethesda, MD 20894. Phone: (800) 638-8480. Monthly.

Psychological Abstracts. American Psychological Association, 1200 17th St. NW, Washington, DC 20036. Phone: (202) 955-7600. Monthly.

PSYSCAN: Clinical Psychology. American Psychological Association, 1200 17th St. NW, Washington, DC 20036. Phone: (202) 955-7600. Quarterly.

Research Alert: Lithium in Psychiatric Therapy. Institute for Scientific Information, 3501 Market St., Philadelphia, PA 19104. Phone: (800) 523-1850. Fax: (215) 386-6362. Weekly.

ANNUALS AND REVIEWS

Adolescent Psychiatry. American Society for Adolescent Psychiatry, 5530 Wisconsin Ave. N.W., Ste. 1149, Washington, DC 20015. Phone: (301) 652-0646. Annual.

Cambridge Medical Reviews: Neurobiology and Psychiatry. Cambridge University Press, 40 W. 20th St., New York, NY 10011. Phone: (800) 431-1580. Irregular.

Child and Adolescent Psychiatric Clinics of North America. W.B. Saunders Co., The Curtis Center, Independence Square W., Philadelphia, PA 19106-3399. Phone: (215) 238-7800. Quarterly.

Current Opinion in Psychiatry. Current Science Ltd., 20 N. Third St., Philadelphia, PA 19106-2199. Phone: (800) 552-5866. Fax: (215) 574-2270. Bimonthly.

Developments in Psychiatry. Elsevier Science Publishing Co., Inc., P.O. Box 882, Madison Square Station, New York, NY 10159-2101. Phone: (212) 989-5800. Fax: (212) 633-3990.

Progress in Psychiatry. American Psychiatric Press, Inc., 1400 K St. NW, Washington, DC 20005. Phone: (202) 682-6268. Fax: (202) 789-2648. Irregular.

Psychiatric Clinics. W.B. Saunders Co., The Curtis Center, Independence Square W., Philadelphia, PA 19106-3399. Phone: (215) 238-7800. Quarterly.

Wiley Series in Clinical Psychology. John Wiley & Sons, Inc., 605 Third Ave., New York, NY 10158-0012. Phone: (212) 850-6000. Fax: (212) 850-6088. Irregular.

Year Book of Psychiatry. Mosby-Year Book, 11830 Westline Industrial Drive, St. Louis, MO 63146. Phone: (800) 325-4177. Fax: (314) 432-1380. Annual.

ASSOCIATIONS, PROFESSIONAL SOCIETIES, ADVOCACY AND SUPPORT GROUPS

American Orthopsychiatric Association (ORTHO). 19 W. 44th St., No. 1616, New York, NY 10036. Phone: (212) 354-5770. Fax: (212) 302-9463.

American Psychiatric Association (APA). 1400 K St. N.W., Washington, DC 20005. Phone: (202) 682-6000. Fax: (202) 682-6114.

Canadian Psychiatric Association. 294 Albert St., Suite 204, Ottawa, ON, Canada K1P 6E6. Phone: (613) 234-2815. Fax: (613) 234-9857.

Canadian Psychological Association. Chemin Vincent, Old Chelsea, PQ, Canada J0X 2N0. Phone: (819) 827-3927. Fax: (819) 827-4639.

National Alliance for the Mentally Ill (NAMI). 2101 Wilson Blvd., Ste. 302, Arlington, VA 22201. Phone: (703) 524-7600. Fax: (703) 524-9094.

National Association of Private Psychiatric Hospitals (NAPPH). 1319 F St. N.W., Ste. 1000, Washington, DC 20004. Phone: (202) 393-6700. Fax: (202) 783-6041.

National Mental Health Association (NMHA). 1021 Prince St., Alexandria, VA 22314-2971. Phone: (703) 684-7722. Fax: (703) 684-5968.

Obsessive Compulsive Disorder Foundation (OCDF). P.O. Box 9573, New Haven, CT 06535. Phone: (203) 772-0565. Fax: (203) 498-8476.

BIBLIOGRAPHIES

National Alliance for the Mentally Ill-Annotated Reading List. National Alliance for the Mentally Ill, 2101 Wilson Blvd., Ste. 302, Arlington, VA 22201. Phone: (703) 524-7600. Fax: (703) 524-9094. Irregular.

CD-ROM DATABASES

Excerpta Medica CD: Psychiatry. SilverPlatter Information, Inc., River Ridge Office Park, 100 River Ridge Rd., Norwood, MA 02062. Phone: (617) 769-2599. Fax: (617) 769-8763. Quarterly.

PC MASS-Psychiatry. Educational Reviews, Inc., 6801 Cahaba Valley Rd., Birmingham, AL 35242. Phone: (800) 633-4743. Fax: (205) 995-1926. Monthly.

PsycLit. SilverPlatter Information, Inc., River Ridge Office Park, 100 River Ridge Rd., Norwood, MA 02062. Phone: (617) 769-2599. Fax: (617) 769-8763. Quarterly.

Year Books on Disc. CMC ReSearch, Inc., 7150 S.W. Hampton, Suite C-120, Portland, OR 97223. Phone: (800) 262-7668. Fax: (503) 639-1796. Annual includes Year Books of Cardiology, Dermatology, Diagnostic Radiology, Drug Therapy, Emergency Medicine, Family Practice, Medicine, Neurology and Neurosurgery, Obstetrics and Gynecology, Oncology, Pediatrics, and Psychiatry and Applied Mental Health.

DIRECTORIES

American Group Psychotherapy Association-Membership Directory. American Group Psychotherapy Association, 25 E. 21st St., 6th Flr., New York, NY 10010. Phone: (212) 477-2677. Biennial.

Directory of Certified Psychiatrists. American Board of Medical Specialties, 1 Rotary Center, Suite 805, Evanston, IL 60201. Phone: (708) 491-9091. Biennial.

ENCYCLOPEDIAS, DICTIONARIES, WORD BOOKS

Psychiatric Dictionary. Robert Jean Campbell. Oxford University Press, 200 Madison Ave., New York, NY 10016. Phone: (212) 679-7300. 1989.

Psychiatry Words. Stedman. Williams & Wilkins, 428 East Preston St., Baltimore, MD 21202. Phone: (800) 638-0672. Fax: (800) 447-8438. 1992.

HANDBOOKS, GUIDES, MANUALS, ATLASES

Concise Guide to Psychodynamic Psychotherapy. Robert J. Ursana, Stephen M. Sonnenberg, Susan Lazar. American Psychiatric Press, Inc., 1400 K St. NW, Washington, DC 20005. Phone: (202) 682-6268. Fax: (202) 789-2648. 1991.

Diagnostic and Statistical Manual of Mental Disorders, Third Edition, Revised. American Psychiatric Association, 1400 K St. N.W., Washington, DC 20005. Phone: (202) 682-6000. Fax: (202) 682-6114. 1987.

Getting Help: A Consumer's Guide to Therapy. Christine Amner. Paragon House Publishers, 90 Fifth Ave., New York, NY 10011. Phone: (800) 727-2466. 1991.

Manual of Clinical Problems in Psychiatry: With Annotated Key References. Steven E. Hyman, Michael Jenike (eds.). Little, Brown and Company, 34 Beacon St., Boston, MA 02108. Phone: (617) 227-0730. 1990.

Manual of Psychiatric Emergencies. Steven E. Hyman (ed.). Little, Brown and Co., 34 Beacon St., Boston, MA 02108. Phone: (617) 227-0730. Fax: (617) 227-0790. Second edition 1988.

JOURNALS

American Journal of Orthopsychiatry. American Orthopsychiatric Association, Inc., 19 W. 44th St., New York, NY 10036. Phone: (212) 354-5770. Fax: (212) 302-9463. Quarterly.

Archives of General Psychiatry. American Medical Association, 515 North State St., Chicago, IL 60610. Phone: (312) 464-0183. Fax: (312) 464-5834. Monthly.

Bulletin of the Menninger Clinic: A Journal for the Mental Health Professions. The Menninger Clinic, Box 829, Topeka, KS 66601-0829. Phone: (913) 273-7500. Fax: (913) 273-8625. Quarterly.

Harvard Review of Psychiatry. Mosby-Year Book, 11830 Westline Industrial Drive, St. Louis, MO 63146. Phone: (800) 325-4177. Fax: (314) 432-1380. Bimonthly.

Journal of Abnormal Psychology. American Psychological Association, 1200 17th St. NW, Washington, DC 20036. Phone: (202) 955-7600. Quarterly.

Journal of Affective Disorders. Elsevier Science Publishing Co., Inc., P.O. Box 882, Madison Square Station, New York, NY 10159-2101. Phone: (212) 989-5800. Fax: (212) 633-3990. 12/year.

Journal of the American Academy of Child and Adolescent Psychiatry. Williams & Wilkins, 428 East Preston St., Baltimore, MD 21202. Phone: (800) 638-0672. Fax: (800) 447-8438.

Journal of Consulting and Clinical Psychology. American Psychological Association, 1200 17th St. NW, Washington, DC 20036. Phone: (202) 955-7600. Bimonthly.

Journal of Nervous and Mental Disease. Williams & Wilkins, 428 E. Preston St., Baltimore, MD 21202. Phone: (800) 638-0672. Fax: (800) 447-8438. Monthly.

Journal of Psychotherapy Practice and Research. American Psychiatric Press, Inc., 1400 K St. NW, Washington, DC 20005. Phone: (202) 682-6268. Fax: (202) 789-2648. Quarterly.

Psychiatric Annals. SLACK Inc., 6900 Grove Rd., Thorofare, NJ 08086-9447. Phone: (800) 257-8290. Fax: (609) 853-5991.

Psychiatric Genetics. Rapid Communications of Oxford Ltd., The Old Malthouse, Paradise St., Oxford OX1 1LD, England. Phone: 44-865-790447. Fax: 44-865-244012. 4/year.

Psychological Medicine. Cambridge University Press, 40 W. 20th St., New York, NY 10011. Phone: (800) 431-1580. Quarterly.

NEWSLETTERS

Harvard Mental Health Letter. Harvard Medical School Publications Group, 164 Longwood Ave., Boston, MA 02115. Monthly.

ONLINE DATABASES

EMBASE. Elsevier Science Publishing Co., Inc., P.O. Box 882, Madison Square Station, New York, NY 10159-2101. Phone: (212) 989-5800. Fax: (212) 633-3990.

MEDLINE. National Library of Medicine, 8600 Rockville Pike, Bethesda, MD 20894. Phone: (800) 638-8480.

Mental Health Abstracts. IFI/Plenum Data Company, 302 Swann Ave., Alexandria, VA 22301. Phone: (800) 368-3093. Monthly.

PsycInfo. SilverPlatter Information, Inc., River Ridge Office Park, 100 River Ridge Rd., Norwood, MA 02062. Phone: (617) 769-2599. Fax: (617) 769-8763. Quarterly.

SciSearch. Institute for Scientific Information, 3501 Market St., Philadelphia, PA 19104. Phone: (215) 386-0100. Fax: (215) 386-6362.

POPULAR WORKS AND PATIENT EDUCATION

The Boy Who Couldn't Stop Washing: The Experience and Treatment of Obsessive-Compulsive Disorder. Judith L. Rapoport. Viking Penguin, 375 Hudson St., New York, NY 10014-3657. Phone: (800) 331-4624. 1990.

The Columbia University College of Physicians and Surgeons Complete Home Guide to Mental and Emotional Health. Frederic I. Kass, John M. Oldham, Herbert Pardes, and others. Holt, Rinehart & Winston, 115 W. 18th St., New York, NY 10011. Phone: (800) 488-5233. 1992.

The Consumer's Guide to Psychotherapy. Louis J. Rosner, Shelley Ross. Simon & Schuster, Inc., 1230 Ave. of the Americas, New York, NY 10020. Phone: (212) 698-7000. 1992.

Family Mental Health Encyclopedia. Frank Bruno. John Wiley & Sons, Inc., 605 Third Ave., New York, NY 10158-0012. Phone: (212) 850-6000. Fax: (212) 850-6088. 1991.

Getting Control: Overcoming Your Obsessions and Compulsions. Lee Baer. Little, Brown and Co., 34 Beacon St., Boston, MA 02108. Phone: (617) 227-0730. 1991.

In Confidence: Four Years of Therapy. Roberta Israeloff. Viking Penguin, 375 Hudson St., New York, NY 10014-3657. Phone: (800) 331-4624. 1991.

Know Your Own Mind: The Comprehensive One-Volume Home Reference Guide to Mental Health. Jane Knowles. HarperCollins Pubs., Inc., 10 E. 53rd St., New York, NY 10022-5299. Phone: (212) 207-7000. 1992.

Psychotherapy Today: A Consumer's Guide to Choosing the Right Therapist. Ronald W. Pies. Skidmore-Roth Publishing, 1001 Wall St., El Paso, TX 79915-1012. Phone: (800) 825-3150. 1991.

Stop Obsessing! How to Control Your Obsessions and Compulsions. Edna Foa. Bantam Books, Inc., 666 Fifth Ave., New York, NY 10103. Phone: (800) 223-6834. 1991.

RESEARCH CENTERS, INSTITUTES, CLEARINGHOUSES

Clarke Institute of Psychiatry. 250 College St., Toronto, ON, Canada M5T 1R8. Phone: (416) 979-0940. Fax: (416) 979-7871.

Eastern Pennsylvania Psychiatric Institute. Medical College of Pennsylvania. 3200 Henry Ave., Philadelphia, PA 19129. Phone: (215) 842-4000. Fax: (215) 843-7384.

Hogg Foundation for Mental Health. University of Texas. Austin, TX 78713-7998. Phone: (512) 471-5041. Fax: (512) 471-9608.

Institute for Mental Health Research. State University of New York at Stony Brook. Dept. of Psychiatry and Behavioral Science, Stony Brook, NY 11794. Phone: (516) 444-2990. Fax: (516) 444-7534.

Institute for Psychosomatic and Psychiatric Research and Training. Humana Hospital Michael Reese, Lake Shore Dr. at 31st St., Chicago, IL 60616. Phone: (312) 791-3877. Fax: (312) 567-7440.

Langley Porter Psychiatric Institute. University of California, San Francisco. 401 Parnassus Ave., San Francisco, CA 94143. Phone: (415) 476-7000.

Menninger Clinic Department of Research. Box 829, Topeka, KS 66601. Phone: (913) 273-7500. Fax: (913) 273-8625.

Missouri Institute of Mental Health. University of Missouri-Columbia. 5247 Fyler Ave., St. Louis, MO 63139-1494. Phone: (314) 644-8787. Fax: (314) 644-8834.

National Clearinghouse on Family Support and Children's Mental Health. Portland State University, P.O. Box 751, Portland, OR 97202-0751. Phone: (800) 628-1696.

National Institute of Mental Health (NIMH). 5600 Fishers Ln., Room 15C-05, Rockville, MD 20857. Phone: (301) 443-4513.

National Resource Center on Homelessness and Mental Illness. 262 Delaware Ave., Delmar, NY 12054. Phone: (800) 444-7415.

Western Psychiatric Institute and Clinic. University of Pittsburgh. 3811 O'Hara St., Pittsburgh, PA 15213. Phone: (412) 624-2360. Fax: (412) 624-1881.

STANDARDS AND STATISTICS SOURCES

Mental Illness in Nursing Homes: United States, 1985. National Center for Health Statistics, 6525 Belcrest Rd., Rm. 1064, Hyattsville, MD 20782. Phone: (301) 436-8500. PHS 91-1766 1991.

Psychiatric Length of Stay. HCIA Inc., P.O. Box 303, Ann Arbor, MI 48106-0303. Annual.

TEXTBOOKS AND MONOGRAPHS

The Art of Psychotherapy. Anthony Storr. Butterworth-Heinemann, 80 Montvale Ave., Stoneham, MA 02180. Phone: (617) 438-8464. Fax: (617) 279-4851. Second edition 1991.

Clinical Aspects of Panic Disorder. James C. Ballenger (ed.). John Wiley & Sons, Inc., 605 Third Ave., New York, NY 10158-0012. Phone: (212) 850-6000. Fax: (212) 850-6088. 1990.

Comprehensive Textbook of Psychiatry. Kaplan. Williams & Wilkins, 428 East Preston St., Baltimore, MD 21202. Phone: (800) 638-0672. Fax: (800) 447-8438. Fifth edition. Two volumes. 1989.

Current Treatments of Obsessive-Compulsive Disorder. Michele Tortora Pato, Joseph Zohar (eds.). American Psychiatric Press, Inc., 1400 K St. NW, Washington, DC 20005. Phone: (202) 682-6268. Fax: (202) 789-2648. 1991.

Dynamic Psychotherapy: An Introductory Approach. Marc H. Hollender, Charles V. Ford. American Psychiatric Press, Inc., 1400 K St. NW, Washington, DC 20005. Phone: (202) 682-6268. Fax: (202) 789-2648. 1990.

Integrating Pharmacotherapy & Psychotherapy. Bernard D. Beitman, Gerald L. Klerman (eds.). American Psychiatric Press, Inc., 1400 K St. NW, Washington, DC 20005. Phone: (202) 682-6268. Fax: (202) 789-2648. 1991.

Mental Health and Illness. R. Kosky, H. Eshkevari, V.J. Carr. Butterworth-Heinemann, 80 Montvale Ave., Stoneham, MA 02180. Phone: (617) 438-8464. Fax: (617) 279-4851. 1991.

Obsessive Compulsive Disorder. S.A. Montgomery (ed.). Rapid Communications of Oxford Ltd., The Old Malthouse, Paradise St., Oxford OX1 1LD, England. Phone: 44-865-790447. Fax: 44-865-244012. 1992.

Obsessive Compulsive Disorders: Theory and Management. M.A. Jenike, L. Baer, W.E. Minichiello. Mosby-Year Book, 11830 Westline Industrial Drive, St. Louis, MO 63146. Phone: (800) 325-4177. Fax: (314) 432-1380. Second edition 1990.

The Practice of Behavioural and Cognitive Psychotherapy. Richard Stern, Lynne M. Drummond. Cambridge University Press, 40 W. 20th St., New York, NY 10011. Phone: (800) 431-1580. 1992.

Psychiatric Disorders in America. L.N. Robins, D.A. Regier. Macmillan Publishing Co., 866 Third Ave., New York, NY 10011. Phone: (800) 257-5755. 1991.

Psychiatry. Waldinger. American Psychiatric Press, Inc., 1400 K St. N.W., Washington, DC 20005. Phone: (202) 682-6268. Fax: (202) 789-2648. Second edition 1990.

Psychobiology of Obsessive-Compulsive Disorder. J. Zohar, T.R. Insel, S. Rasmussen. Springer Publishing Co., Inc., 536 Broadway, 11th Fl., New York, NY 10012. Phone: (212) 431-4370. 1991.

Psychotherapy for the 1990s. J. Scott Rutan (ed.). Guilford Publications, Inc., 72 Spring St., New York, NY 10012. Phone: (800) 365-7006. Fax: (212) 966-6708. 1992.

Treatments of Psychiatric Disorders: A Task Force Report of the American Psychiatric Association. T. Byram Karasu. American Psychiatric Press, Inc., 1400 K St. NW, Washington, DC 20005. Phone: (202) 682-6268. Fax: (202) 789-2648. Four volumes 1989.

PSYCHIATRY

See also: PSYCHOANALYSIS; PSYCHOSOMATIC MEDICINE

ABSTRACTING, INDEXING, AND CURRENT AWARENESS PUBLICATIONS

Digest of Neurology and Psychiatry. Institute of Living, 400 Washington St., Hartford, CT 06106. Phone: (203) 241-6824. Monthly.

Excerpta Medica. Section 32: Psychiatry. Elsevier Science Publishing Co., Inc., P.O. Box 882, Madison Square Station, New York, NY 10159-2101. Phone: (212) 989-5800. Fax: (212) 633-3990. 20/year.

Index Medicus. U.S. National Library of Medicine, 8600 Rockville Pike, Bethesda, MD 20894. Phone: (800) 638-8480. Monthly.

Science Citation Index. Institute for Scientific Information, 3501 Market St., Philadelphia, PA 19104. Phone: (800) 523-1850. Fax: (215) 386-6362. Bimonthly.

ANNUALS AND REVIEWS

Adolescent Psychiatry. American Society for Adolescent Psychiatry, 5530 Wisconsin Ave. N.W., Ste. 1149, Washington, DC 20015. Phone: (301) 652-0646. Annual.

American Psychiatric Press Review of Psychiatry. American Psychiatric Press, Inc., 1400 K St. NW, Washington, DC 20005. Phone: (202) 682-6268. Fax: (202) 789-2648. Annual.

Cambridge Medical Reviews: Neurobiology and Psychiatry. Cambridge University Press, 40 W. 20th St., New York, NY 10011. Phone: (800) 431-1580. Irregular.

Contemporary Psychiatry. Plenum Publishing Co., 233 Spring St., New York, NY 10013-1578. Phone: (212) 620-8000. Fax: (212) 463-0742. Quarterly.

Current Opinion in Psychiatry. Current Science Ltd., 20 N. Third St., Philadelphia, PA 19106-2199. Phone: (800) 552-5866. Fax: (215) 574-2270. Bimonthly.

Developments in Psychiatry. Elsevier Science Publishing Co., Inc., P.O. Box 882, Madison Square Station, New York, NY 10159-2101. Phone: (212) 989-5800. Fax: (212) 633-3990.

Progress in Psychiatry. American Psychiatric Press, Inc., 1400 K St. NW, Washington, DC 20005. Phone: (202) 682-6268. Fax: (202) 789-2648. Irregular.

Psychiatric Clinics. W.B. Saunders Co., The Curtis Center, Independence Square W., Philadelphia, PA 19106-3399. Phone: (215) 238-7800. Quarterly.

Year Book of Psychiatry. Mosby-Year Book, 11830 Westline Industrial Drive, St. Louis, MO 63146. Phone: (800) 325-4177. Fax: (314) 432-1380. Annual.

ASSOCIATIONS, PROFESSIONAL SOCIETIES, ADVOCACY AND SUPPORT GROUPS

American Association of Geriatric Psychiatrists. P.O. Box 376A, Greenbelt, MD 20768. Phone: (301) 220-0952.

American Board of Psychiatry and Neurology (ABPN). 500 Lake Cook Rd., Ste. 335, Deerfield, IL 60015. Phone: (708) 945-7900.

American College of Psychiatrists. P.O. Box 365, Greenbelt, MD 20770. Phone: (301) 345-3534.

American Orthopsychiatric Association (ORTHO). 19 W. 44th St., No. 1616, New York, NY 10036. Phone: (212) 354-5770. Fax: (212) 302-9463.

American Psychiatric Association (APA). 1400 K St. N.W., Washington, DC 20005. Phone: (202) 682-6000. Fax: (202) 682-6114.

Canadian Psychiatric Association. 294 Albert St., Suite 204, Ottawa, ON, Canada K1P 6E6. Phone: (613) 234-2815. Fax: (613) 234-9857.

CD-ROM DATABASES

Excerpta Medica CD: Psychiatry. SilverPlatter Information, Inc., River Ridge Office Park, 100 River Ridge Rd., Norwood, MA 02062. Phone: (617) 769-2599. Fax: (617) 769-8763. Quarterly.

PC MASS-Psychiatry. Educational Reviews, Inc., 6801 Cahaba Valley Rd., Birmingham, AL 35242. Phone: (800) 633-4743. Fax: (205) 995-1926. Monthly.

SCISEARCH. Institute for Scientific Information, 3501 Market St., Philadelphia, PA 19104. Phone: (215) 386-0100. Fax: (215) 386-6362.

Year Books on Disc. CMC ReSearch, Inc., 7150 S.W. Hampton, Suite C-120, Portland, OR 97223. Phone: (800) 262-7668. Fax: (503) 639-1796. Annual includes Year Books of Cardiology, Dermatology, Diagnostic Radiology, Drug Therapy, Emergency Medicine, Family Practice, Medicine, Neurology and Neurosurgery, Obstetrics and Gynecology, Oncology, Pediatrics, and Psychiatry and Applied Mental Health.

DIRECTORIES

American Psychiatric Association Biographical Directory. American Psychiatric Press, Inc., 1400 K St. NW, Washington, DC 20005. Phone: (202) 682-6268. Fax: (202) 789-2648. Irregular.

Directory of Certified Psychiatrists. American Board of Medical Specialties, 1 Rotary Center, Suite 805, Evanston, IL 60201. Phone: (708) 491-9091. Biennial.

Directory of Medical Specialists. Marquis Who's Who, 3002 Glenview Rd., Wilmette, IL 60091. Phone: (800) 621-9669. Fax: (708) 441-2264. Biennial.

Directory of Physicians in the United States. American Medical Association, 515 North State St., Chicago, IL 60610. Phone: (312) 464-0183. Fax: (312) 464-5834. Biennial.

ENCYCLOPEDIAS, DICTIONARIES, WORD BOOKS

Comprehensive Glossary of Psychiatry and Psychology. Harold I. Kaplan, Benjamin J. Saddock. Williams & Wilkins, 428 E. Preston St., Baltimore, MD 21202. Phone: (800) 638-0672. Fax: (800) 447-8438. 1991.

Neurologic and Psychiatric Word Book. Helen E. Littrell. Springhouse Publishing Co., 1111 Bethlehem Pike, Spring House, PA 19477. Phone: (800) 331-3170. Fax: (215) 646-8716. 1992.

Psychiatric Dictionary. Robert Jean Campbell. Oxford University Press, 200 Madison Ave., New York, NY 10016. Phone: (212) 679-7300. 1989.

Psychiatry Words. Stedman. Williams & Wilkins, 428 East Preston St., Baltimore, MD 21202. Phone: (800) 638-0672. Fax: (800) 447-8438. 1992.

HANDBOOKS, GUIDES, MANUALS, ATLASES

Handbook of Psychiatry. Guze. Mosby-Year Book, 11830 Westline Industrial Drive, St. Louis, MO 63146. Phone: (800) 325-4177. Fax: (314) 432-1380. 1990.

Handbook of Studies on General Hospital Psychiatry. F.K. Judd, G.D. Burrows, D.R. Lipsitt (eds.). Elsevier Science Publishing Co., Inc., P.O. Box 882, Madison Square Station, New York, NY 10159-2101. Phone: (212) 989-5800. Fax: (212) 633-3990. 1991.

Pocket Reference for Psychiatrists. Susan C. Jenkins, Timothy P. Gibbs, Sally R. Szymanski. American Psychiatric Press, Inc., 1400 K St. NW, Washington, DC 20005. Phone: (202) 682-6268. Fax: (202) 789-2648. 1990.

Psychiatry: Diagnosis and Therapy. Joseph A. Flaherty, John Davis, Philip Janicak. Appleton & Lange, 25 Van Zant St., East Norwalk, CT 06855. Phone: (800) 423-1359. Fax: (203) 854-9486. Second edition September 1991.

JOURNALS

Academic Psychiatry. American Psychiatric Press, Inc., 1400 K St. NW, Washington, DC 20005. Phone: (202) 682-6268. Fax: (202) 789-2648. Quarterly.

American Journal of Geriatric Psychiatry. American Psychiatric Press, Inc., 1400 K St. NW, Washington, DC 20005. Phone: (202) 682-6268. Fax: (202) 789-2648. Quarterly.

American Journal of Orthopsychiatry. American Orthopsychiatry Association, Inc., 19 W. 44th St., New York, NY 10036. Phone: (212) 354-5770. Fax: (212) 302-9463. Quarterly.

American Journal of Psychiatry. American Psychiatric Press, Inc., 1400 K St. NW, Washington, DC 20005. Phone: (202) 682-6268. Fax: (202) 789-2648. Monthly.

Annals of Clinical Psychiatry. Elsevier Science Publishing Co., Inc., P.O. Box 882, Madison Square Station, New York, NY 10159-2101. Phone: (212) 989-5800. Fax: (212) 633-3990. 4/year.

Archives of General Psychiatry. American Medical Association, 515 North State St., Chicago, IL 60610. Phone: (312) 464-0183. Fax: (312) 464-5834. Monthly.

Arts in Psychotherapy. Pergamon Press, 660 White Plains Rd., Tarrytown, NY 10591-5153. Phone: (914) 592-7700. Fax: (914) 592-3625.

Biological Psychiatry. Elsevier Science Publishing Co., Inc., P.O. Box 882, Madison Square Station, New York, NY 10159-2101. Phone: (212) 989-5800. Fax: (212) 633-3990. 24/year.

British Journal of Psychiatry. Royal Society of Medicine Services Ltd., 1 Wimpole St., London W1M 8AE, England. Phone: 071-408 2119. Fax: 071-355 3198. Monthly.

European Psychiatry. Elsevier Science Publishing Co., Inc., P.O. Box 882, Madison Square Station, New York, NY 10159-2101. Phone: (212) 989-5800. Fax: (212) 633-3990. 6/year.

General Hospital Psychiatry. Elsevier Science Publishing Co., Inc., P.O. Box 882, Madison Square Station, New York, NY 10159-2101. Phone: (212) 989-5800. Fax: (212) 633-3990. 6/year.

Hospital and Community Psychiatry. American Psychiatric Press, Inc., 1400 K St. NW, Washington, DC 20005. Phone: (202) 682-6268. Fax: (202) 789-2648. Monthly.

Journal of Affective Disorders. Elsevier Science Publishing Co., Inc., P.O. Box 882, Madison Square Station, New York, NY 10159-2101. Phone: (212) 989-5800. Fax: (212) 633-3990. 12/year.

Journal of the American Academy of Child and Adolescent Psychiatry. Williams & Wilkins, 428 East Preston St., Baltimore, MD 21202. Phone: (800) 638-0672. Fax: (800) 447-8438.

Journal of Clinical Psychiatry. Physicians Postgraduate Press, Box 240008, Memphis, TN 38124. Phone: (901) 682-1001.

Journal of Nervous and Mental Disease. Williams & Wilkins, 428 E. Preston St., Baltimore, MD 21202. Phone: (800) 638-0672. Fax: (800) 447-8438. Monthly.

Journal of Psychiatric Research. Pergamon Press, 660 White Plains Rd., Tarrytown, NY 10591-5153. Phone: (914) 592-7700. Fax: (914) 592-3625.

Psychiatric Bulletin of the Royal College of Physicians. Royal Society of Medicine Services Ltd., 1 Wimpole St., London W1M 8AE, England. Phone: 071-408 2119. Fax: 071-355 3198. Monthly.

ONLINE DATABASES

EMBASE. Elsevier Science Publishing Co., Inc., P.O. Box 882, Madison Square Station, New York, NY 10159-2101. Phone: (212) 989-5800. Fax: (212) 633-3990.

MEDLINE. National Library of Medicine, 8600 Rockville Pike, Bethesda, MD 20894. Phone: (800) 638-8480.

Mental Health Abstracts. IFI/Plenum Data Company, 302 Swann Ave., Alexandria, VA 22301. Phone: (800) 368-3093. Monthly.

PsycInfo. SilverPlatter Information, Inc., River Ridge Office Park, 100 River Ridge Rd., Norwood, MA 02062. Phone: (617) 769-2599. Fax: (617) 769-8763. Quarterly.

SciSearch. Institute for Scientific Information, 3501 Market St., Philadelphia, PA 19104. Phone: (215) 386-0100. Fax: (215) 386-6362.

RESEARCH CENTERS, INSTITUTES, CLEARINGHOUSES

Clarke Institute of Psychiatry. 250 College St., Toronto, ON, Canada M5T 1R8. Phone: (416) 979-0940. Fax: (416) 979-7871.

Institute for Psychosomatic and Psychiatric Research and Training. Humana Hospital Michael Reese, Lake Shore Dr. at 31st St., Chicago, IL 60616. Phone: (312) 791-3877. Fax: (312) 567-7440.

TEXTBOOKS AND MONOGRAPHS

Comprehensive Textbook of Psychiatry. Kaplan. Williams & Wilkins, 428 East Preston St., Baltimore, MD 21202. Phone: (800) 638-0672. Fax: (800) 447-8438. Fifth edition. Two volumes. 1989.

Introductory Textbook of Psychiatry. Nancy C. Andreasen, Donald W. Black. American Psychiatric Press, Inc., 1400 K St. NW, Washington, DC 20005. Phone: (202) 682-6268. Fax: (202) 789-2648. 1991.

Mental Health and Illness. R. Kosky, H. Eshkevari, V.J. Carr. Butterworth-Heinemann, 80 Montvale Ave., Stoneham, MA 02180. Phone: (617) 438-8464. Fax: (617) 279-4851. 1991.

Oxford Textbook of Psychiatry. Michael Gelder, and others. Oxford University Press, 200 Madison Ave., New York, NY 10016. Phone: (212) 679-7300. 2nd edition, 1989.

Postgraduate Psychiatry. D. Forshaw, Louis Appleby. Butterworth-Heinemann, 80 Montvale Ave., Stoneham, MA 02180. Phone: (617) 438-8464. Fax: (617) 279-4851. 1990.

Psychiatric Ethics. Sidney Bloch, Paul Chodoff (eds.). Oxford University Press, 200 Madison Ave., New York, NY 10016. Phone: (212) 679-7300. Second edition 1991.

Psychiatry for Medical Students. Robert J. Waldinger. American Psychiatric Press, Inc., 1400 K St. NW,

Washington, DC 20005. Phone: (202) 682-6268. Fax: (202) 789-2648. Second edition 1991.

Reflections on Modern Psychiatry. David J. Kupfer (ed.). American Psychiatric Press, Inc., 1400 K St. NW, Washington, DC 20005. Phone: (202) 682-6268. Fax: (202) 789-2648. 1992.

Review of General Psychiatry. Howard H. Goldman. Appleton & Lange, 25 Van Zant St., East Norwalk, CT 06855. Phone: (800) 423-1359. Fax: (203) 854-9486. Second edition 1988.

PSYCHOACTIVE DRUGS

See also: DRUGS

ABSTRACTING, INDEXING, AND CURRENT AWARENESS PUBLICATIONS

Current Contents/Life Sciences. Institute for Scientific Information, 3501 Market St., Philadelphia, PA 19104. Phone: (215) 386-0100. Fax: (215) 386-6362.

Index Medicus. U.S. National Library of Medicine, 8600 Rockville Pike, Bethesda, MD 20894. Phone: (800) 638-8480. Monthly.

Psychological Abstracts. American Psychological Association, 1200 17th St. NW, Washington, DC 20036. Phone: (202) 955-7600. Monthly.

Research Alert: Antidepressants. Institute for Scientific Information, 3501 Market St., Philadelphia, PA 19104. Phone: (800) 523-1850. Fax: (215) 386-6362. Weekly.

Research Alert: Lithium in Psychiatric Therapy. Institute for Scientific Information, 3501 Market St., Philadelphia, PA 19104. Phone: (800) 523-1850. Fax: (215) 386-6362. Weekly.

CD-ROM DATABASES

1993 PDR Library on CD-ROM. Medical Economics, Five Paragon Dr., Montvale, NJ 07645-1742. Phone: (800) 232-7379. Fax: (201) 573-4956. 1993.

PC MASS-Psychiatry. Educational Reviews, Inc., 6801 Cahaba Valley Rd., Birmingham, AL 35242. Phone: (800) 633-4743. Fax: (205) 995-1926. Monthly.

PDR on CD-ROM. Medical Economics, Five Paragon Dr., Montvale, NJ 07645-1742. Phone: (800) 222-3045. Fax: (201) 573-4956. 3/year.

PsycLit. SilverPlatter Information, Inc., River Ridge Office Park, 100 River Ridge Rd., Norwood, MA 02062. Phone: (617) 769-2599. Fax: (617) 769-8763. Quarterly.

ENCYCLOPEDIAS, DICTIONARIES, WORD BOOKS

Psychiatric Dictionary. Robert Jean Campbell. Oxford University Press, 200 Madison Ave., New York, NY 10016. Phone: (212) 679-7300. 1989.

HANDBOOKS, GUIDES, MANUALS, ATLASES

Handbook of Drug Therapy in Psychiatry. Bernstein. Mosby-Year Book, 11830 Westline Industrial Drive, St. Louis, MO 63146. Phone: (800) 325-4177. Fax: (314) 432-1380. Second edition 1988.

Handbook of Psychiatric Drug Therapy. George W. Arana, Steven E. Hyman. Little, Brown and Company, 34 Beacon St., Boston, MA 02108. Phone: (617) 227-0730. Second edition 1991.

Handbook of Psychiatric Drugs. Bernard Salzman. Holt, Rinehart & Winston, 115 W. 18th St., New York, NY 10011. Phone: (800) 488-5233. 1991.

Handbook of Psychotropic Drugs. Springhouse Publishing Co., 1111 Bethlehem Pike, Spring House, PA 19477. Phone: (800) 331-3170. Fax: (215) 646-8716. 1992.

The Practitioner's Guide to Pscyhoactive Drugs. Alan J. Gelenberg, Ellen L. Bassuk, Stephen C. Schoonover. Plenum Publishing Co., 233 Spring St., New York, NY 10013-1578. Phone: (212) 620-8000. Fax: (212) 463-0742. Third edition 1991.

JOURNALS

Journal of Clinical Psychiatry. Physicians Postgraduate Press, Box 240008, Memphis, TN 38124. Phone: (901) 682-1001.

Journal of Clinical Psychopharmacology. Williams & Wilkins, 428 E. Preston St., Baltimore, MD 21202. Phone: (800) 638-0672. Fax: (800) 447-8438. Bimonthly.

ONLINE DATABASES

EMBASE. Elsevier Science Publishing Co., Inc., P.O. Box 882, Madison Square Station, New York, NY 10159-2101. Phone: (212) 989-5800. Fax: (212) 633-3990.

Lithium Index. Center. University of Wisconsin-Madison, Dept. of Psychiatry, Lithium Information Center, 600 Highland Ave., Madison, WI 53792. Phone: (608) 263-6171. Irregular.

Lithium Library. Center. University of Wisconsin-Madison, Dept. of Psychiatry, Lithium Information Center, 600 Highland Ave., Madison, WI 53792. Phone: (608) 263-6171. Irregular.

MEDLINE. National Library of Medicine, 8600 Rockville Pike, Bethesda, MD 20894. Phone: (800) 638-8480.

Mental Health Abstracts. IFI/Plenum Data Company, 302 Swann Ave., Alexandria, VA 22301. Phone: (800) 368-3093. Monthly.

PsycInfo. SilverPlatter Information, Inc., River Ridge Office Park, 100 River Ridge Rd., Norwood, MA 02062. Phone: (617) 769-2599. Fax: (617) 769-8763. Quarterly.

SciSearch. Institute for Scientific Information, 3501 Market St., Philadelphia, PA 19104. Phone: (215) 386-0100. Fax: (215) 386-6362.

POPULAR WORKS AND PATIENT EDUCATION

The Essential Guide to Psychiatric Drugs. Jack M. Gorman. St. Martin's Press, 175 Fifth Ave., New York, NY 10010. Phone: (212) 674-5151. 1991.

Over-50 Guide to Psychiatric Medications. Gary S. Moak, Elliot M. Stein, E.V. Rubin. American Psychiatric Press, Inc., 1400 K St. N.W., Washington, DC 20005. Phone: (202) 682-6268. Fax: (202) 789-2648. 1989.

What You Need to Know About Psychiatric Drugs. Stuart C. Yudofsky, Robert E. Hales, Tom Ferguson. American Psychiatric Press, Inc., 1400 K St. NW, Washington, DC 20005. Phone: (202) 682-6268. Fax: (202) 789-2648. 1991.

TEXTBOOKS AND MONOGRAPHS

Antidepressants: Thirty Years On. B. Leonard, P.S.J. Spencer (eds.). Rapid Communications of Oxford Ltd., The Old Malthouse, Paradise St., Oxford OX1 1LD, England. Phone: 44-865-790447. Fax: 44-865-244012. 1992.

The Anxiolytic Jungle: Where Next?. David Wheatley (ed.). John Wiley & Sons, Inc., 605 Third Ave., New York, NY 10158-0012. Phone: (212) 850-6000. Fax: (212) 850-6088. 1990.

Benzodiazepines in Clinical Practice: Risks and Benfits. Peter Roy-Byrne, Deborah S. Cowley. American Psychiatric Press, Inc., 1400 K St. NW, Washington, DC 20005. Phone: (202) 682-6268. Fax: (202) 789-2648. 1991.

Clinical Pharmacology of Psychotherapeutic Drugs. Leo E. Hollister, John Csernansky. Churchill Livingstone Inc., 650 Avenue of the Americas, New York, NY 10011. Phone: (212) 819-5400. Fax: (212) 302-6598. Third edition 1990.

Comprehensive Textbook of Psychiatry. Kaplan. Williams & Wilkins, 428 East Preston St., Baltimore, MD 21202. Phone: (800) 638-0672. Fax: (800) 447-8438. Fifth edition. Two volumes. 1989.

Psychopharmacology: An Introduction. R. Spiegel. John Wiley & Sons, Inc., 605 Third Ave., New York, NY 10158-0012. Phone: (212) 850-6000. Fax: (212) 850-6088. Second edition 1989.

Psychopharmacology: The Third Generation of Progress. Herbert Y. Meltzer. Raven Press, 1185 Avenue of the Americas, New York, NY 10036. Phone: (212) 930-9500. Fax: (212) 869-3495. 1987.

PSYCHOANALYSIS

See also: PSYCHIATRY

ABSTRACTING, INDEXING, AND CURRENT AWARENESS PUBLICATIONS

Chicago Psychoanalytic Literature Index. Chicago Institute for Psychoanalysis, 180 N. Michigan, Chicago, IL 60601. Phone: (312) 726-6300.

Excerpta Medica. Section 32: Psychiatry. Elsevier Science Publishing Co., Inc., P.O. Box 882, Madison Square Station, New York, NY 10159-2101. Phone: (212) 989-5800. Fax: (212) 633-3990. 20/year.

Index Medicus. U.S. National Library of Medicine, 8600 Rockville Pike, Bethesda, MD 20894. Phone: (800) 638-8480. Monthly.

Psychological Abstracts. American Psychological Association, 1200 17th St. NW, Washington, DC 20036. Phone: (202) 955-7600. Monthly.

PSYSCAN: Psychoanalysis. American Psychological Association, 1200 17th St. NW, Washington, DC 20036. Phone: (202) 955-7600. Quarterly.

ANNUALS AND REVIEWS

Year Book of Psychiatry. Mosby-Year Book, 11830 Westline Industrial Drive, St. Louis, MO 63146. Phone: (800) 325-4177. Fax: (314) 432-1380. Annual.

ASSOCIATIONS, PROFESSIONAL SOCIETIES, ADVOCACY AND SUPPORT GROUPS

American Academy of Psychoanalysis (AAP). 30 E. 40th St., Ste. 206, New York, NY 10016. Phone: (212) 679-4105. Fax: (212) 679-4106.

American College of Psychoanalysts. c/o Harold Mann M.D., 2006 Dwight Way, No. 304, Berkeley, CA 94704. Phone: (415) 845-7957.

American Foundation for Psychoanalysis and Psychoanalysis in Groups. c/o Louis E. DeRosis M.D., 40 E. 89th St., New York, NY 10028. Phone: (212) 348-3500.

American Psychoanalytic Association (APsaA). 309 E. 49th St., New York, NY 10022. Phone: (212) 752-0450.

Association for Advancement of Psychoanalysis. 329 E. 62nd St., New York, NY 10021. Phone: (212) 751-2724.

Canadian Psychiatric Association. 294 Albert St., Suite 204, Ottawa, ON, Canada K1P 6E6. Phone: (613) 234-2815. Fax: (613) 234-9857.

Karen Horney Clinic (KHC). 329 E. 62nd St., New York, NY 10021. Phone: (212) 838-4333. Fax: (212) 838-7158.

CD-ROM DATABASES

PC MASS-Psychiatry. Educational Reviews, Inc., 6801 Cahaba Valley Rd., Birmingham, AL 35242. Phone: (800) 633-4743. Fax: (205) 995-1926. Monthly.

PsycLit. SilverPlatter Information, Inc., River Ridge Office Park, 100 River Ridge Rd., Norwood, MA 02062. Phone: (617) 769-2599. Fax: (617) 769-8763. Quarterly.

DIRECTORIES

American Academy of Psychoanalysis-Membership Roster. American Academy of Psychoanalysis, 30 E. 40th St., Ste. 206, New York, NY 10016. Phone: (212) 679-4105. Fax: (212) 679-4106.

ENCYCLOPEDIAS, DICTIONARIES, WORD BOOKS

Psychiatric Dictionary. Robert Jean Campbell. Oxford University Press, 200 Madison Ave., New York, NY 10016. Phone: (212) 679-7300. 1989.

Psychiatry Words. Stedman. Williams & Wilkins, 428 East Preston St., Baltimore, MD 21202. Phone: (800) 638-0672. Fax: (800) 447-8438. 1992.

JOURNALS

American Journal of Psychoanalysis. Plenum Publishing Co., 233 Spring St., New York, NY 10013-1578. Phone: (212) 620-800. Fax: (212) 463-0742.

Arts in Psychotherapy. Pergamon Press, 660 White Plains Rd., Tarrytown, NY 10591-5153. Phone: (914) 592-7700. Fax: (914) 592-3625.

International Journal of Psychoanalysis. Routledge, Chapman & Hall, Inc., 29 W. 35th St., New York, NY 10001-2291. Phone: (212) 244-3336.

International Review of Psychoanalysis. Routledge, Chapman & Hall, Inc., 29 W. 35th St., New York, NY 10001-2291. Phone: (212) 244-3336.

Psychoanalytic Quarterly. Psychoanalytic Quarterly, 175 Fifth Ave., New York, NY 10010. Phone: (212) 982-9358.

Psychoanalytic Review. Guilford Publications, Inc., 72 Spring St., New York, NY 10012. Phone: (800) 365-7006. Fax: (212) 366-6708.

NEWSLETTERS

The American Psychoanalyst-Newsletter. American Psychoanalytic Association, 309 E. 49th St., New York, NY 10022. Phone: (212) 752-0450. Quarterly.

ONLINE DATABASES

EMBASE. Elsevier Science Publishing Co., Inc., P.O. Box 882, Madison Square Station, New York, NY 10159-2101. Phone: (212) 989-5800. Fax: (212) 633-3990.

MEDLINE. National Library of Medicine, 8600 Rockville Pike, Bethesda, MD 20894. Phone: (800) 638-8480.

Mental Health Abstracts. IFI/Plenum Data Company, 302 Swann Ave., Alexandria, VA 22301. Phone: (800) 368-3093. Monthly.

PsycInfo. SilverPlatter Information, Inc., River Ridge Office Park, 100 River Ridge Rd., Norwood, MA 02062. Phone: (617) 769-2599. Fax: (617) 769-8763. Quarterly.

SciSearch. Institute for Scientific Information, 3501 Market St., Philadelphia, PA 19104. Phone: (215) 386-0100. Fax: (215) 386-6362.

RESEARCH CENTERS, INSTITUTES, CLEARINGHOUSES

Center for Psychoanalytic Training and Research. Columbia University. 722 W. 168th St., New York, NY 10032. Phone: (212) 927-5000.

Institute for Psychoanalysis. 180 N. Michigan Ave., Chicago, IL 60601. Phone: (312) 726-6300.

TEXTBOOKS AND MONOGRAPHS

Comprehensive Textbook of Psychiatry. Kaplan. Williams & Wilkins, 428 East Preston St., Baltimore, MD 21202. Phone: (800) 638-0672. Fax: (800) 447-8438. Fifth edition. Two volumes. 1989.

PSYCHOLOGICAL TESTING

See also: PSYCHOLOGY

ABSTRACTING, INDEXING, AND CURRENT AWARENESS PUBLICATIONS

General Science Index. H.W. Wilson Co., 950 University Ave., Bronx, NY 10452. Phone: (800) 367-6770.

Psychological Abstracts. American Psychological Association, 1200 17th St. NW, Washington, DC 20036. Phone: (202) 955-7600. Monthly.

ANNUALS AND REVIEWS

Mental Measurements Yearbook. Buros Institute of Mental Measurements, 135 Bancroft, University of Nebraska, Lincoln, NE 68588. Phone: (402) 472-6203.

CD-ROM DATABASES

PsycLit. SilverPlatter Information, Inc., River Ridge Office Park, 100 River Ridge Rd., Norwood, MA 02062. Phone: (617) 769-2599. Fax: (617) 769-8763. Quarterly.

HANDBOOKS, GUIDES, MANUALS, ATLASES

Handbook of Psychological Assessment. Gerald Goldstein, Michael Hersen. Pergamon Press, 660 White Plains Rd., Tarrytown, NY 10591-5153. Phone: (914) 592-7700. Fax: (914) 592-3625. 1990.

Psychware Sourcebook. Samuel King (ed.). Gale Research, Inc., 835 Penobscot Bldg., Detroit, MI 48226-4094. Phone: (800) 877-GALE. Fax: (313) 961-6083. 3rd edition, 1989.

Test Critiques. Daniel Keyser, Richard Sweetland. Gale Research, Inc., 835 Penobscot Bldg., Detroit, MI 48226-4094. Phone: (800) 877-4253. Fax: (313) 961-6083. 1992.

Tests. Richard Sweetland, Daniel Keyser. Gale Research, Inc., 835 Penobscot Bldg., Detroit, MI 48226-4094. Phone: (800) 877-4253. Fax: (313) 961-6083. 3rd edition, 1990.

ONLINE DATABASES

PsycInfo. SilverPlatter Information, Inc., River Ridge Office Park, 100 River Ridge Rd., Norwood, MA 02062. Phone: (617) 769-2599. Fax: (617) 769-8763. Quarterly.

TEXTBOOKS AND MONOGRAPHS

The Rorschach: A Comprehensive System. Volume 1: Basic Foundations. John E. Exner Jr.. John Wiley & Sons, Inc., 605 Third Ave., New York, NY 10158-0012. Phone: (212) 850-6000. Fax: (212) 850-6088. Second edition 1986.

The Rorschach: A Comprehensive System. Volume 2: Interpretation. John E. Exner Jr.. John Wiley & Sons, Inc., 605 Third Ave., New York, NY 10158-0012. Phone: (212) 850-6000. Fax: (212) 850-6088. Second edition 1991.

The Rorschach: A Comprehensive System. Volume 3: Assessment of Children and Adolescents. John E. Exner Jr., Irving B. Weiner. John Wiley & Sons, Inc., 605 Third Ave., New York, NY 10158-0012. Phone: (212) 850-6000. Fax: (212) 850-6088. 1982.

PSYCHOLOGY

See also: FAMILY THERAPY; MARITAL THERAPY; PSYCHOLOGICAL TESTING

ABSTRACTING, INDEXING, AND CURRENT AWARENESS PUBLICATIONS

Psychological Abstracts. American Psychological Association, 1200 17th St. NW, Washington, DC 20036. Phone: (202) 955-7600. Monthly.

PSYSCAN: Applied Psychology. American Psychological Association, 1200 17th St. NW, Washington, DC 20036. Phone: (202) 955-7600. Quarterly.

PSYSCAN: Clinical Psychology. American Psychological Association, 1200 17th St. NW, Washington, DC 20036. Phone: (202) 955-7600. Quarterly.

PSYSCAN: Developmental Psychology. American Psychological Association, 1200 17th St. NW, Washington, DC 20036. Phone: (202) 955-7600. Quarterly.

Science Citation Index. Institute for Scientific Information, 3501 Market St., Philadelphia, PA 19104. Phone: (800) 523-1850. Fax: (215) 386-6362. Bimonthly.

ANNUALS AND REVIEWS

Annual Review of Psychology. Annual Reviews Inc., 4139 El Camino Way, P.O. Box 10139, Palo Alto, CA 94303-0897. Phone: (415) 493-4400. Fax: (415) 855-9815. Annual.

Contemporary Psychology. American Psychological Association, 1200 17th St. NW, Washington, DC 20036. Phone: (202) 955-7600. Monthly.

Current Directions in Psychological Science. Cambridge University Press, 40 W. 20th St., New York, NY 10011. Phone: (800) 431-1580. Bimonthly.

Wiley Series in Clinical Psychology. John Wiley & Sons, Inc., 605 Third Ave., New York, NY 10158-0012. Phone: (212) 850-6000. Fax: (212) 850-6088. Irregular.

ASSOCIATIONS, PROFESSIONAL SOCIETIES, ADVOCACY AND SUPPORT GROUPS

American Board of Professional Psychology. 2100 E. Broadway, No. 313, Columbia, MO 65201. Phone: (314) 875-1267.

American Psychological Association (APA). 1200 17th St. N.W., Washington, DC 20036. Phone: (202) 955-7600. Fax: (703) 525-5191.

Canadian Psychological Association. Chemin Vincent, Old Chelsea, PQ, Canada J0X 2N0. Phone: (819) 827-3927. Fax: (819) 827-4639.

C.G. Jung Foundation for Analytical Psychology. 28 E. 39th St., New York, NY 10016. Phone: (212) 697-6430.

Psychonomic Society (PS). c/o Dr. Cynthia H. Null, Dept. of Psychology, Coll. of William and Mary, Williamsburg, VA 23185. Phone: (804) 221-3882. Fax: (804) 221-3896.

CD-ROM DATABASES

PsycLit. SilverPlatter Information, Inc., River Ridge Office Park, 100 River Ridge Rd., Norwood, MA 02062. Phone: (617) 769-2599. Fax: (617) 769-8763. Quarterly.

SCISEARCH. Institute for Scientific Information, 3501 Market St., Philadelphia, PA 19104. Phone: (215) 386-0100. Fax: (215) 386-6362.

DIRECTORIES

American Board of Professional Psychology-Directory of Diplomates. American Board of Professional Psychology, 2100

E. Broadway, Ste. 313, Columbia, MO 65201. Phone: (314) 875-1267. Irregular.

American Psychological Association-Directory. American Psychological Association, 1200 17th St. N.W., Washington, DC 20036. Phone: (202) 955-7600. Fax: (703) 525-5191. Quadrennial.

ENCYCLOPEDIAS, DICTIONARIES, WORD BOOKS

Comprehensive Glossary of Psychiatry and Psychology. Harold I. Kaplan, Benjamin J. Saddock. Williams & Wilkins, 428 E. Preston St., Baltimore, MD 21202. Phone: (800) 638-0672. Fax: (800) 447-8438. 1991.

HANDBOOKS, GUIDES, MANUALS, ATLASES

Developmental Psychology. American Psychological Association, 1200 17th St. NW, Washington, DC 20036. Phone: (202) 955-7600. Bimonthly.

Psychological Bulletin. American Psychological Association, 1200 17th St. NW, Washington, DC 20036. Phone: (202) 955-7600. Bimonthly.

JOURNALS

American Journal of Orthopsychiatry. American Orthopsychiatric Association, Inc., 19 W. 44th St., New York, NY 10036. Phone: (212) 354-5770. Fax: (212) 302-9463. Quarterly.

American Psychologist. American Psychological Association, 1200 17th St. NW, Washington, DC 20036. Phone: (202) 955-7600. Monthly.

Applied and Preventive Psychology: Current Scientific Perspectives. Cambridge University Press, 40 W. 20th St., New York, NY 10011. Phone: (800) 431-1580. Quarterly.

Journal of Abnormal Psychology. American Psychological Association, 1200 17th St. NW, Washington, DC 20036. Phone: (202) 955-7600. Quarterly.

Journal of Clinical Psychology. Clinical Psychology Publishing Co., 4 Corant Sq., Brandon, VT 05733. Phone: (802) 247-6871.

Journal of Consulting and Clinical Psychology. American Psychological Association, 1200 17th St. NW, Washington, DC 20036. Phone: (202) 955-7600. Bimonthly.

Journal of Personality and Social Psychology. American Psychological Association, 1200 17th St. NW, Washington, DC 20036. Phone: (202) 955-7600. Monthly.

Journal of Psychotherapy Practice and Research. American Psychiatric Press, Inc., 1400 K St. NW, Washington, DC 20005. Phone: (202) 682-6268. Fax: (202) 789-2648. Quarterly.

Journal of Social and Clinical Psychology. Guilford Publications, Inc., 72 Spring St., New York, NY 10012. Phone: (800) 365-7006. Fax: (212) 366-6708. Quarterly.

Psychological Science. Cambridge University Press, 40 W. 20th St., New York, NY 10011. Phone: (800) 431-1580. Quarterly.

NEWSLETTERS

APA Monitor. American Psychological Association, 1200 17th St. NW, Washington, DC 20036. Phone: (202) 955-7600. Monthly.

ONLINE DATABASES

Mental Health Abstracts. IFI/Plenum Data Company, 302 Swann Ave., Alexandria, VA 22301. Phone: (800) 368-3093. Monthly.

PsycInfo. SilverPlatter Information, Inc., River Ridge Office Park, 100 River Ridge Rd., Norwood, MA 02062. Phone: (617) 769-2599. Fax: (617) 769-8763. Quarterly.

RESEARCH CENTERS, INSTITUTES, CLEARINGHOUSES

Psychological Consultation Center. Arizona State University, Tempe, AZ 85287. Phone: (602) 965-7296.

Psychological Research Center. Fairleigh Dickinson University, 139 Temple Ave., Hackensack, NJ 07601. Phone: (201) 692-2645.

Psychology Clinic. University of Alabama, Box 6142, Tuscaloosa, AL 35487. Phone: (205) 348-5000.

TEXTBOOKS AND MONOGRAPHS

Mental Health and Illness. R. Kosky, H. Eshkevari, V.J. Carr. Butterworth-Heinemann, 80 Montvale Ave., Stoneham, MA 02180. Phone: (617) 438-8464. Fax: (617) 279-4851. 1991.

PSYCHOPHARMACOLOGY

See also: DRUGS

ABSTRACTING, INDEXING, AND CURRENT AWARENESS PUBLICATIONS

Current Contents/Life Sciences. Institute for Scientific Information, 3501 Market St., Philadelphia, PA 19104. Phone: (215) 386-0100. Fax: (215) 386-6362.

Index Medicus. U.S. National Library of Medicine, 8600 Rockville Pike, Bethesda, MD 20894. Phone: (800) 638-8480. Monthly.

International Pharmaceutical Abstracts. American Society of Hospital Pharmacists, 4630 Montgomery Ave., Bethesda, MD 20814. Phone: (301) 657-3000. Fax: (301) 657-1641. Semimonthly.

Psychological Abstracts. American Psychological Association, 1200 17th St. NW, Washington, DC 20036. Phone: (202) 955-7600. Monthly.

Research Alert: Psychopharmacology. Institute for Scientific Information, 3501 Market St., Philadelphia, PA 19104. Phone: (800) 523-1850. Fax: (215) 386-6362. Weekly.

Science Citation Index. Institute for Scientific Information, 3501 Market St., Philadelphia, PA 19104. Phone: (800) 523-1850. Fax: (215) 386-6362. Bimonthly.

ANNUALS AND REVIEWS

Advances in Biochemical Psychopharmacology. Raven Press, 1185 Ave. of the Americas, New York, NY 10036. Phone: (212) 930-9500. Fax: (212) 869-3495. Irregular.

Progress in Neuro-Psychopharmacology and Biological Psychiatry. Pergamon Press, 660 White Plains Rd., Tarrytown, NY 10591-5153. Phone: (914) 592-7700. Fax: (914) 592-3625. 6/year.

ASSOCIATIONS, PROFESSIONAL SOCIETIES, ADVOCACY AND SUPPORT GROUPS

American College of Neuropsychopharmacology. Box 1823, Station B., Vanderbilt University, Nashville, TN 37235. Phone: (615) 327-7200.

CD-ROM DATABASES

PsycLit. SilverPlatter Information, Inc., River Ridge Office Park, 100 River Ridge Rd., Norwood, MA 02062. Phone: (617) 769-2599. Fax: (617) 769-8763. Quarterly.

SCISEARCH. Institute for Scientific Information, 3501 Market St., Philadelphia, PA 19104. Phone: (215) 386-0100. Fax: (215) 386-6362.

ENCYCLOPEDIAS, DICTIONARIES, WORD BOOKS

Merck Index: An Encyclopedia of Chemicals and Drugs. Merck & Co., Inc., P.O. Box 2000, Rahway, NJ 07065. Phone: (201) 855-4558. Irregular.

HANDBOOKS, GUIDES, MANUALS, ATLASES

Clinical Primer of Psychopharmacology: A Practical Guide. Donald M. Pirodsky, Jerry S. Cohn. McGraw-Hill, Inc., Health Professions Division, 1221 Avenue of the Americas, 28th Floor, New York, NY 10020. Phone: (212) 512-4228. Second edition 1992.

Handbook of Psychotropic Drugs. Springhouse Publishing Co., 1111 Bethlehem Pike, Spring House, PA 19477. Phone: (800) 331-3170. Fax: (215) 646-8716. 1992.

Manual of Clinical Psychopharmacology. Alan F. Schatzberg, Jonathan O. Cole. American Psychiatric Press, Inc., 1400 K St. NW, Washington, DC 20005. Phone: (202) 682-6268. Fax: (202) 789-2648. Second edition 1991.

JOURNALS

Journal of Clinical Psychopharmacology. Williams & Wilkins, 428 E. Preston St., Baltimore, MD 21202. Phone: (800) 638-0672. Fax: (800) 447-8438. Bimonthly.

Neuropharacology. Pergamon Press, 660 White Plains Rd., Tarrytown, NY 10591-5153. Phone: (914) 592-7700. Fax: (914) 592-3625.

Neuropsychopharmacology. Elsevier Science Publishing Co., Inc., P.O. Box 882, Madison Square Station, New York, NY 10159-2101. Phone: (212) 989-5800. Fax: (212) 633-3990. 8/year.

Pharmacopsychiatry. Thieme Medical Publishers, Inc., 381 Park Ave. S., New York, NY 10016. Phone: (212) 683-5088. Fax: (212) 779-9020.

Psychopharmacology. Springer-Verlag New York Inc., 175 Fifth Ave., New York, NY 10010. Phone: (212) 460-1500. Fax: (212) 473-6272.

Psychopharmacology Bulletin. U.S. Alcohol, Drug Abuse & Mental Health Administration, 5600 Fishers Lane, Rockville, MD 20852. Phone: (301) 496-4000.

ONLINE DATABASES

EMBASE. Elsevier Science Publishing Co., Inc., P.O. Box 882, Madison Square Station, New York, NY 10159-2101. Phone: (212) 989-5800. Fax: (212) 633-3990.

International Pharmaceutical Abstracts. American Society of Hospital Pharmacists, 4630 Montgomery Ave., Bethesda, MD 20814. Phone: (301) 657-3000. Fax: (301) 657-1641. Monthly.

MEDLINE. National Library of Medicine, 8600 Rockville Pike, Bethesda, MD 20894. Phone: (800) 638-8480.

Mental Health Abstracts. IFI/Plenum Data Company, 302 Swann Ave., Alexandria, VA 22301. Phone: (800) 368-3093. Monthly.

PsycInfo. SilverPlatter Information, Inc., River Ridge Office Park, 100 River Ridge Rd., Norwood, MA 02062. Phone: (617) 769-2599. Fax: (617) 769-8763. Quarterly.

SciSearch. Institute for Scientific Information, 3501 Market St., Philadelphia, PA 19104. Phone: (215) 386-0100. Fax: (215) 386-6362.

RESEARCH CENTERS, INSTITUTES, CLEARINGHOUSES

Behavioral Pharmacology Research Unit. Johns Hopkins University. School of Medicine, Psychiatry Dept., Francis Scott Key Medical Center, 4940 Eastern Ave., Baltimore, MD 21224. Phone: (410) 550-0035. Fax: (410) 550-0030.

Center for Biomedical Research. University of Kansas. Smissman Research Laboratories, 2099 Constant Ave., Lawrence, KS 66046. Phone: (913) 864-5140.

Nathan S. Kline Institute for Psychiatric Research. Orangeburg, NY 10962. Phone: (914) 365-2000. Fax: (914) 359-7029.

New York State Psychiatric Institute. 722 W. 168th St., New York, NY 10032. Phone: (212) 960-2200. Fax: (212) 795-5886.

Psychopharmacology Research Unit. University of Pennsylvania. 3600 Markey St., Rm. 870, Philadelphia, PA 19104. Phone: (215) 898-4301. Fax: (215) 898-0509.

TEXTBOOKS AND MONOGRAPHS

Clinical Geriatric Psychopharmacology. Salzman. Williams & Wilkins, 428 East Preston St., Baltimore, MD 21202. Phone: (800) 638-0672. Fax: (800) 447-8438. Second edition 1992.

Extra Pharmacopeia. J. Reynolds, W. Martindale. Pharmaceutical Press, Rittenhouse Book Distributors, 511 Feheley Dr., King of Prussia, PA 19406. Phone: (800) 345-6425. 29th edition 1989.

Psychopharmacology: An Introduction. R. Spiegel. John Wiley & Sons, Inc., 605 Third Ave., New York, NY 10158-0012. Phone: (212) 850-6000. Fax: (212) 850-6088. Second edition 1989.

Psychopharmacology of Anxiolytics and Antidepressants. Sandra E. File (ed.). Pergamon Press, 660 White Plains Rd., Tarrytown, NY 10591-5153. Phone: (914) 592-7700. Fax: (914) 592-3625. 1992.

Psychopharmacology: The Third Generation of Progress. Herbert Y. Meltzer. Raven Press, 1185 Avenue of the Americas, New York, NY 10036. Phone: (212) 930-9500. Fax: (212) 869-3495. 1987.

Schizophrenia Research. Carol A. Tamminga, Charles S. Schulz. Raven Press, 1185 Ave. of the Americas, New York, NY 10036. Phone: (212) 930-9500. Fax: (212) 869-3495. 1991.

PSYCHOSES

See: PSYCHIATRIC DISORDERS

PSYCHOSOMATIC MEDICINE

See also: PSYCHIATRY

ABSTRACTING, INDEXING, AND CURRENT AWARENESS PUBLICATIONS

Chicago Psychoanalytic Literature Index. Chicago Institute for Psychoanalysis, 180 N. Michigan, Chicago, IL 60601. Phone: (312) 726-6300.

Excerpta Medica. Section 32: Psychiatry. Elsevier Science Publishing Co., Inc., P.O. Box 882, Madison Square Station, New York, NY 10159-2101. Phone: (212) 989-5800. Fax: (212) 633-3990. 20/year.

Index Medicus. U.S. National Library of Medicine, 8600 Rockville Pike, Bethesda, MD 20894. Phone: (800) 638-8480. Monthly.

Psychological Abstracts. American Psychological Association, 1200 17th St. NW, Washington, DC 20036. Phone: (202) 955-7600. Monthly.

ANNUALS AND REVIEWS

Progress in Psychiatry. American Psychiatric Press, Inc., 1400 K St. NW, Washington, DC 20005. Phone: (202) 682-6268. Fax: (202) 789-2648. Irregular.

Year Book of Psychiatry. Mosby-Year Book, 11830 Westline Industrial Drive, St. Louis, MO 63146. Phone: (800) 325-4177. Fax: (314) 432-1380. Annual.

ASSOCIATIONS, PROFESSIONAL SOCIETIES, ADVOCACY AND SUPPORT GROUPS

Academy of Psychosomatic Medicine (APM). 5824 N. Magnolia, Chicago, IL 60660. Phone: (312) 784-2025.

American Psychosomatic Society (APS). 6728 Old McLean Village Dr., Mc Lean, VA 22101. Phone: (703) 556-9222.

CD-ROM DATABASES

Excerpta Medica CD: Psychiatry. SilverPlatter Information, Inc., River Ridge Office Park, 100 River Ridge Rd., Norwood, MA 02062. Phone: (617) 769-2599. Fax: (617) 769-8763. Quarterly.

PsycLit. SilverPlatter Information, Inc., River Ridge Office Park, 100 River Ridge Rd., Norwood, MA 02062. Phone: (617) 769-2599. Fax: (617) 769-8763. Quarterly.

ENCYCLOPEDIAS, DICTIONARIES, WORD BOOKS

Psychiatric Dictionary. Robert Jean Campbell. Oxford University Press, 200 Madison Ave., New York, NY 10016. Phone: (212) 679-7300. 1989.

JOURNALS

Journal of Psychosomatic Research. Pergamon Press, 660 White Plains Rd., Tarrytown, NY 10591-5153. Phone: (914) 592-7700. Fax: (914) 592-3625.

Journal of Psychotherapy Practice and Research. American Psychiatric Press, Inc., 1400 K St. NW, Washington, DC 20005. Phone: (202) 682-6268. Fax: (202) 789-2648. Quarterly.

Psychosomatic Medicine. Williams & Wilkins, 428 E. Preston St., Baltimore, MD 21202. Phone: (800) 638-0672. Fax: (800) 447-8438. Bimonthly.

Psychosomatics: The Journal of Consultation Liaison Psychiatry. American Psychiatric Press, Inc., 1400 K St. NW, Washington, DC 20005. Phone: (202) 682-6268. Fax: (202) 789-2648. Quarterly.

Psychotherapy and Psychosomatics. S. Karger Publishers, Inc., 26 W. Avon Rd., P.O. Box 529, Farmington, CT 06085. Phone: (203) 675-7834. Fax: (203) 675-7302.

ONLINE DATABASES

EMBASE. Elsevier Science Publishing Co., Inc., P.O. Box 882, Madison Square Station, New York, NY 10159-2101. Phone: (212) 989-5800. Fax: (212) 633-3990.

MEDLINE. National Library of Medicine, 8600 Rockville Pike, Bethesda, MD 20894. Phone: (800) 638-8480.

Mental Health Abstracts. IFI/Plenum Data Company, 302 Swann Ave., Alexandria, VA 22301. Phone: (800) 368-3093. Monthly.

PsycInfo. SilverPlatter Information, Inc., River Ridge Office Park, 100 River Ridge Rd., Norwood, MA 02062. Phone: (617) 769-2599. Fax: (617) 769-8763. Quarterly.

SciSearch. Institute for Scientific Information, 3501 Market St., Philadelphia, PA 19104. Phone: (215) 386-0100. Fax: (215) 386-6362.

POPULAR WORKS AND PATIENT EDUCATION

The Columbia University College of Physicians and Surgeons Complete Home Guide to Mental and Emotional Health. Frederic I. Kass, John M. Oldham, Herbert Pardes, and others. Holt, Rinehart & Winston, 115 W. 18th St., New York, NY 10011. Phone: (800) 488-5233. 1992.

RESEARCH CENTERS, INSTITUTES, CLEARINGHOUSES

Institute for Psychosomatic and Psychiatric Research and Training. Humana Hospital Michael Reese, Lake Shore Dr. at 31st St., Chicago, IL 60616. Phone: (312) 791-3877. Fax: (312) 567-7440.

Psychosomatic Research Program. 450 Clarkson Ave., Box 1203, State University of New York, Brooklyn, NY 11203. Phone: (718) 270-2311.

TEXTBOOKS AND MONOGRAPHS

Comprehensive Textbook of Psychiatry. Kaplan. Williams & Wilkins, 428 East Preston St., Baltimore, MD 21202. Phone: (800) 638-0672. Fax: (800) 447-8438. Fifth edition. Two volumes. 1989.

PSYCHOTHERAPY

See: PSYCHIATRIC DISORDERS; PSYCHOLOGY; PSYCHOSOMATIC MEDICINE

PUBLIC HEALTH

See also: EPIDEMIOLOGY

ABSTRACTING, INDEXING, AND CURRENT AWARENESS PUBLICATIONS

American Statistics Index: A Comprehensive Guide and Index to the Statistical Publications of the United States Government. Congressional Information Service, 4520 East-West Hwy., Bethesda, MD 20814. Phone: (800) 639-8380. 1973-Present Monthly.

Excerpta Medica. Section 17: Public Health, Social Medicine and Epidemiology. Elsevier Science Publishing Co., Inc., P.O. Box 882, Madison Square Station, New York, NY 10159-2101. Phone: (212) 989-5800. Fax: (212) 633-3990. 24/year.

Index to Health Information. Congressional Information Service, 4520 East-West Hwy., Bethesda, MD 20814. Phone: (800) 639-8380. Quarterly.

Index Medicus. U.S. National Library of Medicine, 8600 Rockville Pike, Bethesda, MD 20894. Phone: (800) 638-8480. Monthly.

Science Citation Index. Institute for Scientific Information, 3501 Market St., Philadelphia, PA 19104. Phone: (800) 523-1850. Fax: (215) 386-6362. Bimonthly.

Statistical Reference Index. Congressional Information Service, 4520 East-West Hwy., Bethesda, MD 20814. Phone: (800) 639-8380. 1980-Present Monthly.

ANNUALS AND REVIEWS

Annual Review of Public Health. Annual Reviews Inc., 4139 El Camino Way, P.O. Box 10139, Palo Alto, CA 94303-0897. Phone: (415) 493-4400. Fax: (415) 855-9815. Annual.

Johns Hopkins Series in Contemporary Medicine and Public Health. Johns Hopkins University Press, 701 W. 40th St., Suite 275, Baltimore, MD 21211-2190. Phone: (800) 537-5487. Fax: (410) 516-6998. Irregular.

ASSOCIATIONS, PROFESSIONAL SOCIETIES, ADVOCACY AND SUPPORT GROUPS

American Public Health Association (APHA). 1015 15th St. N.W., Washington, DC 20005. Phone: (202) 789-5600. Fax: (202) 789-5661.

Association of Schools of Public Health (ASPH). 1015 15th St. N.W., Ste. 404, Washington, DC 20005. Phone: (202) 842-4668.

Canadian Public Health Association. 1565 Carling Ave., Suite 400, Ottawa, ON, Canada K1Z 8R1. Phone: (613) 725-3769. Fax: (613) 725-9826.

World Health Organization. Ave. Appia, CH-1211 Geneva 27, Switzerland.

BIBLIOGRAPHIES

Clearinghouse Bibliography on Health Indexes. National Center for Health Statistics, 6525 Belcrest Rd., Hyattsville, MD 20782. Phone: (301) 436-8500. Quarterly.

CD-ROM DATABASES

American Journal of Public Health. MEP, 124 Mt. Auburn St., Cambridge, MA 02138. Phone: (800) 342-1338. Fax: (617) 868-7738. Annual.

Health for All. CD Resources, Inc., 118 W. 74th St., Suite 2A, New York, NY 10023. Phone: (212) 580-2263. Fax: (212) 877-1276. Semiannual.

Morbidity Mortality Weekly Report. MEP, 124 Mt. Auburn St., Cambridge, MA 02138. Phone: (800) 342-1338. Fax: (617) 868-7738. Annual.

SCISEARCH. Institute for Scientific Information, 3501 Market St., Philadelphia, PA 19104. Phone: (215) 386-0100. Fax: (215) 386-6362.

Statistical Masterfile. Congressional Information Service, 4520 East-West Highway, Bethesda, MD 20814-3389. Phone: (800) 638-8380. Quarterly.

DIRECTORIES

American Association of Public Health Physicians-Membership Roster. American Association of Public Health Physicians, Department of Family Medicine and Practice, University of Wisconsin Medical School, 777 S. Mills Rd., Madison, WI 53715. Phone: (405) 271-4476. Annual.

Directory of Medical Specialists. Marquis Who's Who, 3002 Glenview Rd., Wilmette, IL 60091. Phone: (800) 621-9669. Fax: (708) 441-2264. Biennial.

Directory of Physicians in the United States. American Medical Association, 515 North State St., Chicago, IL 60610. Phone: (312) 464-0183. Fax: (312) 464-5834. Biennial.

National Health Directory. Aspen Publishers, Inc., 200 Orchard Ridge Dr., Gaithersburg, MD 20878. Phone: (301) 417-7500. Annual.

JOURNALS

American Journal of Epidemiology. Johns Hopkins University School of Hygiene and Public Health, 2007 E. Monument St., Baltimore, MD 21205. Phone: (301) 955-3441.

American Journal of Public Health. American Public Health Association, 1015 15th St. NW, Washington, DC 20005. Phone: (202) 789-5666. Monthly.

Bulletin of the World Health Organization. World Health Organization, Ave. Appia, CH-1211 Geneva 27, Switzerland. Bimonthly.

Epidemiological Bulletin. Pan American Health Organization, 525 23rd St., N.W., Washington, DC 20037. Phone: (202) 861-3200. Bimonthly.

Journal of Clinical Epidemiology. Pergamon Press, 660 White Plains Rd., Tarrytown, NY 10591-5153. Phone: (914) 592-7700. Fax: (914) 592-3625.

Journal of Epidemiology & Community Health. BMJ Publishing Group, BMA House, Tavistock Square, London WC1H 9JR, England. Phone: 071-383 6244/6638. Fax: 071-383 6662. 6/year.

Morbidity and Mortality Weekly Report. Massachusetts Medical Society, 1440 Main St., Waltham, MA 02154-1649. Phone: (617) 893-3800. Fax: (617) 893-0413. Weekly.

Public Health. Macmillan Publishing Co., 866 Third Ave., New York, NY 10011. Phone: (800) 257-5755.

World Health Statistics Quarterly. World Health Organization, Ave. Appia, CH-1211 Geneva 27, Switzerland. Quarterly.

NEWSLETTERS

Healthy People 2000: Statistical Notes. U.S. Dept. of Health and Human Services. U.S. Govt. Printing Office, Superintendent of Documents, Washington, DC 20402-9325. Phone: (202) 783-3238. Quarterly.

Morbidity and Mortality Weekly Report. Centers for Disease Control, 1600 Clifton Rd. N.E., Atlanta, GA 30333. Phone: (404) 488-4698.

ONLINE DATABASES

EMBASE. Elsevier Science Publishing Co., Inc., P.O. Box 882, Madison Square Station, New York, NY 10159-2101. Phone: (212) 989-5800. Fax: (212) 633-3990.

MEDLINE. National Library of Medicine, 8600 Rockville Pike, Bethesda, MD 20894. Phone: (800) 638-8480.

SciSearch. Institute for Scientific Information, 3501 Market St., Philadelphia, PA 19104. Phone: (215) 386-0100. Fax: (215) 386-6362.

RESEARCH CENTERS, INSTITUTES, CLEARINGHOUSES

California Public Health Foundation. 2001 Addison St., Ste. 210, Berkeley, CA 94704-1103. Phone: (415) 644-8200. Fax: (415) 644-9319.

Center for Public Health Studies. Portland State University. P.O. Box 751, Portland, OR 97207. Phone: (503) 725-3473. Fax: (503) 725-4882.

Division of Epidemiology. University of Minnesota. School of Public Health, 1300 S. Second St., Ste. 300, Minneapolis, MN 55454. Phone: (612) 624-1818. Fax: (612) 624-0315.

Public Health Research Institute. 455 First Ave., New York, NY 10016. Phone: (212) 578-0800. Fax: (212) 578-0804.

Research Triangle Institute. 3040 Cornwallis Rd., P.O. Box 12194, Research Triangle Park, NC 27709-2194. Phone: (919) 541-6000. Fax: (919) 541-7004.

Wadsworth Center for Laboratories and Research. New York State Dept. of Health, Empire State Plaza, Albany, NY 12201. Phone: (518) 474-7592. Fax: (518) 474-8590.

STANDARDS AND STATISTICS SOURCES

Public Health Reports. U.S. Government Printing Office, Superintendent of Documents, P.O. Box 371954, Pittsburgh, PA 15250-7954. Phone: (202) 783-3238. Fax: (202) 512-2250. Bimonthly, No. 717-021-00000-2.

Statistical Abstract of the United States. U.S. Government Printing Office, Superintendent of Documents, Washington, DC 20402. Phone: (202) 783-3238. Annual.

World Health Statistics Annual. World Health Organization, Ave. Appia, CH-1211 Geneva 27, Switzerland. Annual.

TEXTBOOKS AND MONOGRAPHS

Healthy People 2000: National Health Promotion and Disease Prevention Objectives. U.S. Dept. of Health and Human Services. U.S. Government Printing Office, Superintendent of Documents, P.O. Box 371954, Pittsburgh, PA 15250-7954. Phone: (202) 783-3238. Fax: (202) 512-2250. 1991.

Maxcy-Rosenau-Last Public Health and Preventive Medicine. J.M. Last (ed.). Appleton & Lange, 25 Van Zant St., East Norwalk, CT 06855. Phone: (800) 423-1359. Fax: (203) 854-9486. 13th edition, 1992.

Oxford Textbook of Public Health. Walter W. Holland, Sr., Roger Detels, George Knox (eds.). Oxford University Press, 200 Madison Ave., New York, NY 10016. Phone: (212) 679-7300. Second edition. Three volumes. 1991.

Practical Epidemiology. D.J.P. Barker, A.J. Hall. Churchill Livingstone Inc., 650 Ave. of the Americas, New York, NY 10011. Phone: (212) 819-5400. Fax: (212) 302-6598. Fourth edition 1991.

PULMONARY DISEASES

See: LUNG DISEASES

PULMONARY FUNCTION TESTS

See: LUNG DISEASES

PULMONARY HEART DISEASE

See: HEART DISEASES

PYELITIS

See: KIDNEY DISEASES

Q

QUACKERY

See: HEALTH CARE FRAUD AND
QUACKERY

QUALITY ASSURANCE

ABSTRACTING, INDEXING, AND CURRENT AWARENESS PUBLICATIONS

Cumulative Index to Nursing and Allied Health Literature. Glendale Adventist Medical Center, P.O. Box 871, Glendale, CA 91209. Phone: (818) 409-8005. Bimonthly.

Hospital Literature Index. American Hospital Association, 840 N. Lake Shore Dr., Chicago, IL 60611. Phone: (800) 242-2626. Fax: (312) 280-6015. Quarterly.

Index Medicus. U.S. National Library of Medicine, 8600 Rockville Pike, Bethesda, MD 20894. Phone: (800) 638-8480. Monthly.

MEDOC: Index to U.S. Government Publications in the Medical and Health Sciences. Spencer S. Eccles Health Sciences Library, University of Utah, Bldg. 589, Salt Lake City, UT 84112. Phone: (801) 581-5268. Quarterly.

ASSOCIATIONS, PROFESSIONAL SOCIETIES, ADVOCACY AND SUPPORT GROUPS

American Board of Quality Assurance and Utilization Review (ABQAUR). 1777 Tamiami Trail, Ste. 205, Box 12, Port Charlotte, FL 33948. Phone: (813) 743-2425. Fax: (813) 743-2009.

American College of Utilization Review Physicians (ACURP). 1531 S. Tamiami Trail, Ste. 703, Venice, FL 34292. Phone: (813) 497-3340. Fax: (813) 497-5573.

American Medical Peer Review Association (AMPRA). 810 First St. N.E., Ste. 410, Washington, DC 20002. Phone: (202) 371-5610.

National Association of Quality Assurance Professionals (NAQAP). 104 Wilmot, Ste. 201, Deerfield, IL 60015. Phone: (708) 940-8800. Fax: (708) 940-7218.

National Committee for Quality Assurance. 1129 20th St. N.W., No. 600, Washington, DC 20036. Phone: (202) 778-3273.

CD-ROM DATABASES

Health Planning & Administration/EBSCO-CD. EBSCO Publishing, P.O. Box 325, Topsfield, MA 01983. Phone: (800) 221-1826. Fax: (508) 887-3923. Quarterly.

HFCA --On CD-ROM. FD Inc., 600 New Hampshire Ave. NW, Suite 355, Washington, DC 20037. Phone: (800) 332-6623. Fax: (202) 337-0457. Monthly.

Nursing and Allied Health (CINAHL) on CD-ROM. CINAHL, 1509 Wilson Terrace, P.O. Box 871, Glendale, CA 91209-0871. Phone: (818) 409-8005.

HANDBOOKS, GUIDES, MANUALS, ATLASES

The Key to Integrated Quality Management: Improving Nursing Care Quality. Koch. Mosby-Year Book, 11830 Westline Industrial Drive, St. Louis, MO 63146. Phone: (800) 325-4177. Fax: (314) 432-1380. 1992.

JOURNALS

Quality Assurance in Health Care. Pergamon Press, 660 White Plains Rd., Tarrytown, NY 10591-5153. Phone: (914) 592-7700. Fax: (914) 592-3625.

Quality in Health Care. BMJ Publishing Group, BMA House, Tavistock Square, London WC1H 9JR, England. Phone: 071-383 6244/6638. Fax: 071-383 6662. Quarterly.

NEWSLETTERS

Hospital Peer Review. American Health Consultants, P.O. Box 71266, Chicago, IL 60691. Phone: (800) 688-2421. Fax: (404) 352-1971.

ONLINE DATABASES

EMBASE. Elsevier Science Publishing Co., Inc., P.O. Box 882, Madison Square Station, New York, NY 10159-2101. Phone: (212) 989-5800. Fax: (212) 633-3990.

Hospital Database. Urban Decision Systems, Inc., 2040 Armacost Ave., P.O. Box 25953, Los Angeles, CA 90025. Phone: (800) 633-9568. Fax: (213) 826-0933. Irregular.

MEDLINE. National Library of Medicine, 8600 Rockville Pike, Bethesda, MD 20894. Phone: (800) 638-8480.

Nursing and Allied Health (CINAHL). CINAHL, 1509 Wilson Terrace, P.O. Box 871, Glendale, CA 91209-0871. Phone: (818) 409-8005.

SciSearch. Institute for Scientific Information, 3501 Market St., Philadelphia, PA 19104. Phone: (215) 386-0100. Fax: (215) 386-6362.

STANDARDS AND STATISTICS SOURCES

Healthcare Standards. ECRI, 5200 Butler Pike, Plymouth Meeting, PA 19462. Annual.

TEXTBOOKS AND MONOGRAPHS

Excellence in Ambulatory Care: A Practical Guide to Developing Effective Quality Assurance Programs. Dale S. Benson Jr., Peyton G. Townes. Jossey-Bass, Inc., 350 Sansome St., San Francisco, CA 94104. Phone: (415) 433-1740. 1990.

Quality Assurance Policies and Procedures for Health Care. Judith Bulau. Aspen Publishers, Inc., 200 Orchard Ridge Dr., Gaithersburg, MD 20878. Phone: (800) 638-8437. 1989.

Using Practice Parameters in a QA Program. American Medical Association, 515 North State St., Chicago, IL 60610. Phone: (312) 464-0183. Fax: (312) 464-5834. 1992.

QUALITY OF LIFE

See: MEDICAL ETHICS

R

RABIES

See: VIRAL DISEASES

RADIATION EFFECTS

ABSTRACTING, INDEXING, AND CURRENT AWARENESS PUBLICATIONS

Current Contents/Life Sciences. Institute for Scientific Information, 3501 Market St., Philadelphia, PA 19104. Phone: (215) 386-0100. Fax: (215) 386-6362.

Excerpta Medica. Section 14: Radiology. Elsevier Science Publishing Co., Inc., P.O. Box 882, Madison Square Station, New York, NY 10159-2101. Phone: (212) 989-5800. Fax: (212) 633-3990. 24/year.

Excerpta Medica. Section 23: Nuclear Medicine. Elsevier Science Publishers, P.O. Box 882, Madison Square Station, New York, NY 10159-2101. Phone: (212) 633-3950. Fax: (212) 633-3990. 20/year.

Genetics Abstracts. Cambridge Scientific Abstracts, 7200 Wisconsin Ave., Bethesda, MD 20814-4823. Phone: (800) 843-7751. Fax: (301) 961-6720. Monthly.

Index Medicus. U.S. National Library of Medicine, 8600 Rockville Pike, Bethesda, MD 20894. Phone: (800) 638-8480. Monthly.

Science Citation Index. Institute for Scientific Information, 3501 Market St., Philadelphia, PA 19104. Phone: (800) 523-1850. Fax: (215) 386-6362. Bimonthly.

Toxicology Abstracts. Cambridge Scientific Abstracts, 7200 Wisconsin Ave., Bethesda, MD 20814-4823. Phone: (800) 843-7751. Fax: (301) 961-6720. Monthly.

ASSOCIATIONS, PROFESSIONAL SOCIETIES, ADVOCACY AND SUPPORT GROUPS

Health Physics Society. 8000 Westpark Dr., No. 400, Mc Lean, VA 22102. Phone: (703) 790-1745.

International Radiation Protection Association. Postbus 662, NL-5600 Eindhoven AR, Netherlands.

National Committee for Radiation Victims. 6935 Laurel Ave., Takoma Park, MD 20912. Phone: (301) 891-3990.

Radiation Health Information Project. c/o Environmental Policy Institute, 218 D St. S.E., Washington, DC 20003. Phone: (202) 544-2600.

Radiation Research Society. 1101 Market St., Philadelphia, PA 19107. Phone: (215) 574-3153.

BIBLIOGRAPHIES

Radon Gas: Health Risks and Toxicity. National Technical Information Service, 5285 Port Royal Rd., Springfield, VA 22161. Phone: (703) 487-4650. Fax: (703) 321-8547. Mar. 1974-Nov. 1989 PB90-853102/CBY.

CD-ROM DATABASES

SCISEARCH. Institute for Scientific Information, 3501 Market St., Philadelphia, PA 19104. Phone: (215) 386-0100. Fax: (215) 386-6362.

JOURNALS

Health Physicals: The Radiation Protection Journal. Williams & Wilkins, 428 E. Preston St., Baltimore, MD 21202. Phone: (800) 638-0672. Fax: (800) 447-8438. Monthly.

Radiology. Radiological Society of North America, 1415 W. 22nd St., Tower B, Oak Brook, IL 60521. Phone: (708) 571-2670.

ONLINE DATABASES

EMBASE. Elsevier Science Publishing Co., Inc., P.O. Box 882, Madison Square Station, New York, NY 10159-2101. Phone: (212) 989-5800. Fax: (212) 633-3990.

Hazardline. Occupational Health Services Inc., 450 7th Ave., No. 2407, New York, NY 10123. Phone: (212) 967-1100.

MEDLINE. National Library of Medicine, 8600 Rockville Pike, Bethesda, MD 20894. Phone: (800) 638-8480.

SciSearch. Institute for Scientific Information, 3501 Market St., Philadelphia, PA 19104. Phone: (215) 386-0100. Fax: (215) 386-6362.

RESEARCH CENTERS, INSTITUTES, CLEARINGHOUSES

Center for Atomic Radiation Studies. P.O. Box 72, Acton, MA 01720. Phone: (508) 635-0045.

Center for Basic Research in Radiation Bioeffects. University of Texas Health Science Center at San Antonio. Dept. of Radiology, 7703 Floyd Curl Dr., San Antonio, TX 78284. Phone: (512) 567-5560. Fax: (512) 567-6469.

Center for Environmental Toxicology. Colorado State University Center for Environmental Toxicology, Fort Collins, CO 80521. Phone: (303) 491-8522.

Radiation Laboratory. University of Notre Dame. Notre Dame, IN 46556. Phone: (219) 239-7502.

Radiation Science and Engineering Center. Pennsylvania State University. University Park, PA 16802. Phone: (814) 865-6351. Fax: (814) 863-4840.

TEXTBOOKS AND MONOGRAPHS

Biological Effects and Medical Applications of Electromagnetic Energy. Om P. Ghandi. Prentice Hall, Prentice Hall Bldg., 113 Sylvan Ave., Rt. 9W, Englewood Cliffs, NJ 07632. Phone: (201) 767-5937. 1990.

Medical Management of Radiation Accidents. Fred A. Mettler Jr., Charles A. Kelsey, Robert C. Ricks. CRC Press, Inc., 2000 Corporate Blvd. N.W., Boca Raton, FL 33431. Phone: (407) 994-0555. Fax: (407) 997-0949. 1989.

Radiation and Cancer Risk. Tor Brustad, Froydis Langmark, Jon B. Reitan (eds.). Taylor & Francis Inc., 1900 Frost Rd., Suite 101, Bristol, PA 19007-1598. Phone: (800) 821-8312. Fax: (215) 785-5515. 1989.

Radiation Exposure and Occupational Risks. E. Scherer, and others (eds.). Springer-Verlag New York Inc., 175 Fifth Ave., New York, NY 10010. Phone: (212) 460-1500. Fax: (212) 473-6272. 1989.

Radiation Injury to the Nervous System. Philip H. Gutin, Steven A. Leibel, Glenn E. Sheline. Raven Press, 1185 Avenue of the Americas, New York, NY 10036. Phone: (212) 930-9500. Fax: (212) 869-3495. 1991.

Radiation Research. E.M. Fielden, J.F. Fowler, J.H. Hendry, D. Scott (eds.). Taylor & Francis Inc., 1900 Frost Rd., Suite 101, Bristol, PA 19007-1598. Phone: (800) 821-8312. Fax: (215) 785-5515. Two volumes 1988.

RADIATION THERAPY

ABSTRACTING, INDEXING, AND CURRENT AWARENESS PUBLICATIONS

Current Contents/Clinical Medicine. Institute for Scientific Information, 3501 Market St., Philadelphia, PA 19104. Phone: (800) 523-1850. Fax: (215) 386-6362. Weekly.

Excerpta Medica. Section 14: Radiology. Elsevier Science Publishing Co., Inc., P.O. Box 882, Madison Square Station, New York, NY 10159-2101. Phone: (212) 989-5800. Fax: (212) 633-3990. 24/year.

Excerpta Medica. Section 23: Nuclear Medicine. Elsevier Science Publishers, P.O. Box 882, Madison Square Station, New York, NY 10159-2101. Phone: (212) 633-3950. Fax: (212) 633-3990. 20/year.

ICRDB Cancergram: Clinical Treatment of Cancer--Radiation Therapy. U.S. Government Printing Office, Superintendent of Documents, P.O. Box 371954, Pittsburgh, PA 15250-7954. Phone: (202) 783-3238. Fax: (202) 512-2250. Monthly.

Index Medicus. U.S. National Library of Medicine, 8600 Rockville Pike, Bethesda, MD 20894. Phone: (800) 638-8480. Monthly.

Research Alert: Cancer Radiotherapy. Institute for Scientific Information, 3501 Market St., Philadelphia, PA 19104. Phone: (800) 523-1850. Fax: (215) 386-6362. Weekly.

ANNUALS AND REVIEWS

Frontiers of Radiation Therapy and Oncology. S. Karger Publishers, Inc., 26 West Avon Rd., P.O. Box 529, Farmington, CT 06085. Phone: (203) 675-7834. Fax: (203) 675-7302. Irregular.

ASSOCIATIONS, PROFESSIONAL SOCIETIES, ADVOCACY AND SUPPORT GROUPS

American Cancer Society (ACS). 1599 Clifton Rd. N.E., Atlanta, GA 30329. Phone: (404) 320-3333.

American Society for Therapeutic Radiology and Oncology (ASTRO). 1101 Market, 14th Flr., Philadelphia, PA 19107. Phone: (215) 574-3180.

Radiation Therapy Oncology Group. American College of Radiology, 1101 Market St., Philadelphia, PA 19107. Phone: (215) 574-3150.

CD-ROM DATABASES

Excerpta Medica CD: Radiology & Nuclear Medicine. SilverPlatter Information, Inc., River Ridge Office Park, 100 River Ridge Rd., Norwood, MA 02062. Phone: (617) 769-2599. Fax: (617) 769-8763. Quarterly.

ENCYCLOPEDIAS, DICTIONARIES, WORD BOOKS

Radiology Words. Stedman. Williams & Wilkins, 428 East Preston St., Baltimore, MD 21202. Phone: (800) 638-0672. Fax: (800) 447-8438. 1992.

JOURNALS

American Journal of Clinical Oncology. Raven Press, 1185 Ave. of the Americas, New York, NY 10036. Phone: (212) 930-9500. Fax: (212) 869-3495. Bimonthly.

Frontiers of Radiation Therapy and Oncology. S. Karger Publishers, Inc., 26 W. Avon Rd., P.O. Box 529, Farmington, CT 06085. Phone: (203) 675-7834. Fax: (203) 675-7302.

International Journal of Radiation Oncology-Biology-Physics. Pergamon Press, 660 White Plains Rd., Tarrytown, NY 10591-5153. Phone: (914) 592-7700. Fax: (914) 592-3625. 15/year.

Journal of Clinical Oncology. W.B. Saunders Co., The Curtis Center, Independence Square W., Philadelphia, PA 19106-3399. Phone: (215) 238-7800. Monthly.

Radiation Research. Academic Press, Inc., 1250 Sixth Ave., San Diego, CA 92101-4311. Phone: (619) 699-6345. Fax: (619) 699-6715.

Radiotherapy and Oncology. Elsevier Science Publishing Co., Inc., P.O. Box 882, Madison Square Station, New York, NY 10159-2101. Phone: (212) 989-5800. Fax: (212) 633-3990. 12/year.

ONLINE DATABASES

CANCERLIT. U.S. National Cancer Institute, International Cancer Information Center, Building 82, Room 102, Bethesda, MD 20892. Phone: (301) 496-7403. Fax: (301) 480-8105. Monthly.

EMBASE. Elsevier Science Publishing Co., Inc., P.O. Box 882, Madison Square Station, New York, NY 10159-2101. Phone: (212) 989-5800. Fax: (212) 633-3990.

MEDLINE. National Library of Medicine, 8600 Rockville Pike, Bethesda, MD 20894. Phone: (800) 638-8480.

SciSearch. Institute for Scientific Information, 3501 Market St., Philadelphia, PA 19104. Phone: (215) 386-0100. Fax: (215) 386-6362.

POPULAR WORKS AND PATIENT EDUCATION

Everyone's Guide to Cancer Therapy: How Cancer is Diagnosed, Treated, and Managed on a Day to Day Basis. Malin Dollinger, Ernest H. Rosenbaum, Greg Cable. Andrews & McMeel, 4900 Main St., Kansas City, MO 64112. Phone: (800) 826-4216. 1991.

Managing the Side Effects of Chemotherapy and Radiation Therapy. Marilyn J. Dodd. Prentice Hall, 113 Sylvan Ave., Rt. 9W, Prentice Hall Bldg., Englewood Cliffs, NJ 07632. Phone: (201) 767-5937. 1991.

RESEARCH CENTERS, INSTITUTES, CLEARINGHOUSES

Cancer Information Service (CIS). Office of Cancer Communications, National Cancer Institute, Bldg. 31, Rm. 10A24, 9000 Rockville Pike, Bethesda, MD 20892. Phone: (800) 4CA-NCER.

Cancer Research Center. Boston University. 80 E. Concord St., Boston, MA 02118. Phone: (617) 638-4173. Fax: (617) 638-4176.

Dana Farber Cancer Institute. 44 Binney St., Boston, MA 02115. Phone: (617) 732-3000.

Fox Chase Cancer Center. 7701 Burholme Ave., Philadelphia, PA 19111. Phone: (215) 728-6900. Fax: (215) 728-2571.

Joint Center for Radiation Therapy. 50 Binney St., Boston, MA 02115. Phone: (617) 432-2227.

LCF Foundation, Inc.. 41 Mall Rd., Burlington, MA 01805. Phone: (617) 273-5100. Fax: (617) 273-8999.

Mallinckrodt Institute of Radiology. Washington University. 510 S. Kingshighway Blvd., St. Louis, MO 63110. Phone: (314) 362-2866.

Mayo Comprehensive Cancer Center. 200 First St. SW, Rochester, MN 55905. Phone: (507) 284-4718.

Oncology Center. Johns Hopkins University. 600 N. Wolfe St., Baltimore, MD 21205. Phone: (301) 955-8800. Fax: (301) 955-1904.

Radiation Therapy Oncology Center. University of Kentucky Medical Center, Rose St., Lexington, KY 40536. Phone: (606) 233-6486. Fax: (606) 257-3393.

Roswell Park Cancer Institute. 666 Elm St., Buffalo, NY 14263. Phone: (716) 845-2300. Fax: (716) 845-3545.

TEXTBOOKS AND MONOGRAPHS

Advanced Techniques for Radiotherapy. Marco Castiglioni, Argeo A. Benco (eds.). Kluwer Academic Publishers, P.O. Box 358, Accord Station, Hingham, MA 02018-0358. Phone: (617) 871-6600. Fax: (617) 871-6528. 1992.

Introduction to Clinical Radiation Oncology. Coia. Medical Physics Publishing Co., 1300 University Ave., Rm. 27B,

Madison, WI 53706. Phone: (800) 262-6243. Fax: (212) 869-3495. 1991.

Levitt and Tapley's Technological Basis of Radiation Therapy: Practical Clinical Applications. Seymour H. Levitt and others. Williams & Wilkins, 428 East Preston St., Baltimore, MD 21202. Phone: (800) 638-0672. Fax: (800) 447-8438. Second edition 1992.

Medical Radiation Physics. William R. Hendee, E. Russell Ritenour. Mosby-Year Book, 11830 Westline Industrial Drive, St. Louis, MO 63146. Phone: (800) 325-4177. Fax: (314) 432-1380. Third edition 1992.

Principles and Practice of Radiation Oncology. Carlos A. Perez, Luther W. Brady (eds.). J.B. Lippincott Co., 227 East Washington Square, Philadelphia, PA 19106-3780. Phone: (215) 238-4200. Fax: (215) 238-4227. Second edition 1991.

Radiation Oncology. Moss. Mosby-Year Book, 11830 Westline Industrial Drive, St. Louis, MO 63146. Phone: (800) 325-4177. Fax: (314) 432-1380. Sixth edition 1989.

Radiation Therapy Planning. Gunilla C. Bentel. McGraw-Hill, Inc., Health Professions Division, 1221 Avenue of the Americas, 28th Floor, New York, NY 10020. Phone: (212) 512-4228. 1992.

RADIOACTIVE WASTES

See: ENVIRONMENTAL POLLUTANTS; RADIATION EFFECTS

RADIOLOGY

See also: DIAGNOSIS; MAMMOGRAPHY

ABSTRACTING, INDEXING, AND CURRENT AWARENESS PUBLICATIONS

Current Contents/Clinical Medicine. Institute for Scientific Information, 3501 Market St., Philadelphia, PA 19104. Phone: (800) 523-1850. Fax: (215) 386-6362. Weekly.

Current Contents/Life Sciences. Institute for Scientific Information, 3501 Market St., Philadelphia, PA 19104. Phone: (215) 386-0100. Fax: (215) 386-6362.

Excerpta Medica. Section 14: Radiology. Elsevier Science Publishing Co., Inc., P.O. Box 882, Madison Square Station, New York, NY 10159-2101. Phone: (212) 989-5800. Fax: (212) 633-3990. 24/year.

Excerpta Medica. Section 23: Nuclear Medicine. Elsevier Science Publishers, P.O. Box 882, Madison Square Station, New York, NY 10159-2101. Phone: (212) 633-3950. Fax: (212) 633-3990. 20/year.

ICRDB Cancergram: Cancer Detection and Management-- Diagnostic Radiology. U.S. Government Printing Office, Superintendent of Documents, P.O. Box 371954, Pittsburgh, PA 15250-7954. Phone: (202) 783-3238. Fax: (202) 512-2250. Monthly.

ICRDB Cancergram: Cancer Detection and Management-- Nuclear Medicine. U.S. Government Printing Office, Superintendent of Documents, P.O. Box 371954, Pittsburgh, PA 15250-7954. Phone: (202) 783-3238. Fax: (202) 512-2250. Monthly.

Index Medicus. U.S. National Library of Medicine, 8600 Rockville Pike, Bethesda, MD 20894. Phone: (800) 638-8480. Monthly.

Science Citation Index. Institute for Scientific Information, 3501 Market St., Philadelphia, PA 19104. Phone: (800) 523-1850. Fax: (215) 386-6362. Bimonthly.

ANNUALS AND REVIEWS

Advances in Gastrointestinal Radiology. Mosby-Year Book, 11830 Westline Industrial Drive, St. Louis, MO 63146. Phone: (800) 325-4177. Fax: (314) 432-1380. Annual.

Current Opinion in Radiology. Current Science Ltd., 20 N. Third St., Philadelphia, PA 19106-2199. Phone: (800) 552-5866. Fax: (215) 574-2270. Bimonthly.

Current Problems in Diagnostic Radiology. Mosby-Year Book, 11830 Westline Industrial Drive, St. Louis, MO 63146. Phone: (800) 325-4177. Fax: (314) 432-1380. Bimonthly.

Radiologic Clinics. W.B. Saunders Co., The Curtis Center, Independence Square W., Philadelphia, PA 19106-3399. Phone: (215) 238-7800. Bimonthly.

Year Book of Diagnostic Radiology. Mosby-Year Book, 11830 Westline Industrial Drive, St. Louis, MO 63146. Phone: (800) 325-4177. Fax: (314) 432-1380. Annual.

Year Book of Neuroradiology. Mosby-Year Book, 11830 Westline Industrial Drive, St. Louis, MO 63146. Phone: (800) 325-4177. Fax: (314) 432-1380. Annual.

ASSOCIATIONS, PROFESSIONAL SOCIETIES, ADVOCACY AND SUPPORT GROUPS

American Board of Radiology (ABR). 300 Park, Ste. 440, Birmingham, MI 48009. Phone: (313) 645-0600. Fax: (313) 645-0459.

American College of Radiology (ACR). 1891 Preston White Dr., Reston, VA 22091. Phone: (703) 648-8900.

American Roentgen Ray Society (ARRS). 1891 Preston White Dr., Reston, VA 22091. Phone: (703) 648-8992. Fax: (703) 648-9176.

Radiological Society of North America (RSNA). 2021 Spring Rd., Ste. 600, Oak Brook, IL 60521. Phone: (708) 571-2670. Fax: (708) 571-7837.

CD-ROM DATABASES

Excerpta Medica CD: Radiology & Nuclear Medicine. SilverPlatter Information, Inc., River Ridge Office Park, 100 River Ridge Rd., Norwood, MA 02062. Phone: (617) 769-2599. Fax: (617) 769-8763. Quarterly.

RadLine. Aries Systems Corporation, One Dundee Park, Andover, MA 01810. Phone: (508) 475-7200. Fax: (508) 474-8860. Quarterly.

SCISEARCH. Institute for Scientific Information, 3501 Market St., Philadelphia, PA 19104. Phone: (215) 386-0100. Fax: (215) 386-6362.

Year Books on Disc. CMC ReSearch, Inc., 7150 S.W. Hampton, Suite C-120, Portland, OR 97223. Phone: (800) 262-7668. Fax: (503) 639-1796. Annual includes Year Books of

Cardiology, Dermatology, Diagnostic Radiology, Drug Therapy, Emergency Medicine, Family Practice, Medicine, Neurology and Neurosurgery, Obstetrics and Gynecology, Oncology, Pediatrics, and Psychiatry and Applied Mental Health.

DIRECTORIES

Directory of Certified Radiologists. American Board of Medical Specialties, 1 Rotary Center, Suite 805, Evanston, IL 60201. Phone: (708) 491-9091. Biennial.

Directory of Medical Specialists. Marquis Who's Who, 3002 Glenview Rd., Wilmette, IL 60091. Phone: (800) 621-9669. Fax: (708) 441-2264. Biennial.

Directory of Physicians in the United States. American Medical Association, 515 North State St., Chicago, IL 60610. Phone: (312) 464-0183. Fax: (312) 464-5834. Biennial.

ENCYCLOPEDIAS, DICTIONARIES, WORD BOOKS

Radiologic Word Book. Barbara De Lorenzo. Springhouse Publishing Co., 1111 Bethlehem Pike, Spring House, PA 19477. Phone: (800) 331-3170. Fax: (215) 646-8716. 1992.

Radiology Words. Stedman. Williams & Wilkins, 428 East Preston St., Baltimore, MD 21202. Phone: (800) 638-0672. Fax: (800) 447-8438. 1992.

HANDBOOKS, GUIDES, MANUALS, ATLASES

Human Cross-Sectional Anatomy Atlas of Body Section and CT Images. Ellis. Butterworth-Heinemann, 80 Montvale Ave., Stoneham, MA 02180. Phone: (617) 438-8464. Fax: (617) 279-4851. 1991.

Manual of Diagnostic Imaging. Straub. Little, Brown and Co., 34 Beacon St., Boston, MA 02108. Phone: (617) 227-0730. Fax: (617) 227-0790. Second edition 1989.

Pocket Guide to Radiography. Philip W. Ballinger. Mosby-Year Book, 11830 Westline Industrial Drive, St. Louis, MO 63146. Phone: (800) 325-4177. Fax: (314) 432-1380. Second edition 1992.

JOURNALS

American Journal of Roentgenology. American Roentgen Ray Society, 1891 Preston White Dr., Reston, VA 22091. Phone: (800) 438-2777. Monthly.

British Journal of Radiology. Butterworth-Heinemann, 80 Montvale Ave., Stoneham, MA 02180. Phone: (617) 438-8464. Fax: (617) 279-4851.

Clinical Imaging. Elsevier Science Publishing Co., Inc., P.O. Box 882, Madison Square Station, New York, NY 10159-2101. Phone: (212) 989-5800. Fax: (212) 633-3990. 4/year.

European Journal of Radiology. Elsevier Science Publishing Co., Inc., P.O. Box 882, Madison Square Station, New York, NY 10159-2101. Phone: (212) 989-5800. Fax: (212) 633-3990. 6/year.

Journal of Computer Assisted Tomography. Raven Press, 1185 Avenue of the Americas, New York, NY 10036. Phone: (212) 930-9500. Fax: (212) 869-3495. Bimonthly.

Radiology. Radiological Society of North America, 2021 Spring Rd., Ste. 600, Oak Brook, IL 60521. Phone: (708) 571-2670.

NEWSLETTERS

Contemporary Diagnostic Radiology. Williams & Wilkins, 428 E. Preston St., Baltimore, MD 21202. Phone: (800) 638-0672. Fax: (800) 447-8438. Biweekly.

Radiology & Imaging Letter. Quest Publishing Co., 1351 Titan Way, Brea, CA 92621. Phone: (714) 738-6400. Semimonthly.

ONLINE DATABASES

EMBASE. Elsevier Science Publishing Co., Inc., P.O. Box 882, Madison Square Station, New York, NY 10159-2101. Phone: (212) 989-5800. Fax: (212) 633-3990.

MEDLINE. National Library of Medicine, 8600 Rockville Pike, Bethesda, MD 20894. Phone: (800) 638-8480.

SciSearch. Institute for Scientific Information, 3501 Market St., Philadelphia, PA 19104. Phone: (215) 386-0100. Fax: (215) 386-6362.

TEXTBOOKS AND MONOGRAPHS

Clinical Magnetic Resonance Imaging. R.R. Edelman, J.R. Hesselink. W.B. Saunders Co., The Curtis Center, Independence Sqare W., Philadelphia, PA 19106-3399. Phone: (215) 238-7800. 1990.

Computed Body Tomography. Lee. Raven Press, 1185 Ave. of the Americas, New York, NY 10036. Phone: (212) 930-9500. Fax: (212) 869-3495. Second edition 1989.

Diagnostic Radiology. R.G. Grainger, D. Allison. Churchill Livingstone Inc., 650 Ave. of the Americas, New York, NY 10011. Phone: (212) 819-5400. Fax: (212) 302-6598. Second edition 1991.

Diagnostic Radiology in Emergency Medicine. Rosen. Mosby-Year Book, 11830 Westline Industrial Drive, St. Louis, MO 63146. Phone: (800) 325-4177. Fax: (314) 432-1380. 1992.

Differential Diagnosis in Conventional Radiology. F.A. Burgener, M. Kormano. Thieme Medical Publishers, Inc., 381 Park Ave. S., New York, NY 10016. Phone: (212) 683-5088. Fax: (212) 779-9020. Second edition 1991.

Emergency Radiology. Keats. Mosby-Year Book, 11830 Westline Industrial Drive, St. Louis, MO 63146. Phone: (800) 325-4177. Fax: (314) 432-1380. Second edition.

Interventional Radiology. Robert F. Dondelinger, Plinio Rossi, Jean Claud Kurdziel. Thieme Medical Publishers, Inc., 381 Park Ave. S., New York, NY 10016. Phone: (212) 683-5088. Fax: (212) 779-9020. 1990.

Medical Radiation Physics. William R. Hendee, E. Russell Ritenour. Mosby-Year Book, 11830 Westline Industrial Drive, St. Louis, MO 63146. Phone: (800) 325-4177. Fax: (314) 432-1380. Third edition 1992.

Principles of Genitourinary Radiology. Zoran L. Barbaric. Thieme Medical Publishers, Inc., 381 Park Ave. S., New York, NY 10016. Phone: (212) 683-5088. Fax: (212) 779-9020. 1991.

Radiology of Emergency Medicine. Harris. Williams & Wilkins, 428 East Preston St., Baltimore, MD 21202. Phone: (800) 638-0672. Fax: (800) 447-8438. Third edition 1992.

Trauma Radiology. James J. McCort (ed.). Churchill Livingstone Inc., 650 Avenue of the Americas, New York, NY 10011. Phone: (212) 819-5400. Fax: (212) 302-6598. 1990.

RAPE

ABSTRACTING, INDEXING, AND CURRENT AWARENESS PUBLICATIONS

Index Medicus. U.S. National Library of Medicine, 8600 Rockville Pike, Bethesda, MD 20894. Phone: (800) 638-8480. Monthly.

Psychological Abstracts. American Psychological Association, 1200 17th St. NW, Washington, DC 20036. Phone: (202) 955-7600. Monthly.

ASSOCIATIONS, PROFESSIONAL SOCIETIES, ADVOCACY AND SUPPORT GROUPS

Feminist Alliance Against Rape. P.O. Box 21033, Washington, DC 20009. Phone: (202) 686-9463.

Institute for the Study of Sexual Assault. 403 Ashbury St., San Francisco, CA 94116. Phone: (415) 861-2048.

National Coalition Against Sexual Assault. c/o The Sexual Violence Center, 1222 W. 31st St., Minneapolis, MN 55408. Phone: (612) 824-2864.

BIBLIOGRAPHIES

Post-Traumatic Stress Disorder, Rape Trauma, Delayed Stress and Related Conditions: A Bibliography. McFarland & Co., Inc., Box 611, Jefferson, NC 28640. Phone: (919) 246-4460. 1986.

DIRECTORIES

Sexual Assault and Child Sexual Abuse: A Directory of Victim/ Survivor Services and Prevention Programs. Linda Webster (ed.). Oryx Press, 4041 N. Central, Suite 700, Phoenix, AZ 85012. Phone: (800) 279-ORYX. Fax: (800) 279-4663. 1989.

NEWSLETTERS

National Clearinghouse on Marital and Date Rape Newsletter. National Clearinghouse on Marital and Date Rape, 2325 Oak St., Berkeley, CA 94708. Phone: (415) 548-1770.

ONLINE DATABASES

EMBASE. Elsevier Science Publishing Co., Inc., P.O. Box 882, Madison Square Station, New York, NY 10159-2101. Phone: (212) 989-5800. Fax: (212) 633-3990.

MEDLINE. National Library of Medicine, 8600 Rockville Pike, Bethesda, MD 20894. Phone: (800) 638-8480.

PsycInfo. SilverPlatter Information, Inc., River Ridge Office Park, 100 River Ridge Rd., Norwood, MA 02062. Phone: (617) 769-2599. Fax: (617) 769-8763. Quarterly.

SciSearch. Institute for Scientific Information, 3501 Market St., Philadelphia, PA 19104. Phone: (215) 386-0100. Fax: (215) 386-6362.

POPULAR WORKS AND PATIENT EDUCATION

Allies in Healing: When the Person You Love Was Sexually Abused as a Child, a Support Book for Partners. Laura Davis. HarperCollins Pubs., Inc., 10 E. 53rd St., New York, NY 10022-5299. Phone: (212) 207-7000. 1991.

The Courage to Heal: A Guide for Women Survivors of Child Sexual Abuse. Ellen Bass, Laura Davis. HarperCollins Pubs., Inc., 10 E. 53rd St., New York, NY 10022-5299. Phone: (212) 207-7000. Revised edition 1992.

Secret Survivors: Uncovering Incest and Its After Effects. E. Sue Blume. John Wiley & Sons, Inc., 605 Third Ave., New York, NY 10158-0012. Phone: (212) 850-6000. Fax: (212) 850-6088. 1990.

RESEARCH CENTERS, INSTITUTES, CLEARINGHOUSES

National Clearinghouse on Marital and Date Rape. 2325 Oak St., Berkeley, CA 94708. Phone: (415) 548-1770.

National Victims Resource Center. Dept. F., P.O. Box 6000, Rockville, MD 20850. Phone: (800) 627-NVRC.

TEXTBOOKS AND MONOGRAPHS

The Rape Victim: Clinical and Community Interventions. Mary P. Koss, Mary R. Harvey. Sage Publications, Inc., 2455 Teller Road, P.O. Box 5084, Newbury Park, CA 91320. Phone: (805) 499-0721. Fax: (805) 499-0871. 1991.

Theories of Rape: Inquiries into the Causes of Sexual Aggression. Lee Ellis. Taylor & Francis Inc., 1900 Frost Rd., Suite 101, Bristol, PA 19007-1598. Phone: (800) 821-8312. Fax: (215) 785-5515. 1989.

RAYNAUD'S DISEASE

See: VASCULAR DISEASES

RECONSTRUCTIVE SURGERY

See: PLASTIC AND COSMETIC SURGERY

RECTAL CANCER

See: COLORECTAL CANCER

RECTAL DISEASES

See: GASTROINTESTINAL DISORDERS

REHABILITATION

See also: OCCUPATIONAL THERAPY; PHYSICAL THERAPY

ABSTRACTING, INDEXING, AND CURRENT AWARENESS PUBLICATIONS

Cumulative Index to Nursing and Allied Health Literature. Glendale Adventist Medical Center, P.O. Box 871, Glendale, CA 91209. Phone: (818) 409-8005. Bimonthly.

Excerpta Medica. Section 19: Rehabilitation and Physical Medicine. Elsevier Science Publishing Co., Inc., P.O. Box 882, Madison Square Station, New York, NY 10159-2101. Phone: (212) 989-5800. Fax: (212) 633-3990. 8/year.

Index Medicus. U.S. National Library of Medicine, 8600 Rockville Pike, Bethesda, MD 20894. Phone: (800) 638-8480. Monthly.

Physiotherapy Index. Medical Information Service, British Library, Boston Spa, Wetherby, W. Yorkshire LS23 7BQ, England. Phone: 0937-546039. Fax: 0937-546236. Monthly.

Rehabilitation Index. Medical Information Service, British Library, Boston Spa, Wetherby, W. Yorkshire LS23 7BQ, England. Phone: 09375-46039. Fax: 09375-46236. Monthly.

ANNUALS AND REVIEWS

Annual Review of Rehabilitation. Springer Publishing Co., Inc., 536 Broadway, 11th Floor, New York, NY 10012. Phone: (212) 431-4370. Annual.

Critical Reviews in Physical and Rehabilitation Medicine. CRC Press, Inc., 2000 Corporate Blvd. N.W., Boca Raton, FL 33431. Phone: (407) 994-0555. Fax: (407) 997-0949. 4/year.

Physical Medicine and Rehabilitation Clinics of North America. W.B. Saunders Co., The Curtis Center, Independence Square W., Philadelphia, PA 19106-3399. Phone: (215) 238-7800. Quarterly.

Year Book of Rehabilitation. Mosby-Year Book, 11830 Westline Industrial Drive, St. Louis, MO 63146. Phone: (800) 325-4177. Fax: (314) 432-1380. Annual.

ASSOCIATIONS, PROFESSIONAL SOCIETIES, ADVOCACY AND SUPPORT GROUPS

American Academy of Physical Medicine and Rehabilitation (AAPMR). 122 S. Michigan Ave., Ste. 1300, Chicago, IL 60603. Phone: (312) 922-9366. Fax: (312) 922-6754.

American Board of Physical Medicine and Rehabilitation (ABPMR). Norwest Ctr., 21 First St. S.W., Ste. 674, Rochester, MN 55902. Phone: (507) 282-1776.

Canadian Rehabilitation Council for the Disabled. 45 Sheppard Ave. E., Suite 801, Toronto, ON, Canada M4J 3R8. Phone: (416) 250-7490. Fax: (416) 229-1371.

International Rehabilitation Medicine Association (IRMA). Dept. of Physical Medicine, 1333 Moursund Ave., Rm. A-221, Houston, TX 77030. Phone: (713) 799-5086. Fax: (713) 799-5058.

National Rehabilitation Association (NRA). 633 S. Washington St., Alexandria, VA 22314. Phone: (703) 836-0850. Fax: (703) 836-2209.

DIRECTORIES

Directory of Certified Physical Medicine & Rehabilitation Specialists. American Board of Medical Specialties, 1 Rotary Center, Suite 805, Evanston, IL 60201. Phone: (708) 491-9091. Biennial.

Directory of Medical Rehabilitation Programs. Oryx Press, 4041 N. Central, Suite 700, Phoenix, AZ 85012. Phone: (800) 279-6799. Fax: (800) 279-4663. 1990.

Directory of Medical Specialists. Marquis Who's Who, 3002 Glenview Rd., Wilmette, IL 60091. Phone: (800) 621-9669. Fax: (708) 441-2264. Biennial.

Directory of Physicians in the United States. American Medical Association, 515 North State St., Chicago, IL 60610. Phone: (312) 464-0183. Fax: (312) 464-5834. Biennial.

HANDBOOKS, GUIDES, MANUALS, ATLASES

The Home Rehabilitation Program Guide. Paul A. Roggow, Debra K. Berg, Michael D. Lewis. SLACK Inc., 6900 Grove Rd., Thorofare, NJ 08086-9447. Phone: (800) 257-8290. Fax: (609) 853-5991. 1990.

Krusen's Handbook of Physical Medicine and Rehabilitation. Frederic J. Kottke, Justus F. Lehmann. W.B. Saunders Co., The Curtis Center, Independence Square W., Philadelphia, PA 19106-3399. Phone: (215) 238-7800. Fourth edition 1990.

The Rehabilitation Specialist's Handbook. Jules M. Rothstien, Serge H. Roy, Steven L. Wolf. F.A. Davis Co., 1915 Arch St., Philadelphia, PA 19103. Phone: (800) 523-4049. Fax: (215) 568-5065. 1991.

JOURNALS

American Journal of Art Therapy. Vermont College of Norwich University, Montpelier, VT 05602.

American Journal of Physical Medicine & Rehabilitation. Williams & Wilkins, 428 E. Preston St., Baltimore, MD 21202. Phone: (800) 638-0672. Fax: (800) 447-8438. Bimonthly.

American Rehabilitation. U.S. Dept. of Education. Mary E. Switzer Bldg., Rm. 3212, 330 C St. S.W., Washington, DC 20202. Phone: (202) 732-1296. Quarterly.

Archives of Physical Medicine and Rehabilitation. American Congress of Rehabilitation Medicine, 78 E. Adams, Chicago, IL 60603. Phone: (312) 922-9371. Fax: (312) 922-6754. Monthly.

Art Therapy. American Art Therapy Association, Inc., 505 E. Hawley St., Mundelein, IL 60060-2419.

Assistive Technology. Resna Press, 1101 Connecticut Ave. NW, Suite 700, Washington, DC 20036. Phone: (202) 857-1199. Quarterly.

British Journal of Occupational Therapy. College of Occupational Therapists Ltd., 20 Rede Place, Bayswater, London W2 4TU, England. Monthly.

Canadian Journal of Rehabilitation. Canadian Association for Research in Rehabilitation, 13325 St. Albert Trail, Edmonton, AB, Canada T5L 4R3.

Clinical Rehabilitation. Cambridge University Press, 40 W. 20th St., New York, NY 10011. Phone: (800) 431-1580. Quarterly.

International Journal of Rehabilitation Research. Heidelberger Verlagsantalt in Druckerei GmbH, Edition Schindele, Hans-Bunte-Str. 18, D-6900 Heidelberg, Germany.

Journal of Burn Care and Rehabilitation. Mosby-Year Book, 11830 Westline Industrial Drive, St. Louis, MO 63146. Phone: (800) 325-4177. Fax: (314) 432-1380. Bimonthly.

Journal of Occupational Rehabilitation. Plenum Publishing Co., 233 Spring St., New York, NY 10013-1578. Phone: (212) 620-8000. Fax: (212) 463-0742. Quarterly.

Journal of Rehabilitation Administration. AER, 206 N. Washington St., Alexandria, VA 22314.

Journal of Vision Rehabilitation. AER, 206 N. Washington St., Alexandria, VA 22314.

Journal of Visual Impairment and Blindness. AER, 206 N. Washington St., Alexandria, VA 22314.

NEWSLETTERS

The Physiatrist. American Academy of Physical Medicine and Rehabilitation, 122 S. Michigan Ave., Ste. 1300, Chicago, IL 60603. Phone: (312) 922-9366. 10/year.

ONLINE DATABASES

ABLEDATA. Newington Children's Hospital, Adaptive Equipment Center, 181 E. Cedar St., Newington, CT 06111. Phone: (800) 344-5405. Monthly.

EMBASE. Elsevier Science Publishing Co., Inc., P.O. Box 882, Madison Square Station, New York, NY 10159-2101. Phone: (212) 989-5800. Fax: (212) 633-3990.

MEDLINE. National Library of Medicine, 8600 Rockville Pike, Bethesda, MD 20894. Phone: (800) 638-8480.

SciSearch. Institute for Scientific Information, 3501 Market St., Philadelphia, PA 19104. Phone: (215) 386-0100. Fax: (215) 386-6362.

RESEARCH CENTERS, INSTITUTES, CLEARINGHOUSES

Medical Rehabilitation Research and Training Center. New York University, 400 E. 34th St., New York, NY 10016. Phone: (212) 340-6105.

National Rehabilitation Information Center (NARIC). 8455 Colesville Rd., Ste. 935, Silver Spring, MD 20910. Phone: (800) 34N-ARIC.

Office of Special Education and Rehabilitation Services. U.S. Dept. of Education, 330 C St. S.W., Washington, DC 20202. Phone: (202) 732-1265.

Rehabilitation Institute. 261 Mack Blvd., Detroit, MI 48201. Phone: (313) 494-9731.

Rehabilitation Institute of Chicago. 345 E. Superior, Chicago, IL 60611. Phone: (312) 908-4401.

Rehabilitation Research and Development Center. Edward Hines Jr. V.A. Hospital, P.O. Box 20, Hines, IL 60141. Phone: (708) 216-2240.

Rehabilitation Research Institute. Dept. of Rehabilitation and Psychology, University of Wisconsin-Madison, 432 N. Murray St., Madison, WI 53706. Phone: (608) 263-5971.

Sister Kenny Institute. 800 E. 28th St., Minneapolis, MN 55407. Phone: (612) 332-7036.

TEXTBOOKS AND MONOGRAPHS

Art Therapy: In Theory and Practice. Elinor Ulman, Penny Dachinger (eds.). Random House, Inc., 201 E. 50th St., New York, NY 10022. Phone: (800) 726-0600. 1987.

Art Therapy in Practice. Marian Liebmann. Taylor & Francis Inc., 1900 Frost Rd., Suite 101, Bristol, PA 19007-1598. Phone: (800) 821-8312. Fax: (215) 785-5515. 1990.

Geriatric Rehabilitation. B. Kemp, J.K. Brimmel (eds.). Little, Brown and Co., 34 Beacon St., Boston, MA 02108. Phone: (617) 227-0730. Fax: (617) 227-0790. 1990.

Orthopaedic Rehabilitation. Vernon L. Nickel, Michael J. Botte (eds.). Churchill Livingstone Inc., 650 Avenue of the Americas, New York, NY 10011. Phone: (212) 819-5400. Fax: (212) 302-6598. Second edition 1991.

Physical Rehabilitation: Assessment and Treatment. Susan B. O'Sullivan, Thomas J. Schmitz. F.A. Davis Co., 1915 Arch St., Philadelphia, PA 19103. Phone: (800) 523-4049. Fax: (215) 568-5065. Second edition 1988.

Practical Exercise Therapy. M. Hollis and others. Blackwell Scientific Publications, Inc., 3 Cambridge Ctr., Cambridge, MA 02142. Phone: (800) 759-6102. Third edition 1989.

Practicing Rehabilitation with Geriatric Clients. J.D. Frengley, P. Murray (eds.). Springer Publishing Co., Inc., 536 Broadway, 11th Floor, New York, NY 10012. Phone: (212) 431-4370. 1990.

Pulmonary Rehabilitation. Hodgkin. J.B. Lippincott Co., 227 E. Washington Square, Philadelphia, PA 19106-3780. Phone: (215) 238-4200. Fax: (215) 238-4227. 1993.

Rehabilitation of the Coronary Patient. Nanette Kass Wenger, Herman K. Hellerstein. Churchill Livingstone Inc., 650 Ave. of the Americas, New York, NY 10011. Phone: (212) 819-5400. Fax: (212) 302-6598. Third edition 1992.

Rehabilitation Medicine. Fletcher. Williams & Wilkins, 428 East Preston St., Baltimore, MD 21202. Phone: (800) 638-0672. Fax: (800) 447-8438. 1992.

RENAL DISEASES

See: KIDNEY DISEASES

RENAL HYPERTENSION

See: HYPERTENSION

REPRODUCTION

See also: INFERTILITY

ABSTRACTING, INDEXING, AND CURRENT AWARENESS PUBLICATIONS

Current Contents/Life Sciences. Institute for Scientific Information, 3501 Market St., Philadelphia, PA 19104. Phone: (215) 386-0100. Fax: (215) 386-6362.

Excerpta Medica. Section 10: Obstetrics and Gynecology. Elsevier Science Publishing Co., Inc., P.O. Box 882, Madison Square Station, New York, NY 10159-2101. Phone: (212) 989-5800. Fax: (212) 633-3990. 20/year.

General Science Index. H.W. Wilson Co., 950 University Ave., Bronx, NY 10452. Phone: (800) 367-6770.

Index Medicus. U.S. National Library of Medicine, 8600 Rockville Pike, Bethesda, MD 20894. Phone: (800) 638-8480. Monthly.

Research Alert: Reproductive Endocrinology. Institute for Scientific Information, 3501 Market St., Philadelphia, PA 19104. Phone: (800) 523-1850. Fax: (215) 386-6362. Weekly.

ANNUALS AND REVIEWS

Advances in Human Fertility and Reproductive Endocrinology. Raven Press, 1185 Ave. of the Americas, New York, NY 10036. Phone: (212) 930-9500. Fax: (212) 869-3495.

Infertility and Reproductive Medicine Clinics of North America. W.B. Saunders Co., The Curtis Center, Independence Square W., Philadelphia, PA 19106-3399. Phone: (215) 238-7800. Quarterly.

Progress in Reproductive Biology and Medicine. S. Karger Publishers, Inc., 26 West Avon Rd., P.O. Box 529, Farmington, CT 06085. Phone: (203) 675-7834. Fax: (203) 675-7302. Irregular.

Reproductive Medicine Review. Cambridge University Press, 40 W. 20th St., New York, NY 10011. Phone: (800) 431-1580. Semiannual.

ASSOCIATIONS, PROFESSIONAL SOCIETIES, ADVOCACY AND SUPPORT GROUPS

Association of Reproductive Health Professionals. 900 Pennsylvania Ave. S.E., Washington, DC 20003. Phone: (202) 540-6665.

International Society of Reproductive Medicine (ISRM). 11 Furman Ct., Rancho Mirage, CA 92270. Phone: (619) 340-5080. Fax: (619) 773-1425.

Society for the Study of Reproduction. 309 W. Clark St., Champaign, IL 61820. Phone: (217) 356-3182.

JOURNALS

Archives of Andrology. Taylor & Francis Inc., 1900 Frost Rd., Suite 101, Bristol, PA 19007-1598. Phone: (800) 821-8312. Fax: (215) 785-5515. Bimonthly.

Biology of Reproduction. Society for the Study of Reproduction, 309 W. Clark St., Champaign, IL 61820. Phone: (217) 356-3182.

International Journal of Fertility. MSP International, 347 Fifth Ave., No. 706, New York, NY 10016. Phone: (212) 532-9166.

Journal of Andrology. J.B. Lippincott Co., 227 East Washington Square, Philadelphia, PA 19106-3780. Phone: (215) 238-4200. Fax: (215) 238-4227. Bimonthly.

Journal of Reproductive Immunology. Elsevier Science Publishing Co., Inc., P.O. Box 882, Madison Square Station, New York, NY 10159-2101. Phone: (212) 989-5800. Fax: (212) 633-3990. 6/year.

Journal of Reproductive Medicine. Journal of Reproductive Medicine, Inc., P.O. Drawer 12425, 8342 Olive Blvd., St. Louis, MO 63132. Phone: (314) 991-4440. Fax: (314) 991-4654. Monthly.

Seminars in Reproductive Endocrinology. Thieme Medical Publishers, Inc., 381 Park Ave. S., New York, NY 10016. Phone: (212) 683-5088. Fax: (212) 779-9020. Quarterly.

ONLINE DATABASES

EMBASE. Elsevier Science Publishing Co., Inc., P.O. Box 882, Madison Square Station, New York, NY 10159-2101. Phone: (212) 989-5800. Fax: (212) 633-3990.

MEDLINE. National Library of Medicine, 8600 Rockville Pike, Bethesda, MD 20894. Phone: (800) 638-8480.

SciSearch. Institute for Scientific Information, 3501 Market St., Philadelphia, PA 19104. Phone: (215) 386-0100. Fax: (215) 386-6362.

RESEARCH CENTERS, INSTITUTES, CLEARINGHOUSES

Alan Guttmacher Institute. 111 5th Ave., New York, NY 10003. Phone: (212) 254-5656. Fax: (212) 254-9891.

Center for Population and Family Health. Columbia University. Level B-3, 60 Haven Ave., New York, NY 10032. Phone: (212) 305-6960. Fax: (212) 305-7024.

Center for Reproductive Sciences. Columbia University. 630 W. 168th St., New York, NY 10032. Phone: (212) 305-4178. Fax: (212) 305-3869.

Howard and Georgeanne Jones Institute for Reproductive Medicine. 855 W. Brambleton Ave., Norfolk, VA 23510. Phone: (804) 446-5628.

Kinsey Institute for Research in Sex, Gender, and Reproduction, Inc.. Morrison Hall, 3rd. Fl., Bloomington, IN 47405. Phone: (812) 855-7686. Fax: (812) 855-8277.

Laboratory of Human Reproduction and Reproductive Biology. Harvard University. Harvard Medical School, 45 Shattuck, Boston, MA 02115. Phone: (617) 432-2038. Fax: (617) 566-7980.

Male Reproduction and Microsurgery Unit. Cornell University. Infertility Clinic, Division of Urology, 525 E. 68th. St., Rm. 900, New York, NY 10021. Phone: (615) 576-2866.

UCLA Population Research Center. Harbor-UCLA Medical Center, Walter Martin Research Bldg. RB-1, 1124 W. Carson St., Torrance, CA 90509. Phone: (310) 212-1867. Fax: (310) 320-6515.

TEXTBOOKS AND MONOGRAPHS

Clinical Gynecological Endocrinology and Infertility. Leon Speroff, and others. Williams & Wilkins, 428 East Preston St., Baltimore, MD 21202. Phone: (800) 638-0672. Fax: (800) 447-8438. 4th edition, 1988.

Infertility in the Male. Lipshultz. Mosby-Year Book, 11830 Westline Industrial Drive, St. Louis, MO 63146. Phone: (800) 325-4177. Fax: (314) 432-1380. Second edition 1991.

Introduction to Clinical Reproductive Endocrinology. Gillian C.L. Lachelin. Butterworth-Heinemann, 80 Montvale Ave.,

Stoneham, MA 02180. Phone: (617) 438-8464. Fax: (617) 279-4851. 1991.

Reproductive Endocrinology: Physiology, Pathophysiology and Clinical Management. Samuel S.C. Yen, Robert B. Jaffe. W.B. Saunders Co., The Curtis Center, Independence Sqare W., Philadelphia, PA 19106-3399. Phone: (215) 238-7800. 1991.

RESEARCH SUPPORT

ABSTRACTING, INDEXING, AND CURRENT AWARENESS PUBLICATIONS

Biomedical Index to PHS Supported Research. Public Health Service. National Institutes of Health, 5333 Westbard Ave., Rm. 148, Bethesda, MD 20892. Phone: (301) 496-7543. Fax: (301) 496-9975. Annual.

Research Awards Index. U.S. Government Printing Office, Superintendent of Documents, P.O. Box 371954, Pittsburgh, PA 15250-7954. Phone: (202) 783-3238. Fax: (202) 512-2250.

ASSOCIATIONS, PROFESSIONAL SOCIETIES, ADVOCACY AND SUPPORT GROUPS

National Research Council of Canada. Montreal Rd., Bldg. M-58, Ottawa, ON, Canada K1A 0R6. Phone: (613) 993-9101. Fax: (613) 952-9696.

DIRECTORIES

Directory of Biomedical and Health Care Grants. Oryx Press, 4041 N. Central, Suite 700, Phoenix, AZ 85012. Phone: (800) 279-ORYX. Fax: (800) 279-4663. Annual.

Directory of Research Grants. Oryx Press, 4041 N. Central, Suite 700, Phoenix, AZ 85012. Phone: (800) 279-ORYX. Fax: (800) 279-4663. Annual.

Foundation Directory. The Foundation Center, 79 Fifth Ave., New York, NY 10003. Phone: (212) 620-4230.

National Institutes of Health-Research Grants. National Institutes of Health, 5333 Westbard Ave., Bethesda, MD 20892. Phone: (301) 496-7441. Annual.

Research Centers Directory. Karen Hill (ed.). Gale Research, Inc., 835 Penobscot Bldg., Detroit, MI 48226-4094. Phone: (800) 877-GALE. Fax: (313) 961-6083. 1992.

HANDBOOKS, GUIDES, MANUALS, ATLASES

Guidelines for Preparing Proposals. Roy Meador. CRC Press, Inc., 2000 Corporate Blvd. N.W., Boca Raton, FL 33431. Phone: (407) 994-0555. Fax: (407) 997-0949. Second edition 1991.

ONLINE DATABASES

Federal Research in Progress (FEDRIP). U.S. National Technical Information Service, 5285 Port Royal Rd., Springfield, VA 22161. Phone: (703) 487-4650. Fax: (703) 321-8547.

Foundation Directory. The Foundation Center, 79 Fifth Ave., New York, NY 10003. Phone: (212) 620-4230.

Foundation Grants Index. The Foundation Center, 79 Fifth Ave., New York, NY 10003. Phone: (212) 620-4230. Bimonthly.

The Grants Database. Oryx Press, 4041 N. Central, Suite 700, Phoenix, AZ 85012. Phone: (800) 279-ORYX. Fax: (800) 279-4663.

Health Grants & Contracts Weekly. Capitol Publishing Group, P.O. Box 1453, Alexandria, VA 22313-2053. Phone: (703) 683-4100. Fax: (703) 739-6490. Weekly.

Research Centers Directory. Gale Research, Inc., 835 Penobscot Bldg., Detroit, MI 48226-4094. Phone: (800) 877-GALE. Fax: (313) 961-6083.

RESEARCH CENTERS, INSTITUTES, CLEARINGHOUSES

The Grantsmanship Center. 1125 W. Sixth St., Los Angeles, CA 90017. Phone: (213) 482-9863.

The Pew Charitable Trusts. Three Parkway, Ste. 501, Philadelphia, PA 19102-1305. Phone: (215) 568-3330.

Robert Wood Johnson Foundation. P.O. Box 2316, Princeton, NJ 08543-2316. Phone: (609) 452-8701.

W.K. Kellogg Foundation. 400 North Ave., Battle Creek, MI 49017-3398. Phone: (616) 968-1611.

TEXTBOOKS AND MONOGRAPHS

Getting Funded: A Complete Guide to Proposal Writing. Mary Hall. Continuing Education Publications, P.O. Box 1394, Portland State University, Portland, OR 97207. Phone: (503) 464-4891. 3rd edition.

Proposal Writing and Planning. Lynn E. Miner, Jerry Griffith. Oryx Press, 4041 N. Central, Suite 700, Phoenix, AZ 85012. Phone: (800) 279-6799. Fax: (800) 279-4663. 1992.

Research Proposals: A Guide to Success. Thomas E. Ogden. Raven Press, 1185 Avenue of the Americas, New York, NY 10036. Phone: (212) 930-9500. Fax: (212) 869-3495. 1991.

Successful Grant Application. Diane Reif-Lehrer. Jones & Bartlett Publishers, Inc., 20 Park Plaza, Boston, MA 02116. Phone: (800) 832-0034. 2nd edition, 1989.

A Systems Approach to Marketing and Grant Writing. Jean S. Morgenweck, Elnora M. Gilfoyle. SLACK Inc., 6900 Grove Rd., Thorofare, NJ 08086-9447. Phone: (800) 257-8290. Fax: (609) 853-5991. 1992.

RESIDENCY

See: MEDICAL EDUCATION

RESPIRATORY DISTRESS

See: RESPIRATORY TRACT INFECTIONS

RESPIRATORY THERAPY

See also: ALLIED HEALTH EDUCATION;
LUNG DISEASES; RESPIRATORY TRACT
INFECTIONS

ABSTRACTING, INDEXING, AND CURRENT AWARENESS PUBLICATIONS

Cumulative Index to Nursing and Allied Health Literature. Glendale Adventist Medical Center, P.O. Box 871, Glendale, CA 91209. Phone: (818) 409-8005. Bimonthly.

Index Medicus. U.S. National Library of Medicine, 8600 Rockville Pike, Bethesda, MD 20894. Phone: (800) 638-8480. Monthly.

ASSOCIATIONS, PROFESSIONAL SOCIETIES, ADVOCACY AND SUPPORT GROUPS

American Association for Respiratory Care (AARC). 11030 Ables Ln., Dallas, TX 75229. Phone: (214) 243-2272. Fax: (214) 484-2720.

National Board for Respiratory Care (NBRC). 8310 Nieman Rd., Lenexa, KS 66214. Phone: (913) 599-4200.

CD-ROM DATABASES

Nursing and Allied Health (CINAHL) on CD-ROM. CINAHL, 1509 Wilson Terrace, P.O. Box 871, Glendale, CA 91209-0871. Phone: (818) 409-8005.

ENCYCLOPEDIAS, DICTIONARIES, WORD BOOKS

Mosby's Medical, Nursing, and Allied Health Dictionary. Kenneth N. Anderson, Lois Anderson, Walter D. Glanze (eds.). Mosby-Year Book, 11830 Westline Industrial Dr., St. Louis, MO 63146. Phone: (800) 325-4177. Fax: (314) 432-1380. Third edition 1990.

HANDBOOKS, GUIDES, MANUALS, ATLASES

Handbook of Respiratory Care. Robert L. Chatburn, Marvin D. Lough. Mosby-Year Book, 11830 Westline Industrial Drive, St. Louis, MO 63146. Phone: (800) 325-4177. Fax: (314) 432-1380. Second edition 1990.

Manual of Pulmonary Function Testing. Gregg Rupper. Mosby-Year Book, 11830 Westline Industrial Drive, St. Louis, MO 63146. Phone: (800) 325-4177. Fax: (314) 432-1380. 5th edition, 1991.

JOURNALS

Respiration. S. Karger Publishers, Inc., 26 W. Avon Rd., P.O. Box 529, Farmington, CT 06085. Phone: (203) 675-7834. Fax: (203) 675-7302.

Respiratory Medicine. Balliere Tindall, 24-28 Oval Rd., London NW1 7DX, England.

ONLINE DATABASES

Nursing and Allied Health (CINAHL). CINAHL, 1509 Wilson Terrace, P.O. Box 871, Glendale, CA 91209-0871. Phone: (818) 409-8005.

TEXTBOOKS AND MONOGRAPHS

Clinical Application of Respiratory Care. Barry A. Shapiro, and others. Mosby-Year Book, 11830 Westline Industrial Drive, St. Louis, MO 63146. Phone: (800) 325-4177. Fax: (314) 432-1380. 4th edition, 1991.

Egan's Fundamentals of Respiratory Care. Craig L. Scanlan and others (eds.). Mosby-Year Book, 11830 Westline Industrial Drive, St. Louis, MO 63146. Phone: (800) 325-4177. Fax: (314) 432-1380. Fifth edition 1990.

Introduction to Respiratory Care. Michael G. Levitzky, and others. W.B. Saunders Co., The Curtis Center, Independence Square W., Philadelphia, PA 19106-3399. Phone: (215) 238-7800. 1990.

Monitoring in Respiratory Care. Robert M. Kacmarck. Mosby-Year Book, 11830 Westline Industrial Drive, St. Louis, MO 63146. Phone: (800) 325-4177. Fax: (314) 432-1380. 1992.

Principles of Patient Management in Respiratory Care. Robert L. Wilkins, James R. Dexter. F.A. Davis Co., 1915 Arch St., Philadelphia, PA 19103. Phone: (800) 523-4049. Fax: (215) 568-5065. 1992.

Respiratory Care Principles: A Programmed Guide to Entry-Level Practice. Thomas A. Barnes. F.A. Davis Co., 1915 Arch St., Philadelphia, PA 19103. Phone: (800) 523-4049. Fax: (215) 568-5065. Third edition 1991.

Respiratory Therapy Equipment. Steven P. McPherson, Charles B. Spearman. Mosby-Year Book, 11830 Westline Industrial Drive, St. Louis, MO 63146. Phone: (800) 325-4177. Fax: (314) 432-1380. Fourth edition 1990.

RESPIRATORY TRACT INFECTIONS

See also: ASTHMA; LUNG DISEASES

ABSTRACTING, INDEXING, AND CURRENT AWARENESS PUBLICATIONS

Cumulative Index to Nursing and Allied Health Literature. Glendale Adventist Medical Center, P.O. Box 871, Glendale, CA 91209. Phone: (818) 409-8005. Bimonthly.

Current Contents/Clinical Medicine. Institute for Scientific Information, 3501 Market St., Philadelphia, PA 19104. Phone: (800) 523-1850. Fax: (215) 386-6362. Weekly.

Excerpta Medica. Section 15: Chest Diseases, Thoracic Surgery and Tuberculosis. Elsevier Science Publishing Co., Inc., P.O. Box 882, Madison Square Station, New York, NY 10159-2101. Phone: (212) 989-5800. Fax: (212) 633-3990. 20/year.

Index Medicus. U.S. National Library of Medicine, 8600 Rockville Pike, Bethesda, MD 20894. Phone: (800) 638-8480. Monthly.

Science Citation Index. Institute for Scientific Information, 3501 Market St., Philadelphia, PA 19104. Phone: (800) 523-1850. Fax: (215) 386-6362. Bimonthly.

ANNUALS AND REVIEWS

Clinics in Chest Medicine. W.B. Saunders Co., The Curtis Center, Independence Square W., Philadelphia, PA 19106-3399. Phone: (215) 238-7800. Quarterly.

Current Pulmonology. Mosby-Year Book, 11830 Westline Industrial Drive, St. Louis, MO 63146. Phone: (800) 325-4177. Fax: (314) 432-1380.

ASSOCIATIONS, PROFESSIONAL SOCIETIES, ADVOCACY AND SUPPORT GROUPS

American Broncho-Esophageal Association. c/o Loren D. Holinger, 155 N. Michigan Ave., No. 325, Chicago, IL 60601. Phone: (312) 938-1990.

American Lung Association (ALA). 1740 Broadway, New York, NY 10019. Phone: (212) 315-8700. Fax: (212) 265-5642.

American Thoracic Society (ATS). 1740 Broadway, New York, NY 10019-4374. Phone: (212) 315-8700.

CD-ROM DATABASES

SCISEARCH. Institute for Scientific Information, 3501 Market St., Philadelphia, PA 19104. Phone: (215) 386-0100. Fax: (215) 386-6362.

HANDBOOKS, GUIDES, MANUALS, ATLASES

A Color Atlas of Respiratory Diseases. D. Geraint, James Peter, R. Studdy. Mosby-Year Book, 11830 Westline Industrial Drive, St. Louis, MO 63146. Phone: (800) 325-4177. Fax: (314) 432-1380. 1993.

A Laboratory Manual for Legionella. T.G. Harrison, A.G. Taylor (eds.). John Wiley & Sons, Inc., 605 Third Ave., New York, NY 10158-0012. Phone: (212) 850-6000. Fax: (212) 850-6088. 1988.

Manual of Clinical Problems in Pulmonary Medicine: With Annotated Key References. Richard A. Bordow, Kenneth M. Moser (eds.). Little, Brown and Company, 34 Beacon St., Boston, MA 02108. Phone: (617) 227-0730. Third edition 1991.

Pulmonary Diseases & Disorders: Companion Handbook. Alfred P. Fishman. McGraw-Hill, Inc., 1221 Avenue of the Americas, 28th Floor, New York, NY 10020. Phone: (212) 512-4228. Second edition 1992.

JOURNALS

American Review of Respiratory Diseases. American Lung Association, 1740 Broadway, New York, NY 10019. Phone: (212) 315-8700. Fax: (212) 265-5642.

Chest. American College of Chest Physicians, 911 Busse Hwy., Park Ridge, IL 60068. Phone: (708) 698-2200. Fax: (708) 698-1791. Monthly.

Journal of Biomechanics. Pergamon Press, 660 White Plains Rd., Tarrytown, NY 10591-5153. Phone: (914) 592-7700. Fax: (914) 592-3625. Monthly.

Respiration. S. Karger Publishers, Inc., 26 W. Avon Rd., P.O. Box 529, Farmington, CT 06085. Phone: (203) 675-7834. Fax: (203) 675-7302.

Respiratory Care. Daedalus Enterprises Inc., 11030 Ables Lane, Dallas, TX 75229. Phone: (214) 243-2272.

Respiratory Management. Choices Publishing Group, 129 Washington St., Hoboken, NJ 07030. Phone: (201) 792-1900.

Tubercle. Churchill Livingstone Inc., 650 Ave. of the Americas, New York, NY 10011. Phone: (212) 819-5400. Fax: (212) 302-6598.

ONLINE DATABASES

EMBASE. Elsevier Science Publishing Co., Inc., P.O. Box 882, Madison Square Station, New York, NY 10159-2101. Phone: (212) 989-5800. Fax: (212) 633-3990.

MEDLINE. National Library of Medicine, 8600 Rockville Pike, Bethesda, MD 20894. Phone: (800) 638-8480.

SciSearch. Institute for Scientific Information, 3501 Market St., Philadelphia, PA 19104. Phone: (215) 386-0100. Fax: (215) 386-6362.

POPULAR WORKS AND PATIENT EDUCATION

The Chronic Bronchitis and Emphysema Handbook. Francois Haas, Sheila Sperber Haas. John Wiley & Sons, Inc., 605 Third Ave., New York, NY 10158-0012. Phone: (212) 850-6000. Fax: (212) 850-6088. 1990.

Living Well with Chronic Asthma, Bronchitis, and Emphysema: A Complete Guide to Coping with Chronic Lung Disease. Myra B. Shayevitz, Berton R. Shayevitz. Consumer Reports Books, 9180 LeSaint Dr., Fairfield, OH 45014. Phone: (513) 860-1178. 1991.

RESEARCH CENTERS, INSTITUTES, CLEARINGHOUSES

National Jewish Center for Immunology and Respiratory Medicine. 1400 Jackson St., Denver, CO 80206. Phone: (303) 388-4461.

Respiratory Research Group. University of Calgary. 1634 Health Sciences Centre, 3330 Hospital Dr. N.W., Calgary, AB, Canada T2N 4N1. Phone: (403) 220-4516.

TEXTBOOKS AND MONOGRAPHS

Adult Respiratory Distress Syndrome. Artigas. Churchill Livingstone Inc., 650 Ave. of the Americas, New York, NY 10011. Phone: (212) 819-5400. Fax: (212) 302-6598. 1992.

Decision Making in Pulmonary Medicine. Karlinsky. Mosby-Year Book, 11830 Westline Industrial Drive, St. Louis, MO 63146. Phone: (800) 325-4177. Fax: (314) 432-1380. 1991.

Eagan's Fundamentals of Respiratory Care. Scanlan. Mosby-Year Book, 11830 Westline Industrial Drive, St. Louis, MO 63146. Phone: (800) 325-4177. Fax: (314) 432-1380. Fifth editin 1990.

Foundations of Respiratory Care. Pierson. Churchill Livingstone Inc., 650 Ave. of the Americas, New York, NY 10011. Phone: (212) 819-5400. Fax: (212) 302-6598. 1992.

Pulmonary Rehabilitation. Hodgkin. J.B. Lippincott Co., 227 E. Washington Square, Philadelphia, PA 19106-3780. Phone: (215) 238-4200. Fax: (215) 238-4227. 1993.

Respiratory Infections: Diagnosis and Management. James E. Pennington. Raven Press, 1185 Avenue of the Americas, New York, NY 10036. Phone: (212) 930-9500. Fax: (212) 869-3495. Second edition 1989.

Respiratory Medicine. R.A.L. Brewis and others. W.B. Saunders Co., The Curtis Center, Independence Square W., Philadelphia, PA 19106-3399. Phone: (215) 238-7800. 1990.

Synopsis of Clinical Pulmonary Disease. Mitchell. Mosby-Year Book, 11830 Westline Industrial Drive, St. Louis, MO 63146. Phone: (800) 325-4177. Fax: (314) 432-1380. Fourth edition 1989.

Update: Pulmonary Diseases and Disorders. Fishman. McGraw-Hill Inc., 11 West 19th St., New York, NY 10011. Phone: (212) 337-5001. Fax: (212) 337-4092. 1992.

RESUSCITATION

See: CARDIOPULMONARY RESUSCITATION; EMERGENCY MEDICINE

RETARDATION

See: MENTAL RETARDATION

RETINAL DISEASES

See: EYE DISEASES

REYE'S SYNDROME

See also: VIRAL DISEASES

ABSTRACTING, INDEXING, AND CURRENT AWARENESS PUBLICATIONS

Current Contents/Clinical Medicine. Institute for Scientific Information, 3501 Market St., Philadelphia, PA 19104. Phone: (800) 523-1850. Fax: (215) 386-6362. Weekly.

Excerpta Medica. Section 7: Pediatrics and Pediatric Surgery. Elsevier Science Publishing Co., Inc., P.O. Box 882, Madison Square Station, New York, NY 10159-2101. Phone: (212) 989-5800. Fax: (212) 633-3990. 24/year.

Index Medicus. U.S. National Library of Medicine, 8600 Rockville Pike, Bethesda, MD 20894. Phone: (800) 638-8480. Monthly.

ANNUALS AND REVIEWS

Current Problems in Pediatrics. Mosby-Year Book, 11830 Westline Industrial Drive, St. Louis, MO 63146. Phone: (800) 325-4177. Fax: (314) 432-1380. 10/year.

ASSOCIATIONS, PROFESSIONAL SOCIETIES, ADVOCACY AND SUPPORT GROUPS

American Academy of Pediatrics (AAP). 141 Northwest Point Blvd., P.O. Box 927, Elk Grove Village, IL 60009-0927. Phone: (708) 228-5005. Fax: (708) 228-5097.

National Reye's Syndrome Foundation (NRSF). 426 N. Lewis, P.O. Box 829, Bryan, OH 43506. Phone: (419) 626-2679.

CD-ROM DATABASES

Journal of the American Medical Association. Macmillan New Media, 124 Mt. Auburn St., Cambridge, MA 02138. Weekly.

Pediatrics on Disc. CMC ReSearch, Inc., 7150 S.W. Hampton, Suite C-120, Portland, OR 97223. Phone: (800) 262-7668. Fax: (503) 639-1796. Annual.

HANDBOOKS, GUIDES, MANUALS, ATLASES

Handbook of Pediatric Emergencies. Baldwin. Little, Brown and Co., 34 Beacon St., Boston, MA 02108. Phone: (617) 227-0730. Fax: (617) 227-0790. 1989.

JOURNALS

American Journal of Diseases of Children. American Medical Association, 515 North State St., Chicago, IL 60610. Phone: (312) 464-0183. Fax: (312) 464-5834. Monthly.

Archives of Disease in Childhood. BMJ Publishing Group, BMA House, Tavistock Square, London WC1H 9JR, England. Phone: 071-383 6244/6638. Fax: 071-383 6662. Monthly.

Journal of Pediatrics. Mosby-Year Book, 11830 Westline Industrial Drive, St. Louis, MO 63146. Phone: (800) 325-4177. Fax: (314) 432-1380. Monthly.

The New England Journal of Medicine. Massachusetts Medical Society, 1440 Main St., Waltham, MA 02154-1649. Phone: (617) 893-3800. Fax: (617) 893-0413. Weekly.

Pediatrics. American Academy of Pediatrics, 141 Northwest Point Rd., Elk Grove Village, IL 60009-0927. Phone: (708) 228-5005. Fax: (708) 228-5097. Monthly.

NEWSLETTERS

National Reye's Syndrome Foundation-In the News. National Reye's Syndrome Foundation, P.O. Box 829, Bryan, OH 43506. Phone: (313) 987-3625. Semiannual.

ONLINE DATABASES

EMBASE. Elsevier Science Publishing Co., Inc., P.O. Box 882, Madison Square Station, New York, NY 10159-2101. Phone: (212) 989-5800. Fax: (212) 633-3990.

MEDLINE. National Library of Medicine, 8600 Rockville Pike, Bethesda, MD 20894. Phone: (800) 638-8480.

SciSearch. Institute for Scientific Information, 3501 Market St., Philadelphia, PA 19104. Phone: (215) 386-0100. Fax: (215) 386-6362.

POPULAR WORKS AND PATIENT EDUCATION

Childhood Symptoms: Every Parent's Guide to Childhood Illnesses. Edward R. Brace, John P. Pacanaowski. HarperCollins Pubs., Inc., 10 E. 53rd St., New York, NY 10022-5299. Phone: (212) 207-7000. Revised edition 1992.

The Columbia University College of Physicians and Surgeons Complete Guide to Early Child Care. Genell Subak-Sharpe (ed.). Random House, Inc., 201 E. 50th St., New York, NY 10022. Phone: (800) 726-0600. 1990.

TEXTBOOKS AND MONOGRAPHS

Nelson Textbook of Pediatrics. Richard E. Behrman, Victor C. Vaughan. W.B. Saunders Co., The Curtis Center, Independence Sqare W., Philadelphia, PA 19106-3399. Phone: (215) 238-7800. 14th edition, 1992.

Pediatric Emergency Medicine. Barkin. Mosby-Year Book, 11830 Westline Industrial Drive, St. Louis, MO 63146. Phone: (800) 325-4177. Fax: (314) 432-1380. 1992.

RHEUMATIC DISEASES

See: ARTHRITIS; RHEUMATOLOGY

RHEUMATIC FEVER

See: RHEUMATOLOGY

RHEUMATIC HEART DISEASE

See: HEART DISEASES; RHEUMATOLOGY

RHEUMATISM

See: ARTHRITIS

RHEUMATOID ARTHRITIS

See: ARTHRITIS

RHEUMATOLOGY

See also: ARTHRITIS

ABSTRACTING, INDEXING, AND CURRENT AWARENESS PUBLICATIONS

Current Contents/Clinical Medicine. Institute for Scientific Information, 3501 Market St., Philadelphia, PA 19104. Phone: (800) 523-1850. Fax: (215) 386-6362. Weekly.

Excerpta Medica. Section 31. Arthritis and Rheumatism. Elsevier Science Publishing Co., Inc., P.O. Box 882, Madison Square Station, New York, NY 10159-2101. Phone: (212) 989-5800. Fax: (212) 633-3990. 8/year.

Science Citation Index. Institute for Scientific Information, 3501 Market St., Philadelphia, PA 19104. Phone: (800) 523-1850. Fax: (215) 386-6362. Bimonthly.

ANNUALS AND REVIEWS

Current Opinion in Rheumatology. Current Science Ltd., 20 N. Third St., Philadelphia, PA 19106-2199. Phone: (800) 552-5866. Fax: (215) 574-2270. Bimonthly.

Rheumatic Disease Clinics. W.B. Saunders Co., The Curtis Center, Independence Square W., Philadelphia, PA 19106-3399. Phone: (215) 238-7800. Quarterly.

Rheumatology Review. Churchill Livingstone Inc., 650 Avenue of the Americas, New York, NY 10011. Phone: (212) 819-5400. Fax: (212) 302-6598. Quarterly.

ASSOCIATIONS, PROFESSIONAL SOCIETIES, ADVOCACY AND SUPPORT GROUPS

American College of Rheumatology (ACR). 17 Executive Park Dr. N.E., Ste. 480, Atlanta, GA 30329. Phone: (404) 633-3777. Fax: (404) 633-1870.

American Juvenile Arthritis Organization (AJAO). 1314 Spring St. N.W., Atlanta, GA 30309. Phone: (404) 872-7100. Fax: (404) 872-0457.

American Rheumatism Association. 17 Executive Park Dr. N.E., Atlanta, GA 30329. Phone: (404) 633-3777.

Arthritis Foundation (AF). 1314 Spring St. N.W., Atlanta, GA 30309. Phone: (404) 872-2100. Fax: (404) 872-0457.

CD-ROM DATABASES

SCISEARCH. Institute for Scientific Information, 3501 Market St., Philadelphia, PA 19104. Phone: (215) 386-0100. Fax: (215) 386-6362.

DIRECTORIES

Directory of Medical Specialists. Marquis Who's Who, 3002 Glenview Rd., Wilmette, IL 60091. Phone: (800) 621-9669. Fax: (708) 441-2264. Biennial.

Directory of Physicians in the United States. American Medical Association, 515 North State St., Chicago, IL 60610. Phone: (312) 464-0183. Fax: (312) 464-5834. Biennial.

HANDBOOKS, GUIDES, MANUALS, ATLASES

A Color Atlas of Rheumatology. M. Shipley. Mosby-Year Book, 11830 Westline Industrial Drive, St. Louis, MO 63146. Phone: (800) 325-4177. Fax: (314) 432-1380. Third edition 1992.

Handbook of Drug Therapy in Rheumatic Disease: Pharmacology and Clinical Aspects. Joe G. Hardin Jr., Gesina L. Longenecker. Little, Brown and Company, 34 Beacon St., Boston, MA 02108. Phone: (617) 227-0730. 1992.

Manual of Rheumatology and Outpatient Orthopedic Disorders: Diagnosis and Therapy. Stephen Paget, John F. Beary, Charles L. Christian, et. al.. Little, Brown and Company, 34 Beacon St., Boston, MA 02108. Phone: (617) 227-0730. Third edition 1992.

JOURNALS

Annals of the Rheumatic Diseases. BMJ Publishing Group, BMA House, Tavistock Square, London WC1H 9JR, England. Phone: 071-383 6244/6638. Fax: 071-383 6662. Monthly.

Arthritis and Rheumatism. American College of Rheumatology, 17 Executive Park Dr. N.E., Ste. 480, Atlanta, GA 30329. Phone: (404) 633-3777. Fax: (404) 663-1870. Monthly.

British Journal of Rheumatology. Balliere Tindall, 24-28 Oval Rd., London NW1 7DX, England. Bimonthly.

Journal of Rheumatology. Journal of Rheumatology Publishing Co., 920 Yonge St., Ste. 115, Toronto, ON, Canada M4W 3C7. Phone: (416) 967-5155. Fax: (416) 967-7556. Monthly.

Rheumatology International. Springer-Verlag New York Inc., 175 Fifth Ave., New York, NY 10010. Phone: (212) 460-1500. Fax: (212) 473-6272.

Seminars in Arthritis and Rheumatism. W.B. Saunders Co., The Curtis Center, Independence Sqare W., Philadelphia, PA 19106-3399. Phone: (215) 238-7800.

NEWSLETTERS

Bulletin on the Rheumatic Diseases. Arthritis Foundation, 1314 Sprin St., N.W., Atlanta, GA 30309. Phone: (404) 872-7100. Fax: (404) 872-0457. Bimonthly.

ONLINE DATABASES

Combined Health Information Database (CHID). U.S. National Institutes of Health, P.O. Box NDIC, Bethesda, MD 20892. Phone: (301) 496-2162. Fax: (301) 770-5164. Quarterly.

POPULAR WORKS AND PATIENT EDUCATION

Comprehensive Guide to Arthritis. James F. Fries. Addison-Wesley Publishing Co., Rte. 128, Reading, MA 01867. Phone: (800) 447-2226. Third edition 1990.

RESEARCH CENTERS, INSTITUTES, CLEARINGHOUSES

National Arthritis and Musculoskeletal and Skin Diseases Information Clearinghouse (NAMSIC). 9000 Rockville Pike, P.O. Box AMS, Bethesda, MD 20892. Phone: (301) 495-4484. Fax: (301) 587-4352.

National Institute of Arthritis and Musculoskeletal and Skin Diseases. NIH Bldg. 31, 9000 Rockville Pike, Bethesda, MD 20892. Phone: (301) 496-4353.

TEXTBOOKS AND MONOGRAPHS

Arthritis and Allied Conditions. D.J. McCarty. Williams & Wilkins, 428 East Preston St., Baltimore, MD 21202. Phone: (800) 638-0672. Fax: (800) 447-8438.

Arthritis and Rheumatology in Practice. Dieppe. J.B. Lippincott Co., 227 E. Washington Square, Philadelphia, PA 19106-3780. Phone: (215) 238-4200. Fax: (215) 238-4227. 1991.

Current Therapy in Allergy, Immunology and Rheumatology. Lawrence M. Lichtenstein, Anthony Fauci. Mosby-Year Book, 11830 Westline Industrial Drive, St. Louis, MO 63146. Phone: (800) 325-4177. Fax: (314) 432-1380. Fourth edition 1991.

Textbook of Rheumatology. W.N. Kelley. W.B. Saunders Co., The Curtis Center, Independence Sqare W., Philadelphia, PA 19106-3399. Phone: (215) 238-7800.

RHINITIS

See: OTOLARYNGOLOGY

RHINOPLASTY

See: PLASTIC AND COSMETIC SURGERY

RICKETS

See: BONE AND JOINT DISEASES

RINGWORM

See: FUNGAL DISEASES

ROCKY MOUNTAIN SPOTTED FEVER

See: INFECTIOUS DISEASES

S

SALMONELLA

See: FOOD POISONING

SARCOMA

See: CANCER

SCABIES

See: INFECTIOUS DISEASES

SCHIZOPHRENIA

See also: PSYCHIATRIC DISORDERS

ABSTRACTING, INDEXING, AND CURRENT AWARENESS PUBLICATIONS

Current Contents/Clinical Medicine. Institute for Scientific Information, 3501 Market St., Philadelphia, PA 19104. Phone: (800) 523-1850. Fax: (215) 386-6362. Weekly.

Excerpta Medica. Section 32: Psychiatry. Elsevier Science Publishing Co., Inc., P.O. Box 882, Madison Square Station, New York, NY 10159-2101. Phone: (212) 989-5800. Fax: (212) 633-3990. 20/year.

Index Medicus. U.S. National Library of Medicine, 8600 Rockville Pike, Bethesda, MD 20894. Phone: (800) 638-8480. Monthly.

Psychological Abstracts. American Psychological Association, 1200 17th St. NW, Washington, DC 20036. Phone: (202) 955-7600. Monthly.

Research Alert: Schizophrenia/Psychotic Disorders. Institute for Scientific Information, 3501 Market St., Philadelphia, PA 19104. Phone: (800) 523-1850. Fax: (215) 386-6362. Weekly.

Science Citation Index. Institute for Scientific Information, 3501 Market St., Philadelphia, PA 19104. Phone: (800) 523-1850. Fax: (215) 386-6362. Bimonthly.

ANNUALS AND REVIEWS

Progress in Psychiatry. American Psychiatric Press, Inc., 1400 K St. NW, Washington, DC 20005. Phone: (202) 682-6268. Fax: (202) 789-2648. Irregular.

ASSOCIATIONS, PROFESSIONAL SOCIETIES, ADVOCACY AND SUPPORT GROUPS

American Orthopsychiatric Association (ORTHO). 19 W. 44th St., No. 1616, New York, NY 10036. Phone: (212) 354-5770. Fax: (212) 302-9463.

American Psychiatric Association (APA). 1400 K St. N.W., Washington, DC 20005. Phone: (202) 682-6000. Fax: (202) 682-6114.

American Schizophrenia Asociation (ASA). 900 N. Federal Hwy., Ste. 330, Boca Raton, FL 33432. Phone: (407) 393-6167.

Canadian Psychiatric Association. 294 Albert St., Suite 204, Ottawa, ON, Canada K1P 6E6. Phone: (613) 234-2815. Fax: (613) 234-9857.

National Alliance for Research on Schizophrenia and Depression. 60 Cutter Mill Rd., Great Neck, NY 11021. Phone: (516) 829-0091.

CD-ROM DATABASES

Excerpta Medica CD: Psychiatry. SilverPlatter Information, Inc., River Ridge Office Park, 100 River Ridge Rd., Norwood, MA 02062. Phone: (617) 769-2599. Fax: (617) 769-8763. Quarterly.

PC MASS-Psychiatry. Educational Reviews, Inc., 6801 Cahaba Valley Rd., Birmingham, AL 35242. Phone: (800) 633-4743. Fax: (205) 995-1926. Monthly.

PsycLit. SilverPlatter Information, Inc., River Ridge Office Park, 100 River Ridge Rd., Norwood, MA 02062. Phone: (617) 769-2599. Fax: (617) 769-8763. Quarterly.

SCISEARCH. Institute for Scientific Information, 3501 Market St., Philadelphia, PA 19104. Phone: (215) 386-0100. Fax: (215) 386-6362.

ENCYCLOPEDIAS, DICTIONARIES, WORD BOOKS

Encyclopedia of Schizophrenia and the Psychotic Disorders. Richard Noll. Facts on File, Inc., 460 Park Ave. S., New York, NY 10016-7382. Phone: (212) 683-2244. Fax: (212) 683-3633. 1992.

Psychiatry Words. Stedman. Williams & Wilkins, 428 East Preston St., Baltimore, MD 21202. Phone: (800) 638-0672. Fax: (800) 447-8438. 1992.

HANDBOOKS, GUIDES, MANUALS, ATLASES

Getting Help: A Consumer's Guide to Therapy. Christine Amner. Paragon House Publishers, 90 Fifth Ave., New York, NY 10011. Phone: (800) 727-2466. 1991.

Handbook of Schizophrenia. Volume 4: Psychosocial Treatment of Schizophrenia. M.L. Herz, S.J. Keith, J.P. Docherty (eds.). Elsevier Science Publishing Co., Inc., P.O. Box 882, Madison Square Station, New York, NY 10159-2101. Phone: (212) 989-5800. Fax: (212) 633-3990. 1990.

Schizophrenia: A Handbook for Clinical Care. Judy A. Malone (ed.). SLACK Inc., 6900 Grove Rd., Thorofare, NJ 08086-9447. Phone: (800) 257-8290. Fax: (609) 853-5991. 1992.

JOURNALS

American Journal of Psychiatry. American Psychiatric Press, Inc., 1400 K St. NW, Washington, DC 20005. Phone: (202) 682-6268. Fax: (202) 789-2648. Monthly.

Archives of General Psychiatry. American Medical Association, 515 North State St., Chicago, IL 60610. Phone: (312) 464-0183. Fax: (312) 464-5834. Monthly.

Harvard Review of Psychiatry. Mosby-Year Book, 11830 Westline Industrial Drive, St. Louis, MO 63146. Phone: (800) 325-4177. Fax: (314) 432-1380. Bimonthly.

Schizophrenia Bulletin. Center for Studies of Schizophrenia, Alcohol, Drug Abuse and Mental Health Admin., 5600 Fishers Lane, Rockville, MD 20857. Phone: (301) 496-4000.

Schizophrenia Research. Elsevier Science Publishing Co., Inc., P.O. Box 882, Madison Square Station, New York, NY 10159-2101. Phone: (212) 989-5800. Fax: (212) 633-3990. 6/year.

NEWSLETTERS

Harvard Mental Health Letter. Harvard Medical School Publications Group, 164 Longwood Ave., Boston, MA 02115. Monthly.

ONLINE DATABASES

EMBASE. Elsevier Science Publishing Co., Inc., P.O. Box 882, Madison Square Station, New York, NY 10159-2101. Phone: (212) 989-5800. Fax: (212) 633-3990.

MEDLINE. National Library of Medicine, 8600 Rockville Pike, Bethesda, MD 20894. Phone: (800) 638-8480.

Mental Health Abstracts. IFI/Plenum Data Company, 302 Swann Ave., Alexandria, VA 22301. Phone: (800) 368-3093. Monthly.

PsycInfo. SilverPlatter Information, Inc., River Ridge Office Park, 100 River Ridge Rd., Norwood, MA 02062. Phone: (617) 769-2599. Fax: (617) 769-8763. Quarterly.

SciSearch. Institute for Scientific Information, 3501 Market St., Philadelphia, PA 19104. Phone: (215) 386-0100. Fax: (215) 386-6362.

POPULAR WORKS AND PATIENT EDUCATION

The Columbia University College of Physicians and Surgeons Complete Home Guide to Mental and Emotional Health. Frederic I. Kass, John M. Oldham, Herbert Pardes, and others. Holt, Rinehart & Winston, 115 W. 18th St., New York, NY 10011. Phone: (800) 488-5233. 1992.

Surviving Schizophrenia: A Family Manual. E. Fuller Torrey. HarperCollins Publishers, Inc., 10 E. 53rd St., New York, NY 10022-5299. Phone: (800) 242-7737. Revised edition 1988.

RESEARCH CENTERS, INSTITUTES, CLEARINGHOUSES

Clinical Research Center for Schizophrenia and Psychiatric Rehabilitation. VA Medical Center--Brentwood, Wilshire and Sawtell Blvds., Los Angeles, CA 90073. Phone: (213) 824-6620.

Schizophrenic Biologic Research Center. Mount Sinai School of Medicine of City University of New York. VA Medical Center, Psychiatry Service, 116A, 130 W. Kingsbridge Rd., Bronx, NY 10468. Phone: (212) 584-9000. Fax: (212) 933-2121.

Western Psychiatric Institute and Clinic. University of Pittsburgh. 3811 O'Hara St., Pittsburgh, PA 15213. Phone: (412) 624-2360. Fax: (412) 624-1881.

TEXTBOOKS AND MONOGRAPHS

Chronic Schizophrenia and Adult Autism: Issues in Diagnosis, Assessment and Psychological Treatment. Johnny L. Matson (ed.). Springer Publishing Co., Inc., 536 Broadway, 11th Floor, New York, NY 10012. Phone: (212) 431-4370. 1989.

The Concept of Schizophrenia: Historical Perspectives. John G. Howells. American Psychiatric Press, 1400 K St. N.W., Washington, DC 20005. Phone: (202) 682-6000. Fax: (202) 682-6114. 1991.

Fetal Neural Development and Adult Schizophrenia. Sarnoff A. Mednick, Tyrone D. Cannon, Christopher E. Barr. Cambridge University Press, 40 W. 20th St., New York, NY 10011. Phone: (800) 431-1580. 1991.

Schizophrenia Research. Carol A. Tamminga, Charles S. Schulz. Raven Press, 1185 Ave. of the Americas, New York, NY 10036. Phone: (212) 930-9500. Fax: (212) 869-3495. 1991.

Schizophrenia: Treatment of Acute Psychotic Episodes. Steven T. Levy, Philip T. Ninan (eds.). American Psychiatric Press, Inc., 1400 K St. NW, Washington, DC 20005. Phone: (202) 682-6268. Fax: (202) 789-2648. 1990.

SCIATICA

See: NEUROLOGIC DISORDERS

SCLERODERMA

See: BONE AND JOINT DISEASES

SCOLIOSIS

See: SPINAL DISEASES

SEIZURES

See: EPILEPSY; NEUROLOGIC DISORDERS

SENILE DEMENTIA

See: DEMENTIA

SEXUAL ASSAULT

See: RAPE

SEXUAL DEVIATIONS

See: SEXUAL DISORDERS

SEXUAL DISORDERS

ABSTRACTING, INDEXING, AND CURRENT AWARENESS PUBLICATIONS

Index Medicus. U.S. National Library of Medicine, 8600 Rockville Pike, Bethesda, MD 20894. Phone: (800) 638-8480. Monthly.

Psychological Abstracts. American Psychological Association, 1200 17th St. NW, Washington, DC 20036. Phone: (202) 955-7600. Monthly.

ASSOCIATIONS, PROFESSIONAL SOCIETIES, ADVOCACY AND SUPPORT GROUPS

American Association of Sex Educators, Counselors and Therapists (AASECT). 435 N. Michigan Ave., Ste. 1717, Chicago, IL 60611. Phone: (312) 644-0828. Fax: (312) 644-8557.

Impotence Institute of America. 119 S. Ruth St., Maryville, TN 37801. Phone: (615) 983-6064.

Impotents Anonymous (IA). P.O. Box 5299, Maryville, TN 37802-5299. Phone: (615) 983-6064.

Sex Information and Education Council of the U.S. (SIECUS). 130 W. 42nd St., Ste. 2500, New York, NY 10036. Phone: (212) 819-9770. Fax: (212) 819-9776.

Society for the Scientific Study of Sex. P.O. Box 208, Mt. Vernon, IA 52314. Phone: (319) 895-8407. Fax: (319) 895-6203.

CD-ROM DATABASES

PsycLit. SilverPlatter Information, Inc., River Ridge Office Park, 100 River Ridge Rd., Norwood, MA 02062. Phone: (617) 769-2599. Fax: (617) 769-8763. Quarterly.

JOURNALS

Archives of Sexual Behavior. Plenum Publishing Co., 233 Spring St., New York, NY 10013-1578. Phone: (212) 620-800. Fax: (212) 463-0742.

International Journal of Impotence Research. Royal Society of Medicine Services Ltd., 1 Wimpole St., London W1M 8AE, England. Phone: 071-408 2119. Fax: 071-355 3198. Quarterly.

Journal of Sex Education and Therapy. Guilford Publications, Inc., 72 Spring St., New York, NY 10012. Phone: (800) 365-7006. Fax: (212) 966-6708. 4/year.

Journal of Sex and Marital Therapy. Brunner/Mazel Pubs., 19 Union Sq. W., New York, NY 10003. Phone: (212) 924-3344.

Medical Aspects of Human Sexuality. Cahners Publishing Company, 249 W. 17th St., New York, NY 10011. Phone: (212) 645-0067.

Sexuality and Disability. Plenum Publishing Co., 233 Spring St., New York, NY 10013-1578. Phone: (212) 620-8000. Fax: (212) 463-0742. Quarterly.

NEWSLETTERS

SIECUS Report. Sex Information & Education Council of the U.S. (SIECUS), 130 W. 42nd St., New York, NY 10036. Phone: (212) 673-3850. Fax: (212) 673-3850. Bimonthly.

ONLINE DATABASES

EMBASE. Elsevier Science Publishing Co., Inc., P.O. Box 882, Madison Square Station, New York, NY 10159-2101. Phone: (212) 989-5800. Fax: (212) 633-3990.

Human Sexuality. Clinical Communications, Inc., 132 Hutchin Hill, Shady, NY 12409. Phone: (914) 679-2217. Weekly to biweekly.

MEDLINE. National Library of Medicine, 8600 Rockville Pike, Bethesda, MD 20894. Phone: (800) 638-8480.

PsycInfo. SilverPlatter Information, Inc., River Ridge Office Park, 100 River Ridge Rd., Norwood, MA 02062. Phone: (617) 769-2599. Fax: (617) 769-8763. Quarterly.

SciSearch. Institute for Scientific Information, 3501 Market St., Philadelphia, PA 19104. Phone: (215) 386-0100. Fax: (215) 386-6362.

POPULAR WORKS AND PATIENT EDUCATION

When a Woman's Body Says No to Sex: Understanding and Overcoming Vaginismus. Linda Valina. Viking Penguin, 375 Hudson St., New York, NY 10014-3657. Phone: (800) 331-4624. 1992.

RESEARCH CENTERS, INSTITUTES, CLEARINGHOUSES

Johns Hopkins Hospital Sexual Disorders Clinic. Johns Hopkins University. Meyer Bldg., Rm. 101, 600 N. Wolfe St., Baltimore, MD 21205. Phone: (301) 955-6292. Fax: (301) 955-5115.

Kinsey Institute for Research in Sex, Gender, and Reproduction, Inc.. Morrison Hall, 3rd. Fl., Bloomington, IN 47405. Phone: (812) 855-7686. Fax: (812) 855-8277.

Masters & Johnson Institute. 24 S. Kingshighway, St. Louis, MO 63108. Phone: (314) 361-2377. Fax: (314) 361-8390.

TEXTBOOKS AND MONOGRAPHS

Diagnosis and Management of Impotence. Zorgniotti. Mosby-Year Book, 11830 Westline Industrial Drive, St. Louis, MO 63146. Phone: (800) 325-4177. Fax: (314) 432-1380. 1991.

Erectile Disorders: Assessment and Treatment. Raymond Rosen, Sandra Leiblum (eds.). Guilford Publications, Inc., 72 Spring St., New York, NY 10012. Phone: (800) 365-7006. Fax: (212) 366-6708. 1992.

Principles and Practice of Sex Therapy. Sandra Leiblum, Raymond Rosen (eds.). Guilford Publications, Inc., 72 Spring St., New York, NY 10012. Phone: (800) 365-7006. Fax: (212) 366-6708. 1989.

Principles of Trauma Surgery. Moylan. Raven Press, 1185 Ave. of the Americas, New York, NY 10036. Phone: (212) 930-9500. Fax: (212) 869-3495. Second edition 1992.

Sexual Dysfunction: A Guide for Assessment and Treatment. John P. Wincze, Michael P. Carey. Guilford Publications, Inc., 72 Spring St., New York, NY 10012. Phone: (800) 365-7006. Fax: (212) 366-6708. 1991.

World Book of Impotence. Tom F. Lue. Smith-Gordon, Number 1, 16 Gunter Grove, London SW10 0UJ, England. Fax: 44-71-351-1250. 1992.

SEXUALLY TRANSMITTED DISEASES

See also: AIDS; HERPESVIRUS INFECTIONS

ABSTRACTING, INDEXING, AND CURRENT AWARENESS PUBLICATIONS

Current Contents/Clinical Medicine. Institute for Scientific Information, 3501 Market St., Philadelphia, PA 19104. Phone: (800) 523-1850. Fax: (215) 386-6362. Weekly.

Excerpta Medica. Section 13: Dermatology and Venereology. Elsevier Science Publishing Co., Inc., P.O. Box 882, Madison Square Station, New York, NY 10159-2101. Phone: (212) 989-5800. Fax: (212) 633-3990. 16/year.

Index Medicus. U.S. National Library of Medicine, 8600 Rockville Pike, Bethesda, MD 20894. Phone: (800) 638-8480. Monthly.

MEDOC: Index to U.S. Government Publications in the Medical and Health Sciences. Spencer S. Eccles Health Sciences Library, University of Utah, Bldg. 589, Salt Lake City, UT 84112. Phone: (801) 581-5268. Quarterly.

Science Citation Index. Institute for Scientific Information, 3501 Market St., Philadelphia, PA 19104. Phone: (800) 523-1850. Fax: (215) 386-6362. Bimonthly.

Sexually Transmitted Diseases Abstracts and Bibliography. U.S. Centers for Disease Control, 1600 Clifton Rd. NE, Atlanta, GA 30333. Annual.

ASSOCIATIONS, PROFESSIONAL SOCIETIES, ADVOCACY AND SUPPORT GROUPS

American Foundation for the Prevention of Venereal Disease (AFPVD). 799 Broadway, Ste. 638, New York, NY 10003. Phone: (212) 759-2069.

American Social Health Association (ASHA). P.O. Box 13827, Research Triangle Park, NC 27709. Phone: (919) 361-8400. Fax: (919) 361-8425.

American Venereal Disease Association. c/o Edward W. Hook III M.D., Blalock 111, 600 N. Wolfe St., Baltimore, MD 21205. Phone: (301) 955-3150.

Herpes Resource Center (HRC). P.O. Box 13827, Research Triangle Park, NC 27709. Phone: (919) 361-2120. Fax: (919) 361-5736.

National Coalition of Gay Sexually Transmitted Disease Services. P.O. Box 234, Milwaukee, WI 53201. Phone: (414) 277-7671.

BIBLIOGRAPHIES

Chlamydia: Detection Methods. National Technical Information Service, 5285 Port Royal Rd., Springfield, VA 22161. Phone: (703) 487-4650. Fax: (703) 321-8547. Jan. 1978-Oct. 1987 PB88-852082/CBY.

Syphilis and Gonorrhea: Treatment and Therapy. National Technical Information Service, 5285 Port Royal Rd., Springfield, VA 22161. Phone: (703) 487-4650. Fax: (703) 321-8547. Jan. 1978-May 1989 PB89-862239/CBY.

CD-ROM DATABASES

AIDS Compact Library. MEP, 124 Mt. Auburn St., Cambridge, MA 02138. Phone: (800) 342-1338. Fax: (617) 868-7738. Semiannual.

AIDS: Information and Education Worldwide. CD Resources, Inc., 118 W. 74th St., Suite 2A, New York, NY 10023. Phone: (212) 580-2263. Fax: (212) 877-1276. Quarterly.

Morbidity Mortality Weekly Report. MEP, 124 Mt. Auburn St., Cambridge, MA 02138. Phone: (800) 342-1338. Fax: (617) 868-7738. Annual.

The Physician's AIDSLINE. MEP, 124 Mt. Auburn St., Cambridge, MA 02138. Phone: (800) 342-1338. Fax: (617) 868-7738. Annual.

SCISEARCH. Institute for Scientific Information, 3501 Market St., Philadelphia, PA 19104. Phone: (215) 386-0100. Fax: (215) 386-6362.

HANDBOOKS, GUIDES, MANUALS, ATLASES

Color Atlas of Sexually Transmitted Diseases. Anthony Wisdom. Mosby-Year Book, 11830 Westline Industrial Drive, St. Louis, MO 63146. Phone: (800) 325-4177. Fax: (314) 432-1380. 1990.

Color Atlas and Synopsis of Sexually Transmitted Diseases. H. Hunter Handsfield. McGraw-Hill, Inc., Health Professions Division, 1221 Avenue of the Americas, 28th Floor, New York, NY 10020. Phone: (212) 512-4228. 1992.

Sexually Transmitted Diseases: Companion Handbook. Adaora Adimora, Holli Hamilton, King K. Hlmes, et. al.. McGraw-Hill, Inc., Health Professions Division, 1221 Avenue of the Americas, 28th Floor, New York, NY 10020. Phone: (212) 512-4228. Second edition 1992.

JOURNALS

Genitourinary Medicine: The Journal of Sexual Health, STDs and HIV. BMJ Publishing Group, BMA House, Tavistock Square, London WC1H 9JR, England. Phone: 071-383 6244/6638. Fax: 071-383 6662. 6/year.

International Journal of STD and AIDS. Royal Society of Medicine Services Ltd., 1 Wimpole St., London W1M 8AE, England. Phone: 071-408 2119. Fax: 071-355 3198. Bimonthly.

Journal of the European Academy of Dermatology and Venereology. Elsevier Science Publishing Co., Inc., P.O. Box 882, Madison Square Station, New York, NY 10159-2101. Phone: (212) 989-5800. Fax: (212) 633-3990. 4/year.

Medical Aspects of Human Sexuality. Cahners Publishing Company, 249 W. 17th St., New York, NY 10011. Phone: (212) 645-0067.

Morbidity and Mortality Weekly Report. Massachusetts Medical Society, 1440 Main St., Waltham, MA 02154-1649. Phone: (617) 893-3800. Fax: (617) 893-0413. Weekly.

Sexually Transmitted Diseases. J.B. Lippincott Co., 227 E. Washington Square, Philadelphia, PA 19106-3780. Phone: (215) 238-4200. Fax: (215) 238-4227.

NEWSLETTERS

Common Sense about AIDS. American Health Consultants, P.O. Box 71266, Chicago, IL 60691-9987. Phone: (800) 688-2421.

ONLINE DATABASES

EMBASE. Elsevier Science Publishing Co., Inc., P.O. Box 882, Madison Square Station, New York, NY 10159-2101. Phone: (212) 989-5800. Fax: (212) 633-3990.

MEDIS. Mead Data Central, P.O. Box 1830, Dayton, OH 45401. Phone: (800) 227-4908.

MEDLINE. National Library of Medicine, 8600 Rockville Pike, Bethesda, MD 20894. Phone: (800) 638-8480.

SciSearch. Institute for Scientific Information, 3501 Market St., Philadelphia, PA 19104. Phone: (215) 386-0100. Fax: (215) 386-6362.

POPULAR WORKS AND PATIENT EDUCATION

The Essential HIV Treatment Fact Book. Laura Pinsky, Paul Harding Douglas, Craig Metroka. Pocket Books, Inc., 1230 Ave. of the Americas, New York, NY 10020. Phone: (800) 223-2348. Fax: (800) 284-0735. 1992.

The HIV Test: What You Need to Know to Make an Informed Decision. Marc Vargo. Pocket Books, Inc., 1230 Ave. of the Americas, New York, NY 10020. Phone: (800) 223-2348. Fax: (800) 284-0735. 1992.

RESEARCH CENTERS, INSTITUTES, CLEARINGHOUSES

National Herpes Hotline. P.O. Box 13827, Research Triangle Park, NC 27709. Phone: (919) 361-8488.

National STD Hotline. American Social Health Association, P.O. Box 13827, Research Triangle Park, NC 27709. Phone: (800) 227-8922.

STANDARDS AND STATISTICS SOURCES

Sexually Transmitted Disease Surveillance, 1990. Centers for Disease Control, 1600 Clifton Rd. N.E., Atlanta, GA 30333. Phone: (404) 488-4698. July 1991.

TEXTBOOKS AND MONOGRAPHS

ABC of Sexually Transmitted Diseases. M.W. Adler. BMJ Publishing Group, BMA House, Tavistock Square, London WC1H 9JR, England. Phone: 071-383 6244/6638. Fax: 071-383 6662. Second edition 1990.

AIDS and Alcohol/Drug Abuse: Psychosocial Research. Dennis G. Fisher (ed.). Haworth Press, 10 Alice Street, Binghamton,

NY 13904-1580. Phone: (800) 342-9678. Fax: (607) 722-1424. 1991.

AIDS, Drugs, and Sexual Risk. McKegany. Taylor & Francis Inc., 1900 Frost Rd., Suite 101, Bristol, PA 19007-1598. Phone: (800) 821-8312. Fax: (215) 785-5515. 1992.

AIDS and the Hospice Community. Madalon O'Rawe, Amenta Claire Tehan (eds.). Haworth Press, 10 Alice Street, Binghamton, NY 13904-1580. Phone: (800) 342-9678. Fax: (607) 722-1424. 1991.

The AIDS Knowledge Base. P.T. Cohen, Merle A. Sande, Paul A. Volberding (eds.). Massachusetts Medical Society, 1440 Main St., Waltham, MA 02154-1649. Phone: (617) 893-3800. Fax: (617) 893-0413. 1992.

AIDS and Other Manifestations of HIV Infection. G. Wormser (ed.). Noyes Publications, Mill Rd. at Grand Ave., Park Ridge, NJ 07656. Phone: (201) 391-8484. 1987.

Chlamydia. Per-Anders Mardh, Jorma Paavonen, Mirja Puolakkainen. Plenum Publishing Co., 233 Spring St., New York, NY 10013-1578. Phone: (212) 620-8000. Fax: (212) 463-0742. 1989.

Cocaine, AIDS and Intravenous Drug Use. Samuel R. Friedman, Douglas S. Lipton (eds.). Haworth Press, 10 Alice Street, Binghamton, NY 13904-1580. Phone: (800) 3HA-WORTH. Fax: (607) 722-1424. 1991.

The Medical Management of AIDS. Merle A. Sande, Paul A. Volberding. W.B. Saunders Co., The Curtis Center, Independence Square W., Philadelphia, PA 19106-3399. Phone: (215) 238-7800. Second edition 1991.

Sexually Transmitted Diseases. King K. Holmes, Per-Anders Mardh, P. Frederick, et. al.. McGraw-Hill, Inc., Health Professions Division, 1221 Avenue of the Americas, 28th Floor, New York, NY 10020. Phone: (212) 512-4228. Second edition 1990.

SHINGLES

See: HERPESVIRUS INFECTIONS

SHOCK

See: EMERGENCY MEDICINE; WOUNDS AND INJURIES

SHOTS

See: IMMUNIZATION

SICKLE CELL ANEMIA

See also: HEMATOLOGIC DISORDERS

ABSTRACTING, INDEXING, AND CURRENT AWARENESS PUBLICATIONS

Current Contents/Clinical Medicine. Institute for Scientific Information, 3501 Market St., Philadelphia, PA 19104. Phone: (800) 523-1850. Fax: (215) 386-6362. Weekly.

Excerpta Medica. Section 25: Hematology. Elsevier Science Publishers, P.O. Box 882, Madison Square Station, New York, NY 10159-2101. Phone: (212) 633-3950. Fax: (212) 633-3990. 24/year.

Index Medicus. U.S. National Library of Medicine, 8600 Rockville Pike, Bethesda, MD 20894. Phone: (800) 638-8480. Monthly.

Research Alert: Hematology-Hemoglobinpathies, Sickle Cell Anemia & Thalassemia. Institute for Scientific Information, 3501 Market St., Philadelphia, PA 19104. Phone: (800) 523-1850. Fax: (215) 386-6362. Weekly.

ANNUALS AND REVIEWS

Current Studies in Hematology and Blood Transfusion. S. Karger Publishers, Inc., 26 West Avon Rd., P.O. Box 529, Farmington, CT 06085. Phone: (203) 675-7834. Fax: (203) 675-7302. Irregular.

Year Book of Hematology. Mosby-Year Book, 11830 Westline Industrial Drive, St. Louis, MO 63146. Phone: (800) 325-4177. Fax: (314) 432-1380. Annual.

ASSOCIATIONS, PROFESSIONAL SOCIETIES, ADVOCACY AND SUPPORT GROUPS

National Association for Sickle-Cell Disease (NASCD). 3345 Wilshire Blvd., Ste. 1106, Los Angeles, CA 90010-1880. Phone: (800) 421-8453.

BIBLIOGRAPHIES

Sickle Cell Disease. National Technical Information Service, 5285 Port Royal Rd., Springfield, VA 22161. Phone: (703) 487-4650. Fax: (703) 321-8547. Apr. 1978-Jul. 1989 PB90-856394/CBY.

JOURNALS

American Journal of Hematology. John Wiley & Sons, Inc., 605 Third Ave., New York, NY 10158-0012. Phone: (212) 850-6000. Fax: (212) 850-6088. 12/year.

International Journal of Hematology. Elsevier Science Publishing Co., Inc., P.O. Box 882, Madison Square Station, New York, NY 10159-2101. Phone: (212) 989-5800. Fax: (212) 633-3990. 6/year.

NEWSLETTERS

Center for Sickle Cell Disease-Newsletter. Center for Sickle Cell Disease. Howard University, 2121 Georgia Ave. N.W., Washington, DC 20059. Phone: (202) 636-7930. Quarterly.

ONLINE DATABASES

Combined Health Information Database (CHID). U.S. National Institutes of Health, P.O. Box NDIC, Bethesda, MD 20892. Phone: (301) 496-2162. Fax: (301) 770-5164. Quarterly.

EMBASE. Elsevier Science Publishing Co., Inc., P.O. Box 882, Madison Square Station, New York, NY 10159-2101. Phone: (212) 989-5800. Fax: (212) 633-3990.

MEDLINE. National Library of Medicine, 8600 Rockville Pike, Bethesda, MD 20894. Phone: (800) 638-8480.

SciSearch. Institute for Scientific Information, 3501 Market St., Philadelphia, PA 19104. Phone: (215) 386-0100. Fax: (215) 386-6362.

RESEARCH CENTERS, INSTITUTES, CLEARINGHOUSES

Boston Sickle Cell Center. Boston City Hospital, 818 Harrison Ave., Boston, MA 02118. Phone: (617) 424-5727.

Center for Sickle Cell Disease. Howard University, 2121 Georgia Ave. N.W., Washington, DC 20059. Phone: (202) 636-7930.

Comprehensive Sickle Cell Center. Children's Hospital and Research Foundation. Elland and Bethesda Aves., Cincinnati, OH 45229. Phone: (513) 559-4543.

Comprehensive Sickle Cell Center. University of Illinois at Chicago. 1919 West Taylor St., Chicago, IL 60612. Phone: (312) 996-7013.

TEXTBOOKS AND MONOGRAPHS

Hematology: Basic Principles and Practice. Ronald Hoffman, Edward J. Benz Jr., Sanford J. Shattil. Churchill Livingstone Inc., 650 Avenue of the Americas, New York, NY 10011. Phone: (212) 819-5400. Fax: (212) 302-6598. 1991.

Hematology of Infancy and Childhood. David G. Nathan, Frank A. Oski. W.B. Saunders Co., The Curtis Center, Independence Square W., Philadelphia, PA 19106-3399. Phone: (215) 238-7800. Fourth edition. Two volumes. 1991.

Wintrobe's Clinical Hematology. G. Richard Lee, Thomas C. Bithell, John Foerster, and others. Williams & Wilkins, 428 E. Preston St., Baltimore, MD 21202. Phone: (800) 638-0672. Fax: (800) 447-8438. Ninth edition. Two volumes. 1992.

SIDS

See: SUDDEN INFANT DEATH SYNDROME

SIGMOIDOSCOPY

See: ENDOSCOPY

SILICOSIS

See: LUNG DISEASES

SINUSITIS

See: RESPIRATORY TRACT INFECTIONS

SJOGREN'S SYNDROME

See: ARTHRITIS

SKIN CANCER

See also: CANCER; DERMATOLOGY

ABSTRACTING, INDEXING, AND CURRENT AWARENESS PUBLICATIONS

Current Contents/Clinical Medicine. Institute for Scientific Information, 3501 Market St., Philadelphia, PA 19104. Phone: (800) 523-1850. Fax: (215) 386-6362. Weekly.

Excerpta Medica. Section 16: Cancer. Elsevier Science Publishing Co., Inc., P.O. Box 882, Madison Square Station, New York, NY 10159-2101. Phone: (212) 989-5800. Fax: (212) 633-3990. 32/year.

ICRDB Cancergram: Melanoma and Other Skin Cancer-- Diagnosis, Treatment. U.S. Government Printing Office, Superintendent of Documents, P.O. Box 371954, Pittsburgh, PA 15250-7954. Phone: (202) 783-3238. Fax: (202) 512-2250. Monthly.

Index Medicus. U.S. National Library of Medicine, 8600 Rockville Pike, Bethesda, MD 20894. Phone: (800) 638-8480. Monthly.

Science Citation Index. Institute for Scientific Information, 3501 Market St., Philadelphia, PA 19104. Phone: (800) 523-1850. Fax: (215) 386-6362. Bimonthly.

ANNUALS AND REVIEWS

Advances in Dermatology. Mosby-Year Book, 11830 Westline Inustrial Drive, St. Louis, MO 63146. Phone: (800) 325-4177. Fax: (314) 432-1380. Annual.

In Development New Medicines for Older Americans. 1991 Annual Survey. More Medicines in Testing for Cancer Than for Any Other Disease of Aging. Pharmaceutical Manufacturers Association, 1100 15th St. N.W., Washington, DC 20005. Phone: (202) 835-3400. 1991.

ASSOCIATIONS, PROFESSIONAL SOCIETIES, ADVOCACY AND SUPPORT GROUPS

American Cancer Society (ACS). 1599 Clifton Rd. N.E., Atlanta, GA 30329. Phone: (404) 320-3333.

American Society for Dermatologic Surgery (ASDS). P.O. Box 3116, Evanston, IL 60204. Phone: (312) 869-3954.

Skin Cancer Foundation. 245 Fifth Ave., Suite 2402, New York, NY 10016. Phone: (212) 725-5176.

Skin Cancer Foundation (SCF). 245 Fifth Ave., Ste. 2402, New York, NY 10016. Phone: (212) 725-5176.

CD-ROM DATABASES

Cancer-CD. SilverPlatter Information, Inc., River Ridge Office Park, 100 River Ridge Rd., Norwood, MA 02062. Phone: (617) 769-2599. Fax: (617) 769-8763. Quarterly.

SCISEARCH. Institute for Scientific Information, 3501 Market St., Philadelphia, PA 19104. Phone: (215) 386-0100. Fax: (215) 386-6362.

Year Books on Disc. CMC ReSearch, Inc., 7150 S.W. Hampton, Suite C-120, Portland, OR 97223. Phone: (800) 262-

7668. Fax: (503) 639-1796. Annual includes Year Books of Cardiology, Dermatology, Diagnostic Radiology, Drug Therapy, Emergency Medicine, Family Practice, Medicine, Neurology and Neurosurgery, Obstetrics and Gynecology, Oncology, Pediatrics, and Psychiatry and Applied Mental Health.

ENCYCLOPEDIAS, DICTIONARIES, WORD BOOKS

Oncology Words. Stedman. Williams & Wilkins, 428 East Preston St., Baltimore, MD 21202. Phone: (800) 638-0672. Fax: (800) 447-8438. 1992.

HANDBOOKS, GUIDES, MANUALS, ATLASES

Color Atlas of Dermatology. G.M. Levene, D.C. Calnan. Mosby-Year Book, 11830 Westline Industrial Drive, St. Louis, MO 63146. Phone: (800) 325-4177. Fax: (314) 432-1380. 1984.

A Color Atlas of Skin Tumors. S.K. Goolamali, G.M. Levene. Mosby-Year Book, 11830 Westline Industrial Drive, St. Louis, MO 63146. Phone: (800) 325-4177. Fax: (314) 432-1380. 1993.

JOURNALS

CA - A Cancer Journal for Clinicians. J.B. Lippincott Co., 227 E. Washington Square, Philadelphia, PA 19106-3780. Phone: (215) 238-4200. Fax: (215) 238-4227. Bimonthly.

Cancer Causes and Control. Rapid Communications of Oxford Ltd., The Old Malthouse, Paradise St., Oxford OX1 1LD, England. Phone: 44-865-790447. Fax: 44-865-244012. 6/year.

Journal of the American Academy of Dermatology. Mosby-Year Book, 11830 Westline Industrial Drive, St. Louis, MO 63146. Phone: (800) 325-4177. Fax: (314) 432-1380. Monthly.

Journal of Dermatologic Surgery and Oncology. Journal of Dermatologic Surgery, Inc., 245 Fifth Ave., New York, NY 10016. Phone: (212) 721-5175. Monthly.

Journal of the National Cancer Institute. Superintendent of Documents, P.O. Box 371954, Pittsburgh, PA 15250-7954. Fax: (202) 512-2233. Semimonthly.

Melanoma Research. Rapid Communications of Oxford Ltd., The Old Malthouse, Paradise St., Oxford OX1 1LD, England. Phone: 44-865-790447. Fax: 44-865-244012. 6/year.

Skin Cancer Foundation Journal. Skin Cancer Foundation, 245 Fifth Ave., Suite 2402, New York, NY 10016. Phone: (212) 725-5176.

NEWSLETTERS

The Melanoma Letter. Skin Cancer Foundation, 245 Fifth Ave., Ste. 2402, New York, NY 10016. Phone: (212) 725-5176. Quarterly.

Sun & Skin News. Skin Cancer Foundation, 245 Fifth Ave., Ste. 2402, New York, NY 10016. Phone: (212) 725-5176. Quarterly.

ONLINE DATABASES

Cancer Weekly. CDC AIDS Weekly/NCI Cancer Weekly, 206 Rogers St. NE, Suite 104, P.O. Box 5528, Atlanta, GA 30317. Phone: (404) 377-8895. Weekly.

CANCERLIT. U.S. National Cancer Institute, International Cancer Information Center, Building 82, Room 102, Bethesda,

MD 20892. Phone: (301) 496-7403. Fax: (301) 480-8105. Monthly.

Clinical Protocols. U.S. National Cancer Institute, International Cancer Information Center, Building 82, Room 102, Bethesda, MD 20892. Phone: (301) 496-7403. Fax: (301) 480-8105.

EMBASE. Elsevier Science Publishing Co., Inc., P.O. Box 882, Madison Square Station, New York, NY 10159-2101. Phone: (212) 989-5800. Fax: (212) 633-3990.

MEDLINE. National Library of Medicine, 8600 Rockville Pike, Bethesda, MD 20894. Phone: (800) 638-8480.

Physician Data Query (PDQ) Cancer Information File. U.S. National Cancer Institute, International Cancer Information Center, Building 82, Room 102, Bethesda, MD 20892. Phone: (301) 496-7403. Fax: (301) 480-8105. Monthly.

Physician Data Query (PDQ) Directory File. U.S. National Cancer Institute, International Cancer Information Center, Building 82, Room 102, Bethesda, MD 20892. Phone: (301) 496-7403. Fax: (301) 480-8105. Monthly.

Physician Data Query (PDQ) Protocol File. U.S. National Cancer Institute, International Cancer Information Center, Building 82, Room 102, Bethesda, MD 20892. Phone: (301) 496-7403. Fax: (301) 480-8105. Monthly.

SciSearch. Institute for Scientific Information, 3501 Market St., Philadelphia, PA 19104. Phone: (215) 386-0100. Fax: (215) 386-6362.

POPULAR WORKS AND PATIENT EDUCATION

Cancervive: The Challenge of Life After Cancer. Susan Nessim, Judith Ellis. Houghton Mifflin Co., 1 Beacon St., Boston, MA 02108. Phone: (800) 225-3362. 1991.

Safe in the Sun. Mary-Ellen Siegel. Walker Publishing Co., Inc., 720 Fifth Ave., New York, NY 10019. Phone: (212) 265-3532. 1990.

RESEARCH CENTERS, INSTITUTES, CLEARINGHOUSES

Cancer Information Service (CIS). Office of Cancer Communications, National Cancer Institute, Bldg. 31, Rm. 10A24, 9000 Rockville Pike, Bethesda, MD 20892. Phone: (800) 4CA-NCER.

TEXTBOOKS AND MONOGRAPHS

Andrews' Diseases of the Skin: Clinical Dermatology. Harry L. Arnold, Richard B. Odom, William D. James. W.B. Saunders Co., The Curtis Center, Independence Square W., Philadelphia, PA 19106-3399. Phone: (215) 238-7800. Eighth edition 1990.

Cancer: Principles and Practice of Oncology. Vincent T. DeVita. J.B. Lippincott Co., 227 E. Washington Square, Philadelphia, PA 19106-3780. Phone: (215) 238-4200. Fax: (215) 238-4227. 1989 3rd edtion.

Cancer Treatment. Charles M. Haskell. W.B. Saunders Co., The Curtis Center, Independence Square W., Philadelphia, PA 19106-3399. Phone: (215) 238-7800. Third edition 1990.

Cutaneous Melanoma. Charles M. Balch, ALan Houghton, Gerald Milton, and others. J.B. Lippincott Co., 227 East

Washington Square, Philadelphia, PA 19106-3780. Phone: (215) 238-4200. Fax: (215) 238-4227. Second edition 1991.

Dermatology: Diagnosis and Therapy. Edward E. Bondi, Brian V. Jegasothy, Gerald S. Lazarus (eds.). Appleton & Lange, 25 Van Zant Street, East Norwalk, CT 06855. Phone: (800) 423-1359. Fax: (203) 854-9486. 1991.

Hereditary Malignant Melanoma. Henry T. Lynch, Ramon M. Fusaro. CRC Press, Inc., 2000 Corporate Blvd. N.W., Boca Raton, FL 33431. Phone: (407) 994-0555. Fax: (407) 997-0949. 1991.

Melanoma of the Head and Neck. John Conley. Thieme Medical Publishers, Inc., 381 Park Ave. S., New York, NY 10016. Phone: (212) 683-5088. Fax: (212) 779-9020. 1990.

Principles and Practice of Dermatology. W. Mitchell Sams Jr., Peter J. Lynch (eds.). Churchill Livingstone Inc., 650 Avenue of the Americas, New York, NY 10011. Phone: (212) 819-5400. Fax: (212) 302-6598. 1990.

SKIN DISEASES

See: DERMATOLOGIC DISEASES

SLEEP APNEA

See: SLEEP DISORDERS

SLEEP DISORDERS

ABSTRACTING, INDEXING, AND CURRENT AWARENESS PUBLICATIONS

Current Contents/Life Sciences. Institute for Scientific Information, 3501 Market St., Philadelphia, PA 19104. Phone: (215) 386-0100. Fax: (215) 386-6362.

Index Medicus. U.S. National Library of Medicine, 8600 Rockville Pike, Bethesda, MD 20894. Phone: (800) 638-8480. Monthly.

Psychological Abstracts. American Psychological Association, 1200 17th St. NW, Washington, DC 20036. Phone: (202) 955-7600. Monthly.

Research Alert: Sleep Disorders. Institute for Scientific Information, 3501 Market St., Philadelphia, PA 19104. Phone: (800) 523-1850. Fax: (215) 386-6362. Weekly.

Science Citation Index. Institute for Scientific Information, 3501 Market St., Philadelphia, PA 19104. Phone: (800) 523-1850. Fax: (215) 386-6362. Bimonthly.

ANNUALS AND REVIEWS

Sleep Research. Brain Information Service, Brain Research Institute, University of California, Los Angeles, No. 43-367 CHS, Los Angeles, CA 90024-1746. Phone: (213) 825-3417. Annual.

ASSOCIATIONS, PROFESSIONAL SOCIETIES, ADVOCACY AND SUPPORT GROUPS

American Narcolepsy Association (ANA). P.O. Box 1187, San Carlos, CA 94070. Phone: (800) 222-6085. Fax: (415) 591-4934.

American Sleep Disorders Association (ASDA). 604 2nd St. S.W., Rochester, MN 55902. Phone: (507) 287-6006. Fax: (507) 287-6008.

American Sleep Disorders Foundation. 112 Massachusetts Ave., Arlington, MA 02174. Phone: (617) 648-8805.

Association of Professional Sleep Societies (APSS). 604 2nd St. S.W., Rochester, MN 55902. Phone: (507) 287-6006. Fax: (507) 287-6008.

Better Sleep Council. 2233 Wisconsin Ave. N.W., Ste. 500, Washington, DC 20007. Phone: (202) 333-0700.

Narcolepsy and Cataplexy Foundation of America (NCFA). Mail Box # 22, 1410 York Ave., Ste. 2D, New York, NY 10021. Phone: (212) 628-6315.

Narcolepsy Network. 155 Van Brackle Rd., Aberdeen, NJ 07747.

CD-ROM DATABASES

SCISEARCH. Institute for Scientific Information, 3501 Market St., Philadelphia, PA 19104. Phone: (215) 386-0100. Fax: (215) 386-6362.

DIRECTORIES

American Sleep Disorders Association Roster of Member Centers and Laboratories. American Sleep Disorders Association, 604 2nd St. S.W., Rochester, MN 55902. Phone: (507) 287-6006. Fax: (507) 287-6008. Quarterly.

ENCYCLOPEDIAS, DICTIONARIES, WORD BOOKS

Encyclopedia of Sleep and Sleep Disorders. Michael Thorpy, Jan Yager. Facts on File, Inc., 460 Park Ave. S., New York, NY 10016-7382. Phone: (212) 683-2244. Fax: (212) 683-3633. 1991.

HANDBOOKS, GUIDES, MANUALS, ATLASES

Atlas of Sleep Medicine. Shepard. Futura Publishing Co., Inc., P.O. Box 330, Mount Kisco, NY 10549. Phone: (914) 666-7528. 1991.

Concise Guide to the Evaluation and Management of Sleep Disorders. Martin Reite, Kim Nagel, John Ruddy. American Psychiatric Press, Inc., 1400 K St. NW, Washington, DC 20005. Phone: (202) 682-6268. Fax: (202) 789-2648. 1990.

JOURNALS

Sleep. Raven Press, 1185 Ave. of the Americas, New York, NY 10036. Phone: (212) 930-9500. Fax: (212) 869-3495. Bimonthly.

Sleep Research. Brain Research Institute, UCLA Center for Health Sciences, University of California, Los Angeles, CA 90024. Phone: (213) 825-5061.

ONLINE DATABASES

EMBASE. Elsevier Science Publishing Co., Inc., P.O. Box 882, Madison Square Station, New York, NY 10159-2101. Phone: (212) 989-5800. Fax: (212) 633-3990.

MEDLINE. National Library of Medicine, 8600 Rockville Pike, Bethesda, MD 20894. Phone: (800) 638-8480.

PsycInfo. SilverPlatter Information, Inc., River Ridge Office Park, 100 River Ridge Rd., Norwood, MA 02062. Phone: (617) 769-2599. Fax: (617) 769-8763. Quarterly.

SciSearch. Institute for Scientific Information, 3501 Market St., Philadelphia, PA 19104. Phone: (215) 386-0100. Fax: (215) 386-6362.

POPULAR WORKS AND PATIENT EDUCATION

How to Fight Insomnia. Peter Hauri, Shirley Linde. John Wiley & Sons, Inc., 605 Third Ave., New York, NY 10158-0012. Phone: (212) 850-6000. Fax: (212) 850-6088. 1990.

No More Sleepless Nights: The Complete Program for Ending Insomnia. Peter Hauri, Shirley Linde. John Wiley & Sons, Inc., 605 Third Ave., New York, NY 10158-0012. Phone: (212) 850-6000. Fax: (212) 850-6088. 1990.

Sleep and Its Secrets. Michael S. Aronoff. Plenum Publishing Co., 233 Spring St., New York, NY 10013-1578. Phone: (212) 620-800. Fax: (212) 463-0742. 1991.

Sleep: Problems and Solutions. Quentin Regestein, David Ritchie. Consumer Reports Books, 9180 LeSaint Dr., Fairfield, OH 45014. Phone: (513) 860-1178. 1990.

Stop Your Husband from Snoring. Rodale Press, Inc., 33 E. Minor St., Emmaus, PA 18098. Phone: (800) 527-8200. 1990.

RESEARCH CENTERS, INSTITUTES, CLEARINGHOUSES

Center for Research on Sleep and Circadian Rhythm. Stanford University. 701 Welch Rd., Ste. 2226, Palo Alto, CA 94304. Phone: (415) 723-8131.

Sleep Disorders Center. Columbia-Presbyterian Medical Center, 161 Fort Washington Ave., New York, NY 10032. Phone: (212) 305-1860.

Sleep Disorders Center of Henry Ford Hospital. 2921 W. Grand Blvd., Detroit, MI 48202. Phone: (313) 972-1800. Fax: (313) 874-7158.

Sleep Disorders and Research Center. Baylor College of Medicine. 1 Baylor Plaza, Houston, TX 77030. Phone: (713) 798-4886. Fax: (713) 796-9718.

STANDARDS AND STATISTICS SOURCES

The Treatment of Sleep Disorders of Older People. Consensus Statement. NIH Consensus Development Conference. March 20-26, 1990. National Institutes of Health, Office of Medical Applications of Research, Federal Bldg., Rm. 618, Bethesda, MD 20892. 1990.

TEXTBOOKS AND MONOGRAPHS

Epilepsy, Sleep and Sleep Deprivation. Rolf Degen, Ernst Rodin (eds.). Elsevier Science Publishing Co., Inc., P.O. Box 882, Madison Square Station, New York, NY 10159-2101. Phone: (212) 989-5800. Fax: (212) 633-3990. 1991.

Obstructive Sleep Apnea Syndrome: Clinical Research and Treatment. Christian Guilleminault, Markku Partinen. Raven Press, 1185 Avenue of the Americas, New York, NY 10036. Phone: (212) 930-9500. Fax: (212) 869-3495. 1990.

Sleep and Alertness: Chronobiological, Behavioral, and Medical Aspects of Napping. David F. Dinges, Roger J. Broughton.

Raven Press, 1185 Avenue of the Americas, New York, NY 10036. Phone: (212) 930-9500. Fax: (212) 869-3495. 1989.

Sleep Disorders: Diagnosis and Treatment. Robert Williams, and others (eds.). John Wiley & Sons, Inc., 605 Third Ave., New York, NY 10158-0012. Phone: (212) 850-6000. Fax: (212) 850-6088. 2nd edition, 1987.

SMALLPOX

See: INFECTIOUS DISEASES

SMOKING

ABSTRACTING, INDEXING, AND CURRENT AWARENESS PUBLICATIONS

Index Medicus. U.S. National Library of Medicine, 8600 Rockville Pike, Bethesda, MD 20894. Phone: (800) 638-8480. Monthly.

MEDOC: Index to U.S. Government Publications in the Medical and Health Sciences. Spencer S. Eccles Health Sciences Library, University of Utah, Bldg. 589, Salt Lake City, UT 84112. Phone: (801) 581-5268. Quarterly.

Research Alert: Smoking-Pathology & Addiction. Institute for Scientific Information, 3501 Market St., Philadelphia, PA 19104. Phone: (800) 523-1850. Fax: (215) 386-6362. Weekly.

ASSOCIATIONS, PROFESSIONAL SOCIETIES, ADVOCACY AND SUPPORT GROUPS

Action on Smoking and Health. 2013 H St. N.W., Washington, DC 20006. Phone: (202) 659-4310.

American Cancer Society (ACS). 1599 Clifton Rd. N.E., Atlanta, GA 30329. Phone: (404) 320-3333.

American Heart Association (AHA). 7320 Greenville Ave., Dallas, TX 75231. Phone: (214) 373-6300.

American Lung Association (ALA). 1740 Broadway, New York, NY 10019. Phone: (212) 315-8700. Fax: (212) 265-5642.

Citizens Against Tobacco Smoke. P.O. Box 36236, Cincinnati, OH 45236. Phone: (513) 984-8834.

Coalition of Smoking or Health (CSH). 1614 New Hampshire Ave. N.W., 2nd Flr., Washington, DC 20009. Phone: (202) 234-9375.

National Interagency Council on Smoking and Health. 7320 Greenville Ave., Dallas, TX 75231. Phone: (214) 750-5359.

Smoking Policy Institute. 914 E. Jefferson, P.O. Box 20271, Seattle, WA 98102. Phone: (206) 324-4444.

BIBLIOGRAPHIES

Bibliography on Smoking and Health. U.S. Public Health Service, Office on Smoking and Health, Park Bldg., Room 116, 5600 Fishers Lane, Rockville, MD 20857. Phone: (301) 443-1575. Annual.

Cigarette Smoking. National Technical Information Service, 5285 Port Royal Rd., Springfield, VA 22161. Phone: (703) 487-4650. Fax: (703) 321-8547. Jan. 1970-Feb. 1989 PB89-857189/CBY.

Cigarette Smoking: Health Effects of Passive Smoking. National Technical Information Service, 5285 Port Royal Rd., Springfield, VA 22161. Phone: (703) 487-4650. Fax: (703) 321-8547. Jan. 1970-Feb. 1989 PB89-857346.

DIRECTORIES

Alcohol, Drug Abuse, Mental Health Research Grant Awards. Alcohol, Drug Abuse, and Mental Health Administration, 5600 Fishers Lane, Rockville, MD 20857. Phone: (301) 443-1596.

Drug, Alcohol, and Other Addictions: A Directory of Treatment Centers and Prevention Programs Nationwide. Oryx Press, 4041 N. Central, Suite 700, Phoenix, AZ 85012. Phone: (800) 279-ORYX. Fax: (800) 279-4663.

HANDBOOKS, GUIDES, MANUALS, ATLASES

How to Help Your Patients Stop Smoking. U.S. National Cancer Institute, International Cancer Information Center, Building 82, Room 102, Bethesda, MD 20892. Phone: (301) 496-7403. Fax: (301) 480-8105. NIH Pub. No. 89-3064, 1989.

NEWSLETTERS

Addictions Alert. American Health Consultants, Department C1290, P.O. Box 740060, Atlanta, GA 30374. Phone: (800) 559-1032. Monthly.

Smoking and Health Newsletter. National Interagency Council on Smoking and Health, 7320 Greenville Ave., Dallas, TX 75231. Phone: (214) 750-5359.

ONLINE DATABASES

Combined Health Information Database (CHID). U.S. National Institutes of Health, P.O. Box NDIC, Bethesda, MD 20892. Phone: (301) 496-2162. Fax: (301) 770-5164. Quarterly.

EMBASE. Elsevier Science Publishing Co., Inc., P.O. Box 882, Madison Square Station, New York, NY 10159-2101. Phone: (212) 989-5800. Fax: (212) 633-3990.

MEDLINE. National Library of Medicine, 8600 Rockville Pike, Bethesda, MD 20894. Phone: (800) 638-8480.

SciSearch. Institute for Scientific Information, 3501 Market St., Philadelphia, PA 19104. Phone: (215) 386-0100. Fax: (215) 386-6362.

Smoking and Health. Information Center. U.S. Centers for Disease Control, Office on Smoking and Health, Technical Information Center, Rhodes Bldg., Mailstop K12, 1600 Clifton Rd. NE, Atlanta, GA 30333. Phone: (404) 488-5080. Fax: (301) 443-1194. Bimonthly.

POPULAR WORKS AND PATIENT EDUCATION

The Facts about Smoking. C. Barr Taylor, Joel D. Killen, and others. Consumer Reports Books, 101 Truman Ave., Yonkers, NY 10703. Phone: (914) 378-2000. 1991.

RESEARCH CENTERS, INSTITUTES, CLEARINGHOUSES

Office on Smoking and Health (OSH). Centers for Disease Control, Dept. of Health and Human Services, Park Bldg., Rm. 1-16, 5600 Rishers Ln., Rockville, MD 20857. Phone: (301) 443-1690.

Smokenders. 18551 Von Karman Ave., Irvine, CA 92715. Phone: (714) 851-2273.

Tobacco and Health Research Institute. University of Kentucky, Cooper and Alumni Drives, Lexington, KY 40546. Phone: (606) 257-2816.

Tobacco Institute. 1875 I St. N.W., No. 800, Washington, DC 20006. Phone: (202) 457-4800.

STANDARDS AND STATISTICS SOURCES

Health Benefits of Smoking Cessation: A Report of the Surgeon General. Centers for Disease Control, 1600 Clifton Rd. N.E., Atlanta, GA 30333. Phone: (404) 488-4698. Annual.

Smoking and Health: A National Status Report. Centers for Disease Control, 1600 Clifton Rd. N.E., Atlanta, GA 30333. Phone: (404) 488-4698. Biennial.

Tuberculosis Statistics in the U.S. Centers for Disease Control, 1600 Clifton Rd. N.E., Atlanta, GA 30333. Phone: (404) 488-4698. Annual.

TEXTBOOKS AND MONOGRAPHS

Tobacco Smoking and Atherosclerosis: Pathogenesis and Cellular Mechanisms. John N. Diana (ed.). Plenum Publishing Co., 233 Spring St., New York, NY 10013-1578. Phone: (212) 620-8000. Fax: (212) 463-0742. 1990.

SNAKEBITE

See: EMERGENCY MEDICINE

SPASTIC COLON

See: GASTROINTESTINAL DISORDERS

SPEECH DISORDERS

See: COMMUNICATION DISORDERS

SPEECH THERAPY

See: AUDIOLOGY; COMMUNICATION DISORDERS

SPERM BANKS

See: INFERTILITY

SPINA BIFIDA

See also: BIRTH DEFECTS

ABSTRACTING, INDEXING, AND CURRENT AWARENESS PUBLICATIONS

Excerpta Medica. Section 8: Neurology and Neurosurgery. Elsevier Science Publishers, P.O. Box 882, Madison Square Station, New York, NY 10159-2101. Phone: (212) 633-3950. Fax: (212) 633-3990. 32/year.

ANNUALS AND REVIEWS

Annual Review of Neuroscience. Annual Reviews Inc., 4139 El Camino Way, P.O. Box 10139, Palo Alto, CA 94303-0897. Phone: (415) 493-4400. Fax: (415) 855-9815. Annual.

Current Opinion in Neurology & Neurosurgery. Current Science Ltd., 20 N. Third St., Philadelphia, PA 19106-2199. Phone: (800) 552-5866. Fax: (215) 574-2270. Bimonthly.

ASSOCIATIONS, PROFESSIONAL SOCIETIES, ADVOCACY AND SUPPORT GROUPS

Spina Bifida Association of America (SBAA). 1700 Rockville Pike, Ste. 250, Rockville, MD 20852. Phone: (800) 621-3141. Fax: (301) 881-3392.

HANDBOOKS, GUIDES, MANUALS, ATLASES

Manual of Neurologic Therapy. Samuels. Little, Brown and Co., 34 Beacon St., Boston, MA 02108. Phone: (617) 227-0730. Fax: (617) 227-0790. Fourth edition 1991.

JOURNALS

Developmental Medicine and Child Neurology. MacKeith Press, 5A Netherall Gardens, London NW3, England.

Journal of Child Neurology. Mosby-Year Book, 11830 Westline Industrial Drive, St. Louis, MO 63146. Phone: (800) 325-4177. Fax: (314) 432-1380. Quarterly.

Journal of Spinal Disorders. Raven Press, 1185 Avenue of the Americas, New York, NY 10036. Phone: (212) 930-9500. Fax: (212) 869-3495. Quarterly.

Spine. J.B. Lippincott Co., 227 E. Washington Square, Philadelphia, PA 19106-3780. Phone: (215) 238-4200. Fax: (215) 238-4227. 11/year.

NEWSLETTERS

Spina Bifida Insights. Spina Bifida Association of America, 1700 Rockville PIke, Ste. 540, Rockville, MD 20852. Phone: (800) 621-3141. Bimonthly.

TEXTBOOKS AND MONOGRAPHS

Current Concepts in Spina Bifida and Hydrocephalus. Carys Bannister, Brian Tew (eds.). Cambridge University Press, 40 W. 20th St., New York, NY 10011. Phone: (800) 431-1580. 1992.

Diagnosis and Management of Lumbar Spine Disease. Neil Kahanovitz. Raven Press, 1185 Avenue of the Americas, New York, NY 10036. Phone: (212) 930-9500. Fax: (212) 869-3495. 1991.

Disorders of the Cervical Spine. Martin B. Camins, Patrick F. O'Leary (eds.). Williams & Wilkins, 428 East Preston St., Baltimore, MD 21202. Phone: (800) 638-0672. Fax: (800) 447-8438. 1992.

Surgery of the Spinal Cord. Holtzman. Springer-Verlag New York Inc., 175 Fifth Ave., New York, NY 10010. Phone: (212) 460-1500. Fax: (212) 473-6272. 1992.

SPINAL CORD INJURIES

See also: PARALYSIS

ABSTRACTING, INDEXING, AND CURRENT AWARENESS PUBLICATIONS

Current Contents/Clinical Medicine. Institute for Scientific Information, 3501 Market St., Philadelphia, PA 19104. Phone: (800) 523-1850. Fax: (215) 386-6362. Weekly.

Excerpta Medica. Section 8: Neurology and Neurosurgery. Elsevier Science Publishers, P.O. Box 882, Madison Square Station, New York, NY 10159-2101. Phone: (212) 633-3950. Fax: (212) 633-3990. 32/year.

Index Medicus. U.S. National Library of Medicine, 8600 Rockville Pike, Bethesda, MD 20894. Phone: (800) 638-8480. Monthly.

Science Citation Index. Institute for Scientific Information, 3501 Market St., Philadelphia, PA 19104. Phone: (800) 523-1850. Fax: (215) 386-6362. Bimonthly.

ANNUALS AND REVIEWS

Spine: State of the Art Reviews. Hanley & Belfus, Inc., 210 S. 13th St., Philadelphia, PA 19107. Phone: (215) 546-7293.

ASSOCIATIONS, PROFESSIONAL SOCIETIES, ADVOCACY AND SUPPORT GROUPS

American Paralysis Association (APA). P.O. Box 187, Short HillS, NJ 07078. Phone: (201) 379-2690.

American Paraplegia Society (APS). 75-20 Astoria Blvd., Jackson Heights, NY 11370. Phone: (718) 803-3782.

American Spinal Injury Association (ASIA). 250 E. Superior, Rm. 619, Chicago, IL 60611. Phone: (312) 908-3425.

National Spinal Cord Injury Association (NSCIA). 600 W. Cummings Park, Ste. 2000, Woburn, MA 01801. Phone: (800) 962-9629. Fax: (617) 935-8369.

Spinal Cord Society (SCS). Wendell Rd., Fergus Falls, MN 56537. Phone: (218) 739-5252. Fax: (218) 739-5262.

CD-ROM DATABASES

SCISEARCH. Institute for Scientific Information, 3501 Market St., Philadelphia, PA 19104. Phone: (215) 386-0100. Fax: (215) 386-6362.

DIRECTORIES

Directory of Organizations Serving People with Disabilities. Commission on Accreditation of Rehabilitation Facilities, 101 N. Wilmot Rd., Ste. 500, Tucson, AZ 85711. Phone: (602) 748-1212. Annual.

Spinal Network: The Total Resource for the Wheelchair Community. Spinal Associates, 1911 11th St., No. 307, P.O. Box 4162, Boulder, CO 80306. Annual.

JOURNALS

Archives of Physical Medicine and Rehabilitation. American Congress of Rehabilitation Medicine, 78 E. Adams, Chicago, IL 60603. Phone: (312) 922-9371. Fax: (312) 922-6754. Monthly.

Brain Research. Elsevier Science Publishing Co., Inc., P.O. Box 882, Madison Square Station, New York, NY 10159-2101. Phone: (212) 989-5800. Fax: (212) 633-3990. 101/year.

Journal of Neurology. Springer-Verlag New York Inc., 175 Fifth Ave., New York, NY 10010. Phone: (212) 460-1500. Fax: (212) 473-6272.

Neurology. Edgell Communications, 7500 Old Oak Blvd., Cleveland, OH 44130. Phone: (216) 826-2839. Fax: (216) 891-2726. Monthly.

Paraplegia. Churchill Livingstone Inc., 650 Ave. of the Americas, New York, NY 10011. Phone: (212) 819-5400. Fax: (212) 302-6598. 9/year.

Spine. J.B. Lippincott Co., 227 E. Washington Square, Philadelphia, PA 19106-3780. Phone: (215) 238-4200. Fax: (215) 238-4227. 11/year.

NEWSLETTERS

Spinal Cord Injury Life. National Spinal Cord Injury Association, 600 W. Cummings Park, Woburn, MA 01801. Phone: (617) 935-2722. Fax: (617) 932-8369. Quarterly.

Spinal Cord Society Newsletter. Spinal Cord Society (SCS), Wendell Rd., Box 22A, Fergus Falls, MN 56537-9805. Phone: (218) 739-5252. Fax: (218) 739-5262. Monthly.

ONLINE DATABASES

EMBASE. Elsevier Science Publishing Co., Inc., P.O. Box 882, Madison Square Station, New York, NY 10159-2101. Phone: (212) 989-5800. Fax: (212) 633-3990.

MEDLINE. National Library of Medicine, 8600 Rockville Pike, Bethesda, MD 20894. Phone: (800) 638-8480.

SciSearch. Institute for Scientific Information, 3501 Market St., Philadelphia, PA 19104. Phone: (215) 386-0100. Fax: (215) 386-6362.

POPULAR WORKS AND PATIENT EDUCATION

Spinal Cord Injury: A Guide for Patient and Family. Lynn Phillips, Mark N. Ozer, Peter Axelson, and others. Raven Press, 1185 Avenue of the Americas, New York, NY 10036. Phone: (212) 930-9500. Fax: (212) 869-3495. 1987.

RESEARCH CENTERS, INSTITUTES, CLEARINGHOUSES

Medical Rehabilitation Research and Training Center in Spinal Cord Dysfunction. University of Alabama at Birmingham. University Sta., Birmingham, AL 35294. Phone: (205) 934-3334.

TEXTBOOKS AND MONOGRAPHS

Ailing Spine. Tilscher. Springer-Verlag New York Inc., 175 Fifth Ave., New York, NY 10010. Phone: (212) 460-1500. Fax: (212) 473-6272. 1991.

MRI of the Spine. Modic. Mosby-Year Book, 11830 Westline Industrial Drive, St. Louis, MO 63146. Phone: (800) 325-4177. Fax: (314) 432-1380. Second edition 1992.

Spinal Cord Compression: Diagnosis and Principles of Management. Thomas N. Byrne, Stephen G. Waxman. F.A. Davis Co., 1915 Arch St., Philadelphia, PA 19103. Phone: (800) 523-4049. Fax: (215) 568-5065. Contemporary Neurology. Series No. 33. 1990.

Surgery of the Spine: A Combined Orthopedic Neurosurgical Approach. Findlay. Blackwell Scientific Publications, Inc., 3 Cambridge Ctr., Cambridge, MA 02142. Phone: (800) 759-6102. 1992.

The Total Care of Spinal Cord Injuries. Donald S. Pierce (ed.). Little, Brown and Company, 34 Beacon St., Boston, MA 02108. Phone: (617) 227-0730. Second edition 1992.

SPINAL DISEASES

ABSTRACTING, INDEXING, AND CURRENT AWARENESS PUBLICATIONS

Current Contents/Clinical Medicine. Institute for Scientific Information, 3501 Market St., Philadelphia, PA 19104. Phone: (800) 523-1850. Fax: (215) 386-6362. Weekly.

Excerpta Medica. Section 8: Neurology and Neurosurgery. Elsevier Science Publishers, P.O. Box 882, Madison Square Station, New York, NY 10159-2101. Phone: (212) 633-3950. Fax: (212) 633-3990. 32/year.

Index Medicus. U.S. National Library of Medicine, 8600 Rockville Pike, Bethesda, MD 20894. Phone: (800) 638-8480. Monthly.

ANNUALS AND REVIEWS

Spine: State of the Art Reviews. Hanley & Belfus, Inc., 210 S. 13th St., Philadelphia, PA 19107. Phone: (215) 546-7293.

ASSOCIATIONS, PROFESSIONAL SOCIETIES, ADVOCACY AND SUPPORT GROUPS

National Scoliosis Foundation (NSF). 72 Mt. Auburn St., Watertown, MA 02172. Phone: (617) 926-0397. Fax: (617) 926-0398.

North American Spine Society (NASS). 222 S. Prospect Ave., Park Ridge, IL 60068. Phone: (708) 698-1628. Fax: (708) 823-0536.

Scoliosis Association (SA). P.O. Box 51353, Raleigh, NC 27609-1353. Phone: (919) 846-2639.

CD-ROM DATABASES

Excerpta Medica CD: Neurosciences. SilverPlatter Information, Inc., River Ridge Office Park, 100 River Ridge Rd., Norwood, MA 02062. Phone: (617) 769-2599. Fax: (617) 769-8763. Quarterly.

HANDBOOKS, GUIDES, MANUALS, ATLASES

Atlas of Spinal Surgery. Donlin M. Long. Williams & Wilkins, 428 E. Preston St., Baltimore, MD 21202. Phone: (800) 638-0672. Fax: (800) 447-8438. 1992.

MRI Atlas of the Spine. Kenneth R. Maravilla, Wendy A. Cohen. Raven Press, 1185 Avenue of the Americas, New York, NY 10036. Phone: (212) 930-9500. Fax: (212) 869-3495. 1991.

JOURNALS

Journal of Spinal Disorders. Raven Press, 1185 Avenue of the Americas, New York, NY 10036. Phone: (212) 930-9500. Fax: (212) 869-3495. Quarterly.

Neurology. Edgell Communications, 7500 Old Oak Blvd., Cleveland, OH 44130. Phone: (216) 826-2839. Fax: (216) 891-2726. Monthly.

Paraplegia. Churchill Livingstone Inc., 650 Ave. of the Americas, New York, NY 10011. Phone: (212) 819-5400. Fax: (212) 302-6598. 9/year.

Spine. J.B. Lippincott Co., 227 E. Washington Square, Philadelphia, PA 19106-3780. Phone: (215) 238-4200. Fax: (215) 238-4227. 11/year.

NEWSLETTERS

Backtalk. Scoliosis Association, Inc., P.O. Box 51353, Raleigh, NC 27609. Phone: (919) 846-2639. Irregular.

Spina Bifida Insights. Spina Bifida Association of America, 1700 Rockville Pike, Ste. 540, Rockville, MD 20852. Phone: (800) 621-3141. Bimonthly.

The Spinal Connection. National Scoliosis Foundation, 93 Concord Ave., P.O. Box 547, Belmont, MA 02178. Phone: (617) 489-0880. Fax: (617) 489-0888. Biennial.

Spinal Cord Society Newsletter. Spinal Cord Society (SCS), Wendell Rd., Box 22A, Fergus Falls, MN 56537-9805. Phone: (218) 739-5252. Fax: (218) 739-5262. Monthly.

ONLINE DATABASES

EMBASE. Elsevier Science Publishing Co., Inc., P.O. Box 882, Madison Square Station, New York, NY 10159-2101. Phone: (212) 989-5800. Fax: (212) 633-3990.

MEDLINE. National Library of Medicine, 8600 Rockville Pike, Bethesda, MD 20894. Phone: (800) 638-8480.

SciSearch. Institute for Scientific Information, 3501 Market St., Philadelphia, PA 19104. Phone: (215) 386-0100. Fax: (215) 386-6362.

TEXTBOOKS AND MONOGRAPHS

Adult Spine: Principles and Practice. Frymoyer. Raven Press, 1185 Ave. of the Americas, New York, NY 10036. Phone: (212) 930-9500. Fax: (212) 869-3495. Two volumes 1991.

The Aging Spine: Essentials of Pathophysiology, Diagnosis and Treatment. Scott D. Boden, Sam W. Wiesel. W.B. Saunders Co., The Curtis Center, Independence Square W., Philadelphia, PA 19106-3399. Phone: (215) 238-7800. 1991.

Ailing Spine. Tilscher. Springer-Verlag New York Inc., 175 Fifth Ave., New York, NY 10010. Phone: (212) 460-1500. Fax: (212) 473-6272. 1991.

Diagnosis and Management of Lumbar Spine Disease. Neil Kahanovitz. Raven Press, 1185 Avenue of the Americas, New York, NY 10036. Phone: (212) 930-9500. Fax: (212) 869-3495. 1991.

Disorders of the Cervical Spine. Martin B. Camins, Patrick F. O'Leary (eds.). Williams & Wilkins, 428 East Preston St., Baltimore, MD 21202. Phone: (800) 638-0672. Fax: (800) 447-8438. 1992.

Fractures of the Thoracic and Lumbar Spine. Gertzbein. Williams & Wilkins, 428 East Preston St., Baltimore, MD 21202. Phone: (800) 638-0672. Fax: (800) 447-8438. 1992.

Low Back Pain: Mechanisms, Diagnosis, and Treatment. Jamel M. Cox. Williams & Wilkins, 428 East Preston St., Baltimore, MD 21202. Phone: (800) 638-0672. Fax: (800) 447-8438. 1990.

Lumbar Spine and Back Pain. Jayson. Churchill Livingstone Inc., 650 Ave. of the Americas, New York, NY 10011. Phone: (212) 819-5400. Fax: (212) 302-6598. Fourth edition 1992.

MRI of the Spine. Modic. Mosby-Year Book, 11830 Westline Industrial Drive, St. Louis, MO 63146. Phone: (800) 325-4177. Fax: (314) 432-1380. Second edition 1992.

Spinal MRI: A Teaching File Approach. John H. Bisese. McGraw-Hill, Inc., Health Professions Division, 1221 Avenue of the Americas, 28th Floor, New York, NY 10020. Phone: (212) 512-4228. 1992.

Spinal Surgery: Science and Practice. Robert A. Dickson. Butterworth-Heinemann, 80 Montvale Ave., Stoneham, MA 02180. Phone: (617) 438-8464. Fax: (617) 279-4851. 1990.

Surgery of the Spinal Cord. Holtzman. Springer-Verlag New York Inc., 175 Fifth Ave., New York, NY 10010. Phone: (212) 460-1500. Fax: (212) 473-6272. 1992.

Textbook of Spinal Surgery. Bidwell. J.B. Lippincott Co., 227 E. Washington Square, Philadelphia, PA 19106-3780. Phone: (215) 238-4200. Fax: (215) 238-4227. Two volumes 1991.

SPORTS MEDICINE

See also: ORTHOPEDICS; WOUNDS AND INJURIES

ABSTRACTING, INDEXING, AND CURRENT AWARENESS PUBLICATIONS

Current Contents/Clinical Medicine. Institute for Scientific Information, 3501 Market St., Philadelphia, PA 19104. Phone: (800) 523-1850. Fax: (215) 386-6362. Weekly.

Index Medicus. U.S. National Library of Medicine, 8600 Rockville Pike, Bethesda, MD 20894. Phone: (800) 638-8480. Monthly.

Physical Education Index. BenOak Publishing Co., P.O. Box 474, Cape Girardeau, MO 63702-0474. Phone: (314) 334-8789. Quarterly.

Physical Fitness/Sports Medicine. President's Council on Physical Fitness and Sports, 450 Fifth St. NW, Suite 7130, Washington, DC 20001. Phone: (202) 272-3421. Quarterly.

Research Alert: Sports Medicine. Institute for Scientific Information, 3501 Market St., Philadelphia, PA 19104. Phone: (800) 523-1850. Fax: (215) 386-6362. Weekly.

Science Citation Index. Institute for Scientific Information, 3501 Market St., Philadelphia, PA 19104. Phone: (800) 523-1850. Fax: (215) 386-6362. Bimonthly.

ANNUALS AND REVIEWS

Advances in Sports Medicine and Fitness. Mosby-Year Book, 11830 Westline Industrial Drive, St. Louis, MO 63146. Phone: (800) 325-4177. Fax: (314) 432-1380. Annual.

Clinics in Sports Medicine. W.B. Saunders Co., The Curtis Center, Independence Square W., Philadelphia, PA 19106-3399. Phone: (215) 238-7800. Quarterly.

Current Opinion in Orthopaedics. Current Science Ltd., 20 N. Third St., Philadelphia, PA 19106-2199. Phone: (800) 552-5866. Fax: (215) 574-2270. Bimonthly.

Current Therapy in Sports Medicine. Mosby-Year Book, 11830 Westline Industrial Drive, St. Louis, MO 63146. Phone: (800) 325-4177. Fax: (314) 432-1380. Irregular.

Orthopaedic Physical Therapy Clinics of North America. W.B. Saunders Co., The Curtis Center, Independence Square W., Philadelphia, PA 19106-3399. Phone: (215) 238-7800. Quarterly.

Orthopedic Clinics. W.B. Saunders Co., The Curtis Center, Independence Square W., Philadelphia, PA 19106-3399. Phone: (215) 238-7800. Quarterly.

Year Book of Sports Medicine. Mosby-Year Book, 11830 Westline Industrial Drive, St. Louis, MO 63146. Phone: (800) 325-4177. Fax: (314) 432-1380. Annual.

ASSOCIATIONS, PROFESSIONAL SOCIETIES, ADVOCACY AND SUPPORT GROUPS

American Academy of Orthopedic Surgeons (AAOS). 222 S. Prospect Ave., Park Ridge, IL 60068-4058. Phone: (708) 823-7186. Fax: (708) 823-8125.

American College of Sports Medicine (ACSM). P.O. Box 1440, Indianapolis, IN 46206-1440. Phone: (317) 637-9200. Fax: (317) 634-7817.

American Orthopaedic Society for Sports Medicine (AOSSM). 2250 E. Devon Ave., Ste. 115, Des Plaines, IL 60018. Phone: (708) 836-7000. Fax: (708) 803-8653.

American Osteopathic Academy of Sports Medicine (AOASM). 7611 Elmwood Ave., Ste. 201, Middleton, WI 53562. Phone: (608) 831-4400. Fax: (608) 831-5122.

Canadian Academy of Sport Medicine. 1600 James Naismith Dr., Gloucester, ON, Canada K1B 5N4. Phone: (613) 748-5671. Fax: (613) 748-5729.

BIBLIOGRAPHIES

Nutri-Topics: Sports Nutrition. Food and Nutrition Center, National Agricultural Library, 10301 Baltimore Blvd., Beltsville, MD 20705.

CD-ROM DATABASES

Ortholine. Aries Systems Corporation, One Dundee Park, Andover, MA 01810. Phone: (508) 475-7200. Fax: (508) 474-8860. Monthly or quarterly.

SCISEARCH. Institute for Scientific Information, 3501 Market St., Philadelphia, PA 19104. Phone: (215) 386-0100. Fax: (215) 386-6362.

SPORT Discus. SilverPlatter Information, Inc., River Ridge Office Park, 100 River Ridge Rd., Norwood, MA 02062. Phone: (617) 769-2599. Fax: (617) 769-8763. Semiannual.

DIRECTORIES

Directory of Medical Specialists. Marquis Who's Who, 3002 Glenview Rd., Wilmette, IL 60091. Phone: (800) 621-9669. Fax: (708) 441-2264. Biennial.

Directory of Physicians in the United States. American Medical Association, 515 North State St., Chicago, IL 60610. Phone: (312) 464-0183. Fax: (312) 464-5834. Biennial.

ENCYCLOPEDIAS, DICTIONARIES, WORD BOOKS

Handbook of Orthopedic Terminology. Kilcoyne. CRC Press, Inc., 2000 Corporate Blvd. N.W., Boca Raton, FL 33431. Phone: (407) 994-0555. Fax: (407) 997-0949. 1991.

Orthopedic Word Book. Thomas J. Cittadine. Springhouse Publishing Co., 1111 Bethlehem Pike, Spring House, PA 19477. Phone: (800) 331-3170 Fax: (215) 646-8710. 1992.

Orthopedic Words. Stedman. Williams & Wilkins, 428 East Preston St., Baltimore, MD 21202. Phone: (800) 638-0672. Fax: (800) 447-8438. 1992.

HANDBOOKS, GUIDES, MANUALS, ATLASES

A Color Atlas of Injury in Sport. J.G.P. Williams. Mosby-Year Book, 11830 Westline Industrial Drive, St. Louis, MO 63146. Phone: (800) 325-4177. Fax: (314) 432-1380. Second edition 1989.

Pocket Picture Guide to Sports Injuries. Brooks. Gower Publishing Co., Inc., Old Post Rd., Brookfield, VT 05036. Phone: (802) 276-3162. Second edition 1992.

Practical Joint Assessment: A Sports Medicine Manual. Hartley. Mosby-Year Book, 11830 Westline Industrial Drive, St. Louis, MO 63146. Phone: (800) 325-4177. Fax: (314) 432-1380. 1990.

Therapeutic Modalities in Sports. Drez. Mosby-Year Book, 11830 Westline Industrial Drive, St. Louis, MO 63146. Phone: (800) 325-4177. Fax: (314) 432-1380. 1988.

JOURNALS

American Journal of Sports Medicine. American Orthopedic Society for Sports Medicine, P.O. Box 9517, Columbus, GA 31995. Phone: (404) 576-3340.

Annals of Sports Medicine. Raven Press, 1185 Avenue of the Americas, New York, NY 10036. Phone: (212) 930-9500. Fax: (212) 869-3495. Bimonthly.

British Journal of Sports Medicine. Butterworth-Heinemann, 80 Montvale Ave., Stoneham, MA 02180. Phone: (617) 438-8464. Fax: (617) 279-4851. Quarterly.

Chiropractic Sports Medicine. Williams & Wilkins, 428 E. Preston St., Baltimore, MD 21202. Phone: (800) 638-0672. Fax: (800) 447-8438. Quarterly.

Clinical Journal of Sports Medicine. Raven Press, 1185 Avenue of the Americas, New York, NY 10036. Phone: (212) 930-9500. Fax: (212) 869-3495. Quarterly.

International Journal of Sports Medicine. Thieme Medical Publishers, Inc., 381 Park Ave. S., New York, NY 10016. Phone: (212) 683-5088. Fax: (212) 779-9020. Bimonthly.

Journal of Bone and Joint Surgery: American Volume. Journal of Bone and Joint Surgery, Inc., 10 Shattuck St., Boston, MA 02115. Phone: (617) 734-2835. 10/year.

Journal of Orthopaedic and Sports Physical Therapy. Williams & Wilkins, 428 E. Preston St., Baltimore, MD 21202. Phone: (800) 638-0672. Fax: (800) 447-8438. Monthly.

Journal of Osteopathic Sports Medicine. American Osteopathic Academy of Sports Medicine, P.O. Box 623, Middleton, WI 53562-0623.

Medicine and Science in Sports and Exercise. Williams & Wilkins, 428 E. Preston St., Baltimore, MD 21202. Phone: (800) 638-0672. Fax: (800) 447-8438. Monthly.

NEWSLETTERS

Sports Medicine Bulletin. American College of Sports Medicine (ACSM), P.O. Box 1440, Indianapolis, IN 46206-1440. Phone: (317) 637-9200. Quarterly.

Sports Medicine Digest. PM, Inc., P.O. Box 2468, Van Nuys, CA 91404. Phone: (818) 873-4399. Monthly.

ONLINE DATABASES

EMBASE. Elsevier Science Publishing Co., Inc., P.O. Box 882, Madison Square Station, New York, NY 10159-2101. Phone: (212) 989-5800. Fax: (212) 633-3990.

MEDLINE. National Library of Medicine, 8600 Rockville Pike, Bethesda, MD 20894. Phone: (800) 638-8480.

The Physician and Sportsmedicine. McGraw-Hill Inc., 11 West 19th St., New York, NY 10011. Phone: (212) 337-5001. Fax: (212) 337-4092. Monthly.

SciSearch. Institute for Scientific Information, 3501 Market St., Philadelphia, PA 19104. Phone: (215) 386-0100. Fax: (215) 386-6362.

Sport and Leisure Database. Faculty of Human Kinetics and Leisure Studies, University of Waterloo, Waterloo, ON, Canada N2L 3G1. Phone: (519) 885-1211.

POPULAR WORKS AND PATIENT EDUCATION

The Complete Sports Medicine Book for Women: Revised for the '90s. Mona Shangold, Gabe Mirkin. Simon & Schuster, Inc., 1230 Ave. of the Americas, New York, NY 10020. Phone: (212) 698-7000. Revised edition.

Fitness and Sports Medicine: An Introduction. David C. Nieman. Bull Publishing Co., 110 Gilbert Ave., Menlo Park, CA 94025. Phone: (800) 676-2855. 1990.

The Sports Injury Handbook: Professional Advice for Amateur Athletes. Allan M. Levy, Mark L. Fuerst. John Wiley & Sons,

Inc., 605 Third Ave., New York, NY 10158-0012. Phone: (212) 850-6000. Fax: (212) 850-6088. 1992.

Sports Medicine: Health and Medication. Bengt O. Eriksson, Tore Mellstrand, Lars Peterson, and others. Facts on File, Inc., 460 Park Ave. S., New York, NY 10016-7382. Phone: (212) 683-2244. Fax: (212) 683-3633. 1990.

RESEARCH CENTERS, INSTITUTES, CLEARINGHOUSES

Center for Sports Medicine and Science. Temple University, Broad and Tioga Sts., Philadelphia, PA 19140. Phone: (215) 221-2111.

National Center for Catastrophic Sports Injury Research. 311 Woollen Gymnasium, Campus Box #8600, University of North Carolina at Chapel Hill, Chapel Hill, NC 27599. Phone: (919) 962-2021.

Sports Injuries/Therapeutic Exercise Research Unit. University of Illinois, 906 S. Goodwin, Urbana, IL 61801. Phone: (217) 333-7699.

TEXTBOOKS AND MONOGRAPHS

Athletic Injuries to the Head, Neck and Face. Torg. Mosby-Year Book, 11830 Westline Industrial Drive, St. Louis, MO 63146. Phone: (800) 325-4177. Fax: (314) 432-1380. Second edition 1991.

Knee Ligaments. Jack C. Hughston. Mosby-Year Book, 11830 Westline Industrial Drive, St. Louis, MO 63146. Phone: (800) 325-4177. Fax: (314) 432-1380. 1993.

Medical Issues for Active and Athletic Women. Agostini. Mosby-Year Book, 11830 Westline Industrial Drive, St. Louis, MO 63146. Phone: (800) 325-4177. Fax: (314) 432-1380. 1993.

Prevention of Athletic Injuries. Mueller. F.A. Davis Co., 1915 Arch St., Philadelphia, PA 19103. Phone: (800) 523-4049. Fax: (215) 568-5065. 1991.

Prevention and Treatment of Running Injuries. Robert D. D'Ambrosia, David Drez (eds.). SLACK Inc., 6900 Grove Rd., Thorofare, NJ 08086-9447. Phone: (800) 257-8290. Fax: (609) 853-5991. Second edition 1989.

Sports Injuries. M.A. Hutson. Oxford University Press, 200 Madison Ave., New York, NY 10016. Phone: (212) 679-7300. 1990.

Sports Injury Assessment and Rehabilitation. David C. Reid. Churchill Livingstone Inc., 650 Avenue of the Americas, New York, NY 10011. Phone: (212) 819-5400. Fax: (212) 302-6598. 1991.

Sports Medicine. Richard H. Strauss. W.B. Saunders Co., The Curtis Center, Independence Square W., Philadelphia, PA 19106-3399. Phone: (215) 238-7800. Second edition 1991.

Sports, Medicine, and Health. G.P. Hermans, W.L. Mostrerd. Elsevier Science Publishing Co., Inc., P.O. Box 882, Madison Square Station, New York, NY 10159-2101. Phone: (212) 989-5800. Fax: (212) 633-3990. 1991.

Sports Medicine: Health Care for Young Athletes. American Academy of Pediatrics, 141 Northwest Point Blvd., P.O. Box 927, Elk Grove Village, IL 60009-0927. Phone: (800) 433-9016. Fax: (708) 228-1281. Second edition 1991.

Sports Medicine for the Primary Care Physician. Richard B. Birrer. Appleton & Lange, 25 Van Zant St., East Norwalk, CT 06855. Phone: (800) 423-1359. Fax: (203) 854-9486. 1983.

SPOUSE ABUSE

ABSTRACTING, INDEXING, AND CURRENT AWARENESS PUBLICATIONS

Psychological Abstracts. American Psychological Association, 1200 17th St. NW, Washington, DC 20036. Phone: (202) 955-7600. Monthly.

ASSOCIATIONS, PROFESSIONAL SOCIETIES, ADVOCACY AND SUPPORT GROUPS

American Psychological Association (APA). 1200 17th St. N.W., Washington, DC 20036. Phone: (202) 955-7600. Fax: (703) 525-5191.

CD-ROM DATABASES

American Journal of Public Health. MEP, 124 Mt. Auburn St., Cambridge, MA 02138. Phone: (800) 342-1338. Fax: (617) 868-7738. Annual.

Journal of the American Medical Association. Macmillan New Media, 124 Mt. Auburn St., Cambridge, MA 02138. Weekly.

PsycLit. SilverPlatter Information, Inc., River Ridge Office Park, 100 River Ridge Rd., Norwood, MA 02062. Phone: (617) 769-2599. Fax: (617) 769-8763. Quarterly.

JOURNALS

American Journal of Nursing. American Journal of Nursing Co., 555 W. 57th St., New York, NY 10019. Phone: (212) 582-8820. Monthly.

American Journal of Obstetrics and Gynecology. Mosby-Year Book, 11830 Westline Industrial Drive, St. Louis, MO 63146. Phone: (800) 325-4177. Fax: (314) 432-1380. Monthly.

American Journal of Orthopsychiatry. American Orthopsychiatric Association, Inc., 19 W. 44th St., New York, NY 10036. Phone: (212) 354-5770. Fax: (212) 302-9463. Quarterly.

American Journal of Public Health. American Public Health Association, 1015 15th St. NW, Washington, DC 20005. Phone: (202) 789-5666. Monthly.

ONLINE DATABASES

PsycInfo. SilverPlatter Information, Inc., River Ridge Office Park, 100 River Ridge Rd., Norwood, MA 02062. Phone: (617) 769-2599. Fax: (617) 769-8763. Quarterly.

POPULAR WORKS AND PATIENT EDUCATION

Trauma and Recovery: The Aftermath of Violence--from Domestic Abuse to Political Terror. Judith Lewis Herman. Basic Books, 10 E. 53rd St., New York, NY 10022. Phone: (800) 242-7737. 1993.

TEXTBOOKS AND MONOGRAPHS

The Battered Woman and Shelters: The Social Construction of Wife Abuse. Donileen R. Loseke. State University of New York

Press, State University Plaza, Albany, NY 12246-0001. Phone: (800) 666-2211. 1992.

SPRAINS

See: WOUNDS AND INJURIES

STAPHYLOCOCCAL INFECTIONS

See: INFECTIOUS DISEASES

STATISTICS

See: VITAL STATISTICS

STERILITY

See: INFERTILITY

STERILIZATION

See: CONTRACEPTION

STEROIDS

See: HORMONES

STOMA

See also: COLORECTAL SURGERY

ASSOCIATIONS, PROFESSIONAL SOCIETIES, ADVOCACY AND SUPPORT GROUPS

Crohn's & Colitis Foundation of America, Inc.. 444 Park Ave. S., 11th Flr., New York, NY 10016-7374. Phone: (800) 343-3637.

International Association for Enterostomal Therapy. 2081 Business Circle Dr., No. 290, Irvine, CA 92715. Phone: (714) 476-0268.

United Ostomy Association (UOA). 36 Executive Park, Ste. 120, Irvine, CA 92714. Phone: (714) 660-8624. Fax: (714) 660-9262.

JOURNALS

British Journal of Surgery. Butterworth-Heinemann, 80 Montvale Ave., Stoneham, MA 02180. Phone: (617) 438-8464. Fax: (617) 279-4851. Monthly Monthly.

Diseases of the Colon and Rectum. Williams & Wilkins, 428 E. Preston St., Baltimore, MD 21202. Phone: (800) 638-0672. Fax: (800) 447-8438. Monthly.

Gut. BMJ Publishing Group, BMA House, Tavistock Square, London WC1H 9JR, England. Phone: 071-383 6244/6638. Fax: 071-383 6662. Monthly.

Journal of Laryngology and Otology. Headley Bros. Ltd., Invicta Press, Ashford, Kent TN24 8HH, England. Monthly.

Journal of Urology. Williams & Wilkins, 428 E. Preston St., Baltimore, MD 21202. Phone: (800) 638-0672. Fax: (800) 447-8438. Monthly.

Surgery: Gynecology & Obstetrics. American College of Surgeons, 55 East Erie St., Chicago, IL 60611-2797. Phone: (312) 664-4050. Monthly.

ONLINE DATABASES

EMBASE. Elsevier Science Publishing Co., Inc., P.O. Box 882, Madison Square Station, New York, NY 10159-2101. Phone: (212) 989-5800. Fax: (212) 633-3990.

MEDLINE. National Library of Medicine, 8600 Rockville Pike, Bethesda, MD 20894. Phone: (800) 638-8480.

SciSearch. Institute for Scientific Information, 3501 Market St., Philadelphia, PA 19104. Phone: (215) 386-0100. Fax: (215) 386-6362.

POPULAR WORKS AND PATIENT EDUCATION

The Ostomy Book: Living Comfortably with Colostomies, Ileostomies & Urostomies. Barbara D. Mullen, Kerry A. McGinn. Bull Publishing Co., 110 Gilbert Ave., Menlo Park, CA 94025. Phone: (800) 676-2855. 1992.

TEXTBOOKS AND MONOGRAPHS

Methods in Stomatal Research. Jonathan Weyers, Hans Meidner. John Wiley & Sons, Inc., 605 Third Ave., New York, NY 10158-0012. Phone: (212) 850-6000. Fax: (212) 850-6088. 1991.

STRABISMUS

See: EYE DISEASES; VISION DISORDERS

STREP THROAT

See: INFECTIOUS DISEASES

STREPTOCOCCAL INFECTIONS

See: INFECTIOUS DISEASES

STRESS

See also: POST-TRAUMATIC STRESS DISORDER

ABSTRACTING, INDEXING, AND CURRENT AWARENESS PUBLICATIONS

Excerpta Medica. Section 32: Psychiatry. Elsevier Science Publishing Co., Inc., P.O. Box 882, Madison Square Station, New York, NY 10159-2101. Phone: (212) 989-5800. Fax: (212) 633-3990. 20/year.

Index Medicus. U.S. National Library of Medicine, 8600 Rockville Pike, Bethesda, MD 20894. Phone: (800) 638-8480. Monthly.

Psychological Abstracts. American Psychological Association, 1200 17th St. NW, Washington, DC 20036. Phone: (202) 955-7600. Monthly.

PSYSCAN: Clinical Psychology. American Psychological Association, 1200 17th St. NW, Washington, DC 20036. Phone: (202) 955-7600. Quarterly.

ASSOCIATIONS, PROFESSIONAL SOCIETIES, ADVOCACY AND SUPPORT GROUPS

American Institute of Stress (AIS). 124 Park Ave., Yonkers, NY 10703. Phone: (914) 963-1200. Fax: (914) 965-6267.

American Psychological Association (APA). 1200 17th St. N.W., Washington, DC 20036. Phone: (202) 955-7600. Fax: (703) 525-5191.

Society for Traumatic Stress Studies (STSS). 435 N. Michigan Ave., Ste. 1717, Chicago, IL 60611. Phone: (312) 644-0828. Fax: (312) 644-8557.

BIBLIOGRAPHIES

Occupational Health: Stress. National Technical Information Service, 5285 Port Royal Rd., Springfield, VA 22161. Phone: (703) 487-4650. Fax: (703) 321-8547. Jan. 1985-May 1989 PB89-862304/CBY.

A Selected Bibliography on Stress and Stress Management. National Heart, Lung, and Blood Institute Education-Programs Information Center, 4733 Bethesda Ave., Ste. 530, Bethesda, MD 20814. Phone: (301) 951-3260. Monthly.

CD-ROM DATABASES

PsycLit. SilverPlatter Information, Inc., River Ridge Office Park, 100 River Ridge Rd., Norwood, MA 02062. Phone: (617) 769-2599. Fax: (617) 769-8763. Quarterly.

JOURNALS

Stress and Anxiety. Taylor & Francis Inc., 1900 Frost Rd., Suite 101, Bristol, PA 19007-1598. Phone: (800) 821-8312. Fax: (215) 785-5515.

Stress Medicine. John Wiley & Sons, Inc., 605 Third Ave., New York, NY 10158-0012. Phone: (212) 850-6000. Fax: (212) 850-6088. Quarterly.

NEWSLETTERS

American Institute of Stress-Newsletter. American Institute of Stress, Inc., 124 Park Ave., Yonkers, NY 10703. Phone: (914) 963-1200. Annual.

ONLINE DATABASES

EMBASE. Elsevier Science Publishing Co., Inc., P.O. Box 882, Madison Square Station, New York, NY 10159-2101. Phone: (212) 989-5800. Fax: (212) 633-3990.

MEDLINE. National Library of Medicine, 8600 Rockville Pike, Bethesda, MD 20894. Phone: (800) 638-8480.

Mental Health Abstracts. IFI/Plenum Data Company, 302 Swann Ave., Alexandria, VA 22301. Phone: (800) 368-3093. Monthly.

PsycInfo. SilverPlatter Information, Inc., River Ridge Office Park, 100 River Ridge Rd., Norwood, MA 02062. Phone: (617) 769-2599. Fax: (617) 769-8763. Quarterly.

SciSearch. Institute for Scientific Information, 3501 Market St., Philadelphia, PA 19104. Phone: (215) 386-0100. Fax: (215) 386-6362.

POPULAR WORKS AND PATIENT EDUCATION

Living with Stress and Anxiety. Bob Whitmore. St. Martin's Press, 175 Fifth Ave., New York, NY 10010. Phone: (212) 674-5151. 1992.

RESEARCH CENTERS, INSTITUTES, CLEARINGHOUSES

Center for Stress and Anxiety Disorders. State University of New York at Albany. 1535 Western Ave., Albany, NY 12203. Phone: (518) 456-4143.

Center for Study of Trauma. University of California, San Francisco. Dept. of Psychiatry, 401 Parnassus, San Francisco, CA 94143-0984. Phone: (415) 476-7344. Fax: (415) 388-4913.

TEXTBOOKS AND MONOGRAPHS

Post-Traumatic Stress Disorder: Assessment, Differential Diagnosis, and Forensic Evaluation. Carroll L. Meek (ed.). Professional Resource Exchange, P.O. Box 15560, 2033 Wood St., Ste. 215, Sarasota, FL 34237-1560. Phone: (800) 443-3364. 1990.

STROKE

See: CEREBROVASCULAR DISEASES

STUTTERING

See: COMMUNICATION DISORDERS

SUBSTANCE ABUSE

See: ALCOHOLISM; DRUG ABUSE

SUDDEN INFANT DEATH SYNDROME

ABSTRACTING, INDEXING, AND CURRENT AWARENESS PUBLICATIONS

Current Contents/Clinical Medicine. Institute for Scientific Information, 3501 Market St., Philadelphia, PA 19104. Phone: (800) 523-1850. Fax: (215) 386-6362. Weekly.

Excerpta Medica. Section 7: Pediatrics and Pediatric Surgery. Elsevier Science Publishing Co., Inc., P.O. Box 882, Madison Square Station, New York, NY 10159-2101. Phone: (212) 989-5800. Fax: (212) 633-3990. 24/year.

Index Medicus. U.S. National Library of Medicine, 8600 Rockville Pike, Bethesda, MD 20894. Phone: (800) 638-8480. Monthly.

Science Citation Index. Institute for Scientific Information, 3501 Market St., Philadelphia, PA 19104. Phone: (800) 523-1850. Fax: (215) 386-6362. Bimonthly.

ASSOCIATIONS, PROFESSIONAL SOCIETIES, ADVOCACY AND SUPPORT GROUPS

American Sudden Infant Death Syndrome Institute (ASIDSI). 275 Carpenter Dr. N.E., Atlanta, GA 30328. Phone: (800) 232-SIDS.

The Danny Foundation. 3160-F Danville Blvd., P.O. Box 680, Alamo, CA 94507. Phone: (800) 833-2669.

National Sudden Infant Death Syndrome Foundation (NSIDSF). 10500 Little Patuxent Pkwy., No. 420, Columbia, MD 21044. Phone: (800) 221-SIDS.

SIDS Alliance. 10500 Little Patuxent Pkwy., Ste. 420, Columbia, MD 21044. Phone: (800) 221-SIDS.

BIBLIOGRAPHIES

Sudden Infant Death Syndrome (SIDS). National Technical Information Service, 5285 Port Royal Rd., Springfield, VA 22161. Phone: (703) 487-4650. Fax: (703) 321-8547. Jan. 1978-May 1989 PB89-862833/CBY.

CD-ROM DATABASES

Pediatrics on Disc. CMC ReSearch, Inc., 7150 S.W. Hampton, Suite C-120, Portland, OR 97223. Phone: (800) 262-7668. Fax: (503) 639-1796. Annual.

SCISEARCH. Institute for Scientific Information, 3501 Market St., Philadelphia, PA 19104. Phone: (215) 386-0100. Fax: (215) 386-6362.

DIRECTORIES

Directory of Sudden Infant Death Syndrome Programs and Resources. National Sudden Infant Death Syndrome Clearinghouse, 8201 Greensboro Dr., Ste. 600, Mc Lean, VA 22102. Phone: (703) 821-8955. Fax: (703) 506-0384. 1988.

JOURNALS

American Journal of Diseases of Children. American Medical Association, 515 North State St., Chicago, IL 60610. Phone: (312) 464-0183. Fax: (312) 464-5834. Monthly.

Journal of Pediatrics. Mosby-Year Book, 11830 Westline Industrial Drive, St. Louis, MO 63146. Phone: (800) 325-4177. Fax: (314) 432-1380. Monthly.

Pediatrics. American Academy of Pediatrics, 141 Northwest Point Rd., Elk Grove Village, IL 60009-0927. Phone: (708) 228-5005. Fax: (708) 228-5097. Monthly.

NEWSLETTERS

The Leaflet. National Sudden Infant Death Syndrome Foundation, Inc., 10500 Little Patuxent Parkway, Ste. 420, Columbia, MD 21044. Phone: (800) 221-7437. Fax: (301) 964-8009. 4/year.

ONLINE DATABASES

EMBASE. Elsevier Science Publishing Co., Inc., P.O. Box 882, Madison Square Station, New York, NY 10159-2101. Phone: (212) 989-5800. Fax: (212) 633-3990.

MEDLINE. National Library of Medicine, 8600 Rockville Pike, Bethesda, MD 20894. Phone: (800) 638-8480.

SciSearch. Institute for Scientific Information, 3501 Market St., Philadelphia, PA 19104. Phone: (215) 386-0100. Fax: (215) 386-6362.

POPULAR WORKS AND PATIENT EDUCATION

The Baby Book: The Most Comprehensive Guide to Infant Care. William Sears, Martha Sears. Little, Brown and Co., 34 Beacon St., Boston, MA 02108. Phone: (617) 227-0730. Fax: (617) 227-0790. 1992.

The Columbia University College of Physicians and Surgeons Complete Guide to Early Child Care. Genell Subak-Sharpe (ed.). Random House, Inc., 201 E. 50th St., New York, NY 10022. Phone: (800) 726-0600. 1990.

Sudden Infant Death: Enduring the Loss. John DeFrain, and others. D.C. Heath & Co., 125 Spring St., Lexington, MA 02173. Phone: (800) 235-3565. 1991.

RESEARCH CENTERS, INSTITUTES, CLEARINGHOUSES

National Center for the Prevention of Sudden Infant Death Syndrome. 330 N. Charles St., Baltimore, MD 21201. Phone: (301) 547-0300.

National Sudden Infant Death Syndrome Clearinghouse (NSIDSC). 8201 Greensboro Dr., Ste. 600, Mc Lean, VA 22102. Phone: (703) 821-8955. Fax: (703) 506-0384.

Sudden Infant Death Syndrome Institute. 22 S. Greene St., Baltimore, MD 21201. Phone: (301) 538-3363.

TEXTBOOKS AND MONOGRAPHS

Nelson Textbook of Pediatrics. Richard E. Behrman, Victor C. Vaughan. W.B. Saunders Co., The Curtis Center, Independence Sqare W., Philadelphia, PA 19106-3399. Phone: (215) 238-7800. 14th edition, 1992.

SUICIDE

ABSTRACTING, INDEXING, AND CURRENT AWARENESS PUBLICATIONS

Excerpta Medica. Section 32: Psychiatry. Elsevier Science Publishing Co., Inc., P.O. Box 882, Madison Square Station, New York, NY 10159-2101. Phone: (212) 989-5800. Fax: (212) 633-3990. 20/year.

Index Medicus. U.S. National Library of Medicine, 8600 Rockville Pike, Bethesda, MD 20894. Phone: (800) 638-8480. Monthly.

Psychological Abstracts. American Psychological Association, 1200 17th St. NW, Washington, DC 20036. Phone: (202) 955-7600. Monthly.

Research Alert: Suicide. Institute for Scientific Information, 3501 Market St., Philadelphia, PA 19104. Phone: (800) 523-1850. Fax: (215) 386-6362. Weekly.

Science Citation Index. Institute for Scientific Information, 3501 Market St., Philadelphia, PA 19104. Phone: (800) 523-1850. Fax: (215) 386-6362. Bimonthly.

ASSOCIATIONS, PROFESSIONAL SOCIETIES, ADVOCACY AND SUPPORT GROUPS

American Association of Suicidology. 2459 S. Ash St., Denver, CO 80222.

American Psychiatric Association (APA). 1400 K St. N.W., Washington, DC 20005. Phone: (202) 682-6000. Fax: (202) 682-6114.

Hemlock Society. P.O. Box 11830, Eugene, OR 97440. Phone: (503) 342-5748.

National Alliance for the Mentally Ill (NAMI). 2101 Wilson Blvd., Ste. 302, Arlington, VA 22201. Phone: (703) 524-7600. Fax: (703) 524-9094.

Samaritans. 500 Commonwealth Ave., Kenmore Square, Boston, MA 02215. Phone: (617) 247-0220.

Seasons: Suicide Bereavement. c/o Joan Clark, 1358 Sunset Dr., Salt Lake City, UT 84116. Phone: (801) 596-2341.

Society for the Right to Die. 250 W. 57th St., New York, NY 10107. Phone: (212) 246-6973.

CD-ROM DATABASES

Morbidity Mortality Weekly Report. MEP, 124 Mt. Auburn St., Cambridge, MA 02138. Phone: (800) 342-1338. Fax: (617) 868-7738. Annual.

SCISEARCH. Institute for Scientific Information, 3501 Market St., Philadelphia, PA 19104. Phone: (215) 386-0100. Fax: (215) 386-6362.

ENCYCLOPEDIAS, DICTIONARIES, WORD BOOKS

Encyclopedia of Suicide. Glen Evans, Norman L. Farberow. Facts on File, Inc., 460 Park Ave. S., New York, NY 10016-7382. Phone: (212) 683-2244. Fax: (212) 683-3633. 1988.

JOURNALS

Journal of Clinical Psychiatry. Physicians Postgraduate Press, Box 240008, Memphis, TN 38124. Phone: (901) 682-1001.

Morbidity and Mortality Weekly Report. Massachusetts Medical Society, 1440 Main St., Waltham, MA 02154-1649. Phone: (617) 893-3800. Fax: (617) 893-0413. Weekly.

Suicide and Life-Threatening Behavior. Guilford Publications, Inc., 72 Spring St., New York, NY 10012. Phone: (800) 365-7006. Fax: (212) 366-6708.

ONLINE DATABASES

EMBASE. Elsevier Science Publishing Co., Inc., P.O. Box 882, Madison Square Station, New York, NY 10159-2101. Phone: (212) 989-5800. Fax: (212) 633-3990.

MEDLINE. National Library of Medicine, 8600 Rockville Pike, Bethesda, MD 20894. Phone: (800) 638-8480.

PsycInfo. SilverPlatter Information, Inc., River Ridge Office Park, 100 River Ridge Rd., Norwood, MA 02062. Phone: (617) 769-2599. Fax: (617) 769-8763. Quarterly.

SciSearch. Institute for Scientific Information, 3501 Market St., Philadelphia, PA 19104. Phone: (215) 386-0100. Fax: (215) 386-6362.

Suicide Information and Education. Suicide Information Education Center, 1615 10th Ave. S.W., Calgary, AB, Canada. Phone: (403) 245-3900.

POPULAR WORKS AND PATIENT EDUCATION

Dying with Dignity: Understanding Euthanasia. Derek Humphry. Carol Publishing Group, 600 Madison Ave., 11th Flr., New York, NY 10022. Phone: (212) 486-2200. 1992.

Final Exit: The Practicalities of Self-Deliverance and Assisted Suicide for the Dying. Derek Humphry. Bantam Books, Inc., 666 Fifth Ave., New York, NY 10103. Phone: (800) 223-6834. 1993.

Prescription Medicine: The Goodness of Planned Death. Jack Kevorkian. Prometheus Books, 700 E. Amherst St., Buffalo, NY 14215. Phone: (800) 421-0351. 1991.

Survivors of Suicide. Rita Robinson. Borgo Press, P.O. Box 2845, San Bernardino, CA 92406-2845. Phone: (909) 884-5813. Fax: (909) 888-4942. 1989.

RESEARCH CENTERS, INSTITUTES, CLEARINGHOUSES

Center for the Study of Suicide and Life Threatening Behavior. 228 Callcott Bldg., University of South Carolina at Columbia, Columbia, SC 29208. Phone: (803) 777-6870.

Youth Suicide National Center. 445 Virginia Ave., San Mateo, CA 94402. Phone: (415) 347-3961.

TEXTBOOKS AND MONOGRAPHS

Suicidal Behaviour. S.A. Montgomery (ed.). Rapid Communications of Oxford Ltd., The Old Malthouse, Paradise St., Oxford OX1 1LD, England. Phone: 44-865-790447. Fax: 44-865-244012. 1992.

Suicide Intervention in the Schools. Scott Polard. Guilford Publications, Inc., 72 Spring St., New York, NY 10012. Phone: (800) 365-7006. Fax: (212) 366-6708. 1989.

Suicide and the Older Adult. Antoon A. Leenars, and others. Guilford Publications, Inc., 72 Spring St., New York, NY 10012. Phone: (800) 365-7006. Fax: (212) 366-6708. 1992.

Suicide Over the Life Cycle: Risk Factors, Assessment, and Treatment of Suicidal Patients. Susan J. Blumenthal, David J. Kupfer (eds.). American Psychiatric Press, Inc., 1400 K St. NW, Washington, DC 20005. Phone: (202) 682-6268. Fax: (202) 789-2648. 1990.

Suicide: Right or Wrong? John Donnelly. Prometheus Books, 700E. Amherst St., Buffalo, NY 14215. Phone: (800) 421-0351. 1990.

SUNSTROKE

See: EMERGENCY MEDICINE

SURGERY

See also: CARDIOVASCULAR SURGERY;
COLORECTAL SURGERY; EYE SURGERY;
LASER SURGERY; ORTHOPEDICS; PLASTIC
AND COSMETIC SURGERY; THORACIC
SURGERY

ABSTRACTING, INDEXING, AND CURRENT AWARENESS PUBLICATIONS

Current Contents/Clinical Medicine. Institute for Scientific Information, 3501 Market St., Philadelphia, PA 19104. Phone: (800) 523-1850. Fax: (215) 386-6362. Weekly.

Excerpta Medica. Section 9: Surgery. Elsevier Science Publishing Co., Inc., P.O. Box 882, Madison Square Station, New York, NY 10159-2101. Phone: (212) 989-5800. Fax: (212) 633-3990. 24/year.

Excerpta Medica. Section 18: Cardiovascular Disease and Cardiovascular Surgery. Elsevier Science Publishing Co., Inc., P.O. Box 882, Madison Square Station, New York, NY 10159-2101. Phone: (212) 989-5800. Fax: (212) 633-3990. 24/year.

Index Medicus. U.S. National Library of Medicine, 8600 Rockville Pike, Bethesda, MD 20894. Phone: (800) 638-8480. Monthly.

Science Citation Index. Institute for Scientific Information, 3501 Market St., Philadelphia, PA 19104. Phone: (800) 523-1850. Fax: (215) 386-6362. Bimonthly.

ANNUALS AND REVIEWS

Advances in Surgery. Mosby-Year Book, 11830 Westline Industrial Drive, St. Louis, MO 63146. Phone: (800) 325-4177. Fax: (314) 432-1380. Annual.

Chest Surgery Clinics of North America. W.B. Saunders Co., The Curtis Center, Independence Square W., Philadelphia, PA 19106-3399. Phone: (215) 238-7800. Quarterly.

Current Practice in Surgery. Churchill Livingstone Inc., 650 Avenue of the Americas, New York, NY 10011. Phone: (212) 819-5400. Fax: (212) 302-6598. Quarterly.

Current Problems in Surgery. Mosby-Year Book, 11830 Westline Industrial Drive, St. Louis, MO 63146. Phone: (800) 325-4177. Fax: (314) 432-1380. Monthly.

Surgical Clinics. W.B. Saunders Co., The Curtis Center, Independence Square W., Philadelphia, PA 19106-3399. Phone: (215) 238-7800. Bimonthly.

Surgical Oncology Clinics of North America. W.B. Saunders Co., The Curtis Center, Independence Square W., Philadelphia, PA 19106-3399. Phone: (215) 238-7800. Quarterly.

Year Book of Surgery. Mosby-Year Book, 11830 Westline Industrial Drive, St. Louis, MO 63146. Phone: (800) 325-4177. Fax: (314) 432-1380. Annual.

Yearbook of the American College of Surgeons. American College of Surgeons, 55 East Erie St., Chicago, IL 60611-2797. Phone: (312) 664-4050. Triennial.

ASSOCIATIONS, PROFESSIONAL SOCIETIES, ADVOCACY AND SUPPORT GROUPS

American Board of Surgery (ABS). 1617 John F. Kennedy Blvd., Ste. 860, Philadelphia, PA 19103. Phone: (215) 568-4000.

American College of Surgeons (ACS). 55 E. Erie St., Chicago, IL 60611. Phone: (312) 664-4050. Fax: (312) 440-7014.

International College of Surgeons (ICS). 1516 N. Lake Shore Dr., Chicago, IL 60610. Phone: (312) 642-3555. Fax: (312) 787-1624.

Royal College of Physicians and Surgeons of Canada. 74 Stanley, Ottawa, ON, Canada K1M 1P4.

CD-ROM DATABASES

SCISEARCH. Institute for Scientific Information, 3501 Market St., Philadelphia, PA 19104. Phone: (215) 386-0100. Fax: (215) 386-6362.

DIRECTORIES

Directory of Certified Orthopaedic Surgeons. American Board of Medical Specialties, 1 Rotary Center, Suite 805, Evanston, IL 60201. Phone: (708) 491-9091. Biennial.

Directory of Certified Surgeons. American Board of Medical Specialties, 1 Rotary Center, Suite 805, Evanston, IL 60201. Phone: (708) 491-9091. Biennial.

Directory of Certified Thoracic Surgeons. American Board of Medical Specialties, 1 Rotary Center, Suite 805, Evanston, IL 60201. Phone: (708) 491-9091. Biennial.

Directory of Medical Specialists. Marquis Who's Who, 3002 Glenview Rd., Wilmette, IL 60091. Phone: (800) 621-9669. Fax: (708) 441-2264. Biennial.

Directory of Physicians in the United States. American Medical Association, 515 North State St., Chicago, IL 60610. Phone: (312) 464-0183. Fax: (312) 464-5834. Biennial.

ENCYCLOPEDIAS, DICTIONARIES, WORD BOOKS

Surgery on File: General Surgery. The Diagram Group. Facts on File, Inc., 460 Park Ave. S., New York, NY 10016-7382. Phone: (212) 683-2244. 1988.

Surgical Word Book. Sam McMillan. Springhouse Publishing Co., 1111 Bethlehem Pike, Spring House, PA 19477. Phone: (800) 331-3170. Fax: (215) 646-8716. 1992.

HANDBOOKS, GUIDES, MANUALS, ATLASES

Atlas of Hernia Surgery. George E. Wantz. Raven Press, 1185 Avenue of the Americas, New York, NY 10036. Phone: (212) 930-9500. Fax: (212) 869-3495. 1991.

Atlas of Surgical Operations. Robert M. Zollinger Jr., Robert M. Zollinger. McGraw-Hill, Inc., Health Professions Division, 1221 Avenue of the Americas, 28th Floor, New York, NY 10020. Phone: (212) 512-4228. Seventh edition 1992.

Atlas of Surgical Techniques. Marvin L. Gliedman. McGraw-Hill, Inc., Health Professions Division, 1221 Avenue of the Americas, 28th Floor, New York, NY 10020. Phone: (212) 512-4228. 1990.

Handbook of Surgery. Schrock. Mosby-Year Book, 11830 Westline Industrial Drive, St. Louis, MO 63146. Phone: (800) 325-4177. Fax: (314) 432-1380. Ninth edition 1989.

Handbook of Surgical Intensive Care. Lyerly. Mosby-Year Book, 11830 Westline Industrial Drive, St. Louis, MO 63146. Phone: (800) 325-4177. Fax: (314) 432-1380. Third edition 1992.

Manual of Medical Care of the Surgical Patient. Coussons. Little, Brown and Co., 34 Beacon St., Boston, MA 02108. Phone: (617) 227-0730. Fourth edition 1990.

Manual of Surgical Therapeutics. Lloyd M. Nyhus, Robert E. Condon. Little, Brown and Company, 34 Beacon St., Boston, MA 02108. Phone: (617) 227-0730. Eighth edition 1992.

Mont Reid Surgical Handbook. Hiyama. Mosby-Year Book, 11830 Westline Industrial Drive, St. Louis, MO 63146. Phone: (800) 325-4177. Fax: (314) 432-1380. Second edition 1990.

Principles of Surgery: Companion Handbook. Seymour I. Schwartz. McGraw-Hill, Inc., Health Professions Division, 1221 Avenue of the Americas, 28th Floor, New York, NY 10020. Phone: (212) 512-4228. Fifth edition 1990.

Surgery: Diagnosis and Therapy. Stillman. Appleton & Lange, 25 Van Zant St., East Norwalk, CT 06855. Phone: (800) 423-1359. Fax: (203) 854-9486. Second edition 1992.

JOURNALS

American Journal of Surgery. Cahners Publishing Company, 249 W. 17th St., New York, NY 10011. Phone: (212) 645-0067.

American Surgeon. J.B. Lippincott Co., 227 E. Washington Square, Philadelphia, PA 19106-3780. Phone: (215) 238-4200. Fax: (215) 238-4227.

Annals of Surgery. J.B. Lippincott Company, 227 E. Washington Square, Philadelphia, PA 19106-3780. Phone: (215) 238-4200. Fax: (215) 238-4227. Monthly.

Archives of Surgery. American Medical Association, 515 North State St., Chicago, IL 60610. Phone: (312) 464-0183. Fax: (312) 464-5834. Monthly.

British Journal of Surgery. Butterworth-Heinemann, 80 Montvale Ave., Stoneham, MA 02180. Phone: (617) 438-8464. Fax: (617) 279-4851. Monthly Monthly.

Canadian Journal of Surgery/Le Journal Canadien de Chirurgie. Canadian Medical Association, 1867 Alta Vista Drive, Box 8650, Ottawa, ON, Canada K1G 0G8. Phone: (613) 731-9331. Fax: (613) 731-4797. Bimonthly.

Current Surgery. J.B. Lippincott Co., 227 E. Washington Square, Philadelphia, PA 19106-3780. Phone: (215) 238-4200. Fax: (215) 238-4227.

Journal of Gynecologic Surgery. Mary Ann Liebert, Inc., 1651 Third Ave., New York, NY 10128. Phone: (212) 289-2300. Fax: (212) 289-4697. Quarterly.

Journal of Investigative Surgery. Taylor & Francis Inc., 1900 Frost Rd., Suite 101, Bristol, PA 19007-1598. Phone: (800) 821-8312. Fax: (215) 785-5515. Quarterly.

Journal of Surgical Research. Academic Press, Inc., 1250 Sixth Ave., San Diego, CA 92101-4311. Phone: (619) 699-6345. Fax: (619) 699-6715.

Microsurgery. John Wiley & Sons, Inc., 605 Third Ave., New York, NY 10158-0012. Phone: (212) 850-6000. Fax: (212) 850-6088. Bimonthly.

Obesity Surgery. Rapid Communications of Oxford Ltd., The Old Malthouse, Paradise St., Oxford OX1 1LD, England. Phone: 44-865-790447. Fax: 44-865-244012. 4/year.

Surgery. Mosby-Year Book, 11830 Westline Industrial Drive, St. Louis, MO 63146. Phone: (800) 325-4177. Fax: (314) 432-1380. Monthly.

Surgery: Gynecology & Obstetrics. American College of Surgeons, 55 East Erie St., Chicago, IL 60611-2797. Phone: (312) 664-4050. Monthly.

NEWSLETTERS

Surgery Alert. American Health Consultants, Department C1290, P.O. Box 740060, Atlanta, GA 30374. Phone: (800) 559-1032. Fax: (404) 352-1971. Monthly.

ONLINE DATABASES

EMBASE. Elsevier Science Publishing Co., Inc., P.O. Box 882, Madison Square Station, New York, NY 10159-2101. Phone: (212) 989-5800. Fax: (212) 633-3990.

MEDIS. Mead Data Central, P.O. Box 1830, Dayton, OH 45401. Phone: (800) 227-4908.

MEDLINE. National Library of Medicine, 8600 Rockville Pike, Bethesda, MD 20894. Phone: (800) 638-8480.

SciSearch. Institute for Scientific Information, 3501 Market St., Philadelphia, PA 19104. Phone: (215) 386-0100. Fax: (215) 386-6362.

POPULAR WORKS AND PATIENT EDUCATION

So Your Doctor Recommended Surgery. John Lewis. Holt, Rinehart & Winston, 115 W. 18th St., New York, NY 10011. Phone: (800) 488-5233. 1992.

Surgery: A Complete Guide for Patients and Their Families. Allen Gross, and others. HarperCollins Publishers, Inc., 10 E. 53rd St., New York, NY 10022-5299. Phone: (212) 207-7000. Fax: (800) 242-7737.

RESEARCH CENTERS, INSTITUTES, CLEARINGHOUSES

Harrison Department of Surgical Research. University of Pennsylvania. 313 Medical Education Bldg., Margarett M. Clark Laboratories, Philadelphia, PA 19104-6070. Phone: (215) 898-8081.

National Second Surgical Opinion Program. Health Care Financing Administration, 200 Independence Ave. S.W., Washington, DC 20201. Phone: (800) 638-6833.

Surgical Research Institute. St. Louis University. 3635 Vista Ave. at Grand Blvd., P.O. Box 15250, St. Louis, MO 63110-0250. Phone: (314) 577-8561. Fax: (314) 771-1945.

STANDARDS AND STATISTICS SOURCES

Socio-Economic Factbook for Surgery. American College of Surgeons, 55 E. Erie St., Chicago, IL 60611. Phone: (312) 664-4050. Annual.

TEXTBOOKS AND MONOGRAPHS

Clinical Thinking in Surgery. Sterns. Appleton & Lange, 25 Van Zant St., East Norwalk, CT 06855. Phone: (800) 423-1359. Fax: (203) 854-9486. 1988.

Current Surgical Diagnosis and Treatment. L.W. Way. Appleton & Lange, 25 Van Zant St., East Norwalk, CT 06855. Phone: (800) 423-1359. Fax: (203) 854-9486. Ninth edition 1990.

High Tech Surgery. John G. Hunter, Jonathan M. Sackler. McGraw-Hill, Inc., Health Professions Division, 1221 Avenue of the Americas, 28th Floor, New York, NY 10020. Phone: (212) 512-4228. 1992.

Mastery of Surgery. Lloyd M. Nyhus, Robert J. Baker (eds.). Little, Brown and Company, 34 Beacon St., Boston, MA 02108. Phone: (617) 227-0730. Second edition Two volumes 1992.

Principles of Surgery. Seymour I. Schwartz, G. Tom Shires, Frank C. Spencer. McGraw-Hill, Inc., Health Professions Division, 1221 Avenue of the Americas, 28th Floor, New York, NY 10020. Phone: (212) 512-4228. Fifth edition 1989.

Principles of Trauma Surgery. Moylan. Raven Press, 1185 Ave. of the Americas, New York, NY 10036. Phone: (212) 930-9500. Fax: (212) 869-3495. Second edition 1992.

Surgery: Scientific Principles and Practice. Greenfield. J.B. Lippincott Co., 227 E. Washington Square, Philadelphia, PA 19106-3780. Phone: (215) 238-4200. Fax: (215) 238-4227. 1992.

Textbook of Surgery: The Biological Basis of Modern Surgical Practice. David C. Sabiston (ed.). W.B. Saunders Co., The Curtis Center, Independence Sqare W., Philadelphia, PA 19106-3399. Phone: (215) 238-7800. 14th edition, 1992.

Therapeutic Drugs. Sir Colin Dollery (ed.). Churchill Livingstone Inc., 650 Avenue of the Americas, New York, NY 10011. Phone: (212) 819-5400. Fax: (212) 302-6598. Two volumes 1991.

Urologic Surgery. Hector Bensimon. McGraw-Hill, Inc., Health Professions Division, 1221 Avenue of the Americas, 28th Floor, New York, NY 10020. Phone: (212) 512-4228. 1991.

SYPHILIS

See: SEXUALLY TRANSMITTED DISEASES

SYSTEMIC LUPUS ERYTHEMATOSUS

See: LUPUS ERYTHEMATOSUS

T

TACHYCARDIA

See: ARRHYTHMIA; HEART DISEASES

TARDIVE DYSKINESIA

See: NEUROMUSCULAR DISORDERS

TAY-SACHS DISEASE

See also: GENETIC DISEASES

ABSTRACTING, INDEXING, AND CURRENT AWARENESS PUBLICATIONS

Current Contents/Clinical Medicine. Institute for Scientific Information, 3501 Market St., Philadelphia, PA 19104. Phone: (800) 523-1850. Fax: (215) 386-6362. Weekly.

Current Contents/Life Sciences. Institute for Scientific Information, 3501 Market St., Philadelphia, PA 19104. Phone: (215) 386-0100. Fax: (215) 386-6362.

Excerpta Medica. Section 22: Human Genetics. Elsevier Science Publishers, P.O. Box 882, Madison Square Station, New York, NY 10159-2101. Phone: (212) 633-3950. Fax: (212) 633-3990. 24/year.

Index Medicus. U.S. National Library of Medicine, 8600 Rockville Pike, Bethesda, MD 20894. Phone: (800) 638-8480. Monthly.

ASSOCIATIONS, PROFESSIONAL SOCIETIES, ADVOCACY AND SUPPORT GROUPS

National Foundation for Jewish Genetic Diseases (NFJGD). 250 Park Ave., Ste. 1000, New York, NY 10017. Phone: (212) 371-1030.

National Tay-Sachs and Allied Diseases Association (NTSAD). 385 Elliot St., Newton, MA 02164. Phone: (617) 964-5508.

DIRECTORIES

Tay-Sachs Test Center Directory. National Tay-Sachs & Allied Diseases Association, Inc., 385 Elliot St., Newton, MA 02164. Phone: (617) 964-5508. Annual.

ENCYCLOPEDIAS, DICTIONARIES, WORD BOOKS

Encyclopedia of Genetic Disorders and Birth Defects. Mark D. Ludman, James Wynbrandt. Facts on File, Inc., 460 Park Ave.

S., New York, NY 10016-7382. Phone: (212) 683-2244. Fax: (212) 683-3633. 1991.

Glossary of Genetics. Rieger. Springer-Verlag New York Inc., 175 Fifth Ave., New York, NY 10010. Phone: (212) 460-1500. Fax: (212) 473-6272. Fifth edition 1991.

JOURNALS

American Journal of Human Genetics. University of Chicago Press, P.O. Box 37005, Chicago, IL 60637. Phone: (312) 753-3347. Fax: (312) 753-0811. Monthly.

Annals of Neurology. Little, Brown and Co., 34 Beacon St., Boston, MA 02108. Phone: (617) 227-0730. Fax: (617) 227-0790. Monthly.

Clinical Biochemistry. Pergamon Press, 660 White Plains Rd., Tarrytown, NY 10591-5153. Phone: (914) 592-7700. Fax: (914) 592-3625. 6/year.

Journal of Genetic Counseling. Human Sciences Press, 233 Spring St., New York, NY 10013-1578. Phone: (800) 221-9369. Fax: (212) 807-1047. Quarterly.

Journal of Medical Genetics. BMJ Publishing Group, BMA House, Tavistock Square, London WC1H 9JR, England. Phone: 071-383 6244/6638. Fax: 071-383 6662. Monthly.

Lancet. Williams & Wilkins, 428 East Preston St., Baltimore, MD 21202. Phone: (800) 638-0672. Fax: (800) 447-8438. Weekly.

NEWSLETTERS

National Tay-Sachs & Allied Diseases Association-Breakthrough. National Tay-Sachs & Allied Diseases Association, Inc., 385 Elliot St., Newton, MA 02164. Phone: (617) 964-5508. 2/year.

ONLINE DATABASES

EMBASE. Elsevier Science Publishing Co., Inc., P.O. Box 882, Madison Square Station, New York, NY 10159-2101. Phone: (212) 989-5800. Fax: (212) 633-3990.

MEDLINE. National Library of Medicine, 8600 Rockville Pike, Bethesda, MD 20894. Phone: (800) 638-8480.

SciSearch. Institute for Scientific Information, 3501 Market St., Philadelphia, PA 19104. Phone: (215) 386-0100. Fax: (215) 386-6362.

RESEARCH CENTERS, INSTITUTES, CLEARINGHOUSES

Center for Jewish Genetic Disease. Div. of Medical Genetics of Mt. Sinai Medical Ctr., 100th St. at Fifth Ave., New York, NY 10029. Phone: (212) 241-6947.

TEXTBOOKS AND MONOGRAPHS

The Metabolic Basis of Inherited Disease. Charles R. Scriver, Arthur L. Beaudet, William S. Sly, et. al.. McGraw-Hill Inc., 11 West 19th St., New York, NY 10011. Phone: (212) 337-5001. Fax: (212) 337-4092. Two volumes 1989.

Therapy for Genetic Disease. Theodore Friedmann. Oxford University Press, 200 Madison Ave., New York, NY 10016. Phone: (212) 679-7300. 1991.

Treatment of Genetic Diseases. Robert J. Desnick (ed.). Churchill Livingstone Inc., 650 Avenue of the Americas, New York, NY 10011. Phone: (212) 819-5400. Fax: (212) 302-6598. 1991.

TEETH

See: DENTISTRY; MOUTH DISEASES; ORAL SURGERY

TEMPOROMANDIBULAR JOINT SYNDROME

ABSTRACTING, INDEXING, AND CURRENT AWARENESS PUBLICATIONS

Dental Abstracts. Mosby-Year Book, 11830 Westline Industrial Drive, St. Louis, MO 63146. Phone: (800) 325-4177. Fax: (314) 432-1380. Bimonthly.

Index to Dental Literature. American Dental Association, 211 E. Chicago Ave., Chicago, IL 60611-2678. Phone: (800) 947-4746. Fax: (312) 440-3542. Quarterly.

Index Medicus. U.S. National Library of Medicine, 8600 Rockville Pike, Bethesda, MD 20894. Phone: (800) 638-8480. Monthly.

ANNUALS AND REVIEWS

Oral and Maxillofacial Surgery Clinics. W.B. Saunders Co., The Curtis Center, Independence Square W., Philadelphia, PA 19106-3399. Phone: (215) 238-7800. Quarterly.

Year Book of Dentistry. Mosby-Year Book, 11830 Westline Industrial Drive, St. Louis, MO 63146. Phone: (800) 325-4177. Fax: (314) 432-1380. Annual.

ASSOCIATIONS, PROFESSIONAL SOCIETIES, ADVOCACY AND SUPPORT GROUPS

American Association of Oral and Maxillofacial Surgeons (AAOMS). 9700 W. Bryn Mawr, Rosemont, IL 60018. Phone: (800) 822-6637. Fax: (708) 678-6286.

American Board of Oral and Maxillofacial Surgery (ABOMS). 625 N. Michigan Ave., Ste. 1820, Chicago, IL 60611. Phone: (312) 642-0070.

American Dental Association (ADA). 211 E. Chicago Ave., Chicago, IL 60611. Phone: (312) 440-2500.

HANDBOOKS, GUIDES, MANUALS, ATLASES

Arthroscopyic Atlas of the Temporomandibular Joint. David I. Blaustein, Leslie B. Heffez. Williams & Wilkins, 428 East Preston St., Baltimore, MD 21202. Phone: (800) 638-0672. Fax: (800) 447-8438. 1990.

Color Atlas and Textbook of the Temporomandibular Joint Diseases, Disorders, Surgery. John E. DeBurgh, Norman Paul Bramley (eds.). Mosby-Year Book, 11830 Westline Industrial Drive, St. Louis, MO 63146. Phone: (800) 325-4177. Fax: (314) 432-1380. 1990.

TMJ Arthroscopy: Diagnostic and Surgical Atlas. Allen W. Tarro. J.B. Lippincott Co., 227 East Washington Square, Philadelphia, PA 19106-3780. Phone: (215) 238-4200. Fax: (215) 238-4227. 1992.

JOURNALS

Cranio: The Journal of Craniomandibular Practice. Williams & Wilkins, 428 E. Preston St., Baltimore, MD 21202. Phone: (800) 638-0672. Fax: (800) 447-8438. Quarterly.

Journal of Oral and Maxillofacial Surgery. W.B. Saunders Co., The Curtis Center, Independence Square W., Philadelphia, PA 19106-3399. Phone: (215) 238-7800. Monthly.

Journal of Prosthetic Dentistry. Mosby-Year Book, 11830 Westline Industrial Drive, St. Louis, MO 63146. Phone: (800) 325-4177. Fax: (314) 432-1380. Monthly.

Oral Surgery, Oral Medicine, Oral Pathology. Mosby-Year Book, 11830 Westline Industrial Drive, St. Louis, MO 63146. Phone: (800) 325-4177. Fax: (314) 432-1380. Monthly.

ONLINE DATABASES

EMBASE. Elsevier Science Publishing Co., Inc., P.O. Box 882, Madison Square Station, New York, NY 10159-2101. Phone: (212) 989-5800. Fax: (212) 633-3990.

MEDLINE. National Library of Medicine, 8600 Rockville Pike, Bethesda, MD 20894. Phone: (800) 638-8480.

SciSearch. Institute for Scientific Information, 3501 Market St., Philadelphia, PA 19104. Phone: (215) 386-0100. Fax: (215) 386-6362.

POPULAR WORKS AND PATIENT EDUCATION

Relief of Pain from Headaches and TMJ. Paula Mackowiak. Solomon Books, 3095 Elmwood Ave., Buffalo, NY 14217. Phone: (716) 874-5155. 1989.

TMJ Book. Andrew Kaplan, Gray Williams, Jr.. Pharos Books, 200 Park Ave., New York, NY 10166. Phone: (212) 692-3830. 1988.

TMJ Syndrome: The Overlooked Diagnosis. Richard Goldman, Virginia McCullough. Pocket Books, Inc., 1230 Ave. of the Americas, New York, NY 10020. Phone: (800) 223-2348. Fax: (800) 284-0735. 1989.

TMJ: The Self Help Program. John J. Taddy, Constance Schrader, James Dillon. Surrey Park Press, P.O. Box 2887, La Jolla, CA 92038-2887. Phone: (619) 454-9333. Revised edition 1991.

RESEARCH CENTERS, INSTITUTES, CLEARINGHOUSES

American Equilibration Society. 8726 N. Ferris Ave., Morton Grove, IL 60053. Phone: (312) 965-2888.

TEXTBOOKS AND MONOGRAPHS

Diagnostic and Operative Arthroscopy of the Temporomandibular Joint. McCain. Mosby-Year Book, 11830 Westline Industrial Drive, St. Louis, MO 63146. Phone: (800) 325-4177. Fax: (314) 432-1380. 1991.

Magnetic Resonance of the Temporomandibular Joint. E. Palacios, G.E. Valvassori, M. Shannon, C.F. Reed. Thieme Medical Publishers, Inc., 381 Park Ave. S., New York, NY 10016. Phone: (212) 683-5088. Fax: (212) 779-9020. 1990.

Principles of Oral and Maxillofacial Surgery. Larry J. Peterson, A. Thomas Indresano, Robert Marciani. J.B. Lippincott Co., 227 East Washington Square, Philadelphia, PA 19106-3780. Phone: (215) 238-4200. Fax: (215) 238-4227. Three volumes 1992.

Temporomandibular Disorders: Classification, Diagnosis, Management. Welden E. Bell. Mosby-Year Book, 11830 Westline Industrial Drive, St. Louis, MO 63146. Phone: (800) 325-4177. Fax: (314) 432-1380. 3rd edition, 1990.

Temporomandibular Disorders: Diagnosis and Treatment. Andrew S. Kaplan, Leon A. Assael. W.B. Saunders Co., The Curtis Center, Independence Square W., Philadelphia, PA 19106-3399. Phone: (215) 238-7800. 1992.

The Temporomandibular Joint: A Biological Basis for Clinical Practice. Bernard G. Sarnat, Daniel M. Laskin. W.B. Saunders Co., The Curtis Center, Independence Square W., Philadelphia, PA 19106-3399. Phone: (215) 238-7800. Fourth edition 1992.

Textbook of Temporomandibular Disorders. Kaplan. W.B. Saunders Co., The Curtis Center, Independence Square W., Philadelphia, PA 19106-3399. Phone: (215) 238-7800. 1991.

TERATOGENS

See: BIRTH DEFECTS

TERMINAL CARE

See also: DEATH AND DYING; HOSPICES

ABSTRACTING, INDEXING, AND CURRENT AWARENESS PUBLICATIONS

Cumulative Index to Nursing and Allied Health Literature. Glendale Adventist Medical Center, P.O. Box 871, Glendale, CA 91209. Phone: (818) 409-8005. Bimonthly.

Index Medicus. U.S. National Library of Medicine, 8600 Rockville Pike, Bethesda, MD 20894. Phone: (800) 638-8480. Monthly.

Palliative Care Index. Medical Information Service, British Library, Boston Spa, Wetherby, W. Yorkshire LS23 7BQ, England. Phone: 0937-546039. Fax: 0937-546236. Monthly.

ASSOCIATIONS, PROFESSIONAL SOCIETIES, ADVOCACY AND SUPPORT GROUPS

Children's Hospice International. 1101 King St., No. 131, Alexandria, VA 22314. Phone: (703) 684-0330.

Concern for Dying. 250 W. 57th St., New York, NY 10107. Phone: (212) 246-6962.

Foundation for Hospice and Homecare (FHH). 519 C St. NE, Stanton Park, Washington, DC 20002. Phone: (202) 547-6586.

Foundation of Thanatology. 630 W. 168th St., New York, NY 10032. Phone: (212) 928-2066.

Hemlock Society. P.O. Box 11830, Eugene, OR 97440. Phone: (503) 342-5748.

Society for the Right to Die. 250 W. 57th St., New York, NY 10107. Phone: (212) 246-6973.

CD-ROM DATABASES

Nursing and Allied Health (CINAHL) on CD-ROM. CINAHL, 1509 Wilson Terrace, P.O. Box 871, Glendale, CA 91209-0871. Phone: (818) 409-8005.

DIRECTORIES

Guide to the Nation's Hospices. National Hospice Organization, 1901 N. Moore St., Ste. 901, Arlington, VA 22209. Phone: (703) 243-5900. Fax: (703) 525-5762. Annual.

Home Health Care and Hospice Directory. National Association of Home Care, 519 C St. NE, Washington, DC 20002. Phone: (202) 547-7424. Fax: (202) 547-3540. Annual.

Hospices Directory. American Business Directories, Inc., 5711 S. 86th Circle, Omaha, NE 68127. Phone: (402) 593-4600. Fax: (402) 331-1505. Annual.

National Home Care and Hospice Directory. National Association of Home Care, 519 C St. N.E., Washington, DC 20002. Phone: (202) 547-7424. Fax: (202) 547-3540. Annual.

JOURNALS

Hospice Journal. Haworth Press, 10 Alice Street, Binghamton, NY 13904-1580. Phone: (800) 429-6784. Fax: (607) 722-1424. Quarterly.

Palliative Medicine. Cambridge University Press, 40 W. 20th St., New York, NY 10011. Phone: (800) 431-1580. Quarterly.

NEWSLETTERS

Concern for Dying Newsletter. Concern for Dying, 250 W. 57th St., New York, NY 10107. Phone: (212) 246-6962.

Hospice Letter. Health Resources Publishing, Brinley Professional Plaza, 3100 Hwy. 138, Wall, NJ 07719-1442. Phone: (201) 681-1133. Monthly.

Hospice Newsletter. Sovereign Hospitaller Order of Saint John, Villa Anneslie, 529 Dunkirk Rd., Baltimore, MD 21212. Phone: (301) 377-4352. Annual.

NHO Hospice News. National Hospice Organization, 1901 N. Moore St., Ste. 901, Arlington, VA 22209. Phone: (703) 243-5900. Fax: (703) 525-5762. Monthly.

ONLINE DATABASES

EMBASE. Elsevier Science Publishing Co., Inc., P.O. Box 882, Madison Square Station, New York, NY 10159-2101. Phone: (212) 989-5800. Fax: (212) 633-3990.

MEDLINE. National Library of Medicine, 8600 Rockville Pike, Bethesda, MD 20894. Phone: (800) 638-8480.

Nursing and Allied Health (CINAHL). CINAHL, 1509 Wilson Terrace, P.O. Box 871, Glendale, CA 91209-0871. Phone: (818) 409-8005.

SciSearch. Institute for Scientific Information, 3501 Market St., Philadelphia, PA 19104. Phone: (215) 386-0100. Fax: (215) 386-6362.

POPULAR WORKS AND PATIENT EDUCATION

The Complete Guide to Hospice Care. Larry Beresford. Little, Brown and Co., 34 Beacon St., Boston, MA 02108. Phone: (617) 227-0730. Fax: (617) 227-0790. 1992.

Dying at Home: A Family Guide for Caregiving. Andrea Sankar. Johns Hopkins University Press, 701 W. 40th St., Suite 275, Baltimore, MD 21211-2190. Phone: (800) 537-5487. 1991.

The Hospice Movement: A Better Way of Caring for the Dying. Sandol Stoddard. Random House, Inc., 201 E. 50th St., New York, NY 10022. Phone: (800) 726-0600. Expanded edition 1991.

When a Loved One Is Ill: How to Take Better Care of Your Loved One, Your Family and Yourself. Leonard Felder. Viking Penguin, 375 Hudson St., New York, NY 10014-3657. Phone: (800) 331-4624. 1990.

TEXTBOOKS AND MONOGRAPHS

Caring for the Dying Patient and the Family. J. Robbins. HarperCollins Pubs., Inc., 10 E. 53rd St., New York, NY 10022-5299. Phone: (212) 207-7000. Fax: (800) 242-7737. 2nd edition 1989.

Social Work Theory and Practice with the Terminally Ill. Joan K. Parry. Haworth Press, 10 Alice Street, Binghamton, NY 13904-1580. Phone: (800) 3HA-WORTH. Fax: (607) 722-1424. 1989.

TEST TUBE BABIES

See: IN VITRO FERTILIZATION; INFERTILITY

TESTICULAR CANCER

ABSTRACTING, INDEXING, AND CURRENT AWARENESS PUBLICATIONS

Excerpta Medica. Section 16: Cancer. Elsevier Science Publishing Co., Inc., P.O. Box 882, Madison Square Station, New York, NY 10159-2101. Phone: (212) 989-5800. Fax: (212) 633-3990. 32/year.

Index Medicus. U.S. National Library of Medicine, 8600 Rockville Pike, Bethesda, MD 20894. Phone: (800) 638-8480. Monthly.

Science Citation Index. Institute for Scientific Information, 3501 Market St., Philadelphia, PA 19104. Phone: (800) 523-1850. Fax: (215) 386-6362. Bimonthly.

ANNUALS AND REVIEWS

EORTC Genitourinary Gourp Monograph 7: Prostate Cancer and Testicular Cancer. W.G. Jones, Donald W.W. Newling (eds.). John Wiley & Sons, Inc., 605 Third Ave., New York, NY 10158-0012. Phone: (212) 850-6000. Fax: (212) 850-6088. 1990.

Urologic Clinics. W.B. Saunders Co., The Curtis Center, Independence Square W., Philadelphia, PA 19106-3399. Phone: (215) 238-7800. Quarterly.

ASSOCIATIONS, PROFESSIONAL SOCIETIES, ADVOCACY AND SUPPORT GROUPS

American Board of Urology (ABU). 31700 Telegraph Rd., Ste. 150, Birmingham, MI 48010. Phone: (312) 646-9720.

American Cancer Society (ACS). 1599 Clifton Rd. N.E., Atlanta, GA 30329. Phone: (404) 320-3333.

American Urological Association (AUA). 1120 N. Charles St., Baltimore, MD 21201. Phone: (301) 727-1100. Fax: (301) 625-2390.

CD-ROM DATABASES

OncoDisc. J.B. Lippincott Co., 227 East Washington Square, Philadelphia, PA 19106-3780. Phone: (215) 238-4200. Fax: (215) 238-4227. Bimonthly.

SCISEARCH. Institute for Scientific Information, 3501 Market St., Philadelphia, PA 19104. Phone: (215) 386-0100. Fax: (215) 386-6362.

JOURNALS

Journal of Surgical Oncology. John Wiley & Sons, Inc., 605 Third Ave., New York, NY 10158-0012. Phone: (212) 850-6000. Fax: (212) 850-6088. Monthly.

Journal of Urology. Williams & Wilkins, 428 E. Preston St., Baltimore, MD 21202. Phone: (800) 638-0672. Fax: (800) 447-8438. Monthly.

Urology. Cahners Publishing Company, 249 W. 17th St., New York, NY 10011. Phone: (212) 645-0067.

ONLINE DATABASES

CANCERLIT. U.S. National Cancer Institute, International Cancer Information Center, Building 82, Room 102, Bethesda, MD 20892. Phone: (301) 496-7403. Fax: (301) 480-8105. Monthly.

EMBASE. Elsevier Science Publishing Co., Inc., P.O. Box 882, Madison Square Station, New York, NY 10159-2101. Phone: (212) 989-5800. Fax: (212) 633-3990.

MEDLINE. National Library of Medicine, 8600 Rockville Pike, Bethesda, MD 20894. Phone: (800) 638-8480.

Physician Data Query (PDQ) Cancer Information File. U.S. National Cancer Institute, International Cancer Information Center, Building 82, Room 102, Bethesda, MD 20892. Phone: (301) 496-7403. Fax: (301) 480-8105. Monthly.

Physician Data Query (PDQ) Directory File. U.S. National Cancer Institute, International Cancer Information Center, Building 82, Room 102, Bethesda, MD 20892. Phone: (301) 496-7403. Fax: (301) 480-8105. Monthly.

Physician Data Query (PDQ) Protocol File. U.S. National Cancer Institute, International Cancer Information Center, Building 82, Room 102, Bethesda, MD 20892. Phone: (301) 496-7403. Fax: (301) 480-8105. Monthly.

SciSearch. Institute for Scientific Information, 3501 Market St., Philadelphia, PA 19104. Phone: (215) 386-0100. Fax: (215) 386-6362.

POPULAR WORKS AND PATIENT EDUCATION

Everyone's Guide to Cancer Therapy: How Cancer is Diagnosed, Treated, and Managed on a Day to Day Basis. Malin Dollinger, Ernest H. Rosenbaum, Greg Cable. Andrews & McMeel, 4900 Main St., Kansas City, MO 64112. Phone: (800) 826-4216. 1991.

RESEARCH CENTERS, INSTITUTES, CLEARINGHOUSES

Cancer Information Service (CIS). Office of Cancer Communications, National Cancer Institute, Bldg. 31, Rm. 10A24, 9000 Rockville Pike, Bethesda, MD 20892. Phone: (800) 4CA-NCER.

TEXTBOOKS AND MONOGRAPHS

Campbell's Urology. Patrick C. Walsh (ed.). W.B. Saunders Co., The Curtis Center, Independence Square W., Philadelphia, PA 19106-3399. Phone: (215) 238-7800. Sixth edition. Three volumes. 1992.

Current Therapy in Genitourinary Surgery. Resnick. Mosby-Year Book, 11830 Westline Industrial Drive, St. Louis, MO 63146. Phone: (800) 325-4177. Fax: (314) 432-1380. Second edition 1992.

Testicular Cancer. Horwich. Williams & Wilkins, 428 East Preston St., Baltimore, MD 21202. Phone: (800) 638-0672. Fax: (800) 447-8438. 1991.

TETANUS

See: IMMUNIZATION; INFECTIOUS DISEASES

TETRACYCLINES

See: ANTIBIOTICS

THALASSEMIA

See: HEMATOLOGIC DISORDERS

THORACIC SURGERY

See also: CARDIOVASCULAR SURGERY;
SURGERY

ABSTRACTING, INDEXING, AND CURRENT AWARENESS PUBLICATIONS

Current Contents/Clinical Medicine. Institute for Scientific Information, 3501 Market St., Philadelphia, PA 19104. Phone: (800) 523-1850. Fax: (215) 386-6362. Weekly.

Excerpta Medica. Section 15: Chest Diseases, Thoracic Surgery and Tuberculosis. Elsevier Science Publishing Co., Inc., P.O. Box 882, Madison Square Station, New York, NY 10159-2101. Phone: (212) 989-5800. Fax: (212) 633-3990. 20/year.

Index Medicus. U.S. National Library of Medicine, 8600 Rockville Pike, Bethesda, MD 20894. Phone: (800) 638-8480. Monthly.

Science Citation Index. Institute for Scientific Information, 3501 Market St., Philadelphia, PA 19104. Phone: (800) 523-1850. Fax: (215) 386-6362. Bimonthly.

ASSOCIATIONS, PROFESSIONAL SOCIETIES, ADVOCACY AND SUPPORT GROUPS

American Association for Thoracic Surgery. 13 Elm St., P.O. Box 1565, Manchester, MA 01944. Phone: (508) 526-8330.

American Board of Thoracic Surgery (ABTS). 1 Rotary Center, Ste. 803, Evanston, IL 60201. Phone: (708) 475-1520. Fax: (708) 475-6240.

American College of Chest Physicians (ACCP). 330 Dundee Rd., Northbrook, IL 60062. Phone: (708) 498-1400.

American Thoracic Society (ATS). 1740 Broadway, New York, NY 10019-4374. Phone: (212) 315-8700.

Society of Thoracic Surgeons (STS). 401 N. Michigan Ave., Chicago, IL 60611-4267. Phone: (312) 644-6610. Fax: (312) 938-1214.

CD-ROM DATABASES

Cardiology MEDLINE. MEP, 124 Mt. Auburn St., Cambridge, MA 02138. Phone: (800) 342-1338. Fax: (617) 868-7738. Quarterly.

Excerpta Medica CD: Cardiology. SilverPlatter Information, Inc., River Ridge Office Park, 100 River Ridge Rd., Norwood, MA 02062. Phone: (617) 769-2599. Fax: (617) 769-8763. Quarterly.

SCISEARCH. Institute for Scientific Information, 3501 Market St., Philadelphia, PA 19104. Phone: (215) 386-0100. Fax: (215) 386-6362.

DIRECTORIES

Directory of Certified Thoracic Surgeons. American Board of Medical Specialties, 1 Rotary Center, Suite 805, Evanston, IL 60201. Phone: (708) 491-9091. Biennial.

JOURNALS

Annals of Thoracic Surgery. Elsevier Science Publishing Co., Inc., P.O. Box 882, Madison Square Station, New York, NY

10159-2101. Phone: (212) 989-5800. Fax: (212) 633-3990. Monthly.

Journal of Thoracic and Cardiovascular Surgery. Mosby-Year Book, 11830 Westline Industrial Drive, St. Louis, MO 63146. Phone: (800) 325-4177. Fax: (314) 432-1380. Monthly.

Thorax. BMJ Publishing Group, BMA House, Tavistock Square, London WC1H 9JR, England. Phone: 071-383 6244/6638. Fax: 071-383 6662. Monthly.

ONLINE DATABASES

EMBASE. Elsevier Science Publishing Co., Inc., P.O. Box 882, Madison Square Station, New York, NY 10159-2101. Phone: (212) 989-5800. Fax: (212) 633-3990.

MEDLINE. National Library of Medicine, 8600 Rockville Pike, Bethesda, MD 20894. Phone: (800) 638-8480.

SciSearch. Institute for Scientific Information, 3501 Market St., Philadelphia, PA 19104. Phone: (215) 386-0100. Fax: (215) 386-6362.

RESEARCH CENTERS, INSTITUTES, CLEARINGHOUSES

Thoracic Research Lab. R-3022 Kresge II, University Medical Center, University of Michigan, Ann Arbor, MI 48109. Phone: (313) 764-0289.

TEXTBOOKS AND MONOGRAPHS

Complications in Cardiothoracic Surgery. John A. Waldhausen, Mark B. Orringer. Mosby-Year Book, 11830 Westline Industrial Drive, St. Louis, MO 63146. Phone: (800) 325-4177. Fax: (314) 432-1380. 1991.

Complications in Thoracic Surgery. Wolfe. Mosby-Year Book, 11830 Westline Industrial Drive, St. Louis, MO 63146. Phone: (800) 325-4177. Fax: (314) 432-1380. 1992.

Current Surgical Diagnosis and Treatment. L.W. Way. Appleton & Lange, 25 Van Zant St., East Norwalk, CT 06855. Phone: (800) 423-1359. Fax: (203) 854-9486. Ninth edition 1990.

Decision Making in Cardiothoracic Surgery. Lawrence H. Cohn, and others. Mosby-Year Book, 11830 Westline Industrial Drive, St. Louis, MO 63146. Phone: (800) 325-4177. Fax: (314) 432-1380. 2nd edition, 1992.

Glenn's Thoracic and Cardiovascular Surgery. Arthur Baue, Alexander S. Geha, Graeme L. Hammond, and others. Appleton & Lange, 25 Van Zant St., East Norwalk, CT 06855. Phone: (800) 423-1359. Fax: (203) 854-9486. Fifth edition 1991.

Surgery of the Chest. David Sabiston, Frank Spencer. W.B. Saunders Co., The Curtis Center, Independence Sqare W., Philadelphia, PA 19106-3399. Phone: (215) 238-7800. 5th edition, 1990.

THROMBOLYTICS

See: VASCULAR DISEASES

THROMBOSIS

See: VASCULAR DISEASES

THYROID CANCER

See: THYROID DISEASES

THYROID DISEASES

See also: ENDOCRINE DISORDERS

ABSTRACTING, INDEXING, AND CURRENT AWARENESS PUBLICATIONS

Current Contents/Life Sciences. Institute for Scientific Information, 3501 Market St., Philadelphia, PA 19104. Phone: (215) 386-0100. Fax: (215) 386-6362.

Excerpta Medica. Section 3: Endocrinology. Elsevier Science Publishing Co., Inc., P.O. Box 882, Madison Square Station, New York, NY 10159-2101. Phone: (212) 989-5800. Fax: (212) 633-3990. 24/year.

Research Alert: Thyroid Function & Disorders. Institute for Scientific Information, 3501 Market St., Philadelphia, PA 19104. Phone: (800) 523-1850. Fax: (215) 386-6362. Weekly.

Science Citation Index. Institute for Scientific Information, 3501 Market St., Philadelphia, PA 19104. Phone: (800) 523-1850. Fax: (215) 386-6362. Bimonthly.

ANNUALS AND REVIEWS

Endocrinology and Metabolism Clinics. W.B. Saunders Co., The Curtis Center, Independence Square W., Philadelphia, PA 19106-3399. Phone: (215) 238-7800. Quarterly.

ASSOCIATIONS, PROFESSIONAL SOCIETIES, ADVOCACY AND SUPPORT GROUPS

American Thyroid Association (ATA). Walter Reed Army Medical Ctr., Endocrine-Metabolic Service, Washington, DC 20307-5001. Phone: (202) 882-7717. Fax: (202) 588-4728.

Endocrine Society (ES). 9650 Rockville Pike, Bethesda, MD 20814. Phone: (301) 571-1802.

Thyroid Foundation of America. Ruth Sleaper Hall, Room 310, Massachussetts General Hospital, Boston, MA 02114. Phone: (617) 426-8500.

CD-ROM DATABASES

SCISEARCH. Institute for Scientific Information, 3501 Market St., Philadelphia, PA 19104. Phone: (215) 386-0100. Fax: (215) 386-6362.

JOURNALS

Clinical Endocrinology. Blackwell Scientific Publications, Inc., 3 Cambridge Ctr., Cambridge, MA 02142. Phone: (800) 759-6102. Monthly.

Journal of Clinical Endocrinology & Metabolism. Williams & Wilkins, 428 E. Preston St., Baltimore, MD 21202. Phone: (800) 638-0672. Fax: (900) 447-8438. Monthly.

Thyroid. Mary Ann Liebert, Inc., 1651 Third Ave., New York, NY 10128. Phone: (212) 289-2300. Fax: (212) 289-4697. Quarterly.

POPULAR WORKS AND PATIENT EDUCATION

Thyroid Disease: The Facts. R.I.S. Bayliss, W.M.G. Tunbridge. Oxford University Press, 200 Madison Ave., New York, NY 10016. Phone: (212) 679-7300. Fax: (212) 725-2972. Second edition 1992.

STANDARDS AND STATISTICS SOURCES

Diagnosis and Management of Asymptomatic Primary Hyperparathyroidism. Consensus Statement. NIH Consensus Development Conference. October 29-31, 199. National Institutes of Health, Office of Medical Applications of Research, Federal Bldg., Rm. 618, Bethesda, MD 20892. 1990.

TEXTBOOKS AND MONOGRAPHS

New Actions of Parathyroid Hormone. Shaul G. Massry, Takuo Fujita (eds.). Plenum Publishing Co., 233 Spring St., New York, NY 10013-1578. Phone: (212) 620-8000. Fax: (212) 463-0742. 1989.

Thyroid Disease in Clinical Practice. McDougall. Oxford University Press, 200 Madison Ave., New York, NY 10016. Phone: (212) 679-7300. 1992.

Thyroid Disease: Endocrinology, Surgery, Nuclear Medicine, and Radiotherapy. Stephen Falk. Raven Press, 1185 Avenue of the Americas, New York, NY 10036. Phone: (212) 930-9500. Fax. (212) 869-3495. 1990.

Thyroid Function and Disease. Gerald N. Burrow, and others. W.B. Saunders Co., The Curtis Center, Independence Sqare W., Philadelphia, PA 19106-3399. Phone: (215) 238-7800.

The Thyroid Gland. Monte Greer. Raven Press, 1185 Avenue of the Americas, New York, NY 10036. Phone: (212) 930-9500. Fax: (212) 869-3495. 1990.

Werner and Ingbar's The Thyroid: A Fundamental and Clinical Text. Lewis E. Braverman, Robert D. Utiger. J.B. Lippincott Co., 227 E. Washington Square, Philadelphia, PA 19106-3780. Phone: (215) 238-4200. Fax: (215) 238-4227. Sixth edition 1992.

TICK INFESTATION

See: PARASITIC DISEASES

TINEA

See: FUNGAL DISEASES

TINNITUS

See also: HEARING DISORDERS

ABSTRACTING, INDEXING, AND CURRENT AWARENESS PUBLICATIONS

Excerpta Medica. Section 11: Otorhinolaryngology. Elsevier Science Publishing Co., Inc., P.O. Box 882, Madison Square

Station, New York, NY 10159-2101. Phone: (212) 989-5800. Fax: (212) 633-3990. 16/year.

ANNUALS AND REVIEWS

Otolaryngologic Clinics. W.B. Saunders Co., The Curtis Center, Independence Square W., Philadelphia, PA 19106-3399. Phone: (215) 238-7800. Bimonthly.

ASSOCIATIONS, PROFESSIONAL SOCIETIES, ADVOCACY AND SUPPORT GROUPS

American Academy of Otolaryngology - Head and Neck Surgery (AAO-HNS). 1 Prince St., Alexandria, VA 22314. Phone: (703) 836-4444. Fax: (703) 683-5100.

American Board of Otolaryngology (ABO). 5615 Kirby Dr., Ste. 936, Houston, TX 77005. Phone: (713) 528-6200.

American Tinnitus Association (ATA). P.O. Box 5, Portland, OR 97207. Phone: (503) 248-9985.

DIRECTORIES

Directory of Certified Otolaryngologists. American Board of Medical Specialties, 1 Rotary Center, Suite 805, Evanston, IL 60201. Phone: (708) 491-9091. Biennial.

ENCYCLOPEDIAS, DICTIONARIES, WORD BOOKS

Encyclopedia of Deafness and Hearing Disorders. Carol Turkington, Allen Sussman. Facts on File, Inc., 460 Park Ave. S., New York, NY 10016-7382. Phone: (212) 683-2244. Fax: (212) 683-3633. 1992.

JOURNALS

Annals of Otology, Rhinology & Laryngology. Annals Publishing Co., 4507 Laclede Ave., St. Louis, MO 63108. Phone: (314) 367-4987. Fax: (314) 367-4988. Monthly.

Archives of Otolaryngology-Head & Neck Surgery. American Medical Association, 515 North State St., Chicago, IL 60610. Phone: (312) 464-0183. Fax: (312) 464-5834. Monthly.

Clinical Otolaryngology. Blackwell Scientific Publications, Inc., 3 Cambridge Ctr., Cambridge, MA 02142. Phone: (800) 759-6102. Bimonthly.

NEWSLETTERS

American Hearing Research Foundation Newsletter. American Hearing Research Foundation, 55 E. Washington St., Ste. 2022, Chicago, IL 60602. Quarterly.

POPULAR WORKS AND PATIENT EDUCATION

Living with Tinnitus. David W. Rees, Simon D. Smith. St. Martin's Press, 175 Fifth Ave., New York, NY 10010. Phone: (212) 674-5151. 1992.

RESEARCH CENTERS, INSTITUTES, CLEARINGHOUSES

House Ear Institute. 2100 W. 3rd St., 5th Fl., Los Angeles, CA 90057. Phone: (213) 483-4431. Fax: (213) 413-6739.

Kresge Hearing Research Institute. University of Michigan. 1301 E. Ann St., Room 5032, Ann Arbor, MI 48109-0506. Phone: (313) 764-8111. Fax: (313) 764-0014.

TEXTBOOKS AND MONOGRAPHS

Tinnitus: Diagnosis/Treatment. Abraham Shulman (ed.). Williams & Wilkins, 428 East Preston St., Baltimore, MD 21202. Phone: (800) 638-0672. Fax: (800) 447-8438. 1991.

TMJ

See: TEMPOROMANDIBULAR JOINT SYNDROME

TOMOGRAPHY

See also: MRI (MAGNETIC RESONANCE IMAGING); NUCLEAR MEDICINE

ABSTRACTING, INDEXING, AND CURRENT AWARENESS PUBLICATIONS

Current Contents/Clinical Medicine. Institute for Scientific Information, 3501 Market St., Philadelphia, PA 19104. Phone: (800) 523-1850. Fax: (215) 386-6362. Weekly.

Excerpta Medica. Section 14: Radiology. Elsevier Science Publishing Co., Inc., P.O. Box 882, Madison Square Station, New York, NY 10159-2101. Phone: (212) 989-5800. Fax: (212) 633-3990. 24/year.

Excerpta Medica. Section 23: Nuclear Medicine. Elsevier Science Publishers, P.O. Box 882, Madison Square Station, New York, NY 10159-2101. Phone: (212) 633-3950. Fax: (212) 633-3990. 20/year.

Index Medicus. U.S. National Library of Medicine, 8600 Rockville Pike, Bethesda, MD 20894. Phone: (800) 638-8480. Monthly.

Research Alert: Imaging Techniques-CT, MR, PET, SPECT. Institute for Scientific Information, 3501 Market St., Philadelphia, PA 19104. Phone: (800) 523-1850. Fax: (215) 386-6362. Weekly.

ANNUALS AND REVIEWS

Critical Reviews in Diagnostic Imaging. CRC Press, Inc., 2000 Corporate Blvd. N.W., Boca Raton, FL 33431. Phone: (407) 994-0555. Fax: (407) 997-0949. Bimonthly.

Neuroimaging Clinics of North America. W.B. Saunders Co., The Curtis Center, Independence Square W., Philadelphia, PA 19106-3399. Phone: (215) 238-7800. Quarterly.

Year Book of Diagnostic Radiology. Mosby-Year Book, 11830 Westline Industrial Drive, St. Louis, MO 63146. Phone: (800) 325-4177. Fax: (314) 432-1380. Annual.

Year Book of Nuclear Medicine. Mosby-Year Book, 11830 Westline Industrial Drive, St. Louis, MO 63146. Phone: (800) 325-4177. Fax: (314) 432-1380. Annual.

ASSOCIATIONS, PROFESSIONAL SOCIETIES, ADVOCACY AND SUPPORT GROUPS

American College of Radiology (ACR). 1891 Preston White Dr., Reston, VA 22091. Phone: (703) 648-8900.

American Society of Neuroimaging (ASN). 2221 University Ave. S.E., Ste. 340, Minneapolis, MN 55414. Phone: (612) 378-7240.

Computerized Medical Imaging Society (CMIS). National Biomedical Research Foundation, Georgetown University Medical Ctr., 3900 Reservoir Rd. N.W., Washington, DC 20007. Phone: (202) 687-2121.

BIBLIOGRAPHIES

Computerized Tomography: Technology and Equipment. National Technical Information Service, 5285 Port Royal Rd., Springfield, VA 22161. Phone: (703) 487-4650. Fax: (703) 321-8547. Mar. 1988-Apr. 1989 PB89-860696/CBY.

CD-ROM DATABASES

Excerpta Medica CD: Radiology & Nuclear Medicine. SilverPlatter Information, Inc., River Ridge Office Park, 100 River Ridge Rd., Norwood, MA 02062. Phone: (617) 769-2599. Fax: (617) 769-8763. Quarterly.

DIRECTORIES

Directory of Certified Nuclear Medicine Specialists. American Board of Medical Specialties, 1 Rotary Center, Suite 805, Evanston, IL 60201. Phone: (708) 491-9091. Biennial.

HANDBOOKS, GUIDES, MANUALS, ATLASES

Human Cross-Sectional Anatomy Atlas of Body Section and CT Images. Ellis. Butterworth-Heinemann, 80 Montvale Ave., Stoneham, MA 02180. Phone: (617) 438-8464. Fax: (617) 279-4851. 1991.

Manual of Diagnostic Imaging. Straub. Little, Brown and Co., 34 Beacon St., Boston, MA 02108. Phone: (617) 227-0730. Fax: (617) 227-0790. Second edition 1989.

Nuclear Medicine. Datz. Mosby-Year Book, 11830 Westline Industrial Drive, St. Louis, MO 63146. Phone: (800) 325-4177. Fax: (314) 432-1380. 1988.

Workbook for MRI and CT of the Head and Neck. Anthony Mancuso, and others. Williams & Wilkins, 428 East Preston St., Baltimore, MD 21202. Phone: (800) 638-0672. Fax: (800) 447-8438. 2nd edition, 1988.

JOURNALS

Clinical Imaging. Elsevier Science Publishing Co., Inc., P.O. Box 882, Madison Square Station, New York, NY 10159-2101. Phone: (212) 989-5800. Fax: (212) 633-3990. 4/year.

Clinical Nuclear Medicine. J.B. Lippincott Co., 227 E. Washington Square, Philadelphia, PA 19106-3780. Phone: (215) 238-4200. Fax: (215) 238-4227.

Journal of Computer Assisted Tomography. Raven Press, 1185 Avenue of the Americas, New York, NY 10036. Phone: (212) 930-9500. Fax: (212) 869-3495. Bimonthly.

Seminars in Ultrasound, CT and MR. W.B. Saunders Co., The Curtis Center, Independence Sqare W., Philadelphia, PA 19106-3399. Phone: (215) 238-7800.

ONLINE DATABASES

EMBASE. Elsevier Science Publishing Co., Inc., P.O. Box 882, Madison Square Station, New York, NY 10159-2101. Phone: (212) 989-5800. Fax: (212) 633-3990.

MEDLINE. National Library of Medicine, 8600 Rockville Pike, Bethesda, MD 20894. Phone: (800) 638-8480.

SciSearch. Institute for Scientific Information, 3501 Market St., Philadelphia, PA 19104. Phone: (215) 386-0100. Fax: (215) 386-6362.

RESEARCH CENTERS, INSTITUTES, CLEARINGHOUSES

Diagnostic Imaging Science Center. University of Washington. Dept. of Radiology, SB-05, Seattle, WA 98195. Phone: (206) 543-0873. Fax: (206) 543-3495.

Mayo Biomedical Imaging Resource. Mayo Clinic. 200 First St. SW, Rochester, MN 55901. Phone: (507) 284-4937. Fax: (507) 284-1632.

TEXTBOOKS AND MONOGRAPHS

Computed Body Tomography. Lee. Raven Press, 1185 Ave. of the Americas, New York, NY 10036. Phone: (212) 930-9500. Fax: (212) 869-3495. Second edition 1989.

Computed Tomography of the Body: With Magnetic Resonance Imaging. W.B. Saunders Co., The Curtis Center, Independence Sqare W., Philadelphia, PA 19106-3399. Phone: (215) 238-7800. 2nd edition, 1992.

Computed Tomography of the Whole Body. John R. Haaga, Ralph J. Alfidi (eds.). Mosby-Year Book, 11830 Westline Industrial Drive, St. Louis, MO 63146. Phone: (800) 325-4177. Fax: (314) 432-1380. 1988.

Diagnostic Radiology. R.G. Grainger, D. Allison. Churchill Livingstone Inc., 650 Ave. of the Americas, New York, NY 10011. Phone: (212) 819-5400. Fax: (212) 302-6598. Second edition 1991.

Magnetic Resonance Imaging and Computed Tomography of the Head and Spine. C. Barrie Grossman. Williams & Wilkins, 428 East Preston St., Baltimore, MD 21202. Phone: (800) 638-0672. Fax: (800) 447-8438. 1990.

TONSILLITIS

See: OTOLARYNGOLOGY

TORTICOLLIS

See: NEUROMUSCULAR DISORDERS

TOURETTE'S SYNDROME

ABSTRACTING, INDEXING, AND CURRENT AWARENESS PUBLICATIONS

Core Journals in Clinical Neurology. Elsevier Science Publishing Co., Inc., P.O. Box 882, Madison Square Station, New York, NY 10159-2101. Phone: (212) 989-5800. Fax: (212) 633-3990. 11/year.

Excerpta Medica. Section 8: Neurology and Neurosurgery. Elsevier Science Publishers, P.O. Box 882, Madison Square Station, New York, NY 10159-2101. Phone: (212) 633-3950. Fax: (212) 633-3990. 32/year.

Index Medicus. U.S. National Library of Medicine, 8600 Rockville Pike, Bethesda, MD 20894. Phone: (800) 638-8480. Monthly.

Psychological Abstracts. American Psychological Association, 1200 17th St. NW, Washington, DC 20036. Phone: (202) 955-7600. Monthly.

ANNUALS AND REVIEWS

Advances in Neurology. Raven Press, 1185 Avenue of the Americas, New York, NY 10036. Phone: (212) 930-9500. Fax: (212) 869-3495. Irregular.

Annual Review of Neuroscience. Annual Reviews Inc., 4139 El Camino Way, P.O. Box 10139, Palo Alto, CA 94303-0897. Phone: (415) 493-4400. Fax: (415) 855-9815. Annual.

Current Neurology. Mosby-Year Book, 11830 Westline Industrial Drive, St. Louis, MO 63146. Phone: (800) 325-4177. Fax: (314) 432-1380. Annual.

Developments in Neurology. Elsevier Science Publishing Co., Inc., P.O. Box 882, Madison Square Station, New York, NY 10159-2101. Phone: (212) 989-5800. Fax: (212) 633-3990. Irregular.

Neurologic Clinics. W.B. Saunders Co., The Curtis Center, Independence Square W., Philadelphia, PA 19106-3399. Phone: (215) 238-7800. Quarterly.

Neuroscience and Biobehavioral Reviews. Pergamon Press, 660 White Plains Rd., Tarrytown, NY 10591-5153. Phone: (914) 592-7700. Fax: (914) 592-3625. Quarterly.

Progress in Neuro-Psychopharmacology and Biological Psychiatry. Pergamon Press, 660 White Plains Rd., Tarrytown, NY 10591-5153. Phone: (914) 592-7700. Fax: (914) 592-3625. 6/year.

Progress in Neuropathology. Raven Press, 1185 Avenue of the Americas, New York, NY 10036. Phone: (212) 930-9500. Fax: (212) 869-3495. Irregular.

Year Book of Neurology and Neurosurgery. Mosby-Year Book, 11830 Westline Industrial Drive, St. Louis, MO 63146. Phone: (800) 325-4177. Fax: (314) 432-1380. Annual.

ASSOCIATIONS, PROFESSIONAL SOCIETIES, ADVOCACY AND SUPPORT GROUPS

Tourette Syndrome Association (TSA). 42-40 Bell Blvd., Bayside, NY 11361. Phone: (718) 224-2999. Fax: (718) 279-9596.

CD-ROM DATABASES

Excerpta Medica CD: Neurosciences. SilverPlatter Information, Inc., River Ridge Office Park, 100 River Ridge Rd., Norwood, MA 02062. Phone: (617) 769-2599. Fax: (617) 769-8763. Quarterly.

PsycLit. SilverPlatter Information, Inc., River Ridge Office Park, 100 River Ridge Rd., Norwood, MA 02062. Phone: (617) 769-2599. Fax: (617) 769-8763. Quarterly.

JOURNALS

American Journal of Psychiatry. American Psychiatric Press, Inc., 1400 K St. NW, Washington, DC 20005. Phone: (202) 682-6268. Fax: (202) 789-2648. Monthly.

Archives of Neurology. American Medical Association, 515 North State St., Chicago, IL 60610. Phone: (312) 464-0183. Fax: (312) 464-5834. Monthly.

British Journal of Psychiatry. Royal Society of Medicine Services Ltd., 1 Wimpole St., London W1M 8AE, England. Phone: 071-408 2119. Fax: 071-355 3198. Monthly.

Journal of Neurology, Neurosurgery & Psychiatry. BMJ Publishing Group, BMA House, Tavistock Square, London WC1H 9JR, England. Phone: 071-383 6244/6638. Fax: 071-383 6662. Monthly.

Neurology. Edgell Communications, 7500 Old Oak Blvd., Cleveland, OH 44130. Phone: (216) 826-2839. Fax: (216) 891-2726. Monthly.

NEWSLETTERS

Tourette Syndrome Association-Newsletter. Tourette Syndrome Association, 42-40 Bell Blvd., Bayside, NY 11361. Phone: (212) 224-2999. Quarterly.

ONLINE DATABASES

EMBASE. Elsevier Science Publishing Co., Inc., P.O. Box 882, Madison Square Station, New York, NY 10159-2101. Phone: (212) 989-5800. Fax: (212) 633-3990.

MEDLINE. National Library of Medicine, 8600 Rockville Pike, Bethesda, MD 20894. Phone: (800) 638-8480.

PsycInfo. SilverPlatter Information, Inc., River Ridge Office Park, 100 River Ridge Rd., Norwood, MA 02062. Phone: (617) 769-2599. Fax: (617) 769-8763. Quarterly.

SciSearch. Institute for Scientific Information, 3501 Market St., Philadelphia, PA 19104. Phone: (215) 386-0100. Fax: (215) 386-6362.

POPULAR WORKS AND PATIENT EDUCATION

Children with Tourette Syndrome: A Parents' Guide. Tracy Haerle (ed.). Woodbine House, 5615 Fishers Ln., Rockville, MD 20852. Phone: (800) 843-7323. 1992.

Ryan: A Mother's Story of Her Hyperactive-Tourette Syndrome Child. Susan Hughes. Hope Press, P.O. Box 188, Duarte, CA 91009-0188. Phone: (818) 303-064. 1990.

TEXTBOOKS AND MONOGRAPHS

Gilles de la Tourette Syndrome. Arthur K. Shapiro, Elaine Shapiro, J. Gerald Young, et. al.. Raven Press, 1185 Ave. of the Americas, New York, NY 10036. Phone: (212) 930-9500. Fax: (212) 869-3495. Second edition 1988.

Merritt's Textbook of Neurology. Lewis P. Rowland (ed.). Williams & Wilkins, 428 E. Preston St., Baltimore, MD 21202. Phone: (800) 638-0672. Fax: (800) 447-8438. Eighth edition 1989.

Tourette Syndrome & Human Behavior. David E. Comings. Hope Press, P.O. Box 188, Duarte, CA 91009-0188. Phone: (818) 303-064. 1990.

Tourette's Syndrome and TIC Disorders: Clinical Understanding and Treatment. Donald J. Cohen, Ruth D. Bruun, James F. Leckman (eds.). John Wiley & Sons, Inc., 605 Third Ave., New York, NY 10158-0012. Phone: (212) 850-6000. Fax: (212) 850-6088. 1988.

TOXEMIA

See: PREGNANCY COMPLICATIONS

TOXIC SHOCK SYNDROME

See: GYNECOLOGIC DISORDERS

TOXICOLOGY

See also: DRUG TOXICITY; INDUSTRIAL TOXICOLOGY; OCCUPATIONAL HEALTH AND SAFETY

ABSTRACTING, INDEXING, AND CURRENT AWARENESS PUBLICATIONS

CA Selects: Chemical Hazards, Health, & Safety. Chemical Abstracts Service, 2540 Olentangy River Road, P.O. Box 3012, Columbus, OH 43210-0012. Phone: (800) 848-6538. Biweekly.

Chemical Abstracts. Chemical Abstracts Service, 2540 Olentangy River Rd., P.O. Box 3012, Columbus, OH 43210-0012. Phone: (800) 848-6538.

Current Contents/Life Sciences. Institute for Scientific Information, 3501 Market St., Philadelphia, PA 19104. Phone: (215) 386-0100. Fax: (215) 386-6362.

Excerpta Medica. Section 52: Toxicology. Elsevier Science Publishing Co., Inc., P.O. Box 882, Madison Square Station, New York, NY 10159-2101. Phone: (212) 989-5800. Fax: (212) 633-3990. 20/year.

Index Medicus. U.S. National Library of Medicine, 8600 Rockville Pike, Bethesda, MD 20894. Phone: (800) 638-8480. Monthly.

Science Citation Index. Institute for Scientific Information, 3501 Market St., Philadelphia, PA 19104. Phone: (800) 523-1850. Fax: (215) 386-6362. Bimonthly.

Toxicology Abstracts. Cambridge Scientific Abstracts, 7200 Wisconsin Ave., Bethesda, MD 20814-4823. Phone: (800) 843-7751. Fax: (301) 961-6720. Monthly.

ANNUALS AND REVIEWS

Annual Review of Pharmacology and Toxicology. Annual Reviews Inc., 4139 El Camino Way, P.O. Box 10139, Palo Alto, CA 94303-0897. Phone: (415) 493-4400. Fax: (415) 855-9815. Annual.

Critical Reviews in Toxicology. CRC Press, Inc., 2000 Corporate Blvd. N.W., Boca Raton, FL 33431. Phone: (407) 994-0555. Fax: (407) 997-0949. Bimonthly.

Reviews of Environmental Contamination and Toxicology. Ware. Springer-Verlag New York, Inc., 175 Fifth Ave., New York, NY 10010. Phone: (212) 460-1500. Fax: (212) 473-6272. 1991.

Year Book of Toxicology. CRC Press, Inc., 2000 Corporate Blvd. N.W., Boca Raton, FL 33431. Phone: (407) 994-0555. Fax: (407) 997-0949. Annual.

ASSOCIATIONS, PROFESSIONAL SOCIETIES, ADVOCACY AND SUPPORT GROUPS

American College of Toxicology. 9650 Rockville Pike, Bethesda, MD 20814. Phone: (301) 571-1840.

American Industrial Health Council. 1330 Connecticut Ave. N.W., Washington, DC 20036. Phone: (202) 659-0060.

Chemical Industry Institute of Technology. P.O. Box 12137, Research Triangle Park, NC 27709. Phone: (919) 541-2070.

Society of Toxicology. 1133 15th St. N.W., No. 1000, Washington, DC 20005. Phone: (202) 293-5935.

Toxicology Forum. 1575 I St. N.W., No. 800, Washington, DC 20005. Phone: (202) 659-0030.

CD-ROM DATABASES

PolTox. Cambridge Scientific Abstracts, 7200 Wisconsin Ave., Bethesda, MD 20814-4823. Phone: (800) 843-7751. Fax: (301) 961-6720. Quarterly.

SCISEARCH. Institute for Scientific Information, 3501 Market St., Philadelphia, PA 19104. Phone: (215) 386-0100. Fax: (215) 386-6362.

TOXLINE. SilverPlatter Information, Inc., River Ridge Office Park, 100 River Ridge Rd., Norwood, MA 02062. Phone: (617) 769-2599. Fax: (617) 769-8763. Quarterly.

TOXLINE Plus. SilverPlatter Information, Inc., River Ridge Office Park, 100 River Ridge Rd., Norwood, MA 02062. Phone: (617) 769-2599. Fax: (617) 769-8763. Quarterly.

HANDBOOKS, GUIDES, MANUALS, ATLASES

Handbook of Medical Toxicology. Peter Viccellio (ed.). Little, Brown and Company, 34 Beacon St., Boston, MA 02108. Phone: (617) 227-0730. 1992.

Handbook of Toxicology. Viccellio. Little, Brown and Co., 34 Beacon St., Boston, MA 02108. Phone: (617) 227-0730. Fax: (617) 227-0790. 1992.

JOURNALS

European Journal of Pharmacology/Environmental Toxicology and Pharmacology Section. Elsevier Science Publishing Co., Inc., P.O. Box 882, Madison Square Station, New York, NY 10159-2101. Phone: (212) 989-5800. Fax: (212) 633-3990. 6/year.

Fundamental and Applied Technology. Academic Press, Inc., 1250 Sixth Ave., San Diego, CA 92101-4311. Phone: (619) 699-6345. Fax: (619) 699-6715.

Human and Experimental Toxicology. Macmillan Publishing Co., 866 Third Ave., New York, NY 10011. Phone: (800) 257-5755.

Journal of the American College of Toxicology. Mary Ann Liebert, Inc., 1651 Third Ave., New York, NY 10128. Phone: (212) 289-2300. Fax: (212) 289-4697. Bimonthly.

Journal of Applied Toxicology. John Wiley & Sons, Inc., 605 Third Ave., New York, NY 10158-0012. Phone: (212) 850-6000. Fax: (212) 850-6088. Bimonthly.

Journal of Toxicology: Clinical Toxicology. Marcel Dekker, Inc., 270 Madison Ave., New York, NY 10016. Phone: (800) 228-1160.

Journal of Toxicology and Environmental Health. Taylor & Francis Inc., 1900 Frost Rd., Suite 101, Bristol, PA 19007-1598. Phone: (800) 821-8312. Fax: (215) 785-5515. Monthly.

Toxicology. Elsevier Science Publishing Co., Inc., P.O. Box 882, Madison Square Station, New York, NY 10159-2101. Phone: (212) 989-5800. Fax: (212) 633-3990. 6/year.

ONLINE DATABASES

CA File (Chemical Abstracts File). Chemical Abstracts Service, 2540 Olentangy River Rd., P.O. Box 3012, Columbus, OH 43210-0012. Phone: (800) 848-6538.

CSA Life Sciences Collection. Cambridge Scientific Abstracts, 7200 Wisconsin Ave., Bethesda, MD 20814-4823. Phone: (800) 843-7751. Fax: (301) 961-6720.

EMBASE. Elsevier Science Publishing Co., Inc., P.O. Box 882, Madison Square Station, New York, NY 10159-2101. Phone: (212) 989-5800. Fax: (212) 633-3990.

MEDLINE. National Library of Medicine, 8600 Rockville Pike, Bethesda, MD 20894. Phone: (800) 638-8480.

Pollution Abstracts. Cambridge Scientific Abstracts, 7200 Wisconsin Ave., Bethesda, MD 20814-4823. Phone: (800) 843-7751. Fax: (301) 961-6720.

SciSearch. Institute for Scientific Information, 3501 Market St., Philadelphia, PA 19104. Phone: (215) 386-0100. Fax: (215) 386-6362.

TOXLINE. U.S. National Library of Medicine, Toxicology Information Program, 8600 Rockville Pike, Bethesda, MD 20894. Phone: (800) 638-8480. Monthly.

RESEARCH CENTERS, INSTITUTES, CLEARINGHOUSES

Center for Environmental Toxicology. Colorado State University Center for Environmental Toxicology, Fort Collins, CO 80521. Phone: (303) 491-8522.

Institute of Toxicology and Environmental Health. University of California, Davis. Davis, CA 95616. Phone: (916) 752-1340. Fax: (916) 752-5300.

Laboratory of Toxicology. Harvard University. 665 Huntington Ave., Boston, MA 02115. Phone: (617) 432-1177.

Toxicology Program. Box 7633, North Carolina State University, Raleigh, NC 27695. Phone: (919) 737-2274.

TEXTBOOKS AND MONOGRAPHS

Advances in Applied Toxicology. A.D. Dayan, A.J. Paine (eds.). Taylor & Francis Inc., 1900 Frost Rd., Suite 101, Bristol, PA 19007-1598. Phone: (800) 821-8312. Fax: (215) 785-5515. 1989.

Casarett and Doull's Toxicology: The Basic Science of Poisons. Mary O. Amdur, John Doull, Curtis D. Klaassen. McGraw-Hill, Inc., 1221 Avenue of the Americas, 28th Floor, New York, NY 10020. Phone: (212) 512-4228. Fourth edition 1991.

Critical Care Toxicology. Lewis Goldfrank, Robert Hoffman (eds.). Churchill Livingstone Inc., 650 Avenue of the

Americas, New York, NY 10011. Phone: (212) 819-5400. Fax: (212) 302-6598. 1991.

Goldfrank's Toxicologic Emergencies. Lewis R. Goldfrank, Neal E. Fomenbaum, Neal A. Lewin, and others. Appleton & Lange, 25 Van Zant St., East Norwalk, CT 06855. Phone: (800) 423-1359. Fax: (203) 854-9486. Fourth edition 1990.

Human Toxicology of Pesticides. Fina Petrova Kaloyanova, M.A. El Batawi. CRC Press, Inc., 2000 Corporate Blvd. N.W., Boca Raton, FL 33431. Phone: (407) 994-0555. Fax: (407) 997-0949. 1992.

Medical Toxicology: Diagnosis and Treatment of Human Poisoning. Ellerhorn. Elsevier Science Publishing Co., Inc., P.O. Box 882, Madison Square Station, New York, NY 10159-2101. Phone: (212) 989-5800. Fax: (212) 633-3990. 1988.

Primer of Environmental Toxicology. Smith. Williams & Wilkins, 428 East Preston St., Baltimore, MD 21202. Phone: (800) 638-0672. Fax: (800) 447-8438. 1992.

Principles of Clinical Toxicology. Thomas A. Gossel, J. Douglas Bricker. Raven Press, 1185 Avenue of the Americas, New York, NY 10036. Phone: (212) 930-9500. Fax: (212) 869-3495. Second edition 1990.

Principles and Practice of Clinical Toxicology. Gossel. Raven Press, 1185 Ave. of the Americas, New York, NY 10036. Phone: (212) 930-9500. Fax: (212) 869-3495. Second edition 1990.

Toxicologic Emergencies. Goldfrank. Appleton & Lange, 25 Van Zant St., East Norwalk, CT 06855. Phone: (800) 423-1359. Fax: (203) 854-9486. Fourth edition 1990.

Toxicology-A Primer on Toxicology Principles and Applications. Michael A. Kamrin. CRC Press, Inc., 2000 Corporate Blvd. N.W., Boca Raton, FL 33431. Phone: (407) 994-0555. Fax: (407) 997-0949. 1988.

TRANQUILIZERS

See: PSYCHOACTIVE DRUGS

TRANSFUSIONS

See also: BLOOD BANKS; HEMATOLOGY

ABSTRACTING, INDEXING, AND CURRENT AWARENESS PUBLICATIONS

Excerpta Medica. Section 25: Hematology. Elsevier Science Publishers, P.O. Box 882, Madison Square Station, New York, NY 10159-2101. Phone: (212) 633-3950. Fax: (212) 633-3990. 24/year.

Index Medicus. U.S. National Library of Medicine, 8600 Rockville Pike, Bethesda, MD 20894. Phone: (800) 638-8480. Monthly.

ANNUALS AND REVIEWS

Current Studies in Hematology and Blood Transfusion. S. Karger Publishers, Inc., 26 West Avon Rd., P.O. Box 529, Farmington, CT 06085. Phone: (203) 675-7834. Fax: (203) 675-7302. Irregular.

ASSOCIATIONS, PROFESSIONAL SOCIETIES, ADVOCACY AND SUPPORT GROUPS

American Association of Blood Banks (AABB). 1117 N. 19th St., Ste. 600, Arlington, VA 22209. Phone: (703) 528-8200. Fax: (703) 527-8036.

Council of Community Blood Centers. 725 15th St. N.W., No. 700, Washington, DC 20005. Phone: (202) 393-5725.

Society for the Study of Blood. 13 Elm St., Manchester, MA 01944. Phone: (508) 526-8330.

JOURNALS

American Journal of Hematology. John Wiley & Sons, Inc., 605 Third Ave., New York, NY 10158-0012. Phone: (212) 850-6000. Fax: (212) 850-6088. 12/year.

Blood. W.B. Saunders Co., The Curtis Center, Independence Sqare W., Philadelphia, PA 19106-3399. Phone: (215) 238-7800.

Transfusion Medicine Reviews. W.B. Saunders Co., The Curtis Center, Independence Sqare W., Philadelphia, PA 19106-3399. Phone: (215) 238-7800.

Transfusion Science. Pergamon Press, 660 White Plains Rd., Tarrytown, NY 10591-5153. Phone: (914) 592-7700. Fax: (914) 592-3625.

ONLINE DATABASES

Combined Health Information Database (CHID). U.S. National Institutes of Health, P.O. Box NDIC, Bethesda, MD 20892. Phone: (301) 496-2162. Fax: (301) 770-5164. Quarterly.

EMBASE. Elsevier Science Publishing Co., Inc., P.O. Box 882, Madison Square Station, New York, NY 10159-2101. Phone: (212) 989-5800. Fax: (212) 633-3990.

MEDLINE. National Library of Medicine, 8600 Rockville Pike, Bethesda, MD 20894. Phone: (800) 638-8480.

SciSearch. Institute for Scientific Information, 3501 Market St., Philadelphia, PA 19104. Phone: (215) 386-0100. Fax: (215) 386-6362.

TEXTBOOKS AND MONOGRAPHS

Clinical Practice of Transfusion Medicine. Petz. Churchill Livingstone Inc., 650 Ave. of the Americas, New York, NY 10011. Phone: (212) 819-5400. Fax: (212) 302-6598. 1989.

Medical Laboratory Haematology. Roger Hall, Bob Malia. Butterworth-Heinemann, 80 Montvale Ave., Stoneham, MA 02180. Phone: (617) 438-8464. Fax: (617) 279-4851. Second edition 1991.

Modern Blood Banking and Transfusion Practice. Denise Harmening. F.A. Davis Co., 1915 Arch St., Philadelphia, PA 19103. Phone: (800) 523-4049. Fax: (215) 568-5065. Second edition 1989.

Principles of Transfusion Medicine. Rossi. Williams & Wilkins, 428 East Preston St., Baltimore, MD 21202. Phone: (800) 638-0672. Fax: (800) 447-8438. 1991.

TRANSPLANTATION

See also: ARTIFICIAL ORGANS; UROLOGY

ABSTRACTING, INDEXING, AND CURRENT AWARENESS PUBLICATIONS

Current Contents/Clinical Medicine. Institute for Scientific Information, 3501 Market St., Philadelphia, PA 19104. Phone: (800) 523-1850. Fax: (215) 386-6362. Weekly.

Current Contents/Life Sciences. Institute for Scientific Information, 3501 Market St., Philadelphia, PA 19104. Phone: (215) 386-0100. Fax: (215) 386-6362.

Current Literature in Nephrology, Hypertension and Transplantation. Current Literature Publications, Inc., 1513 E St., Bellingham, WA 98225. Phone: (206) 671-6664. Monthly.

Excerpta Medica. Section 26: Immunology, Serology and Transplantation. Elsevier Science Publishing Co., Inc., P.O. Box 882, Madison Square Station, New York, NY 10159-2101. Phone: (212) 989-5800. Fax: (212) 633-3990. 32/year.

Index Medicus. U.S. National Library of Medicine, 8600 Rockville Pike, Bethesda, MD 20894. Phone: (800) 638-8480. Monthly.

Research Alert: Transplantation & Histocompatibility. Institute for Scientific Information, 3501 Market St., Philadelphia, PA 19104. Phone: (800) 523-1850. Fax: (215) 386-6362. Weekly.

ANNUALS AND REVIEWS

Advances and Controversies in Thalassemia Therapy: Bone Marrow Transplantation and Other Approaches. C. Dean Buckner, Robert Peter Gale, Guido Lucarelli (eds.). John Wiley & Sons, Inc., 605 Third Ave., New York, NY 10158-0012. Phone: (212) 850-6000. Fax: (212) 850-6088. 1989.

Year Book of Transplantation. Mosby-Year Book, 11830 Westline Industrial Drive, St. Louis, MO 63146. Phone: (800) 325-4177. Fax: (314) 432-1380. Annual.

ASSOCIATIONS, PROFESSIONAL SOCIETIES, ADVOCACY AND SUPPORT GROUPS

American Council on Transplantation. 700 N. Fairfax St., No. 505, Alexandria, VA 22314. Phone: (703) 836-4301.

American Society of Transplant Surgeons (ASTS). 716 Lee St., Des Plaines, IL 60016. Phone: (708) 824-5700. Fax: (708) 824-0394.

International Society for Artificial Organs (ISAO). 8937 Euclid Ave., Cleveland, OH 44106. Phone: (216) 421-0757. Fax: (216) 421-1652.

Medic Alert Organ Donor Program (MAODP). 2323 Colorado Ave., Turlock, CA 95380. Phone: (800) IDA-LERT.

North American Transplant Coordinators Organization (NATCO). P.O. Box 15384, Lenexa, KS 66215. Phone: (913) 492-3600. Fax: (913) 541-0156.

Pittsburgh Transplant Foundation. 5743 Center Ave., Pittsburgh, PA 15206. Phone: (800) 366-6777.

Transplantation Society (TS). Department of Surgery, Means Hall, Rm. 258, 1654 Ugham Dr., Columbus, OH 43210. Phone: (614) 293-8545. Fax: (614) 293-4670.

United Network for Organ Sharing (UNOS). 1100 Boulders Pkwy., Ste. 500, P.O. Box 13770, Richmond, VA 23225. Phone: (804) 330-8500. Fax: (804) 330-8517.

BIBLIOGRAPHIES

Bone Marrow Transplantation as Treatment for Leukemia. National Technical Information Service, 5285 Port Royal Rd., Springfield, VA 22161. Phone: (703) 487-4650. Fax: (703) 321-8547. Jan. 1978-Jul. 1989 PB89-866552/CBY.

Searches on File: Topics in Kidney and Urologic Diseases. Transplantations Professional Materials. National Kidney and Urologic Diseases Information Clearinghouse, P.O. Box NKUDIC, 9000 Rockville Pike, Bethesda, MD 20892. Phone: (301) 468-6345.

HANDBOOKS, GUIDES, MANUALS, ATLASES

Atlas of Heart-Lung Transplantation. Amar S. Kapoor, Hillel Laks. McGraw-Hill, Inc., Health Professions Division, 1221 Avenue of the Americas, 28th Floor, New York, NY 10020. Phone: (212) 512-4228. 1992.

Bone Marrow Processing and Purging: A Practical Guide. Adrian P. Gee. CRC Press, Inc., 2000 Corporate Blvd. N.W., Boca Raton, FL 33431. Phone: (407) 994-0555. Fax: (407) 997-0949. 1992.

Handbook of Kidney Transplantation. Danovitch. Little, Brown and Co., 34 Beacon St., Boston, MA 02108. Phone: (617) 227-0730. Fax: (617) 227-0790. 1992.

JOURNALS

Artificial Organs. Raven Press, 1185 Avenue of the Americas, New York, NY 10036. Phone: (212) 930-9500. Fax: (212) 869-3495. Bimonthly.

The Journal of Heart and Lung Transplantation. Mosby-Year Book, 11830 Westline Industrial Drive, St. Louis, MO 63146. Phone: (800) 325-4177. Fax: (314) 432-1380. Bimonthly.

Nephrology, Dialysis and Transplantation. Springer-Verlag New York Inc., 175 Fifth Ave., New York, NY 10010. Phone: (212) 460-1500. Fax: (212) 473-6272.

Transplantation. Williams & Wilkins, 428 E. Preston St., Baltimore, MD 21202. Phone: (800) 638-0672. Fax: (800) 447-8438. Monthly.

Transplantation Proceedings. Appleton & Lange, 25 Van Zant St., East Norwalk, CT 06855. Phone: (800) 423-1359. Fax: (203) 854-9486. Bimonthly.

Transplantation Reviews. W.B. Saunders Co., The Curtis Center, Independence Sqare W., Philadelphia, PA 19106-3399. Phone: (215) 238-7800.

NEWSLETTERS

Transplant. Northern California Transplant Bank, P.O. Box 7999, San Francisco, CA 94120. Phone: (415) 923-3446. Irregular.

Transplant Action. American Council on Transplantation, 700 N. Fairfax St., No. 505, Alexandria, VA 22314. Phone: (703) 836-4301.

ONLINE DATABASES

EMBASE. Elsevier Science Publishing Co., Inc., P.O. Box 882, Madison Square Station, New York, NY 10159-2101. Phone: (212) 989-5800. Fax: (212) 633-3990.

MEDLINE. National Library of Medicine, 8600 Rockville Pike, Bethesda, MD 20894. Phone: (800) 638-8480.

SciSearch. Institute for Scientific Information, 3501 Market St., Philadelphia, PA 19104. Phone: (215) 386-0100. Fax: (215) 386-6362.

POPULAR WORKS AND PATIENT EDUCATION

A Patient's Guide to Dialysis and Transplantation. Roger Gabriel. Kluwer Academic Publishers, P.O. Box 358, Accord Station, Hingham, MA 02018-0358. Phone: (617) 871-6600. Fax: (617) 871-6528. 1990.

RESEARCH CENTERS, INSTITUTES, CLEARINGHOUSES

Cardiac Transplant Program. Loyola University of Chicago. 2160 S. 1st Ave., Maywood, IL 60153. Phone: (708) 216-4810.

Cleveland Clinic Foundation Research Institute. 9500 Euclid Ave., Cleveland, OH 44195-5210. Phone: (216) 444-3900. Fax: (216) 444-3279.

Laboratory for Transplant Immunology. Stanford University. Stanford, CA 94305-5247. Phone: (415) 723-5641.

McGill Centre for Clinical Immunobiology and Transplantation. McGill University. 687 Ave. des Pins Ouest, Montreal, PQ, Canada H3A 1A1. Phone: (514) 843-1512. Fax: (514) 982-0983.

Organ Transplantation Laboratory. University of Calgary. Health Sciences Centre, 3330 Hospital Dr. N.W., Calgary, AB, Canada T2N 2T9. Phone: (403) 670-1570. Fax: (403) 670-2400.

TEXTBOOKS AND MONOGRAPHS

Bone Marrow Purging and Processing. Samuel Gross, Diane A. Worthinton-White (eds.). John Wiley & Sons, Inc., 605 Third Ave., New York, NY 10158-0012. Phone: (212) 850-6000. Fax: (212) 850-6088. 1990.

Bone Marrow Purging and Processing for Transplantation. Ronald A. Sacher, Ellen Areman, H. Joachim Deeg. F.A. Davis Co., 1915 Arch St., Philadelphia, PA 19103. Phone: (800) 523-4049. Fax: (215) 568-5065. 1992.

Bone Marrow Transplantation: Current Controversies (UCLA Symposia on Molecular and Cellular Biology). Richard E. Champlin, Robert Peter Gale (eds.). John Wiley & Sons, Inc., 605 Third Ave., New York, NY 10158-0012. Phone: (212) 850-6000. Fax: (212) 850-6088. 1988.

Cancer in Organ Transplant Recipients. Schmahl. Springer-Verlag New York Inc., 175 Fifth Ave., New York, NY 10010. Phone: (212) 460-1500. Fax: (212) 473-6272. 1991.

Clinical Management of Renal Transplantation. Mary G. McGeown (ed.). Kluwer Academic Publishers, P.O. Box 358, Accord Station, Hingham, MA 02018-0358. Phone: (617) 871-6600. Fax: (617) 871-6528. 1992.

Heart and Heart-Lung Transplantation. John Wallwork. W.B. Saunders Co., The Curtis Center, Independence Sqare W., Philadelphia, PA 19106-3399. Phone: (215) 238-7800.

New Strategies in Bone Marrow Transplantation. Richard E. Champlin, Robert Peter Gale. John Wiley & Sons, Inc., 605 Third Ave., New York, NY 10158-0012. Phone: (212) 850-6000. Fax: (212) 850-6088. 1990.

Pathology of Organ Transplantation. George E. Sale. Butterworth-Heinemann, 80 Montvale Ave., Stoneham, MA 02180. Phone: (617) 438-8464. Fax: (617) 279-4851. 1990.

Principles of Organ Transplantation. M. Wayne Flye. W.B. Saunders Co., The Curtis Center, Independence Sqare W., Philadelphia, PA 19106-3399. Phone: (215) 238-7800.

TRANSVESTISM

See: SEXUAL DISORDERS

TRAUMA

ABSTRACTING, INDEXING, AND CURRENT AWARENESS PUBLICATIONS

Current Contents/Clinical Medicine. Institute for Scientific Information, 3501 Market St., Philadelphia, PA 19104. Phone: (800) 523-1850. Fax: (215) 386-6362. Weekly.

ANNUALS AND REVIEWS

Advances in Trauma and Critical Care Medicine. Mosby-Year Book, 11830 Westline Industrial Drive, St. Louis, MO 63146. Phone: (800) 325-4177. Fax: (314) 432-1380. Annual.

Current Therapy of Trauma. Mosby-Year Book, 11830 Westline Industrial Drive, St. Louis, MO 63146. Phone: (800) 325-4177. Fax: (314) 432-1380. Irregular.

Year Book of Emergency Medicine. Mosby-Year Book, 11830 Westline Industrial Drive, St. Louis, MO 63146. Phone: (800) 325-4177. Fax: (314) 432-1380. Annual.

ASSOCIATIONS, PROFESSIONAL SOCIETIES, ADVOCACY AND SUPPORT GROUPS

American Association for the Surgery of Trauma (AAST). New York Burn Center, 525 E. 68th St., L-706, New York, NY 10021. Phone: (212) 746-5010.

American Trauma Society (ATS). 1400 Mercantile Ln., Ste. 188, Landover, MD 20785. Phone: (301) 925-8811. Fax: (301) 925-8815.

CD-ROM DATABASES

Emergency Medicine MEDLINE. MEP, 124 Mt. Auburn St., Cambridge, MA 02138. Phone: (800) 342-1338. Fax: (617) 868-7738. Quarterly.

HANDBOOKS, GUIDES, MANUALS, ATLASES

Color Atlas of Trauma Pathology. Fischer. Mosby-Year Book, 11830 Westline Industrial Drive, St. Louis, MO 63146. Phone: (800) 325-4177. Fax: (314) 432-1380. 1991.

The Parkland Trauma Handbook. James Carrico, Irwin Thal, Mike Lopez (eds.). Mosby-Year Book, 11830 Westline Industrial Drive, St. Louis, MO 63146. Phone: (800) 325-4177. Fax: (314) 432-1380. 1993.

JOURNALS

Critical Care Medicine. Williams & Wilkins, 428 E. Preston St., Baltimore, MD 21202. Phone: (800) 638-0672. Fax: (800) 447-8438. Monthly.

Injury: British Journal of Accident Surgery. Butterworth-Heinemann, 80 Montvale Ave., Stoneham, MA 02180. Phone: (617) 438-8464. Fax: (617) 279-4851. 8/year.

Journal of Trauma. Williams & Wilkins, 428 E. Preston St., Baltimore, MD 21202. Phone: (800) 638-0672. Fax: (800) 447-8438. Monthly.

Topics in Emergency Medicine. Aspen Publishers, Inc., 1600 Research Blvd., Rockville, MD 20850. Phone: (301) 251-5554. Quarterly.

RESEARCH CENTERS, INSTITUTES, CLEARINGHOUSES

Shock Trauma Institute. Loyola University of Chicago. 2160 S. 1st Ave., Maywood, IL 60153. Phone: (708) 216-4074. Fax: (708) 216-4024.

TEXTBOOKS AND MONOGRAPHS

Clinical Practice of Emergency Medicine. Harwood. J.B. Lippincott Co., 227 E. Washington Square, Philadelphia, PA 19106-3780. Phone: (215) 238-4200. Fax: (215) 238-4227. 1991.

Clinical Procedures in Emergency Medicine. James R. Roberts, Jerris R. Hedges. W.B. Saunders Co., The Curtis Center, Independence Square W., Philadelphia, PA 19106-3399. Phone: (215) 238-7800. Second edition 1991.

Critical Care. Joseph M. Civetta, Robert W. Taylor, Robert R. Kirby (eds.). J.B. Lippincott Co., 227 E. Washington Square, Philadelphia, PA 19106-3780. Phone: (215) 238-4200. Fax: (215) 238-4227. 1988.

Current Emergency Diagnosis and Treatment. Mary T. Ho, Charles E. Saunders. Appleton & Lange, 25 Van Zant St., East Norwalk, CT 06855. Phone: (800) 423-1359. Fax: (203) 854-9486. Fourth edition 1992.

The Management of Major Trauma. Colin Robertson, Anthony D. Redmond. Oxford University Press, 200 Madison Ave., New York, NY 10016. Phone: (212) 679-7300. 1991.

Pediatric Trauma. Martin R. Eichelberger. Mosby-Year Book, 11830 Westline Industrial Drive, St. Louis, MO 63146. Phone: (800) 325-4177. Fax: (314) 432-1380. 1992.

Trauma: Anesthesia and Intensive Care. levon M. Capan, Sanford Miller, Herman Turndorf (eds.). J.B. Lippincott Co., 227 East Washington Square, Philadelphia, PA 19106-3780. Phone: (215) 238-4200. Fax: (215) 238-4227. 1991.

Trauma Radiology. James J. McCort (ed.). Churchill Livingstone Inc., 650 Avenue of the Americas, New York, NY 10011. Phone: (212) 819-5400. Fax: (212) 302-6598. 1990.

Trauma Surgery. Howard R. Champion, John V. Robbs, Donald D. Trunkey (eds.). Butterworth-Heinemann, 80 Montvale Ave., Stoneham, MA 02180. Phone: (617) 438-8464. Fax: (617) 279-4851. Fourth edition 1989.

TRICHINOSIS

See: PARASITIC DISEASES

TROPICAL DISEASES

See: TROPICAL MEDICINE

TROPICAL MEDICINE

See also: MALARIA; PARASITIC DISEASES

ABSTRACTING, INDEXING, AND CURRENT AWARENESS PUBLICATIONS

Index Medicus. U.S. National Library of Medicine, 8600 Rockville Pike, Bethesda, MD 20894. Phone: (800) 638-8480. Monthly.

Science Citation Index. Institute for Scientific Information, 3501 Market St., Philadelphia, PA 19104. Phone: (800) 523-1850. Fax: (215) 386-6362. Bimonthly.

Tropical Diseases Bulletin. Bureau of Hygiene and Tropical Diseases, Keppel St., London WC1E 7HT, England. Monthly.

ANNUALS AND REVIEWS

Royal Society of Tropical Medicine and Hygiene-Year Book. Bureau of Tropical Medicine and Hygiene, Manson House, 26 Portland Pl., London W1N 4EY, England. Annual.

ASSOCIATIONS, PROFESSIONAL SOCIETIES, ADVOCACY AND SUPPORT GROUPS

American Board of Tropical Medicine (ABTM). P.O. Box 1794, Toledo, OH 43603.

American Society of Tropical Medicine and Hygiene (ASTMH). 8000 Westpark Dr., Ste. 130, Mc Lean, VA 22102. Phone: (703) 790-1745. Fax: (703) 790-9063.

International Leprosy Association. One Broadway, Elmwood Park, NJ 07407. Phone: (201) 794-8650.

BIBLIOGRAPHIES

Quarterly Bibliography of Major Tropical Diseases. World Health Organization, Ave. Appia, CH-1211, Geneva 27, Switzerland. Quarterly.

CD-ROM DATABASES

SCISEARCH. Institute for Scientific Information, 3501 Market St., Philadelphia, PA 19104. Phone: (215) 386-0100. Fax: (215) 386-6362.

DIRECTORIES

Directory of Medical Specialists. Marquis Who's Who, 3002 Glenview Rd., Wilmette, IL 60091. Phone: (800) 621-9669. Fax: (708) 441-2264. Biennial.

Directory of Physicians in the United States. American Medical Association, 515 North State St., Chicago, IL 60610. Phone: (312) 464-0183. Fax: (312) 464-5834. Biennial.

HANDBOOKS, GUIDES, MANUALS, ATLASES

A Color Atlas of Tropical Medicine and Parasitology. W. Peters, H.M. Giles. Mosby-Year Book, 11830 Westline Industrial Drive, St. Louis, MO 63146. Phone: (800) 325-4177. Fax: (314) 432-1380. Third edition 1989.

Tropical & Geographical Medicine: Companion Handbook. Adel A.F. Mahmoud. McGraw-Hill, Inc., Health Professions Division, 1221 Avenue of the Americas, 28th Floor, New York, NY 10020. Phone: (212) 512-4228. Second edition 1992.

JOURNALS

Acta Tropica. Elsevier Science Publishing Co., Inc., P.O. Box 882, Madison Square Station, New York, NY 10159-2101. Phone: (212) 989-5800. Fax: (212) 633-3990. Monthly.

American Journal of Tropical Medicine and Hygiene. American Society of Tropical Medicine and Hygiene, LSU School of Medicine, P.O. Box 33932, Shreveport, LA 71130. Phone: (318) 674-5191. Monthly.

Annals of Tropical Medicine and Parasitology. Academic Press, Inc., 1250 Sixth Ave., San Diego, CA 92101-4311. Phone: (619) 699-6345. Fax: (619) 699-6715. Bimonthly.

Annals of Tropical Pediatrics. Academic Press, Inc., 1250 Sixth Ave., San Diego, CA 92101-4311. Phone: (619) 699-6345. Fax: (619) 699-6715. Quarterly.

Journal of Tropical Medicine and Hygiene. Blackwell Scientific Publications, Inc., 3 Cambridge Ctr., Cambridge, MA 02142. Phone: (800) 759-6102. Bimonthly.

Leprosy Review. British Leprosy Relief Association, Fairfax House, Causton Rd., Colchester, Essex C01 1PU, England.

Transactions of the Royal Society of Tropical Medicine and Hygiene. Manson House, 26 Portland Pl., London W1N 4EY, England. Bimonthly.

Tropical Doctor. Royal Society of Medicine Services Ltd., 1 Wimpole St., London W1M 8AE, England. Phone: 071-408 2119. Fax: 071-355 3198. Quarterly.

Tropical and Geographical Medicine. Foris Publications, Box 509, 3300 AM Amsterdam, Netherlands. Phone: 078-510454.

Tropical Medicine and Parasitology. Thieme Medical Publishers, Inc., 381 Park Ave. S., New York, NY 10016. Phone: (212) 683-5088. Fax: (212) 779-9020. Quarterly.

NEWSLETTERS

Travel Medicine Advisor. American Health Consultants, Department ADI-59, P.O. Box 740060, Atlanta, GA 30374. Phone: (800) 559-1032. Fax: (404) 352-1971.

ONLINE DATABASES

EMBASE. Elsevier Science Publishing Co., Inc., P.O. Box 882, Madison Square Station, New York, NY 10159-2101. Phone: (212) 989-5800. Fax: (212) 633-3990.

MEDLINE. National Library of Medicine, 8600 Rockville Pike, Bethesda, MD 20894. Phone: (800) 638-8480.

SciSearch. Institute for Scientific Information, 3501 Market St., Philadelphia, PA 19104. Phone: (215) 386-0100. Fax: (215) 386-6362.

RESEARCH CENTERS, INSTITUTES, CLEARINGHOUSES

American Academy of Tropical Medicine and Surgery. 16126 E. Warren, Detroit, MI 48224. Phone: (313) 882-5110.

Division of Geographic Medicine. Case Western Reserve University. School of Medicine, 2109 Adelbert Rd., Cleveland, OH 44106. Phone: (216) 368-4818. Fax: (216) 368-4825.

Gorgas Memorial Laboratory. APO, Miami, FL 34002-0012.

Institute of International Health. Michigan State Univeristy. A327 E. Fee Hall, East Lansing, MI 48824-1316. Phone: (517) 353-8992. Fax: (517) 355-1894.

Institute of Tropical Medicine. 1780 N.E. 168th St., North Miami Beach, FL 33162. Phone: (305) 947-1722.

International Health Research Foundation. 3741 LeJeune Rd. S.W., Coconut Grove, FL 33146. Phone: (305) 663-9666. Fax: (305) 663-9671.

McGill Centre for Tropical Diseases. McGill University. Montreal General Hospital, Rm. 787, 1650 Cedar Hospital, Montreal, PQ, Canada H3G 1A4. Phone: (514) 937-6011.

Parasitology and Tropical Diseases Branch. Microbiology and Infections Diseases Program. National Institute of Allergy and Infections Diseases. 5333 Westbard Ave., Bethesda, MD 20892. Phone: (301) 496-2544.

TEXTBOOKS AND MONOGRAPHS

Adams & Maegraith: Clinical Tropical Medicine. Brian Maegraith. Mosby-Year Book, 11830 Westline Industrial Drive, St. Louis, MO 63146. Phone: (800) 325-4177. Fax: (314) 432-1380. Ninth edition 1989.

Clinical Tropical Diseases. A.R.D. Adams, B.G. Maegraith. Blackwell Scientific Publications, Inc., 3 Cambridge Ctr., Cambridge, MA 02142. Phone: (800) 759-6102. Ninth edition 1989.

Hunter's Tropical Medicine. G. Thomas Strickland (ed.). W.B. Saunders Co., The Curtis Center, Independence Square W., Philadelphia, PA 19106-3399. Phone: (215) 238-7800. Seventh edition 1991.

Malaria. Knell. Oxford University Press, 200 Madison Ave., New York, NY 10016. Phone: (212) 679-7300. 1991.

Manson's Tropical Diseases. Philip E.C. Manson-Bahr, Dion R. Bell. W.B. Saunders Co., The Curtis Center, Independence Square W., Philadelphia, PA 19106-3399. Phone: (215) 238-7800. 19th edition 1988.

Oral Disease in the Tropics. Prabhu. Oxford University Press, 200 Madison Ave., New York, NY 10016. Phone: (212) 679-7300. 1992.

Parasitic Disease. Katz. Springer-Verlag New York Inc., 175 Fifth Ave., New York, NY 10010. Phone: (212) 460-1500. Fax: (212) 473-6272. Second edition 1989.

Tropical & Geographical Medicine. Kenneth S. Warren, Adel A.F. Mahmoud. McGraw-Hill, Inc., Health Professions Division, 1221 Avenue of the Americas, 28th Floor, New York, NY 10020. Phone: (212) 512-4228. Second edition 1990.

Tropical Medicine: A Clinical Text. K.M. Cahill, W. O'Brien. Butterworth-Heinemann, 80 Montvale Ave., Stoneham, MA 02180. Phone: (617) 438-8464. Fax: (617) 279-4851. 1990.

Tropical Medicine and Parasitology. Robert Goldsmith, Donald Heyneman. Appleton & Lange, 25 Van Zant St., East Norwalk, CT 06855. Phone: (800) 423-1359. Fax: (203) 854-9486. 1989.

Vaccination Strategies of Tropical Diseases. F.Y. Liew (ed.). CRC Press, Inc., 2000 Corporate Blvd. N.W., Boca Raton, FL 33431. Phone: (407) 994-0555. Fax: (407) 997-0949. 1989.

TUBAL PREGNANCY

See: PREGNANCY COMPLICATIONS

TUBERCULOSIS

ABSTRACTING, INDEXING, AND CURRENT AWARENESS PUBLICATIONS

Current Contents/Clinical Medicine. Institute for Scientific Information, 3501 Market St., Philadelphia, PA 19104. Phone: (800) 523-1850. Fax: (215) 386-6362. Weekly.

Excerpta Medica. Section 15: Chest Diseases, Thoracic Surgery and Tuberculosis. Elsevier Science Publishing Co., Inc., P.O. Box 882, Madison Square Station, New York, NY 10159-2101. Phone: (212) 989-5800. Fax: (212) 633-3990. 20/year.

Index Medicus. U.S. National Library of Medicine, 8600 Rockville Pike, Bethesda, MD 20894. Phone: (800) 638-8480. Monthly.

ASSOCIATIONS, PROFESSIONAL SOCIETIES, ADVOCACY AND SUPPORT GROUPS

American Lung Association (ALA). 1740 Broadway, New York, NY 10019. Phone: (212) 315-8700. Fax: (212) 265-5642.

International Union against Tuberculosis and Lung Disease. 68 Blvd. St. Michel, F-75006 Paris, France.

BIBLIOGRAPHIES

Tuberculosis: Vaccine Development. National Technical Information Service, 5285 Port Royal Rd., Springfield, VA 22161. Phone: (703) 487-4650. Fax: (703) 321-8547. Mar. 1978-July 1989 PB90-857137/CBY.

JOURNALS

Chest. American College of Chest Physicians, 911 Busse Hwy., Park Ridge, IL 60068. Phone: (708) 698-2200. Fax: (708) 698-1791. Monthly.

Tubercle. Churchill Livingstone Inc., 650 Ave. of the Americas, New York, NY 10011. Phone: (212) 819-5400. Fax: (212) 302-6598.

ONLINE DATABASES

EMBASE. Elsevier Science Publishing Co., Inc., P.O. Box 882, Madison Square Station, New York, NY 10159-2101. Phone: (212) 989-5800. Fax: (212) 633-3990.

MEDLINE. National Library of Medicine, 8600 Rockville Pike, Bethesda, MD 20894. Phone: (800) 638-8480.

SciSearch. Institute for Scientific Information, 3501 Market St., Philadelphia, PA 19104. Phone: (215) 386-0100. Fax: (215) 386-6362.

RESEARCH CENTERS, INSTITUTES, CLEARINGHOUSES

Institute for Tuberculosis Research. University of Illinois at Chicago. 904 W. Adams St., Chicago, IL 60607. Phone: (312) 996-3906. Fax: (312) 996-4689.

TUMORS

See: CANCER

TYPHOID

See: INFECTIOUS DISEASES

TYPHUS

See: INFECTIOUS DISEASES

U

ULCERS

ABSTRACTING, INDEXING, AND CURRENT AWARENESS PUBLICATIONS

BIOSIS/CAS Selects: Antiulcer Agents. BIOSIS, 2100 Arch St., Philadelphia, PA 19103-1399. Phone: (215) 587-4800. Fax: (215) 587-2016. Biweekly.

CA Selects: Ulcer Inhibitors. Chemical Abstracts Service, 2540 Olentangy River Road, P.O. Box 3012, Columbus, OH 43210-0012. Phone: (800) 848-6538. Biweekly.

Core Journals in Gastroenterology. Elsevier Science Publishing Co., Inc., P.O. Box 882, Madison Square Station, New York, NY 10159-2101. Phone: (212) 989-5800. Fax: (212) 633-3990. 11/year.

Index Medicus. U.S. National Library of Medicine, 8600 Rockville Pike, Bethesda, MD 20894. Phone: (800) 638-8480. Monthly.

Research Alert: Antiulcer Agents. Institute for Scientific Information, 3501 Market St., Philadelphia, PA 19104. Phone: (800) 523-1850. Fax: (215) 386-6362. Weekly.

ASSOCIATIONS, PROFESSIONAL SOCIETIES, ADVOCACY AND SUPPORT GROUPS

Cure Foundation. 11661 San Vincente Blvd. No. 304, Los Angeles, CA 90049. Phone: (213) 206-6603.

National Ulcer Foundation. 675 Main St., Melrose, MA 02176. Phone: (617) 665-6210.

ONLINE DATABASES

EMBASE. Elsevier Science Publishing Co., Inc., P.O. Box 882, Madison Square Station, New York, NY 10159-2101. Phone: (212) 989-5800. Fax: (212) 633-3990.

MEDLINE. National Library of Medicine, 8600 Rockville Pike, Bethesda, MD 20894. Phone: (800) 638-8480.

SciSearch. Institute for Scientific Information, 3501 Market St., Philadelphia, PA 19104. Phone: (215) 386-0100. Fax: (215) 386-6362.

TEXTBOOKS AND MONOGRAPHS

Helicobacter Pylori, Gastritis and Peptic Ulcer. P. Malfertheiner, H. Ditschuneit (eds.). Springer-Verlag New York Inc., 175 Fifth Ave., New York, NY 10010. Phone: (212) 460-1500. Fax: (212) 473-6272. 1990.

Leg Ulcers: A Practical Approach to Management. D. Negus. Butterworth-Heinemann, 80 Montvale Ave., Stoneham, MA 02180. Phone: (617) 438-8464. Fax: (617) 279-4851. 1991.

Mechanisms of Peptic Ulcer Healing. F. Halter, A. Garner (eds.). Kluwer Academic Publishers, P.O. Box 358, Accord Station, Hingham, MA 02018-0358. Phone: (617) 871-6600. Fax: (617) 871-6528. 1991.

Pharmacology of Peptic Ulcer Disease. M.J. Collen, S.B. Benjamin (eds.). Springer-Verlag New York, Inc., 175 Fifth Ave., New York, NY 10010. Phone: (212) 460-1500. Fax: (212) 473-6272. 1991.

Ulcer Disease: New Aspects of Pathogenesis adn Pharmacology. Sandor Szabo, Carl J. Pfeiffer (eds.). CRC Press, Inc., 2000 Corporate Blvd. N.W., Boca Raton, FL 33431. Phone: (407) 994-0555. Fax: (407) 997-0949. 1989.

ULTRASOUND

See also: DIAGNOSIS

ABSTRACTING, INDEXING, AND CURRENT AWARENESS PUBLICATIONS

Index Medicus. U.S. National Library of Medicine, 8600 Rockville Pike, Bethesda, MD 20894. Phone: (800) 638-8480. Monthly.

Research Alert: Imaging Techniques-Ultrasonic & Echocardiography. Institute for Scientific Information, 3501 Market St., Philadelphia, PA 19104. Phone: (800) 523-1850. Fax: (215) 386-6362. Weekly.

Research Alert: Ultrasound. Institute for Scientific Information, 3501 Market St., Philadelphia, PA 19104. Phone: (800) 523-1850. Fax: (215) 386-6362. Weekly.

ANNUALS AND REVIEWS

Year Book of Ultrasound. Mosby-Year Book, 11830 Westline Industrial Drive, St. Louis, MO 63146. Phone: (800) 325-4177. Fax: (314) 432-1380. Annual.

ASSOCIATIONS, PROFESSIONAL SOCIETIES, ADVOCACY AND SUPPORT GROUPS

American Institute of Ultrasound in Medicine (AIUM). 4405 East-West Hwy., Ste. 504, Bethesda, MD 20814. Phone: (800) 638-5352. Fax: (301) 652-2408.

American Registry of Diagnostic Medical Sonographers (ARDMS). 2368 Victory Pkwy., No. 510, Cincinnati, OH 45206-2810. Phone: (513) 281-7111. Fax: (513) 721-6670.

Society of Diagnostic Medical Sonographers (SDMS). 12225 Greenville Ave., Ste. 434, Dallas, TX 75243. Phone: (214) 235-7980. Fax: (214) 235-7369.

CD-ROM DATABASES

Advanced Fetal Monitoring. Catanzarite. Williams & Wilkins, 428 East Preston St., Baltimore, MD 21202. Phone: (800) 638-0672. Fax: (800) 447-8438. 1990.

Critical Concepts of Fetal Monitoring. Blood. Williams & Wilkins, 428 East Preston St., Baltimore, MD 21202. Phone: (800) 638-0672. Fax: (800) 447-8438. 1990.

DIRECTORIES

American Institute of Ultrasound in Medicine-Membership Roster. American Institute of Ultrasound in Medicine, 4405 East-West Hwy., Ste. 205, Bethesda, MD 20814. Phone: (301) 656-6117. Fax: (301) 652-2408. Biennial.

HANDBOOKS, GUIDES, MANUALS, ATLASES

An Atlas of Ultrasonography in Obstetrics and Gynecology. A. Kurjak (ed.). The Parthenon Publishing Group, Inc., 120 Mill Rd., Park Ridge, NJ 07656. Phone: (201) 391-6796. 1992.

Atlas of Ultrasound Measurement. Goldberg. Mosby-Year Book, 11830 Westline Industrial Drive, St. Louis, MO 63146. Phone: (800) 325-4177. Fax: (314) 432-1380. 1990.

Manual of Diagnostic Imaging. Straub. Little, Brown and Co., 34 Beacon St., Boston, MA 02108. Phone: (617) 227-0730. Fax: (617) 227-0790. Second edition 1989.

Obstetrical Measurements in Ultrasound: A Reference Manual. Alfred B. Kurtz, Barry B. Goldberg. Mosby-Year Book, 11830 Westline Industrial Drive, St. Louis, MO 63146. Phone: (800) 325-4177. Fax: (314) 432-1380. 1988.

Ultrasound in Gynecology and Obstetrics. E. Merz. Thieme Medical Publishers, Inc., 381 Park Ave. S., New York, NY 10016. Phone: (212) 683-5088. Fax: (212) 779-9020. 1991.

JOURNALS

Journal of Clinical Ultrasound. John Wiley & Sons, Inc., 605 Third Ave., New York, NY 10158-0012. Phone: (212) 850-6000. Fax: (212) 850-6088. 9/year.

Journal of Ultrasound in Medicine. American Institute of Ultrasound in Medicine, 11200 Rockville Pike, Suite 205, Rockville, MD 20852-3139. Phone: (800) 638-5352. Fax: (301) 881-7303. Monthly.

Seminars in Ultrasound, CT and MR. W.B. Saunders Co., The Curtis Center, Independence Sqare W., Philadelphia, PA 19106-3399. Phone: (215) 238-7800.

Ultrasound in Medicine and Biology. Pergamon Press, 660 White Plains Rd., Tarrytown, NY 10591-5153. Phone: (914) 592-7700. Fax: (914) 592-3625.

Ultrasound Quarterly. Raven Press, 1185 Avenue of the Americas, New York, NY 10036. Phone: (212) 930-9500. Fax: (212) 869-3495. Quarterly.

ONLINE DATABASES

EMBASE. Elsevier Science Publishing Co., Inc., P.O. Box 882, Madison Square Station, New York, NY 10159-2101. Phone: (212) 989-5800. Fax: (212) 633-3990.

MEDLINE. National Library of Medicine, 8600 Rockville Pike, Bethesda, MD 20894. Phone: (800) 638-8480.

SciSearch. Institute for Scientific Information, 3501 Market St., Philadelphia, PA 19104. Phone: (215) 386-0100. Fax: (215) 386-6362.

RESEARCH CENTERS, INSTITUTES, CLEARINGHOUSES

Mayo Biomedical Imaging Resource. Mayo Clinic. 200 First St. SW, Rochester, MN 55901. Phone: (507) 284-4937. Fax: (507) 284-1632.

TEXTBOOKS AND MONOGRAPHS

Clinical Sonography: A Practical Guide. Roger C. Sanders. Little, Brown and Co., 34 Beacon St., Boston, MA 02108. Phone: (617) 227-0730. Fax: (617) 227-0790. Second edition 1991.

Diagnostic Ultrasonics: Principles and Use of Instruments. W.N. McDicken. Churchill Livingstone Inc., 650 Avenue of the Americas, New York, NY 10011. Phone: (212) 819-5400. Fax: (212) 302-6598. 1991.

Diagnostic Ultrasound: Principles, Instruments, and Exercises. Frederick W. Kremkau. W.B. Saunders Co., The Curtis Center, Independence Square W., Philadelphia, PA 19106-3399. Phone: (215) 238-7800. Third edition 1989.

Fetal Echocardiography. Rudy E. Sabbagha, Samuel Gidding, Janette Strasburger. Appleton & Lange, 25 Van Zant St., East Norwalk, CT 06855. Phone: (800) 423-1359. Fax: (203) 854-9486. 1991.

Principles and Practice of Ultrasonography in Obstetrics and Gynecology. Arthur C. Fleishcer, Roberto Romero, Frank Manning, et. al.. Appleton & Lange, 25 Van Zant St., East Norwalk, CT 06855. Phone: (800) 423-1359. Fax: (203) 854-9486. Fourth edition 1990.

Textbook of Diagnostic Ultrasonography. Sandra L. Hagen-Ansert. Mosby-Year Book, 11830 Westline Industrial Drive, St. Louis, MO 63146. Phone: (800) 325-4177. Fax: (314) 432-1380. Third edition 1989.

Textbook of Ultrasound in Obstetrics and Gynecology. Frank A. Chervenak, Stuart Campbell, Glenn C. Isaacson (eds.). Little, Brown and Company, 34 Beacon St., Boston, MA 02108. Phone: (617) 227-0730. Two volumes 1992.

Transvaginal Ultrasound. Nyberg. Mosby-Year Book, 11830 Westline Industrial Drive, St. Louis, MO 63146. Phone: (800) 325-4177. Fax: (314) 432-1380. Second edition 1992.

Ultrasound in Neurosurgery. Jonathan M. Rubin, William F. Chandler, and others. Raven Press, 1185 Avenue of the Americas, New York, NY 10036. Phone: (212) 930-9500. Fax: (212) 869-3495. 1990.

Ultrasound of the Prostate. Bruno Fornage. John Wiley & Sons, Inc., 605 Third Ave., New York, NY 10158-0012. Phone: (212) 850-6000. Fax: (212) 850-6088. 1988.

UNDERSEA MEDICINE

ABSTRACTING, INDEXING, AND CURRENT AWARENESS PUBLICATIONS

Index Medicus. U.S. National Library of Medicine, 8600 Rockville Pike, Bethesda, MD 20894. Phone: (800) 638-8480. Monthly.

Underwater and Hyperbaric Medicine: Abstracts from the Literature. Undersea & Hyperbaric Medical Society, 9650 Rockville Pike, Bethesda, MD 20814. Phone: (301) 571-1818. Fax: (301) 571-1815. Bimonthly.

ASSOCIATIONS, PROFESSIONAL SOCIETIES, ADVOCACY AND SUPPORT GROUPS

Undersea and Hyperbaric Medical Society (UHMS). 9650 Rockville Pike, Bethesda, MD 20814. Phone: (301) 571-1818. Fax: (301) 571-1815.

DIRECTORIES

Directory-Diving and Hyperbaric Medicine Training Program. Undersea & Hyperbaric Medical Society, 9650 Rockville Pike, Bethesda, MD 20814. Phone: (301) 571-1818. Fax: (301) 571-1815. 1990.

Directory of Hyperbaric Chambers. Undersea and Hyperbaric Medical Society, 9650 Rockville Pike, Bethesda, MD 20814. Phone: (301) 571-1818.

JOURNALS

Journal of Hyperbaric Medicine. Undersea & Hyperbaric Medical Society, 9650 Rockville Pike, Bethesda, MD 20814. Phone: (301) 571-1818. Fax: (301) 571-1815. Quarterly.

Undersea Biomedical Research. Undersea & Hyperbaric Medical Society, 9650 Rockville Pike, Bethesda, MD 20814. Phone: (301) 571-1818. Fax: (301) 571-1815. Bimonthly.

NEWSLETTERS

Pressure. Undersea and Hyperbaric Medical Society, 9650 Rockville Pike, Bethesda, MD 20814. Phone: (301) 571-1818. Bimonthly.

ONLINE DATABASES

EMBASE. Elsevier Science Publishing Co., Inc., P.O. Box 882, Madison Square Station, New York, NY 10159-2101. Phone: (212) 989-5800. Fax: (212) 633-3990.

MEDLINE. National Library of Medicine, 8600 Rockville Pike, Bethesda, MD 20894. Phone: (800) 638-8480.

SciSearch. Institute for Scientific Information, 3501 Market St., Philadelphia, PA 19104. Phone: (215) 386-0100. Fax: (215) 386-6362.

TEXTBOOKS AND MONOGRAPHS

Describing Decompression Illness. Undersea & Hyperbaric Medical Society, 9650 Rockville Pike, Bethesda, MD 20814. Phone: (301) 571-1818. Fax: (301) 571-1815. 1991.

Diving Accident Management. Undersea & Hyperbaric Medical Society, 9650 Rockville Pike, Bethesda, MD 20814. Phone: (301) 571-1818. Fax: (301) 571-1815. 1990.

Diving and Subaquatic Medicine. Carl Edmonds, and others. Butterworth-Heinemann, 80 Montvale Ave., Stoneham, MA 02180. Phone: (617) 438-8464. Fax: (617) 279-4851. 1992.

Fitness to Dive. Undersea & Hyperbaric Medical Society, 9650 Rockville Pike, Bethesda, MD 20814. Phone: (301) 571-1818. Fax: (301) 571-1815. 1990.

Hyperbaric Medicine Procedures. Kindwall Goldmann. Undersea & Hyperbaric Medical Society, 9650 Rockville Pike, Bethesda, MD 20814. Phone: (301) 571-1818. Fax: (301) 571-1815. Revised edition 1988.

Proceedings of the 2nd Swiss Symposium on Hyperbaric Medicine. Undersea & Hyperbaric Medical Society, 9650 Rockville Pike, Bethesda, MD 20814. Phone: (301) 571-1818. Fax: (301) 571-1815. 1990.

Underwater and Hyperbaric Physiology IX. Undersea & Hyperbaric Medical Society, 9650 Rockville Pike, Bethesda, MD 20814. Phone: (301) 571-1818. Fax: (301) 571-1815. 1987.

What is Bends? Undersea & Hyperbaric Medical Society, 9650 Rockville Pike, Bethesda, MD 20814. Phone: (301) 571-1818. Fax: (301) 571-1815. 1991.

UREMIA

See: KIDNEY DISEASES

URINALYSIS

See: DIAGNOSIS

URINARY INCONTINENCE

See: UROLOGIC DISORDERS

UROLOGIC DISORDERS

See also: UROLOGY

ABSTRACTING, INDEXING, AND CURRENT AWARENESS PUBLICATIONS

Current Contents/Clinical Medicine. Institute for Scientific Information, 3501 Market St., Philadelphia, PA 19104. Phone: (800) 523-1850. Fax: (215) 386-6362. Weekly.

Excerpta Medica. Section 28: Urology and Nephrology. Elsevier Science Publishing Co., Inc., P.O. Box 882, Madison Square Station, New York, NY 10159-2101. Phone: (212) 989-5800. Fax: (212) 633-3990. 20/year.

Index Medicus. U.S. National Library of Medicine, 8600 Rockville Pike, Bethesda, MD 20894. Phone: (800) 638-8480. Monthly.

ANNUALS AND REVIEWS

Advances in Urology. Mosby-Year Book, 11830 Westline Industrial Drive, St. Louis, MO 63146. Phone: (800) 325-4177. Fax: (314) 432-1380. Annual.

Contributions to Nephrology. S. Karger Publishers, Inc., 26 West Avon Rd., P.O. Box 529, Farmington, CT 06085. Phone: (203) 675-7834. Fax: (203) 675-7302. Irregular.

Current Problems in Urology. Mosby-Year Book, 11830 Westline Industrial Drive, St. Louis, MO 63146. Phone: (800) 325-4177. Fax: (314) 432-1380. Bimonthly.

Urologic Clinics. W.B. Saunders Co., The Curtis Center, Independence Square W., Philadelphia, PA 19106-3399. Phone: (215) 238-7800. Quarterly.

Year Book of Urology. Mosby-Year Book, 11830 Westline Industrial Drive, St. Louis, MO 63146. Phone: (800) 325-4177. Fax: (314) 432-1380. Annual.

ASSOCIATIONS, PROFESSIONAL SOCIETIES, ADVOCACY AND SUPPORT GROUPS

American Board of Urology (ABU). 31700 Telegraph Rd., Ste. 150, Birmingham, MI 48010. Phone: (312) 646-9720.

American Urological Association (AUA). 1120 N. Charles St., Baltimore, MD 21201. Phone: (301) 727-1100. Fax: (301) 625-2390.

Help for Incontinent People (HIP). P.O. Box 544, Union, SC 29379. Phone: (803) 579-7900. Fax: (803) 579-7902.

Interstitial Cystitis Association (ICA). P.O. Box 1553, Madison Square Sta., New York, NY 10159. Phone: (212) 979-6057.

Simon Foundation. Box 815, Wilmette, IL 60091. Phone: (800) 23S-IMON. Fax: (708) 864-9758.

DIRECTORIES

Directory of Certified Urologists. American Board of Medical Specialties, 1 Rotary Center, Suite 805, Evanston, IL 60201. Phone: (708) 491-9091. Biennial.

HANDBOOKS, GUIDES, MANUALS, ATLASES

Atlas of Surgical Techniques in Urology. Whitehead. J.B. Lippincott Co., 227 E. Washington Square, Philadelphia, PA 19106-3780. Phone: (215) 238-4200. Fax: (215) 238-4227. 1992.

Manual of Clinical Problems in Urology. Resnick. Little, Brown and Co., 34 Beacon St., Boston, MA 02108. Phone: (617) 227-0730. 1989.

Manual of Urology: Diagnosis and Therapy. Mike B. Stroky, Robert J. Krane (eds.). Little, Brown and Company, 34 Beacon St., Boston, MA 02108. Phone: (617) 227-0730. 1990.

Urinary Tract Infections. William Brumfitt, Jeremy M.C. Hamilton-Miller. Mosby-Year Book, 11830 Westline Industrial Drive, St. Louis, MO 63146. Phone: (800) 325-4177. Fax: (314) 432-1380. 1992.

JOURNALS

Contemporary Urology. Medical Economics, Five Paragon Dr., Montvale, NJ 07645-1742. Phone: (800) 222-3045. Fax: (201) 573-4956. 10/year.

Urologic Nursing. Mosby-Year Book, 11830 Westline Industrial Drive, St. Louis, MO 63146. Phone: (800) 325-4177. Fax: (314) 432-1380. Quarterly.

ONLINE DATABASES

Combined Health Information Database (CHID). U.S. National Institutes of Health, P.O. Box NDIC, Bethesda, MD 20892. Phone: (301) 496-2162. Fax: (301) 770-5164. Quarterly.

EMBASE. Elsevier Science Publishing Co., Inc., P.O. Box 882, Madison Square Station, New York, NY 10159-2101. Phone: (212) 989-5800. Fax: (212) 633-3990.

MEDLINE. National Library of Medicine, 8600 Rockville Pike, Bethesda, MD 20894. Phone: (800) 638-8480.

SciSearch. Institute for Scientific Information, 3501 Market St., Philadelphia, PA 19104. Phone: (215) 386-0100. Fax: (215) 386-6362.

POPULAR WORKS AND PATIENT EDUCATION

Male Sexual Health: A Couple's Guide. Richard F. Spark. Consumer Reports Books, 9180 LeSaint Dr., Fairfield, OH 45014. Phone: (513) 860-1178. 1991.

Overcoming Bladder Disorders. Rebecca Chalker, Kristene E. Whitmore. HarperCollins Publishers., Inc., 10 E. 53rd St., New York, NY 10022-5299. Phone: (212) 207-7000. Fax: (800) 242-7737. 1990.

Staying Dry: A Practical Guide to Bladder Control. Kathryn L. Burgio, K. Lynette Pearce, Angelo J. Lucco. Johns Hopkins University Press, 701 W. 40th St., Suite 275, Baltimore, MD 21211-2190. Phone: (800) 537-5487. Fax: (410) 516-6998. 1989.

RESEARCH CENTERS, INSTITUTES, CLEARINGHOUSES

National Kidney and Urologic Diseases Information Clearinghouse (NKUDIC). P.O. Box NKUDIC, 9000 Rockville Pike, Bethesda, MD 20892. Phone: (301) 468-6345.

TEXTBOOKS AND MONOGRAPHS

Campbell's Urology. Patrick C. Walsh (ed.). W.B. Saunders Co., The Curtis Center, Independence Square W., Philadelphia, PA 19106-3399. Phone: (215) 238-7800. Sixth edition. Three volumes. 1992.

Current Therapy in Genitourinary Surgery. Resnick. Mosby-Year Book, 11830 Westline Industrial Drive, St. Louis, MO 63146. Phone: (800) 325-4177. Fax: (314) 432-1380. Second edition 1992.

Diagnosis and Management of Male Erectile Dysfunction. R.S. Kirby, Cully Carson, George D. Webster. Butterworth-Heinemann, 80 Montvale Ave., Stoneham, MA 02180. Phone: (617) 438-8464. Fax: (617) 279-4851. 1991.

Infections of the Female Genital Tract. Richard L. Sweet. Williams & Wilkins, 428 East Preston St., Baltimore, MD 21202. Phone: (800) 638-0672. Fax: (800) 447-8438. Second edition 1990.

Introduction to Clinical Gynecological Urology. John R. Sutherst. Butterworth-Heinemann, 80 Montvale Ave., Stoneham, MA 02180. Phone: (617) 438-8464. Fax: (617) 279-4851. 1991.

Mastery of Surgery: Urologic Surgery. Jackson E. Fowler Jr. (ed.). Little, Brown and Company, 34 Beacon St., Boston, MA 02108. Phone: (617) 227-0730. 1992.

Principles of Genitourinary Radiology. Zoran L. Barbaric. Thieme Medical Publishers, Inc., 381 Park Ave. S., New York, NY 10016. Phone: (212) 683-5088. Fax: (212) 779-9020. 1991.

Stone Therapy in Urology. F. Eisenberger, K. Miller, J. Rassweiler (eds.). Thieme Medical Publishers, Inc., 381 Park Ave. S., New York, NY 10016. Phone: (212) 683-5088. Fax: (212) 779-9020. 1991.

Urinary Tract Pathology. Jay Bernstein, Jacob Churg. Raven Press, 1185 Avenue of the Americas, New York, NY 10036. Phone: (212) 930-9500. Fax: (212) 869-3495. 1992.

Urologic Pathology. Robert Petersen. J.B. Lippincott Co., 227 E. Washington Square, Philadelphia, PA 19106-3780. Phone: (215) 238-4200. Fax: (215) 238-4227. 1992.

Urologic Surgery. Glenn. J.B. Lippincott Co., 227 E. Washington Square, Philadelphia, PA 19106-3780. Phone: (215) 238-4200. Fax: (215) 238-4227. Fourth edition 1991.

Urological Oncology. Alderson Smith. John Wiley & Sons, Inc., 605 Third Ave., New York, NY 10158-0012. Phone: (212) 850-6000. Fax: (212) 850-6088. 1991.

UROLOGY

See also: KIDNEY DISEASES;
TRANSPLANTATION; UROLOGIC
DISORDERS

ABSTRACTING, INDEXING, AND CURRENT AWARENESS PUBLICATIONS

Excerpta Medica. Section 28: Urology and Nephrology. Elsevier Science Publishing Co., Inc., P.O. Box 882, Madison Square Station, New York, NY 10159-2101. Phone: (212) 989-5800. Fax: (212) 633-3990. 20/year.

Index Medicus. U.S. National Library of Medicine, 8600 Rockville Pike, Bethesda, MD 20894. Phone: (800) 638-8480. Monthly.

ANNUALS AND REVIEWS

Advances in Urology. Mosby-Year Book, 11830 Westline Industrial Drive, St. Louis, MO 63146. Phone: (800) 325-4177. Fax: (314) 432-1380. Annual.

Urologic Clinics. W.B. Saunders Co., The Curtis Center, Independence Square W., Philadelphia, PA 19106-3399. Phone: (215) 238-7800. Quarterly.

Year Book of Urology. Mosby-Year Book, 11830 Westline Industrial Drive, St. Louis, MO 63146. Phone: (800) 325-4177. Fax: (314) 432-1380. Annual.

ASSOCIATIONS, PROFESSIONAL SOCIETIES, ADVOCACY AND SUPPORT GROUPS

American Board of Urology (ABU). 31700 Telegraph Rd., Ste. 150, Birmingham, MI 48010. Phone: (312) 646-9720.

American Urological Association (AUA). 1120 N. Charles St., Baltimore, MD 21201. Phone: (301) 727-1100. Fax: (301) 625-2390.

DIRECTORIES

Directory of Certified Urologists. American Board of Medical Specialties, 1 Rotary Center, Suite 805, Evanston, IL 60201. Phone: (708) 491-9091. Biennial.

Directory of Medical Specialists. Marquis Who's Who, 3002 Glenview Rd., Wilmette, IL 60091. Phone: (800) 621-9669. Fax: (708) 441-2264. Biennial.

Directory of Physicians in the United States. American Medical Association, 515 North State St., Chicago, IL 60610. Phone: (312) 464-0183. Fax: (312) 464-5834. Biennial.

HANDBOOKS, GUIDES, MANUALS, ATLASES

Atlas of Endourology. Kurt Amplatz. Mosby-Year Book, 11830 Westline Industrial Drive, St. Louis, MO 63146. Phone: (800) 325-4177. Fax: (314) 432-1380. 1991.

Atlas of Surgical Techniques in Urology. Whitehead. J.B. Lippincott Co., 227 E. Washington Square, Philadelphia, PA 19106-3780. Phone: (215) 238-4200. Fax: (215) 238-4227. 1992.

Manual of Clinical Problems in Urology. Resnick. Little, Brown and Co., 34 Beacon St., Boston, MA 02108. Phone: (617) 227-0730. 1989.

Manual of Urology: Diagnosis and Therapy. Mike B. Stroky, Robert J. Krane (eds.). Little, Brown and Company, 34 Beacon St., Boston, MA 02108. Phone: (617) 227-0730. 1990.

JOURNALS

British Journal of Urology. Churchill Livingstone Inc., 650 Avenue of the Americas, New York, NY 10011. Phone: (212) 819-5400. Fax: (212) 302-6598. Monthly.

Contemporary Urology. Medical Economics, Five Paragon Dr., Montvale, NJ 07645-1742. Phone: (800) 222-3045. Fax: (201) 573-4956. 10/year.

European Urology. S. Karger Publishers, Inc., 26 W. Avon Rd., P.O. Box 529, Farmington, CT 06085. Phone: (203) 675-7834. Fax: (203) 675-7302.

Journal of Urology. Williams & Wilkins, 428 E. Preston St., Baltimore, MD 21202. Phone: (800) 638-0672. Fax: (800) 447-8438. Monthly.

Report on Urologic Techniques. Churchill Livingstone Inc., 650 Avenue of the Americas, New York, NY 10011. Phone: (212) 819-5400. Fax: (212) 302-6598. 10/year.

Seminars in Urology. W.B. Saunders Co., The Curtis Center, Independence Sqare W., Philadelphia, PA 19106-3399. Phone: (215) 238-7800.

Urological Research. Springer-Verlag New York Inc., 175 Fifth Ave., New York, NY 10010. Phone: (212) 460-1500. Fax: (212) 473-6272.

Urology. Cahners Publishing Company, 249 W. 17th St., New York, NY 10011. Phone: (212) 645-0067.

ONLINE DATABASES

EMBASE. Elsevier Science Publishing Co., Inc., P.O. Box 882, Madison Square Station, New York, NY 10159-2101. Phone: (212) 989-5800. Fax: (212) 633-3990.

MEDLINE. National Library of Medicine, 8600 Rockville Pike, Bethesda, MD 20894. Phone: (800) 638-8480.

SciSearch. Institute for Scientific Information, 3501 Market St., Philadelphia, PA 19104. Phone: (215) 386-0100. Fax: (215) 386-6362.

TEXTBOOKS AND MONOGRAPHS

Adult and Pediatric Urology. Gillenwater. Mosby-Year Book, 11830 Westline Industrial Drive, St. Louis, MO 63146. Phone: (800) 325-4177. Fax: (314) 432-1380. Two volumes. Second edition. 1991.

Campbell's Urology. Patrick C. Walsh (ed.). W.B. Saunders Co., The Curtis Center, Independence Square W., Philadelphia, PA 19106-3399. Phone: (215) 238-7800. Sixth edition. Three volumes. 1992.

Current Genitourinary Cancer Surgery. Dana Crawford, Sakvi Dai (eds.). Williams & Wilkins, 428 East Preston St., Baltimore, MD 21202. Phone: (800) 638-0672. Fax: (800) 447-8438. 1990.

Infections of the Female Genital Tract. Richard L. Sweet. Williams & Wilkins, 428 East Preston St., Baltimore, MD 21202. Phone: (800) 638-0672. Fax: (800) 447-8438. Second edition 1990.

Operative Urology. Fray F. Marshall (ed.). W.B. Saunders Co., The Curtis Center, Independence Sqare W., Philadelphia, PA 19106-3399. Phone: (215) 238-7800. 1991.

Smith's General Urology. Emil A. Tanagho, Jack W. McAninch. Appleton & Lange, 25 Van Zant St., East Norwalk, CT 06855. Phone: (800) 423-1359. Fax: (203) 854-9486. Thirteenth edition 1991.

Stone Therapy in Urology. F. Eisenberger, K. Miller, J. Rassweiler (eds.). Thieme Medical Publishers, Inc., 381 Park Ave. S., New York, NY 10016. Phone: (212) 683-5088. Fax: (212) 779-9020. 1991.

Urology. Sokeland. Thieme Medical Publishers, Inc., 381 Park Ave. S., New York, NY 10016. Phone: (212) 683-5088. Fax: (212) 779-9020. Second edition 1989.

UTERINE CANCER

See also: CANCER

ABSTRACTING, INDEXING, AND CURRENT AWARENESS PUBLICATIONS

Current Contents/Clinical Medicine. Institute for Scientific Information, 3501 Market St., Philadelphia, PA 19104. Phone: (800) 523-1850. Fax: (215) 386-6362. Weekly.

ICRDB Cancergram: Gynecologic Tumors--Diagnosis, Treatment. U.S. Government Printing Office, Superintendent of Documents, P.O. Box 371954, Pittsburgh, PA 15250-7954. Phone: (202) 783-3238. Fax: (202) 512-2250. Monthly.

Index Medicus. U.S. National Library of Medicine, 8600 Rockville Pike, Bethesda, MD 20894. Phone: (800) 638-8480. Monthly.

Research Alert: Cancer-Female Reproductive Tract. Institute for Scientific Information, 3501 Market St., Philadelphia, PA 19104. Phone: (800) 523-1850. Fax: (215) 386-6362. Weekly.

Science Citation Index. Institute for Scientific Information, 3501 Market St., Philadelphia, PA 19104. Phone: (800) 523-1850. Fax: (215) 386-6362. Bimonthly.

ANNUALS AND REVIEWS

In Development New Medicines for Older Americans. 1991 Annual Survey. More Medicines in Testing for Cancer Than for Any Other Disease of Aging. Pharmaceutical Manufacturers Association, 1100 15th St. N.W., Washington, DC 20005. Phone: (202) 835-3400. 1991.

ASSOCIATIONS, PROFESSIONAL SOCIETIES, ADVOCACY AND SUPPORT GROUPS

American Cancer Society (ACS). 1599 Clifton Rd. N.E., Atlanta, GA 30329. Phone: (404) 320-3333.

National Foundation for Cancer Research (NFCR). 7315 Wisconsin Ave., Ste. 332W, Bethesda, MD 20814. Phone: (800) 321-2875. Fax: (301) 654-5824.

CD-ROM DATABASES

SCISEARCH. Institute for Scientific Information, 3501 Market St., Philadelphia, PA 19104. Phone: (215) 386-0100. Fax: (215) 386-6362.

ENCYCLOPEDIAS, DICTIONARIES, WORD BOOKS

Oncology Words. Stedman. Williams & Wilkins, 428 East Preston St., Baltimore, MD 21202. Phone: (800) 638-0672. Fax: (800) 447-8438. 1992.

HANDBOOKS, GUIDES, MANUALS, ATLASES

Atlas of Histopathology of the Cervix. G. Dallenbach-Hellweg, H. Poulson (eds.). Springer-Verlag New York Inc., 175 Fifth Ave., New York, NY 10010. Phone: (212) 460-1500. Fax: (212) 473-6272. 1990.

JOURNALS

Cancer Causes and Control. Rapid Communications of Oxford Ltd., The Old Malthouse, Paradise St., Oxford OX1 1LD, England. Phone: 44-865-790447. Fax: 44-865-244012. 6/year.

Journal of the National Cancer Institute. Superintendent of Documents, P.O. Box 371954, Pittsburgh, PA 15250-7954. Fax: (202) 512-2233. Semimonthly.

Journal of Surgical Oncology. John Wiley & Sons, Inc., 605 Third Ave., New York, NY 10158-0012. Phone: (212) 850-6000. Fax: (212) 850-6088. Monthly.

Journal of Women's Health. Mary Ann Liebert, Inc., 1651 Third Ave., New York, NY 10128. Phone: (212) 289-2300. Fax: (212) 289-4697. Quarterly.

ONLINE DATABASES

Clinical Protocols. U.S. National Cancer Institute, International Cancer Information Center, Building 82, Room 102, Bethesda, MD 20892. Phone: (301) 496-7403. Fax: (301) 480-8105.

EMBASE. Elsevier Science Publishing Co., Inc., P.O. Box 882, Madison Square Station, New York, NY 10159-2101. Phone: (212) 989-5800. Fax: (212) 633-3990.

MEDLINE. National Library of Medicine, 8600 Rockville Pike, Bethesda, MD 20894. Phone: (800) 638-8480.

SciSearch. Institute for Scientific Information, 3501 Market St., Philadelphia, PA 19104. Phone: (215) 386-0100. Fax: (215) 386-6362.

POPULAR WORKS AND PATIENT EDUCATION

Cancervive: The Challenge of Life After Cancer. Susan Nessim, Judith Ellis. Houghton Mifflin Co., 1 Beacon St., Boston, MA 02108. Phone: (800) 225-3362. 1991.

Every Woman's Medical Handbook. Marie Stoppard. Ballantine Books, Inc., 201 E. 50th St., New York, NY 10022. Phone: (800) 733-3000. 1991.

Everyone's Guide to Cancer Therapy: How Cancer is Diagnosed, Treated, and Managed on a Day to Day Basis. Malin Dollinger, Ernest H. Rosenbaum, Greg Cable. Andrews & McMeel, 4900 Main St., Kansas City, MO 64112. Phone: (800) 826-4216. 1991.

If It Runs In Your Family: Ovarian and Uterine Cancer. Sherilynn J. Hummel. Bantam Books, Inc., 666 Fifth Ave., New York, NY 10103. Phone: (800) 223-6834. 1992.

Women Talk about Gynecological Surgery: From Diagnosis to Recovery. Amy Gross, Dee Ito. HarperCollins Pubs., Inc., 10 E. 53rd St., New York, NY 10022-5299. Phone: (212) 207-7000. Fax: (800) 242-7737. 1992.

Women's Cancers: How to Prevent Them, How to Treat Them, How to Beat Them. Donna Dawson, Marlene Mersch (eds.). Hunter House, Inc., 2200 Central, Ste. 202, Alameda, CA 94501-4451. Phone: (510) 865-5282. 1992.

RESEARCH CENTERS, INSTITUTES, CLEARINGHOUSES

Cancer Information Service (CIS). Office of Cancer Communications, National Cancer Institute, Bldg. 31, Rm. 10A24, 9000 Rockville Pike, Bethesda, MD 20892. Phone: (800) 4CA-NCER.

TEXTBOOKS AND MONOGRAPHS

Cancer: Principles and Practice of Oncology. Vincent T. DeVita. J.B. Lippincott Co., 227 E. Washington Square, Philadelphia, PA 19106-3780. Phone: (215) 238-4200. Fax: (215) 238-4227. 1989 3rd edtion.

Gynecologic Oncology. Robert C. Knapp, Ross Berkowitz. McGraw-Hill Inc., 11 West 19th St., New York, NY 10011. Phone: (212) 337-5001. Fax: (212) 337-4092. Second edition 1992.

UTERINE FIBROIDS

See: GYNECOLOGIC DISORDERS

V

VACCINES

See: IMMUNIZATION

VAGINAL DISEASES

See: GYNECOLOGIC DISORDERS

VASCULAR DISEASES

See also: HEART DISEASES

ABSTRACTING, INDEXING, AND CURRENT AWARENESS PUBLICATIONS

CA Selects: Atherosclerosis & Heart Disease. Chemical Abstracts Service, 2540 Olentangy River Road, P.O. Box 3012, Columbus, OH 43210-0012. Phone: (800) 848-6538. Biweekly.

Current Contents/Clinical Medicine. Institute for Scientific Information, 3501 Market St., Philadelphia, PA 19104. Phone: (800) 523-1850. Fax: (215) 386-6362. Weekly.

Index Medicus. U.S. National Library of Medicine, 8600 Rockville Pike, Bethesda, MD 20894. Phone: (800) 638-8480. Monthly.

Research Alert: Cardiovascular Diseases-Coronary Disease & Myocardial Infarction. Institute for Scientific Information, 3501 Market St., Philadelphia, PA 19104. Phone: (800) 523-1850. Fax: (215) 386-6362. Weekly.

ANNUALS AND REVIEWS

Vascular Medicine Review. Cambridge University Press, 40 W. 20th St., New York, NY 10011. Phone: (800) 431-1580. Semiannual.

ASSOCIATIONS, PROFESSIONAL SOCIETIES, ADVOCACY AND SUPPORT GROUPS

American College of Angiology (ACA). 1044 Northern Blvd., Ste. 103, Roslyn, NY 11576. Phone: (516) 484-6880. Fax: (516) 625-1174.

International College of Angiology (ICA). 1044 Northern Blvd., Ste. 103, Roslyn, NY 11576. Phone: (516) 484-6880. Fax: (516) 625-1174.

International Society on Thrombosis and Hemostasis. 9650 Rockville Pike, Bethesda, MD 20814. Phone: (301) 530-7120.

CD-ROM DATABASES

Cardiology MEDLINE. MEP, 124 Mt. Auburn St., Cambridge, MA 02138. Phone: (800) 342-1338. Fax: (617) 868-7738. Quarterly.

Hyperlipidemia. Hoffer. Williams & Wilkins, 428 East Preston St., Baltimore, MD 21202. Phone: (800) 638-0672. Fax: (800) 447-8438. 1992.

ENCYCLOPEDIAS, DICTIONARIES, WORD BOOKS

Cardiology Words. Stedman. Williams & Wilkins, 428 East Preston St., Baltimore, MD 21202. Phone: (800) 638-0672. Fax: (800) 447-8438. 1992.

HANDBOOKS, GUIDES, MANUALS, ATLASES

Atlas of Venous Surgery. John J. Bergan , Robert L. Kistner. W.B. Saunders Co., The Curtis Center, Independence Sqare W., Philadelphia, PA 19106-3399. Phone: (215) 238-7800. 1992.

JOURNALS

Arteriosclerosis and Thrombosis: A Journal of Vascular Biology. American Heart Association, 7320 Greenville Ave., Dallas, TX 75231. Phone: (214) 706-1310. Fax: (214) 691-6342. Bimonthly.

Catheterization and Cardiovascular Diagnosis. John Wiley & Sons, Inc., 605 Third Ave., New York, NY 10158-0012. Phone: (212) 850-6000. Fax: (212) 850-6088. Monthly.

Heart and Vessels. Springer-Verlag New York Inc., 175 Fifth Ave., New York, NY 10010. Phone: (212) 460-1500. Fax: (212) 473-6272.

Journal of Vascular Nursing. Mosby-Year Book, 11830 Westline Industrial Drive, St. Louis, MO 63146. Phone: (800) 325-4177. Fax: (314) 432-1380. Quarterly.

Microvascular Research. Academic Press, Inc., 1250 Sixth Ave., San Diego, CA 92101-4311. Phone: (619) 699-6345. Fax: (619) 699-6715.

Thrombosis and Haemostasis. F.K. Schattauer Verlagsgesellschaft, Lenzhalde 3, W-7000 Stuttgart, Germany. Phone: 0711-22987-0.

Thrombosis Research. Pergamon Press, 660 White Plains Rd., Tarrytown, NY 10591-5153. Phone: (914) 592-7700. Fax: (914) 592-3625.

Vascular Surgery. Westminster Publications, 1044 Northern Blvd., Roslyn, NY 11576. Phone: (516) 484-6880.

ONLINE DATABASES

EMBASE. Elsevier Science Publishing Co., Inc., P.O. Box 882, Madison Square Station, New York, NY 10159-2101. Phone: (212) 989-5800. Fax: (212) 633-3990.

MEDLINE. National Library of Medicine, 8600 Rockville Pike, Bethesda, MD 20894. Phone: (800) 638-8480.

SciSearch. Institute for Scientific Information, 3501 Market St., Philadelphia, PA 19104. Phone: (215) 386-0100. Fax: (215) 386-6362.

POPULAR WORKS AND PATIENT EDUCATION

The Cooper Clinic Cardiac Rehabilitation Program: Featuring the Unique Heart Points System. Neil F. Gordon, Larry W. Gibbons. Pocket Books, Inc., 1230 Ave. of the Americas, New York, NY 10020. Phone: (800) 223-2348. Fax: (800) 284-0735. 1990.

Yale University School of Medicine Heart Book. Barry L. Zaret, Lawrence S. Cohen, Marvin Moser, and others. William Morrow & Company, Inc., 1350 Ave. of the Americas, New York, NY 10019. Phone: (800) 237-0657. 1992.

RESEARCH CENTERS, INSTITUTES, CLEARINGHOUSES

Center for Thrombosis and Hemostasis. University of North Carolina at Chapel Hill. Campus Box 7015, UNC-CH School of Medicine, Chapel Hill, NC 27599-7015. Phone: (919) 966-3704. Fax: (919) 966-6012.

Cleveland Clinic Foundation Research Institute. 9500 Euclid Ave., Cleveland, OH 44195-5210. Phone: (216) 444-3900. Fax: (216) 444-3279.

Sol Sherry Thrombosis Research Center. Temple University. 3400 N. Broad St., Philadelphia, PA 19140. Phone: (215) 221-4665. Fax: (215) 221-2783.

TEXTBOOKS AND MONOGRAPHS

Endovascular Surgery. Wesley S. Moore, Samuel S. Ahn. W.B. Saunders Co., The Curtis Center, Independence Sqare W., Philadelphia, PA 19106-3399. Phone: (215) 238-7800. 2nd edition, 1993.

Noninvasive Diagnostics in Vascular Disease. Amost Fronek. McGraw-Hill, Inc., Health Professions Division, 1221 Avenue of the Americas, 28th Floor, New York, NY 10020. Phone: (212) 512-4228. 1989.

Vascular Diseases in the Limbs: Mechanisms and Principles of Treatment. Denis Clement, John T. Shepherd. Mosby-Year Book, 11830 Westline Industrial Drive, St. Louis, MO 63146. Phone: (800) 325-4177. Fax: (314) 432-1380. 1992.

Vascular Injuries in Surgical Practice. Fred Bangard, and others. Appleton & Lange, 25 Van Zant St., East Norwalk, CT 06855. Phone: (800) 423-1359. Fax: (203) 854-9486. 1990.

Vascular Medicine. Joseph Loscalzo, Mark A. Creager, Victor J. Dzau (eds.). Little, Brown and Company, 34 Beacon St., Boston, MA 02108. Phone: (617) 227-0730. 1992.

Vascular Surgery. Robert Rutherford. W.B. Saunders Co., The Curtis Center, Independence Sqare W., Philadelphia, PA 19106-3399. Phone: (215) 238-7800. 3rd edition, 1989.

Venous Thrombosis. V.V. Kakkar. Butterworth-Heinemann, 80 Montvale Ave., Stoneham, MA 02180. Phone: (617) 438-8464. Fax: (617) 279-4851. 1991.

VASCULAR HEADACHE

See: HEADACHE

VASCULAR SURGERY

See: CARDIOVASCULAR SURGERY

VASECTOMY

See: CONTRACEPTION

VENEREAL DISEASES

See: HERPESVIRUS INFECTIONS; SEXUALLY TRANSMITTED DISEASES

VENTRICULAR FIBRILLATION

See: ARRHYTHMIA; HEART DISEASES

VETERINARY MEDICINE

ABSTRACTING, INDEXING, AND CURRENT AWARENESS PUBLICATIONS

CAB Abstracts. C.A.B. International, 845 N. Park Ave., Tucson, AZ 85719. Phone: (800) 528-4841.

Index Medicus. U.S. National Library of Medicine, 8600 Rockville Pike, Bethesda, MD 20894. Phone: (800) 638-8480. Monthly.

Index Veterinarius. C.A.B. International, 845 N. Park Ave., Tucson, AZ 85719. Phone: (800) 528-4841. Monthly.

Science Citation Index. Institute for Scientific Information, 3501 Market St., Philadelphia, PA 19104. Phone: (800) 523-1850. Fax: (215) 386-6362. Bimonthly.

Veterinary Bulletin. C.A.B. International, 845 N. Park Ave., Tucson, AZ 85719. Phone: (800) 528-4841. Monthly.

Veterinary Update Clinical Abstract Service. American Veterinary Publications, Inc., 5782 Thornwood Dr., Goleta, CA 93117-3896. Phone: (805) 967-5988. Monthly.

ANNUALS AND REVIEWS

Review of Medical and Veterinary Mycology. C.A.B. International, 845 N. Park Ave., Tucson, AZ 85719. Phone: (800) 528-4841. Quarterly.

Veterinary Clinics: Equine Practice. W.B. Saunders Co., The Curtis Center, Independence Square W., Philadelphia, PA 19106-3399. Phone: (215) 238-7800. 3/year.

Veterinary Clinics: Food Animal Practice. W.B. Saunders Co., The Curtis Center, Independence Square W., Philadelphia, PA 19106-3399. Phone: (215) 238-7800. 3/year.

Veterinary Clinics: Small Animal Practice. W.B. Saunders Co., The Curtis Center, Independence Square W., Philadelphia, PA 19106-3399. Phone: (215) 238-7800. Bimonthly.

ASSOCIATIONS, PROFESSIONAL SOCIETIES, ADVOCACY AND SUPPORT GROUPS

American Animal Hospital Association (AAHA). Denver West Office Park, P.O. Box 150899, Denver, CO 80215. Phone: (303) 279-2500. Fax: (303) 279-1816.

American College of Veterinary Internal Medicine (ACVIM). 620 N. Main St., Ste. C-1A, Blacksburg, VA 24060. Phone: (703) 951-8543. Fax: (703) 951-4268.

American College of Veterinary Surgeons. 405 Park Ln., Champaign, IL 61820. Phone: (217) 356-6736.

American Veterinary Medical Association (AVMA). 930 N. Meacham Rd., Schaumburg, IL 60196. Phone: (708) 605-8070. Fax: (708) 330-2862.

Canadian Council on Animal Care. 151 Slater St., Suite 1000, Ottawa, ON, Canada K1P 5H3. Phone: (613) 238-4031. Fax: (613) 563-7739.

Canadian Veterinary Medical Association. 339 Booth St., Ottawa, ON, Canada K1R 7K1.

CD-ROM DATABASES

CABCD (CAB Abstracts on CD-ROM). C.A.B. International, 845 N. Park Ave., Tucson, AZ 85719. Phone: (800) 528-4841.

SCISEARCH. Institute for Scientific Information, 3501 Market St., Philadelphia, PA 19104. Phone: (215) 386-0100. Fax: (215) 386-6362.

VETCD. SilverPlatter Information, Inc., River Ridge Office Park, 100 River Ridge Rd., Norwood, MA 02062. Phone: (617) 769-2599. Fax: (617) 769-8763. Annual.

ENCYCLOPEDIAS, DICTIONARIES, WORD BOOKS

Black's Veterinary Dictionary. Geoffrey West (ed.). Barnes & Noble Books, 4270 Boston Way, Lanham, MD 20706. Phone: (800) 462-6420. 17th edition 1992.

JOURNALS

British Veterinary Journal. Balliere Tindall, 24-28 Oval Rd., London NW1 7DX, England.

Preventive Veterinary Medicine. Elsevier Science Publishing Co., Inc., P.O. Box 882, Madison Square Station, New York, NY 10159-2101. Phone: (212) 989-5800. Fax: (212) 633-3990. Monthly.

Research in Veterinary Science. British Veterinary Association, 7 Mansfield St., London W1M 0AT, England. Phone: 01-636-6541.

Seminars in Veterinary Medicine and Surgery: Small Animal. W.B. Saunders Co., The Curtis Center, Independence Sqare W., Philadelphia, PA 19106-3399. Phone: (215) 238-7800.

Veterinary Immunology and Immunopathology. Elsevier Science Publishing Co., Inc., P.O. Box 882, Madison Square Station, New York, NY 10159-2101. Phone: (212) 989-5800. Fax: (212) 633-3990. 16/year.

Veterinary Medicine. Medical Economics, Five Paragon Dr., Montvale, NJ 07645-1742. Phone: (800) 222-3045. Fax: (201) 573-4956. Monthly.

Veterinary Microbiology. Elsevier Science Publishing Co., Inc., P.O. Box 882, Madison Square Station, New York, NY 10159-2101. Phone: (212) 989-5800. Fax: (212) 633-3990. 16/year.

The Veterinary Quarterly. Kluwer Academic Publishers, P.O. Box 358, Accord Station, Hingham, MA 02018-0358. Phone: (617) 871-6600. Fax: (617) 871-6528. 4/year.

Veterinary Record. British Veterinary Association, 7 Mansfield St., London W1M 0AT, England. Phone: 01-636-6541. Weekly.

Veterinary Research Communications. Kluwer Academic Publishers, P.O. Box 358, Accord Station, Hingham, MA 02018-0358. Phone: (617) 871-6600. Fax: (617) 871-6528. 6/year.

Veterinary Surgery. J.B. Lippincott Co., 227 E. Washington Square, Philadelphia, PA 19106-3780. Phone: (215) 238-4200. Fax: (215) 238-4227.

ONLINE DATABASES

EMBASE. Elsevier Science Publishing Co., Inc., P.O. Box 882, Madison Square Station, New York, NY 10159-2101. Phone: (212) 989-5800. Fax: (212) 633-3990.

MEDLINE. National Library of Medicine, 8600 Rockville Pike, Bethesda, MD 20894. Phone: (800) 638-8480.

SciSearch. Institute for Scientific Information, 3501 Market St., Philadelphia, PA 19104. Phone: (215) 386-0100. Fax: (215) 386-6362.

RESEARCH CENTERS, INSTITUTES, CLEARINGHOUSES

J.A. Baker Institute for Animal Health. Cornell University, Ithaca, NY 14853. Phone: (607) 277-3044.

TEXTBOOKS AND MONOGRAPHS

Equine Practice. Sue Dyson (ed.). Mosby-Year Book, 11830 Westline Industrial Drive, St. Louis, MO 63146. Phone: (800) 325-4177. Fax: (314) 432-1380. 1992.

Farm Animal Practice. Roger Blowey. Mosby-Year Book, 11830 Westline Industrial Drive, St. Louis, MO 63146. Phone: (800) 325-4177. Fax: (314) 432-1380. 1992.

Kirk's Current Veterinary Therapy 11: Small Animal Practice. Robert W. Kirk, John D. Bonagard. W.B. Saunders Co., The Curtis Center, Independence Sqare W., Philadelphia, PA 19106-3399. Phone: (215) 238-7800. 1992.

Small Animal Practice. Raymond Long (ed.). Mosby-Year Book, 11830 Westline Industrial Drive, St. Louis, MO 63146. Phone: (800) 325-4177. Fax: (314) 432-1380. 1992.

Veterinary Emergency Medicine and Critical Care. Robert J. Murtaugh, Paul Kaplan. Mosby-Year Book, 11830 Westline Industrial Drive, St. Louis, MO 63146. Phone: (800) 325-4177. Fax: (314) 432-1380. 1991.

Veterinary Medicine: A Textbook of the Diseases of Cattle, Sheep, Pigs, Goats and Horses. D.C. Blood, O.M. Radostis. Balliere Tindall, 24-28 Oval Rd., London NW1 7DX, England. 1989.

Veterinary Practice Management. McCurnin. J.B. Lippincott Co., 227 E. Washington Square, Philadelphia, PA 19106-3780. Phone: (215) 238-4200. Fax: (215) 238-4227. 1989.

VIRAL DISEASES

See also: INFECTIOUS DISEASES; REYE'S SYNDROME; VIROLOGY

ABSTRACTING, INDEXING, AND CURRENT AWARENESS PUBLICATIONS

BIOSIS/CAS Selects: Antiviral Agents. BIOSIS, 2100 Arch St., Philadelphia, PA 19103-1399. Phone: (215) 587-4800. Fax: (215) 587-2016. Biweekly.

CA Selects: Virucides & Virustats. Chemical Abstracts Service, 2540 Olentangy River Road, P.O. Box 3012, Columbus, OH 43210-0012. Phone: (800) 848-6538. Biweekly.

Current Contents/Clinical Medicine. Institute for Scientific Information, 3501 Market St., Philadelphia, PA 19104. Phone: (800) 523-1850. Fax: (215) 386-6362. Weekly.

Excerpta Medica. Section 4: Microbiology, Mycology, Parasitology and Virology. Elsevier Science Publishers, P.O. Box 882, Madison Square Station, New York, NY 10159-2101. Phone: (212) 633-3950. Fax: (212) 633-3990. 32/year.

Index Medicus. U.S. National Library of Medicine, 8600 Rockville Pike, Bethesda, MD 20894. Phone: (800) 638-8480. Monthly.

Research Alert: Antiviral Agents. Institute for Scientific Information, 3501 Market St., Philadelphia, PA 19104. Phone: (800) 523-1850. Fax: (215) 386-6362. Weekly.

Research Alert: Infections Diseases-Viral. Institute for Scientific Information, 3501 Market St., Philadelphia, PA 19104. Phone: (800) 523-1850. Fax: (215) 386-6362. Weekly.

Virology & AIDS Abstracts. Cambridge Scientific Abstracts, 7200 Wisconsin Ave., Bethesda, MD 20814-4823. Phone: (800) 843-7751. Fax: (301) 961-6720. Monthly.

ANNUALS AND REVIEWS

Advances in Virus Research. Academic Press, Inc., 1250 Sixth Ave., San Diego, CA 92101-4311. Phone: (619) 699-6345. Fax: (619) 699-6715. Irregular.

CD-ROM DATABASES

Infectious Diseases MEDLINE. MEP, 124 Mt. Auburn St., Cambridge, MA 02138. Phone: (800) 342-1338. Fax: (617) 868-7738. Quarterly.

HANDBOOKS, GUIDES, MANUALS, ATLASES

Atlas of Infectious Disease. Edmond. Mosby-Year Book, 11830 Westline Industrial Drive, St. Louis, MO 63146. Phone: (800) 325-4177. Fax: (314) 432-1380. Second edition 1987.

JOURNALS

Antiviral Research. Elsevier Science Publishing Co., Inc., P.O. Box 882, Madison Square Station, New York, NY 10159-2101. Phone: (212) 989-5800. Fax: (212) 633-3990. 12/year.

Papillomavirus Report. Royal Society of Medicine Services Ltd., 1 Wimpole St., London W1M 8AE, England. Phone: 071-408 2119. Fax: 071-355 3198. Bimonthly.

ONLINE DATABASES

EMBASE. Elsevier Science Publishing Co., Inc., P.O. Box 882, Madison Square Station, New York, NY 10159-2101. Phone: (212) 989-5800. Fax: (212) 633-3990.

MEDLINE. National Library of Medicine, 8600 Rockville Pike, Bethesda, MD 20894. Phone: (800) 638-8480.

SciSearch. Institute for Scientific Information, 3501 Market St., Philadelphia, PA 19104. Phone: (215) 386-0100. Fax: (215) 386-6362.

POPULAR WORKS AND PATIENT EDUCATION

A Dancing Matrix: Voyages Along the Viral Frontier. Robin Marantz Henig. Alfred A. Knopf, 201 E. 50th St., New York, NY 10022. Phone: (800) 733-3000. 1993.

Virus Hunting: AIDS, Cancer and the Human Retrovirus. Robert Gallo. HarperCollins Pubs., Inc., 10 E. 53rd St., New York, NY 10022-5299. Phone: (212) 207-7000. 1991.

RESEARCH CENTERS, INSTITUTES, CLEARINGHOUSES

Acute Viral Respiratory Disease Unit. Baylor College of Medicine. 1 Baylor Plaza, Houston, TX 77030. Phone: (713) 799-4469.

Center for Immunization Research. Johns Hopkins University. School of Hygiene & Public Health, Hampton House 125, 624 N. Broadway, Baltimore, MD 21205. Phone: (301) 955-4376. Fax: (301) 955-2791.

Division of Vector-Borne Infectious Diseases. Centers for Disease Control. U.S. Public Health Service, P.O. Box 2087, Fort Collins, CO 80522-2087. Phone: (303) 221-6400. Fax: (303) 221-6476.

TEXTBOOKS AND MONOGRAPHS

Cytomegalovirus: Biology and Infection. Monto Ho. Plenum Publishing Co., 233 Spring St., New York, NY 10013-1578. Phone: (212) 620-8000. Fax: (212) 463-0742. Second edition 1991.

Infectious Diseases. Farrar. Raven Press, 1185 Ave. of the Americas, New York, NY 10036. Phone: (212) 930-9500. Fax: (212) 869-3495. 1992.

The Natural History of Rabies. George M. Baer. CRC Press, Inc., 200 Corporate Blvd. N.W., Boca Raton, FL 33431. Phone: (407) 994-0555. Fax: (407) 997-0949. Second edition 1991.

Viral Infections of Humans: Epidemiology and Control. Alfred S. Evans (ed.). Plenum Publishing Co., 233 Spring St., New York, NY 10013-1578. Phone: (212) 620-8000. Fax: (212) 463-0742. Third edition 1991.

Virology. Dulbecco. J.B. Lippincott Co., 227 E. Washington Square, Philadelphia, PA 19106-3780. Phone: (215) 238-4200. Fax: (215) 238-4227. Second edition 1988.

VIRAL HEPATITIS

See: HEPATITIS

VIROLOGY

See also: VIRAL DISEASES

ABSTRACTING, INDEXING, AND CURRENT AWARENESS PUBLICATIONS

BIOSIS/CAS Selects: Bacterial & Viral Genetics. BIOSIS, 2100 Arch St., Philadelphia, PA 19103-1399. Phone: (215) 587-4800. Fax: (215) 587-2016. Biweekly.

Current Contents/Life Sciences. Institute for Scientific Information, 3501 Market St., Philadelphia, PA 19104. Phone: (215) 386-0100. Fax: (215) 386-6362.

Excerpta Medica. Section 4: Microbiology, Mycology, Parasitology and Virology. Elsevier Science Publishers, P.O. Box 882, Madison Square Station, New York, NY 10159-2101. Phone: (212) 633-3950. Fax: (212) 633-3990. 32/year.

ICRDB Cancergram: Antitumor and Antiviral Agents--Mechanism of Action. U.S. Government Printing Office, Superintendent of Documents, P.O. Box 371954, Pittsburgh, PA 15250-7954. Phone: (202) 783-3238. Fax: (202) 512-2250. Monthly.

Index Medicus. U.S. National Library of Medicine, 8600 Rockville Pike, Bethesda, MD 20894. Phone: (800) 638-8480. Monthly.

Science Citation Index. Institute for Scientific Information, 3501 Market St., Philadelphia, PA 19104. Phone: (800) 523-1850. Fax: (215) 386-6362. Bimonthly.

Virology & AIDS Abstracts. Cambridge Scientific Abstracts, 7200 Wisconsin Ave., Bethesda, MD 20814-4823. Phone: (800) 843-7751. Fax: (301) 961-6720. Monthly.

ANNUALS AND REVIEWS

Advances in Virus Research. Academic Press, Inc., 1250 Sixth Ave., San Diego, CA 92101-4311. Phone: (619) 699-6345. Fax: (619) 699-6715. Irregular.

Applied Virology Research. Plenum Publishing Co., 233 Spring St., New York, NY 10013-1578. Phone: (212) 620-8000. Fax: (212) 463-0742. Irregular.

Current Topics in Clinical Virology. Peter Morgan-Capner (ed.). Cambridge University Press, 40 W. 20th St., New York, NY 10011. Phone: (800) 431-1580. 1992.

Medical Virology. Plenum Publishing Co., 233 Spring St., New York, NY 10013-1578. Phone: (212) 620-8000. Fax: (212) 463-0742. Irregular.

Reviews in Medical Virology. John Wiley & Sons, Inc., 605 Third Ave., New York, NY 10158-0012. Phone: (212) 850-6000. Fax: (212) 850-6088. Quarterly.

CD-ROM DATABASES

SCISEARCH. Institute for Scientific Information, 3501 Market St., Philadelphia, PA 19104. Phone: (215) 386-0100. Fax: (215) 386-6362.

HANDBOOKS, GUIDES, MANUALS, ATLASES

Manual of Clinical Virology. P. Taylor, Christopher J. Ronalds (eds.). Butterworth-Heinemann, 80 Montvale Ave., Stoneham, MA 02180. Phone: (617) 438-8464. Fax: (617) 279-4851. 1991.

A Practical Guide to Clinical Virology. G.C. Haukenes, L.R. Haaheim, J.R. Pattison (eds.). John Wiley & Sons, Inc., 605 Third Ave., New York, NY 10158-0012. Phone: (212) 850-6000. Fax: (212) 850-6088. 1989.

JOURNALS

Archives of Virology. Springer-Verlag New York Inc., 175 Fifth Ave., New York, NY 10010. Phone: (212) 460-1500. Fax: (212) 473-6272.

Journal of General Virology. Society for Gernal Microbiology, Harvest House, 62 London Rd., Reading, Berks. RG1 5AS, England. Phone: 07348-61345. Fax: 07343-14112. Monthly.

Journal of Medical Virology. John Wiley & Sons, Inc., 605 Third Ave., New York, NY 10158-0012. Phone: (212) 850-6000. Fax: (212) 850-6088. Monthly.

Journal of Virology. American Society for Microbiology, 1325 Massachusetts Ave. N.W., Washington, DC 20005. Phone: (202) 737-3600. Monthly.

Research in Virology. Elsevier Science Publishing Co., Inc., P.O. Box 882, Madison Square Station, New York, NY 10159-2101. Phone: (212) 989-5800. Fax: (212) 633-3990. 6/year.

Virology. Academic Press, Inc., 1250 Sixth Ave., San Diego, CA 92101-4311. Phone: (619) 699-6345. Fax: (619) 699-6715. Monthly.

Virus Genes. Kluwer Academic Publishers, P.O. Box 358, Accord Station, Hingham, MA 02018-0358. Phone: (617) 871-6600. Fax: (617) 871-6528. 4/year.

Virus Research. Elsevier Science Publishing Co., Inc., P.O. Box 882, Madison Square Station, New York, NY 10159-2101. Phone: (212) 989-5800. Fax: (212) 633-3990. 12/year.

ONLINE DATABASES

EMBASE. Elsevier Science Publishing Co., Inc., P.O. Box 882, Madison Square Station, New York, NY 10159-2101. Phone: (212) 989-5800. Fax: (212) 633-3990.

MEDLINE. National Library of Medicine, 8600 Rockville Pike, Bethesda, MD 20894. Phone: (800) 638-8480.

SciSearch. Institute for Scientific Information, 3501 Market St., Philadelphia, PA 19104. Phone: (215) 386-0100. Fax: (215) 386-6362.

RESEARCH CENTERS, INSTITUTES, CLEARINGHOUSES

Coriell Institute for Medical Research (Camden). 401 Haddon Ave., Camden, NJ 08103. Phone: (609) 966-7377. Fax: (609) 964-0254.

Department of Microbiology and Immunology. University of Rochester. 601 Elmwood Ave., Box 672, Rochester, NY 14642. Phone: (716) 275-3402. Fax: (716) 473-9573.

Institute for Molecular Virology. St. Louis University. 3681 Park Ave., St. Louis, MO 63110. Phone: (314) 577-8403. Fax: (314) 577-8406.

Wistar Institute of Anatomy and Biology. 36th and Spruce Streets, Philadelphia, PA 19104. Phone: (215) 898-3700. Fax: (215) 573-2097.

Yale Arbovirus Research Unit. Yale University. 60 College St., Box 3333, New Haven, CT 06510. Phone: (203) 785-2901. Fax: (203) 785-4782.

TEXTBOOKS AND MONOGRAPHS

Clinical Virology in Oral Medicine and Dentistry. Crispian Scully, Lakshman Samaranayake. Cambridge University Press, 40 W. 20th St., New York, NY 10011. Phone: (800) 431-1580. 1992.

Fields Virology. Bernard N. Fields, David M. Knipe (eds.). Raven Press, 1185 Avenue of the Americas, New York, NY 10036. Phone: (212) 930-9500. Fax: (212) 869-3495. Second edition. Two volumes. 1990.

Fundamental Virology. Bernard N. Fields, David M. Knipe (eds.). Raven Press, 1185 Avenue of the Americas, New York, NY 10036. Phone: (212) 930-9500. Fax: (212) 869-3495. Second edition 1991.

The Human Retroviruses. Robert C. Gallo, Gilbert Jay (eds.). Academic Press, Inc., 1250 Sixth Ave., San Diego, CA 92101-4311. Phone: (619) 699-6345. Fax: (619) 699-6715. 1991.

Medical Virology. Morag Timbury. Churchill Livingstone Inc., 650 Avenue of the Americas, New York, NY 10011. Phone: (212) 819-5400. Fax: (212) 302-6598. Ninth edition 1991.

Principles and Practice of Clinical Virology. A.J. Zuckerman. John Wiley & Sons, Inc., 605 Third Ave., New York, NY 10158-0012. Phone: (212) 850-6000. Fax: (212) 850-6088. 2nd edition 1990.

Textbook of Human Virology. Robert B. Belshe. Mosby-Year Book, 11830 Westline Industrial Drive, St. Louis, MO 63146. Phone: (800) 325-4177. Fax: (314) 432-1380. Second edition 1991.

Virology. Dulbecco. J.B. Lippincott Co., 227 E. Washington Square, Philadelphia, PA 19106-3780. Phone: (215) 238-4200. Fax: (215) 238-4227. Second edition 1988.

VISION DISORDERS

See also: BLINDNESS; CATARACTS; EYE DISEASES; EYE SURGERY; GLAUCOMA; OPHTHALMOLOGY; OPTOMETRY

ABSTRACTING, INDEXING, AND CURRENT AWARENESS PUBLICATIONS

Excerpta Medica. Section 12: Ophthalmology. Elsevier Science Publishing Co., Inc., P.O. Box 882, Madison Square Station, New York, NY 10159-2101. Phone: (212) 989-5800. Fax: (212) 633-3990. 16/year.

Index Medicus. U.S. National Library of Medicine, 8600 Rockville Pike, Bethesda, MD 20894. Phone: (800) 638-8480. Monthly.

ASSOCIATIONS, PROFESSIONAL SOCIETIES, ADVOCACY AND SUPPORT GROUPS

American Council of the Blind (ACB). 1155 15th St. N.W., Ste. 720, Washington, DC 20005. Phone: (800) 424-8666. Fax: (202) 467-5085.

American Foundation for the Blind (AFB). 15 W. 16th St., New York, NY 10011. Phone: (212) 620-2000. Fax: (212) 727-7418.

Associated Services for the Blind (ASB). 919 Walnut St., Philadelphia, PA 19107. Phone: (215) 627-0600. Fax: (215) 922-0692.

Association for Education and Rehabilitation of the Blind and Visually Impaired (AER). 206 N. Washington St., Ste. 320, Alexandria, VA 22314. Phone: (703) 548-1884.

Braille Institute (BI). 741 N. Vermont Ave., Los Angeles, CA 90029. Phone: (213) 663-1111.

Canadian Association of Optometrists. 1785 Alta Vista Dr., Suite 301, Ottawa, ON, Canada K1G 3Y6. Phone: (613) 738-4412. Fax: (613) 738-7161.

Canadian National Institute for the Blind. 1931 Bayview Ave., Toronto, ON, Canada M4G 4C8. Phone: (416) 480-7580.

Canadian Ophthalmological Society. 1525 Carling Ave., No. 610, Ottawa, ON, Canada K1Z 8R9. Phone: (613) 729-6779. Fax: (613) 729-7209.

Helen Keller National Center for Deaf-Blind Youths and Adults (HKNC). 111 Middle Neck Rd., Sands Point, NY 11050. Phone: (516) 944-8900. Fax: (516) 944-7302.

National Braille Association (NBA). 1290 University Ave., Rochester, NY 14607. Phone: (716) 473-0900.

BIBLIOGRAPHIES

Library Resources for the Blind and Physically Handicapped. National Library Service for the Blind and Physically Handicapped, Library of Congress, 1291 Taylor St. N.W., Washington, DC 20542. Phone: (800) 424-8567. Fax: (202) 707-0712. Annual.

DIRECTORIES

Directory of Certified Ophthalmologists. American Board of Medical Specialties, 1 Rotary Center, Suite 805, Evanston, IL 60201. Phone: (708) 491-9091. Biennial.

ENCYCLOPEDIAS, DICTIONARIES, WORD BOOKS

Encyclopedia of Blindness and Vision Impairment. Jill Sardegna, T. Otis Paul. Facts on File, Inc., 460 Park Ave. S., New York, NY 10016-7382. Phone: (212) 683-2244. Fax: (212) 683-3633. 1992.

Ophthalmic Terminology. Stein. Mosby-Year Book, 11830 Westline Industrial Drive, St. Louis, MO 63146. Phone: (800) 325-4177. Fax: (314) 432-1380. Third edition 1992.

Ophthalmology Words. Stedman. Williams & Wilkins, 428 East Preston St., Baltimore, MD 21202. Phone: (800) 638-0672. Fax: (800) 447-8438. 1992.

JOURNALS

American Journal of Ophthalmology. Ophthalmic Publishing Co., 435 N. Michigan Ave., Chicago, IL 60611. Phone: (312) 787-3853.

Archives of Ophthalmology. American Medical Association, 515 North State St., Chicago, IL 60610. Phone: (312) 464-0183. Fax: (312) 464-5834. Monthly.

Clinical Eye and Vision Care. Butterworth-Heinemann, 80 Montvale Ave., Stoneham, MA 02180. Phone: (617) 438-8464. Fax: (617) 279-4851. Quarterly.

The Journal of the British Contact Lens Association. Mosby-Year Book, 11830 Westline Industrial Drive, St. Louis, MO 63146. Phone: (800) 325-4177. Fax: (314) 432-1380. Quarterly.

Journal of Rehabilitation Administration. AER, 206 N. Washington St., Alexandria, VA 22314.

Journal of Vision Rehabilitation. AER, 206 N. Washington St., Alexandria, VA 22314.

Journal of Visual Impairment and Blindness. AER, 206 N. Washington St., Alexandria, VA 22314.

Ophthalmology. J.B. Lippincott Co., 227 E. Washington Square, Philadelphia, PA 19106-3780. Phone: (215) 238-4200. Fax: (215) 238-4227.

ONLINE DATABASES

EMBASE. Elsevier Science Publishing Co., Inc., P.O. Box 882, Madison Square Station, New York, NY 10159-2101. Phone: (212) 989-5800. Fax: (212) 633-3990.

MEDLINE. National Library of Medicine, 8600 Rockville Pike, Bethesda, MD 20894. Phone: (800) 638-8480.

SciSearch. Institute for Scientific Information, 3501 Market St., Philadelphia, PA 19104. Phone: (215) 386-0100. Fax: (215) 386-6362.

POPULAR WORKS AND PATIENT EDUCATION

20/20: A Total Guide to Improving Your Vision and Preventing Eye Disease. Mitchell H. Friedlaender. Rodale Press, Inc., 33 E. Minor St., Emmaus, PA 18098. Phone: (800) 527-8200. Fax: (215) 967-6263. 1991.

Better Sight Without Glasses. Harry Benjamin. HarperCollins Pubs., Inc., 10 E. 53rd St., New York, NY 10022-5299. Phone: (212) 207-7000. Fax: (800) 242-7737. 1984.

Sudden Vision. John Crater. SLACK Inc., 6900 Grove Rd., Thorofare, NJ 08086-9447. Phone: (800) 257-8290. Fax: (609) 853-5991. 1989.

RESEARCH CENTERS, INSTITUTES, CLEARINGHOUSES

W.K. Kellogg Eye Center. University of Michigan. 1000 Wall St., Ann Arbor, MI 48105-1994. Phone: (313) 763-1415. Fax: (313) 936-2340.

TEXTBOOKS AND MONOGRAPHS

Age-Related Cataract. Richard W. Young. Oxford University Press, 200 Madison Ave., New York, NY 10016. Phone: (212) 679-7300. 1991.

Ambylopia: Basic and Clinical Aspects. Kenneth J. Ciuffreda, Dennis M. Levi, Arkady Selenow. Butterworth-Heinemann, 80 Montvale Ave., Stoneham, MA 02180. Phone: (617) 438-8464. Fax: (617) 279-4851. 1991.

The Art and Practice of Low Vision. Paul B. Freeman, Randall T. Jose. Butterworth-Heinemann, 80 Montvale Ave., Stoneham, MA 02180. Phone: (617) 438-8464. Fax: (617) 279-4851. 1991.

Binocular Vision Anomalies: Investigation and Treatment. W.D. Pickwell. Butterworth-Heinemann, 80 Montvale Ave., Stoneham, MA 02180. Phone: (617) 438-8464. Fax: (617) 279-4851. Second edition 1989.

A Text and Atlas of Strabismus Surgery. Renee Richards. Williams & Wilkins, 428 East Preston St., Baltimore, MD 21202. Phone: (800) 638-0672. Fax: (800) 447-8438. 1991.

VITAL STATISTICS

ABSTRACTING, INDEXING, AND CURRENT AWARENESS PUBLICATIONS

American Statistics Index: A Comprehensive Guide and Index to the Statistical Publications of the United States Government. Congressional Information Service, 4520 East-West Hwy., Bethesda, MD 20814. Phone: (800) 639-8380. 1973-Present Monthly.

Excerpta Medica. Section 17: Public Health, Social Medicine and Epidemiology. Elsevier Science Publishing Co., Inc., P.O. Box 882, Madison Square Station, New York, NY 10159-2101. Phone: (212) 989-5800. Fax: (212) 633-3990. 24/year.

Hospital Literature Index. American Hospital Association, 840 N. Lake Shore Dr., Chicago, IL 60611. Phone: (800) 242-2626. Fax: (312) 280-6015. Quarterly.

Index to Health Information. Congressional Information Service, 4520 East-West Hwy., Bethesda, MD 20814. Phone: (800) 639-8380. Quarterly.

Index Medicus. U.S. National Library of Medicine, 8600 Rockville Pike, Bethesda, MD 20894. Phone: (800) 638-8480. Monthly.

MEDOC: Index to U.S. Government Publications in the Medical and Health Sciences. Spencer S. Eccles Health Sciences Library, University of Utah, Bldg. 589, Salt Lake City, UT 84112. Phone: (801) 581-5268. Quarterly.

Statistical Reference Index. Congressional Information Service, 4520 East-West Hwy., Bethesda, MD 20814. Phone: (800) 639-8380. 1980-Present Monthly.

BIBLIOGRAPHIES

Catalog of Publications, 1980-1989. National Center for Health Statistics, 6525 Belcrest Rd., Hyattsville, MD 20782. Phone: (301) 436-8500. PHS90-1301.

Catalog of Publications, 1990-1991. National Center for Health Statistics, 6525 Belcrest Rd., Hyattsville, MD 20782. Phone: (301) 436-8500. PHS92-1301.

Catalog of Publications of the National Center for Health Statistics, 1962-1979. National Center for Health Statistics, 6525 Belcrest Rd., Hyattsville, MD 20782. Phone: (301) 436-8500. PHS80-1301.

Vital and Health Statistics Series: An Annotated Checklist and Index to the Publications of the Rainbow Series. Jim Walsh, A. James Bothmer. Greenwood Publishing Group, Inc., 88 Post Rd. W., P.O. Box 5007, Westport, CT 06881. Phone: (203) 226-3571. 1991.

CD-ROM DATABASES

Morbidity Mortality Weekly Report. MEP, 124 Mt. Auburn St., Cambridge, MA 02138. Phone: (800) 342-1338. Fax: (617) 868-7738. Annual.

Statistical Masterfile. Congressional Information Service, 4520 East-West Highway, Bethesda, MD 20814-3389. Phone: (800) 638-8380. Quarterly.

JOURNALS

Morbidity and Mortality Weekly Report. Massachusetts Medical Society, 1440 Main St., Waltham, MA 02154-1649. Phone: (617) 893-3800. Fax: (617) 893-0413. Weekly.

NEWSLETTERS

Healthy People 2000: Statistical Notes. U.S. Dept. of Health and Human Services. U.S. Govt. Printing Office, Superintendent of Documents, Washington, DC 20402-9325. Phone: (202) 783-3238. Quarterly.

Healthy People 2000: Statistics and Surveillance. U.S. Dept. of Health and Human Services. U.S. Govt. Printing Office, Superintendent of Documents, Washington, DC 20402-9325. Phone: (202) 783-3238. Quarterly.

Morbidity and Mortality Weekly Report. Centers for Disease Control, 1600 Clifton Rd. N.E., Atlanta, GA 30333. Phone: (404) 488-4698.

ONLINE DATABASES

EMBASE. Elsevier Science Publishing Co., Inc., P.O. Box 882, Madison Square Station, New York, NY 10159-2101. Phone: (212) 989-5800. Fax: (212) 633-3990.

MEDLINE. National Library of Medicine, 8600 Rockville Pike, Bethesda, MD 20894. Phone: (800) 638-8480.

SciSearch. Institute for Scientific Information, 3501 Market St., Philadelphia, PA 19104. Phone: (215) 386-0100. Fax: (215) 386-6362.

RESEARCH CENTERS, INSTITUTES, CLEARINGHOUSES

National Center for Health Statistics. 6525 Belcrest Rd., Rm. 1064, Hyattsville, MD 20782. Phone: (301) 436-8500.

STANDARDS AND STATISTICS SOURCES

Advance Data from Vital and Health Statistics. National Center for Health Statistics, 6525 Belcrest Rd., Rm. 1064, Hyattsville, MD 20782. Phone: (301) 436-8500. Irregular.

Birth and Fertility Rates by Education: 1980 and 1985. National Center for Health Statistics, 6525 Belcrest Rd., Rm. 1064, Hyattsville, MD 20782. Phone: (301) 436-8500. PHS 91-1927 1991.

Health United States. U.S. National Center for Health Statistics, Federal Center Bldg. No. 2, 3700 East-West Hwy., Hyattsville, MD 20782. Phone: (301) 436-7016. Annual.

Monthly Vital Statistics Report. National Center for Health Statistics, 6525 Belcrest Rd., Rm. 1064, Hyattsville, MD 20782. Phone: (301) 436-8500. Monthly.

Statistical Abstract of the United States. U.S. Government Printing Office, Superintendent of Documents, Washington, DC 20402. Phone: (202) 783-3238. Annual.

Vital & Health Statistics: 3. Analytical and Epidemiological Studies. National Center for Health Statistics, 6525 Belcrest Rd., Hyattsville, MD 20782. Phone: (301) 436-8500.

Vital & Health Statistics: 11. Data from the National Health and Nutrition Examination Series. National Center for Health Statistics, 6525 Belcrest Rd., Hyattsville, MD 20782. Phone: (301) 436-8500.

Vital & Health Statistics: 12. Data from the Institutionalized Population Surveys. National Center for Health Statistics, 6525 Belcrest Rd., Hyattsville, MD 20782. Phone: (301) 436-8500.

Vital & Health Statistics: 22. Data from the National Mortality and Natality Surveys. National Center for Health Statistics, 6525 Belcrest Rd., Hyattsville, MD 20782. Phone: (301) 436-8500.

Vital & Health Statistics: 23. Data from the National Survey of Family Growth. National Center for Health Statistics, 6525 Belcrest Rd., Hyattsville, MD 20782. Phone: (301) 436-8500.

Vital and Health Statistics. Series 1. Programs and Collection Procedures. National Center for Health Statistics, 6525 Belcrest Rd., Rm. 1064, Hyattsville, MD 20782. Phone: (301) 436-8500. Irregular.

Vital and Health Statistics. Series 2. Data Evaluation and Methods Research. National Center for Health Statistics, 6525 Belcrest Rd., Rm. 1064, Hyattsville, MD 20782. Phone: (301) 436-8500. Irregular.

Vital and Health Statistics. Series 4. Documents and Committee Reports. National Center for Health Statistics, 6525 Belcrest Rd., Rm. 1064, Hyattsville, MD 20782. Phone: (301) 436-8500. Irregular.

Vital and Health Statistics. Series 5. Comparative International Vital and Health Statistics Reports. National Center for Health Statistics, 6525 Belcrest Rd., Rm. 1064, Hyattsville, MD 20782. Phone: (301) 436-8500. Irregular.

Vital and Health Statistics. Series 6. Cognition and Survey Measurement. National Center for Health Statistics, 6525 Belcrest Rd., Rm. 1064, Hyattsville, MD 20782. Phone: (301) 436-8500. Irregular.

Vital and Health Statistics. Series 10. Data from the National Health Interview Survey. National Center for Health Statistics, 6525 Belcrest Rd., Rm. 1064, Hyattsville, MD 20782. Phone: (301) 436-8500. Irregular.

Vital and Health Statistics. Series 13. Data on Health Resources Utilization. National Center for Health Statistics, 6525 Belcrest

Rd., Rm. 1064, Hyattsville, MD 20782. Phone: (301) 436-8500. Irregular.

Vital and Health Statistics. Series 16. Compilations of Advance Data from Vital and Health Statistics. National Center for Health Statistics, 6525 Belcrest Rd., Rm. 1064, Hyattsville, MD 20782. Phone: (301) 436-8500. Irregular.

Vital and Health Statistics. Series 20. Data on Mortality. National Center for Health Statistics, 6525 Belcrest Rd., Rm. 1064, Hyattsville, MD 20782. Phone: (301) 436-8500. Irregular.

Vital and Health Statistics. Series 21. Data on Natality, Marriage, and Divorce. National Center for Health Statistics, 6525 Belcrest Rd., Rm. 1064, Hyattsville, MD 20782. Phone: (301) 436-8500. Irregular.

Vital and Health Statistics. Series 24. Compilations of Data on Natality, Mortality, Marriage, Divorce, and Induced Terminations of Pregnancy. National Center for Health Statistics, 6525 Belcrest Rd., Rm. 1064, Hyattsville, MD 20782. Phone: (301) 436-8500. Irregular.

Vital Statistics of the United States. Volume I, Natality, 1988. National Center for Health Statistics, 6525 Belcrest Rd., Rm. 1064, Hyattsville, MD 20782. Phone: (301) 436-8500. PHS 90-1100. 1990.

Vital Statistics of the United States. Volume II, Mortality, Part A, 1987. National Center for Health Statistics, 6525 Belcrest Rd., Rm. 1064, Hyattsville, MD 20782. Phone: (301) 436-8500. PHS 90-1101. 1990.

Vital Statistics of the United States. Volume II, Mortality, Part A, 1988. National Center for Health Statistics, 6525 Belcrest Rd., Rm. 1064, Hyattsville, MD 20782. Phone: (301) 436-8500. PHS 91-1101. 1991.

Vital Statistics of the United States. Volume II, Mortality, Part B, 1988. National Center for Health Statistics, 6525 Belcrest Rd., Rm. 1064, Hyattsville, MD 20782. Phone: (301) 436-8500. PHS 90-1102. 1990.

Vital Statistics of the United States. Volume III, Marriage and Divorce, 1986. National Center for Health Statistics, 6525 Belcrest Rd., Rm. 1064, Hyattsville, MD 20782. Phone: (301) 436-8500. PHS 90-1103. 1990.

Vital Statistics of the United States. Volume III, Marriage and Divorce , 1987. National Center for Health Statistics, 6525 Belcrest Rd., Rm. 1064, Hyattsville, MD 20782. Phone: (301) 436-8500. PHS 91-1103. 1991.

World Health Statistics Annual. World Health Organization, Ave. Appia, CH-1211, Geneva 27, Switzerland. Annual.

VITAMINS AND MINERALS

See also: NUTRITION; NUTRITIONAL
DISORDERS

ABSTRACTING, INDEXING, AND CURRENT AWARENESS PUBLICATIONS

Consumer Health and Nutrition Index. Alan Rees. Oryx Press, 4041 N. Central, Suite 700, Phoenix, AZ 85012. Phone: (800) 279-6799. Fax: (800) 279-4663. Quarterly.

Index Medicus. U.S. National Library of Medicine, 8600 Rockville Pike, Bethesda, MD 20894. Phone: (800) 638-8480. Monthly.

Research Alert: Vitamins. Institute for Scientific Information, 3501 Market St., Philadelphia, PA 19104. Phone: (800) 523-1850. Fax: (215) 386-6362. Weekly.

ANNUALS AND REVIEWS

Advances in Food and Nutrition Research. Academic Press, Inc., 1250 Sixth Ave., San Diego, CA 92101-4311. Phone: (619) 699-6345. Fax: (619) 699-6715. Irregular.

Annual Review of Nutrition. Annual Reviews Inc., 4139 El Camino Way, P.O. Box 10139, Palo Alto, CA 94303-0897. Phone: (415) 493-4400. Fax: (415) 855-9815. Annual.

ASSOCIATIONS, PROFESSIONAL SOCIETIES, ADVOCACY AND SUPPORT GROUPS

American Dietetic Association (ADA). 216 W. Jackson Blvd., Ste. 800, Chicago, IL 60606. Phone: (312) 899-0040. Fax: (312) 899-1979.

American Society for Clinical Nutrition (ASCN). 9650 Rockville Pike, Bethesda, MD 20814. Phone: (301) 530-7110.

ENCYCLOPEDIAS, DICTIONARIES, WORD BOOKS

Vitamin and Mineral Encyclopedia. Shelson S. Hendler. Simon & Schuster, 1230 Ave. of the Americas, New York, NY 10020. Phone: (800) 223-2348. Fax: (800) 284-0735. 1990.

JOURNALS

Journal of the American Dietetic Association. American Dietetic Association, 216 W. Jackson Blvd., Suite 800, Chicago, IL 60606-6995. Phone: (312) 899-0040. 12/year.

NEWSLETTERS

Environmental Nutrition. Environmental Nutrition, Inc., 52 Riverside Dr., New York, NY 10024. Phone: (212) 362-0424. Monthly.

Nutrition Forum. George F. Stickley Co., P.O. Box 1747, Allentown, PA 18105. Phone: (215) 437-1795. Bimonthly.

Nutrition & the M.D.. PM, Inc., P.O. Box 2468, Van Nuys, CA 91404-2160. Phone: (800) 365-2468. Monthly.

ONLINE DATABASES

EMBASE. Elsevier Science Publishing Co., Inc., P.O. Box 882, Madison Square Station, New York, NY 10159-2101. Phone: (212) 989-5800. Fax: (212) 633-3990.

MEDLINE. National Library of Medicine, 8600 Rockville Pike, Bethesda, MD 20894. Phone: (800) 638-8480.

SciSearch. Institute for Scientific Information, 3501 Market St., Philadelphia, PA 19104. Phone: (215) 386-0100. Fax: (215) 386-6362.

POPULAR WORKS AND PATIENT EDUCATION

Complete Guide to Vitamins, Minerals and Supplements. H. Winter Griffith. Fisher Books, P.O. Box 38040, Tucson, AZ 85740. Phone: (602) 292-9080.

Good Health with Vitamins and Minerals: A Complete Guide to a Lifetime of Safe and Effective Use. John Gallagher. Simon & Schuster, 1230 Ave. of the Americas, New York, NY 10020. Phone: (800) 223-2348. Fax: (800) 284-0735. 1990.

Mount Sinai School of Medicine Complete Book of Nutrition. Victor Herbert. St. Martin's Press, 175 Fifth Ave., New York, NY 10010. Phone: (212) 674-5151. 1990.

The Tufts University Guide to Total Nutrition. Stanley Gershoff, Catherine Whitney. HarperCollins Publishers., Inc., 10 E. 53rd St., New York, NY 10022-5299. Phone: (212) 207-7000. Fax: (800) 242-7737. 1990.

VOCATIONAL REHABILITATION

See: OCCUPATIONAL THERAPY

VOYEURISM

See: SEXUAL DISORDERS

VULVAR DISEASES

See: GYNECOLOGIC DISORDERS

W

WARTS

See: VIRAL DISEASES

WATER POLLUTION

See: ENVIRONMENTAL POLLUTANTS

WEIGHT CONTROL DIETS

See also: OBESITY

ABSTRACTING, INDEXING, AND CURRENT AWARENESS PUBLICATIONS

Consumer Health and Nutrition Index. Alan Rees. Oryx Press, 4041 N. Central, Suite 700, Phoenix, AZ 85012. Phone: (800) 279-6799. Fax: (800) 279-4663. Quarterly.

Index Medicus. U.S. National Library of Medicine, 8600 Rockville Pike, Bethesda, MD 20894. Phone: (800) 638-8480. Monthly.

ASSOCIATIONS, PROFESSIONAL SOCIETIES, ADVOCACY AND SUPPORT GROUPS

The Obesity Foundation (TOF). 5600 S. Quebec, Ste. 160-D, Englewood, CO 80111. Phone: (303) 779-4833.

Overeaters Anonymous. 1246 S. LaCienega Blvd., Rm. 203, Los Angeles, CA 90035. Phone: (213) 618-8835.

BIBLIOGRAPHIES

Nutri-Topics: Weight Control. Food and Nutrition Center, National Agricultural Library, 10301 Baltimore Blvd., Beltsville, MD 20705.

Weight Control, Diet, and Physical Activity. National Technical Information Service, 5285 Port Royal Rd., Springfield, VA 22161. Phone: (703) 487-4650. Fax: (703) 321-8547. Sept. 1970-Nov. 1989.

DIRECTORIES

American Society of Bariatric Physicians-Directory. American Society of Bariatric Physicians, 5600 S. Quebec, Ste. 160-D, Englewood, CO 80111. Phone: (303) 779-4833. Fax: (303) 779-4834. Annual.

JOURNALS

Journal of the American Dietetic Association. American Dietetic Association, 216 W. Jackson Blvd., Suite 800, Chicago, IL 60606-6995. Phone: (312) 899-0040. 12/year.

Journal of Nutrition. American Institute of Nutrition, 9650 Rockville Pike, Bethesda, MD 20814. Phone: (301) 530-7027.

ONLINE DATABASES

EMBASE. Elsevier Science Publishing Co., Inc., P.O. Box 882, Madison Square Station, New York, NY 10159-2101. Phone: (212) 989-5800. Fax: (212) 633-3990.

MEDLINE. National Library of Medicine, 8600 Rockville Pike, Bethesda, MD 20894. Phone: (800) 638-8480.

SciSearch. Institute for Scientific Information, 3501 Market St., Philadelphia, PA 19104. Phone: (215) 386-0100. Fax: (215) 386-6362.

POPULAR WORKS AND PATIENT EDUCATION

American Heart Association Cookbook. Ballantine Books, 201 E. 50th St., New York, NY 10022. Phone: (800) 733-3000.

Diet Right! The Consumer's Guide to Diet and Weight Loss Programs. Matthew Quincy. Borgo Press, P.O. Box 2845, San Bernardino, CA 92406-2845. Phone: (909) 884-5813. Fax: (909) 888-4942. 1991.

How Many Calories? How Much Fat? Guide to Calculating the Nutritional Content of the Foods You Eat. Rosemary Baskin. Consumer Reports Books, 9180 LeSaint Dr., Fairfield, OH 45014. Phone: (513) 860-1178. 1992.

Now That You've Lost It: How to Maintain Your Best Weight. Joyce D. Hash. Bull Publishing Co., 110 Gilbert Ave., Menlo Park, CA 94025. Phone: (800) 676-2855. 1992.

Prevention: Lose Weight Guidebook 1992. Mark Bricklin, Anne Remondi Inmhoff (eds.). Rodale Press, Inc., 33 E. Minor St., Emmaus, PA 18098. Phone: (800) 527-8200. 1992.

The Wellness Way to Weight Loss. Elizabeth M. Gallup. Plenum Publishing Co., 233 Spring St., New York, NY 10013-1578. Phone: (212) 620-8000. Fax: (212) 463-0742. 1990.

TEXTBOOKS AND MONOGRAPHS

Essentials of Nutrition and Diet Therapy. S.R. Williams. Mosby-Year Book, 11830 Westline Industrial Drive, St. Louis, MO 63146. Phone: (800) 325-4177. Fax: (314) 432-1380. Fifth edition 1990.

Obesity. Bjorntarp. J.B. Lippincott Co., 227 E. Washington Square, Philadelphia, PA 19106-3780. Phone: (215) 238-4200. Fax: (215) 238-4227. 1992.

WHOOPING COUGH

See: INFECTIOUS DISEASES

WIFE ABUSE

See: SPOUSE ABUSE

WILM'S TUMOR

See: CANCER

WOUNDS AND INJURIES

See also: SPORTS MEDICINE

ABSTRACTING, INDEXING, AND CURRENT AWARENESS PUBLICATIONS

Index Medicus. U.S. National Library of Medicine, 8600 Rockville Pike, Bethesda, MD 20894. Phone: (800) 638-8480. Monthly.

ASSOCIATIONS, PROFESSIONAL SOCIETIES, ADVOCACY AND SUPPORT GROUPS

Family Interest Group-Head Trauma. 5034 Oliver Ave. S., Minneapolis, MN 55430. Phone: (612) 521-2266.

National Head Injury Foundation (NHIF). 333 Turnpike Rd., Southborough, MA 01772. Phone: (508) 485-9950. Fax: (508) 488-9893.

CD-ROM DATABASES

Emergency Medicine MEDLINE. MEP, 124 Mt. Auburn St., Cambridge, MA 02138. Phone: (800) 342-1338. Fax: (617) 868-7738. Quarterly.

HANDBOOKS, GUIDES, MANUALS, ATLASES

A Color Atlas of Injury in Sport. J.G.P. Williams. Mosby-Year Book, 11830 Westline Industrial Drive, St. Louis, MO 63146. Phone: (800) 325-4177. Fax: (314) 432-1380. Second edition 1989.

JOURNALS

Archives of Emergency Medicine. Blackwell Scientific Publications, Inc., 3 Cambridge Ctr., Cambridge, MA 02142. Phone: (800) 759-6102. Quarterly.

Emergency Medicine. Reed Publishing USA, 249 W. 17th St., New York, NY 10011. Phone: (212) 645-0067. Fax: (212) 242-6987. 21/year.

Injury: British Journal of Accident Surgery. Butterworth-Heinemann, 80 Montvale Ave., Stoneham, MA 02180. Phone: (617) 438-8464. Fax: (617) 279-4851. 8/year.

Journal of Trauma. Williams & Wilkins, 428 E. Preston St., Baltimore, MD 21202. Phone: (800) 638-0672. Fax: (800) 447-8438. Monthly.

Wound Repair and Regeneration. Mosby-Year Book, 11830 Westline Industrial Drive, St. Louis, MO 63146. Phone: (800) 325-4177. Fax: (314) 432-1380. Quarterly.

ONLINE DATABASES

EMBASE. Elsevier Science Publishing Co., Inc., P.O. Box 882, Madison Square Station, New York, NY 10159-2101. Phone: (212) 989-5800. Fax: (212) 633-3990.

MEDLINE. National Library of Medicine, 8600 Rockville Pike, Bethesda, MD 20894. Phone: (800) 638-8480.

SciSearch. Institute for Scientific Information, 3501 Market St., Philadelphia, PA 19104. Phone: (215) 386-0100. Fax: (215) 386-6362.

POPULAR WORKS AND PATIENT EDUCATION

The American Red Cross First Aid and Safety Handbook. Kathleen A. Handal. Little, Brown and Co., 34 Beacon St., Boston, MA 02108. Phone: (617) 227-0730. 1992.

Childhood Emergencies-What to Do: A Quick Reference Guide. Project Care for Children Staff. Bull Publishing Co., 110 Gilbert Ave., Menlo Park, CA 94025. Phone: (800) 676-2855. 1989.

Head Injury: The Facts, A Guide for Families and Care-Givers. Dorothy Gronwall, Philip Wrightson, Peter Waddell. Oxford University Press, 200 Madison Ave., New York, NY 10016. Phone: (212) 679-7300. 1991.

The Sports Injury Handbook: Professional Advice for Amateur Athletes. Allan M. Levy, Mark L. Fuerst. John Wiley & Sons, Inc., 605 Third Ave., New York, NY 10158-0012. Phone: (212) 850-6000. Fax: (212) 850-6088. 1992.

RESEARCH CENTERS, INSTITUTES, CLEARINGHOUSES

National Injury Information Clearinghouse. U.S. Consumer Product Safety Commission, 5401 Westbard Ave., Rm. 625, Washington, DC 20207. Phone: (301) 492-6424.

STANDARDS AND STATISTICS SOURCES

Impairments Due to Injuries: United States, 1985-87. National Center for Health Statistics, 6525 Belcrest Rd., Rm. 1064, Hyattsville, MD 20782. Phone: (301) 436-8500. PHS 91-1505 1991.

Types of Injuries by Selected Characteristics: United States, 1985-1987. National Center for Health Statistics, 6525 Belcrest Rd., Rm. 1064, Hyattsville, MD 20782. Phone: (301) 436-8500. PHS 91-1503 1991.

TEXTBOOKS AND MONOGRAPHS

The Anatomy of Injury: Its Surgical Implications. P.S. London. Butterworth-Heinemann, 80 Montvale Ave., Stoneham, MA 02180. Phone: (617) 438-8464. Fax: (617) 279-4851. 1991.

Athletic Injuries to the Head, Neck and Face. Torg. Mosby-Year Book, 11830 Westline Industrial Drive, St. Louis, MO 63146. Phone: (800) 325-4177. Fax: (314) 432-1380. Second edition 1991.

Critical Care. Joseph M. Civetta, Robert W. Taylor, Robert R. Kirby (eds.). J.B. Lippincott Co., 227 E. Washington Square, Philadelphia, PA 19106-3780. Phone: (215) 238-4200. Fax: (215) 238-4227. 1988.

Head Injury. Cooper. Williams & Wilkins, 428 East Preston St., Baltimore, MD 21202. Phone: (800) 638-0672. Fax: (800) 447-8438. Third edition 1992.

Prevention of Athletic Injuries. Mueller. F.A. Davis Co., 1915 Arch St., Philadelphia, PA 19103. Phone: (800) 523-4049. Fax: (215) 568-5065. 1991.

Shock Resuscitation: Principles and Practice. Evan R. Geller. McGraw-Hill, Inc., 1221 Avenue of the Americas, 28th Floor, New York, NY 10020. Phone: (212) 512-4228. 1992.

Sports Injuries. M.A. Hutson. Oxford University Press, 200 Madison Ave., New York, NY 10016. Phone: (212) 679-7300. 1990.

Sports Injury Management Series. Terry R. Malone. Williams & Wilkins, 428 East Preston St., Baltimore, MD 21202. Phone: (800) 638-0672. Fax: (800) 447-8438. 1990.

Wound Healing: Biochemical and Clinical Aspects. I. Kelman Cohen, and others. W.B. Saunders Co., The Curtis Center, Independence Sqare W., Philadelphia, PA 19106-3399. Phone: (215) 238-7800. 1992.

Wound Management and Dressing. Thomas. Pharmaceutical Press, Rittenhouse Book Distributors, 511 Feheley Dr., King of Prussia, PA 19406. Phone: (800) 345-6425. Fax: (800) 223-7488. 1990.

Wounds and Lacerations: Emergency Care and Closure. Alexander Trott. Mosby-Year Book, 11830 Westline Industrial Drive, St. Louis, MO 63146. Phone: (800) 325-4177. Fax: (314) 432-1380. Second edition 1991.

X-Y-Z

X-RAYS

See: RADIOLOGY

YEAST INFECTIONS

See: FUNGAL DISEASES

YELLOW FEVER

See: INFECTIOUS DISEASES